Planning and Designing of Specialty Healthcare Facilities

Planning and Designing of Specialty Healthcare Facilities

Shakti Kumar Gupta
MBBS MHA FNAMS FIMSA FIHE FAHA MACHE (USA)
Medical Superintendent
Dr RP Centre for Ophthalmic Sciences
All India Institute of Medical Sciences
New Delhi, India

Lt Gen Sunil Kant, SM, VSM
MBBS DIT MBA MHA MNAMS M Phil
Director General Hospital Services (Armed Forces)
Office of Director General Armed Forces Medical Services
New Delhi, India

Prof (Dr) R Chandrashekhar
B Arch HFP PhD FIIA FIHE MAHA FIHEEM SFIGBC
Chairman, IGBC Green Healthcare Rating
Consultant- World Bank, Consultant- IUIH (Indo UK Institute of Health)
Vice President RFHHA
Vice President IBIMA (India BIM Association)
Former Chief Architect, Ministry of Health and Family Welfare
Government of India
New Delhi, India

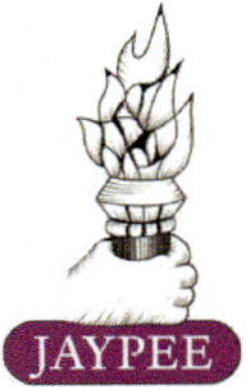

JAYPEE BROTHERS MEDICAL PUBLISHERS
The Health Sciences Publisher
New Delhi | London

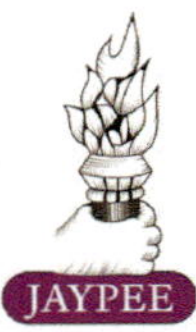

Jaypee Brothers Medical Publishers (P) Ltd

Headquarters
EMCA House
23/23-B, Ansari Road, Daryaganj
New Delhi 110 002, India
Landline: +91-11-23272143, +91-11-23272703
+91-11-23282021, +91-11-23245672
E-mail: jaypee@jaypeebrothers.com

Overseas Office
J.P. Medical Ltd.
83, Victoria Street, London
SW1H 0HW (UK)
Phone: +44-20 3170 8910
E-mail: info@jpmedpub.com

Corporate Office
4838/24, Ansari Road, Daryaganj
New Delhi 110 002, India
Phone: +91-11-43574357
Fax: +91-11-43574314
E-mail: jaypee@jaypeebrothers.com

EU GPSR Authorised Representative
Logos Europe, 9 rue Nicolas Poussin
17000, La Rochelle, France
Phone: +33 (0) 6 67 93 73 78
E-mail: contact@logoseurope.eu

Website: www.jaypeebrothers.com
Website: www.jaypeedigital.com

Planning and Designing of Specialty Healthcare Facilities

First Edition: 2021, *Reprint:* **2025**

ISBN: 978-93-89188-98-1

Printed in India

Dedicated to

My Parents
for their guidance and moral support
My students - past, present and future and teachers
who always inspired me for academic excellence
My beautiful and brilliant wife Madhu
who provides me with unwavering love and support
Our affectionate daughter and Son-in-Law - Shilpa and Rachit
for their undaunting patience and understanding while I pursued my dreams
and our granddaughter, Nysha—our bundle of joy

Shakti Kumar Gupta

My wife, Sheeba
for being my steady anchor and omnipresent sublime loec
Our extraordinarily affectionate and supportive daughter,
Dakshita
and
The eternal memory and divine blessings of
my father, mother and brother

Lt Gen Sunil Kant, SM, VSM

My mother
for her constant encouragement and belief in me
Gowri, my ever supportive wife
for her patience and unflinching support through every stage of my life
My Son Saurabh and Gaurav
For their vital and thought stirring inputs
and moral support of my daughter in law Brinda
and my grandchildren Naina and Dhruv
and to the memory of my father

Prof (Dr) R Chandrashekhar

CONTRIBUTORS

Aarti Vij MBBS MHA
Professor, Department of Hospital Administration and Professor I/C ORBO
Chairperson, Media Cell and Protocol Division
AIIMS, New Delhi, India

Angel Rajan Singh MBBS PGDHHM MHA
Associate Professor
Department of Hospital Administration
AIIMS, New Delhi, India

Anil Sain MBBS MHA
Chief Medical Officer, (SAG), CGHS

Anki Reddy Jangamreddy MBBS DPH MHA
Medical Superintendent and Head Quality Organization
Nuterna Hospital
Meerut, Uttar Pradesh, India

Anoop Saraya MD DM
Professor of Gastroenterology and Human Nutrition
AIIMS, New Delhi, India

Col Arvind Kushal MBBS MHA
Col (Med) Army

AS Rana MBBS MS MHA
MY Hospital
Indore, Madhya Pradesh, India

Brig Balakrishan Jayan BDS MDS
Commandant, Army Dental Centre
Research and Referral
New Delhi, India

Biplab Kumar GBC AP ECBC
Master Trainer
Senior Energy Associate
Green Tree Building Energy Pvt Ltd
Noida, Uttar Pradesh, India

Dibakar Rakshit PhD
Assistant Professor
Centre for Energy Studies
IIT Delhi

Dinesh Negi MBBS MHA
OIVS and Assistant Chief Registrar (Birth and Death)
Bureau of Health Intelligence
North Delhi Municipal Corporation
New Delhi, India

Diwakar Thimmappa MBBS MHA
Medical Officer, Indian Armed Forces
New Delhi, India

IB Singh MBBS MHA
Professor
Department of Hospital Administration
AIIMS, New Delhi, India

Jitender Mehta MBBS MHA
National Health Mission
Government of Jammu and Kashmir
Jammu and Kashmir, India

Jitender Sodhi MBBS MHA
Assistant Professor
Department of Hospital Administration
AIIMS, New Delhi, India

Col Jitesh V MBBS MHA
Commanding Officer
181, MH, Arunachal Pradesh, India

Kanika Jain MBBS DNB
Assistant Professor
Hospital Administration
AIIMS, New Delhi, India

Khalid Mehmood MBBS MHA
Senior Resident Administrator
Department of Hospital Administration
AIIMS, New Delhi, India

Kumari Shweta MBBS MHA
Medical Services
Manipal Health Enterprises
Bengaluru, Karnataka, India

Laxmi Tej Wundavalli MBBS MHA
Assistant Professor
Department of Hospital Administration
AIIMS, New Delhi, India

Maneesh Rathee MBBS MD MHA
Medical Superintendent
Civil Hospital
Gurugram, Haryana, India

Maj Meeta Tyagi MD DHHM DMLS QM and AHO MHA
Senior Consultant
Hospital Management
PMU, AIIMS, New Delhi, India

Col MM Singh MBBS MHA MBA PhD PGD (Law)
Commanding Officer
322 Field Hospital

Mohd Kausar MBBS MHA
Senior Consultant
Hospital Management
AIIMS, New Delhi, India

Mukunda Chandra Sahoo MBBS MHA MSc
Associate Professor
Department of Hospital Administration
AIIMS, Bhubaneswar, Odisha, India

Col Neeraj Garg MBBS MHA
Classified Specialist and
Associate Professor (Hospital Administration)
AFMC, Pune, Maharashtra, India

NP Gupta MD
Professor and Head
Department of Urology
AIIMS, New Delhi, India

Pankaj Arora MBBS MHA DNB
Associate Professor
Department of Hospital Administration
PGIMER
Chandigarh, India

Maj Parmeshwar Kumar MBBS MHA DNB
Associate Professor
Department of Hospital Administration
AIIMS, New Delhi, India

Brig Pawan K Singh BDS
Commandant
Command Military Dental Centre
Udhampur, Jammu and Kashmir, India

Pramod Garg MD DM
Professor
Department of Gastroenterology and Human Nutrition
AIIMS, New Delhi, India

Priti Goel MBBS MHA
Assistant Professor
Hospital Administration
Subharti Medical College
Meerut, Uttar Pradesh, India

Rajesh Gupta MD
Director and CMO
AFC Urgent Care Centres
3379 Crompond Road
Yorktown Heights, NY, 10598

Rajesh Harsvardhan MBBS MHA (AIIMS) DNB MPH DGM DMLE MNAMS LLB-I
Head, Department of Hospital Administration
SGPGI and Medical Superintendent
Super-specialty Cancer Institute and Hospital
Lucknow, Uttar Pradesh, India

Rajiv Kumar Pathni MBBS MHA PGDHHM
Consultant (Healthcare and Hospitals)

Col Rakesh Verma MBBS MHA PGDHHM PGDMLS
Resident Administrator
Department of Hospital Administration
AIIMS, New Delhi, India

Ravi Prakash Narayan MS MCh
Professor and Consultant
Department of Burns and Reconstructive Surgery
VMMC and Safdarjung Hospital
New Delhi, India

R Chandrashekhar B Arch HFP PhD FIIA FIHE MAHA FIHEEM SFIGBC
Chairman, IGBC Green Healthcare Rating
Consultant- World Bank, Consultant- IUIH (Indo UK Institute of Health)
Vice President RFHHA
Vice President IBIMA (India BIM Association)
Former Chief Architect, Ministry of Health and Family Welfare, Government of India
New Delhi, India

RY Asangi MBBS MHA
Chief Medical Officer, CGHS, GoI

Samarpita Dutta MBBS MD MHA
Deputy Medical Superintendent
Agartala Govt Medical College
and GB Pant Hospital
Agartala, Tripura, India

Sandeep Guleria MS DNB FRCS FRCSEd FRCS (Glas) FRCP
Senior Consultant Surgeon and
Lead Clinical Coordinator, Apollo Hospital
New Delhi, India

Gp Capt Sanjeev Sood MBBS MD M Phil (HHSM) PGDHHM PGCQMHC FCGP AFeISAM
Hospital and Health Systems Administrator

Sapna Ramani PGDHHM MBA MHA
Chief Medical Administrator

Saroj Kumar Patnaik MBBS (Hons) MHA
Associate Professor
Department of Hospital Administration
AFMC
Pune, Maharashtra, India

Shakti Kumar Gupta MBBS MHA FNAMS FIMSA FIHE FAHA MACHE (USA)
Medical Superintendent
Dr RP Centre for Ophthalmic Sciences
AIIMS, New Delhi, India

Shalini Kumar Bhalla MBBS MHA Fulbright-Nehru Fellow
Medical Director Fortis
Noida, Uttar Pradesh, India

Sheetal Singh MBBS MHA
Assistant Professor
Department of Hospital Administration
National Cancer Institute
AIIMS, New Delhi, India

Shilpi Verma MBBS MHA PGDHHM PGDMLS
Director of AEON Health

Shrish Kumar BE MHA Big Data Analyst XLRI
Chief Information Officer

Col SK Dutt MBBS MHA
Commanding Officer
Military Hospital
Leimakhong (Manipur) India
Ministry of Defence; Army Medical Corps

S Satpathy MBBS MD MHA
Professor and Head
Department of Hospital Administration
AIIMS, New Delhi, India

Sudharshan Kumar MSc PhD
Former Director General, DRDO
Ministry of Defence, Government of India

Col Sudhin Kurien MBBS MHA
Directing Staff, Officers Training College
Army Medical Corps Centre and College

Sujata Mohanty PhD
Professor
Centre of Excellence for Stem Cell Research
AIIMS, New Delhi, India

Lt Gen Sunil Kant, SM, VSM MBBS DIT MBA MHA MNAMS M Phil
Director General Hospital Services (Armed Forces)
Office of Director General Armed Forces Medical Services
New Delhi, India

Sunil Seth PG Diploma in Journalism and Mass Communication, MA in Mass Communication, Bachelor of Law
Dr RP Centre
AIIMS, New Delhi, India

Lt Col Sunil Verma MBBS MHA
Director, Medical Services (Hospital Projects)
DGMS (ARMY)

Surajeet Kr Barua MBBS (AMC) MHA (AIIMS) PGDHHM (AHA) PGDHHM (IGNOU)
Head of Medical Services

Col Uma Shankar Garg MBBS MHA
Commanding Officer, Military Hospital
Bhuj-Kutch, Gujarat, India

Vijaydeep Siddharth MBBS DHA MHA
Associate Professor
Department of Hospital Administration
AIIMS, New Delhi, India

Vijay Kumar Tadia MBBS MHA PGDMLE MIMSA
Senior Resident Administrator
Department of Hospital Administration
AIIMS, New Delhi, India

PREFACE

Hospitals today face rapidly changing population of patients with differing needs who require a range of new communication links that are transforming our concept of the hospital spaces and create a set of new and complex challenges for those delivering healthcare services. Hospital buildings may never be perfect as these are continuously impacted by resource availability, technological advancements, skills levels, user needs, and expectations of the society, various insurance models in vogue, government, and private stakeholder's priority to healthcare provisioning and the globalization. However, a well-designed hospital building enables the local acceptance and eases the process of securing planning permission.

Hospital needs to be cost-effective to build, run and maintain, support the organization's objectives well and offers an improved service to the user and make an impact on the community. Paradigm shift in the provisioning of healthcare services in terms of hospital stays, diagnostics and superspecialty care has led to the emergence of newer concepts such as Daycare, Integrated Care and standalone facilities with a resultant increase in both the need as well as demand of superspecialty healthcare facilities such as Hybrid OTs, Urgent Care Centers, Birthing Centers, Transplantation Centers and the like.

The authors as the teacher-medical administrator-architect trio have spent more than 30 years in the field of hospital administration, planning and designing of varied specialty and general hospitals and having published their research work profusely and written more than a dozen books on core areas of the specialty, including but not limited to different aspects, of hospital planning and management, feels obliged to share their knowledge, experiences and exposures. Writing is essential to disseminate evidence, share initiatives and innovations, to provide information about new dimensions to professionals to keep them updated. The authors have practiced a holistic and integrated approach to all facets related to the planning and designing of specialty healthcare facilities.

The book comprises 51 chapters. Chapters on Wellness Center, Green and Smart Hospitals, Telemedicine, Assisted Reproductive Technology Facility, Critical Care Unit, Sleep Center, Nanomedicine and Nanotechnology, Stem Cell Center and Facility for Robotic Surgery may be appropriately and optimally utilized as standalone or add on centers with existing healthcare institutions. Chapter 50 titled "COVID-19: Planning Premises and Design Considerations for Healthcare Facilities" incorporates metamorphic changes in the planning and designing of specialty healthcare facilities necessitated by the global emergence of COVID-19 disease. Last Chapter 51, "Laws Applicable to Hospitals" provides a comprehensive brief of the diverse legal and statutory norms applicable to hospitals.

This book is envisaged to be a useful guide and reference source and complement another title by the authors "Modern Trends in Planning and Designing of Hospitals—Principles and Practice", that has already been a resource for policy makers, academicians, hospital planners, architects, administrators, clinicians, engineers and students associated with planning, designing, construction, maintenance and administration of hospitals. The book is intended to facilitate the planning and designing of new superspecialty hospitals and to steer a clear path for hospital administrators, planners and medical architects through the systems and processes that they need to understand as members of a team overseeing the planning of new hospital building projects, major refurbishment or remodeling of an existing hospital. It will aid the students of hospital administration and medical architecture to understand and implement the principles and practice of hospital planning and designing. It will also be of great relevance to architects unfamiliar with hospital building requirements.

Although, we have many expert colleagues who helped us with sourcing, writing and structuring the material but we wish to greatly acknowledge the contributions of Ar. Subodh Malasi who developed and fine-tuned CADD Line diagrams for various chapters. We sincerely appreciate the valuable inputs, encouragement, guidance and support of Group Chairman of M/s Jaypee Brothers Medical Publishers Pvt Ltd, Mr Jitendar P Vij and acknowledge the exemplary commitment and professionalism of his team.

The authors welcome the suggestions and feedback of our esteemed and revered readers which will definitely aid in further improving and enriching the subsequent editions of this book.

Shakti Kumar Gupta
Sunil Kant
R Chandrashekhar

CONTENTS

ABBREVIATIONS

A&E : Accident and Emergency
AASM : American Academy of Sleep Medicine
AAUCM : American Academy of Urgent Care Medicine
ABG : Arterial Blood Gas
ABS : Acrylonitrile Butadiene Styrene
ACC : American College of Cardiology
ACH : Air Changes per hour
ACRS : Advisory Committee on Radiological Safety
ACSCOT : American College of Surgeons Committee on Trauma
ADL : Activities of Daily Living
ADT : Admission, Discharge, Transfer
AERB : Atomic Energy Regulatory Board
AFM : Atomic Force Microscope
AGVs : Automated-guided Vehicles
AHA : America Heart Association
AHRs : Animal Housing Rooms
AHU : Air Handling Unit
AI : Artificial Intelligence
AIA : American Institute of Architects
AID : Artificial Insemination with Donor
AIHA : America Industrial Hygiene Association
AII : Airborne Infection Isolation
ALOE : Average Length of Encounter
ANSI : American National Standards Institute
ART : Assisted Reproductive Technology
ASHRAE : American Society of Heating Refrigerating and Air Conditioning Engineer
ASRM : American Society for Reproductive Medicine
ATS : Automatic Transfer Switches
AVMs : Arteriovenous Malformations
BAL : Bronchoalveolar Lavage
BARC : Bhabha Atomic Research Center
BAS : Building Automation Systems
BBV : Blood Borne Viral
BHU : Bed Head Unit
BIM : Building Information Modelling
BIPV : Building Integrated Photovoltaics
BMBL : Biosafety in Microbiology and Biomedical Laboratories
BMD : Bone Mineral Density
BMI : Body Mass Index
BMS : Building Management System
BOS : Building Operating System
BRDAB : Bariatric Room Design Advisory Board
BREEAM : Building Research Establishment Environment Assessment Method
BSS : Basic Safety Standards
CASBEE : Comprehensive Assessment System of Building Environmental Efficiency
CBCT : Cone Beam Computed Tomography
CBRN : Chemical, Biological, Radiological and Nuclear
CCA : Critical Care Anaesthesia
CCRAS : Central Council for Research in Ayurveda and Shiddha
CCRH : Central Council for Research in Homoeopathy
CCRUM : Central Council for Research in Unani Medicine
CCRYN : Central Council for Research in Yoga and Naturopathy
CCU : Critical Care Unit
CDC : Center for Disease Control
CFC : Chloro Floro Carbon
CFM : Cubic Feet per Minute
CII : Confederation of Indian Industry
CKD : Chronic Kidney Disease
CLIA : Chemiluminescence Immunoassay
CNG : Compressed Natural Gas
COC : Chain of Custody
CPAP : Continuous Positive Airway Pressure
CPM : Continuous Passive Motion
CRI : Color Rendering Index
CSICU : Cardiac Surgery Intensive Care Unit
CSSD : Central Sterile Services Department
CT : Computed Tomography
CTVS : Cardiothoracic and Vascular Surgery
CVD : Cardiovascular Disease
CWS : Clinic Workstation
DA : Differently Abled
DDC : Direct Digital Control
DDLT : Dead Donor Liver Transplantation
DGCA : Director General of Civil Aviation
DI : Deionization
DICOM : Digital Imaging and Communications in Medicine
DIS : Diagnostic Information System
DM : Disaster Management
DMSO : Di Methyl Sulfoxide
DNA : Deoxyribonucleic Acid
DVT : Deep Vein Thrombosis
DXA/DEXA : Dual-Energy X-Ray Absorptiometry
EBD : Evidence-based Design
ECA : Essential Complementary Accommodation
ECBC : Energy Conservation Building Code
ECG : Electrocardiography
ECT : Electro convulsive Therapy
ED : Emergency Department
ELISA : Enzyme-linked Immunosorbent Assay
EMCAPS : Emergency Mass Casualty Assessment and Planning Scenario
EMG : Electromyography
EMR : Electronic Medical Record
EMS : Equipment Maintenance System
ENT : Ear, Nose and Throat
EPS : Electrophysiological Studies

ESCs : Embryonic Stem Cells
ESHRE : European Society of Human Reproductive and Embryology
ESS : Epworth Sleeping Scale, Electric Substation
ESWL : Extracorporeal Shock Wave Lithotripsy
FCU : Fan Coil Units
FEMS : Federal Emergency Management Series
FGI : Facility Guidelines Institute
FISH : Fluorescence in Situ Hybridization
FNAC : Fine Needle Aspiration Cytology
FSC : Forest Stewardship Council
FTIR : Fourier Transform Infrared Spectroscopy
GA : General Anesthesia
GC : Gas Chromatography
GE : Gastroenterology
GFCLs : Ground Fault Circuit Interrupters
GIFT : Gamete Intrafallopian Tube Transfer
GLP : Good Laboratory Practice
GMP : Good Manufacturing Process
GRIHA : Green Rating for Integrated Habitat Assessment
HACs : Housekeeping Aides Closets
HAI : Hospital Acquired Infection
HBOT : Hyperbaric Oxygen Therapy
HBV : Hepatitis B Virus
HCG : Human Chorionic Gonadotropin
HD : Hemodialysis
HDR : High Dose Rate
HDU : High Dependency Unit
HEPA : High Efficiency Particulate Arrestance
HEPA-MD : High Efficiency Particulate Arrestance Microbial Destruction
HER : Electronic Health Record
HID : High Intensive Discharge
HLA : Human Leukocyte Antigen
HMIS : Hospital Management Information System
HOST : Hypo-osmotic Swelling Test
HPL : High Pressure Laminates
hPSC : Human pluripotent stem cell
HSCT : Hematopoietic System Cell Transplant
HSDU : Hospital Sterilization and Decontamination Unit
HTK : Histidine Tryptophan Ketoglutarate
HVAC : Heating, ventilating and air conditioning
IBD : Inflammatory Bowel Disease
IBMS : Integrated Building Management System
ICF : International Classification of Functioning
ICM : Inner Cell Mass
ICMR : Indian Council of Medical Research
ICP : Inductively Coupled Plasma
ICPD : International Conference on Population and Development
ICSI : Intra Cytoplasmic Sperm Injection
ICT : Information and Communication Technologies
ICU : Intensive Care Unit
IED : Improvised Explosive Device
IFFS : International Federation of Fertility Societies
IGBC : Indian Green Building Council
IMV : Intubation Mechanical Ventilation
IOT : Internet of Things
IPD : In-Door Patient Department
IPHS : Indian Public Health Standards
IPL : Intense Pulse Light
IPSCs : Induct Pluripotent Stem Cells
ISMH : Indian System of Medicine and Homeopathy
IT : Information Technology
IUI : Intrauterine Insemination
IVF : In Vitro Fertilization
JIT : Just in Time
KMC : Kangaroo Mother Care
LAN : Local Area Network
LCA : Life Cycle Analysis
LDLT : Living Donor Liver Transplantation
LDRP : Labor, Delivery, Recovery and Postpartum
LEED : Leadership In Energy and Environmental Design
LIS : Laboratory Information System
M2M : Machine to Machine
MAR : Medicine Administration Record
MARS : Molecular Adsorbent Recycling System
MHUs : Mobile Health Units
MIP : Maximal Implantation Potential
MIS : Management Information System
MLOP : Mid Level Ophthalmic Personnel
MPI : Master Patent Index
MRD : Medical Records Department
MRI : Magnetic Resonance Imaging
MS : Mass Spectrometry
MSSO : Medical Social Service Officer
NBC : Nuclear, Biological or Chemical
NDMA : National Disaster Management Authority
NICU : Neonatal Intensive Care Unit
NIH : National Institute of Health
NIMHANS : National Institute of Mental Health and Neurosciences
NIV : Non Invasive Ventilation
NMR : Nuclear Magnetic Resonance
NOC : No Objection Certificate
NPCB & VI : National Programme for Control of Blindness and Visual Impairment
NPHCE : National Programme for Health Care of Elderly
NREM : Non-rapid Eye Movement
NRHM : National Rural Health Mission
NSF : Net Square Feet
NSIC : National Spinal Injuries Centre
NSM : Net Square Meter
NST : Non Stress Test
NVR : Network Video Recording
O&M : Operation and Maintenance
OEM : Original Equipment Manufacture
OES : Occupational Exposure Standard
OPC : Ordinary Portland Cement
OPD : Outpatient Department
Ors : Operating Rooms
OSA : Obstructive Sleep Apnea
OSHA : Occupational Safety & Health Administration
OSP : Other Service Provider
OT : Operation Theatre
PAC : Preanaesthesia Check-up
PACG : Primary Angle Closure Glaucoma
PACS : Picture Archive and Communication System
PAI : Percutaneous Alcohol Injection
PBPU : Prefabricated Beside Patient Unit
PBT : Persistent, Bio-Accumulative and Toxic
PCIs : Percutaneous Coronary Interventions
PCR : Polymerase Chain Reaction
PD : Peritoneal Dialysis
PDF : Portable Document Format
PESA : Percutaneous Epididymal Sperm Aspiration
PET : Positron Emission Tomography
PFT : Positron Function Testing
PGD : Preimplantation Genetic Diagnosis

PHAMA : Patient Handling and Movement Assessment
PHI : Photo Hydro Ionization
PM : Preventive Maintenance
PMR : Physical Medicine and Rehabilitation
PNC : Post Natal Clinical
PPE : Personal Protective Equipment
PPP : Public Private Partnership
PRD : Patient Relation Department
PVC : Poly vinyl chloride
PVD : Physical Vapor Deposition
PVDF : Poly Vinyli Dence Fluoride
PZD : Partial Zona Dissection
QTLYs : Quality Adjusted Life Years
REM : Rapid Eye Movement
RF : Radio Frequency
RFA : Radio Frequency Ablation
RFID : Radio Frequency Identification
RIA : Radio Immuno Assay
RICU : Respiratory Intensive Care Unit
RIS : Radiology Information System
RME : Reusable Medical Equipment
RO : Reverse Osmosis
RPR : Radiation Protection Rules
RSD : Radiological Safety Officer
RTIs : Reproductive Tract Infections
RT-PCR : Reverse Transcription Polymerase increase Chain Reaction
SBS : Sick Building Syndrome
SCMT : Sperm Cervical Mucus Test
SIC : Spinal Injury Centre
SNVT : Standard Network Variable Types
SOPs : Standard Operating Procedures
SPD : Supply, Processing and Distribution
SRR : Skylight to Roof Ratio
SRS : Stereotactic Radio Surgery
STM : Scanning Tunneling Microscope
SUZI : Sub Zonal Insemination
SV : Sheet Vinyl
SVS : Society of Vascular Surgery
SWL : Safe Working Load
TB : Tuberculosis
TBI : Total Body Irradiation
TCA : Tri Chloroacetic Acid
TCC : Tele Consulting Center
TDS : Total Dissolved Solids
TECAB : Total Endoscopic Coronary Artery Bypass
TEEs : Tran esophageal Echocardiograms
TENS : Transcutaneous Electrical Nerve Stimulation
TESA : Testicular Sperm Aspiration
TET : Tubal Embryo Transfer
TIM : Toxic Industrial Material
TLD : Thermo Luminescent Dosimetry
TRAMAH : Trauma Resource Allocation Model for Ambulances and Hospitals
TSC : Tele Specialist Centre
TVOR : Trans Vaginal Oocyte Retrieval
TVS : Trans Vaginal Sonography
UCAoA : Urgent Care Association of America
UCV : Ultra Clean Ventilation
UDIFI : Urban Development Plans Formulation and Implementation
ULPA : Ultra Low Particulate Air
UPS : Uninterruptible Power Supply
USG : Ultrasonography
USGBC : United State Green Building Council
UV : Ultraviolet
UVGI : Ultraviolet Germicidal Irradiation
VAS : Value Added Services
VAV : Variable Air Value
VCF : Urgent Care Facilities
VCT : Vinyl Composite tile
VDP : Visual Display Terminal
VOCs : Volatile Organic Compounds
VPN : Virtual Private Network
VSDs : Ventricular Septal Defects
VZV : Varicella Zoster Virus
WCs : Water Closets
WHB : Wash Hand Basin
WHO : World Health Organization
WRIS : Water Resources Information System
WWR : Window to Wall Ratio
ZIFR : Zygote Intrafallopian Transfer

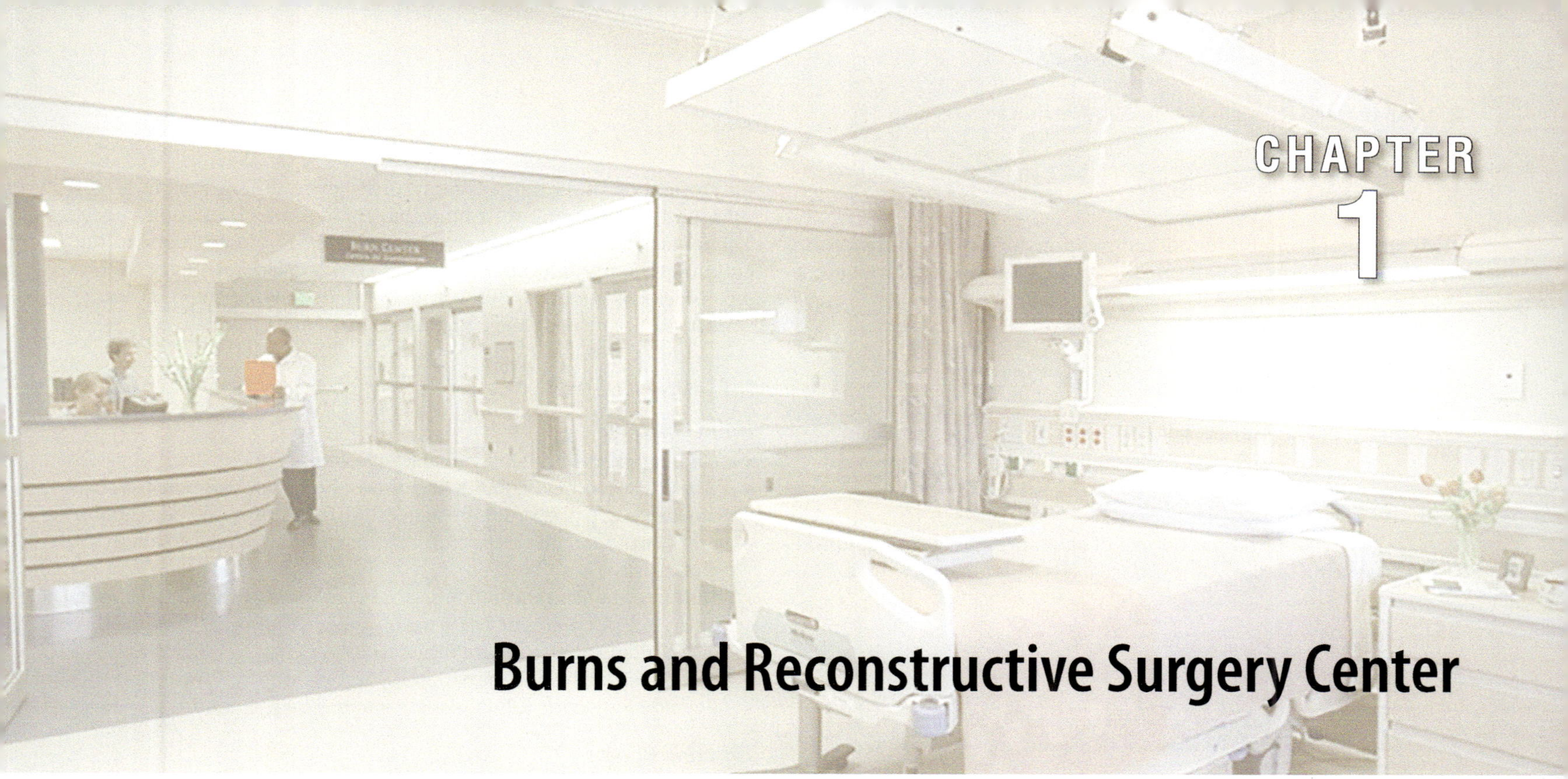

CHAPTER 1

Burns and Reconstructive Surgery Center

Rakesh Verma, Ravi Prakash Narayan, Shakti Kumar Gupta, Sunil Kant, R Chandrashekhar

INTRODUCTION

The high proportion of burns cases, among all causes of injuries, underlines the need for specialized treatment facilities of a burns center. As burns patients require intensive life support, expert medical and nursing care and complex treatment protocols, the burns centers are accordingly designed, equipped and staffed. The recovery from burns injury among other factors also depends upon the level of healthcare facility where the victim is being treated and expertise of the medical team. The clinical outcomes in burns cases are intimately linked with the design of the facility. The facility may be standalone or integrated burns center (Box 1).

FUNCTIONS

The primary function of the burns and reconstructive surgery unit is to provide specialized care to the burns patients and those requiring reconstructive surgical interventions in order to ensure fast recovery, subsequent rehabilitation and return to vocation/society.

KEY PLANNING AND DESIGN PARAMETERS

The key planning and design parameters for emergency care unit, ICU, OT, wards, OPD and physical and rehabilitation unit for burns center are same as for any such generic unit. Special requirements have been detailed below.

Box 1: Standalone or integrated burns center.

> Burns units treat only burns patients. It may however be established with trauma/emergency units. The advantages of an integrated burns center are:
> - Cases to burns care facility get filtered at the emergency department allowing only those requiring specialized burns management to reach there
> - Needs of a burns facility for large quantum of sterile supplies, blood and blood products are met
> - Burns is a complex problem in clinical terms. Multidisciplinary approach is best suited for its care
> - Reconstructive surgery facility is functionally related to the burns center. Planning of the reconstructive surgery center should be within the ambit of burns center

COMPONENTS OF BURNS CENTER

- Emergency care unit
- Intensive care unit (Fig. 1)
- Operation theater
- Ward unit
- Outpatient department
- Physical medicine and rehabilitation unit
- *Special facilities:* Saline bath unit and skin/amnion banking facility.

The description of these components is limited to the extent that pertains to the specific requirements for burns and reconstructive surgery unit.

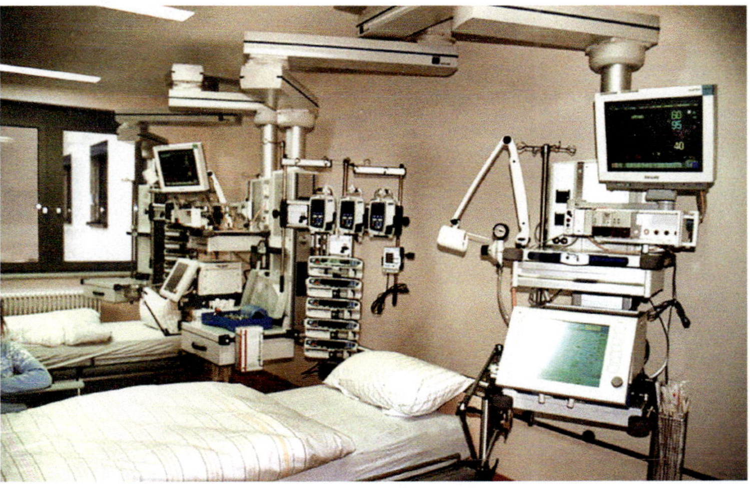

Fig. 1: Burns ICU.

BURNS CENTER—SPECIFIC REQUIREMENTS

The stack diagram and functional relationships of the burns unit is depicted in Figures 2A and 2B. The saline bath features are enumerated in Box 2 and Figure 3.

Weight Measurement Facility

This should be provided in the emergency unit and allow accurate weighing of the patient along with trolley.

Skin/Amnion Banking Facility

This facility is required for storage of skin and amniotic membranes used as dressing for the burnt surfaces. It is a tissue bank with facilities for storage of amnion at very low/ultra-low temperatures in large-refrigeration equipment. It must have adequate circulation space. The space required for the equipment would be equivalent to the cumulative footprint of all equipment to be installed. An area of 16 sqm is considered adequate. The room must have adequate lighting, ergonomic workstations, and separate air handling unit (AHU).

Box 2: Saline bath unit.

- Specialized area for cleaning of the affected body surface of the patient
- Unit may either be integral part of ICU or it may be located adjacent to ICU
- Provision for manifold outlets for sedated/anesthetized patients
- Provision of ample supply of saline, warming facilities and flexible hose with pumps
- Effective drainage is essential

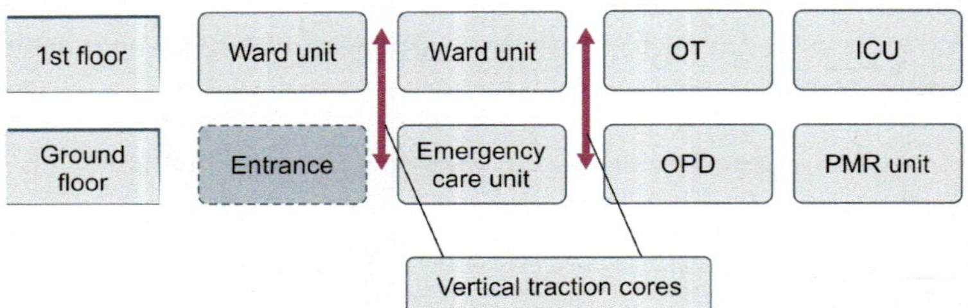

Fig. 2: Stack diagram of burns unit.

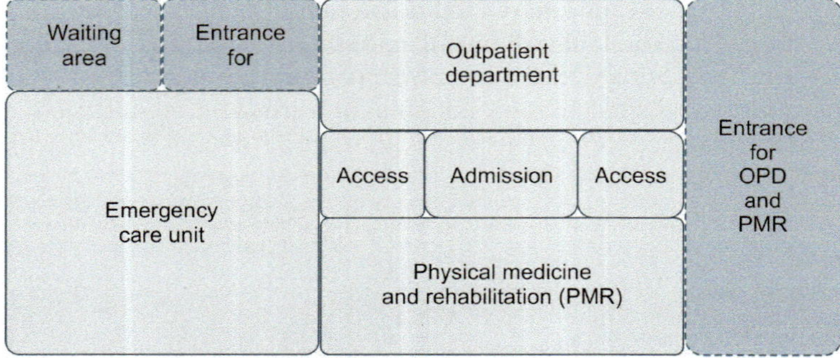

Fig. 2A: Level-I functional relationships.

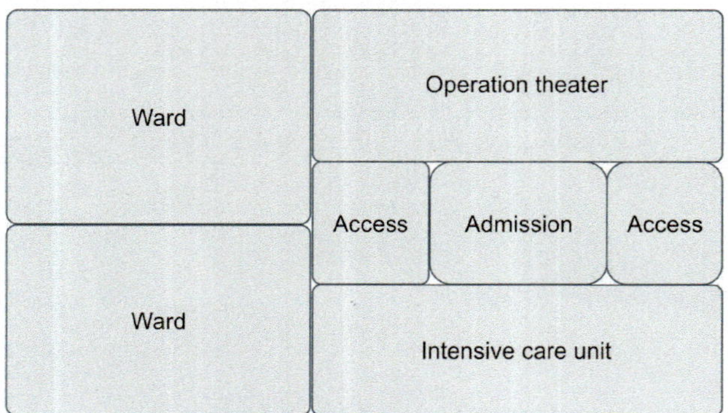

Fig. 2B: Level-II functional relationships.

Infection Control

Hand Washing

- Dedicated hand-basins for each treatment area
- These should be available at a ratio of one per every four beds/one for every procedure/resuscitation/consulting room. Type of units could be surgical scrub station or hand wash basins in all clinical areas
- Number of units required are—for ICUs—one per enclosed room, one per bed; emergency care unit—one per four open bays; OPD—one per consultant and for other areas. A person requiring to use a hand wash unit should be within 10-12 meters away from a wash unit
- Bedside antiseptic lotion dispensers may be provided.

Isolation Rooms

These are required on a scale up to 20% of total beds. Class 'P' Isolation rooms ensure that burns patients are protected from infection. These rooms must have its own independent AHU for meaningful isolation in terms of heating, ventilating, and air conditioning (HVAC). Positive pressure ensures unidirectional movement of air so that all airborne contaminants are carried away. The requirements of Class 'P' room are shown in Box 3 and the layout of isolation room in Figure 4.

Box 3: Requirements for Class 'P' isolation room.

- Hand wash basin in each room
- Ensuite comprising of shower, toilet and hand wash basin
- Sealed room, door grills for controlled airflow
- 8–10 air changes/hour
- + 30 Pa air pressure inside room
- + 15 Pa air pressure inside ensuite
- Pan sanitizer

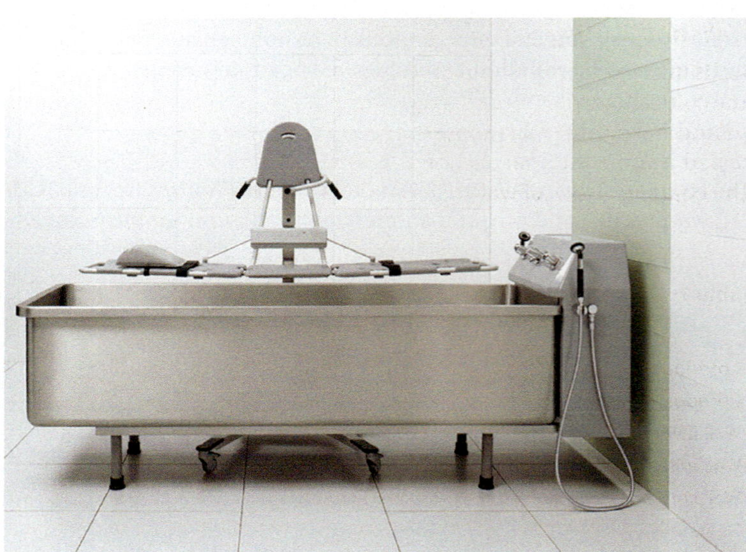

Fig. 3: Saline bath unit.

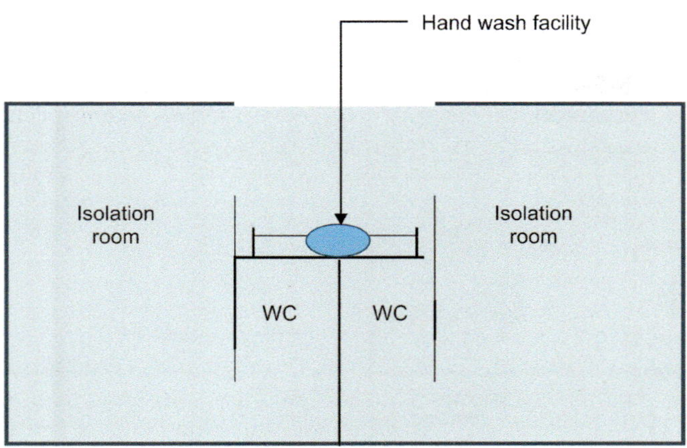

Fig. 4: Layout of isolation room.

Ultraviolet Germicidal Irradiation

Ultraviolet germicidal irradiation (UVGI) is a sterilization method that uses ultraviolet (UV) light at short wavelength that is harmful to life at the microorganism level. The characteristics are given in Box 4.

Photohydroionization

Photohydroionization (PHI) is a combination of safe, low levels of ozone, UV light and metal ions that produce safe oxidizers that neutralize odors and destroy airborne bacteria and mold. These oxidizers travel through a room by natural air movement. An advantage of PHI is there are no harmful byproducts, as the oxidizers revert back to oxygen and water vapor. Commonly used oxidizer is hydrogen peroxide.[1]

Air Pressure Gradients

Isolation rooms provided with pressurized air ensure unidirectional movement of air and thereby airborne contaminants are carried away.

Surfaces and Finishes

Floors

Flooring should be impervious, smooth, nonstainable and should allow easy movement. These should be jointless and antistatic in operation theaters.

Walls and Skirting

Walls in clinical areas should be water resistant, smooth and joint free. The color should be nonreflecting type and of soothing shades. Skirting should have same finish as floors, be integral with floors, be tightly sealed against the wall and constructed without any voids or cracks. The characteristics of walls and floors are given in Box 5.

Box 4: Ultraviolet germicidal irradiation (UVGI).

- Lethal effect is by destruction of nucleic acids in microorganisms by UV light
- UV exposure comes from UV lamps and forced flow of air/water through this environment ensures the exposure
- These systems can be freestanding units
- Key to this form of sterilization is placement of the UV lamps, a good filtration system to remove the dead microorganisms

Box 5: Materials for walls and floors.

- Floor-epoxy, vitrified tiles or marble, antibacterial vinyl
- Walls/skirting—ceramic wall tiles, PVC wall cladding systems, resin wall coatings, and epoxy based finishes with antibacterial paints

Ceilings

All exposed ceilings and ceiling structures in areas occupied by patients or staff, and in food preparation or food storage areas, should have finishings so as to be readily cleanable with equipment routinely used in daily housekeeping activities. In areas where dust fallout would present a potential problem, such as clinical areas, supply and storage areas and sterile stock storage, there should be a finished ceiling that covers all conduits, piping, ductwork and open construction systems.[2,3]

Ceilings in operating, isolation rooms should be monolithic from wall to wall without fissures, open joints, or crevices that may retain or permit passage of dirt particles. Light fittings should also be recessed and flush fitting and sealed to prevent dust ingress. Lay-in ceilings should not be used where particulate matter may interfere with infection control; however, acoustical parameters must be kept in mind.[2,3]

Space Standards and Dimensions

Corridors

All corridors should be at least 2.7 meters wide. Where doors have been provided in the corridors, *the effective usable width is reduced by at least 25 cm*. Where storage bays have been provided to store trolleys/wheel chairs, etc., these should be outside the corridor width, i.e. should be recessed. Corridor dimensions and usage are given in Table 1.

Ceiling Heights

- Operation theaters : 3.0 meters clear height
- All other areas : 2.7 meters height
- Recesses/storage bays : Up to 2.25 meters

Schedule of Accommodation and Floor Plans

The schedule of accommodation is given in Table 2. The floor plans for ground and 1st floor plan for the center are given in Figures 5 and 6.

Table 1: Corridor dimensions.

Category	*Usage*	*Dimension*	*Specification*	*Remarks*
Corridor	Patient on trolley/bed/regular use	Width	2700 mm	Width between hand grab rails
Corridor	Only staff, no trolley	Width	1000 mm	
Wall low protection	Wheelchairs	Height of protection	150–350 mm	Kick boards required
Wall mid protection	Trolleys	Height of protection	900 mm	Trolley protection
Wall corners protection	Trolleys	Height of protection	150–900 mm	Trolley protection
Hand rails	For patients	Height	900 mm	32 mm thick
Equipment bays	For equipment	Recessed bays	On one side only	–
Wall phones in long corridors	–	–	–	As required

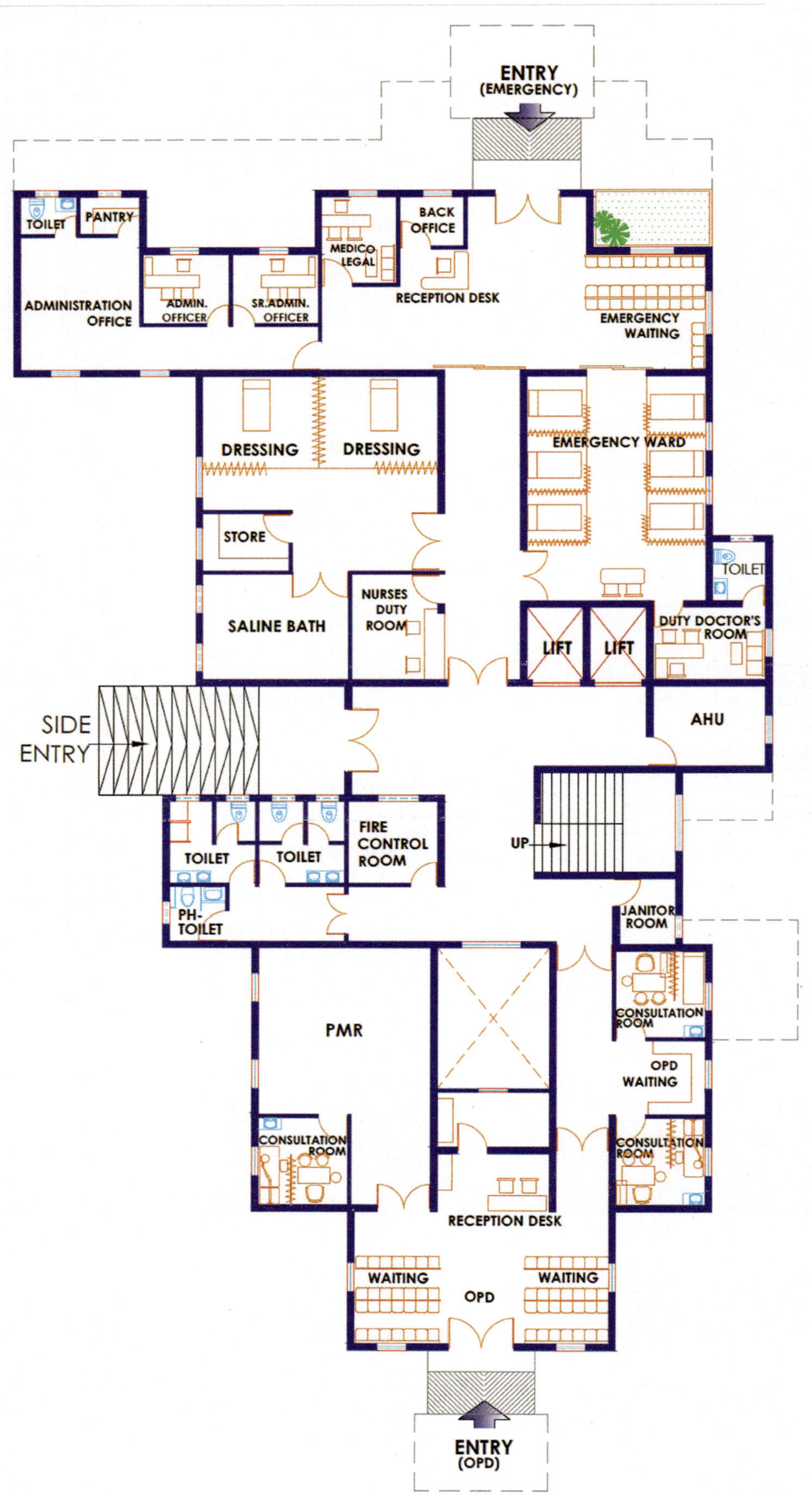

Fig. 5: Ground floor plan.
(PH Toilet: toilet for differently abled)

Table 2: Schedule of accommodation.

Type of area/space/room	Area (sqm)	Remarks
1 bed room isolation + anteroom	15 + 8	–
Bay for mobile equipment	4	For X-ray equipment it is to be 6 sqm
Saline bath unit	16	–
Amnion banking facility	16	To house equipment and work stations
Toilet–disabled/patient/public/ staff	5/4/3/2	–
Waiting area	@ 0.5 sqm per able bodied and 1.0 sqm per disabled person	

Note: Spaces for areas specific to burns center have been included.

Ergonomics and Human Engineering Aspects

At all places principles of ergonomics should be considered. For ensuring the facility *disabled friendly and barrier free* it is important to consider this issue at the time of planning. For this, ramps and rails, etc. should thus be provided. Adequate number of lifts should also be provided. The height of each step on a staircase should be such that enables easy climbing and descend. Recommended measurements are staircase width 1500 mm, tread 300 mm and riser of *150 mm.*[4]

Signages: Signages required are—*External signages*—for indicating the layout of the facility and various blocks, wards, etc.; *Internal signages*—to indicate fire exits, specific patient care areas, offices, etc. and

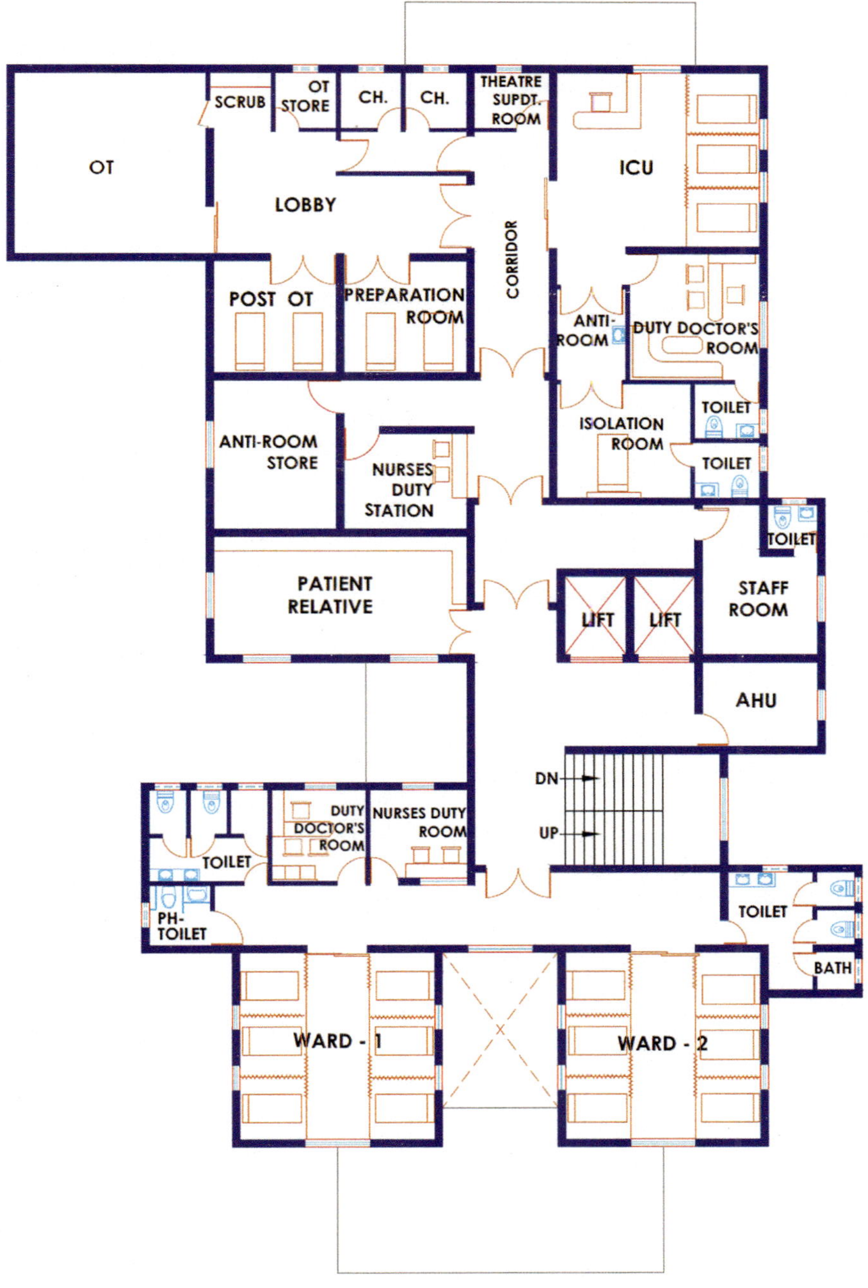

Fig. 6: First floor plan.
(PH Toilet: toilet for differently abled; CH: change room)

Box 6: Control of noise.

- Absorbent floor, wall and ceiling materials
- Least intrusive level for alarms
- Ceiling baffles
- Offsetting of doors
- Using counters and partitions

safety/escape signages. These should be prominently displayed and lighted at night or should be self glow type.[4]

Acoustics

Without reducing their importance or sense of urgency, such signals should be modulated to a level that will alert staff members, yet be rendered less intrusive. The variables for control of noise is given in Box 6.

Security

The building plan should facilitate secured housing of the patients, staff and equipment. It must cater the requirements of access control and should have provisions for preventing thefts and other such incidents. Intruder/duress alarms should be provided in suitable places. In critical areas online camera based monitoring can be considered. Adequate guard posts should be built-in in the plan.

Communication System

The requirement of a robust communication system is essential. It should consist of multiple means of communications to have redundancy in the system.

Building Codes/Regulations

Building codes and regulations to be complied with are local and National Building Code and norms for safety.

Air Conditioning

Air-treatment plants are required to fulfill two unrelated set of requirements: firstly guaranteeing ideal microclimatic conditions (temperature, humidity, dilution of smells, etc.) while keeping noise to a minimum, and second that of reaching and maintaining required levels of asepsis in the air, as required in the burns center. The recommended system for the airflow is directed vertical flow (Fig. 7 and Box 7). This ensures adequate air changes and sterility.[1,2,5]

In the wards and other direct patient care areas, there should be a separate exhaust system for quick evacuation of foul air in case of requirement. This system should have its activation switch-cum-damper in the nurses' duty station. The damper ensures that there is no need to deactivate the switch (i.e. auto-switch-off of the quick exhaust system). This system should be capable of evacuation of foul air as quickly as possible.[1,2,5]

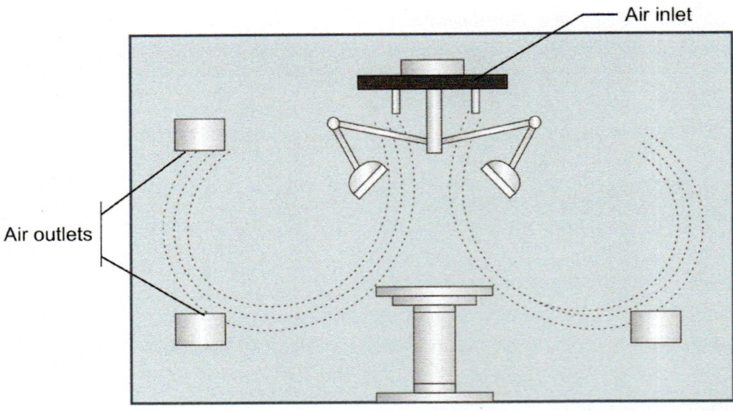

Fig. 7: Directed vertical flow.

Box 7: Air conditioning.

- Directed vertical flow is recommended method of airflow
- 100% fresh air, 22° ± 40° C; 4°–55% RH, 20–25 air changes per hour
- Separate AHUs for isolation rooms
- Heat-recovery wheel may be used for energy saving
- Regular monitoring and maintenance for good quality of indoor environment

Lighting

Adequate lighting is an essential requirement. In the management of burns patients for various bedside procedures both emergency and non-emergency require adequate lighting. Therefore glare free lighting should be provided as follows:

- General illumination : 100 lux
- Nursing station : 300 lux
- Examination area : 500 lux

CONCLUSION

The burns and reconstructive surgery center is a specialized facility which is essential to be established for management of burns. The special considerations must be taken into consideration for ensuring its appropriate utilization and effectiveness.

REFERENCES

1. www.expert-air-purifier-reviews.com
2. www.healthdesign.com.au
3. www.fgiguidelines.org
4. Gupta SK, Kant S, Chandrashekhar R, Satpathy S. Modern Trends in Planning and Designing of Hospitals—Principle and Practice. New Delhi: Jaypee Brothers Medical Publishers (P) Ltd, 2006.
5. Inzani F, Azienda Ospedaliera A.S.O., Restructuring and realization of the new burns centre at the Celio Military Polyclinic in Rome, in the light of new criteria in the control of infection, Annals of Burns and Fire Disasters—Vol XV–No. 4-December 2002.

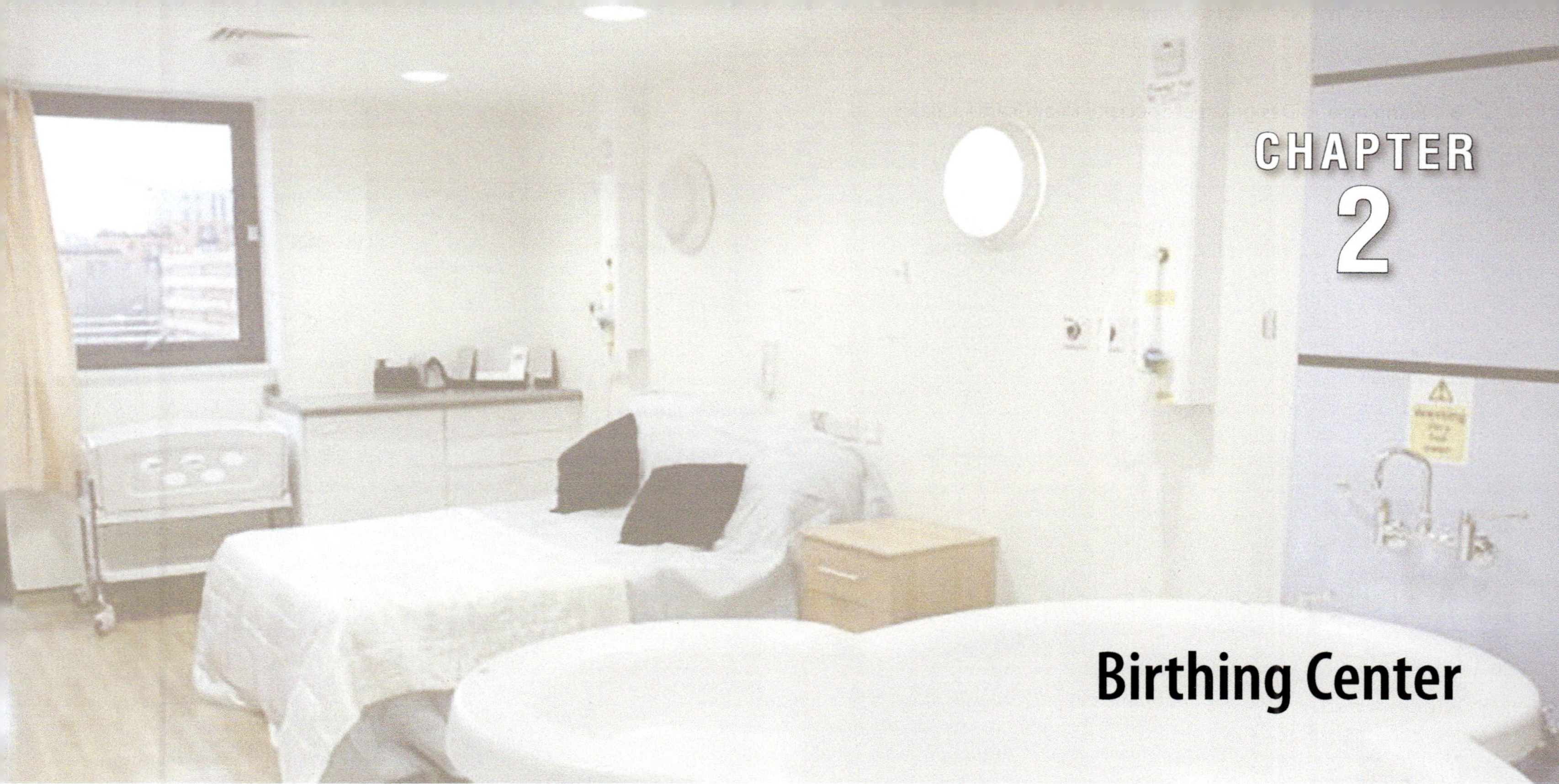

CHAPTER 2

Birthing Center

Pankaj Arora, Shakti Kumar Gupta, Sunil Kant, R Chandrashekhar

INTRODUCTION

A birth center is a home like facility existing within a healthcare system with a program of care designed in the wellness model of pregnancy and birth. Birth centers are guided by principles of prevention, sensitivity, safety, appropriate medical intervention, and cost-effectiveness. Birth centers provide family-centered care for healthy women before, during and after normal pregnancy, *labor* and birth.[1]

It needs to be emphasized that giving birth to a child is a natural process and that it is not a disease which needs to be cured. There are complications associated with this normal event on occasions wherein the expertise of an obstetrician is required. Hence, the natural process of normal labor needs to take place under the watchful eyes but it need not always be in the premises of a stressful place like a tertiary care hospital. Herein lays the origin of the concept of the *birthing center.*

The birthing center can be a place where deliveries take place in the safest manner by possibly reducing the MMR and NMR.[2] For women thought to be at low risk for obstetrical complications, labor and delivery at a birth center can result in higher patient satisfaction, cost savings, and equivalent or better outcomes than in-hospital birth.[3,4]

COMPONENTS OF THE BIRTHING CENTER

- Outpatient department (OPD)
- Diagnostic services
- Inpatient department
- Operation theater complex
- Obstetric intensive care unit (ICU)
- Neonatal intensive care unit (NICU)
- Support services.

There should be provisions for the support services, e.g. dietary services, sterile supply, laundry, security, parking, etc. If the center is located within a hospital campus then the services of central sterile services department (CSSD), laundry, kitchen, blood bank may be utilized. If it is a standalone center then these have to be considered. These may be outsourced or catered for in-house depending upon the policy of the facility or controlling authority and the size of the facility. This should essentially take into consideration the economic viability of establishing such support services in-house.

LOCATION OF THE BIRTHING CENTER

The decision regarding the location of the birthing center will depend on the following factors:

- State of the healthcare delivery system in the community
- Connectivity among the healthcare institutions
- Availability of the suitable land
- Policies governing the establishment of birthing center.

It may be located far from the hospital but easily connected to it so that the patient can be transferred in a minimum time at any stage without any problem. In conditions where this prerequisite is not always met, it may be established near the hospital or may be within the hospital campus but far from the main hospital building. In such a scenario, it should have a separate approach, entry and exit and different ambience without compromising its separate identity. There should be a buffer zone comprising of landscape or a garden, etc. between the hospital and the birthing center if the birthing center is located within the hospital campus. The buffer zone will:

- Add to the aesthetics of the place
- Give distinct look to the center
- Create a healing environment.

Healing is better and faster in the natural environment and such healthy environment leads to a general well-being of the patients. The functional relationship of birthing center with other facilities is shown in Figure 1.

Fig. 1: Relationship of birthing center with other facilities.
(ART: assisted reproductive technology; CSSD: central sterile services department; ICU: intensive care unit; OPD: outpatient department; OT: operation theater)

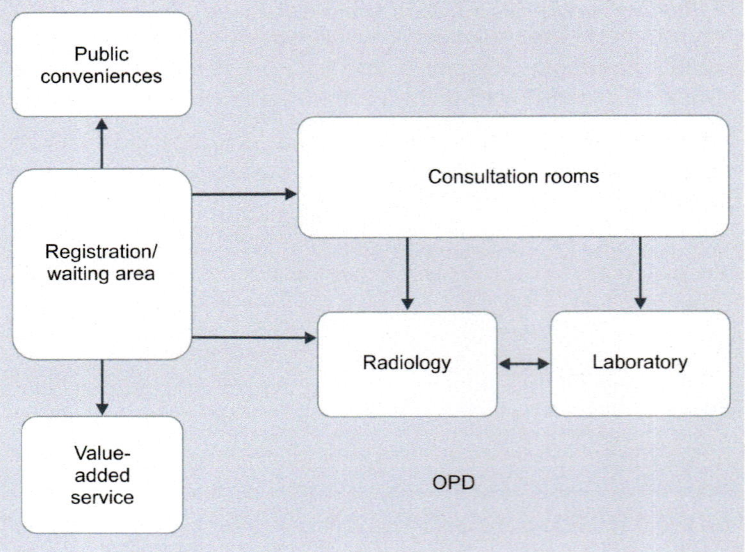

Fig. 2: Functional relationship in the OPD.
(OPD: outpatient department)

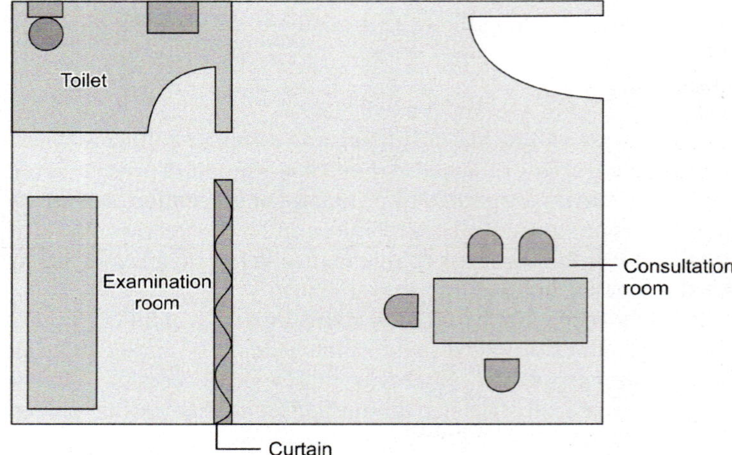

Fig. 3: Consultation room.

OUTPATIENT DEPARTMENT

Planning Considerations

The OPD is the first point of contact between the patient (client) and the center (provider). The OPD should provide the following services:

- Antenatal clinics
- Physiotherapy services
- Counseling services
- Immunization services.

The OPD should have the following:

- Consultation chambers
- Waiting spaces
- Public conveniences
- Value added services like ATM, book shop, gift shop, cafeteria, communication facility including internet cafe, pharmacy store, etc.

The functional relationships in the OPD are shown in Figure 2.

Design Considerations

Entrance: It should have ramps, wide doors (1.8 m) as well as steps.

Waiting area: Antenatal clinics generally have significant number of patients attending the facility. To reduce the waiting time and crowding in the facility appointment system should be followed but the waiting area cannot be done away with completely.

- Comfortable sitting arrangement should be made considering the fact the client is a pregnant woman
- A music system which can play "soft music" to ease the stress of waiting and any apprehension regarding visiting a health facility
- Alternatively it can have television to show programs related to pregnancy and delivery, family planning program, etc.
- *Space requirement*: An area of 0.5–0.8 sqm is required per patient
- Any other feature which can relieve the patient of apprehensions, e.g. paintings, aquarium, etc.

Consultation chamber: Depending upon the expected workload a number of consultation rooms have to be planned.

- Each consultation room should have the anteroom or a partition where the pregnant female can be examined in privacy (Fig. 3)
- *Space requirement*: A typical consultation room requires an area of 14 sqm, including the examination room and a toilet.

Physiotherapy room: Pregnancy causes certain changes in the female including hormonal and muscular changes. Hence, to support the antenatal as well as postnatal program, an physiotherapy room with at least four couches and instructors table should be provided.

Counseling room: During the period of pregnancy a woman may need counseling on a number of issues hence, counseling services should be provided.

Immunization facility: An immunization room manned by a trained nurse should be located in the OPD.

Nonstress test (NST)/fetal cardiotocography: An area/room to carry out NST/fetal cardiotocography should be provided in the OPD.

Reception and registration: A reception counter/help counter at the entry will help those visiting the facility for the first time especially the illiterate people. One registration desk per 20 patients should be provided. Counter should be 100 cm high with 60 cm wide work area.

Public conveniences: Toilets should be separate for male and female at the scale of one per 200 patients/visitors. It must include atleast one toilet for the disabled and children.

Access and circulation: The doors, wherever provided, should be wide enough (2 m) for easy movement of equipment, furniture and patient trolleys/wheelchairs.

Heating, Ventilating and Air-conditioning System (Table 1)

To economize, forced mechanical ventilation with a minimum 12 air changes may be provided.

Lighting: Whenever possible natural light is to be utilized as it promotes healing. Otherwise in patient examination area— 300–500 lux while in corridors and waiting area—200 lux.

DIAGNOSTIC SERVICES

The diagnostic facility should be housed on the same level as the OPD for the ease of patient movement. It should comprise predominantly of:

- Radiology services
- Laboratory services
- Sample collection room.

Radiology Services

The diagnostic radiology services should consist of X-ray, ultrasonography (USG) and color Doppler.

Planning Considerations

- Easy access for the patients
- Adequate sub-waiting area and having washrooms in close proximity
- Efficient recordkeeping.

Design Considerations

- Flexibility in design to cater for future expansion in view of rapid advancements in technology
- Wide entrance and wide doors for the movement of trolleys and equipment
- Safety features as X-ray room is part of the complex. The design and construction of the X-ray room must cater to the guidelines issued by Atomic Energy Regulatory Board (AERB) and Bhabha Atomic Research Center (BARC) such as thickness of the wall, lead lining and measurement of exposure to the staff, etc.

Table 1: Heating, ventilating and air-conditioning in outpatient department.

Parameter	*Specification*
Air pressure relationship to adjacent area	Standard, i.e. normal pressure
Minimum air changes per hour	8–10
Relative humidity	45 ± 5 normal filters
Temperature	24 ± 2°C

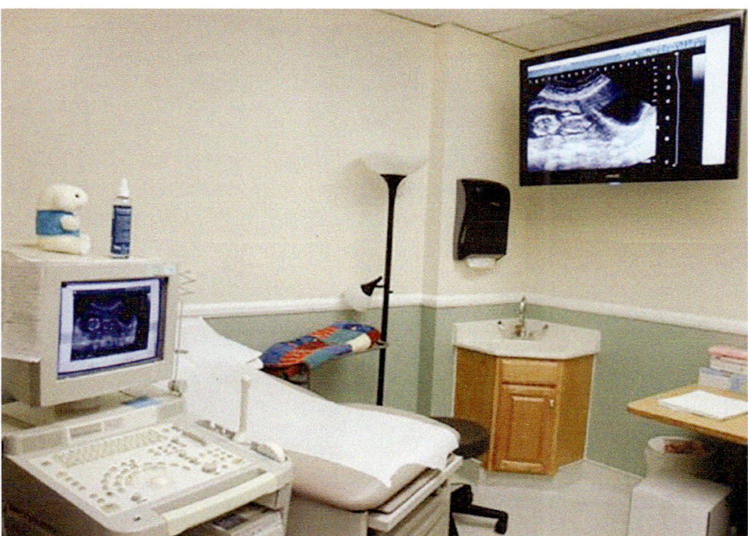

Fig. 4: Ultrasonography room.

Ultrasonography Room

Any obstetric set up will have predominantly USG facilities as far as radiology services are concerned. Multiple USG rooms have to be planned to cater for the expected workload. The USG room (Fig. 4) should have an area of 12 sqm.

X-ray Room

Though X-ray exposure is not advised during pregnancy but still an X-ray facility should be built to cater for those few indications that require such investigation. In such a scenario adequate lead protection must be given to the patient to minimize the exposure.

- Optimum size of X-ray room is 5.5 m × 6.0 m
- Ceiling height should be 3.0 m
- Thickness of the walls and ceiling will depend upon the construction material
- Film processing area should be 10–30 sqm depending upon the workload and the kind of equipment used
- Computer processing area should be 50 sqm and network connectivity should be provided to integrate with the picture archive and communication system (PACS) and telemedicine facility.

LABORATORY

Key features are:

- Comprehensive laboratory to conduct investigations, i.e. biochemical, hematological, microbiological and pathological should be built
- Adequate work space to be provided for smooth operations. Safe storage of all kind of materials, e.g. acidic, inflammable and radioactive, etc has to be thought of when planning a laboratory
- Flooring and work benches to be seamless and chemical resistant
- Pneumatic tube system for transport of samples from the indoor area
- Entry to the laboratory should be strictly regulated.

Sample Collection Area

Sample collection area should be a part of the laboratory complex. *Key features are:*

- Sample collection window and inquiry window (help counter)
- Adequate waiting area with easy access to washrooms.

Lighting

- *Radiology*: Specific lighting requirements in USG and X-ray room
- *Laboratory*: About 500 lux in the area of work
- *Waiting area and corridors*: About 200 lux.

Heating, Ventilating and Air-conditioning: Different areas will have different requirement, e.g. temperature should be between 20°C and 24°C in the laboratory but in the area having hot air oven in the laboratory it may not be so. Lab area should have 8–10 air changes per hour.

SEMINAR ROOM

A seminar room to address a gathering of around 30–50 people with advanced audiovisual aids should be constructed where teaching and educational activity may be carried out for the patients as well as the staff (if the birthing center also has teaching mandate, i.e. to train resident doctors, midwives, etc.). The seminar room must have a telemedicine node for connectivity for teleconsultation, education, etc.

Indoor/Inpatient Area

For ease of description it may be divided into three sub-units:
- Antenatal ward
- Labor, delivery, recovery, and postpartum (LDRP) suite
- Postnatal ward.

BIRTHING SUITE/LABOR, DELIVERY, RECOVERY AND POSTPARTUM CARE SUITE (FIGS. 5 AND 6)

The LDRP suites may be located on one level. Birthing suite or LDRP suite, i.e. labor, delivery, recovery, postpartum care suite is so called because the whole process of the childbirth, that is labor, delivery, recovery, postpartum care takes place in one room. Hence, these suites are to be built in such a way that they are equipped for labor and delivery. The facility offers the best of the two worlds, i.e. comfort and assurance of the homely environment plus the confidence of the health care setting. Any expectant mother who is admitted in the LDRP suite moves only once at the time of discharge, with the baby. This is an excellent example of patient focus care.

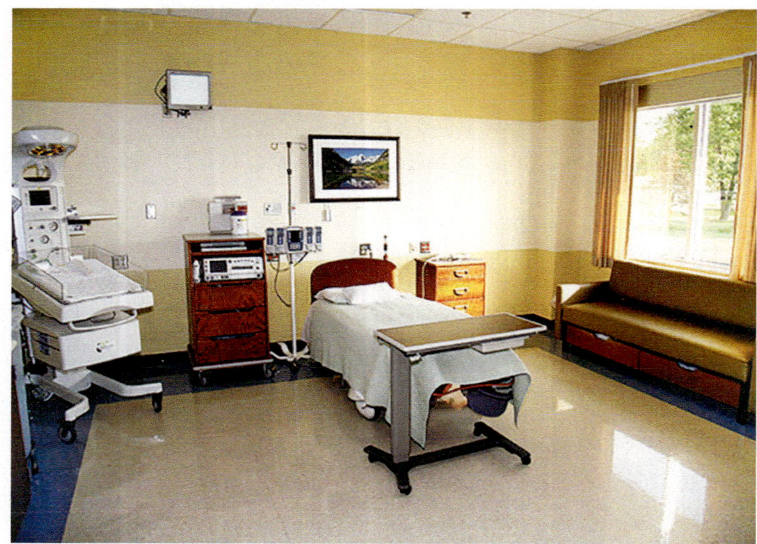

Fig. 5: Birthing suite/labor, delivery, recovery, and postpartum care suite.

Planning Parameters

- Provision of homely environment
- Provision of modern medical care
- Privacy of the patient
- Patient safety.

Design Parameters

- The room provides the resemblance of a home on a miniature scale having a bed for the patient as well as a sofa cum bed/settee for an attendant
- Cupboards are provided for the convenience of the patient and the relative. These cupboards are also used to keep the equipment required for the delivery and recovery, e.g. the portable delivery table light, etc.
- Entertainment facilities in the form of television/audio system add to the pleasure of the patient and helps in making her stress free
- *Communication facilities*: In the modern era of communication a telephone and a computer may also be provided as a part of value-added service
- Space and HVAC requirements are listed in Tables 2 and 3, respectively.

Architectural Considerations

- The interiors should be such that they have a soothing effect on the patient and the relatives
- The room can be decorated with works of art but attention should be given to the fact that these in no way should make the task of keeping the environment clean

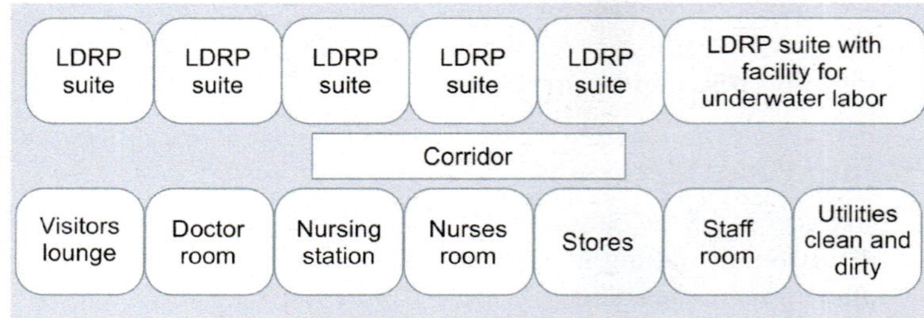

Fig. 6: Bubble diagram of a ward.
(LDRP: labor, delivery, recovery and postpartum)

Table 2: Space requirement—Labor, delivery, recovery and postpartum suite.

Parameter	Specification
Total area for LDRP suite	28 sqm
Area for toilet	5 sqm
Area for bassinet	3 sqm
Lighting	300–500 lux

Table 3: Heating, ventilating and air-conditioning—Labor, delivery, recovery and postpartum suite.

Parameter	Specification
Temperature	24°C ± 2°C
Relative humidity	45 ± 5%
Air changes	8–10 air changes per hour
Filtration efficiency	HEPA filters

- The room is also provided with attached toilet and may be a small pantry but the furniture in the room may be arranged in such a fashion that the entry is not in the line of direct vision. This will improve the aesthetics of the room. The door of the toilet should open outward into the patient room in view of patient safety
- The manifold or medical gases system is hidden, may be behind a painting or inside a cupboard, and is brought out only at the time of need.

LABOR, DELIVERY, RECOVERY AND POSTPARTUM BED

A very vital part of the furniture is the patient's bed. The specialty of the LDRP bed (Figs. 7A to E) is that it can be modified/converted to a delivery bed whenever required. Hence, there is no need to shift the patient to a delivery table at the time of delivery. A monitoring panel at the *head board* of the bed with maternal and fetal monitoring equipment can be provided. Provision should be made for the cradle with medical gases for neonatal care.

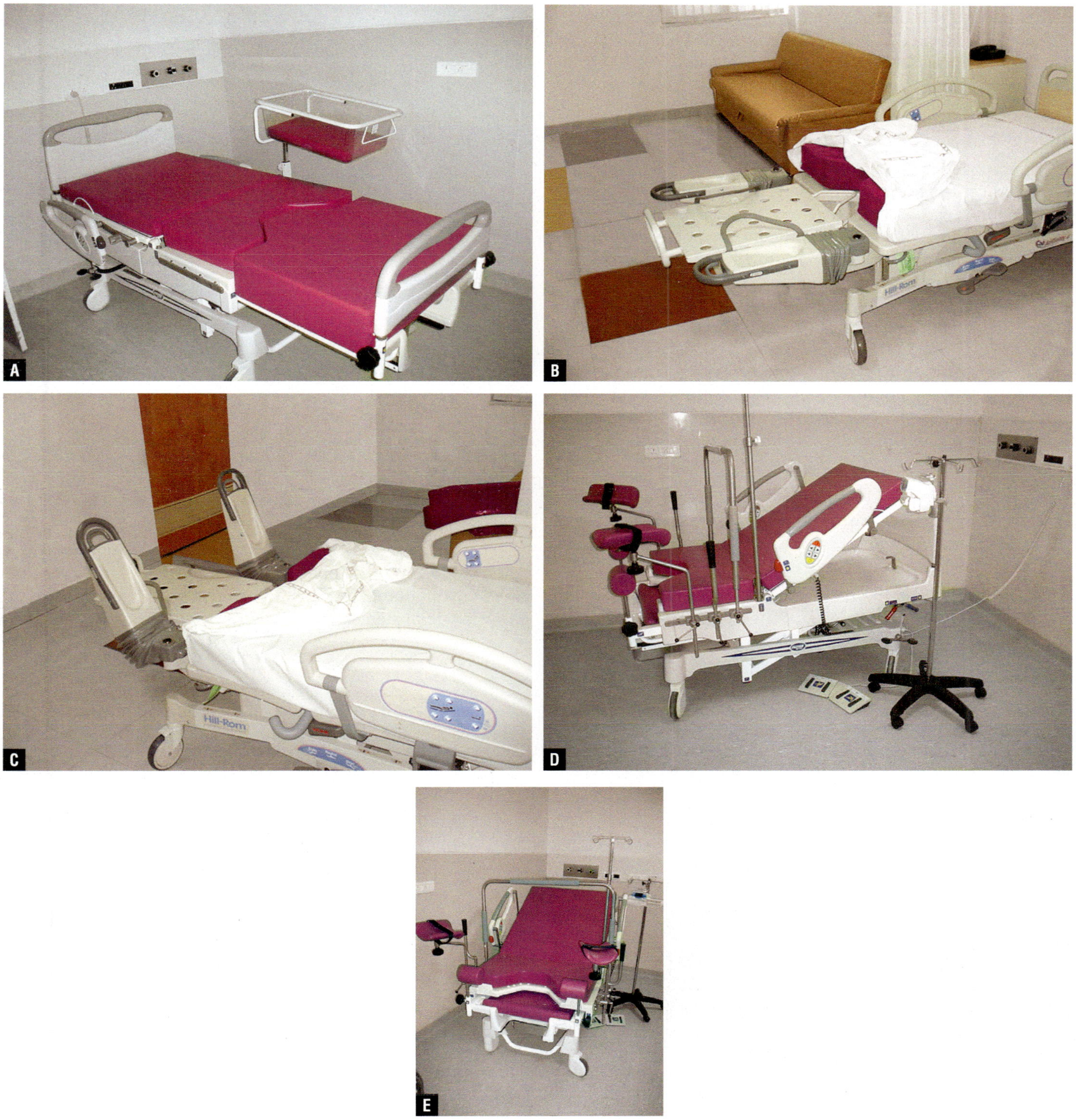

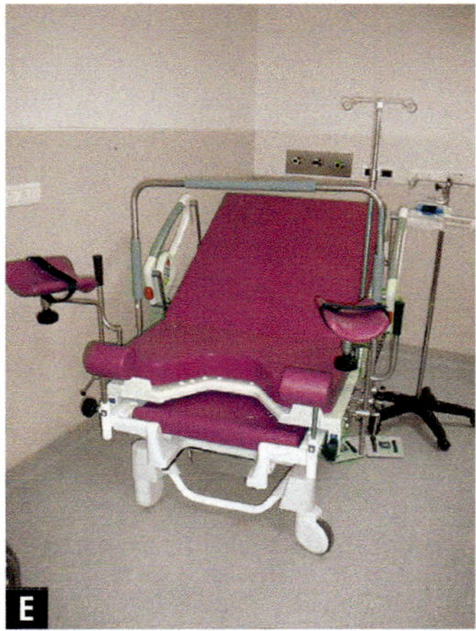

Figs. 7A to E: Conversion of a labor, delivery, recovery and postpartum bed to a delivery table.

UNDERWATER DELIVERY

A *concept* that has caught the attention is of "underwater delivery" (Fig. 8). It is said that the benefit of such a delivery is that warm water imparts elasticity to the tissues of the perineum reducing the incidence of tearing. The buoyancy of the water relaxes the female thereby reducing the pain and stress-related hormones, easing the process of delivery. A special wider birthing suite can be constructed to cater for such a birthing requirement. In addition to the facilities described above peninsular bath, with access to both sides of the bath, has to be provided which may be portable or a permanent feature of the suite. The area of such a bathroom should be 15 sqm. The temperature of the pool should be between 35°C and 37°C. The infrastructural requirements protocol for such a delivery has to be rigorously followed.[5,6]

Antenatal Area

Though the emphasis is on safe delivery and minimal stay of patients in the birthing center, there will be a few patients who will require prolonged monitoring. Such patients should be housed in the antenatal ward. It has to be ensured that the environment is as homely as possible within the constraints and the patient is provided as much privacy as is possible. The ward should have a small recreation room with facility for reading the books, indoor games and such other things. The privacy should be provided with the use of curtains or movable low height partitions.[5,6]

In case of anticipated normal delivery the patient can be shifted to a LDRP suite or in case of operative intervention to the OT. Each ward should have atleast two isolation rooms to cater for the cases suffering from some infectious comorbidity.

Postoperative Area

On the lines of an antenatal ward, a postnatal ward will take care of the patients who have undergone an operative procedure, i.e. cesarean section. The considerations and parameters are more or less same for both the antenatal and postnatal ward.

Some of the key parameters while designing a ward (antenatal/postnatal) are at Table 4.

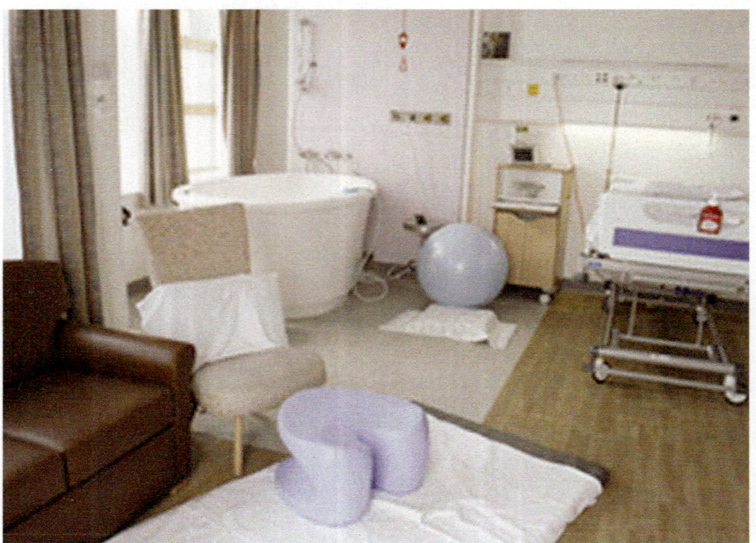

Fig. 8: Underwater delivery.

Table 4: Parameters for antenatal ward.

Parameters	Specification
Area per bed space (min)	7 sqm
Isolation room/one bed room with attached toilet and bath	15 sqm
2 beds room	24 sqm
4 beds room	36 sqm
Nursing station	16 sqm
Space at the head end	0.25 m
Space at the foot end	0.9 m
Corridor width	2.7 m
Distance between two bed centers	2.25 m
Door width	1.2 m
Water closet/bath	1 per 8 beds/attached with each room
Lighting	300–500 lux
Lighting in corridors	150–200 lux

Heating, Ventilating and Air-conditioning System

Temperature	: 24°C ± 2°C
Relative humidity	: 45 ± 5%
Air changes	: 8–10 air changes per hour; 100% fresh air preferred in isolation room
Filtration efficiency	: HEPA filters

CRITICAL AREAS

The critical areas of a hospital should be housed on one level. These are:
- Operation theater/suite including a labor room
- Obstetric ICU
- Nursery/NICU

The advantage of keeping these units on one floor is close relationship with each other and minimization of traffic resulting in ease of maintaining the sterility required in such an area and ease in providing dedicated mechanical services.

OPERATION THEATER COMPLEX

The operating unit provides a controlled climatic environment for the operative and perioperative care of patients undergoing a surgical procedure under anesthesia.

Number: An operation theater complex consisting of two or more OTs, depending on the workload and the policy of the birthing center needs to be constructed.

Location: While planning for an OT complex the objectives are to ensure highest standards of asepsis, safety and flexibility including future expansion. To achieve these objectives all nonessential traffic in this area should be avoided. Hence the location should be such so as to achieve this objective. When the birthing center is located within a major hospital complex, it is preferable to match with the hospital OT floor for easy connectivity for any major/specialized nature of surgical procedure.

Planning: All the norms that are followed while designing any other OT viz. pressure zoning, lighting, spaces, rooms and equipment are to be followed.

Space requirement: An area of 36–48 sqm per major OT is required for the theater itself while the complex requires a far larger area as it houses other facilities, e.g. the space requirement for support areas which include stores, anesthetic room, clean up room, etc. can be 150 sqm and above depending upon the scale of operations. Corridors should be wide and in no case less than 2.85 m in width to allow movement of stretchers and trolleys.

Medical gases: A manifold system must be provided for medical gases in the operation theater complex. Outlets should be provided in all patient care areas. Cylinders should be kept for emergency in case the backup manifold points also fail or due to some other reason there is disruption in piped gas supply.

Heating, Ventilating and Air-conditioning System

Heating, ventilating and air-conditioning system parameters are summarized in Table 5.

Labor Room

A *labor* room/delivery room should be planned alongside OT where a trial of labor is given in cases where some difficulty to normal *labor* is expected so that the patient may be shifted to OT without delay in case of exigency.

OBSTETRIC INTENSIVE CARE UNIT (FIG. 9)

The ICU provides the critical care needed due to the serious condition of the patients, e.g. puerperal sepsis, PPH, etc.

Location: An ICU is to be located in close proximity to the OT away from the traffic zones with 6–12 beds depending upon the expected workload. It must be easily connected to other areas with controlled access.

Patient care area: Each bed should have adequate circulation space (preferably 360°C) for each patient. Every bed should have arrangements for adequate lights for examination/emergent intervention. Nursing station should be planned in such a way that all the beds are visible from the station. A central multisign monitoring system is to be provided.

Manifold: Bed head panel should have manifold outlets in the form of:

Oxygen outlets—2, vacuum—1, medical air—1.

The panel also contains holder for vacuum collection jar, nurse call switch, infusion pump mount pole and one head light. There must be atleast 6 electrical points for:

Ventilator—1, infusion pumps—2, multisign monitor —1, defibrillator—1, reserve—1. Out of these 6 points at least 3 should be power backed and differently colored for easy identification.

Table 5: Heating, ventilating and air-conditioning system parameter and specification.

Parameter	*Specification*
Air pressure relationship to adjacent area	Positive
Air changes per hour	Preferably 100% fresh air to be provided; otherwise 15–20 changes per hour
Filtration efficiency	HEPA filters
Relative humidity	45 ± 5%
Temperature	22 ± 2°C

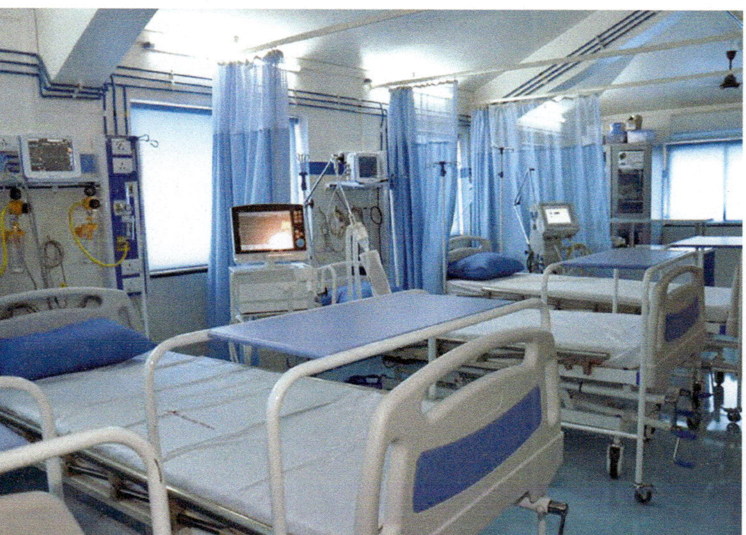

Fig. 9: Obstetric intensive care unit.

Table 6: Heating, ventilating and air-conditioning system—Obstetric intensive care unit.

Parameter	*Specification*
Air pressure relationship to adjacent area	Positive
Air changes per hour	15–20 changes per hour
Filtration efficiency	HEPA filters
Relative humidity	45 ± 5%
Temperature	22 ± 2°C

Space requirement: An area of 12–15 sqm per bed is required which is larger than a general ward bed and is exclusive of the space requirement for service areas.

Heating, Ventilating and Air-conditioning System

Parameters recommended are listed in Table 6.

Eclampsia Room

Two isolation rooms should be earmarked as eclampsia rooms at one end of the ICU. These rooms should have all the facilities of an ICU. Additionally these must also be capable for the delivery to take place. The rooms should be readily connected to OT in case an operative intervention is required. Alternatively such rooms can be planned alongside the labor room which will save on the cost of creating facilities for the delivery as required in the previous setting (Fig. 10).

NURSERY/NEONATAL INTENSIVE CARE UNIT

The NICU (Fig. 11) is meant to take care of sick neonates who require long-term life support/advanced life support.

The neonatal ICU should be manned by trained staff at all the times, i.e. pediatrician, nursing staff and even the house keeping staff should be accustomed to the peculiar requirements of the area.

Each patient treatment area in the NICU is to be 12 sqm. This floor area excludes the areas meant for support facilities, e.g. staff station, store, and hand washing, etc. which are to be provided when designing a NICU.

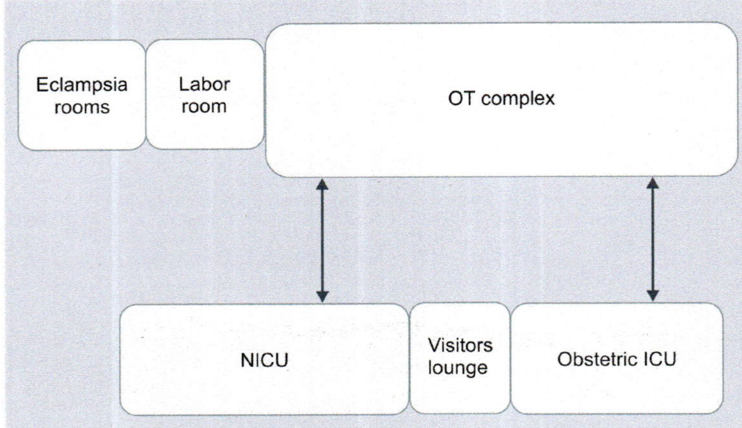

Fig. 10: Relationship of a delivery complex in the intensive care unit.
(ICU: intensive care unit; NICU: neonatal intensive care unit; OT: operation theater)

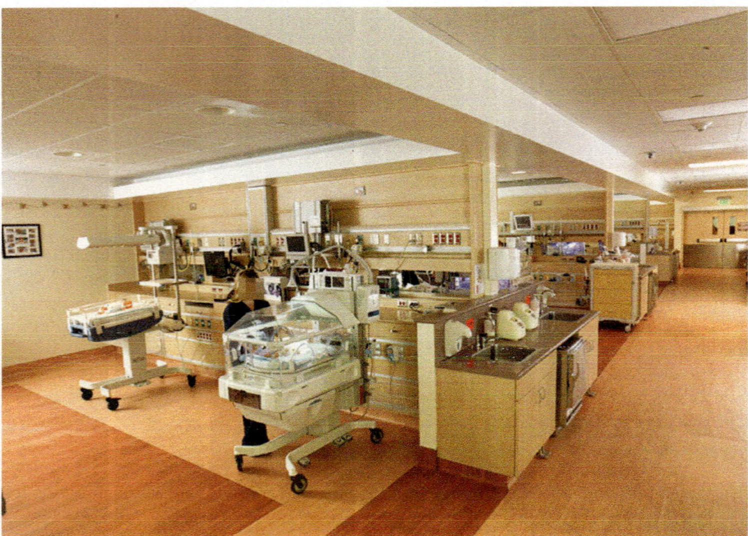

Fig. 11: Neonatal intensive care unit.

There should be a consult/breastfeeding room of an area of 9 sqm with the facilities for the mothers to feed their babies, e.g. breast pump, etc. Depending upon the amount of medical and general supplies to be stocked, stores may occupy an area of 20–50 sqm. The width of the door of the NICU should be such that it allows the entry of investigative apparatus, i.e. X-ray machine, etc.

Special Provision for Asepsis

The NICU can have a large glass window for the relatives of the patient to view the neonate as it may provide them some amount of emotional support. Alternatively, aid of audiovisual system can be taken. The NICU should have multiple closed circuit cameras and the images are fed into a screen (television) placed in the visitor's lounge. This will serve the emotional needs of the parents and also help in maintaining the sterility. Whenever the healthcare worker needs to contact the parents the help of the audio aid can be taken.

OTHER CONSIDERATIONS FOR THE BIRTHING CENTER

Infection Control

General Considerations

Infection control should aim at prevention of spread of infection by any means within the facility.

Infection control measures should be a part of planning and designing. LDRP suite is one step in this direction.

The most effective and efficient, yet simplest, measure of preventing infection is hand washing.

Hand Washing

- Wash basins for hand washing should be available within each treatment area and should be accessible without traversing any other clinical area
- Number of hand washing units required are:
  - ICU—one per bed
  - Ward—one per four beds
  - OPD—one per consultant.
- Under no circumstances a person requiring to use a hand wash unit should be 10–12 m away from a wash unit.
- To avoid some of the disadvantages associated with wash basins (plumbing issues), a sterilizing liquid can be used instead of soap and water. This sterilizing liquid has to be used without water and it evaporates with rubbing the hands.

Floor Plans

These are depicted at Figures 12 to 16.

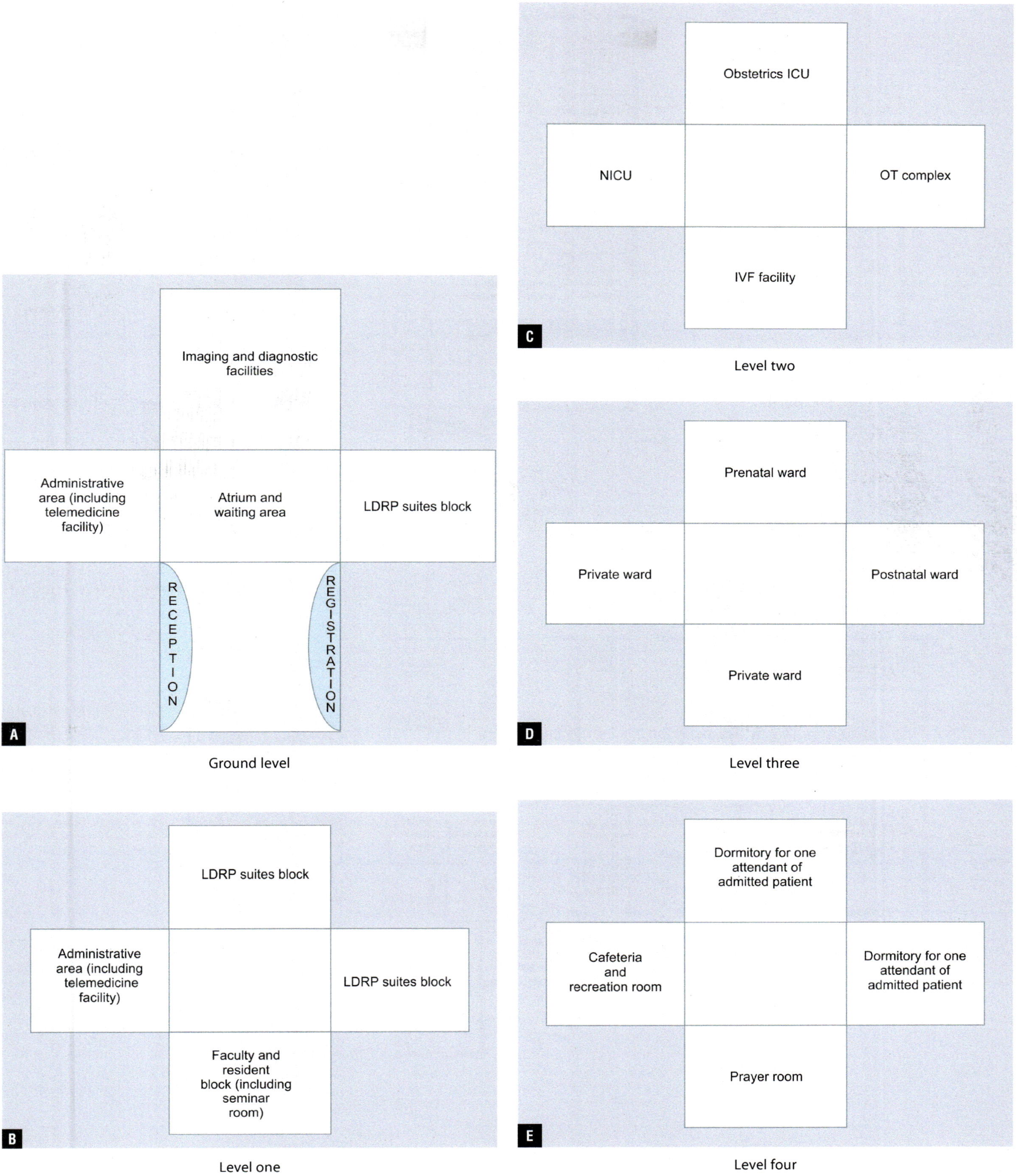

Figs. 12A to E: Floor-wise space distribution for a birthing center.

(ICU: intensive care unit; ICU: intensive care unit; IVF: *in vitro* fertilization; LDRP: labor, delivery, recovery and postpartum; NICU: neonatal intensive care unit; OT: operation theater)

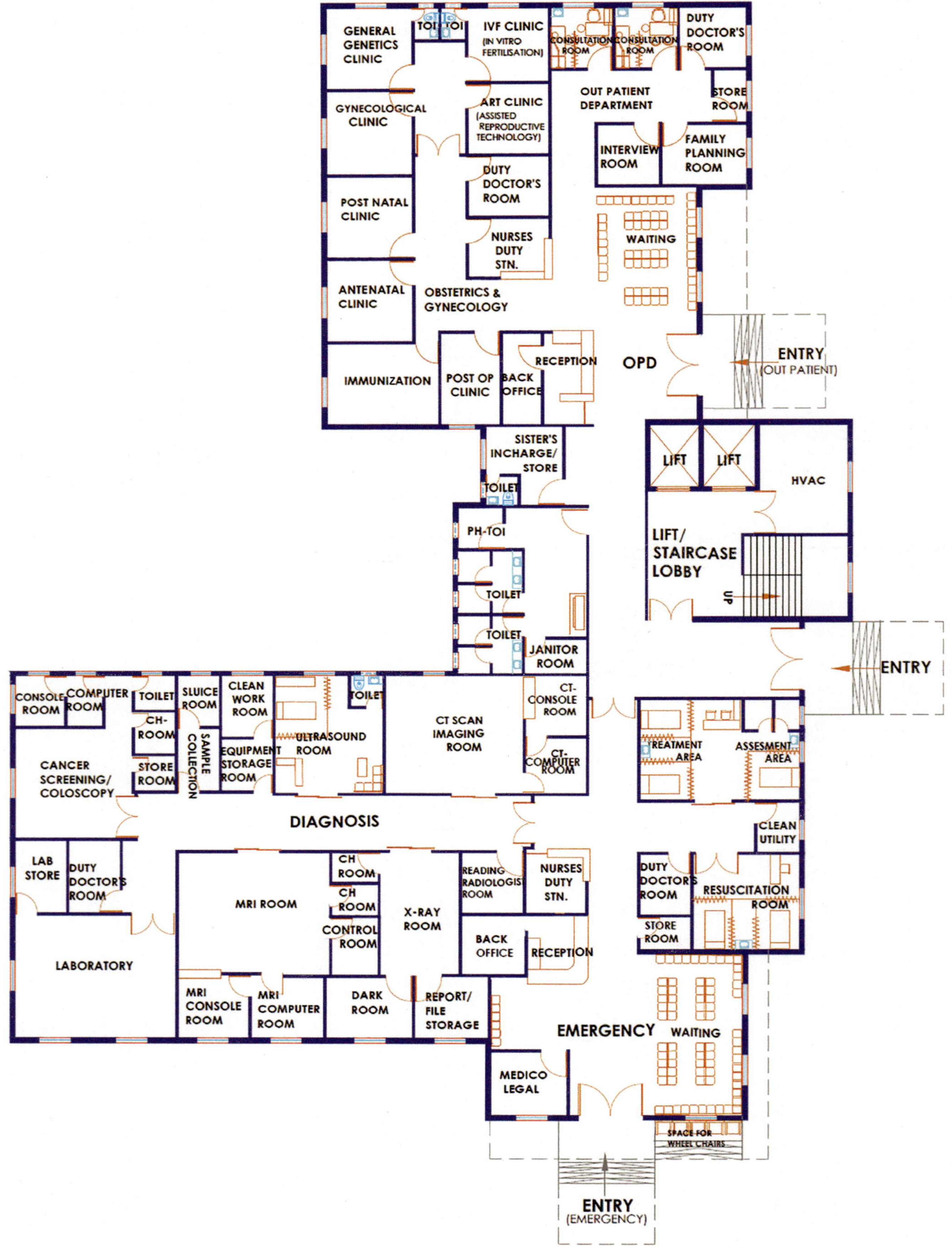

Fig. 13: Ground floor plan.

(CH: change room; PH-TOI: toilet for differently abled)

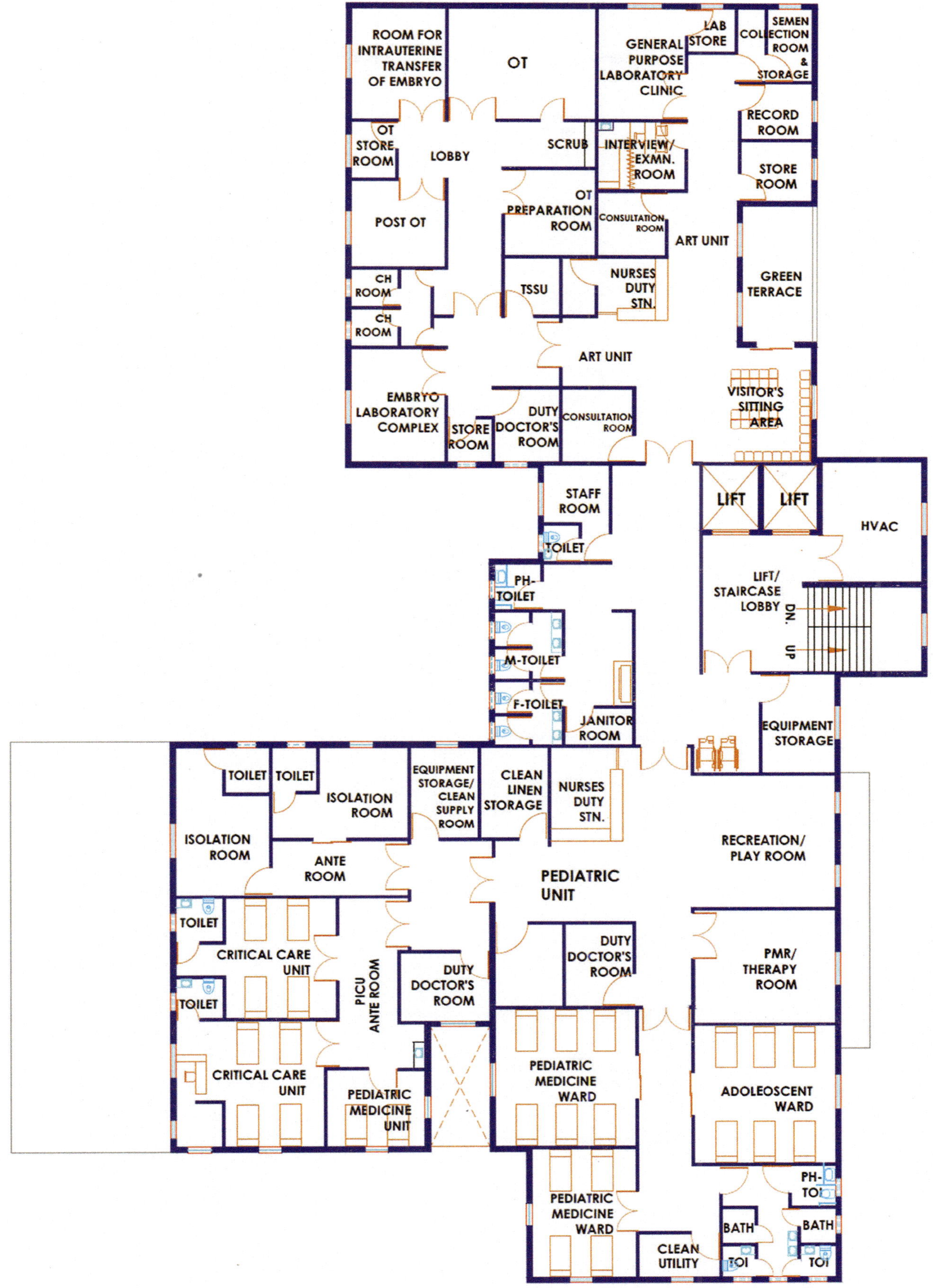

Fig. 14: First floor plan.

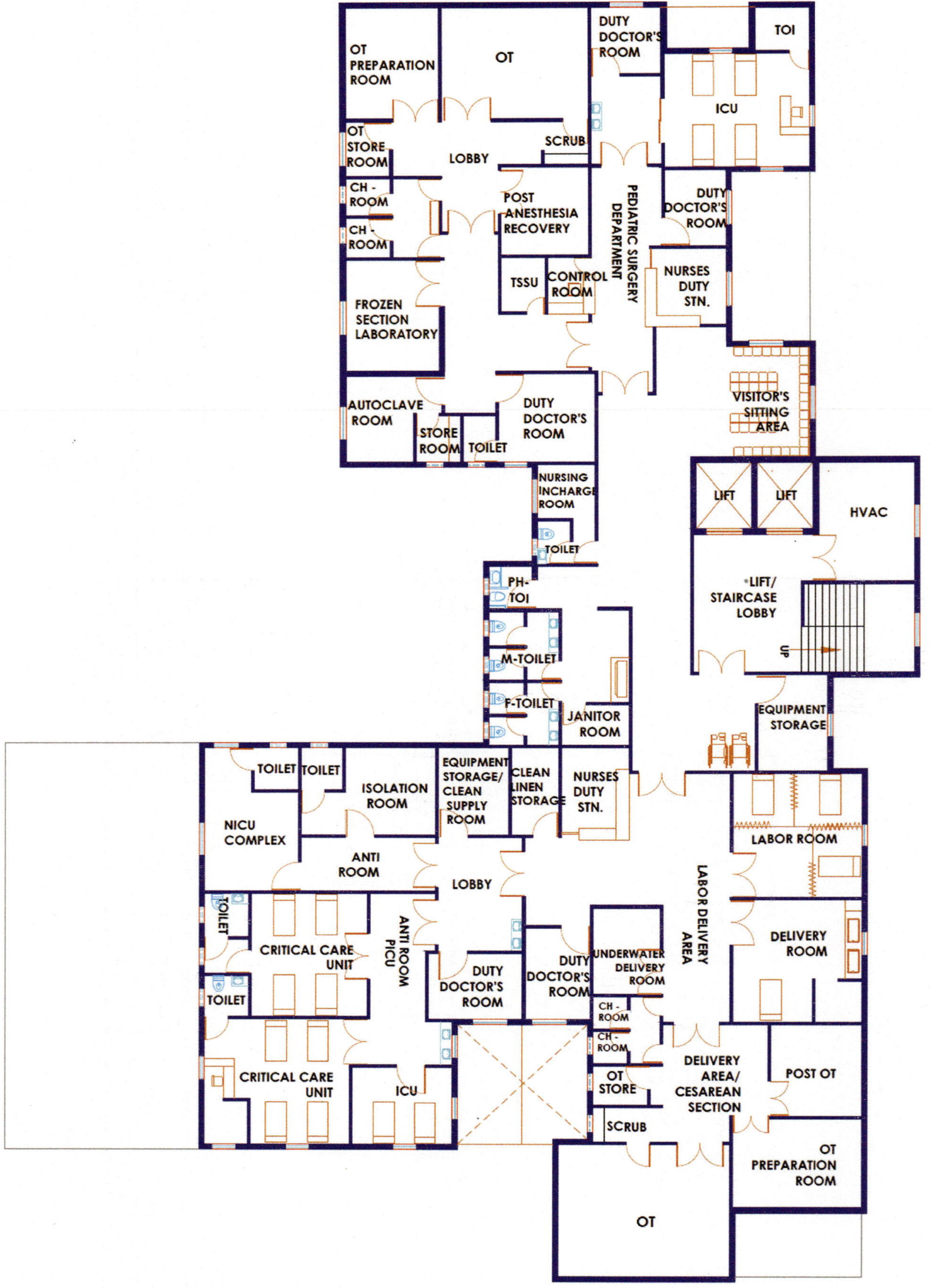

Fig. 15: Second floor plan.

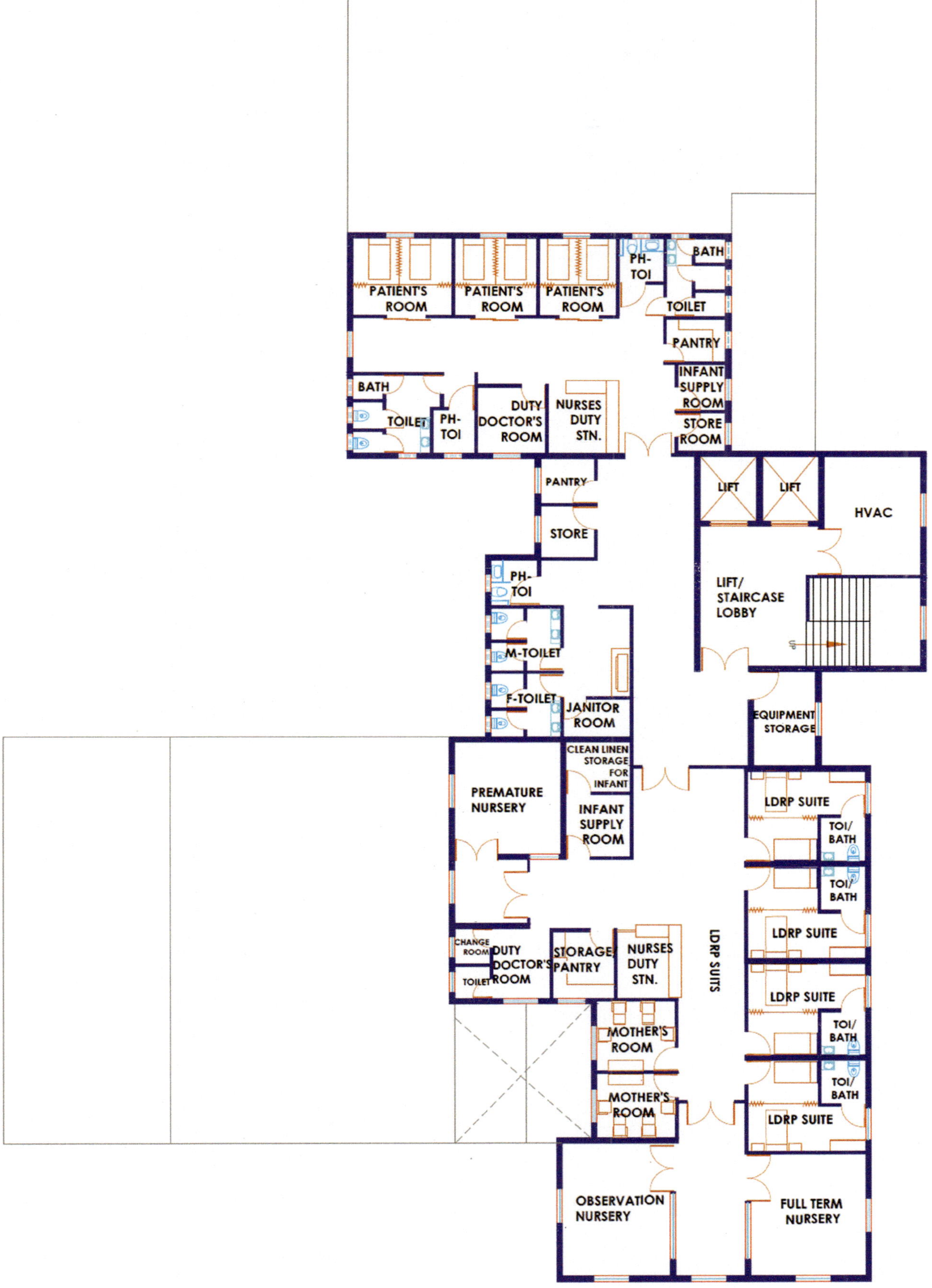

Fig. 16: Third floor plan.

CONCLUSION

The intent behind the birthing center is to give due importance to this area of medical science as it is often seen that it is neglected by the planners while allocating funds and space. As per the necessities of the community and various constraints, e.g. space, finances, manpower, etc. a birthing center can be planned and designed. The eventual birthing center may be a stand alone facility with its own support services or it may be a part of an existing hospital as a satellite center.

REFERENCES

1. American Association of Birth Centers. Position Statements. [online] Available from: http://www.birthcenters.org/about-aabc/position-statements/definition-of-birth-center 2016.
2. Martin JA, Hamilton BE, Ventura SJ, et al. Births: Final data for 2010. Natl Vital Stat Rep. 2012; 61:1-72.
3. Swartz W, Jackson D, Lang J, et al. The BirthPlace collaborative practice model: results from the San Diego Birth Center Study. Prim Care Update Ob Gyns. 1998;5(4):207.
4. www.uptodate.com
5. American Association of Birth Centers: http:/www.birthcenters.org/about-aabc/positionstatments/immersion-in-water.
6. Henderson J, Burns EE, Regalia AL, et al. Labouring women who used a birthing pool in obstetric units in italy: prospective observational study. BMC Pregnancy and Childbirth. 2014;14:17.

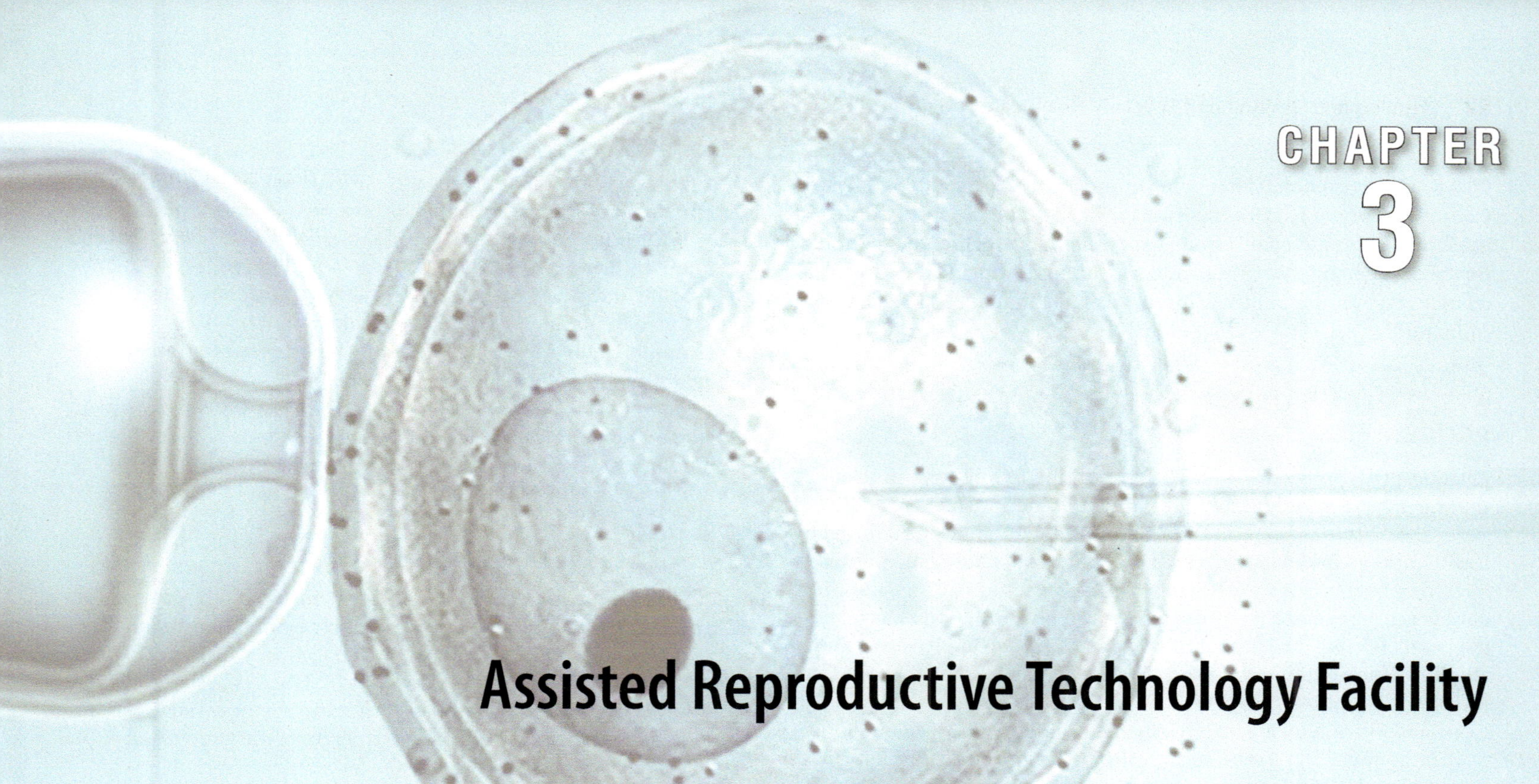

CHAPTER 3

Assisted Reproductive Technology Facility

Sheetal Singh, Shakti Kumar Gupta, Sunil Kant, R Chandrashekhar

INTRODUCTION

Assisted reproductive technology (ART) *clinic*[1] means any premises used for procedures related to *assisted reproductive technology*. *Assisted reproductive technology*,[2] with its grammatical variations and cognate expressions, means all techniques that attempt to obtain a pregnancy by handling or manipulating the sperm or the oocyte outside the human body, and transferring the gamete or the embryo into the uterus. Assisted reproductive technology according to the WHO definition[1-4] refers to infertility treatments, where both eggs (oocytes) and sperm are handled to achieve a live birth. In conventional ART procedures the oocytes and sperm are combined in a laboratory (*in vitro*) and the resulting embryo is transferred to a woman. ARTs include *in vitro* fertilization (IVF) with or without injection of a sperm into the oocyte intracytoplasmic sperm injection (ICSI).

Infertility, though not life threatening, causes intense mental agony and trauma that can only be best described by infertile couples themselves. There are no detailed figures of the extent of infertility prevalent in India but a multinational study carried out by WHO[1] that included India, places the incidence of infertility between 10% and 15%. *Out of a population of 1,000 million Indians*, an estimated 25% (250 million individuals) may be conservatively estimated to be attempting parenthood at any given time; by extrapolating the WHO estimate, approximately 13–19 million couples are likely to be infertile in the country at any given time.

Prevention and appropriate treatment of infertility has been included in the ICPD (International Conference on Population and Development) Program of Action; it follows that alleviation of infertility should be included as a component of the primary healthcare system. Most types of infertility, such as reproductive tract infections (RTIs) and genital tuberculosis, are preventable and amenable to treatment. About 8% of infertile couples, however, need serious medical intervention involving the use of advanced ART procedures, such as IVF ICSI. Such advanced treatment is expensive and not easily affordable to the majority of Indians. Further, the successful practice of ART requires considerable technical expertise and expensive infrastructure. Moreover, the success rate of any ART procedure is below 30% under the best of circumstances.[4]

Infertility, especially in our country, also has far-reaching societal implications. Therefore, with the rapidly increasing use of ART in our country, it has become imperative to ensure their safety and have safeguards against their possible misuse.[5]

Scientific societies around the world, such as the American Society for Reproductive Medicine (ASRM), European Society of Human Reproductive and Embryology (ESHRE), and International Federation of Fertility Societies (IFFS), have drawn up guidelines for the safe and ethical practice of ART. The European Union and the Governments of several countries, such as Australia, the UK and the USA have taken steps to accredit and supervise the performance of infertility clinics.[5]

HISTORY OF IN VITRO FERTILIZATION

The world's first IVF baby, Louise Brown, was born on July 25, 1978 in UK through the efforts of Dr Robert G Edwards and Dr Patrick Steptoe. The world's second and India's first IVF baby, Kanupriya, alias Durga, was born 67 days later on October 3, 1978, through the efforts of Dr Subhas Mukherjee and his two colleagues in Kolkata. Dr Mukherjee and his colleagues published a short note on their above work, in the Indian Journal of Cryogenics. The techniques used by Mukherjee were markedly different from those used by Edwards and Steptoe.[6]

Dr Mukherjee was the first person in the world to use:

- Gonadotropins for ovarian stimulation prior to ovum pick-up in an IVF treatment cycle
- The transvaginal route by colpotomy for harvesting oocytes
- Freezing and thawing of human embryos before transferring them into the uterus that led to the successful birth of Durga.

India's first scientifically documented IVF baby, Harsha, was born on August 6, 1986, in Mumbai, through the collaborative efforts of the Indian Council of Medical Research's (ICMRs), Institute for Research in Reproduction and the King Edward's Memorial Hospital (KEM).

This work was executed after being approved by the Scientific Advisory Committee of the ICMR's Institute for Research in Reproduction and the Ethics Committee for Human Experimentation of the KEM Hospital. Births of IVF babies were reported subsequently during the same year by two other clinics in India. There are an estimated 250 IVF clinics in India today.[7]

ASSISTED REPRODUCTIVE TECHNOLOGY: PROCEDURES

A variety of ART procedures have been described. Only those procedures that have been widely tested and proven to be satisfactory are listed here. The National Accreditation Committee[1] or a body appointed by it will approve or disapprove the new procedure within six months of its having been made aware of in writing—if this is not done, the clinic could continue to use the procedure until the above body has taken a decision on it. No new procedure that has not been approved as above should be permitted to be used by an infertility clinic for more than the period mentioned above.[3,6]

If a clinic is offering an ART that is not listed in these guidelines now or as modified in the future, the procedure must be approved by the clinics ethics committee, constituted as recommended by the ICMR Ethical Guidelines, 2000, justifying the need for the procedure and explaining why alternatives are not suitable. Only clinics of Level 2 or Level 3 would be required to have an ethics committee.[3,5]

Artificial Insemination with Husband's Semen

The technique consists in placing in the interior of the vagina a sample of the unprocessed semen.

Artificial Insemination with Donor Semen

The indications for Artificial Insemination with Donor Semen (AID) are when there is (a) nonobstructive azoospermia; (b) the husband has a hereditary genetic defect; or (c) when the couples have Rh incompatibility.

The main advantage of AID is that it enables a couple to achieve pregnancy even though the husband is not the biological father. However, the possible transmission of diseases from the donor to the future child and the risk of consanguinity, constitute some drawbacks that must be brought to the notice of the patients.[7,8]

Intrauterine Insemination with either Husband's or Donor Semen

Intrauterine insemination (IUI) involves the processing of semen in the laboratory so as to yield pure, activated sperm, devoid of seminal plasma, which are then directly placed into the uterus.

In Vitro Fertilization and Embryo Transfer

The technique of IVF consists of bringing about the fertilization of the oocyte and the spermatozoa in the laboratory instead of in the woman's fallopian tube. IVF involves induction of ovulation in order to obtain multiple oocytes, thus making available more embryos with which higher pregnancy rates can be achieved. Serial determination of plasma estradiol levels and daily monitoring of ovarian follicular growth by ultrasonography would indicate the response to ovarian stimulation. At the appropriate moment of follicular growth, the follicles are aspirated to obtain the oocytes. The oocytes are mixed with appropriately capacitated spermatozoa from the husband (or the donor, if the medical condition indicates the use of donor sperm) and kept in an incubator for fertilization which is observed microscopically after 16–18 hours. Embryos are transferred into the uterine cavity between days 2 and 6 after oocyte aspiration. If implantation ensues, pregnancy can be confirmed by 14–16 days after embryo transfer by determining the presence of human chorionic gonadotropin (HCG) in a blood or urine sample. Such a test is reliable only when progesterone is used for luteal supplementation instead of hCG.

The success rate of IVF is approximately one in every 4–5 women. IVF is the therapeutic option of reproductive medicine with the highest yield per attempt, coming close on many occasions to that achieved by fertile couples conceiving naturally.

IVF-associated Techniques (Fig. 1)

Gamete intrafallopian tube transfer (GIFT) or tubal embryo transfer (TET) has been recommended for patients with undamaged fallopian tubes. Access to the tube is gained by laparoscopy or by retrograde catheterization through the uterine cervix. GIFT is associated with higher levels of pregnancy than IVF, but it has the drawback that it is unable to demonstrate the fertilizing capacity of the gametes.

Intracytoplasmic Sperm Injection with Ejaculated, Epididymal or Testicular Spermatozoa

It is well known that the incidence of fertilization with suboptimal semen is much lower in contrast to normal semen samples. It has been argued that since a sizable number of couples are not suitable for IVF because their sperm count is far below 10 million/mL with less than 30% sperm being motile and more than 30% having abnormal morphology, alternate methods must be found to facilitate fertilization. Several approaches have been developed to circumvent the barriers (the zona pellucida and the ooplasmic membrane) that prevent the sperm reaching the ooplasm. Notable amongst these are—partial zona dissection (PZD), subzonal insemination (SUZI), and ICSI.

Live births have been reported using all these methods. The use of PZD or SUZI must be discouraged, as they do not offer any distinct advantage. ICSI is the most widely accepted choice of treatment for male factor infertility. ICSI can be carried out with fresh or frozen-thawed ejaculated or epididymal/testicular motile or live spermatozoa.

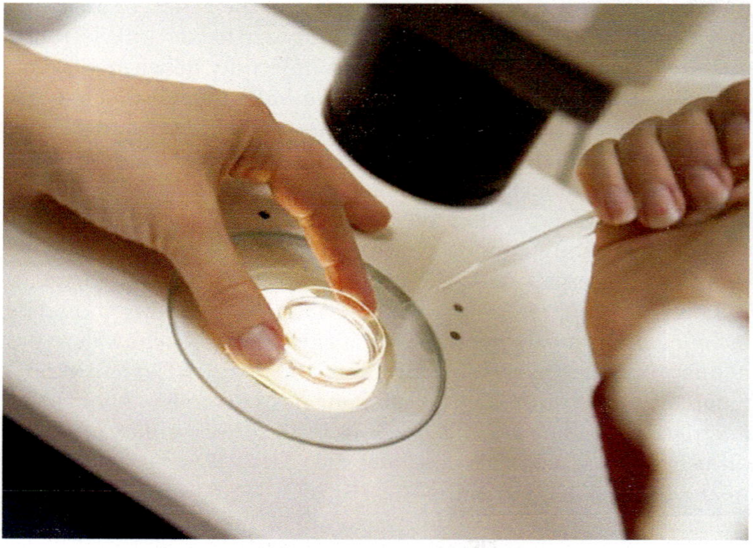

Fig. 1: *In vitro* fertilization-associated techniques.

Oocyte Donation or Embryo Donation

Oocyte donation would necessitate using the husband's semen for fertilization and transferring the resultant embryo to the infertile female partner. Embryo donation would obviate the necessity of using the husband's semen. The choice of oocytes and embryos for oocyte or embryo donation would depend entirely on the circumstances prevalent at the time the infertile couple comes for treatment, and the access of the infertility clinic to frozen oocytes or embryos.

Cryopreservation (Fig. 2)

Facilities for cryopreservation are an essential component of an ART clinic as they are to be used under a variety of conditions, such as those described below.[7,8]

Freezing Semen (Fig. 3)

Men, who are likely to suffer from psychological stress at the time of ovum pick-up or those who cannot be present at the time of ovum pick-up, are recommended to have their semen frozen for use at the appropriate time. One of the important reasons for freezing semen from donors is that any donor semen has to be quarantined for six months. The safety of using frozen sperm has been abundantly proven, both by experimental work and the actual results in humans. Matters of concern are the donor's health and the necessity to avoid donors who are infected with venereal diseases, hepatitis B or C, or HIV. One of the drawbacks of sperm freezing is an approximate 20% loss in motility after thawing. Donors whose semen is frozen for future use are required to report to the semen bank six months after donation to be checked for HIV, HBV or HCV infection/disease status.[1]

Freezing Embryos (Fig. 4)

Embryos are routinely cryopreserved to enable storage of supernumerary embryos, as up to a maximum of only three embryos are allowed for transfer to avoid the risk of multiple pregnancies. Embryo freezing is a widespread routine procedure to increase cumulative pregnancy rates. Human embryos can be successfully cryopreserved at any stage from zygote to blastocyst, using 1, 2 propanediol (PROH) or dimethyl sulfoxide (DMSO) for zygotes and cleaved embryos and glycerol for blastocysts. The formation of ice crystals is of concern during embryo freezing. Using programmed, slow freezers reduces this problem considerably, and slow cooling is the most widely employed method. Human embryos are known to survive a simple ultrarapid procedure of fast cooling but there is not much data on the efficacy of these techniques when used routinely. Straws or ampoules used for freezing embryos should be carefully and permanently labeled for identification purpose.[1,9]

Patients should be fully informed before the treatment cycle on the procedure of cryopreservation, the risks and, particularly, what is to be done with their embryos if they do not use them. They should sign a consent form concerning the agreement for embryo freezing as well as for the future use of the embryos.

Oocyte Cryopreservation

This procedure has been successfully used in cases where a large number of immature oocytes have been retrieved during ovum pick-up. The oocyte can be thawed at a later date, matured *in vitro* and used for oocyte

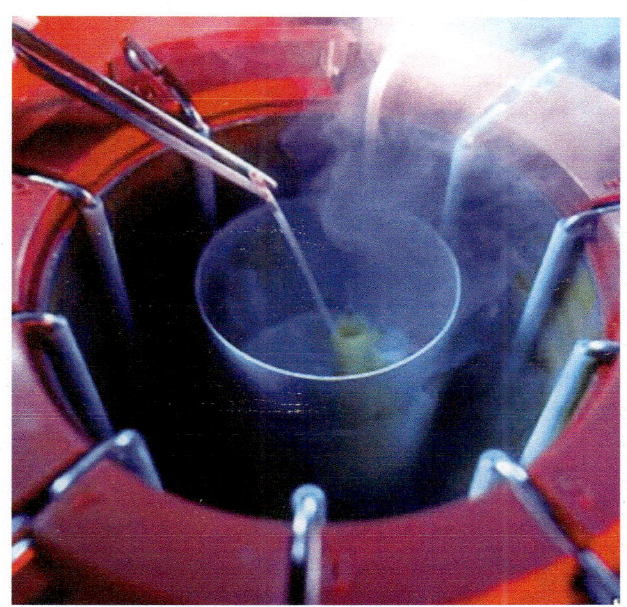

Fig. 3: Freezing semen.

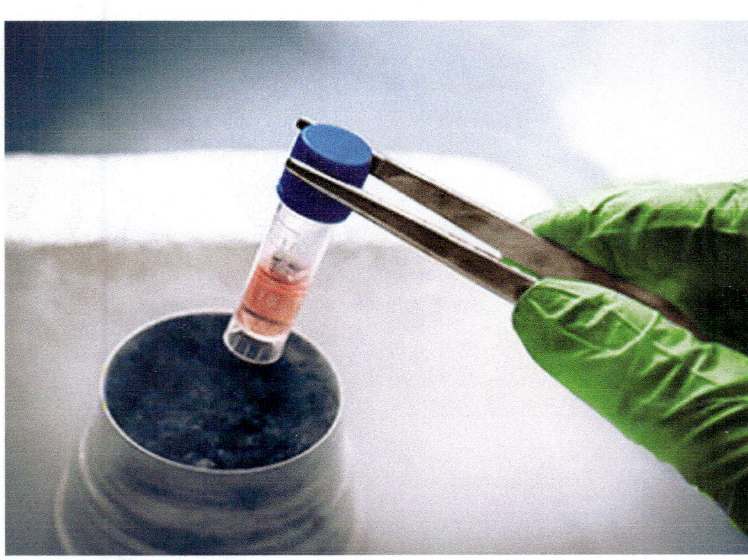

Fig. 2: Cryopreservation.

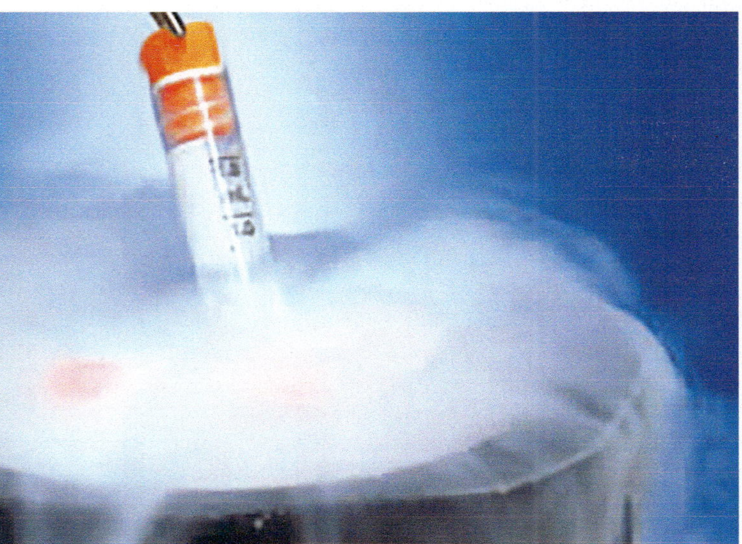

Fig. 4: Freezing embryos.

donation or similar procedures either on the person from whom the oocytes were retrieved or on other prospective recipients. However, the success rates in terms of fertilization, pregnancy and live births with the use of cryopreserved oocytes are not very encouraging. Much remains to be learnt on identifying the optimal stage of oocyte development when cryopreservation would be of value.

In Vitro Culture Media

There has been a spurt of new media introduced for *in vitro* culture of gametes and embryos. If one takes a close look at these media, they are products that have evolved over the years. However, some manufacturers do not give the exact composition of their media but merely state that for reasons of patent protection or as trade secret they are constrained to give full details of the composition of their media. This is an undesirable situation. Infertility clinics that deal with human embryos and the future life of the products they create in the laboratory must be privy to the knowledge about the media they use, if need be by signing an appropriate confidentiality agreement which would prohibit the clinic from using or passing on the proprietary information provided by the manufactures of the media to any other organization that may commercially exploit this information.[1,5,6,9]

When a serum supplementation has to be used in the preparation of media, one must carefully avoid the risk of viral transmission to the embryo through the serum.[1,5,6,9]

Selection Criteria for Assisted Reproductive Technology

The choice of the procedure used, e.g. IVF-ET, GIFT, ZIFT, or ICSI, is made depending upon the needs, resources and circumstances of the couple, availability of the facilities, and experience and expertise of the gynecologist/embryologist.[1,6,7]

PLANNING PREMISES AND DESIGN CONSIDERATIONS

Planning Premises

When planning the provision of ART facilities, it may be useful to consider modular construction methods (Fig. 5). There is a range of modular methods which leads to varying degrees of standardization and preassembly. Layout of IVF center and functional relationships are shown in Figures 6 and 7. Schedule of accommodation is shown in Table 1.

Functional Relationships[6,10,11]

External[11-13]

The ART unit may have a close working relationship (Fig. 7) with:

- Pathology laboratories
- Pharmacy
- Medical imaging.

The ART unit should be ideally located on the ground floor. If located on an upper floor, there must be a stretcher carrying lift available.

Internal[6,10,11]

Within the ART unit; the following relationships are significant:

- Laboratory areas should be located with a direct adjacent relationship to the operating rooms for egg collection and reimplantation laboratories should be located in a separate zone away from the outpatient/consult area and secured

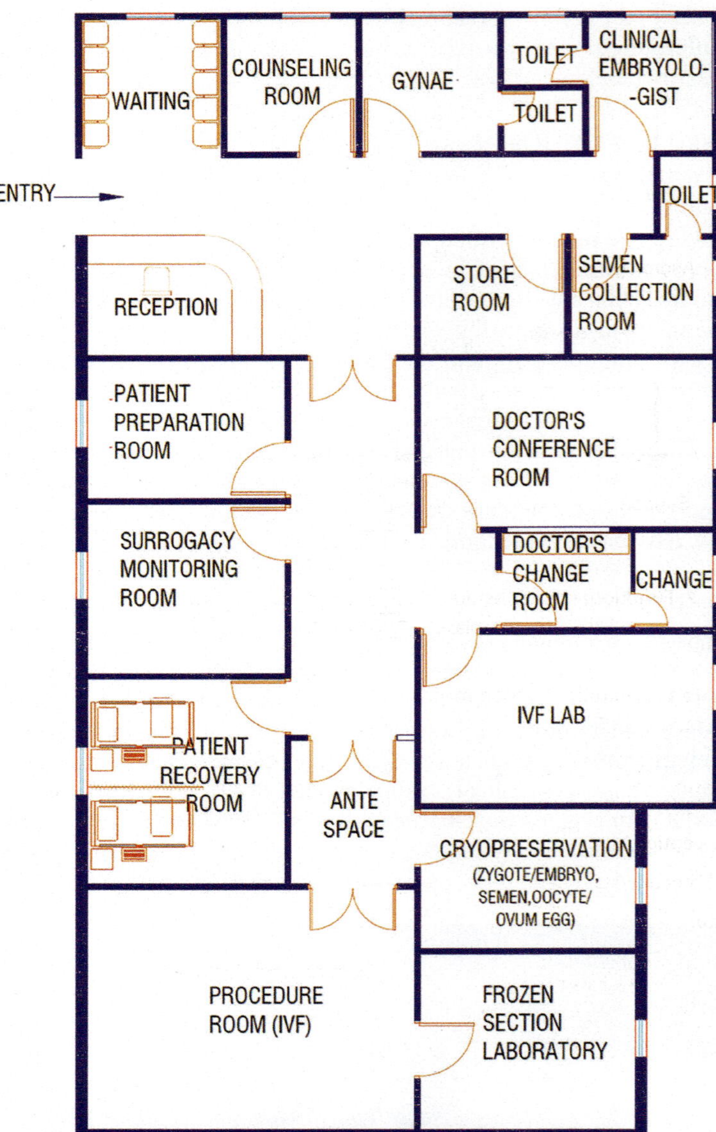

Fig. 6: Layout of assisted reproductive technology (ART) facility.
(IFV: *in vitro* fertilization)

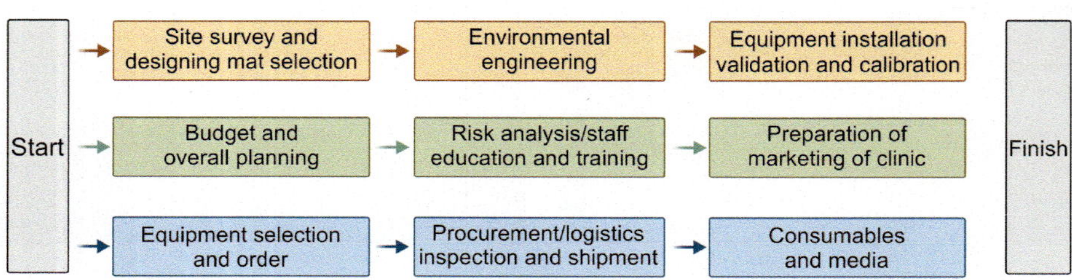

Fig. 5: Action plan for setting up of *in vitro* fertilization facility.

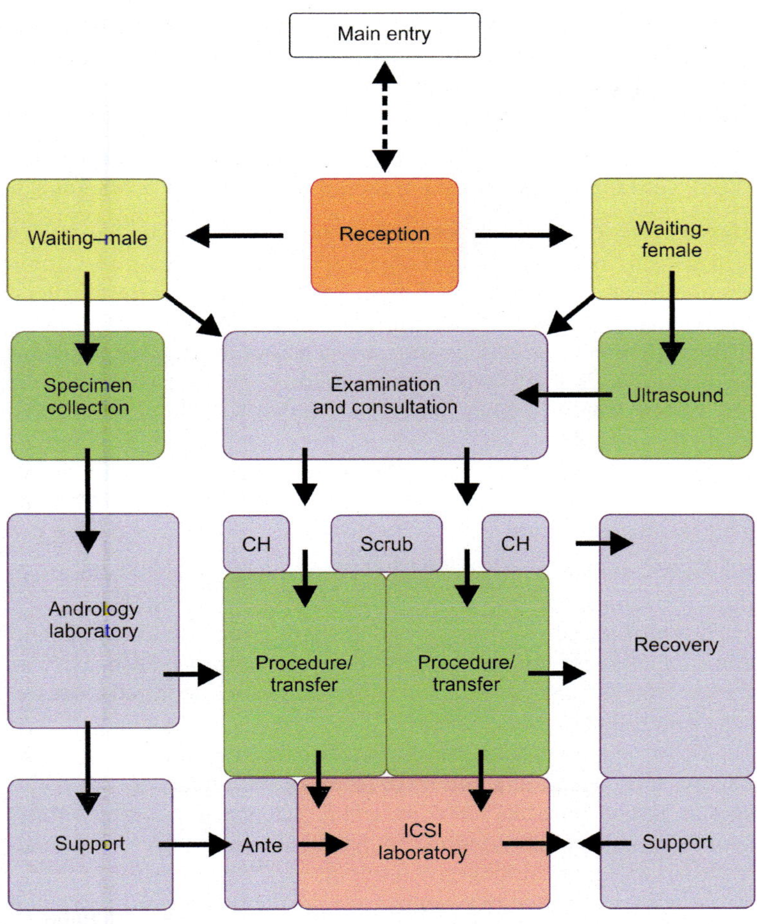

Fig. 7: Functional relationship—assisted reproductive technology (ART) facility. (ICSI: intracytoplasmic sperm injection; CH: change room)

Table 1: Schedule of accommodation.

Room/Space	Recommended areas in sqm	Remarks
Entry/consulting area		
Reception/clerical	15	
Photocopy/stationery	8	
Store—files	8	
Waiting male/female	10	Separate waiting areas for male and female
Waiting family	25	
Toilet—visitors, accessible	2 × 5	Located adjacent to male and female waiting
Interview room—family	12	
Consult/examination/ treatment room	15	
Collection room	6	Semen samples
En suite	5	Adjacent to semen collection rooms
Blood collection bay	5	
Ultrasound room	14	
Patient procedural area		

Contd...

Contd...

Room/Space	Recommended areas in sqm	Remarks
Operating room—general	42	
Patient change cubicle	4	1 adjacent to each procedure room
Patient toilet	3	1 adjacent to each procedure room; 1 adjacent to recovery
Change—staff (male/female)	2 × 10	
Scrub up	6	Maybe shared between 2 procedure rooms
Patient bay—recovery	10	
Bay-handwashing, type b	1 × 1	
Bay—beverage	5	
Bay—linen	2	
Bay—resuscitation trolley	2	
Clean utility	8	
Dirty utility	8	
Staff station	5	
Store—general	8	
Circulation	35%	
Laboratory areas		
IVF/ICSI laboratory	40	Size will depend on service plan
Andrology laboratory	30	Size will depend on service plan
Genetics laboratory	15	PGD functions
Cryopreservation store	30	
Store-gas bottle	10	
Change-staff (male/female)	6	Includes toilets and change facilities
Circulation	35%	
Support areas		
Clean-up room	10	
Cleaners room	5	
Disposal room	5	
Sterilizing/packing	15	Locate adjacent to clean up
Store—sterile stock	8	
Staff areas		
Meeting room—medium	20	
Office—manager	12	
Office—single person	9	Physician
Office—single person	9	Nursing
Security room		Security guard
Staff room	15	
Property bay-staff	2	

(ICSI: intracytoplasmic sperm injection; IVF: *in vitro* fertilization; PGD: preimplantation genetic diagnosis)

- Sperm collection rooms have a close functional relationship with the andrology laboratory; specimens require rapid transfer to the laboratory to avoid deterioration
- Office areas should be separate from the treatment and laboratory zone.

Compliance with Statuary and Other Requirements

Compliance with statuary and other requirements of the country, e.g. Building Laws and Regulations, Environment Protection Act, etc.

Design Consideration

The design of the unit should create a pleasant, reassuring atmosphere for patients whilst retaining the necessary functional requirements associated with clinical spaces and laboratories. Consideration may be given to a private and discreet entry area for patients, away from general public view.[3,6,11]

Parking Area

Parking area should be accessible and must have mobility assistance for patient to move from the parking to the facility. Approach from the parking area to the entrance of the facility should be well thought and laid as per the user profile. The area must have earmarked space for the staff.

Security

Security aspect for the parking area must be kept in mind during the planning stage, including the surveillance camera and structural features like boom barriers and access control.

Signposting

Signposting should be clear and keeping the user profile in mind. In addition it is to be kept in mind that the visitors will have multiple disabilities and, therefore, should be factored in the design consideration. The provision of wheel chair or assistive devices for mobility of patients within the facility should be catered for.

Ramps and Patient Lifts

The design of the ramps and patients lifts need special mention here.

Ramped Approach

Ramp should be finished with nonslip material to enter the building. Minimum width or ramp should be 1,800 mm with maximum gradient 1:12, length of ramp should not exceed 9.0 m having double handrail at a might of 800 and 900 mm on both sides extending 300 mm beyond top and bottom of the ramp. Minimum gap from the adjacent wall to the hand rail should be 50 mm.[10, 12, 13]

Environmental Considerations[3,12-20]

Growing embryos can be very frustrating. Embryos are extremely sensitive. A deep concern should be involved when they are exposed to laboratory environment.

Volatile organic compounds (VOCs) are emitted as gases from certain solids or liquids. VOCs include a variety of chemicals, some of which may have short- and long-term adverse health effects.

Here are some points for concern:

VOC: It is responsible for lack of success during the first years of any lab life. "Off-gas" process along with a proper ventilation pattern could dramatically reduce the negative effects of VOC on embryo survival.

Ultraviolet radiation: Fluorescent lamps, the microscope lamp, sun light are all "contaminated"with ultraviolet (UV) light spectrum. UV is an excellent disinfectant, but we do not want to disinfect our embryos. Replacing the lamps with truly "UV free" lamps can solve this problem.

CO_2 quality: Compressed gases contain dangerous levels of organic (VOC) contamination. Use of prefiltered CO_2 VOC free, is essential.

Magnetic flux: It is probably responsible for many failures in the "*In vitro* fertilization" process. Modern equipment contains heavy electronic circuits. Electronic heaters and fans increase dramatically the magnetic flux in incubators and on laminar work stations. Studies showed that embryos in their first 24 hours are most sensitive to magnetic radiation from heated work surfaces and incubators. The deoxyribonucleic acid (DNA) might be damaged at as low as 0.1 A/M magnetic field, while the magnetic flux inside incubators reaches levels as strong as 10 A/M. Until manufacturers will be more aware of that problem you can use a "Safety Box" that stops the magnetic flux and gives embryos a better chance to live.

Bio-Safe: It shields embryos against the strong magnetic flux found in most IVF equipment.

A major source of disease and contamination in hospitals and clinics is in the air-conditioning systems and in the quality of air. Sore throat, red eyes, headaches, "lack of air syndrome" acquired diseases, are all part of the same problem.

Airborne concentrations of microbes and nanoparticles pose a hazard both to patients and staff. In many hospitals, this source of contamination looks like a new, unfamiliar science. A simple air sample usually reveals contamination that has been associated with human health problems in indoor environments.

Base maintenance personnel have no regular access to provide periodic professional disease preventive maintenance (PM) on the hospital heating, ventilation and air-conditioning (HVAC) systems.

Periodical Examination and Tests for IVF Clinics[4-7,12-24]

- Air quality measurements
  - Monitoring of air cleanliness according to ISO 14644-1
  - Humidity and temperature patterns
  - CO_2 ppm in the air CO ppm in the air
  - O_2 percentage in the air
  - VOC levels in the air
  - VOC levels in compressed CO_2.
- Measuring and evaluating the effective number of air changes in the room
  - Evaluating the tightness factor
  - Measuring the number of air changes
  - Evaluating the air movement pattern in the room
  - Inspection of the AHU and filters, measuring the quality and efficiency of the HEPA filters
  - Measuring the differential pressure between the room and the surrounding relevant area.
- Evaluating sterile qualities of the room and surroundings
  - Evaluating airborne microorganisms in the room
  - Evaluating the cleanliness of the room and equipment (protein test and adenosine triphosphate test)
  - Total microorganism count in samples taken from room surface and equipment
  - Evaluating the sterilization effectiveness of autoclave sterilizer and the way materials are being handled.

- Physical environment hazards
  - Monitoring the intensity of electromagnetic fields in the room
  - Monitoring the intensity of ultraviolet light
  - Monitoring the sound levels
  - Monitoring the quantity of positive ions in the air.

These series of tests, which last no more than a few hours, provide a clear and accurate picture of the room and of the maintenance quality. Thereafter one can determine what measures have to be taken in order to bring the room condition to an acceptable level. These series of tests determine the Room Grade according to the EN-GMP.[6,7,18]

Natural Lighting

Natural light is highly desirable where achievable, particularly for laboratory areas where staff will spend a majority of their time.[6,10]

Artificial Lighting

The general lighting design approach is a common strategy used to provide a fairly uniform amount of light throughout a room. This approach usually results in a regular pattern of light fixtures that produces very even light levels, slightly higher than the average value in the center of the room, and slightly lower in the outer corners of the room.[16, 17, 21]

The Handbook of Facilities Planning (1990) notes that the "Lighting requirements in a laboratory environment generally are the same as for an office: 75–150 foot-candles [fc or lux] at the bench top [usually 30 inches or 760 mm from the floor]. However, some lab functions require higher or lower levels." One hundred fc usually requires an energy expenditure of approximately four watts/square foot. Most of that energy is ultimately converted to heat in the laboratory. The required color of the light (in terms of wavelength in nanometers) should also be considered.[16,17, 21]

With the diversity of tasks performed in any given space of a research facility, standard practice has been to design the general lighting system to a 500 lux maintained level of illumination. This lighting is typically provided by 2 × 4 lens troffers installed in a uniform grid pattern. This pattern is easiest to install and least expensive in terms of first cost. If the space configuration remains the same with no modifications to work stations, no repositioning of walls and modular furniture, and the same task being performed throughout the space, this lighting system will perform adequately.[16, 17, 21]

Although this design provides sufficient light for most clerical-type tasks, it often interferes with computer station operation. The disruption is a result of glare on video display terminals, produced by the ceiling-mounted fluorescent fixtures. Individual requirements of the occupants of the space are also not considered. The brightness and intensity of lighting that an occupant requires is contingent on the particular task being performed, the occupant's age, and the overall reflectivity of the space. Simply installing a fluorescent troffer system with a 50 fc maintained light level is not an acceptable choice for laboratory lighting designers.[16, 17, 21]

The general lighting design described above may also require additional fixtures where instruments and specialized equipment require higher ranges of illumination, such as in a gross tissue review room or a chemistry room. A more efficient design might be to examine the potential for using both low ambient and specific task area sources to provide the levels of illumination required.[16, 17, 21]

Acoustics

Confidential patient information is exchanged between patients and staff, therefore the interview, consult, collection and treatment rooms should be acoustically treated to maximize privacy. In acoustically treated rooms, return air grilles should be acoustically treated to avoid transfer of conversations to adjacent areas. Door grilles and undercuts to these areas should be avoided.[10,11]

Space Standards and Components

Laboratories and storage areas should be sized to suit the design requirements of the equipment to be used, to provide a safe working environment and to allow the effective movement of staff.[3,6,10,11]

Ergonomics

Laboratories should be designed with consideration to ergonomics to ensure an optimal working environment. Aspects for consideration will include height of benches and chairs, height of equipment in constant use such as microscopes and biosafety cabinets.[6,10,11]

Safety and Security

Zones within the unit will require access control to prevent unauthorized access, particularly laboratory areas, cryopreservation areas and staff office areas. A separate room or a fume hood should be available for procedures requiring use of fixatives.[6,10,11]

Finishes

Floor finishes should be appropriate to the function of the space. Consideration must be given to the appearance and quality of environment required, e.g. acoustic performance, slip resistance, infection control, movement of trolleys and maintenance.[6,10,11]

Laboratory, storage and procedural areas should have vinyl or similar impervious floors. Ceiling and wall finishes, laboratory cabinetry and bench tops must be easily cleaned.[6,10,11]

Fixtures and Fittings[6,10]

Critical items of equipment, including incubators and liquid nitrogen storage should be temperature alarmed and monitored.

Building Service Requirements

Laboratories will require air-conditioning with controlled humidity and temperature to provide an environment that minimizes staff distraction and fatigue. Procedure rooms will require temperature regulation to assist in maintaining patient temperature at 37°C and prevent deterioration of oocytes. Power supplies to critical equipment, such as incubators, refrigerators, biosafety cabinets should be on emergency supply with generator back-up.[6,10,11]

Infection Control[6,10,11, 17, 18, 22-34]

Infection control teams should be taken into consideration from the outset and should remain integral planning team member throughout. Since the inception of IVF, questions about contamination and the transmission of infection have been raised. All assisted reproductive techniques involve handling of biological material and; therefore, pose a potential infection control risk to staff and to other patients' reproductive cells (gametes, zygotes, embryos). Strict infection control measures are required within the unit to protect laboratory staff from potentially contaminated body fluids (follicular fluid, etc.) and to ensure aseptic environment for reproductive cells, preventing cross infection.

Transmission of infectious diseases to laboratory personnel can be prevented by adherence to strict safety guidelines, wearing of protective clothing, hepatitis B virus (HBV) vaccination, prohibition of mouth pipetting, and developing a plan for the disposal of biohazardous material.[1]

Measures will include:
- Hand basins for staff hand washing in all patient areas and laboratories
- Use of laboratory clothing in laboratories
- Use of theater clothing in procedure rooms
- Use of laminar flow biosafety cabinets in laboratories (a Class II cabinet should be available for handling of contaminated samples)
- A class II laminar flow cabinet that protects both the operator and the specimen should be used when contaminated samples are handled.

Sterilization Practices

Infection control society should be followed to prevent any postoperative infection or any hospital-acquired infection. High level sterilization practices are required as this lab deals with embryos.[5]

Protecting Patients' Privacy and Dignity[3, 15-18]

Privacy is essential for confidential conversations and interviews and will minimize stress and discomfort for patients. Patient's privacy and confidentiality may be enhanced by provision of private interview rooms for personal discussions between staff and patient.[2,3,6,10,11]

Protective Measures[6,17, 18, 23-27]

All body fluids (follicular fluid, semen, etc.) should be treated as potentially contaminated. The purpose of the protective measures is both to protect laboratory staff and to ensure aseptic conditions for gametes, zygotes, and embryos. The procedures should deal with, but not be limited to, the following:
- Strict observation of staff hygiene regulations
- Use of laboratory clothing
- Use of nontoxic (nonpowdered) gloves and masks where appropriate
- Use of eye and face protection, and of cryogloves if cryogenic materials are handled
- Use of vertical laminar-flow benches
- Use of mechanical pipetting devices
- Use of fume hood in case of fixatives
- Use of disposable material; after usage, discard it immediately in the proper waste containers. Potential infectious materials must be disposed of in a manner that protects laboratory workers and maintenance, service, and housekeeping staff from exposure to infectious materials in the course of their work
- Needles and other sharps should be handled with extreme caution and discarded in special containers. If possible, omit glassware in the laboratory; otherwise discard the Pasteur pipettes and broken glassware in special containers
- Food, drinks, cigarettes and cigars are strictly forbidden
- The use of make-up and strong perfumes should be limited.

Planning for ART Center[1-6,11-21]

Planning Team

A qualified medical technology planning firm should be brought on board at the earliest planning stage to coordinate with all stakeholders. Planning team should consists of:
- Gynecologist
- Andrologist
- Embryologist
- IT department
- Biomedical engineering
- Architects
- Contractors
- Hospital administrators
- Other stakeholders.

All successful hospitals are built on the triad of good planning, efficient design and good construction. *"Design should follow function"*.

General Design Consideration

This section describes general design requirements for the ART clinic.

The IVF Unit may be developed as:
- A stand-alone unit
- A dedicated unit within a general hospital.

Indian Council of Medical Research in its Guidelines on ART has Classified ART Facility into Four Levels

Primary Infertility Clinics (Level IA)

- Clinics where preliminary investigations are carried out and type and cause of infertility diagnosed
- Primary infertility care unit or clinics could be a doctor's consulting room, such as a gynecologist's or a physician's consulting room, or even a general hospital
- These clinics will not require registration under the Act
- The gynecologist or the physician in charge of a Level 1A infertility care unit and should have an appropriate post-graduate degree
- In case a Level 1A clinics engaged in AIH and IUI it must maintain records of the use of the requisitioned semen and of all AIH and IUI done, appropriately and confidentially; these records will be liable to inspection by an appropriate Review Committee.

The responsibilities of a Level 1A primary infertility care unit would be:[5]
- Completion of the basic investigations
- Treatment of minor anatomical defects like tough imperforate hymen
- Treatment of mild endometriosis
- Introduction of ovulation in nonovulatory women (especially PCOS) with clomiphene citrate, with or without adjuncts like bromocriptine, eltroxin, dexamethasone or spironolactone (gonadotropin should not be used at a primary infertility care unit level)
- Correcting minor endocrine disorders such as thyroid disorders or hyperprolactinemia, by prescribing appropriate corrective medications
- Treatment of oligozoospermia without asthenozoospermia
- Detecting infection of the reproductive tract using appropriate diagnostic tests, followed by normal healthcare steps after carrying out appropriate antibiotic sensitivity tests (particular care must be taken to treat the couple and not the female or the male patient alone)
- Ability to carry out AIH
- Ability to carry out IUI using processed semen of husband or donor obtained from an accredited laboratory or semen bank which must maintain a record of complete details including the name, qualification and complete address of the gynecologist/clinic requesting the processed semen and carrying out the IUI
- Referral of the couple to Level 1B, Level 2 or Level 3 infertility care unit as appropriate, especially when the woman's age is more than

35, or when the couple has a multifactorial defect, or when patients with single treatable defect have not responded to conventional therapy.

Primary Infertility Clinics (Level IB)

These clinics would be required to have, in addition to what has been stated in Primary Infertility Clinic (Level IA). Infertility clinics falling into this category shall need accreditation. The IUI in such clinics must be done under the supervision of a gynecologist with a postgraduate degree.[5]

Facilities for Investigations[1]

- Immunological tests for infertility, sperm cervical mucus penetration test (SCMPT), sperm cervical mucus test (SCMT), and test for antibodies (IgG, IgA) against sperm antigen in cervical mucus
- Sperm function tests like hypo-osmotic swelling test (HOST), and assessment for improvement of sperm motility potential with pentoxifylline coculture
- Assessment of follicular growth and ovulation by serial transvaginal sonography (TVS)
- Hysteroscopy, laparoscopy and transvaginal sonography.

Treatment Facilities

- Facilities for semen preparation for IUI, including an appropriate clean room for IUI
- Provision for semen collection in men with a vibrator or an electroejaculator in functional erectile and ejaculatory problems[1]
- Conservative surgery either through a laparoscope, hysteroscope or via laparotomy. It should be possible to perform hysteroscopic cannulation of blocked tubes, and resection of submucous myoma or uterine septum.[1]

Secondary (Level 2) Infertility Clinics

- These clinics will require registration under the Act
- They must have infrastructure for further in-depth investigation and extended treatment of infertility except where oocytes are handled outside the body.[1]

Facilities for Investigations

- Immunological tests for infertility, SCMPT, SCMT, and tests for antibodies (IgG, IgA) against sperm antigen in cervical mucus
- Sperm function tests like HOST, and assessment for improvement of sperm motility potential with pentoxifylline coculture
- Assessment of follicular growth and ovulation by serial TVS
- Hysteroscopy, laparoscopy and transvaginal sonography.

Treatment Facilities[1,5]

- Facilities for semen preparation and IUI
- Provision for semen collection in men with a vibrator or an electroejaculator in functional erectile and ejaculatory problems
- Conservative surgery either through a laparoscope, hysteroscope or via laparotomy. It should be possible to perform hysteroscopic cannulation of blocked tubes, and resection of submucous myoma or uterine septum
- Combined medical-surgical therapy by a coordinate team as in endometriosis or in some cases of polycystic ovaries (ovarian drilling)
- Provision for extended treatment of infertility except for oocyte pick-up and IVF, ICSI, etc.

Tertiary (Level 3) Infertility Care Units[1,5]

Such units will have three functions to perform:

- Diagnostic
- Therapeutic at the highest level of specialization and with the best of facilities
- Research.

If any of the facilities mentioned below does not exist in the clinic, the clinic should have access to such a facility in another appropriately accredited clinic, semen bank, or laboratory.

Facilities Available[1,5]

Diagnostic procedures for male infertility

- Endocrine assay (Fig. 8)
- Further tests for sperm function and integrity, such as a Croome reaction and sperm-oocyte interaction *in vitro*
- Assessment of cell contaminants, debris and infection
- Karyotyping when sperm density, morphology and motility are abnormal
- Assessment of seminal plasma for viscosity, thinness, blood contamination and biochemical constituents.

Diagnostic procedures for female infertility[1,5]

- Endocrine assay
- Karyotyping in premature ovarian failure in Kallmann's syndrome
- Color Doppler for checking growing follicles, functional integrity of corpus luteum, and developing endometrium in stimulated or unstimulated cycle
- GnRH challenge test in nonovulation due to hypothalamic pituitary failure
- Clomiphene challenge tests to ascertain ovarian reserves before ovulation induction or controlled ovarian hyperstimulation.

Therapeutic procedures

- Induction of ovulation in refractory nonovulation due to PCO-downregulation with a GnRH-agonist followed by induction with gonadotropin
- All varieties of assisted reproductive technologies, including ICSI
- Procedures for IUI using split ejaculate, pooled ejaculate or sperm recovered from postcoital specimen of urine in retrograde ejaculation
- Embryo freezing.

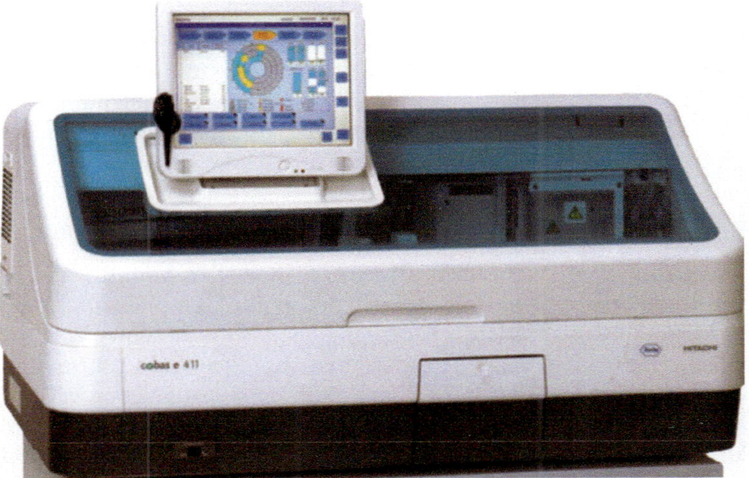

Fig. 8: Endocrine assay.

Location

The IVF unit may be developed as:

- A stand-alone unit
- A dedicated unit within a general hospital.

The ART facility is a part of a general hospital should ideally be located in ground floor, and if not, should be connected by vertical means of transportation.

This section describes general design requirements for the ART clinic.

Functional Areas

The ART facility may consist of a number of functional zones:[10]

Entry/Consult zone

- Entry
- Reception
- Waiting area
- Administration
- Records
- Interview room
- Consult/Examination
- Treatment room
- Ultrasound room/s
- Collection room/s with ensuite shower and toilet
- Public toilets.

Patient procedural zone

- Operating room/s for oocyte (egg) collection and reimplantation
- Recovery areas
- Change areas and toilets for staff and patients.

Laboratory zone

- Laboratories (Embryology, IVF, ICSI, andrology, genetics)
- Cryopreservation facilities
- Gas bottle store.

Staff and support zone

- Clean-up and disposal room
- Store rooms and sterile store
- Offices, meeting rooms, staff room
- *Sterilizing area*: If the IVF unit is a stand-alone building, dedicated sterilizing facilities will be required.

ENTRY/CONSULT ZONE

Entry

Patients and staff will all use the main entrance to the department. Parking facilities should be considered. Covered area for alighting from vehicle should be considered. The powered doors with access control (Fig. 9) may be a value addition at the facility.

Reception

Reception should cater for the needs of wheelchair bound patients, which would entail a lower desk height, in addition to ensuring the privacy of the interaction. A reception desk with a low counter top is welcoming to all patients. The assistance should include information dissemination, certificate issue, appointments, guidance on various aspects of help and facility available. Desk-height writing surfaces with knee space for use by wheelchair users and others who cannot stand while transacting business should be made available.

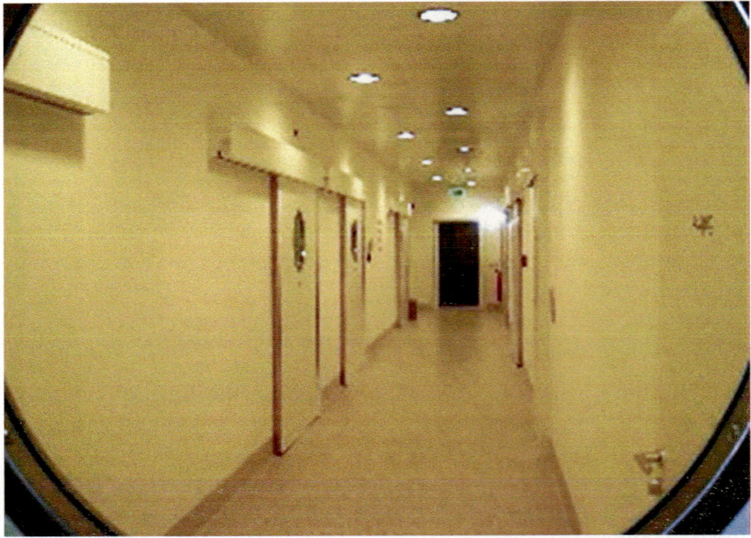

Fig. 9: Restricted access area for operating theater and *in vitro* fertilization laboratory.

Waiting Area

Waiting areas should be calm, comforting and relaxing. They should be divided for gender separation. The waiting area at the reception wing should form the major place for social interaction between the visitors.

Administrative Room

This office should be large enough to accommodate two people along with computer and telecommunication equipment.

Record Room

Record keeping must be computerized as far as possible, so that data is accessible retrospectively for analysis or when called upon by the supervisory agency. There are many software programs for this purpose, which are commercially available today. Besides containing essential details of the patient's records, it must contain history of the cause of infertility as diagnosed earlier, results of new diagnosis if relevant, the treatment option best suited for the particular patient, the treatment carried out and the outcome of treatment, and follow-up if any.

Room with Privacy/Interview Room

A room with privacy for interviewing and examining male and female partners independently is essential. Evaluation of infertility necessitates history taking of the most intimate sexual practices between the couples. This is followed by close examination of the reproductive tract and sexual organs. Adequate measures must be taken to ensure that history taking and examination are carried out in strict privacy, maintaining the dignity of the patients.

Consultant Room/Examination Room

The room must be equipped with an examination table and gynecological instruments for examining the female per vaginum, an appropriate ultrasonographic machine with a probe for transvaginal examination of the female and examination of the testes and excurrent male reproductive tract. A color Doppler would be useful but not essential.

Ultrasonography Room

The ultrasonography room (Fig. 10) should be located with access to patient toilet facilities.

Collection Room(s)

This must be a well-appointed room with privacy and an appropriate environment; it should be located in a secluded area close to the laboratory. Such a facility must be available in-house rather than having the patient collect the sample and bring it to the laboratory for analysis as, in the latter case, semen quality and identity is likely to be compromised. Procedures for collection of semen, as described in the WHO Semen Analysis Manual must be followed with special reference to the type of container used; these containers must be sterile, maintained at body temperature and nontoxic.

Description and Function

The collection rooms are private and enclosed rooms used for collection of sperm specimens from patients.[10]

Location and Relationships

The collection rooms have a close functional relationship with the andrology laboratory; rapid delivery of specimens is required to prevent cell deterioration. The collection rooms will require an ensuite shower/toilet.[10]

Considerations

The rooms should include:[10]

- Comfortable seating
- Hand basin and fittings including soap and paper towel dispenser
- TV, DVD player
- Acoustic treatment
- A pass-through hatch for specimens.

Rest Room

The rest room should be catering to the needs of the visitors and plan should include that the whole of the facility if barrier free and easily accessible to all forms of the visitors using the facility. Space must be planned for the storage of housekeeping stores and wares for the smooth running of the reception center.

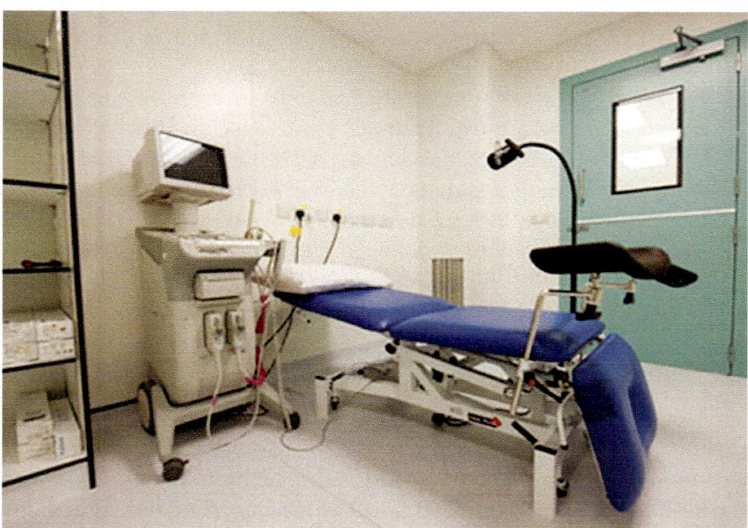

Fig. 10: Ultrasonography room.

PATIENT PROCEDURAL ZONE

Operation Theater

This must be well-equipped with facilities for carrying out surgical endoscopy and transvaginal ovum pick-up. The operation theater must be equipped for emergency resuscitative procedures:

- Transvaginal oocyte retrieval (TVOR) is performed in an operating room or a physician's office, with the (female) subject in the lithotomy position. TVOR is usually performed under procedural sedation, general anesthesia, paracervical block, or sometimes spinal anesthesia, local anesthesia is not typically used because local anesthetic agents interfere with follicular cleavage and the technique requires multiple needle punctures[34]
- Percutaneous epididymal sperm aspiration (PESA) is a procedure performed for men who have obstructive azoospermia from either a prior vasectomy or infection. In this procedure, a needle is inserted into the epididymis and sperm is withdrawn. It is done under local anesthesia in the operating room or office and is coordinated with their female partner's egg retrieval[34]
- If sperm cannot be found in the epididymis, testicular sperm aspiration (TESA) is used to extract sperm from testicular tissue, and the needle is inserted directly into the testis. TESA is a procedure performed for men where sperm are being retrieved for IVF/ICSI. This procedure is performed on the male under local anesthesia in the operating room. In this procedure a needle is inserted directly into the testicles and the tissue or sperms are aspirated from there. TESA is performed for men with obstructive azoospermia. TESA at times may not provide enough tissue or sperms and an open testis biopsy may be required.[34]

The essential principle that should be followed while planning the physical layout of an operating room suite are the exclusion of contamination from outside the suite, with proper traffic patterns within the suite and separation of the clean areas from contaminated within the suite.

Room for Intrauterine Transfer of Embryo

The room (Fig. 11) must be a sterile area having an examination table on which the patient can be placed for carrying out the procedure and rest undisturbed for a period of time.

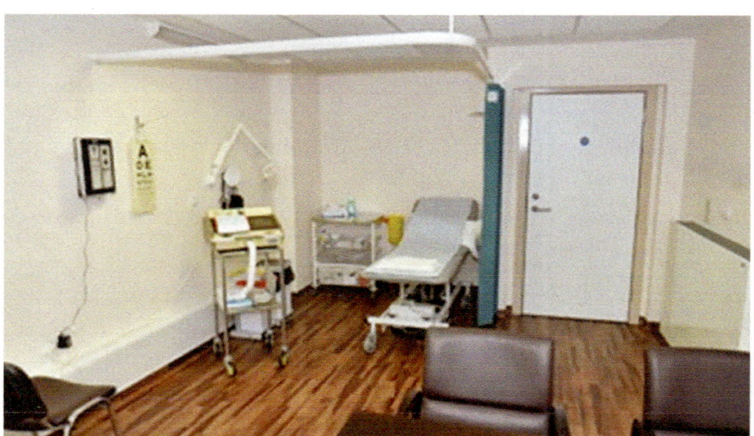

Fig. 11: Room for intrauterine transfer of embryo.

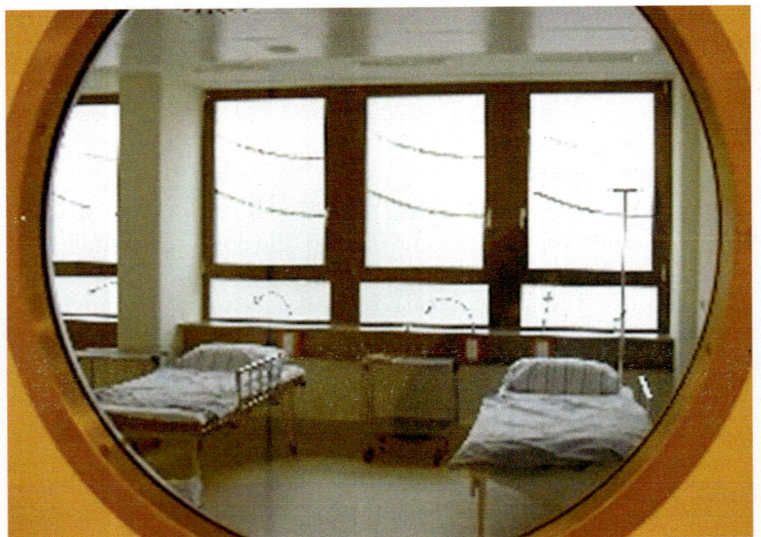

Fig. 12: Recovery area.

The embryo transfer procedure starts by placing a speculum in the vagina to visualize the cervix, which is cleansed with saline solution or culture media. A soft-transfer catheter is loaded with the embryos and handed to the clinician after confirmation of the patient's identity. The catheter is inserted through the cervical canal and advanced into the uterine cavity.[35]

There is good and consistent evidence of benefit in *ultrasound guidance*, that is, making an abdominal ultrasound to ensure correct placement, which is 1-2 cm from the uterine fundus. Anesthesia is generally not required. Single embryo transfers in particular require accuracy and precision in placement within the uterine cavity. The optimal target for embryo placement, known as the maximal implantation potential (MIP) point, is identified using 3D/4D ultrasound. However, there is limited evidence that supports deposition of embryos in the midportion of the uterus.[35]

After insertion of the catheter, the contents are expelled and the embryos are deposited. Limited evidence supports making trial transfers before performing the procedure with embryos. After expulsion, the duration that the catheter remains inside the uterus has no effect on pregnancy rates. Limited evidence suggests avoiding negative pressure from the catheter after expulsion. After withdrawal, the catheter is handed to the embryologist, who inspects it for retained embryos.[34]

In the process of zygote intrafallopian transfer (ZIFT), eggs are removed from the woman, fertilized, and then placed in the woman's fallopian tubes rather than the uterus.[34]

Recovery area (Fig. 12): Postprocedure patients are kept in recovery area.

Change area for staff and patient: Separate areas/rooms should be provided for male and female staff containing lockers, showers, toilets and space for donning surgical attire. These areas should be designed to allow one way traffic and move inside.[34]

Duty room for nurses and doctors: There should be duty room for nurses and doctors.

LABORATORY ZONE

Laboratories[5]

Ancillary Laboratory Facilities

The infertility clinic need not have in-house facilities to perform all the procedures necessary to diagnose infertility, such as those mentioned below. They can be farmed out to specialty laboratories specializing in delivering such services, as long as they are located in the neighborhood.

Hormone and other assays: The infertility clinic must have ready access to laboratories that are able to carry out immunoassays of hormones (FSH, LH, prolactin, hCG, TSH, insulin, estradiol, progesterone, testosterone and DHEA) and tests, such as for HIV and Hepatitis B.[5]

Microbiology and histopathology: Another important facility in an ART clinic (or easily accessible to it) would be that of a microbiology laboratory that can carry out rapid tests for any infection and a clinical chemistry laboratory. Facilities for carrying out histopathological studies on specimens obtained from the operation theater would also be desirable.[5]

Maintenance of the laboratories: Each laboratory should maintain in writing, standard-operating manuals for the different procedures carried out in the laboratory. It should be ensured that there is no "mix up" of gametes or embryos. The patient's name should be clearly labeled on all the tubes, dishes and pipettes containing the gametes and embryos. All pipettes should be immediately discarded after use.[5]

Quality of consumable used in the laboratory: All disposable plastic ware must be procured from reliable sources after ensuring that they are not toxic to the embryo. Culture media used for processing gametes or growing embryos *in vitro* should be preferably procured from reliable manufacturers. Each batch of culture medium needs to be tested for sterility, endotoxins, osmolality and pH. The embryologist should know the composition of the media that are being used. Most media are supplemented with serum; they should, therefore, be tested for antibodies to HIV 1 and 2, Hepatitis B surface antigen and Hepatitis C RNA.[5]

Embryology Laboratory Complex: (IVF/ICSI) Laboratory[5]

Description and function

The embryology laboratory provides facilities for the handling, preparation, culture and storage of human gametes (sperm and oocytes). The laboratory is responsible for identifying oocytes in ovarian fluid, culturing these eggs with the partner's sperm, and embryo examination prior to embryo implantation into the patient.[4,10]

The Intracytoplasmic sperm injection (ICSI) laboratory involves the process of injecting a single sperm into the nucleus of the egg using a microscopic needle without affecting the viability of the egg. The zygote (fertilized egg) is then monitored until it starts to divide forming a small cluster of cells known as the blastocyst (in approximately 5 days in the lab) which is then reimplanted to form an embryo.

The embryology laboratory (Figs. 13 to 16) must have facilities for the control of temperature and humidity and must have filtered air with an appropriate number of air exchanges per hour. Walls and floors must be composed of materials that can be easily washed and disinfected; use of carpeting must be strictly avoided, laboratory equipment will require emergency power, temperature monitoring and alarms. The construction of the lab should ensure aseptic and optimal handling of reproductive tissue during all stages of the process. Air-conditioning for the laboratory will include HEPA filters, controlled humidity (20%) and controlled temperature (22–24°C). Access to the laboratory should be limited.[5,10]

Location and relationships

Due to the sensitive nature of its functions, the embryology laboratory should be located in a secure and sterile area away from the outpatient/clinic facilities but in close proximity to the procedure room where the oocytes (eggs) are collected.[11]

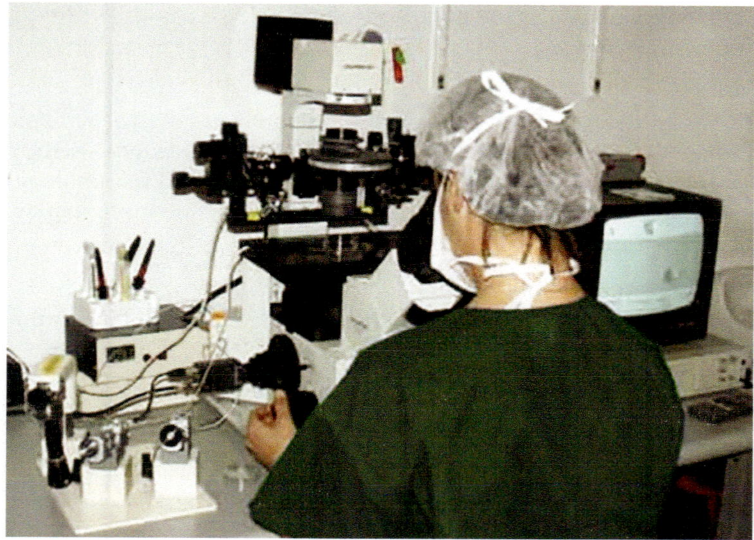

Fig. 13: Embryologist at work at embryos on the inverted microscope.

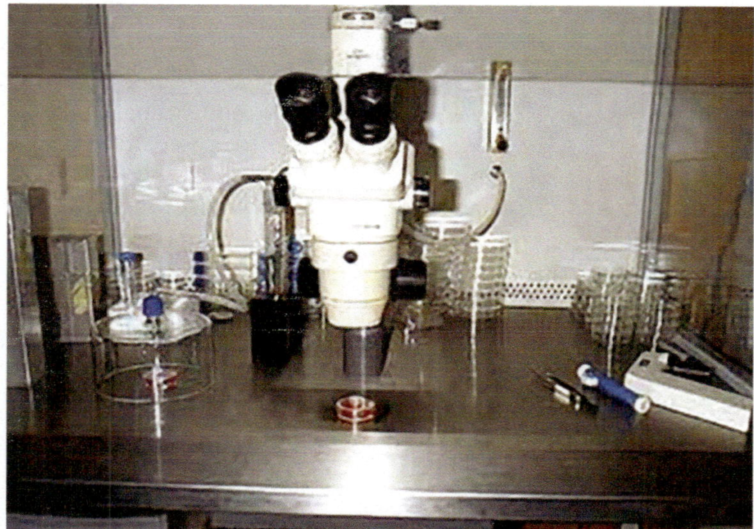

Fig. 14: A hood.

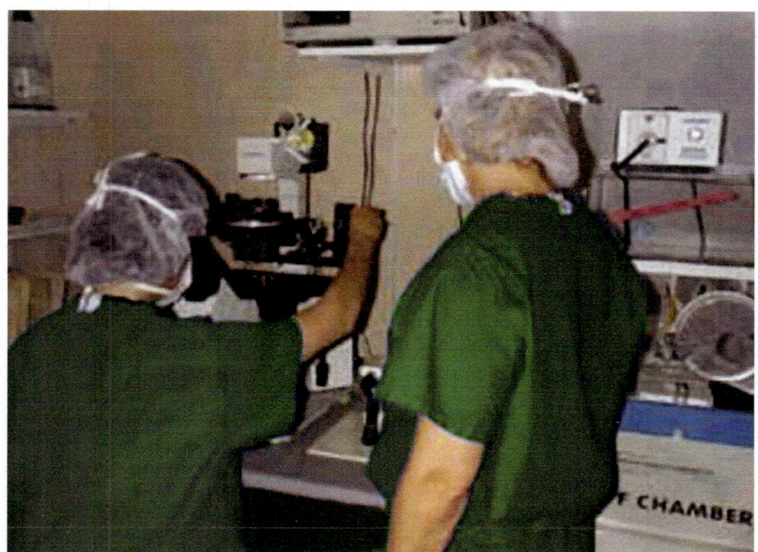

Fig. 15: Performing micromanipulation intracytoplasmic sperm injection.

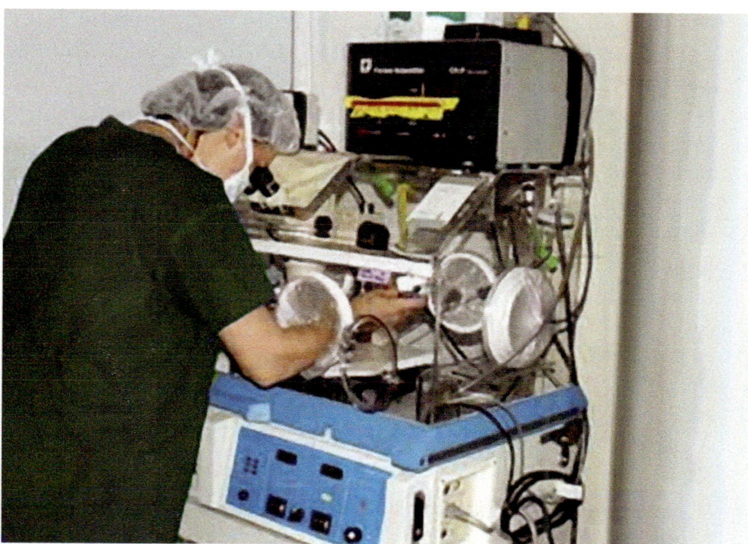

Fig. 16: Preparing embryo for the transfer procedure.

The IVF/ICSI laboratory should be located with a direct relationship to the operating room/s for oocyte collection and reimplantation. A pass-through hatch from the laboratory to each operating room is recommended. Staff change and hand wash areas should be located at the laboratory entry.[10]

Considerations

Fittings and equipment to be located in this laboratory will include:[10,11]

- Laboratory benches and storage units
- Laminar flow IVF workstation cabinets
- Benchtop microscopes, inverted microscope, stereo-microscope
- CO_2 incubators preferably with a back-up
- Electrical pipettes
- Variable pipettes
- Fyrite analyzer (CO_2 and O_2 gas analyzer)
- Laboratory refrigerator
- Hand basin and staff change area at entry
- Stereomicroscope
- Routine high-powered binocular light microscope
- 'High resolution' inverted microscope with phase contrast or Hoffman optics, preferably with facilities for video recording
- Micromanipulator (if ICSI is done)
- A hot air oven
- A laboratory centrifuge
- Equipment for freezing embryos in a programmed manner
- Liquid nitrogen cans.

Handling of Embryos, Zygotes, Oocytes and Spermatozoa

- The laboratory procedures regarding the handling of embryos, zygotes and gametes for ART have been standardized. The procedures should be easy, simple and effective and should be performed in a laminar flow hood equipped with heating stages and prewarmed heating blocks
- Class II hoods should be used for documented contaminated samples, since they provide protection also to the operator
- Aseptic technique should be used at all times

- Appropriate measures should be taken to ensure that oocytes, zygotes and embryos are maintained at 378°C during handling/ observation
- Whenever possible, tissue culture grade disposables should be used for handling body fluids/cells
- Pipetting devices (pasteurs, drawn pipettes, tips, etc.) should be used for one procedure only, must never be used for more than one patient, and should be disposed of immediately after use
- Simultaneous treatment of more than one patient should never be done in the same working place. Each sample should be handled individually and its treatment should be completed before moving to the following sample
- Identifying information marked on the culture dish/tube should be cross referenced to the patient and the patient's documentation
- At each stage of the procedure, date, time and identity of the operator should be recorded. This is especially useful in cases of recalls
- Before receiving samples, the identity of the corresponding patients should be confirmed
- All the above points are also to be applied during freezing and to thawed gametes, zygotes and embryos with the exception of temperature requirement during thawing that may vary according to the used protocol.

Laboratory Design[4,5, 17-19]

The embryology laboratory must have adequate space to allow good laboratory practice and should be as close as possible to the operating room in which the clinical procedures are performed.

- When commissioning the laboratory, thought should be given to the most recent developments in equipment and facilities
- Attention should be given to the ergonomics of the operator—bench height, adjustable chairs, microscope eye, height, efficient use of space and surfaces, sufficient air-condition with controlled humidity and temperature, all contributing to a working environment that minimizes distraction and fatigue. Consideration should also be given to local health and safety requirements
- Construction of the laboratory should ensure aseptic and optimal handling of gametes, zygotes and embryos during all phases of the treatment
- High-efficiency particulate air and volatile organic compounds filtration of the air supplied to the laboratory and clinical procedure rooms should be considered to maintain clean conditions. In addition, overpressure of the laboratory could contribute to exclude contamination from external areas
- Rooms for changing clothes should be located close to the laboratory, having hand washing facilities
- Access to the laboratory should be limited to authorized personnel only
- Pass-throughs for all materials and disposables coming into the laboratory are recommended
- Location of storage areas and equipment such as incubators, centrifuges and cryoequipment should be logically planned for efficiency and safety within each working area
- Separate office space should be provided for administrative work, such as record keeping and data entry
- A general wet area in which washing of equipment, sterilization, etc. is performed must be separate from the embryo laboratory
- Analyses in which fixatives are applied must be performed in a separate room, preferably in a fume hood.

Semen Processing Laboratory/Andrology Laboratory (Fig. 17)

Description and function

The andrology laboratory performs the evaluation, testing, preparation and storage of sperm specimens. Diagnostic procedures include—semen analysis determine sperm count, motility, viability and morphology, preparation of sperm for fertilization and intrauterine insemination (IUI) and thawing of frozen specimens.[11]

Location and relationships

The andrology laboratory has a close working relationship with the IVF/ICSI laboratories.[10]

The collection room/s should be located in close proximity.

Considerations

Fittings and equipment to be located in this laboratory will include:[10]

- Laboratory benches and storage units
- Laminar flow IVF workstation cabinets
- Benchtop microscopes
- Automatic sperm analyzing units
- CO_2 incubators
- Electrical pipettes
- Variable pipettes
- Mackler cell
- Fyrite analyzer (CO_2 and O_2 gas analyzer)
- Laboratory refrigerator
- Hand basin and staff change area at entry.

Laboratory equipment will require emergency power, temperature monitoring and alarms.

The construction of the lab should ensure aseptic and optimal handling of reproductive tissue during all stages of the process. Air-conditioning for the laboratory will include HEPA filters, controlled humidity (20%) and controlled temperature (22–24°C). Access to the laboratory should be limited. Care must be taken for the safe disposal of biological waste and other materials (syringes, glass slides, etc.). Laboratory workers should be immunized against hepatitis B and tetanus.[5,11]

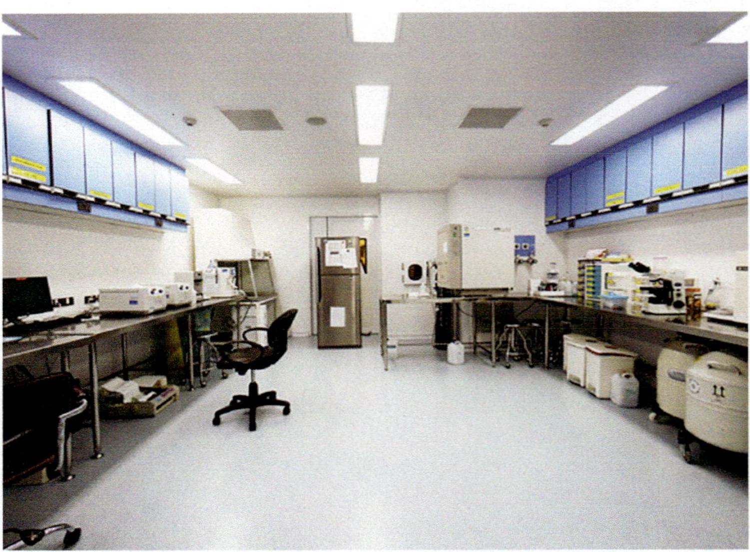

Fig. 17: Andrology laboratory.

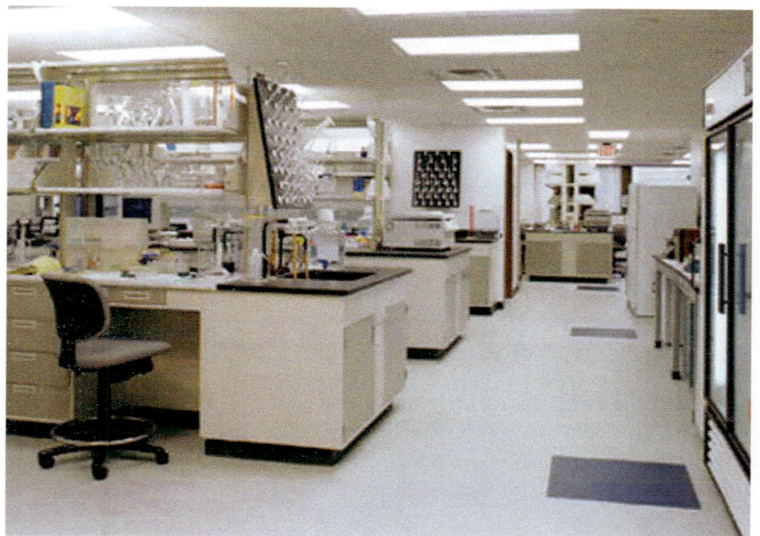

Fig. 18: Genetics laboratory.

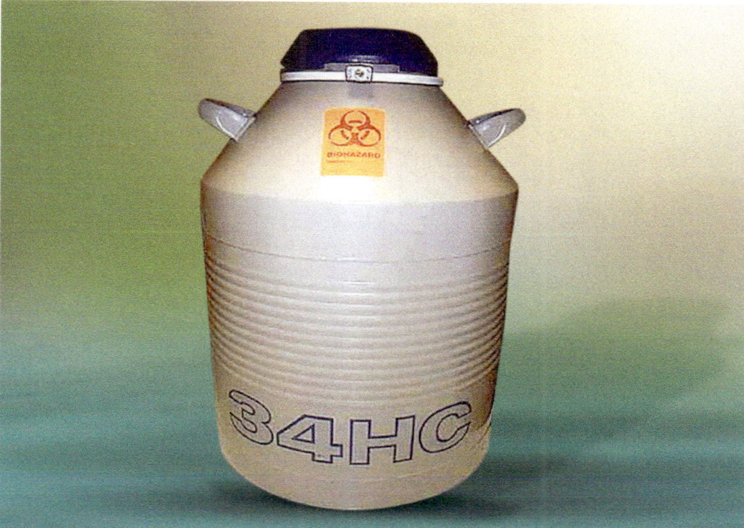

Fig. 19: Nitrogen cylinder.

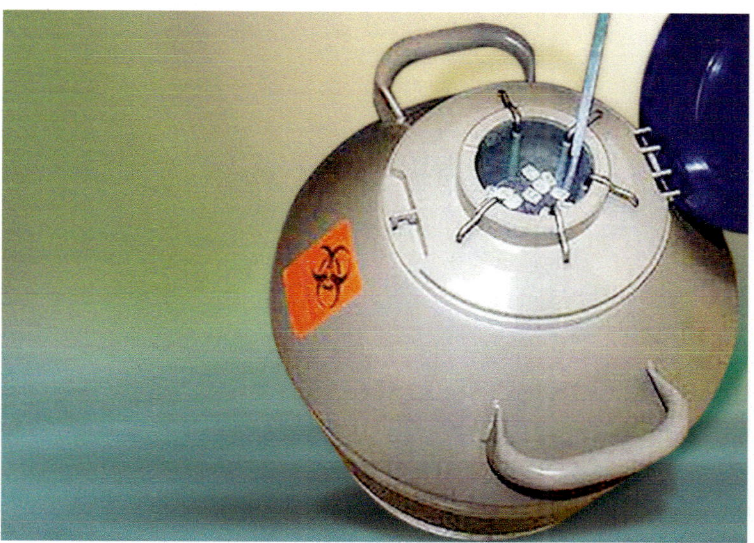

Fig. 20: Cane with frozen embryo is being plunged into the storage tank. The tank contains liquid nitrogen at 196°C (minus 320°F).

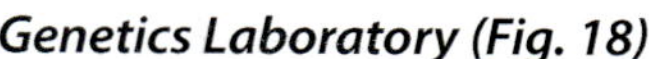

Genetics Laboratory (Fig. 18)

Description and function[11]

The genetics laboratory undertakes cytogenetics studies of the embryo cells, particularly the nucleus which contains the chromosomes that carry genes and their DNA to determine the status of the embryo after IVF and before reimplantation, also referred to as preimplantation genetic diagnosis (PGD). This process can also identify and diagnose abnormalities and genetic diseases that may accompany the pregnancy by the use of sophisticated techniques, such as fluorescence in situ hybridization (FISH) or polymerase chain reaction (PCR).

Location and relationships

The genetics laboratory has a close working relationship with the IVF/ICSI laboratory.

Considerations

Fittings and equipment to be located in this laboratory will include:[10]

- Laboratory benches and storage units
- Laminar flow IVF workstation cabinets
- Benchtop microscopes
- Laboratory refrigerator
- Hand basin and staff change area at entry.

Laboratory equipment will require emergency power, temperature monitoring and alarms.

The construction of the lab should ensure aseptic and optimal handling of reproductive tissue during all stages of the process. Air-conditioning for the laboratory will include HEPA filters, controlled humidity (20%) and controlled temperature (22-24°C). Access to the laboratory should be limited.

Cryopreservation Store

Description and function

Storage room for liquid nitrogen tanks containing frozen gametes (Figs. 19 to 21) nitrogen tanks should be stored in an enclosed space in case of nitrogen leakage. Strict protocols on the method of storage and specimen labeling are required for this process.[11]

Location and relationships

The cryopreservation storage area should be located in close proximity to the laboratory areas, in an area with controlled access.

Considerations

A monitoring system is required for low levels of liquid nitrogen in the storage tanks and for high levels of nitrogen in the air.[10]

Strict cryopreservation protocols are required and will include:[10]

- Infection control (minimizing the risk of cross contamination of frozen gametes, zygotes and embryos
- Labeling, packaging and documentation of tissue frozen
- Provide controlled access to the room.

For "slow freezing" the embryos are frozen in small straws in a controlled rate freezer (Fig. 22). Straws are put in a liquid nitrogen tank for storage.

Incubators are often stacked like this to save lab space. The colored tape on the door of the upper unit is used to identify the location of a patient's eggs or embryos in the incubator before the door is opened (Fig. 23). This reduces the amount of time that the door has to remain open.[10]

Sudden drastic temperature losses, recovery times and change in pH are minimized when using Warming Blocks.

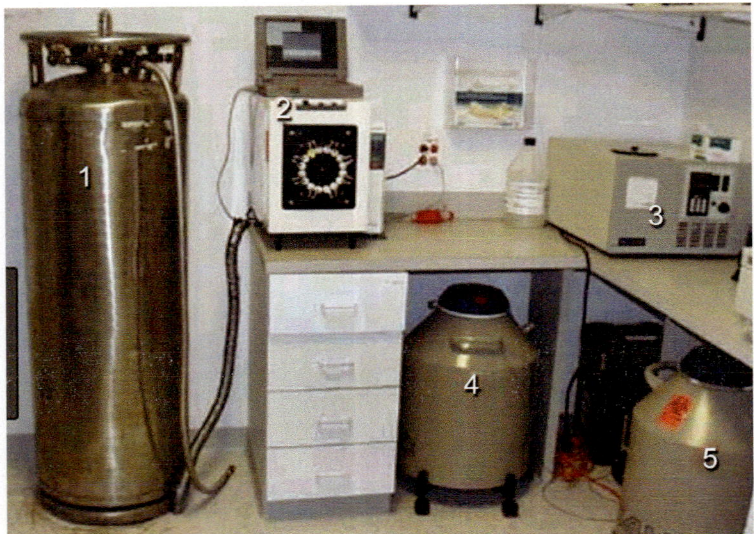

Fig. 21: Cryopreservation area of lab. (1) Liquid nitrogen supply tank; (2) Back-up embryo freezer; (3) Main embryo freezer; (4) and (5) Storage tanks for frozen embryos and sperm.

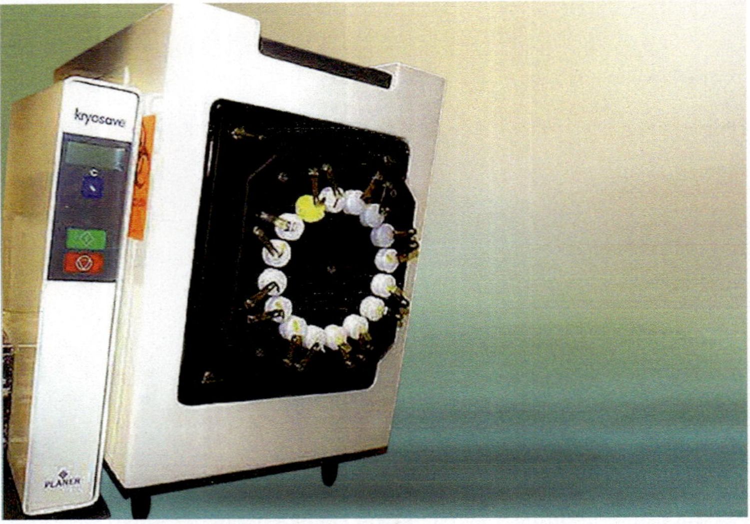

Fig. 22: "Slow freezing" embryos are frozen in small straws in a controlled rate freezer.

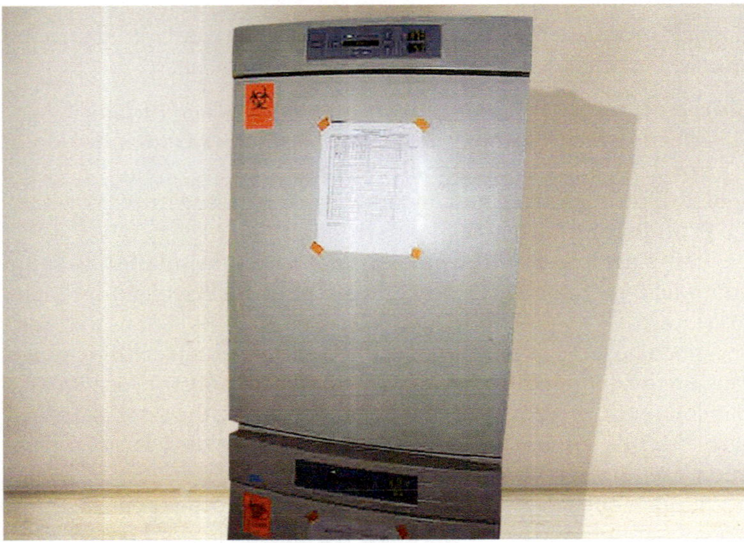

Fig. 23: Incubators.

STAFF AND SUPPORT ZONE

Disposal Room/Clean-up Room

Store Room

A well-stocked store for keeping essential stock of especially those items that have to be imported, precluding the need to be caught short in the middle of treatment. Facilities must be available for storing sterile (media, needles, catheters, petri dishes and such-like items) and nonsterile material under refrigerated and nonrefrigerated conditions as appropriate.[1]

Sterile Room

Sterile storage is the instrumentation and equipment warehouse. If a product is disinfected and/or sterilized it will have a home in this room. Like a warehouse, orders are packed and sent to other locations for use on specific patients undergoing specific procedures.

Meeting Room/Staff Room

Sterilizing/Packing

- *Description and function*: An area where cleaned and dried instruments are sorted, assembled into sets, packaged, and then sterilized in an autoclave[10]
- *Location and relationships*: The sterilizing/packing room will be located adjacent to the clean-up room where the instruments are cleaned and decontaminated[10]
- *Considerations*: Fittings and equipment located in this room will include:[10]
  - Hand basin
  - Benches and cupboards
  - Instrument packing table
  - Heat sealing device
  - Autoclave
  - Cooling trolleys.

The room requires a defined unidirectional workflow for instruments from clean to sterile and then to sterile store. Sterile stock should not be stored in this.

CONCLUSION

Infertility is a complex medicosocial problem. In a number of societies there is stigma attached to infertility, ART is an art and science process which has produced effective results to overcome this issue. ART is a technology intensive, infrastructure specific and skill driven.

There are statutory and regulatory and accreditation requirements which must be fulfilled the optimization of this complex yet essential facility.

REFERENCES

1. www.ivftraining.com.
2. The Assisted Reproductive Technology (Regulation) Bill, 2008. 2008.pp.1-135.
3. Technologies AR, Committee R. Independent Review.
4. www.health.gov.au.
5. www.scribd.com.
6. www.icmr.nic.in.
7. lrd.yahooapis.com.
8. Unit LO, Models P, Areas F. 22.0 IVF Unit (Fertilisation Centres) 22.1. 2011. pp.158-69.
9. https://kwa.kerala.gov.in/
10. www.healthdesign.com.au.
11. www.health.vic.gov.au.

12. urbanindia.nic.in.
13. www.nfs.scot.nhs.uk.
14. www.ivf.net.
15. www.buildingindustry.org.
16. www.rutibarsinai.com.
17. Izquierdo EG, Ángel C, Velasco B, Vicente J, Escudero M, Rodríguez AG. The Design of an In Vitro Fertilization (IVF) Laboratory and its Importance in Risk Prevention : Applicability of UV Radiation. 2009;52:1579-86.
18. Steyaert SR, Leroux-Roels GG, Dhont M. Infections in IVF: review and guidelines. [Internet]. Human reproduction update. p. 432–41. Available from: http://www.ncbi.nlm.nih.gov/pubmed/19040462.
19. Magli MC, Van den Abbeel E, Lundin K, Royere D, Van der Elst J, Gianaroli L. Revised guidelines for good practice in IVF laboratories. Human reproduction (Oxford, England) [Internet]. 2008 Jun [cited 2012 Dec 30];23(6):1253-62. Available from: http://www.ncbi.nlm.nih.gov/pubmed/18375408.
20. Section R. Designing and Testing Clean Rooms for Biocontamination Control and Compliance. 2003;46001 1996.pp.1-4.
21. ateam.lbl.gov.
22. aaucm.org.
23. www.sismer.it.
24. www.oup.co.uk.
25. humrep.oxfordjournals.org.
26. www.fpg.unc.edu.
27. www.indmedica.com.
28. Practical Manual of In Vitro Fertilization, Springer Publishers 2012
29. medlibrary.org.
30. www.eshre.com.
31. advancedfertility.com.
32. www.bizviet.net.
33. www.advancedfertility.com.
34. www.dus.at.gov
35. www.fgiguidelines.org

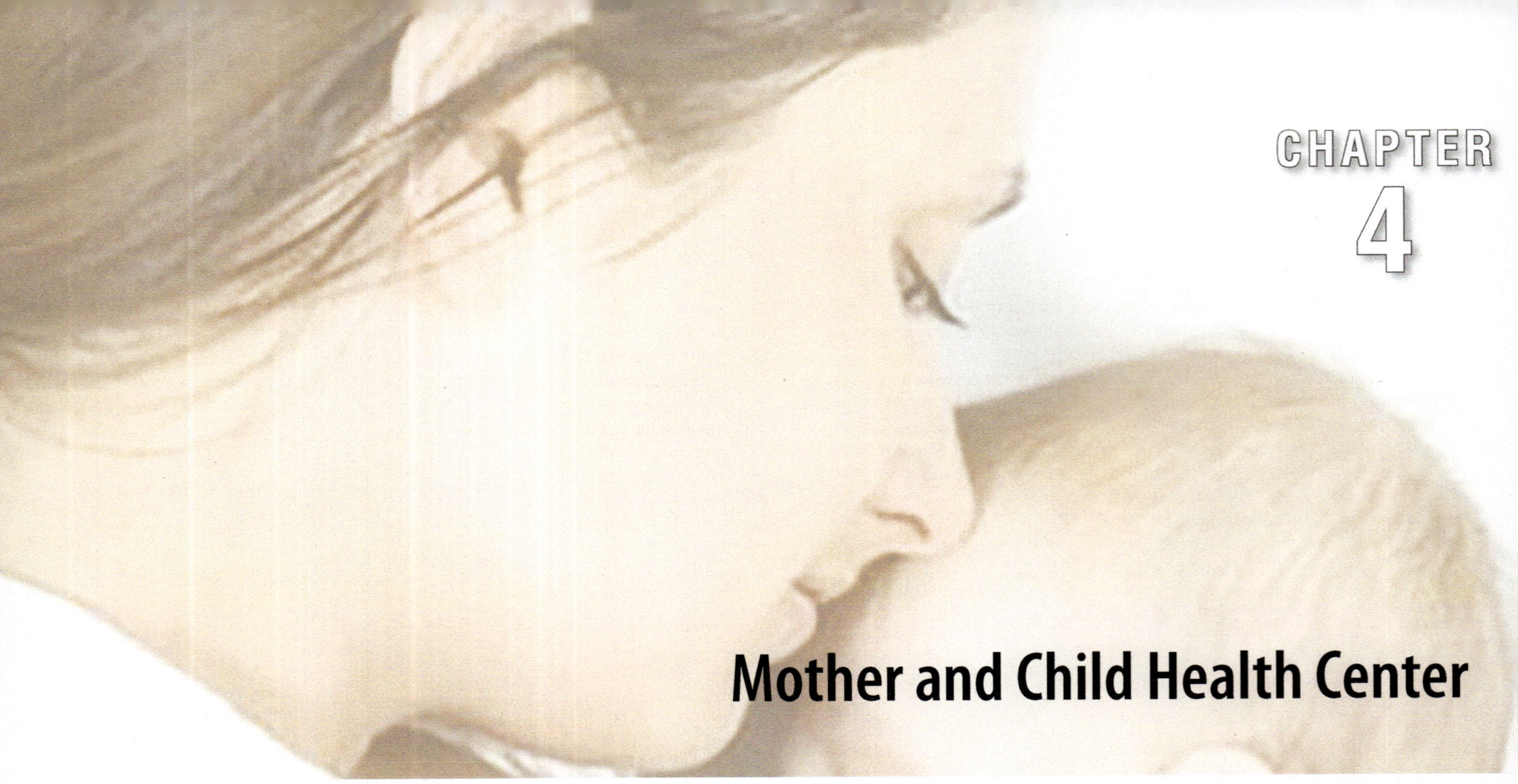

CHAPTER 4

Mother and Child Health Center

Parmeshwar Kumar, Shakti Kumar Gupta, Sunil Kant, R Chandrashekhar

INTRODUCTION

The special bond that a mother and her child share right from the womb continues, even as the umbilical cord gets severed at birth. While the health of the community is intimately linked to that of the female, it is also noteworthy that the women and children form a substantial and vulnerable group of society. Recognizing this, the Government of India has launched the *Reproductive and Child Health* initiative which is currently in its second phase. The main objective of the program is to bring about a change in three critical health indicators, i.e. reducing the total fertility rate, infant mortality rate and maternal mortality rate.

FUNCTIONS OF THE FACILITY

The aim of the mother and child health facility would be to act as a center for excellence in caring for the health of women and children including neonates and adolescents. Following are the objectives of the facility:

- To provide comprehensive care in obstetrics including assisted reproductive therapy
- To cater to patients with gynecological conditions but excluding malignancies
- To provide complete medical and surgical care to pediatric patients
- To address problems related to the adolescent population including their mental health
- To act as an advanced center for imparting education and research in the field of pediatrics, obstetrics and gynecology.

GENERAL PLANNING CONSIDERATIONS

Stack Diagram of Mother and Child Center

Stack diagram may be designed as a six storeyed structure shown in Figure 1.

OUTPATIENT SERVICES

Special Planning Considerations

The important factors are:

- OPD should be at the ground floor and must be accessible from the main center entrance. It should be integrated with the IPD physically, functionally and from the clinical and administrative points of view.
- Signage should be scientific.

Entrance and parking: The space around the entrance has to be slip free and sized to allow the simultaneous setting down or picking up of patients from two cars. Multilevel car parking is desirable.

Special Design Considerations

Public Area

In the OPD, the waiting spaces for pediatric and adult patients should be separate. Creative waiting areas should be provided for pediatric patient (Fig. 2) Subwaiting areas in the immediate vicinity of various clinics should be provided.

- Lobby and lounge to provide seating.
- Multipurpose room(s) for conferences, meetings, health education programs, etc.

Clinical Facilities

General purpose examination rooms—minimum floor area 7.43 sqm (80 sqft) excluding vestibules, toilets, closets, etc. Wash basin and a counter top for writing. At least 80 cm (30 inch) clearance on either side and at the foot end of the examination table.

Ancillary Area

Public conveniences: Separate for males and females with 1 per 50 patients. At least one toilet must be there for the disabled and children.

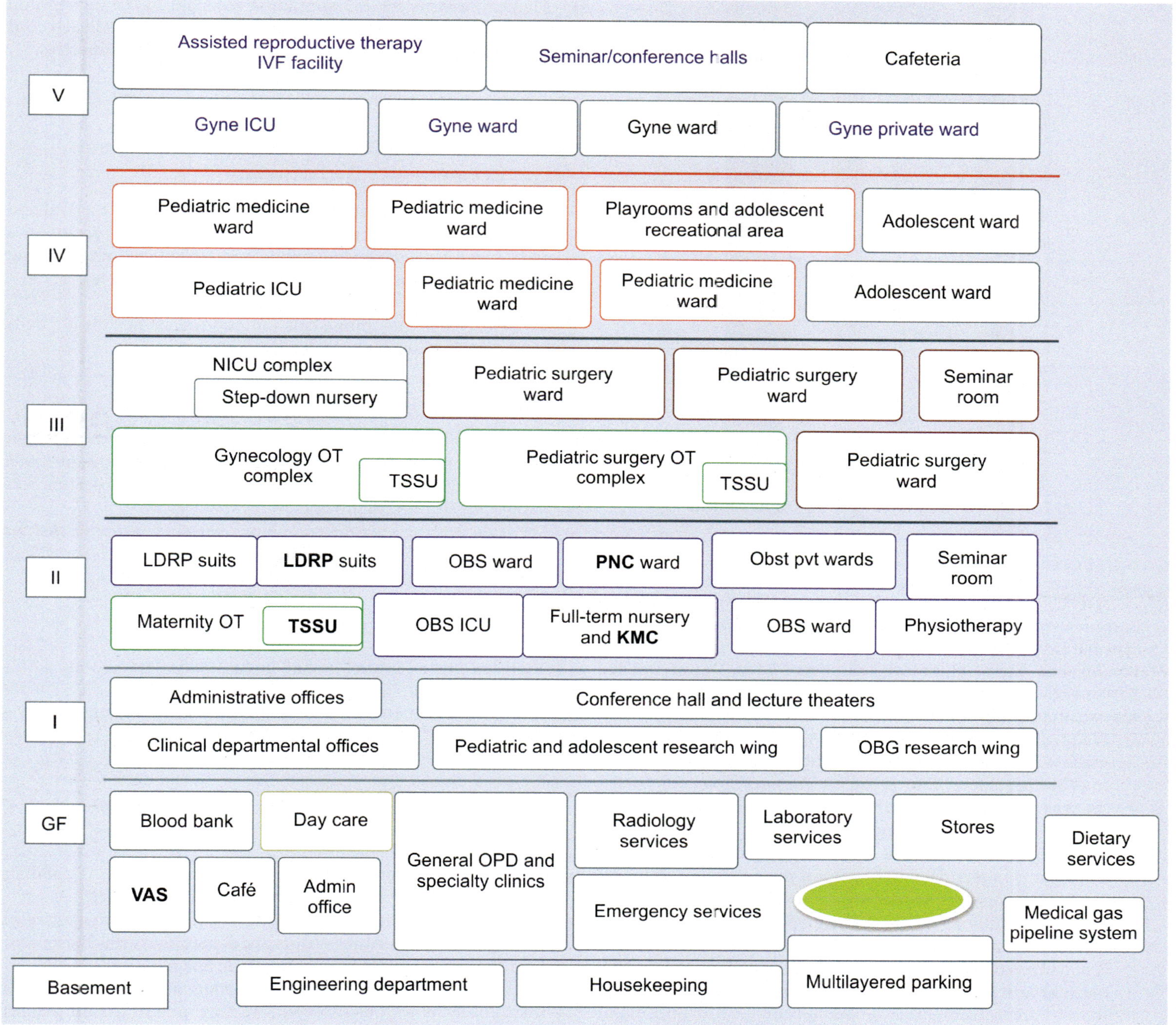

Fig. 1: Stack diagram of mother and child center.

(TSSU: theater steriple supply unit; LDRP: labor delivery, recovery and postpartum; KMC: Kangaroo mother care; VAS: value added services; PNC: postnatal clinical)

- Coffee shop/snack bar in the vicinity
- Gift shop. Best location is off the lobby in a conspicuous location with adequate display space
- Meditation room/retiring facility—for meditation or for use by anxious or bereaved relatives.

OBSTETRICS AND GYNECOLOGY

The OPD should have the following services:

- Antenatal clinic
- Postnatal clinic
- ART/IVF clinic
- Genetics
- Physiotherapy/Exercise service
- Counseling services
- Immunization services
- MTP clinic
- Gynecological clinic
- Postoperative clinic
- Cancer screening and colposcopy
- Ultrasound clinic
- Family planning clinic.

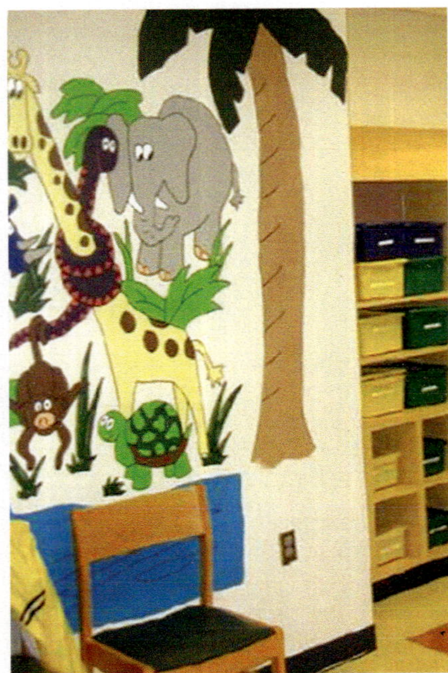

Fig. 2: Creative waiting areas for the pediatric patients.

Design Considerations Special to Gynecology and Obstetrics

- Entrance should have ramps, with door width being 1.8 m and likewise for steps.
- *Waiting area*: Antenatal clinics usually have a heavy load of patients. To reduce the waiting time and crowding in the facility, *appointment system* should be followed
  - Waiting area should have piped or otherwise soft music which while not hampering the functioning of the OPD would serve to allay the anxiety of the pregnant women.
  - Alternatively, it should also have *television programs* related to antenatal and delivery, family planning.
  - *Space requirement*: An *area of 0.5–0.8 sqm* per patient.
- *Consultation chamber*: Depending upon the expected workload, the number of consultation rooms may be planned:
  - Each consultation room should have a partition or an anteroom where the expectant mother can be examined in privacy.
  - A consultation room should have a couch, furniture for the consultant/residents and the patient, cupboard for documents, the relevant instruments, examination lamp and an ultrasound machine.
  - *Space requirement*: A consultation room requires an area of 14 sqm including the examination room and toilet.
- *Physiotherapy room*: A room with at least 4 couches and instructors tables should be provided for antenatal and postnatal programs.
- *Counseling room*: This is required for the parents pregnancy counseling and consent for preoperative patients.
- *Immunization facility*: For routine immunization, injectable preparations and immediate post-delivery injections to be given to the newborn.
- Nonstress test/fetal cardiotocography: An area/room for NST must be provided in the OPD.
- *Reception and registration*: A counter at the entry should be present to help the patients. One desk per 20 patients should be provided. Counter should be 100 cm high and 60 cm wide.
- Medical records section should be adjacent to the registration office within the complex. Alternatively, electronic medical record (EMR) system may be used to make the entire MRD paperless.

EMERGENCY SERVICES

Special Physical Facilities and Space Requirements Access to Emergency Department

The directional signs to the ED should be unmistakably marked and clearly visible, day and night. Weatherproof fittings and accessories should be used in all external situations. Per 100,000 annual visits about 6 parking spaces should be provided in a nearby parking lot.

Space requirement: The thumb rule for total special need is— a daily patient load of 100 patients requires about 1,000 sqm.

Public Area

- *Stretcher, trolley, wheelchair store*: A trolley, stretcher, and wheelchair store or bay should be located immediately adjacent to the entrance. Usually, a wheelchair per about 800 annual visits is needed. Stretchers should, be sturdy and provided with wheel-locks.
- Separate waiting area for emergency patients and relatives, for accompanying children a separate waiting area should be provided. A pram bay of about 6 sqm is needed.

Administrative Area

- There may be a requirement of an ambulance attendants, police and a mass media room.
- A room of about 10 sqm near the entrance hall equipped with a desk, chairs and telephones may serve the purpose.

ADMITTING DEPARTMENT

Location

- It would be adjacent or close to emergency service, outpatient department, medical records, laboratory and radiology.
- As obstetric patients may sometimes require immediate care in areas quickly reached by elevators, the department would be located near the main vertical circulation of the hospital.
- The admitting department should be contiguous with the hospital's main lobby as well as the main waiting area of the outpatient department.

PLANNING AND DESIGNING OF NURSING SERVICES

Certain features common to nursing units are enumerated in Figure 3.

GENERAL NURSING UNIT: ADULT

Location

Nursing units have a close relationship with the operating rooms, pharmacy, central stores, laboratory and the dietary. In maintaining this relationship, they are highly dependent on vertical transportation and an efficient communication system (Fig. 3).

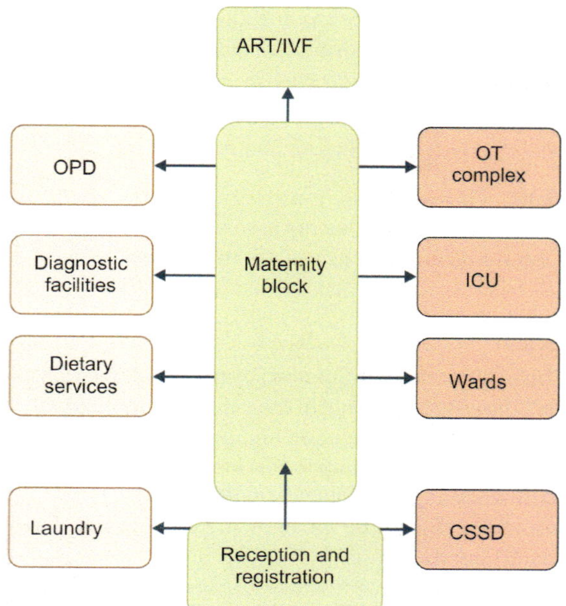

Fig. 3: Functional relationship of the components.
(ART: assisted reproductive technology; IVF: *in vitro* fertilization; CSSD: central sterile supply department OPD: outpatient department; OT: operation theater; ICU: intensive care unit)

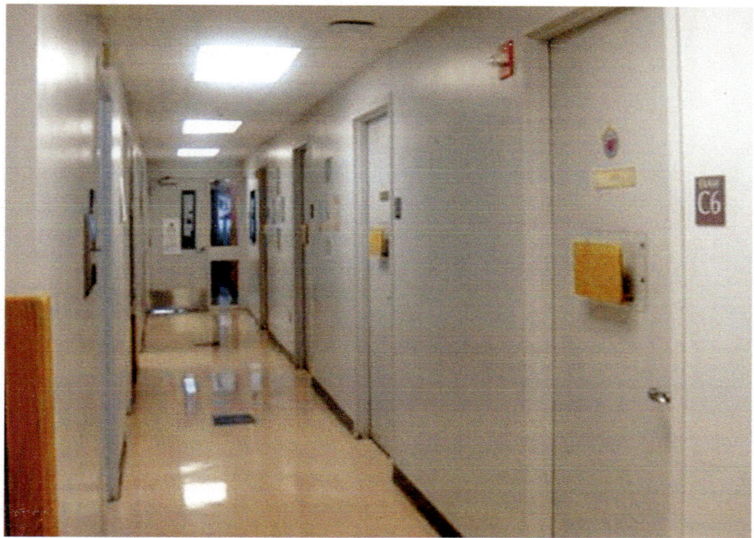

Fig. 4: Private ward should be segregated as for the floor plan—The obstetric private ward on the same floor as the labor room and maternity OT.

Design (Fig. 4)

- The most common size of a nursing unit is between 20 and 40 beds.
- *Double corridor*: A double corridor system in which a nursing floor with double corridors resembles a racetrack, is widely used.
- The nurses' station, utilities and supply rooms, treatment and procedure rooms, doctors' rooms, etc. are located in the central core.
- Patient rooms are situated outside the track.
- Double corridors not only serve to shorten horizontal travel and save steps, they also facilitate patient segregation.

Patient Rooms (Fig. 5)

- Paying patients may use the two-bed rooms, dimensions of which would be a minimum of 15 sqm in size and provided with cubicle curtains for visual privacy.

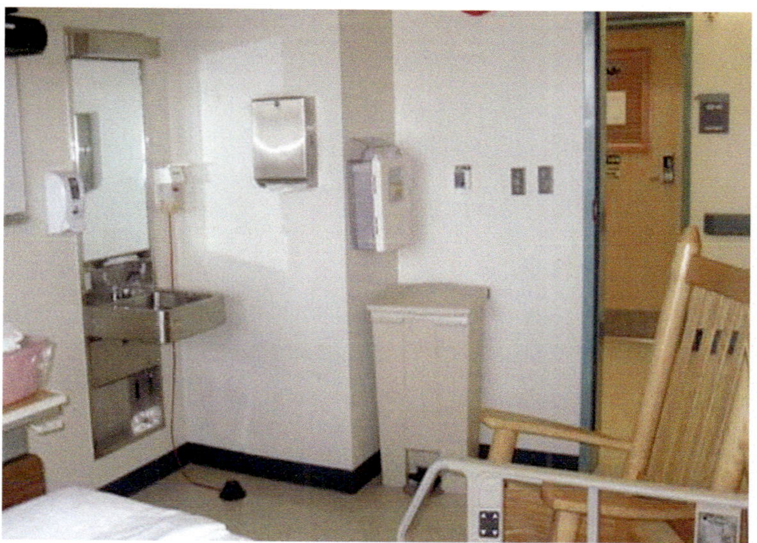

Fig. 5: Patient rooms.

- The four-bed rooms should have a minimum floor area of 30 sqm.
- There should be sufficient space between the beds, and between the bed and the wall to allow the nurse and equipment to pass.
- The patient room toilet should be provided with a grab bar, an emergency call button within easy reach, and a flush valve for bedpan cleaning.
- Bed should have a built-in wardrobe and the regular furniture. Doors should open outward towards the corridor with an outside lock.
- The height of the window-sill should not exceed 0.9 m to allow the patient an outside view.

The Nursing Station

Facilities and Space Requirements

It must be proximal to the elevator, stairway and the corridor. In addition to facilities like patients' rooms, nurses' station, etc. the following additional facilities are also required:

- Examination and treatment room with wash basin, counter, shelf, etc.
- Clean workroom or clean holding room.
- Soiled workroom with clinical sink, work top, waste receptacle, etc.
- Clean linen store.
- Equipment storage room.
- Recessed space for storing stretchers and wheelchairs.
- Staff facilities such as lockers, etc. for staff's personal effects.
- Pantry with sink, work top, storage cabinets and space for temporary storage of dietary trays.
- A multipurpose room for staff and patient conference, education, demonstration, etc.

DAY SPACE

- Solarium—a day room. The room should have large windows, a table, individual seating, magazine and bookracks, storage cabinets, emergency call button connected to nurses' station, etc.

PEDIATRIC UNIT

General Planning for Pediatric Wards

Playrooms and outdoor play areas for children must be provided (Fig. 6). The playrooms would be in the sunny areas accommodating

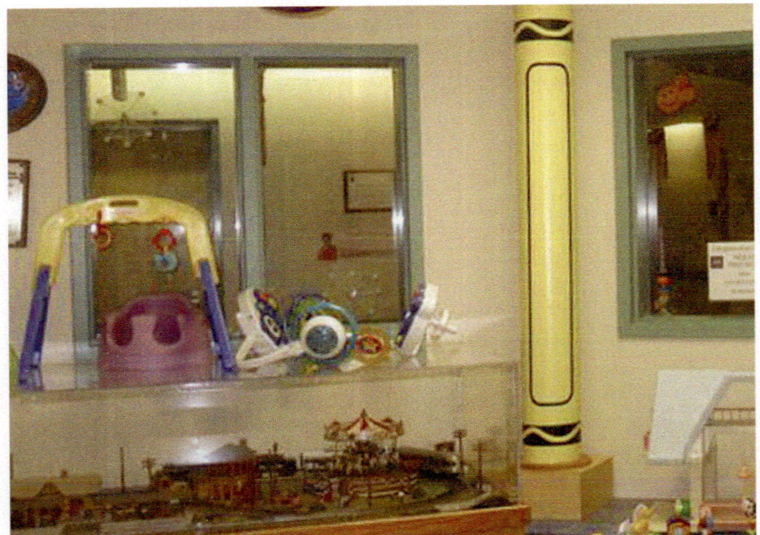

Fig. 6: Playroom.

about 25 children. It would be furnished with low stationary tables and child sized chairs.

Location

The pediatric nursing unit is generally noisy. It should therefore be located in a quiet area, away from the main stream of hospital traffic, ensuring natural sunlight into the rooms, and if possible, adjacent to an enclosed terrace which may be used as a play area.

Unique Design Requirements

This unit has some special requirements besides those mentioned above, these are:

- In view of the size variation and the need to change from cribs to beds, and vice versa, space provided for cribs should be the same as for the beds.
- Minimum floor area for a one-bed room be 10 sqm and for a two-bed room 15 sqm. Recommended areas including space for working around the patient and moving beds and stretchers are 12 sqm for single rooms and 18 sqm for two-bed rooms.
- Every pediatric nursing unit should have its own nurses' station, preferably situated centrally within the unit. As a general rule, rooms designed for the use of the sickest patients and for young infants should be nearest the nurses' station.
- It is essential that each pediatric unit be provided with one or more isolation rooms for patients with known or suspected infection. The room should have only one bed and should have an anteroom with gowning and masking facilities, sink with hand washing facilities without the use of hands, foot-operated waste receptacle, and small cabinet for clean gowns, masks, etc.
- At least 25% of the beds should be in single rooms for critically-ill patients for those who are disturbing to other patients.
- A recreation room/playroom should be provided for group activities and recreation. This room should serve as a playroom for the younger children, for games, occupational therapy and school work for the older children, and a social room and library for the adolescents. The room should be so designed structurally as to minimize the transmission of noise and impact through the floor, walls and ceilings.
- Walls between patient rooms and the corridors should have clear glass panels so that children can see activities around them, and nurses can see the children easily.

NEWBORN NURSERIES (FIGS. 7A AND B)

Traditionally, what was only a nursery has now given place to the concept of nurseries like the newborn, suspect (observation), premature, isolation, high-risk and intensive care nurseries.

Location

The location of nurseries is influenced by many factors such as especially trained staff, the advances made in the field and professional philosophy. This is particularly true of isolation and premature nurseries. The trend is to locate these in the pediatric service with the premature nursery as part of the neonatal intensive care unit (ICU).

- The nurseries should be close to the mothers in the obstetrical (postnatal) nursing unit.
- They should also be close to the labor-delivery suite so as to minimize travel distance and exposure of the newborn infants.

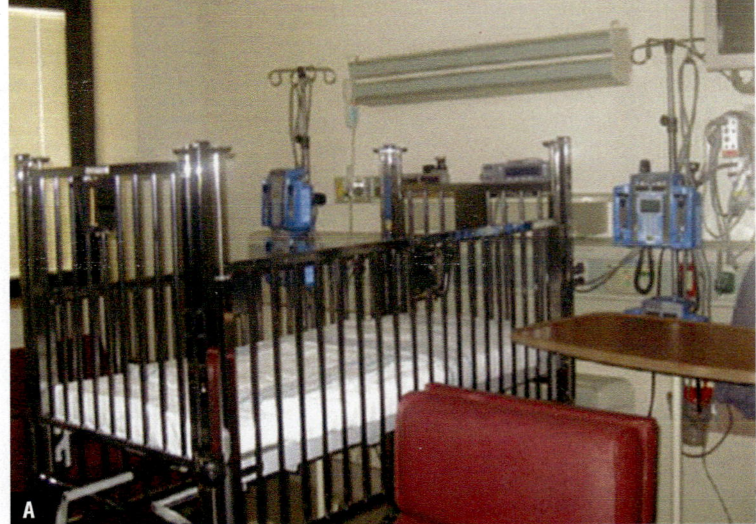

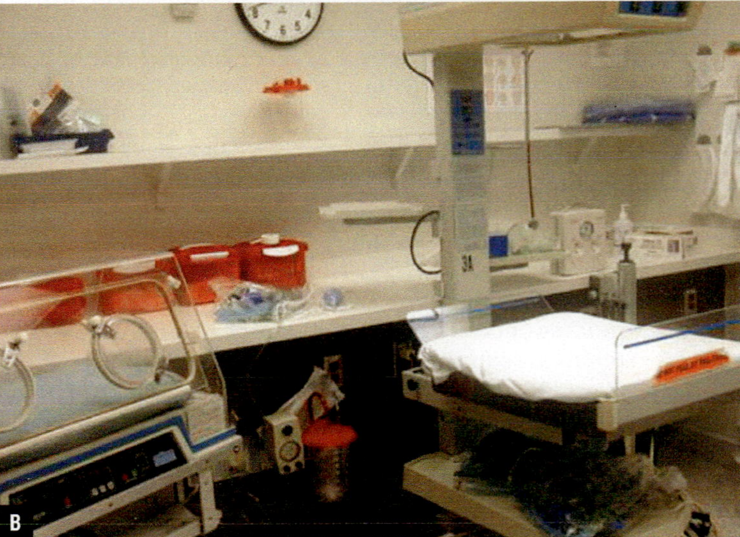

Figs. 7A and B: Preterm nursery.

Design

The intensive therapy units have been designed predominantly for adults.

One ICU-bed for 20 pediatric beds, including subspecialities, has been recommended. It has also been assumed that the beds in pediatric intensive care units should constitute 6% of all beds in the pediatric clinic.

Recent evidence suggests that newborn infants are especially interested in face-like configurations. It is therefore important that planning premises be such that it can maximize parent-infant involvement. The following guidelines are to be used:

- The number of infants in each nursery should be limited.
- Separate bassinets by cubicle partitions to prevent crowding.
- Wide spacing of bassinets within each nursery should be allowed.
- The use of aseptic techniques and individual care and hand-washing facilities should be promoted.
- Optimum conditions of temperature, relative humidity and ventilation.
- Premature infants from infected infants or those suspected of infection should be separate.
- In a full-scale nursery, the maximum number of bassinets would be 12.

Some Special Design Elements and Facilities

Every nursery would contain the following in addition to those in regular ICUs:

- Glazed observation windows which allow the viewing of infants by visitors from the public areas and viewing by the staff from their workrooms.
- Provision for storing linen, nursery equipment and infant supplies
- Provision for storage of emergency carts and equipment out of traffic but at an easily accessible place.
- Mothers' room or area for breastfeeding with a table, infant scales and a rocking chair.
- Facilities for the preparation of infant formulas or milk mixtures with work counter, sink and a small refrigerator, refrigerated storage and provision for warming infant formula must be available at all times.
- A Kangaroo Mother Care (KMC) ward should be at close proximity to the NICU.

Full-term Nursery

The full-term nursery is intended for normal infants, and should be located in the postpartum nursing unit, as close to the mothers as possible. An area of 3 sqm per infant or bassinet is recommended exclusive of the nurses' station, with a provision for at least 0.9 m between bassinets and on all sides.

Observation Nursery

An observation or suspect nursery should be provided for infants suspected of infection. A minimum of 4 sqm per infant or bassinet is recommended.

Premature Nursery

The premature nursery is used for infants "born too soon" and "born too less". Premature infants need more specialized care. So the nursery should accommodate no more than five infants and would have a minimum of 4 sqm of space per incubator or bassinet.

OBSTETRICS NURSING UNIT

Location

- Ideally, the obstetrical unit should be located on the same floor as the labor-delivery suite and in close proximity to it.
- The unit should also be adjacent or close to the nursery to minimize the distance of travel and consequent exposure of babies between the nursery and the mother's room.
- The obstetrical unit should also be close to the vertical transport.

Facilities and Space Requirements

- Ultrasound scanning is a routine procedure during the antenatal period, a scanning room should be provided. Many obstetric patients prefer double rooms because of the social interaction they provide.
- A conference room is necessary for patient education programs and prenatal classes.

Isolation Rooms

Location

Isolation rooms may be located within the individual nursing units and placed at the end of the corridor. They should be available for normal acute care when not required for isolation cases. Isolation rooms may be grouped as a separate isolation unit.

Special Design Considerations

- Each isolation room should contain only one bed and would have all the facilities of the acute care patient room.
- Viewing panel(s) may be provided to allow staff to observe patients from the anteroom.
- Each isolation room should have a toilet, bath and hand washing facilities so arranged as to permit access from the bed without passing through the anteroom or the work area.

INTENSIVE CARE UNITS

Location

- ICUs should be in a centralized place and be close to the emergency department, labor room, operating rooms, recovery rooms, respiratory therapy, laboratory and radiology.
- The ICUs should not be too far away from the general nursing units. This will reduce to a minimum the movement and time required to transfer patients from one unit to the other, especially from the nursing unit to the ICU, in an emergency.
- ICUs should be located away from heavy traffic and noise. In deciding the location, the electrical influence of equipment like elevator motors and X-ray equipment on the displays of monitors would be kept in mind.
- Intensive care now encompasses many disciplines; it is recommended that a minimum of 5% of the total beds be designated to ICUs. However, for practical purposes, 10% may be a better figure considering a woman and child hospital.

Facilities and Space Requirements[1]

- The entrance door to rooms should be at least 1.2 m wide, for easy movement of beds and large equipment.

- Rooms should be at least 12 sqm with free movable space surrounding the bed.
- Outlets should be no lower than 750 mm off the floor.
- In the non-cubicled curtained area, there should be a clear space of at least 1350 mm between beds, and 1050 mm between the end bed and the wall. There should be a clear space of at least 900 mm between head end of the wall, and 1200 mm (4 ft) at the foot end to permit resuscitation procedures.
- The central control station should be designed to seat two or three persons only. This will discourage staff from idling in that area.
- Multipurpose room for conferences, training sessions, demonstrations for staff, patients, and patients' families.
- Family waiting room with toilet and pay phone facilities. There should be a gowning area and storage for clean gowns, masks, etc.

ICU BED

- The spatial need for an ICU bed in a single-bed room is 17–20 sqm.
- The comfortable working height should be 975 mm for female staff and 1075 mm for male staff. For the patient to get safely in and out of the bed, the compressed mattress height would need to be as low as 325 mm.
- Studies have shown that the space around the bed in a single-bled accommodation can be used most efficiently when the shape of the floor is close to a square.
- For each bed in the open ICU an average of about 20 sqm should be allowed, with about 3.5 m between the centers. About 15 sqm per bed is the minimum.
- The pediatric ICU should be designed to have at least 12 sqm allotted for each bed space. There must be at least 6 electrical outlets per bed space (Fig. 8).

CLINICAL LABORATORY SERVICES

Laboratory Elements

Modular unit: To obtain a multifunctional use, laboratories need to be modular. A module unit choice is 3.0 m. Each pathological assistant needs a functional area of 25 sqm. If traffic and technical areas are included this amounts to about 35 sqm. An acceptable laboratory room height should be between 2.7 m and 3.0 m.

RADIOLOGICAL SERVICES

Diagnostic Radiology

- The CT scan facility must follow Bhabha Atomic Research Center (BARC) guidelines and Atomic Energy Regulatory Board (AERB) in planning and designing.
- In terms of spatial needs, the total area per X-ray room including all the auxiliary and ancillary facilities should be 200 sqm.
- The planning of the CT and MRI facility should ensure that the problem of closed treatment rooms with large and intimidating equipment causing anxiety, claustrophobia, abnormal fear is addressed. This can be creatively done by ensuring that skyline is visible and the view through the bore of the machine is a pleasing piece of art.
- A floor area of about 1.3 sqm should be allowed for each waiting patient. Parking area for trolleys and beds must be provided. A particular waiting area for children and accompanying mothers should be provided. The corridors must be 2.8 m wide for bed traffic.

Location

The diagnostic radiology department should be located on the ground floor, conveniently accessible to inpatients, outpatient and emergency patients. The department should be located close to the elevators and other diagnostic and treatment facilities.

Design

The planning must consult experts who will be familiar with the mandatory regulations of the Atomic Energy Regulatory Board (AERB) and the Division of Radiological Protection, BARC, in designing the department.

There is a definite need for a mammography facility in a mother and child hospital and should be close to the OPD where gynecological cases are being reviewed (Fig. 9).

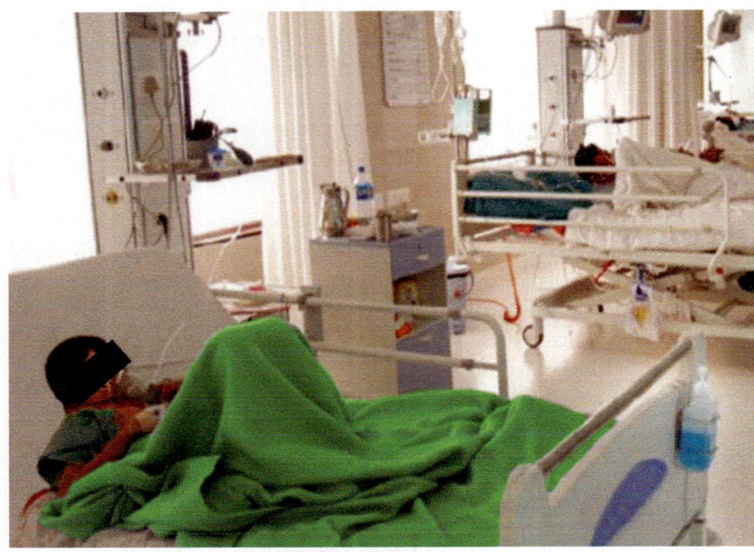

Fig. 8: Pediatric ICU.

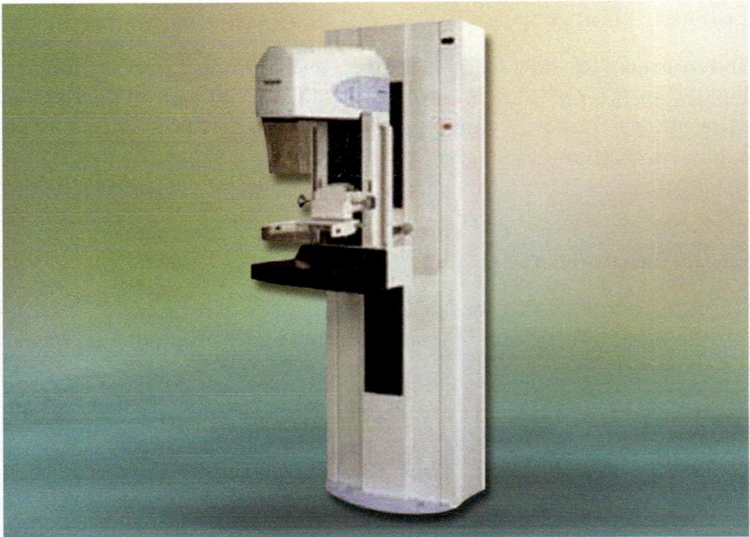

Fig. 9: Force field mammogram.

PEDIATRIC SURGERY DEPARTMENT

Location[2]

- The best location for the pediatric surgery department is one which permits a convenient and uncomplicated flow of patients, staff and clean supplies traffic.
- Surgery receives inpatients from the floors through non-public corridors, elevators and ramps. Convenient access to elevators is, therefore, essential.
- With regard to services, ideal adjacencies should be emergency, radiology, clinical laboratories, intensive care units, central sterile and supply department and delivery suite.

Design

The design depends on the number and type of operating rooms.

Some key factors to be considered relate to size, usage, lighting (surgical and general illumination), intercommunication and signal systems, electronic equipment and monitoring system, medical gas system (suction, oxygen, nitrous oxide and compressed air) and other service lines, fixtures, safety precautions such as grounding for X-ray, TV camera, and against static electricity, storage, supply cabinets, environmental control, etc.

- Post anesthesia recovery
- The frozen section laboratory
- Changing area
- Scrubbing area.

Dimensions

It is recommended that surgical corridors should be 3 m to 3.5 m wide.

Operating rooms must have a minimum clear area of 36 sqm, excluding fixed cabinets and built-in shelves. Many surgeons, however, recommend larger space, i.e. 45 sqm for major operating rooms and 56 sqm for special procedure rooms. Each operating room should have X-ray film illuminators which will handle at least two films at the same time, and an emergency communication system.

Major operating rooms size should be 48 sqm and special procedure rooms 72 sqm.

Prefabricated Surgical Suite and Stainless Steel Panels

A prefabricate surgical suite is a structural steel shell with a jointless sealed sterile coating. An especially designed steel frame will accept a variety of wall panels. These may be seamless stainless steel or zintex sheets, powder-coated demountable stainless steel or high density compact laminated panels or solid mineral sheets.

Ceiling Pendants and OT Control Panels

Ceiling pendants or ceiling supply units-motorized arm ceiling mounted pendants increase efficiency by keeping medical gases and electrical cables off the floor thereby easing the congestion.

Facilities and Space Requirements

Special facilities and space are required for:

- Control station should be so located as to permit visual observation of all traffic into and within the department.
- *Operating rooms*: Total number of OR for 100 beds in pediatrics surgery—04 (1 OR for every 25 surgical beds).
- *Sterilizing facilities*: High speed autoclave conveniently located to serve all operating rooms. Dumb waiters should be brought to use.
- Laboratory for preparation and examination of frozen section. This can be done in the main laboratory if the distance and time needed do not delay the completion of surgery.
- Provision for refrigerated blood bank.
- Consultation and conference room.

OBSTETRICS DEPARTMENT

Labor and Delivery Suite[1]

Location

- The clinical section of the obstetrical department should be located in a convenient but secluded area. Within the clinical facilities, the labor and delivery suites should be as remote as practicable but easily accessible from the entrance to the department so as to avoid unnecessary traffic and to provide privacy to patients.
- The facility should be close to the nursery, obstetrical nursing unit, and to the vertical transport so that patients can access it easily
- The department should be close to the operating rooms.

Preparation Room

Patients have to be prepared for labor and delivery. The preparation room should be located within the labor delivery suite but away from labor and delivery rooms. The room must have facilities for carrying out the procedures in connection with preparation such as an examining table, bath, wash basin, kit for giving enema and preparation tray. A locker to keep the patient's clothes is desirable.

Labor Rooms

This is the room in which the patient remains during the first stage of labor, i.e. from the time the pains commence till she is ready to be moved to the delivery room (Fig. 10).

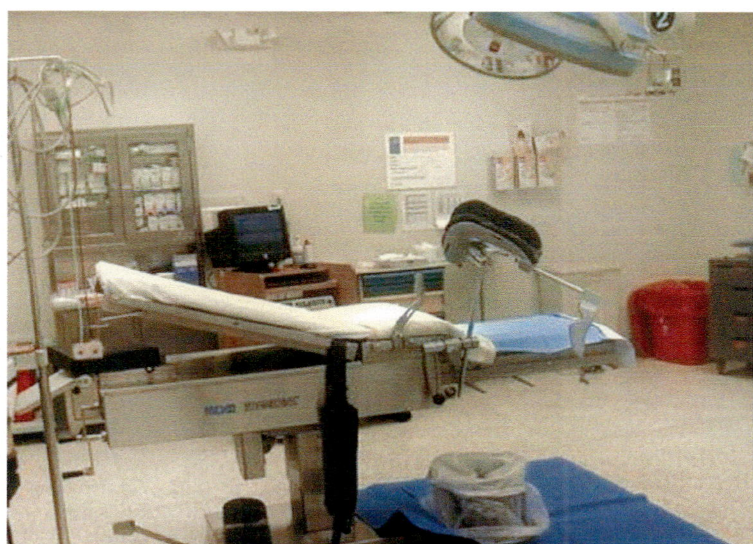

Fig. 10: Delivery room.

The total number of labor rooms should be as follows:
- High dependency unit labor rooms—10
- Delivery rooms—5.

Design Considerations

- Labor rooms must be designed in such a way that they can serve as emergency delivery rooms. The preferred size is 5.5 by 5.5 meters. Single rooms are recommended. They should be equipped with electronic fetal heart monitors.
- The labor rooms should be close to the delivery rooms, but not so close that the two areas are almost one or that the patients can overhear or view delivery room procedures. Both rooms are noisy and so should be sound-proofed, if possible.
- Lighting and color should be conducive to patients' relaxation.
- There would be a good extension light so that the patient can be properly examined by the obstetrician or the nurse. The other auxiliary facilities are as with other parts of the hospital.
- Doors would be 1.2 m wide to permit passage of the bed or stretcher with attendants.
- The bed must be furnished with oxygen, suction and compressed air outlets, nurse call system, and lighting controls.
- Piped music and a lockable locker for patient's personal belongings are desirable.
- Delivery rooms would be similar to operating rooms in their design with finishes that promote maximum aseptic conditions. Facilities provided in the delivery room are essentially the same as for the surgical suite. A delivery room would accommodate only one patient at a time.
- The delivery room would also contain a designated area to receive the newborn baby immediately after birth. This area would have a baby receiving tray, warmer, suction, oxygen and other resuscitating facilities like an Ambu bag. There would be adequate lighting around the area. Each delivery room would have a foot or elbow-operated emergency call system with a dome light and buzzer on the corridor over each delivery room. Similar light signals and buzzers must be installed in the lounge and at the nurses' station.

Cesarean Section Room

These should be an operating room in the department where major obstetrical surgeries are performed.

Scrub Facilities

Two scrub positions should be provided near the entrance to each delivery room. One area with three positions may serve two adjacent delivery rooms.

Recovery Rooms[1]

Modern maternity departments should have a recovery room where all postpartum patients are observed during the first 6 hours after delivery.

Each recovery room may have two or more beds. It would have a nurses' station with charting facilities and visual control of all beds. Provision must be made for dispensing medicine, washing hands, clinical sink with bedpan flushing device and storage for supplies.

Fathers' Wait

This would be located near the labor rooms but outside the labor-delivery suite, with toilet facilities, pay telephone and drinking water facilities.

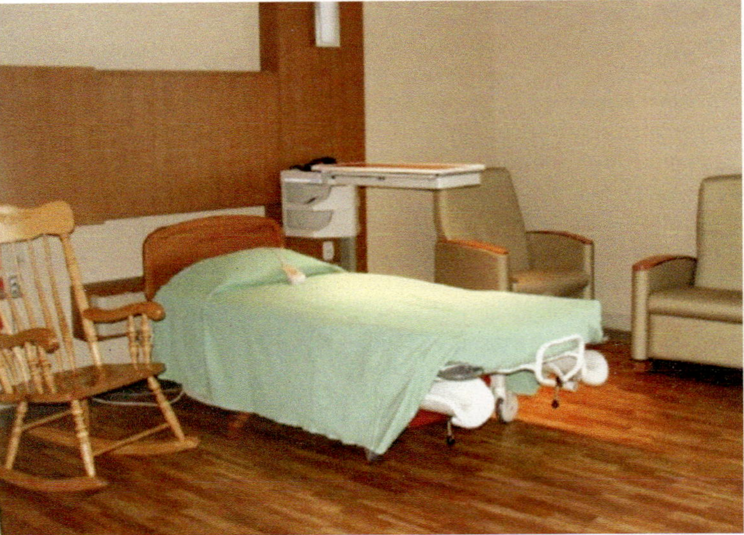

Fig. 11: Labor, delivery, recovery and postpartum (LDRP) suite.

Birthing suite or labor, delivery, recovery and postpartum (LDRP) suite (Fig. 11), i.e. labor, delivery, recovery, postpartum care suite is so-called because the whole process of child birth can take place in one room. These suites, built and equipped for labor and delivery, ensures that the expectant mother moves only once, at the time of discharge, with the baby. The focus has shifted to the family. Some studies recommend LDRP suites, where patient is moved to the postpartum room. It is thus an example of patient focussed care.

Planning Premises

- Provisioning of a homely environment
- Provision of modern medical care
- Privacy to the patient
- Patient safety.

Design Parameters

- The feel as well as the decor would be akin to a miniature home with a bed for the patient and a sofa cum bed/settee for the attendant.
- Cupboards are used, both for the convenience of the patient, the relatives and also to store equipment. The equipments remain hidden from view allaying the anxiety of a patient and at the same time saving space while being available conveniently at the time of need.
- The infant warmer is either built-in or freestanding and is placed where emergency care teams have quick access to it without being too close to the bed.
- Entertainment facilities like televisions and communication facilities like telephones and computers may also be used.

Architectural Consideration

- The interiors should have a healing effect on the patient
- The room may be decorated with works of art but should not make the room resemble a museum.
- The room should be provided with a pantry, and would be furnished in such a way that entry is not in direct line of vision.
- The manifold system should be hidden behind a painting or inside a cupboard.

Labor, Delivery Recovery and Postpartum Beds

The most important furniture is the patient's bed. This can be modified or converted to a delivery whenever required. A monitoring panel with maternal and fetal monitoring would be there at the head end. Provision would be made for a bassinet/cradle with medical gases for neonatal care.

Space requirement:

- Total area for LDRP suite: 28 sqm
- Area for toilets: 5 sqm
- Area for bassinet: 3 sqm

Lighting

The lighting should be adjustable with dimming facility, the range being 300–500 lux.

HEATING, VENTILATION AND AIR-CONDITION

- Temperature: 24°C ± 2°C
- Relative humidity: 45 ± 5%
- Air changes: 8 to 10 air changes per hour
- Filter: HEPA filter

Underwater Delivery

The birthing suite needs to be wider, a peninsular bath with double-sided access is required. The area should be 15 sqm. The temperature of the pool should be strictly maintained between 35°C and 37°C.

Patient's Lounge

- It is important to have a lounge for the first stage of labor patients
- Allowing women in early labor to move around freely and socialize with others will help to minimize problems created by anxiety during labor.

Delivery Room

- The delivery table is equipped with stirrups and footplates, and is also equipped with handgrips. At each delivery bed, there should be oxygen outlets, also for the babies, suction points, and wall-mounted sphygmomanometers.
- An overhead mirror should be available.
- Since the newborn does not tolerate even brief episodes of hypoxia, oxygen warmed to 32–34°C with 60–80% relative humidity is administered.
- When a premature baby is anticipated, the delivery room temperature should be increased to 32°C or higher.
- Storage space is important, hence wall cabinets for resuscitation equipment, measured 650 × 600 × 220 mm, have been recommended.
- A delivery room should have a floor area of about 30 sqm. For obstetrical or surgical lamps a ceiling height of at least 3 m is required. A door width of 1.2 m allows the patients to be moved to the delivery room on a labor bed.

Operation Room

If the obstetric suite is a section of the surgical department, the occasional need for immediate surgical intervention is easily met. In an independent delivery suite, an operation unit should be included as about 20% of deliveries require a surgical intervention.

Recovery Room

- For rest, observation, and care 12 sqm recovery rooms are needed.
- The recovery room should be placed adjacent to the delivery room and be equipped as a postanesthetic recovery room.

Prenatal and Lamaze Classes

Space must be provided for conducting prenatal classes for expectant mothers. Lamaze classes where relaxation and breathing techniques along with movement and positions are taught.

FACILITY GUIDELINES FOR AN ASSISTED REPRODUCTIVE THERAPY FACILITY (ICMR GUIDELINES)

Minimal Physical Requirements for an ART[3,4]

- It should have a non-sterile and a strictly sterile with the space provision for the sterile area not being combined with those for the non-sterile area and vice-versa.
- A reception and waiting room for patients.
- *A room with privacy*: This is for interviewing and examining male and female partners independently is essential.
- A general-purpose clinical laboratory.
- *Store room*: A well-stocked store for keeping essential stock of especially those items that have to be imported.
- *Record room*: Record keeping must be computerized as far as possible.
- *Autoclave room*: A separate facility must be available for sterilizing and autoclaving all surgical items as well as some of those to be used in the *in vitro* culture laboratory.
- *Steps for vermin proofing*: This essential detail should be planned at an early stage because no pesticide can be used in a fully functional IVF clinic, as it could be toxic to the gametes and embryos.
- Semen collection room.
- Semen processing laboratory.
- Clean room for IUI.
- The sterile area.
- The operation theater.
- Room for intrauterine transfer of embryo.
- The embryology laboratory complex.
- Ancillary laboratory facilities.
- Hormone and other assays.
- Microbiology and histopathology laboratory.
- Back-up power supply a power back-up in the form of UPS systems and/or a captive power generation system is available in the ART clinic.

OPERATION THEATER IN GYNECOLOGY AND OBSTETRICS

Operation Department Size and Locating

The number of operation rooms in a hospital has been related to the number of surgical beds. The guidelines recommend one operation room for every 50 general beds, for 25 surgical beds.

The proper number of operation rooms has also been indicated to be 5% of the total number of surgical beds.

As a thumb rule, 0.1 operations per bed and day, has been used in the past for calculation. It has been assumed that approximately one hour's operation time is required per surgical bed per week.

Up to 35% of operation time has been kept available for emergencies, etc. although usually the emergency operations represent only about 15% of the work load, also in terms of time.

When a hospital requires over ten operation rooms, two or more separated surgery departments may be preferred. The total number of operations-T- is determined by the formula

- T = B × 365 × P
- L × 100
- B—No. of beds in the surgical block
- P—Percentage of bed occupancy
- L—Average length of stay in days
- 50% of obstetrics beds can be considered as surgical beds and all the beds of gynecology should be considered as surgical beds. Therefore, 2 OTs for obstetrics and 4 OTs for gynecology should be planned.

Surgical Department Build-up

Zoning Concept

Areas within the OT should be divided into zones where the bacteriological count progressively diminishes from outer to the inner zone and is maintained by a differential decreasing positive pressure ventilation gradient from the inner to the outer to the outer zone. Four types of zones must be planned:

- *Protective zone*: Includes the reception, waiting area, trolley bay and changing room.
- *Clean zone*: Includes the preoperative room, recovery room, plaster room, staff room and the store.
- *Sterile zone*: The areas included are the operating suite, scrub room, anesthesia induction room and the set-up room.
- *Disposal zone*: The areas included in this zone are the dirty utility and the disposal corridor.

Departmental Planning Approaches

Surgical department corridors should be not less than 2.85 m, preferably 3 m wide.

Spatial Elements

Special waiting rooms for children and accompanying mothers should be provided.

Children need recognizable individuals. They should be accompanied to the anesthetic room, if parents not available, a nurse or attendant with whom they are familiar.

The children's waiting area must be closed to all traffic, and extraneous conversation should not be allowed.

Transfer Areas, Patient Bed in the Pediatric Surgery Department

- To keep the patient bed outside the anesthetic room during the operation special transfer areas or rooms of at least 16 sqm of size, adjacent the holding area have been suggested for transferring the patient from her bed to the operation table or operation table top or from a ward trolley to an operation room trolley.
- A considerable total transfer area is needed in a major surgical department, as each transfer may take 6–10 minutes.
- A technical refinement of the transfer room idea is the patient transfer hatchway between the holding area and the operation room suite area.

Procedure Area

Anesthetic room: In an anesthetic room, also called preparation or induction room the patient is transferred to the OT table.

The anesthetic table requires a space of 0.6 × 1.8 m. The dimensions 5 × 4 m can be recommended for an anesthetic room as they cover the needs of the majority of the anesthesiologists. All stimuli unpleasant to the patient should be eliminated. The anesthetic room should be both visually and acoustically well screened from the surgical department so that the patient is not in any way disturbed.

A temperature of not less than 23°C should be maintained.

For the sake of consistency of quality and intensity, artificial light has been considered more satisfactory.

Egress Room

Instead of using the anesthetic room for terminating anesthesia and for extubation the provision of an egress room with an area of 10–20 sqm has been suggested.

The egress rooms may increase the capacity of surgical departments by about 5%.

Scrubbing and Gowning Area

An area of about 3.0 sqm is required for donning a gown. A scrub-up and gowning area to serve one operation room equipped with three scrub-up places required about 10 sqm.

Operation Room Size

Mostly only about 1/3rd of the operation room space is planned for surgical intervention. The reminder is for support system. Activities around the operation table require 3 × 1.5 m. The circulation needs increase the required area to 4.25 × 2.65 m.

The minimum area of a contemporary operation room for pediatric/gynecological surgery, where standard aseptic techniques can be easily applied is 30 sqm. A suitable size for an operation room for most forms of surgery has been for some time in the region of 40–42 sqm.

A rectangular oblong operation room with rounded internal corners to ease the cleaning procedures meets most of the surgeons' needs.

The free ceiling, with/without a suspended ceiling, would preferably be 3.6 m high and not less than 3 m.

Maximum height for the operation room is about 3.6 m when the ceiling light is considered.

Auditory Effects

The reverberation time in operation rooms should be reduced to below 1 second.

Measured sound from ventilation systems should not exceed 35 dB in anesthetic rooms and 40 dB in operation rooms.

SUPPORT SERVICES

Blood Bank

The provisions of the *Drugs and Cosmetics Rules* (GoI) relevant to planning and designing of blood banks must be followed.

PHYSICAL MEDICINE AND REHABILITATION

Facilities and Space Requirements

- Reception-control room
- Waiting area
- Speech pathologist's and speech therapist's offices
- Audiologists' offices
- Sound treatment rooms
- Therapy room
- Storage room.

CENTRAL STERILIZATION AND SUPPLY DEPARTMENT

The parameters as applicable for a 500 bedded unit should be applicable. Ordinarily an area of 500 sqm (at 1 sqm per bed) would suffice.

LAUNDRY

The laundry should be a centralized facility which feed the center along with the other satellite centers of the main hospital.

DIETETICS DEPARTMENT[1]

Location

- A ground floor location is preferable, and is also convenient to deliver supplies as one in the basement should be difficult to maintain.
- The department should be close to the materials management department. The storage area should be close to the unloading dock.
- Easy access to vertical transportation system serving patient care units is important to facilitate delivery of patient meals and return of used trays and utensils.
- It can be a cafeteria conveniently located close to the OTs and the private ward.

Design

The design and layout of the dietetics department have a large role to play in the standard of food service, the preparation, the delivery and quality. The area are enumerated:

- Receiving area and control station
- Storage and refrigeration room(s)
- Preparation and production areas
- Serving room
- Special diet kitchen
- Dishwashing area
- Cafeteria.

Admission Office

Creation of an independent medical records department (MRD) for a center may lead to administrative difficulties. Therefore, it is proposed to centralize the MRD at the main hospital with an admission counter being an extension which is electronically linked so that e-records may be facilitated.

The front office of medical records—the registration together with the enquiry—is often the patient's first point of contact with the hospital.

ENGINEERING CONSIDERATIONS

Lighting: Light impacts biological function since it is related to the circadian rhythm, the important factors are:

- The illuminance needed for bedside medical and nursing tasks should not exceed 500 lux. A higher level is considered to be a stress factor.
- The contrast between illuminants and the ceiling should be minimal. Indirect lighting is preferred. For internal rooms, a two level lighting system should be employed: 400 lux during the day and 200 lux during the evening.

Lighting in Operation Theater

General lighting in operation room should attain a minimum of 400 lux. Illumination within the special field a disparity not greater than 10:1 should be permitted between the centrum and the periphery of the visual field.

Intensity: It would be realistic to require an intensity of about 40,000 lux at the plane of incision. The lamp should give an intensity of 8,000 lux at the bottom of an about 13 cm deep and 5 cm wide incision. The intensity at source must be 1.5 lakh lux

Luminance: The normal luminance brightness for the central field during an operation should be 2,000-3,000 cd/sqm. Within the central field of the view of the surgeon the relationship between the maximum and minimum brightness—the wound and the surrounding drapes—should be less than 2.5:1, the relation between maximum and minimum luminance should not exceed 1:10 within a base of a 60° cone.

Reflectance: It is the measure of light reflected from the surface of an object and expressed as a percentage of the light striking the surface.

Reflectance values: Recommended values are—ceiling reflectance 80%, wall reflectance 70%, surgical wound 9%, surgical drape 30%, light pastel colored wall 60%, retractors and instruments up to 90%, and white plaster 90%.

Operating Lamp Characteristics

- An illumination adjustable between 30,000 lux and 1,35,000 lux without any change of the spectral characteristics in the red is offered.
- The color temperature should be at least 5000 K.
- The color reproduction index should be RI-70. The heat radiation should be as small as possible.
- The maximum temperature of outer surfaces of luminaires should be less than 58°C to avoid injury to the hands of the surgeon or ancillary staff.
- The operation lamp should have no part hanging lower than 2.0 m above the floor.

ICU lighting: General illumination must be of adequate intensity—300 lux would suffice.

In neonatal intensive care units, the general lighting intensity 100 lux is usually adapted as well as the intensity of 500 lux at the incubators and 1,000 lux for some examinations.

Casualty lighting: High visual requirements in emergency departments warrant 600–1000 lux. Basic lighting level may be 400 lux of indirect lighting.

Radiodiagnostic facility: X-ray rooms lighting has to be indirect and not ceiling fixed. In the radiodiagnostic room, 400–500 lux is recommended. In the processing rooms, the illumination level ought to be 100 to 200 lux. These values are applicable at 1 m above floor level.

Laboratory lighting: With precision instruments, the illumination should be 1,000 lux and with regular instruments 500 to 600 lux. The level of illumination at work with microscopes is about 3,000 lux.

Tungsten lighting has been recommended for radioactive counting rooms.

Heating, Ventilating and Air-conditioning Systems

To maintain oxygenation for ten persons in the operation room, a volume of about 28 m^3 of air will be required per hour. This means that less than one-tenth of the air volume in a regular operation room—sized 6.2 × 6.2 × 3.2 m—has to be replaced every hour.

Fifteen to twenty air changes an hour is required in an operation room of the size of about 40 sqm if an average surgical team is involved.

The use of filters would hinder the outside pathogenic particles over the 1 μm range to enter the operation room.

Ventilation in patient care areas: It is advisable for the benefit of comfort to limit the air velocity to 0.15 m/s. It is probably desirable that the ICU has 15–20 air changes per hour.

Recirculation of air: At least partial recirculation may be permitted in all areas desirable in fresh air.

Isolation rooms: These rooms would be protected with HEPA filters at 99.97% efficiency for a 0.3 μm sized particle in the supply airstream.

Air-conditioning system: Operating rooms, labor-delivery suites, ICUs, nurseries and sophisticated medical equipment are sensitive to temperature and humidity

Hospital air-conditioning should be more attuned to patient and patient treatment rather than comfort. They need cooled and dehumidified air that requires dry bulb temperature of 20°C ± 1°C and RH 50 ± 5%.

- All the return air to be through duct only.

Operating rooms: Some of the design parameters considered for the operating rooms are:

- Temperature range should be between 23°C and 24°C.
- Positive pressure to be maintained with respect to adjacent areas.
- Air turbulence in the room should be reduced by supplying air at velocity of not more than 200–250 ft per min (fpm) near the operating table. Low level exhaust air pick-up points should be placed at peripheral walls for a scavenging effect.
- Ducting material should be aluminum. Care must be taken during duct fabrication, and joints must be properly sealed to avoid collection of dust particles and growth of bacteria.
- "Laminar flow" is preferred in the OTs.
- Twenty to thirty air changes in the OTs reduce the incidence of contamination.
- There should be horizontal and vertical separation in fresh intake and exhaust of ORs.
- It is recommended that individual air handling systems be provided for each operating room along with its changing rooms.
- The relative humidity should be maintained at 55 ± 5%.

Labor delivery suites: Unlike surgery, the labor-delivery suites operate on a 24-hour schedule. These suites are air-conditioned at the same temperature as the operating rooms, usually 23°C.

Protection of heating, ventilating and air-conditioning systems against chemical, biological, and radiological attack should be considered.

Noncentral air-handling systems (i.e. individual room units used for heating and cooling purposes, such as fan-coil units) should be used as recirculating units only. All outdoor air requirements should be met by a separate central air-handling system with proper filtration.

Water and steam supplies: The general estimate of water supply needs is about 400–650 liters per day and bed. Hospitals require a two temperature range for hot water. Low temperature; about 43.5°C is required patient washroom. Higher temperatures between 71°C and 90°C account for the majority of hospital requirements for hot water including physiotherapy, kitchen and cafeteria requirements. The temperature of hot water supplied to the clinical departments would be 40°C and 44°C.

Electrical installations: All electrical power should be connected to an isolation transformer. The power outlets in various area are:

- Operation room—20 outlets. It is preferred to have the control panel hanging from the ceiling.
- Anesthetic room—6 electrical outlets.
- General postanesthetic units—8 electrical points per bed.
- ICUs—10 electrical points per bed.
- Neonatal ICUs—10 to 12 electrical outlets per bed.
- Corridors electrical outlets with protective ground would be spaced at 10–12 m intervals.

Signages, identification signs: Signage along with architectural features like skylights, atriums, ceremonial stairs, and sufficient reinforcement form wayfinding. Wayfinding also includes, in main arterial corridors, easily understood signs and numbers coordinated with lighting and interior finishes.

PHYSICAL ENVIRONMENT

Color

Operation room walls and ceilings: With high level of illumination warm colors such as yellow, orange, and pink, the body tends to increase its activation in general. With softer surroundings, lower brightness and color hues such as gray, blue, green and turquoise, there is less distraction, and good inward orientation is furthered.

FLOOR PLANS

Floor plans are depicted in Figures 12 to 15.

CONCLUSION

There is a need of creating an independent woman and child center as there is an overarching need to address the health concerns of two special section of patient clientele together. Contemporary evidence-based designing, therapeutic healing and state-of-the-art technology must be amalgamated to give the hospital a less clinical look.

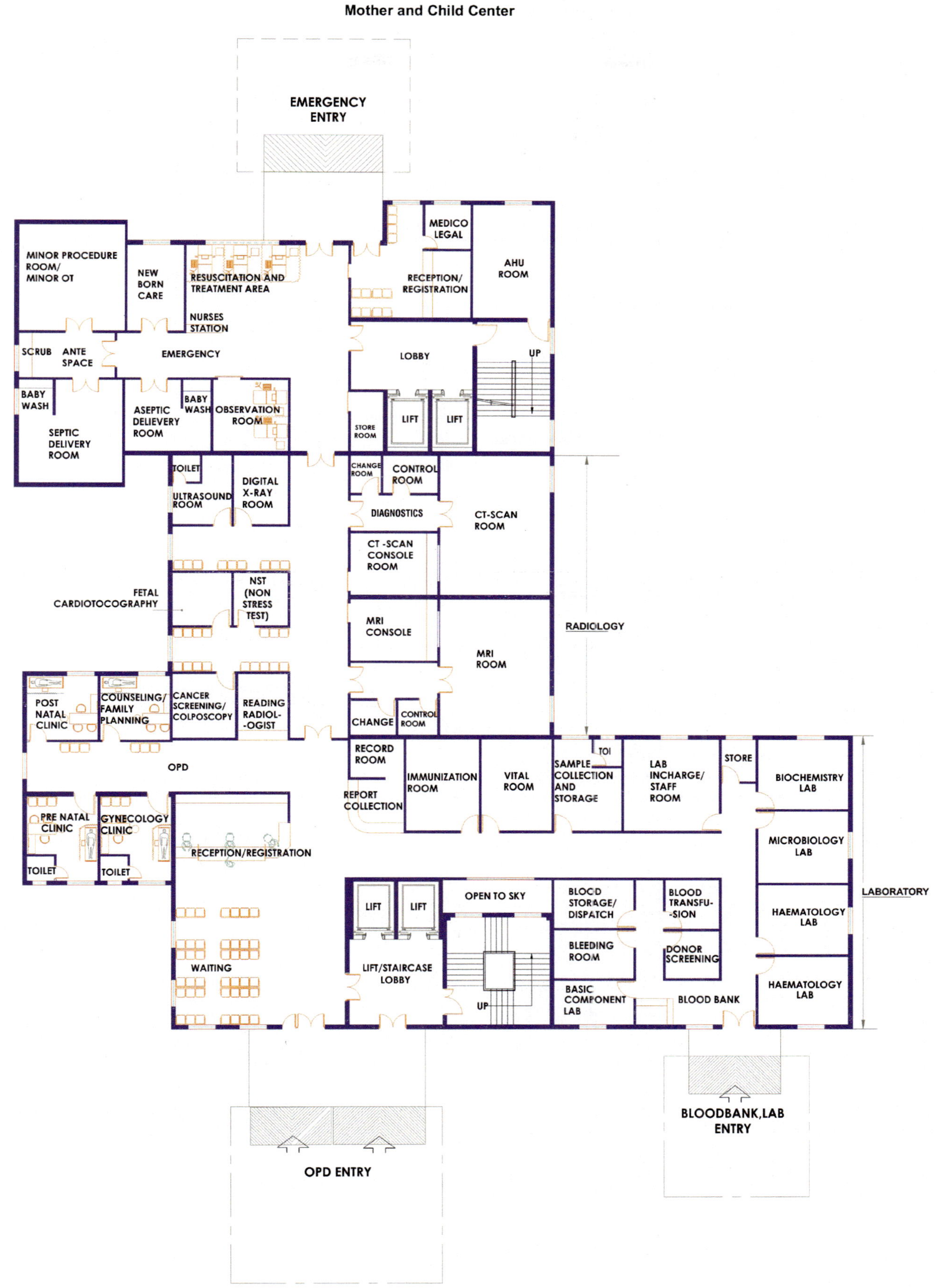

Fig. 12: Ground floor plan.

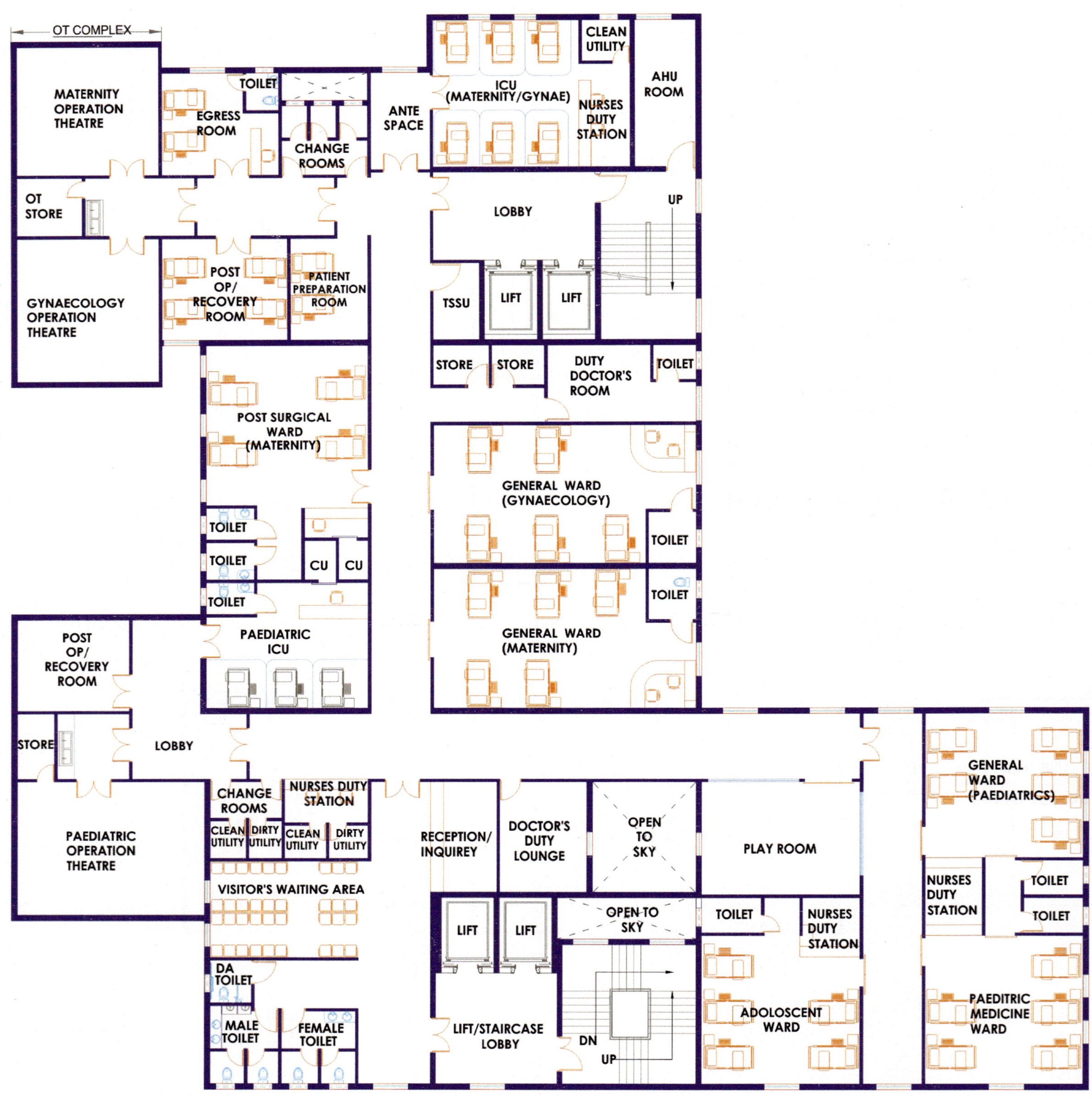

Fig. 13: First floor plan.
(DA: differently abled)

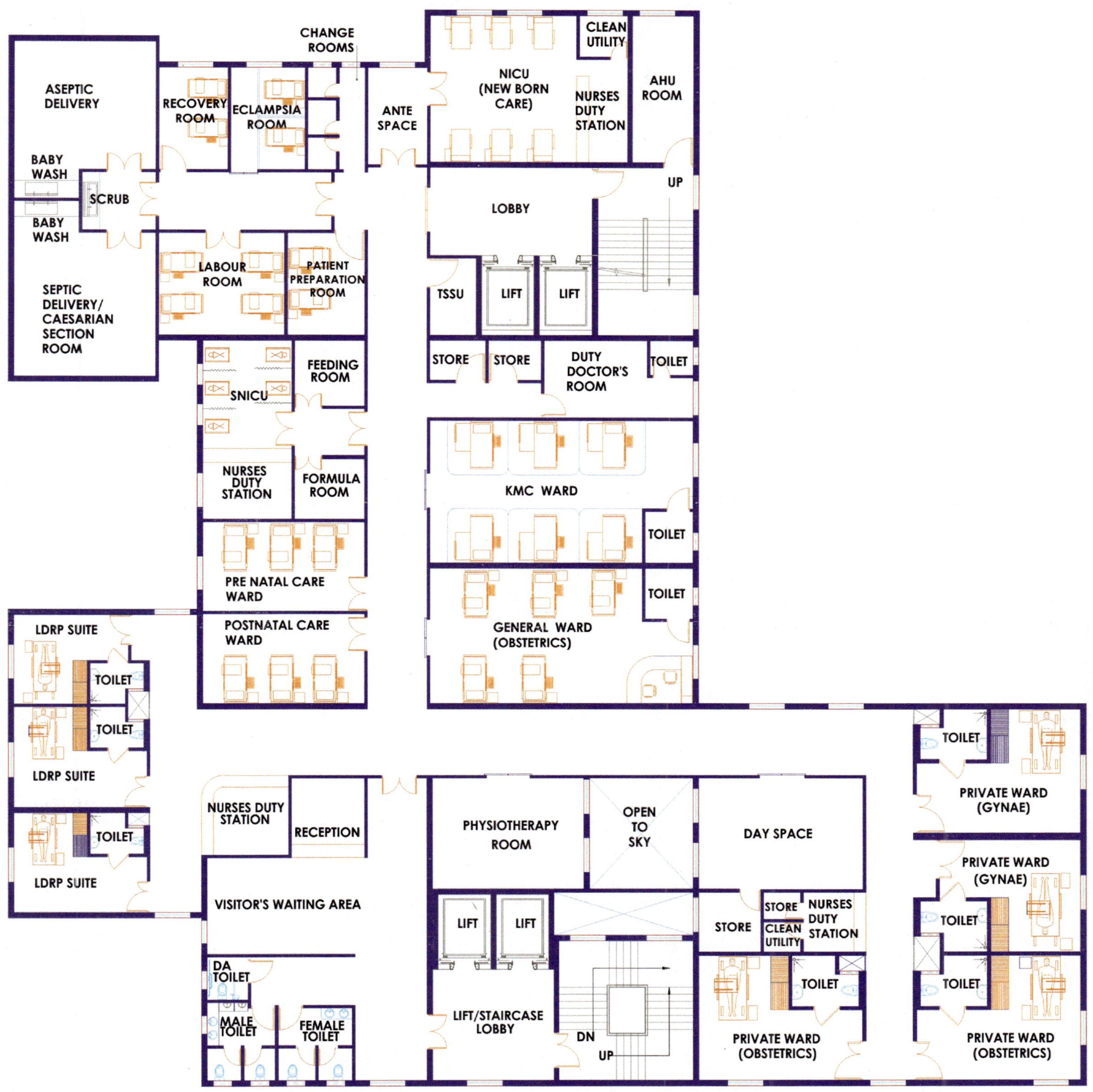

Fig. 14: Second floor plan.
(DA: differently abled)

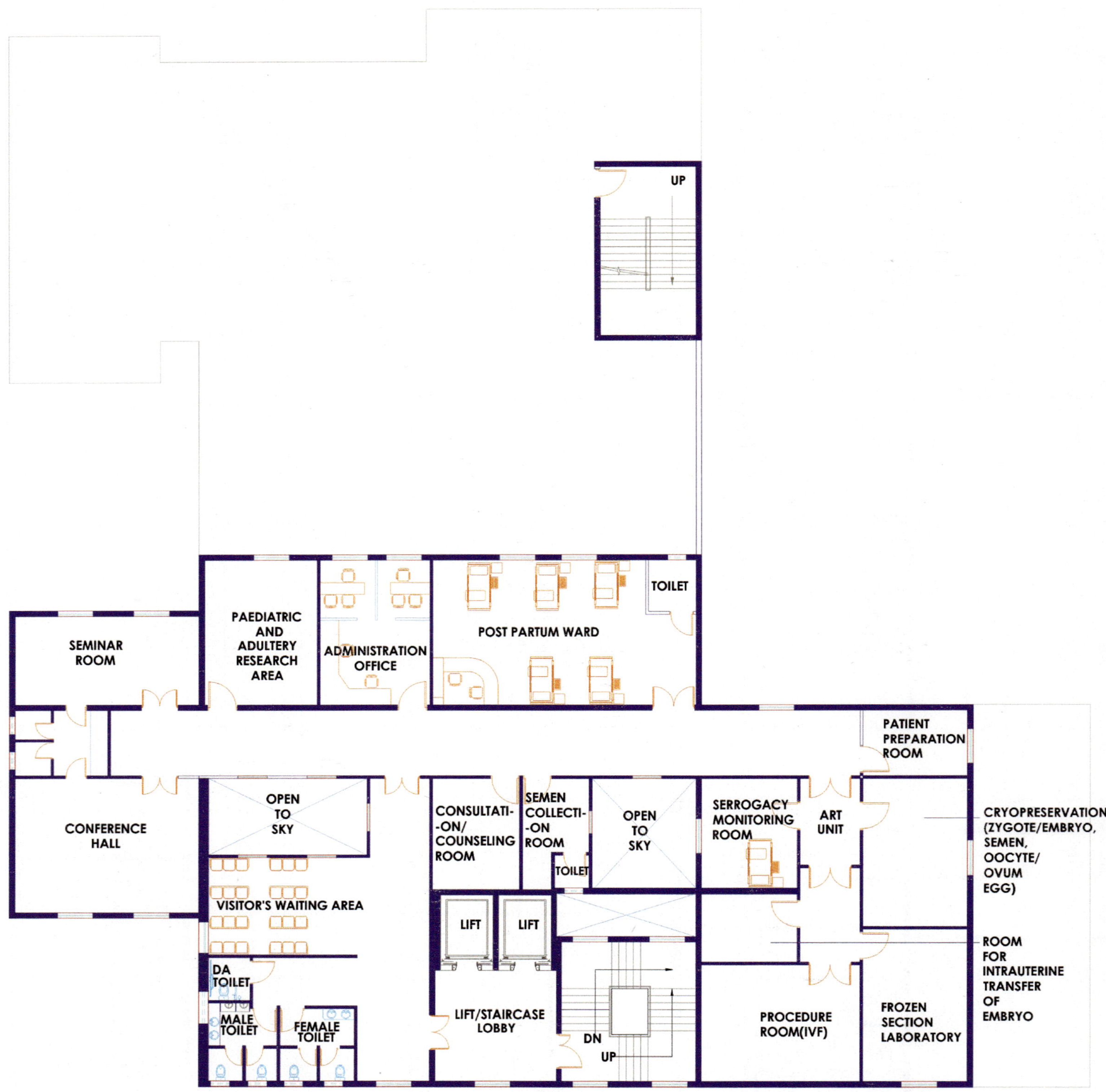

Fig. 15: Third floor plan.
(DA: differently abled)

The challenge, despite constraints, should also be to integrate interdependent functional areas so that the idiom-design follows function, is validated.

REFERENCES

1. Ervin P. nternational Planning Practices, 1st edition. London: Lloyd-luke Ltd; 1979.
2. www.medvarsity.com
3. www.cedengineering.com
4. www.kwa.kerala.gov.in

OTHER REFERENCES

- Gupta SK, Kant S, Chandrashekhar R, et al. Modern trends in planning and designing of hospitals. Delhi: Jaypee Brothers Medical Publishers Pvt. Ltd; 2007.
- Kunders GD. Facilities Planning and Management, 2nd edition. Delhi: Tata McGraw-Hill Publishing Company Limited; 2009.
- Jain M. A Visual Reference for Evidence-based Design. California: Center for Health Design; 2008.
- MacEachern Malcom T. Hospital organisation and Management. Chicago: Physicians' Record Company; 1957.
- McGibony JR. Principles of Hospital administration. New York: GP Putnam's Sons; 1969.
- Aldis Guy. Hospital Planning and Requirement. London: Sir Isaac Pitman & Sons; 1957.
- Malkin Jain. Medical and dental space planning: a comprehensive guide to design, equipment and clinical procedures, 3rd edition. New York: John Wiley and Sons; 2002.
- Facilities guidelines Institute. Guidelines for Design and Construction of Health Care facilities. New York American Institute of Architecture; 2006.
- Natalie Z, Amy K. The Pebble report: a pebble payoff. Healthcare design. 2009;9(11):20-23.
- http://www.publichealth.va.gov/womenshealth/ .
- Veterans health administration: childcare/development center *www.cfm.va.gov/til/space/SPchapter420.doc.*
- icmr.nic.in.
- www.fgiguide ines.org.
- Ascher BH. "Maternal Anxiety in Pregnancy and Fetal Homeostasis", Journal of Obstetric Gynecologic & Neonatal Nursing, 5/1978

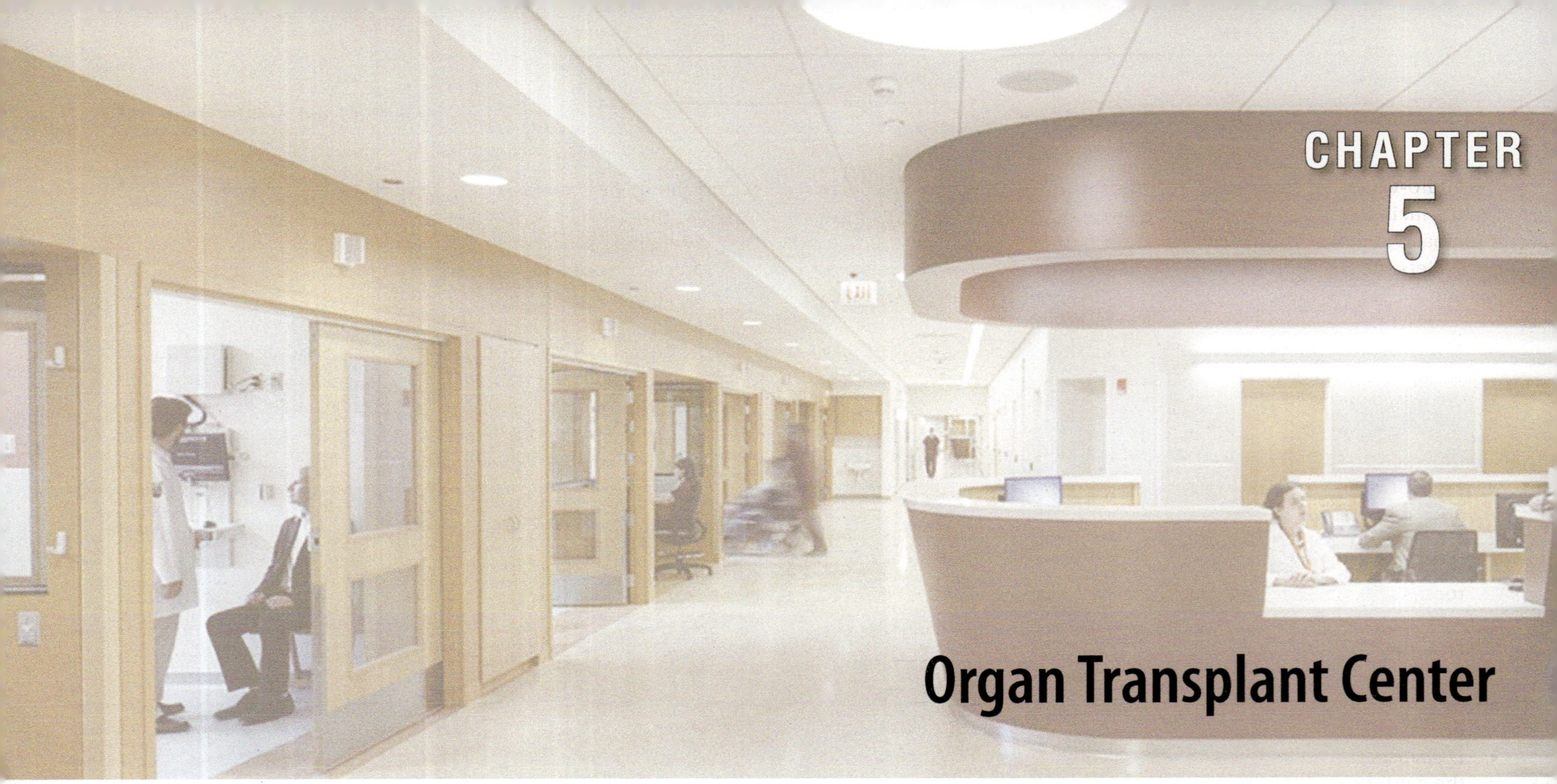

CHAPTER 5

Organ Transplant Center

Diwakar Thimmappa, Sandeep Guleria, Aarti Vij, Shakti Kumar Gupta, Sunil Kant, R Chandrashekhar

INTRODUCTION

Organ transplant is a surgical operation in which the surgeon places an organ from another person into a recipient's body. The transplanted organ does the functions of failed organs. The transplants may come from cadaveric organ, i.e. from people who have recently died and whose organs have been donated for transplantation or living (related/nonrelated) organ, i.e. from family members/spouses, etc., who are living and donate one part of the organs. The organ transplant in India is to be done as per directives of the Organ Transplantation Act. The first heart transplant in India was done at AIIMS, New Delhi, India in 1994 by Professor P Venugopal and his team and the first lung transplant at Madras Medical Mission Hospital, Chennai, Tamil Nadu, India. Non-availability of organs is a major issue in India.[1]

DESIGN AND PLANNING CONSIDERATIONS

The transplant center should be designed according to the modern standards, including wide doors, spacious rooms, bright surroundings, underground parking, and designated areas for nursing care instead of nursing stations. The outpatient transplant clinic should be close to other outpatient clinics and physicians' offices. Comfortable, affordable accommodations should be available for follow-up care and for patients from out of town. In some cases, patients will need to stay in these facilities for a considerable time.[2-5]

OUTPATIENT UNIT

Functional Areas

The functional relationship of OPD to other areas/departments are shown in Figure 1. The recommended area are:

- *Entrance*: There should be an entrance, which is entry to the hospital, drop off and collection area, patient reception, patient and an attendant enquires. In addition, door with width of 1500 mm and the floor should be nonslippery. Vehicle access is required at all times and the facility should be suitable for people with disabilities.
- *Reception*: The reception counter should be provided which may also function as registration/appointment counter. It should be well ventilated, lighted (general illumination 300 lux) and adequately furnished with furniture.
- *Waiting area*: There should be waiting area for visitors and patients to wait in comfort prior to or during visits to center. A waiting area may be for the use of the public, patients, families and other visitors to the center. The waiting area should be planned to accommodate more than the number of people expected during peak hours. Sub-waiting area may be shared between the various consultation rooms. To facilitate movement of patients, an audiovisual system should be provided, which directs the patient to appropriate consultation room and also can be utilized for education of the patients/relatives of the procedures and also the organ donation programs of the center. The

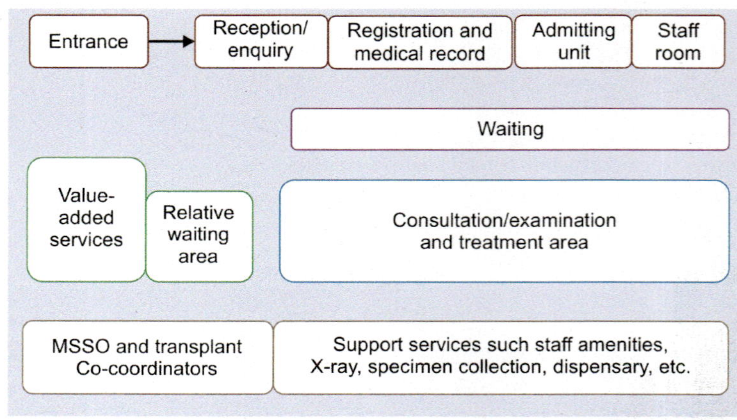

Fig. 1: Functional relationship of outpatient department.
(MSSO: medical social service officer)

audio-visual aid can also utilized to depict the patients' rights and the facilities available in the center. The distance from the waiting area to the consultation room should be short and clearly marked. Toilets should be close to the waiting area. Male and female toilets should be separate. Waiting areas must be 0.1 sqm per patient and sub-waiting areas to be 0.8 sqm per patient.[6]

- *Consultation room*: A room of about 15 sqm is adequate for a consultation as well as examination. This also includes space for examination tables, a washbasin, instrument trolley, an X-ray viewing screen, desk and chair for doctor as well as two chairs for patients/attendants. The lighting should be about 500 lux.
- *Board room:* A multipurpose room for staff meetings, training or educational purposes, of approximate dimension 20 sqm is adequate. The board room should be located in a low traffic area. A room minimum of 15 sqm should be located with OPD consultation rooms, which may be used as treatment room with adequate lighting and furniture.
- *Specimen collection*: A specimen collection point that is the extension of laboratory services should be provided.
- *Staff amenities*: Adequate staff amenities with toilet facilities should be provided.
- *Dispensary*: A well-stocked dispensary with medicines related to the center should be made available 24 × 7.
- *Allied services*: The OPD may have allied services such as X-ray, laboratory, medical social service officer (MSSO), transplant coordinators, social guides, etc.
- *Value added services* like books shop, telephone facility, air booking, ATM, cafeteria, etc. may be provided.

Intensive Care Unit

Functional Areas

- *Reception*: The reception in the ICU (Fig. 2) acts as enquiry office, clerical office as well as center for coordination. It is to be provided with means of communication and separate work force for staffing it on 24 × 7 basis. Attached with the ICU is a waiting area where the attendants of critically-ill patients can stay. It should be provided with collapsible beds chairs and basic amenities of water, toilets and a television. The waiting area is important, as the attendants cannot be with the patient in the ICU. In India usually one attendant is permitted with each patient, therefore the waiting area should have appropriate space.

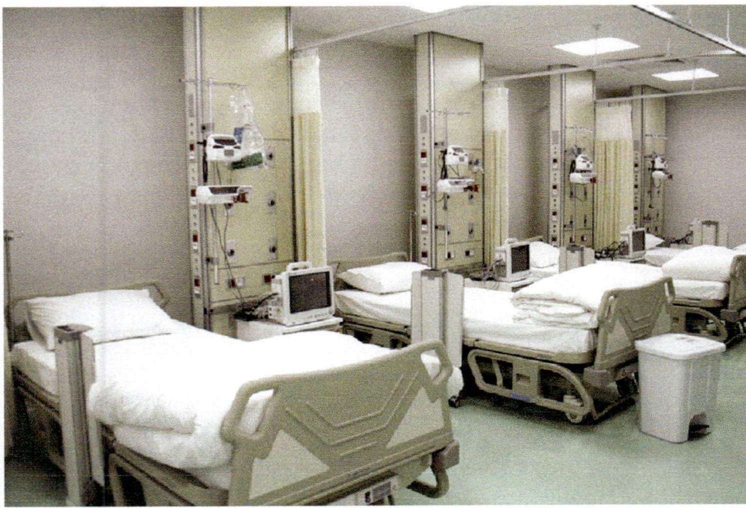

Fig. 2: Intensive care unit.

- *The patient care area*: Each bed should have adequate circulation space for 360° access to the patient. Space between the beds to be wide enough to accommodate large size trolleys typically required for dressing and movements for equipment such as X-ray. Each bed should be clearly visible from the doctors/nurses' duty station. Each bed should have dedicated equipment such as monitors, ventilators, etc. with manifold outlets and brackets for positioning monitoring equipment. Distress call system should be installed on every bed. At least 15 sqm floor area for single bed accommodation exclusive of service areas. At least 24 sqm floor area for multiple bed accommodation. The beds can be segregated for donor and recipients. A few beds should be earmarked for brain dead patients who are potential donors.[5,6]
- *Nursing station* in the patient area is to be on a raised platform for unhindered visibility. A common station for doctors and nurses should be made with separate tables for both. The station must have spaces for central monitoring system, clinical records, storage for frequently used medicines, consumables, equipment and an attached treatment bay. This bay is for housing various trolleys and resuscitation equipment. Monitoring equipment of each ICU bed should be independent in terms of equipment such as ventilator, cardiac monitor, medical gases, BP apparatus, etc.
- *Electrical panels*: Each bed should have at least 8 electrical points (Ventilator—1, two infusion pumps—3, multisign monitor—1, defibrillator—1, reserve—2). All the points in the panel must have 100% power backup, however at least 4 points should be power backed up, i.e. always powered. The points should be composite type, i.e. should be able to take both 5 amp and 15 amp plugs. If all points do not have power backup then the backed up points should be colored differently so that they are easily identifiable. All the plug points must be properly earthed.
- *Bed-head panel*: It should comprise of outlets viz. Two oxygen outlets, two vacuum outlets, one compressed air at 4 bars, one reading light, eight multipin 15 amps, switch socket outlet combine (four to be backed up), one arm lamp 60 W with adapter holder for vacuum collection jar, one infusion pump rail mount pole with adapter, two spare spaces, one nurse call switch (with remote).
- *Allied and support services* including utility rooms, store rooms, linen, disposal room, cleaner's room, pantry, staff amenities areas. These should be out of traffic paths but conveniently located outside the patient care area and should have independent access.
- *Equipment room*: Mobile equipment and mobile X-ray units that are located within the ICU require storage areas that are out of traffic paths but conveniently located for easy access by staff. Consideration should be given to the ever-increasing number of equipment used.[5,6]
- *Communications*: The ICU should have communications facilities for communication with hospital staff, lab, blood bank and other key hospital departments. In addition to a standard telephone service, there should be a mechanism for emergency internal and external communications when normal systems fail such as mobile/paging. Plasma screen and telecom in waiting areas linked up with ICU, so that entry to ICU is restricted and relatives can see their patients in waiting area, which not only prevents infection it also prevents overcrowding and security problems of the area.
- *Lighting*: The requirement is to have 300 lux light illumination in patient care areas. The patient care areas should be uniformly lit especially near the floor for easy monitoring of drainage seal and suction equipment. Windows are an important aspect of sensory orientation to reinforce day/night orientation. Natural lighting

Table 1: HVAC requirements in ICU.

Place	Patient area	Treatment room	Pantry	Corridor	Disposal room
Air pressure	Positive	Positive	Negative	Negative	Negative
Air changes per hour	8–10	10–12	10	6	10
Relative humidity (%)	45 ± 5	45 ± 5	45 ± 5	45 ± 5	45 ± 5
Temperature °C	22 ± 2	22 ± 2	22 ± 2	22 ± 2	22 ± 2

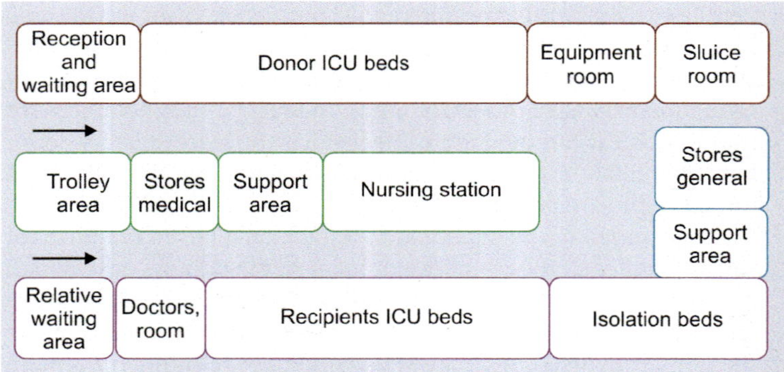

Fig. 3: Functional relationship of ICU.

should be provided in abundance. Drapes or shades of fireproof fabric can make attractive window coverings and absorb sound. If windows cannot be provided in each room, an alternate option is to allow a remote view of an outside window or skylight. The color shades of the walls and ceiling should not affect perception of skin color. Adequate and appropriate lighting about 200 lux for corridors and 500 lux for clinical observation.

- *Hand wash facilities*: Hand washing facilities should be provided convenient to the staff station and patient bed areas. A minimum of one hand wash unit per two beds is required though one such unit per bed is preferable. Along with this there must also be alcohol-based hand rub disinfectants placed near each bed and in the areas easily accessible by the staff and attendants.[8]
- *Circulation space*: When an open plan arrangement is provided, a circulation space of 2.4 sqm minimum clear widths should be provided beyond dedicated cubicle space. Separate cubicles and isolation rooms should be minimum 3.9 sqm. All doors and openings should be minimum 2 m wide to permit transit of heavy equipment, patient beds and trolleys. These should permit hassle-free movement and easy maneuverability.
- *HVAC*: The air-conditioning requirements recommended for ICU are depicted in Table 1.
- The functional relationship of ICU is shown in Figure 3.

OPERATION THEATER (FIG. 4)[6-11]

The operating unit provides a controlled climatic environment for the operative and postoperative care of patients undergoing organ transplant and retrieval procedures under anesthesia. The number of operating rooms and recovery beds and the sizes of the service areas should be based on the expected surgical workload. In the brief, the size, location, and configuration of the surgical suite and support service departments should reflect the projected volume of patients.[6,7]

Distribution of Operating Rooms

For a standalone center multiple operation rooms are required viz.

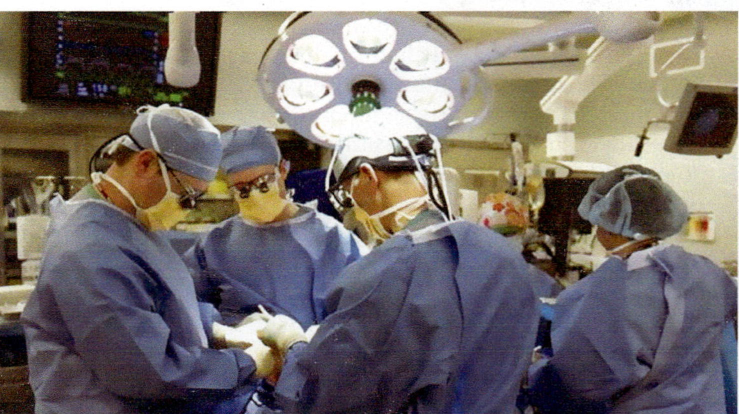

Fig. 4: Operation theater.

1—Organ retrieval, 1—Heart transplant, 2—Liver transplant, 4—Kidney transplant, 2—Cadaver, 2—Liver, 1—Bone marrow transplant, 1—Stem cell facility, 1—Infectious OT (Septic OT).

However, if the center is part of a multispecialty/tertiary care hospital than it should share the operation theater facility of that hospital, then there should be at least 2 operating suites for 20 beds dedicated for only organ transplant procedures.

Functional Areas

Planning Parameters

An operating unit design with a sterile core should provide for no cross traffic of staff and supplies from the decontaminated/soiled areas to the sterile/clean areas. The use of facilities outside the operating room for soiled decontaminated processing and clean assembly and sterile processing should be designed to move the flow of goods and personnel without compromising universal precautions or aseptic techniques in both departments. The operating unit should be located and arranged to prevent nonrelated traffic through the suite.

Operating Suite (Fig. 5)

Preference of modular theater for procedures area which consists of prefabricated units for operating suites complete with integrated mechanical and electrical service including air-conditioning should be utilized. In addition, the operating room should integrate with the telemedicine department of the center.

- It should be a prefabricated joint less operation theater with all structural steel.
- The floor should be of the type that does not promote bacteriological growth and the finish should be 2 mm static conductive PVC tiles, laid on a semiconductive adhesive base. The floor finish should be smooth, nonslip impervious material, seamless, welded and washable and terminate at the room perimeter passing over a concealed cover and continuing up the wall for 100 mm. The doors of the OT should be 2100 mm height and 1500 mm width for patient

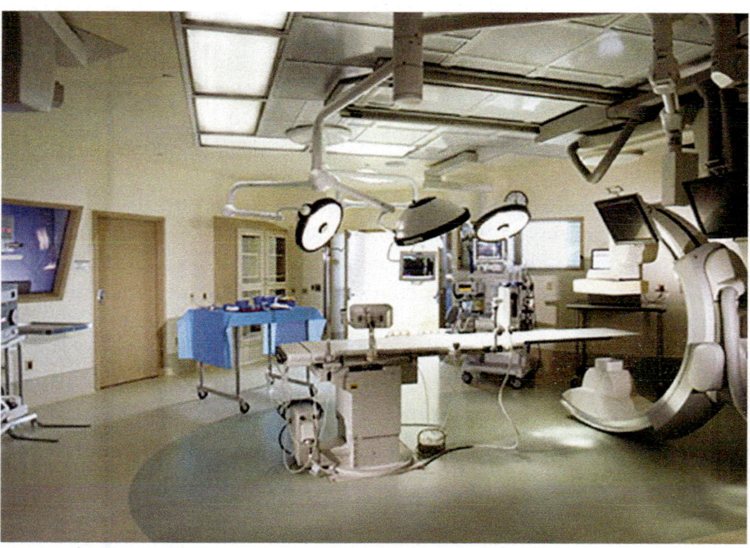

Fig. 5: Operating suite.

entry, and 2100 mm height and 1000 mm width where staffs enter. The doors should be of sliding type; it should slide within tracks with nylon wheels and fitted with proper vision panels. All doors should be hermetically sealed to maintain sterility, correct air pressure and the edges should get sealed in closed position. All doors should be able to be operated manually in the event of power failure.

- The ceiling smooth, impervious, soundproof and seamless, height should be 3.0 m. The ceiling should provide optimum air distribution over the patient area, integrated with shadow less lighting. The ceiling should be constructed with a plenum box supplied with central air-conditioning system via "S" class 8 Nos. High efficiency particulate air (HEPA) filters mounted on the exit from the supply ducting. It should include integral lighting and composite air/light diffuser. The laminar flow ceiling should have illumination across its total area.[8]
- The lighting should be evenly distributed throughout the room. General illumination is furnished by ceiling lights. To minimize eye fatigue, the ratio of intensity of general room lighting to that at the surgical site should not exceed 1:5, preferably 1:3. It should be sufficient to provide an illumination level of 1500 lux (with 40 illumination lights) at the wound site and should be dimmable down to 3% of full lighting, without flicker. It is a combination of one major and one satellite light-head with intensity of about 1,10,000 for major and 1,00,000 for satellite lighthead with an individual intensity control arrangements for each lightheads. The color temperature is 3300 K and color rendering index is 95 Ra. Shadow reduction is to be achieved by prismatic optical system.[8]
- *The panels*: All controls within the theater should be located on a membrane control panel mounted in the theater wall. It should consist of time elapse clock, standard clock, temperature and humidity indicators, temperature and humidity set points adjust, plenum lighting controls, medical gas alarms.
- *Medical gases*: Main storage of medical gases should be outside the facility and reticulated internally to gas outlets. Provision should be made for additional separate storage of reserve gas cylinders necessary to complete at least one-day's procedures.
- *Others*: These include the equipment storage unit, pressure stabilizer and surgical scrub system.

Reception Area

Its function is to receive patients to the unit, with general overseeing of day-to-day operations, control of entry and exit from the unit and completion of general administrative tasks.

Holding Areas

Holding areas for holding and management of patients prior to donation and transplant and should facilitate the movement of both stretchers as well as ambulatory patients not requiring stretchers. This area should be located away from the operation theater complex and preferably it can be located in the ward floor area. The area should be 7.5 sqm and should have a clearance of 1.22 m which can hold a trolley/bed for the patient.

Patient Transfer Area

The patient from the holding area should be under direct supervision of the staff and who can be kept ready for transfer on request from the reception of the operating theater. There should be an earmarked route for transfer of patient from holding area and the operating theater and this can also be used for transfer of patients from different area of the hospital and operating room. It will be convenient to have a separate route/corridor for transfer of patients from all areas of the hospital to operating theater. This will not only reduce the infection, but also will be easy to segregate the unnecessary traffic movements towards OT.

Anesthesia Workroom

An anesthesia workroom may be provided for cleaning, testing and storing of anesthesia equipment. It should be located with direct access to circulation corridors and ready access to the operating rooms. The anesthetic workroom should contain workbenches, sink/s and racks for cylinders. Provisions should be made for separate storage of clean and soiled items. The room will require sufficient power and data outlets and a medical gas panel for testing of equipment. A clinical hand washing basin should be provided within the room. The area should be 15 sqm per operating suite and should have a clearance of 1.22 m.

Storage (Fig. 6)

Adequate equipment store room/s for equipment and supplies used in the operating unit should be provided. Equipment stores should be provided at the minimum rate of 10 sqm per operating room. Store rooms are best designed in an elongated rectangular to allow easy access to all items. Storage bays should be provided for equipment such as portable X-ray equipment, stretchers, warming devices and auxiliary lamps. Storage bays should be provided at the minimum rate of 5 sqm

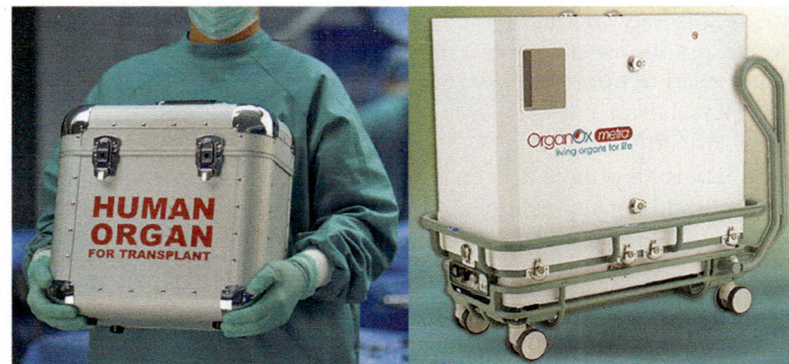

Fig. 6: Storage.

per operating room and minimum dimension of 0.8 m (1 m preferred). These areas should be out of corridors and traffic. This can be satisfied by recessing the bay the corridor width. Adequate storage facility must be provided in the theater in the form of adjustable open shelving systems.

Equipment Room

An area for testing operating equipment also requires consideration in the planning stage of an operating unit to determine on-site facility needs. Part of the operating unit general store may be used for this function, or a dedicated room for this purpose may be necessary.

Recovery Areas

Areas where patients are assisted through the process of recovering from the effects of anesthetic should have medication station, hand washing station, nurse station, storage space for stretchers, supplies and equipment. The area should be 7.5 sqm and should have a clearance of 1.22 m to accommodate a trolley/bed. Administrative and staff areas including change rooms, staff room, offices and administrative space for clinical staff should also be present.[5]

Change Rooms

Appropriate change rooms should be provided for male and female personnel (nurse, doctors and technicians) working within the operating unit. The change rooms should contain adequate lockers, showers, toilets, hand basins and space for donning surgical attire and booting. These staff change rooms should be arranged to encourage a one-way traffic pattern so that personnel entering from outside the surgical suite can change and move directly into the operating unit. Alternatively, the entrance to the change rooms may be planned in direct view of a staff station at the entrance to the operating unit and the entry must be from nonsterile area with proper infection control measures. The change room entrance door should be provided with locks or electronic access devices to prevent the entry of unauthorized persons into the operating unit.

Coffee Room/Lounge

Coffee room/lounge should be provided within the unit for staff to relax and prepare beverages. Inclusion of a window to the outside is desirable. Staff room may be made separately for various categories of staff like doctors, nurses, paramedical staff, etc. the air-conditioning of this area must be segregated by proper compartmentalization and connected to exhaust system.

Sterilizing Facilities

Sterilizing facilities with high-speed sterilizers or other sterilizing equipment for immediate or emergency use must be grouped to several operating rooms for convenient, efficient use. A workspace and hand-washing facility should be included. The facilities for processing and sterilizing reusable instruments may be located in another area of hospital unit such as Central Sterilizing Supply Department (CSSD).

Infection Control

A room must be provided for an infection control nurse with appropriate furniture and also for taking samples for testing. A clinical hand washing basin should be provided within the room. The room must be of 9 sqm.

Preparation/Lay-up Room

This room in the operating unit where clean or sterile materials are held and arranged prior to use in the operating rooms.

The main functions for which facilities should be provided are:

- Flash sterilization
- Storage of instruments and materials
- Holding of sterile supplies and packs
- Storage of lotions in a special purpose warming cabinet
- Preparation of dressing and instrument trolleys
- A clean room, with direct access to the operating room may be provided. Sharing of one clean room between two or more operating rooms is acceptable provided layout and size of the room facilitates such sharing. If provided, clean room should be a minimum of 20 sqm.

Clean Utility Room

The clean utility is for the storage and preparation of clean and sterile consumables and equipment for operations, secure storage and preparation of medications, including intravenous fluids. It also functions as an alternative storage area for the medication trolley. The room may also provide storage for dangerous drugs. The clean utility should be a minimum of 12 sqm or 14 sqm when access is required from two sides of the room. The clean utility is to have direct access from the unit corridor, with close proximity to the staff station and ready access to patient areas. Doors to the clean utility should be lockable.

Dirty Utility Room

The dirty utility room may be combined with a disposal room for space efficiency. The dirty utility should be a minimum of 10 sqm or 12 sqm when access is required from two sides of the room. If combined with disposal room, the combined dirty utility/disposal should be minimum of 14 sqm. The dirty utility positioned centrally to allow for ready access from the operating suite and have easy access to hand washing facilities. The dirty utility should have direct access to the unit corridor and close proximity to the clean utility.

Equipment and Special Fluids

Since the center is being a surgical oriented, all the operation theaters should be fully equipped with basic equipment such as anesthetic machines, cell shaver, rapid infusers, diathermy, cardiopulmonary bypass machine, venovenous bypass machine, central line Hickman catheters, cell separator, irradiators, flow cytometry, ABG machine with lactate test, thromboelastic graph, AR gun, C-arm, intraoperative USG machine, Doppler, cardiac output monitor, patient warming devices, intermittent pneumatic calf compression, ice maker machine, refrigerator, defreezers, and special perfusion/preservative fluids such as renogram for kidney transplant and histidine histidine-tryptophan-ketoglutarate (HTK) for liver transplant. An ice machine and cold storage facilities should be provided to provide storage, transportation of organs, for treatments and patient use. These equipment must be provided with a room of 20 sqm with good lighting and storage shelves should be retrieved easily as whenever required.

Operating Table

The OT table should be an electrohydraulic, operated on high storage capacity batteries and also must work on 220/240V AC single-phase power supply, it must be disinfectant resistant, radiolucent table top, with no crevices for ingress of liquids so as to enable proper infection control.

The air-conditioning is required for operation theater is depicted in Table 2.

Table 2: HVAC operating theater.

Place	Operating suite	Preparation room	Recovery room	Corridor	Disposal room	TSSU
Air pressure	Positive	Positive	Positive	Negative	Negative	Negative
Air changes per hour	20	15	6–8	6	10	10
Relative humidity (%)	45 ± 5	45 ± 5	45 ± 5	45 ± 5	45 ± 5	45 ± 5
Temperature °C	22 ± 2	22 ± 2	22 ± 2	22 ± 2	22 ± 2	22 ± 2

Note: The operating suite must be fitted with high efficiency particulate air (HEPA) filters and minimum 50% of air exhausted outdoors, facility of heat recovery wheel for energy parameter.

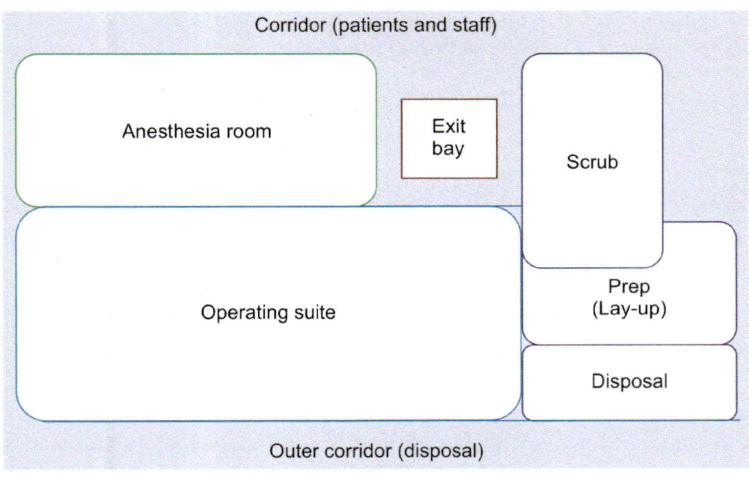

Fig. 7: Functional relationship of an operating suite.

Functional Relationship of an Operating Suit

These are depicted in Figure 7.

Functional Relationship of Operation Theater

These are depicted in Figure 8.

Inpatient Unit (Ward)

The inpatient accommodation unit is for all types of organ transplants pre- and post-transplant patients. Patients awaiting placement elsewhere may also be accommodated in this type of facility. The prime function of the inpatient unit is to provide appropriate accommodation for the delivery of healthcare services including diagnosis, care and treatment to inpatients. The unit should also provide facilities and conditions to meet the needs of patients and visitors as well as the workplace requirements of staff.[5,6]

FUNCTIONAL AREAS

Bed Complement

A transplant center wherein patients are prone for post-transplant infections maximum bed complement should be provided as single bedrooms.

Isolation Rooms

All transplanted patients such as renal, cardiac, liver, bone marrow, etc. require staying in isolation postoperatively. In addition, the patients undergoing liver and bone marrow transplant stay for longer duration. Minimum space requirement of a single bed isolation room is 15 sqm. The isolation rooms must have attached toilets, washbasin and a self-closing door. All the isolation rooms must have nurse call bell, medical gas connections and dedicated equipment such as cardiac monitors, ventilators, infusion pumps, etc. The rooms must be connected with air-conditioning system, with negative air pressure, HEPA filters with minimum 12 air changes/hour and temperature of 24°C. In addition, no air is circulated back into the room from other areas. All the air-conditioned area of the ward must have air-condition duct connected with exhaust system and a dampener to control and regulate the air to be exhausted during the removal of foul air.

Wards

The inpatient ward unit may consist of two-bed rooms with minimum space of 25 sqm with one toilet and bath facility where it may be used for recovery stage of transplanted and donor patients. In addition, these rooms can be used for patients waiting for transplant and patients with post-transplant complications. The facilities in the room may include medical gases and basic equipment such as BP apparatus, infusion pumps, etc. The rooms should be provided with furniture for patient attendants. The inpatient ward unit may consist of 4–6 bedrooms with common toilet facilities and other supportive services. There should be a clearance of 1200 mm available at the foot of each bed to allow for easy movement of equipment and beds. In multiple-bed rooms, the minimum distance between bed center lines should be 2400 mm. Visual privacy from casual observation by other patients and attendants shall be provided in two- and four-bedded rooms. The design for privacy should not restrict patient access to the entrance, toilet or shower. These rooms may be connected with main air-conditioning of the center and adequate lighting and electrical points must be provided.

Drug Storage

Each inpatient accommodation unit should have drug storage space with a lockable storage area or cupboard. Lockable cupboards for the storage of restricted substances, a lockable steel cabinet for the storage of drugs of addiction, a refrigerator to store restricted substances, it must be lockable or housed within a lockable storage area, space for medication trolley.[5,6]

Access and Allied Services

The inpatient wards must have easy access from the main entrance of a facility, access from one unit to another, easy access to critical care units, diagnostic facilities such as medical imaging and laboratory and easy access to staff amenities. There must be treatment room, sluice room, changing room for staff with toilet facilities in each ward.

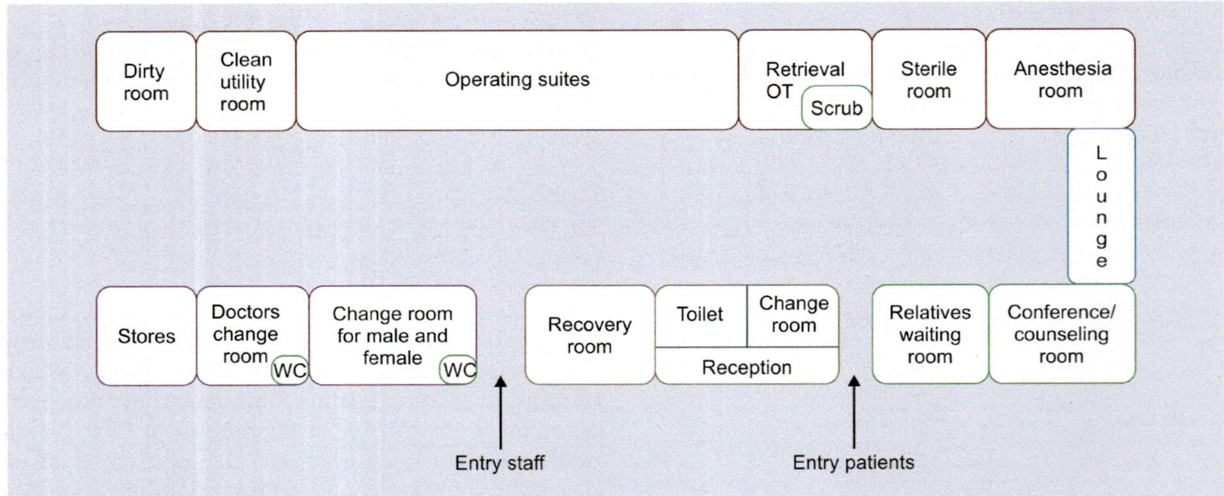

Fig. 8: Functional relationship of operation theater.

Table 3: HVAC in wards.

Place	*Wards*	*Treatment room*	*Pantry*	*Corridor*	*Disposal room*
Air pressure	Positive	Positive	Negative	Negative	Negative
Air changes per hour	6–8	6–8	10	6	10
Relative humidity (%)	45 ± 5	45 ± 5	45 ± 5	45 ± 5	45 ± 5
Temperature °C	22 ± 2	22 ± 2	22 ± 2	22 ± 2	22 ± 2

Lighting

The corridors of the inpatient area must have 200–300 lux and examination and nursing station of the area must have 500 lux. All support areas must have 200–300 lux illumination.

Air-conditioning

The air-conditioning required for various areas is depicts in Table 3.

FUNCTIONAL RELATIONSHIP OF INPATIENT AREA (FIG. 9)[5,6]

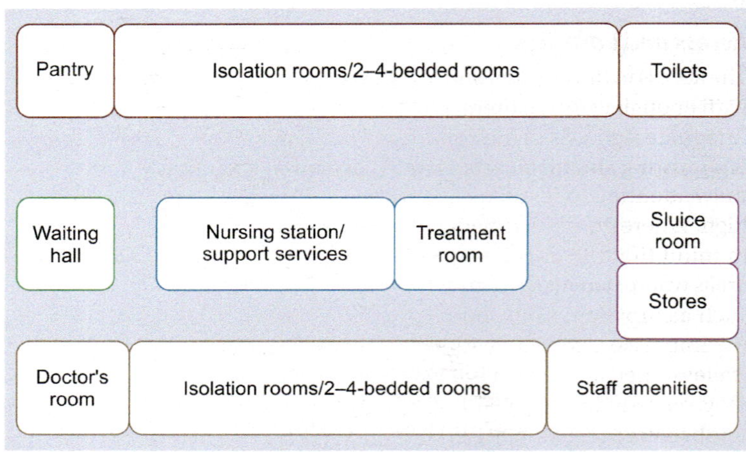

Fig. 9: Functional relationship of inpatient area.

Laboratory

The laboratory provides facilities and equipment for the examination of blood and fluids. Involving receipt of donors and patient specimens, testing and issue of reports. The laboratory of the center may be divided into two main categories—Routine laboratory and HLA laboratory.

Routine Laboratory

The routine laboratory includes four main departments viz:
- Biochemistry
- Hematology
- Microbiology
- Histopathology.

The lab must be provided with modules with each workstation consisting of space for equipment, microscopes, incubators, centrifuge, etc. Each workstation must be provided with below and overhead cabinets. The workstations should be equipped with vacuum, gas, electrical services, sinks and water. A revolving adjustable stool/chair must be provided along with each workstation. Adequate storage facilities for reagents, standards, supplies, stained specimen microscopic slides and separate for chemicals and flammable liquids. The floor must be made of moisture resistant such as quarry or vitreous tiles. The junctions of walls must be coved and washable.

The room must be provided with proper air-conditioning system, so that the windows may be closed, but important it is to ensure that the air circulation from the lab is not connected in any way with that of the reminder of the hospital. The lab must consist of areas for media preparation, cold storage, facilities for washing, sterilization and storage. The lab department must have offices for staff. Staff facilities must include a tearoom, library, conference room, changing rooms and toilets facilities. Moreover, sample collection room for patients, waiting rooms and toilet facilities for patients and attendants. The reporting system must be completely computerized for easy retrieving and maintenance.

Human Leukocyte Antigen Laboratory

The human leukocyte antigen (HLA) laboratory provides specialized histocompatibility testing for patients awaiting organ transplantation. These labs being a specialized area the facility must have areas designated for different tests such as DNA, RNA separator and cytogenesis. The room must be spacious with stainless steel topped tables along with revolving stools. The overall space requirement is 2 rooms of 20 sqm with UV light fumigation facility and positive pressured air conditioning and lighting of 1000 lux. At the entrance of the HLA lab, change room for staff before going inside the room and the two entry doors (one for entry of staff after changing which is fitted with automatic air shower for cleaning of dust particles and the second door for entry for cleaning and maintenance only should be provided). The room requires to be fumigated daily. A washbasin at the entry of the lab is mandatory. The lighting of the lab should be about 500 lux and separate extendable focus lights on each workstation should be provided.

The following air-conditioning are required for laboratory:

- *Air-pressure relationship to adjacent area*: Negative except biochemistry and HLA lab both require positive air pressure.
- Minimum total air changes per hour 6–8
- *Relative humidity*: 45 ± 5%
- *Temperature*: 22 ± 2°C.

FUNCTIONAL RELATIONSHIP OF LABORATORY (FIG. 10)

General Considerations of the Center

Access and Corridors

The access to the hospital and any department must be free and provided with enough width so there is free movement of patient and attendants. Adequate signages in the common language of the place must be used. Signposting should clearly identify staff, patient and visitor areas, and draw attention to restricted areas. All corridors should be at least 2.7 m high. Where doors have been provided in the corridors it must be borne in mind that the effective usable width reduces by at least 25 cm. In areas where patient beds, trolleys and stretchers will be moved regularly, such as inpatient units, operating units, and intensive care units, the minimum clear corridor width shall be 2500 mm. In areas where irregular trolley or bed movement is expected, such as radiology, corridor widths may be reduced to 1800 mm. Corridor widths should mean clear, unobstructed widths. Items such as handrails, drinking fountains, hand basins, telephone booths, vending machines and portable/mobile equipment of any type should not reduce the minimum width or impede traffic flow. The walls of the corridors must be protected from damage due to trolleys and equipment movements by kick boards and bed/trolley protection. Doors should not swing into corridors in a manner that might obstruct traffic flow or reduce the required corridor width. Clear door openings to rooms that may be accessed by stretchers, wheeled bed stretchers, wheelchairs or handicapped persons, should be a minimum of 900 mm.[5-7]

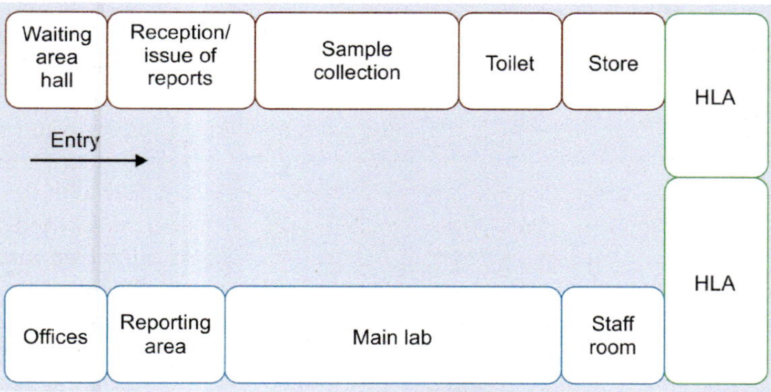

Fig. 10: Functional relationship of laboratory.
(HLA: human leukocyte antigen)

Fixtures and Furnishers

Furniture's both fixed and mobile should be provided in sufficient quantity and quality to satisfy safety requirements. All furniture and equipment is to be maintained in a clean, safe and serviceable condition. Cubicle screens, bed screens and curtains/window treatments should be noncombustible or rendered flame retardant. Grab rails, handrails, vertical adjustable shower supports, towel rails, soap holders, footrests and any other fixture which may be used for support, should have sufficient anchorage and strength to resist the sustained concentrated load of a falling heavy human.

Space Standards

Floor areas given are recommended spaces and increases or decreases must be justified. The schedule of accommodation is depicted in Table 4.

Table 4: Schedule of accommodation.

Type of room	*Area in Sqm*
1 bed isolation (positive/negative pressure)	15
Ultra isolation	25
1 bed ICU	18
2 bed inpatient	25
4 bed inpatient	42
Anesthesia room	15
Change cubicle-patient	2
Change cubicle-staff	8
Clean utility	12–14
Consultation room	12
Dirty utility	12–14
Disposal room	8
Board room	15
Office-1 person	9
Office-2 person shared	12
Office-4 person shared	20
Office consultant	12
Operating room	42
Pantry	8
Scrub room	6
Shower—patient	4
Shower—staff	2
Store—equipment	20
Store—general	10
Toilet—disabled/patient/public/staff	5/4/4/2
Treatment room	15
Waiting—inpatient	10
Waiting—general	0.5 sqm per able bodied and 1.0 sqm per disabled person
X-ray viewing and reporting	12

INFECTION CONTROL[5-12]

Infection control requirements are critical for organ transplant center and need to be incorporated in the plans and specifications. All areas of the facility should be designed, constructed, furnished and equipped in keeping with the principles of infection control. A number of strategies contribute to the control of infection, such as hand washing, careful aseptic technique and the observance of 'standard precautions'. Hand-washing facilities should be installed in all patient care areas, and also in all areas where careful attention to hygiene is essential, such as kitchens, laundries, pharmacies and laboratories. Staff amenities areas, such as bathrooms, toilets and change rooms should also be equipped with hand washing facilities. These must include ventilation; floor coverings; waste management; provision for ease of cleaning; provision for sterilization and disinfection of equipment and instruments; and provision for the isolation of infectious patients as required.[5-7]
Hand wash bays should be provided in the following ratios:

- Intensive/critical care units—one per enclosed room, one per two open bays.
- Ambulatory care areas—one per four open bays
- Other patient treatment areas—generally staff should not be more than 10-12 m from a hand wash bay.
- Alcohol-based hand rubs must be placed in various place of patient care areas, near each bed and in the corridors of ICU, isolation rooms and support services.

COMMON FACILITIES

The services which may be outsourced are housekeeping, security, engineering maintenance and repairs, laundry centralized medical gas system, pharmacy and cafeteria. The layout of a transplant center is shown in Figure 11 and floor plans in Figures 12 to 14.

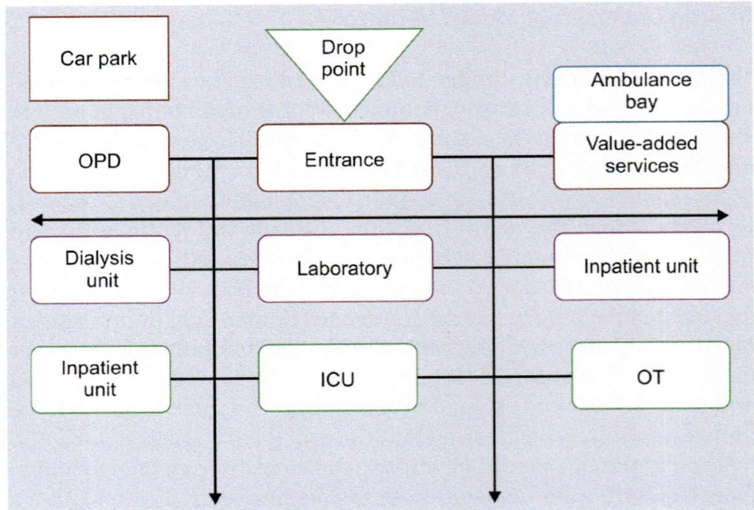

Fig. 11: Layout of transplant center.

CONCLUSION

A transplant center requires meticulous planning and implementation so as to ensure that the structure, processes and outcomes are as per the requirements of all the stakeholders.

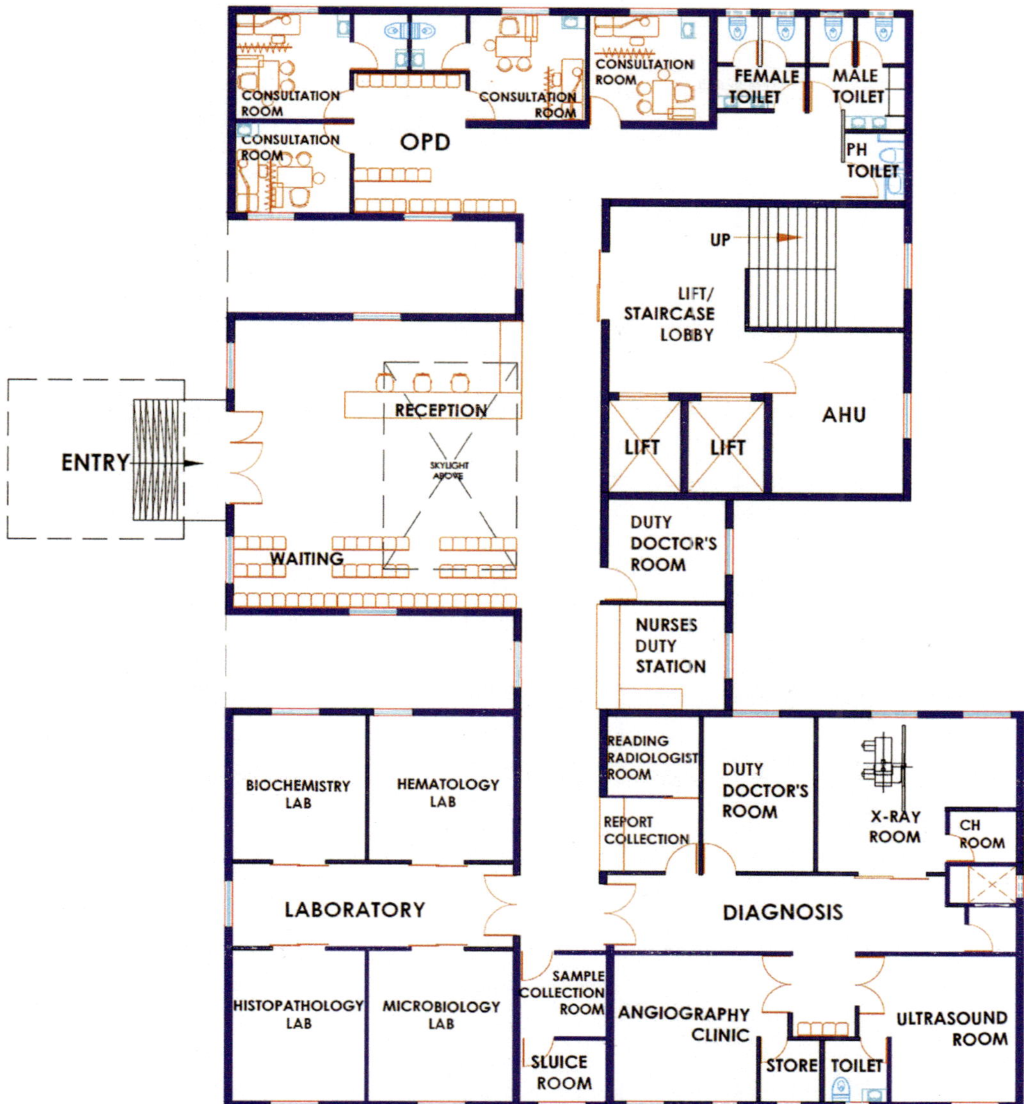

Fig. 12: Ground floor plan.

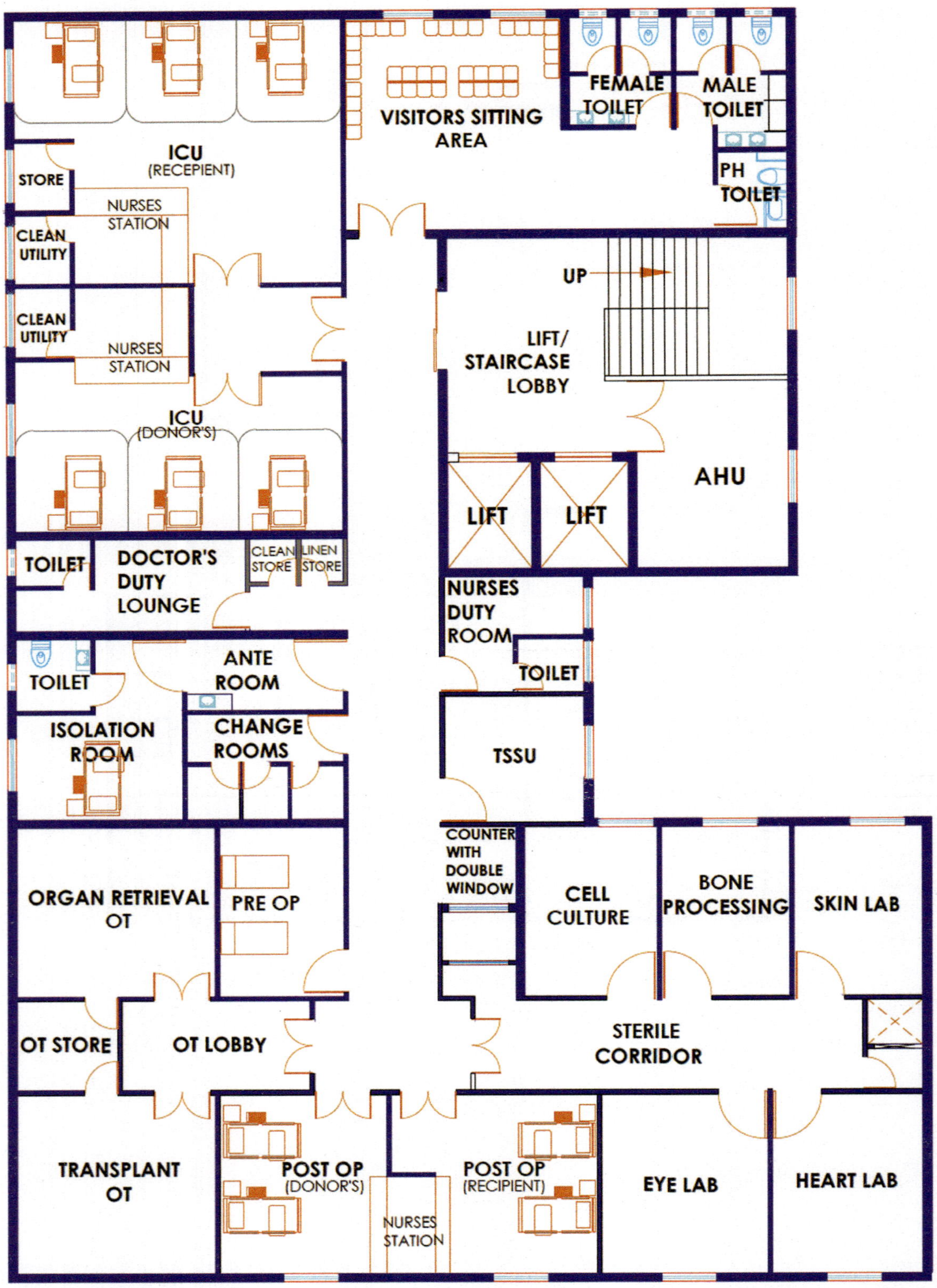

Fig. 13: First floor plan.

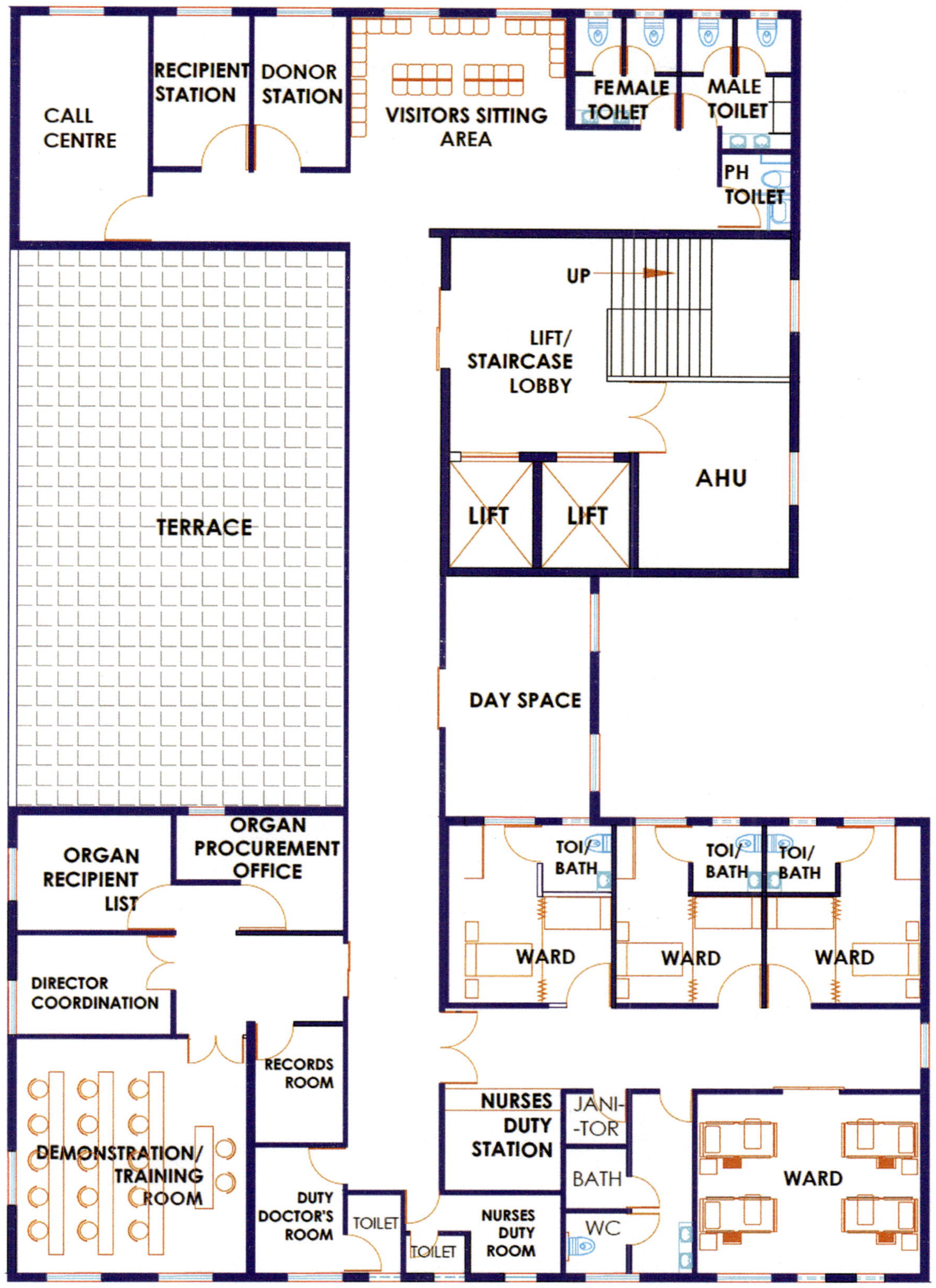

Fig. 14: Second floor plan.

REFERENCES

1. urbanindia.nic.in
2. Elizabeth J. Tuttle-Newhall. Building a modern transplant center, NC Med J.
3. Design Guidelines for Hospitals and Daycare Procedure Center, Department of Human Services, Victoria; 2004.
4. www.muhc.mcgill.ca
5. www.fgiguidelines.org
6. www.healthdesign.com.au
7. aushfg-prod-com-au.s3.amazonaws.com
8. www.statehealthsocietybihar.org
9. www.health.wa.gov.au
10. www.indmedica.com
11. www.health.state.ok.us
12. www.iussonline.co.za

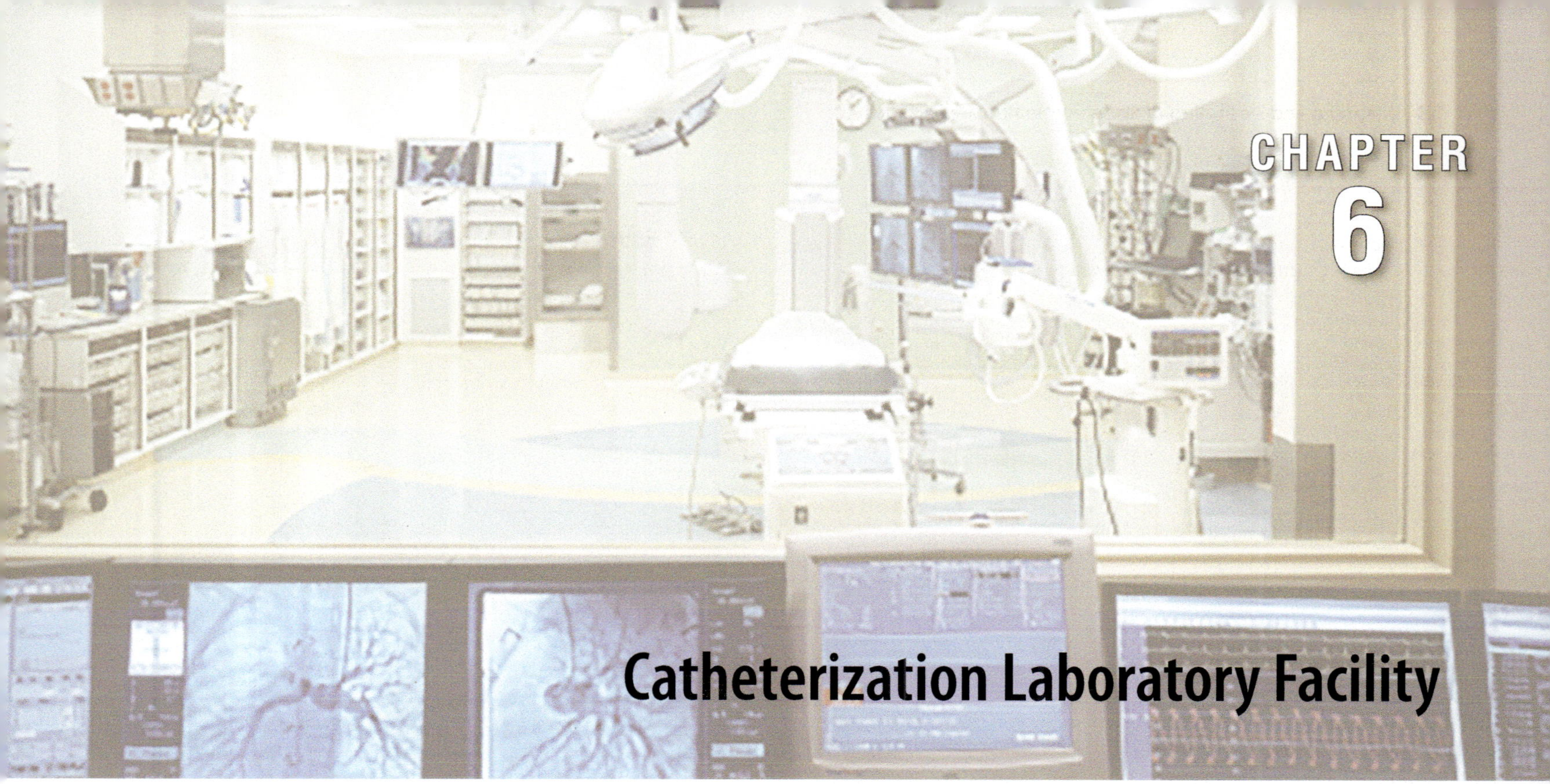

CHAPTER 6

Catheterization Laboratory Facility

Rajesh Harsvardhan, Shakti Kumar Gupta, Sunil Kant, R Chandrashekhar

INTRODUCTION

Cardiovascular diseases (CVD) are one of the major causes of premature mortality, morbidity and disability in most of the countries. Coronary heart disease is the cause of 25–30% deaths in most industrialized countries. The World Health Organization (WHO) has drawn attention to the fact that coronary heart disease is our modern "epidemic", i.e. a disease that affects populations, not an unavoidable attribute of aging.[1,2]

PLANNING PREMISES FOR CARDIAC CATHETERIZATION LABORATORY[3]

The coronary angiography of modern times is performed in a well-organized hospital laboratory called cardiac catheterization laboratory or cath lab.

Location of Cath Lab Services

Population Base

Criteria such as age, sex and disease prevalence of residents and the volume needed to ensure quality must be considered.

DESIGN CONSIDERATIONS FOR CARDIAC CATHETERIZATION LABORATORY (FIG. 1)

Laboratory Design[4,5]

An angiographic and interventional suite must have adequate space for radiographic equipment, ancillary and monitoring equipment, and any emergency care equipment as well as adequate space for patient access and care during the procedure. The optimum size is 70 sqm, not including the control room and additional space, for necessary supportive facilities. Block plan is shown in Figure 1.

Oversized 2 mm lead-lined doors are required at patient entrance and exit points, with a minimum door width of 1.2 m. The ideal ceiling height is 3.6 m, with at least a 900 m mechanical access space above the ceiling. This ceiling height permits adequate focal spot-to-patient distance and focal spot-to-distance for long-leg cut film imaging. In newly constructed facilities the ceiling should be washable. The facility should be equipped with the following utility features:

- Three-phase 150 kVA, 220 V and 440 V air-conditioning power supply with a minimum of 100 amperes per phase.
- Hot and cold water in the room with scrub sink in or very near the room.
- A "dirty" sink just outside the room.
- Manifold system for piped gas and suction.
- Provision is needed to make available suction and 100% oxygen/ any inhalational anesthetic gases on the anesthesia cart, and a scavenging system for medical gases may be appropriate.
- Ceiling-mounted surgical lights.
- Fully rheostated ceiling lights for infinite control of the room lighting during fluoroscopy (fluorescent lighting does not provide the range of lighting adjustments required in these rooms, and fluoroscopic activation of dimming is desirable).
- Ample counter and cupboard space in the room for preparation of equipment and materials used during a procedure, and glass-fronted storage cabinets on the available free wall space.
- Sealed floor and walls; or the floor and walls should have a continuous, hard, washable surface (floor electrical troughs should be avoided whenever possible to allow for appropriate cleaning).
- Adequate electrical receptacles around the room and angiographic table for ancillary equipment.

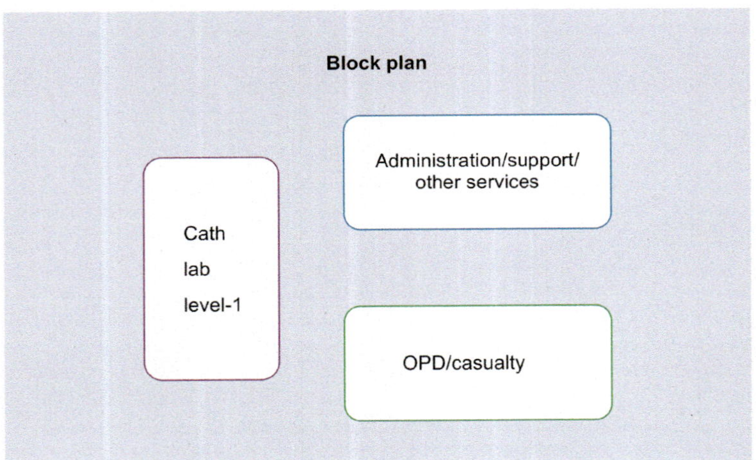

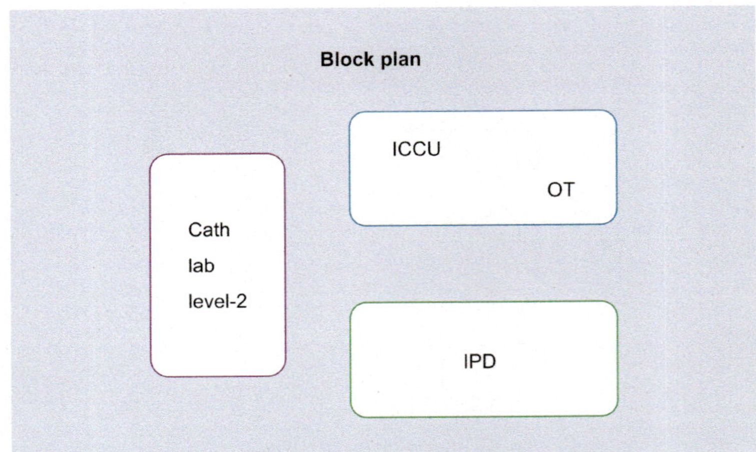

Fig. 1: Block plan for catheterization laboratory.

OPD: outpatient department; ICCU: intensive cardiac care unit; OT: operation theatre; IPD: inpatient departments

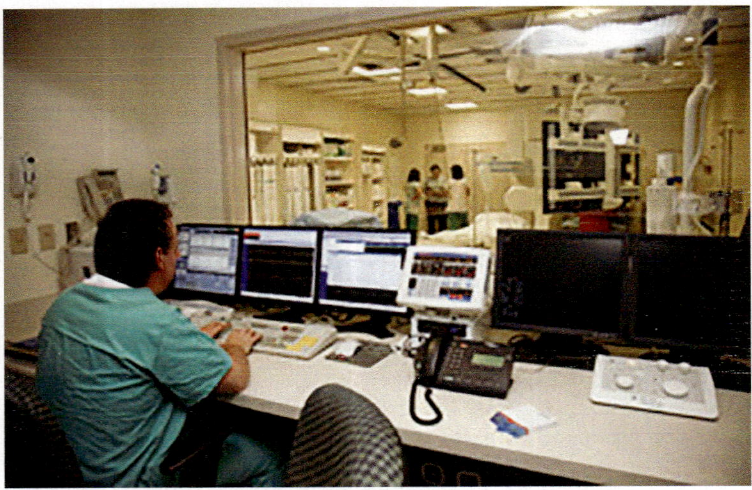

Fig. 2: Control room.

Control Room (Fig. 2)[4]

Ideally, at least 12 sqm are provided for this area. The design should allow ready access to all instrumentation. The control room (Fig. 2) should have leaded glass to allow visual communication with the laboratory. Blinds should be considered to inhibit viewing when necessary. A two-way intercom system is essential.[3,4]

Equipment Room[4,5]

Transformers, power modules, and other related electrical equipment may be placed in the procedure room, the control room, or preferably, in a separate, cooled room with adequate air flow around the electronic cabinets and computer fitting. If placed in the control room or the laboratory itself, the equipment should be enclosed in a space with adequate cooling and ventilation. There should be adequate access for maintenance. If equipment is placed in the control room, the room should be appropriately larger.

The equipment should be positioned so that high voltage cables do not exceed 15 m in length. Ready access to the equipment should be provided, and the room should be fully air-conditioned. The recommended size for the equipment room is 8–10 sqm (i.e. on an average 15 sqm).

Treatment Room

Treatment room is different from the recovery room. It houses the patient immediately before and after the procedure. It should be equipped with the monitoring panel and manifold points.[3,4]

Recovery Room

A recovery room should be in close proximity to the laboratory. The area should be divided into individual patient bays with at least one more bay than the number of laboratories. Hence, a single cardiac cath lab should have minimum two patient bays in the recovery room. At least 6 sqm should be allocated for each bay.[4,5]

Storage Room

Adequate storage space for catheters, wires, and other equipment is essential. Each peripheral vascular and interventional laboratory should have ample in-room storage space for frequently used catheters, wires, interventional devices, and ancillary support equipment. The out-of-room storage space should be at least 25 sqm per procedure room. The storage space should be close to laboratory.[4,5]

FLOOR PLAN TO SHOW FUNCTIONAL RELATIONSHIP AT LEVEL 1

Refer Figure 3.

FLOOR PLAN TO SHOW FUNCTIONAL RELATIONSHIP AT LEVEL 2

Refer Figure 4.

Ancillary Space[4,5]

The procedure, control, equipment, storage and recovery rooms do not constitute a total functioning laboratory unit. Additional support

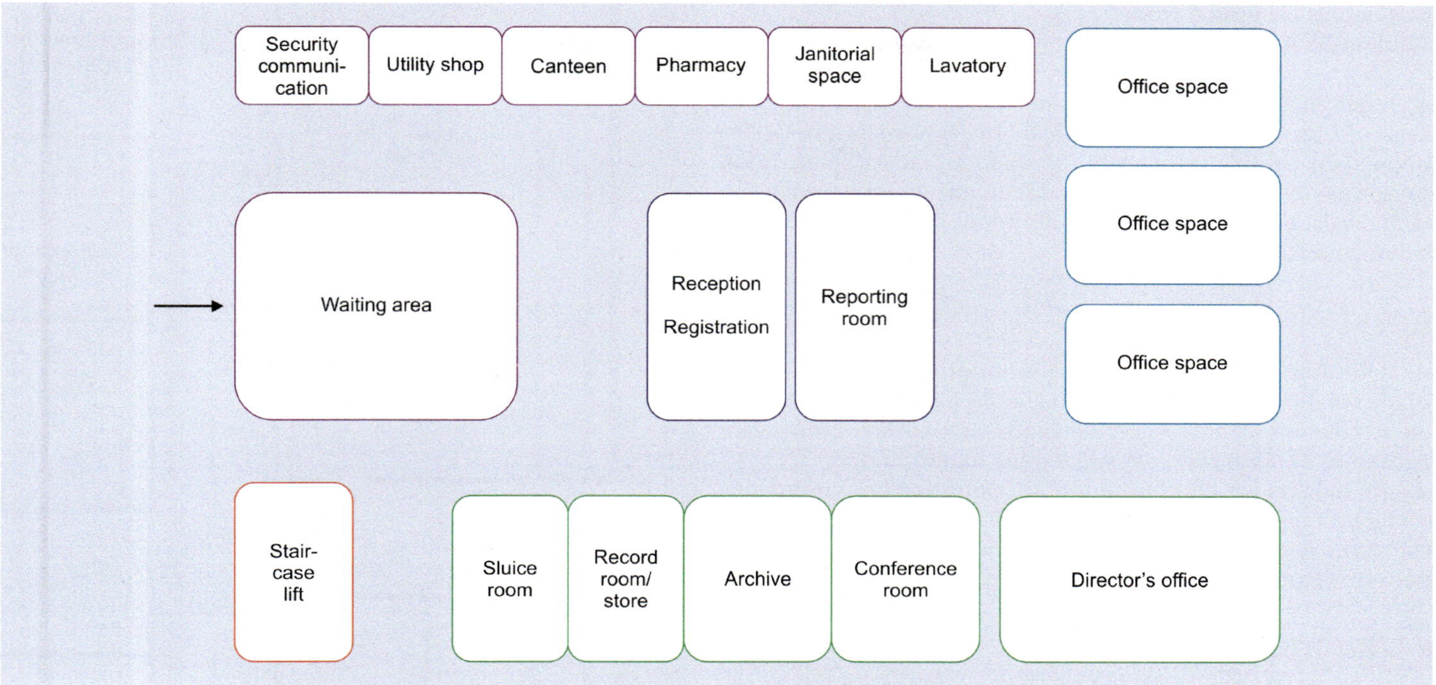

Fig. 3: Floor plan to show functional relationship at cath lab—level 1.

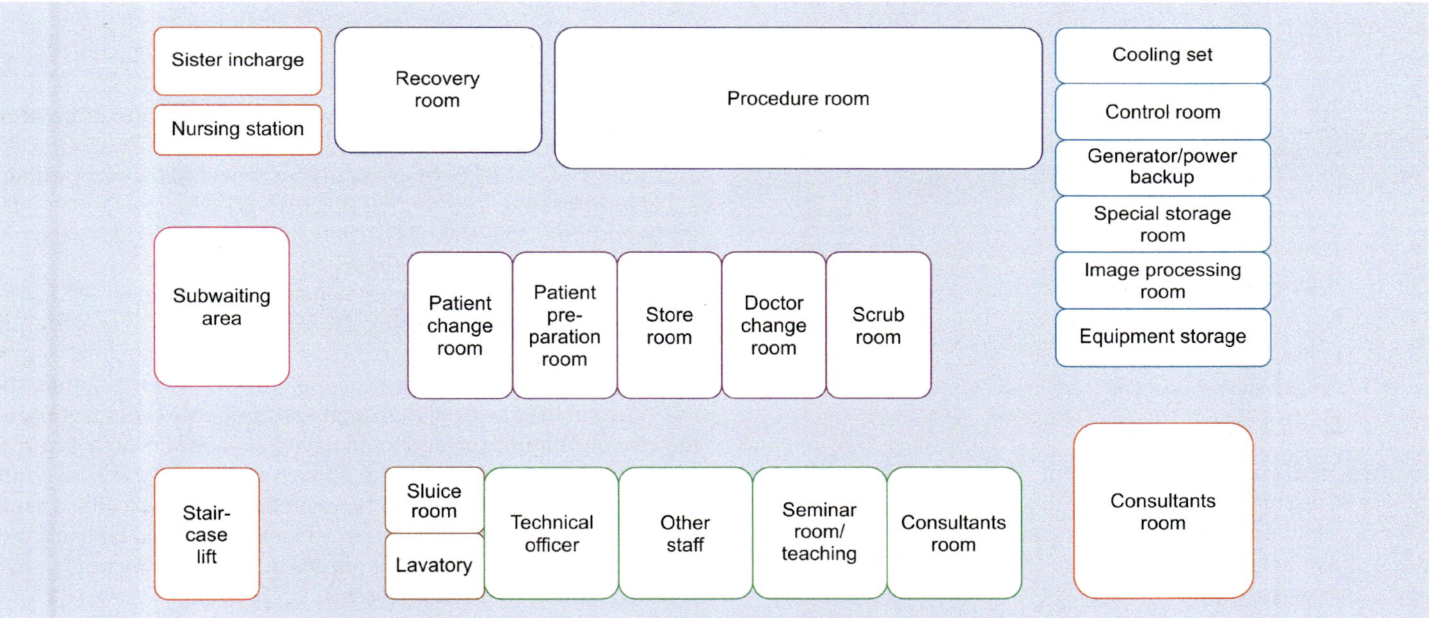

Fig. 4: Floor plan to show functional relationship at cath lab—level 2.

space is required. The following facilities should be available in the immediate vicinity.

- Waiting and holding areas
- Image processing room
- Reception area
- Changing rooms for outpatients and staff
- Viewing and reporting areas
- Office space for the director, staff, and allied health personnel
- Storage space for general supplies, linen, etc.
- Soiled-laundry utility room
- Secretarial resources
- Blood gas and coagulation factor area
- Wash room/lavatory.

Additional facilities may be shared with other services at more remote locations:

- Conference room
- Library and study room
- Room for teaching aids and files

- Additional office space
- Staff lounge, janitorial space
- Equipment storage.

These requirements are similar to those enunciated in the American College of Cardiology (ACC)/American Heart Association (AHA) guidelines for cardiac catheterization and cardiac catheterization laboratories. As per the consensus document on catheterization lab standards, the suggested minimum room sizes for the cardiac catheterization laboratory.

SPACE STANDARDS[3-6]

Table 1 outlines some suggested minimum room sizes for the cardiac catheterization laboratory. It should be obvious that these recommendations are only suggestions and that space for development and access to newer technology will require modification.

Room heights are commensurate to room-need requirements. Procedure rooms require a minimum height of 3.0 m. Heights of the control room and most other rooms are generally 2.7 m. Layout plan is shown in Figure 5.

AIR-CONDITIONING[4]

American Heart Association (AHA) Intercouncil Report on Peripheral and Visceral Angiographic and Interventional laboratories gives the details of air-conditioning requirements. There should be adequate capacity for humidification and dehumidification of the facility.

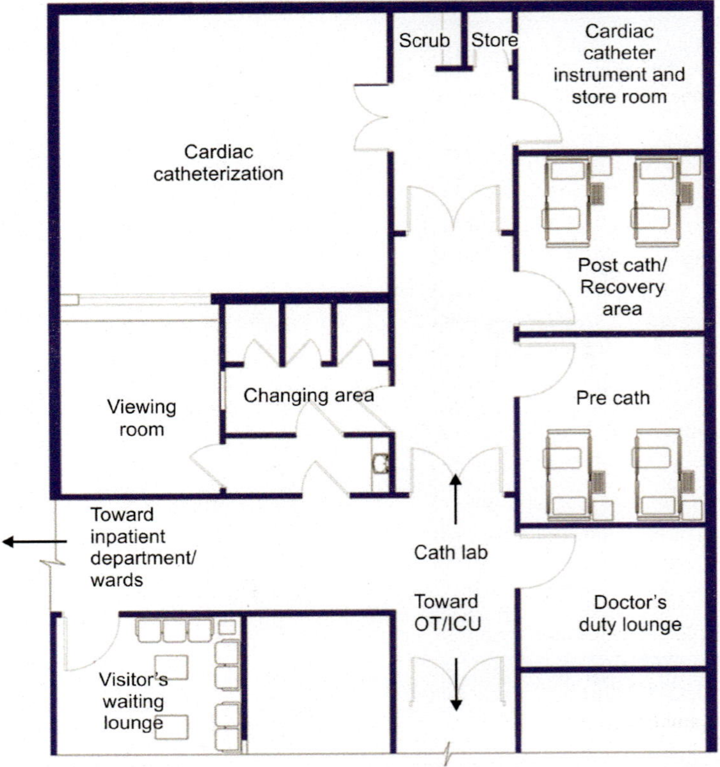

Fig. 5: Layout plan.
(OT: operation theater; ICU: intensive care unit)

Table 1: Schedule of accommodation

Catheterization suite		
Sl. No.	Name of the area	Area in sqm
1.	Procedure room	50–60
2.	Control room	15–20
3.	Equipment room	10–12
4.	Scrub facility	3
5.	Holding room	12
6.	Patient preparation room	12
7.	Recovery room	12
8.	Catheter and other storage room	10
9.	Patient dressing room	7
10.	Staff dressing room	7
11.	Wash room one each for staff and patients	3
12.	Pharmacy space	3
13.	Blood gas analysis	2
14.	Staff lounge	7
15.	Reception area	7
16.	Film viewing area	7
17.	Archival area	7
18.	Processing room	7
19.	Soiled utility	7
20.	Janitorial space	2
21.	Offices (space per office)	7
22.	Conference room	12
23.	Library	7

Three factors are important in determining air-conditioning requirements:

1. Cooling of 3–4 BTU/hour should be provided for every cubic foot of interior space.
2. In addition, 400–1500 BTU/hour should be added for each person continuously present in the room.
3. For equipment that generates heat, the number of BTU/ hour is determined by multiplying the kilowatt-hours of the equipment by 3420.

The total load is the sum from these three calculations. In general, the air-conditioning units should have a capacity 30–50% greater than needed.

Air-conditioning units are often specified in tons of cooling capacity; one ton equals 12,000 BTUs/hour. A laboratory would typically require 40,000–70,000 BTUs of cooling per hour. The best way out is to go for centralized air-conditioning system.

POWER SUPPLY

Refer Table 2.

ENVIRONMENT

Refer Table 3.

TRANSPORT

The transport route doors and hallway requires sufficient dimension for the following parts:

Table 2: Power supply.

	Non-connection voltage (V)	*Frequency (Hz)*	*Internal fuse (A)*	*External fuse (A)*	*Maximum-power consumption (kVA)*	*Connection value (kVA)*
Angiogenerator-M	3ph 400	50/60	63	63 Slow blow	18 with fluoro	43.6
	ph 415	50				
	3ph 420	50/60	80	80 Slow blow	160 with exposure	
	3ph 480	60				52.4
Polydrops–a100	3ph 380	50/60	63	63 Slow blow	18 with fluoro	32.0
	3ph 400					34.6
	3ph 420				160 with exposure	36.4
	3ph 440					38.1
	3ph 480					41.6
System control cabinet	3ph 380	50/60	35	50 Slow blow		23.0
	3ph 400	50/60				24.2
	3ph 440	50/60				26.7
	3ph 480	60				29.1

Table 3: Environment requirements.

Facility	*Variables*	*Range*
Examination and control room	Temperature range and relative humidity	15–30°C 20–75% noncondensing
Image system	Temperature range and relative humidity Maximum temperature gradient Air flow volume Maximum noise generation	10–35°C 20–75% noncondensing 10°C/h 657 cubic m/h 50 db
Angiogenerator-M/polydrops–a100	Temperature range and relative humidity Maximum temperature gradient Air flow volume Maximum noise generation	10–35°C 20–75% noncondensing 5°C/h 800 cubic m/h 55 db
System control cabinet	Temperature range and relative humidity Maximum temperature gradient Air flow volume Maximum noise generation	10–30°C 20–75% noncondensing 5°C/h 500 cubic m/h 48 db
Cooling set	Cooling air Air flow volume Maximum noise generation	5–30°C (frost free room) 1100 cubic m/h 55 db at 50 Hz 59 db at 60 Hz
Digital control system	Temperature range and relative humidity	10–40°C 20–75% noncondensing

- Largest single part—250 × 82 × 190 cm ($w \times d \times h$) with weight—760 kg
- Largest crate—276 × 102 × 209 cm ($w \times d \times h$) with weight—1200 kg.

The door must have final clearance of 125 cm if bed entrance is requested.

FLOOR SPACE AND HEIGHT OF THE SYSTEM COMPONENT[7]

- Generator cabinet, system control cabinet and cooling set should be located in the equipment room (due to generation of noise and heat).
- Generator cabinet and system control cabinet are located in the examination room and the cooling set in the equipment room.
- *Image system*: It is regularly positioned within the control room (as standard).

ROOM LIGHTING[7]

Ambient light in rooms where diagnosis takes place on image display devices (monitors). It must meet the following requirements:

- Free of dazzle, controllable and reproducible setting of the light intensity (dimmer with scale).
- No reflection from window, lamps and viewing boxes in the usual operating position of the image display device should be allowed.
- In general, the nominal lighting intensity should be 500 Lux.

- If only X-ray exposures are produced, the lighting need not meet any special requirements.
- When images are displayed on a monitor, the general lighting must be reduced to 10–30 LUX.

REFERENCES

1. ahca.myflorida.com.
2. www.ypab.com.
3. www.irjpas.com.
4. www.jvir.org.
5. www.scai.org.
6. www.ccn.on.ca.
7. www.partnershipsbc.ca

OTHER REFERENCES

- ACC/SCA&I Expert Consensus Document on Cath Lab Standards, 2001:2170-214.
- Cardiac Care Network Guidelines, Ontario, Canada.

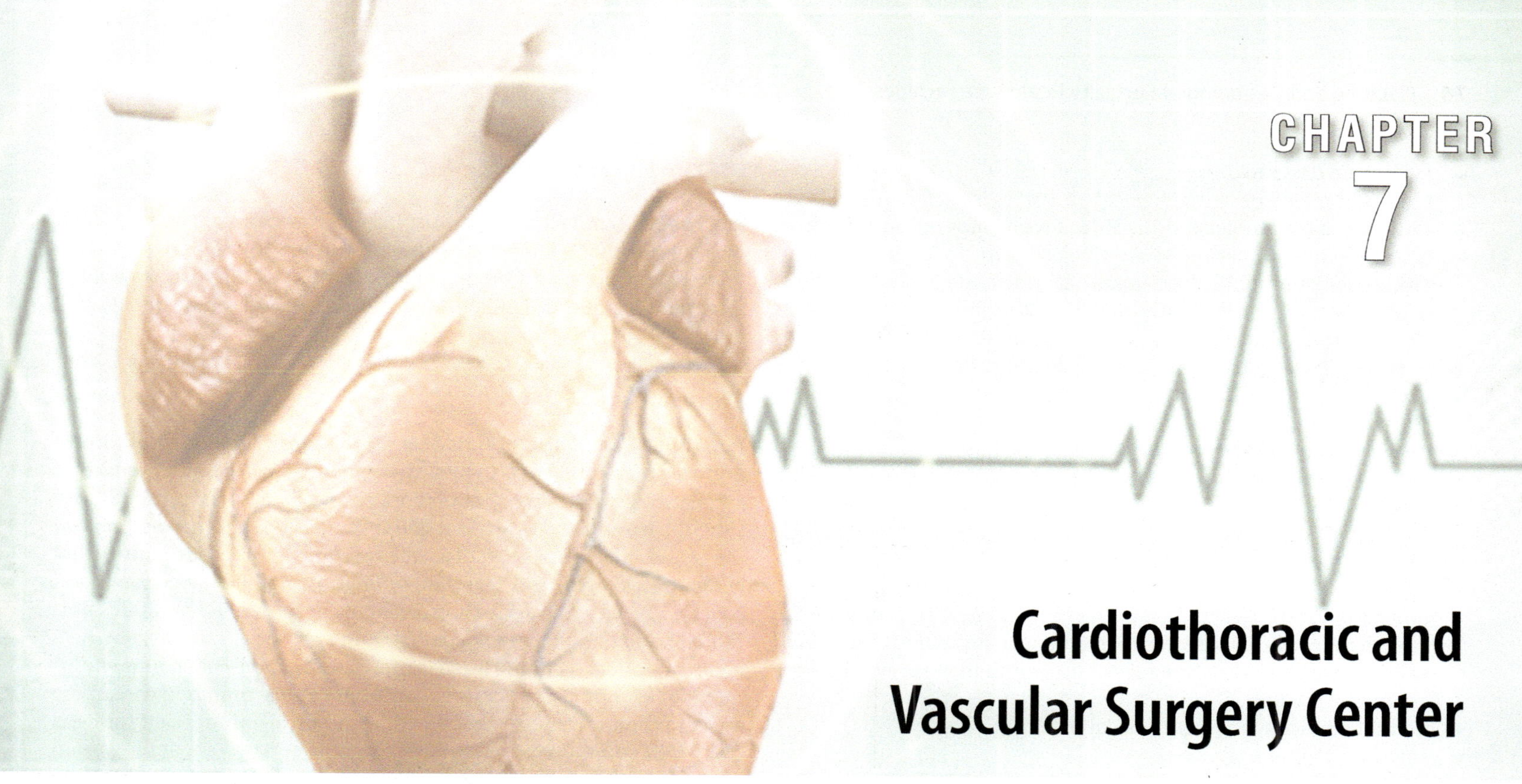

Cardiothoracic and Vascular Surgery Center

MM Singh, Shakti Kumar Gupta, Sunil Kant, R Chandrashekhar

INTRODUCTION

The cardiothoracic and vascular center is a superspecialty center, which is dedicated to effective diagnosis and comprehensive treatment of disease of heart, chest and vascular origin. The center is manned by a highly qualified team of cardiologist, cardiothoracic and vascular surgeon and is supported by cardioradiologist, dietician and cardiointensive care team. They work collaboratively with a skilled, multidisciplinary team of nurses, rehabilitation specialist and support staff who are specialized in cardiothoracic and vascular care.

Cardiac surgery is changing at a very fast pace. With better living conditions and better healthcare the incidence of rheumatic heart diseases are decreasing. Hence, valvular heart diseases have decreased by 10–15%. The incidence of congenital heart disease has been the same. Survival of the patients with congenital heart disease has however improved due to early detection and better surgical correction. Atherosclerosis and its effect on the heart has resulted in more cases of coronary heart diseases. More cases are presenting with ischemic heart diseases at a younger age. With better survival rates, more cases are coming up for coronary artery intervention. Wherever cardiac catheterization lab exists, it is a mandatory requirement to have cardiac surgery back for any emergency.

Prevalence of coronary artery disease (CAD) has increased in India over the years from 0.4% to 12% of population, essentially because of changing lifestyles and increased life expectancy. Increased availability of diagnostic modalities and awareness among the population has also contributed to the increased in number of cardiac procedures that are being carried out. Rheumatic heart disease continues to contribute towards morbidity and mortality among the population.

FUNCTIONS

- The primary function is to provide accurate cardiac and vascular disease diagnosis and deliver a rational and effective therapy for patients suffering from any cardiovascular disease.
- Responsible for all invasive procedures, both diagnostic and therapeutic, e.g. cardiac catheterization and electrophysiologic studies, percutaneous coronary intervention, valvular intervention, intervention with congenital heart disease.
- To contribute to the provision of patient care by decreasing the level of risk factors of patients at risk for cardiovascular diseases through health education and medical intervention.
- To train cardiology, vascular surgery fellows, clinical research fellows, and community healthcare providers on the prevention and control of cardiovascular diseases (CVD).
- To undertake epidemiological studies and use the finding as basis for planning and implementing programs and services for CVD prevention and control.
- To establish hospital and community-based registry system for CVD
- To perform data processing and analysis of research project/activities.
- To render consultancy services to other units of the hospital on research designs, data processing, statistical analysis of results, and data presentation.
- To disseminate cardiovascular health information to population groups through development and distribution of information, education, and communication materials, seminars and lectures.

KEY PLANNING AND DESIGN PARAMETERS[1-4]

The following parameters should merit consideration:

- Dedicated outpatients unit (for provision of consultation/examination and patient support/information services).
- Noninvasive investigations unit (for undertaking electrocardiograms, blood pressure monitoring, echocardiography, and analysis of pacemakers and other implantable devices).
- Catheter laboratories and associated facilities (for undertaking invasive cardiac investigations and treatments and implanting devices).
- Minor cardiac procedures room.

- Dedicated daycare unit.
- Cardiothoracic operating theaters and associated facilities.
- Children with congenital disorders who undergo any form of interventional procedure should be cared for in an environment tailored for children. This may take the form of a dedicated children's cardiac unit or designated children's facilities within a cardiac unit treating both adults and children. It should provide facilities for parents and families, including overnight accommodation. This should not jeopardize the security of the unit.
- The needs of patients with learning difficulties and multiple health problems should be considered.

The following services and facilities should be immediately available on a 24-hour basis:

- Surgical and cardiological team appropriate for age group served.
- Cardiac intensive care unit.
- Inpatient services for intermediate and convalescent care.
- Emergency room with full time director, staffed 24 hours for cardiac emergencies with acute coronary suspect surveillance area and voice communication linkage to the ambulance service and the coronary care unit.
- Catheterization—angiographic laboratory.
- Nuclear medicine laboratory.
- Cardiographic laboratory, electrocardiography including exercise stress testing, continuous ECG monitoring and phonocardiography.
- Echocardiographic services.
- Hematology laboratory.
- Microbiology laboratory.
- Blood gas and electrolyte laboratory with microtechniques for pediatric patients.
- Blood bank and coagulation laboratory.
- Coronary care unit with intermediate step-down area.
- Pulmonary care unit.
- Installation of pacemaker facility.
- Organized cardiopulmonary resuscitation team or capability.
- Bioengineering department.
- Ambulatory service for pre- and postoperative cardiac patients.

It is essential that all these administrative units, laboratories and services be available on an inpatient basis in the hospital with a cardiac surgical program, some may be shared with one or more adjacent community hospitals. There should be an organized administrative structure for each with full time professional director to ensure control and accountability and to facilitate the integration of function essential to a quality program.

The facilities should

- Embrace newer technology and innovation.
- Be supportive to patient and family requirements.
- Enhance operational efficiency.
- Be designed for future flexibility.
- Be staff-friendly.
- Be differently abled friendly.
- Be ergonomically designed.
- Create a sense of confidence in a comfortable environment.
- Develop an effective plan that provides a clear sense of entry as well as convenient and accessible parking.
- Utilize natural features, "green" architecture.
- Integrate value added services.
- Minimize disruption during expansion construction.

OUTPATIENT DEPARTMENT PLANNING

It is a point of contact between hospital and community. Cardiovascular disease hospital performs a number of functions, which are highly selective for heart and thorax. Early diagnosis is the mainstay of the treatment for cure and limitation of the disease. Screening of high-risk group is a special function.

Clinical Area

It includes consulting rooms (Fig. 1) for cardiology, cardiothoracic and vascular surgery (CTVS) surgery, pediatric cardiology, vascular surgeon, administrative control room and medical social service officer (MSSO). Number of outpatient department (OPD) rooms depends on the workload, type of heart disease prevalent in the community of that geographical area, and mandate of the hospital. Single consultation room with shared examination facility is desirable. It should accommodate doctor's chair, table, patient's chair, patient's trolley, or wheel chair, attendant's chairs, wash basin, examination couch and equipment for examination. For inter communicating combined consulting and examination room, an area of 15 sqm is recommended for each room. For common examination room between two consulting room and more consulting rooms, size of each consulting room should be 12 sqm and size of examination room should be 9 sqm. Size should be little larger than the usual consulting room to provide the space for more number of attendants and trolleys/wheel chair, i.e. 15 sqm. Special equipment required in certain departments for examination needs separate space.

Noninvasive Investigation Unit

Ideally this unit should be adjacent to OPD with which it may share common facilities, e.g. reception and waiting facilities and many of the support services. It should be close to the catheter laboratories and cardiac operating theaters. The number of ECG and echocardiography rooms will depend on the workload of the unit. Where children attend

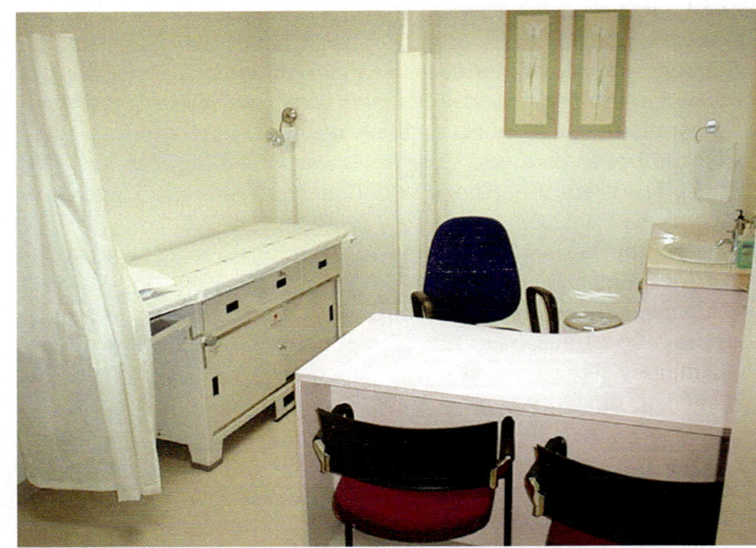

Fig. 1: Consulting room in OPD.

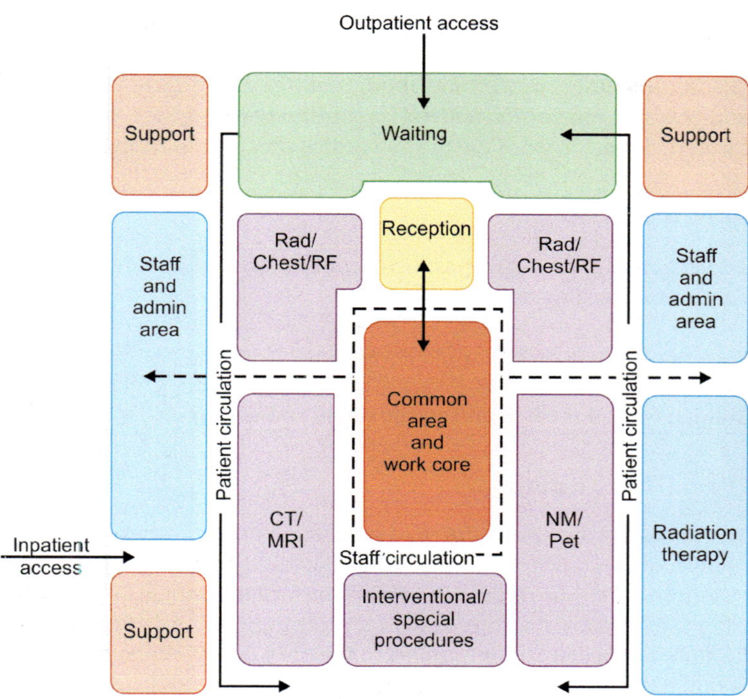

Fig. 2: Functional diagram of radiology department.

the unit, a number of ECG and echocardiography rooms should be designated for pediatric use.[1-5]

Components[1]

- *Patient changing room*: Ideally separate changing room for ECG/Echo with storage for clean and used gowns.
- Resting ECG room.
- Stress ECG room.
- Holter fitting room/cubicles.
- *Echocardiography room*: With space for trolley mounted equipment and a free standing, specialist echocardiography fully adjustable couch offering all-round access to patient.
- *Stress echocardiography room*: With treadmill or exercise *bike* and trolley mounted 12 lead ECG monitor and recorder, sphygmomanometer and stands/pumps for administering drugs.
- Transesophageal echocardiography room.
- Interview room.
- Tilt room.
- Rhythm analysis room.
- Echocardiography reporting room.
- Implantable devices clinic room.
- Storage space for pacemaker programmers.
- Radiology department (Fig. 2).

CATHETER LABORATORY AND ASSOCIATED FACILITIES (FIG. 3)

This unit should be contiguous with daycare unit sharing common facilities, e.g. reception, patient changing, waiting and recovery facilities. It should also be close to cardiac wards [including critical care areas (CCAs)] and cardiac operating theaters with direct access for emergency patients. These laboratories will be used for range of invasive investigations and treatments including cardioversion; coronary angiography, electrophysiological studies (EPS); percutaneous coronary interventions (PCIs); radiofrequency ablation (RFAs); closure of atrial septal defects (ASDs) and ventricular septal defects (VSDs); mitral valvuloplasty and insertion of implantable devices (including complex devices). Coronary angiography and electrophysiology studies will usually be undertaken in a catheter laboratory. Congenital malformation of the heart can be diagnosed by noninvasive investigations such as cross-sectional and color Doppler echocardiography, computerized tomographic scanning, and magnetic resonance imaging.[1,6]

Physical arrangements and space requirements have been suggested for a cardiac catheterization laboratory in Table 1.

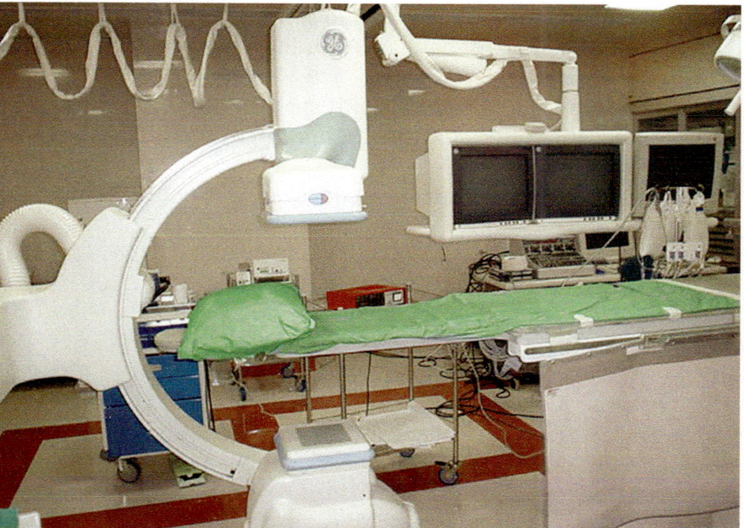

Fig. 3: Catheter laboratory and associated facilities.

Table 1: Space requirements of cardiac catheterization laboratory.[1,6-8]

Sl. No.	Facility	Size sqm
1.	Procedure room	50
2.	Control room	15
3.	Equipment room	12
4.	Clean utility room	9
5.	Soiled utility room	7
6.	Staff dressing room	7
7.	Dark room and film processing	6
8.	Patient preparation room	12
9.	Recovery/observation room	12
10.	Holding room	12
11.	Reception/secretarial room	7
12.	Scrub facility	3
13.	Film/record storage	6
14.	Toilet facility	3
15.	Patient dressing room	1.2
16.	Janitorial space	2
17.	Equipment storage room	9
18.	Pharmacy area	3
19.	Blood gas area	2
20.	Staff lounge	7
21.	Conference room	12
22.	Library	7
23.	Office space (per office)	7

A sterile environment comparable with that expected in the operating room must be maintained in the catheterization theater, with frequent changes of air at the rate of 15 to 22 room cycles per hour. The theater should be sufficiently spacious to permit conversion into an emergency surgical theater. Appropriate control of the room temperature is essential.[1,6]

The procedure room should be constructed to contain radiations and ensure electric safety.[2,7]

MINOR CARDIAC PROCEDURES ROOM AND ASSOCIATED FACILITIES (FIG. 4)

Area of 28 sqm for each minor procedure is recommended. It should accommodate a moveable, fully-adjustable and long axis tilting couch, a mobile single C arm X-ray imaging system, controls and trolley mounted monitor, ceiling mounted minor operating light and a small surgical procedure trolley. It should have medical *services* with gas scavenging system and lead aprons and their storage. Medical *services* should be provided from ceiling or wall-mounted outlets and should comprise medical oxygen, medical compressed air and medical vacuum, together with nitrous oxide and active anesthetic gas scavenging. Alternatively, a pendant solution to medical gases provision may be preferred. Wall-mounted fixtures and fittings, where provided, should have 'easy clean', nondust-collecting surfaces. Lead aprons and their storage hangers should be located adjacent to the entrance to the minor procedures room.[1,9]

Lighting[10]

- LED light fixtures 600 mm × 1200 mm
- Lux level is averagely maintained
- Provide ballasts per fixture for desired switching configuration
- To provide a uniform lighting level, switch inner lamp(s) on first switch and outer lamps on second switch
- Exact quantity, location, and lamping of light fixtures should be chosen to meet the lux-candle requirement.

Heating, Ventilating and Air-conditioning[10]

- *Inside design conditions*: 21°C to 24°C
- *Minimum air changes per hour*: 10
- *Room air balance*: Positive (+).

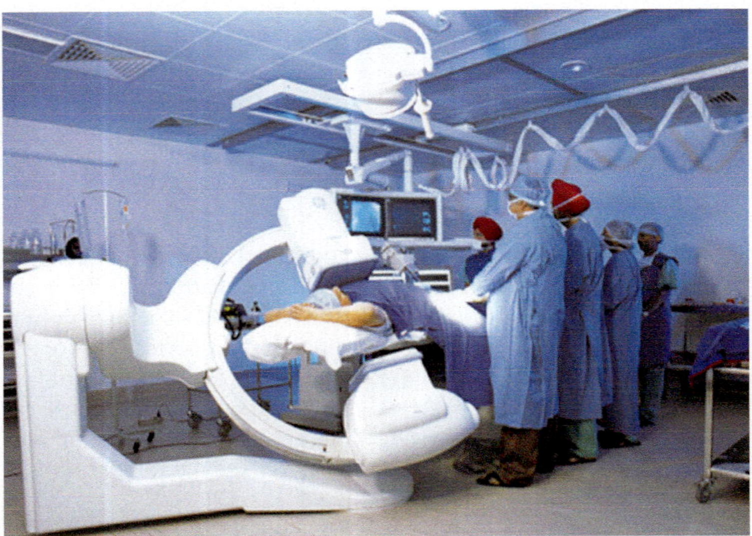

Fig. 4: Minor cardiac procedures room and associated facilities.

Scrub and Gowning Room

The minor cardiac procedures room requires direct access to a scrub and gowning room. Alternatively, scrub and gowning facilities may be located in the corner of the minor cardiac procedures room.[1]

Preparation Room

There should be a preparation room, located in an adjacent communicating space.[1]

Bulk Store

Storage space for clean and sterile items and equipment is required.[1]

Dirty Utility Room

The minor cardiac procedures room requires direct access to a dirty utility room. A disposal unit consisting of sink and hopper with concealed cistern should be provided. Hand-washing facilities should be provided. After use, reusable instruments (used when implanting devices) should be stored on a distribution trolley in the dirty utility. When the trolley is full, it should be taken to the disposal hold prior to dispatch to the Central Sterile Services Department (CSSD).[1]

Disposal Hold

A locked room should be provided to hold bagged refuse, clinical waste, soiled linen and recyclable materials awaiting collection. The room should be accessible from the hospital street.[1]

NONINVASIVE INVESTIGATION UNIT

- It should also be close to the catheter laboratories and cardiac operating theaters.[1,11]
- The purpose of this unit is to investigate cardiorespiratory status using:[1,11]
  - 24-hours ambulatory blood pressure monitoring
  - Resting, stress and ambulatory ECGs
  - Resting, stress and transesophageal echocardiograms
  - ECG and continuous blood pressure monitoring, whilst tilting patient at an angle (tilt test)
  - Analysis of implantable devices.

Components

- Patient changing rooms.
- *Resting ECG rooms*: A standard exam room (2 × 4 m) can be used for ECG studies.
- *Stress ECG rooms*: These will also need space for the equipment with the addition of a treadmill or exercise bike (for exercise stress), trolley-mounted sphygmomanometer (for blood pressure measurement) and stands/pumps for administering drugs (for pharmacological stress).[1,11]
- *Holter fitting rooms/cubicles*: Facilities are required for fitting patients with Holter leads and recording packs (for the purpose of undertaking ambulatory ECGs and 24-hour, blood pressure monitoring). Holter monitoring is a noninvasive procedure for recording cardiac activity on a 24-hour basis.[1,11]
- *Echocardiography rooms*: Echocardiography is a noninvasive procedure that images the heart with ultrasound technology. It will

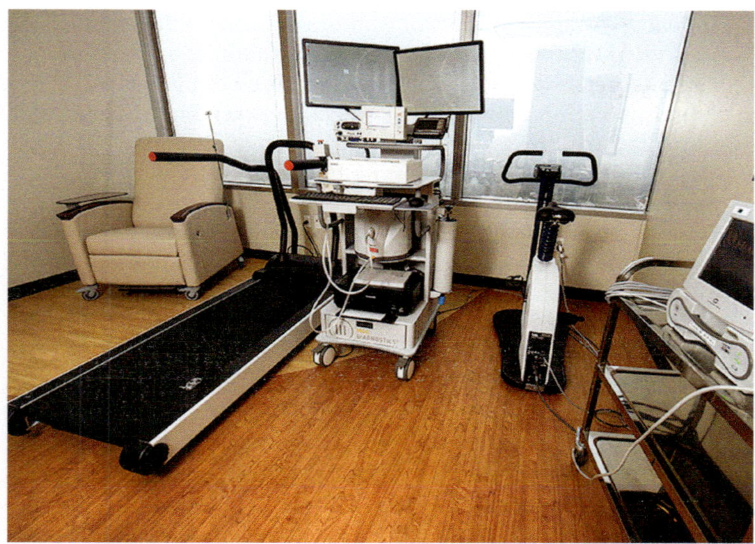

Fig. 5: Stress echocardiography room.

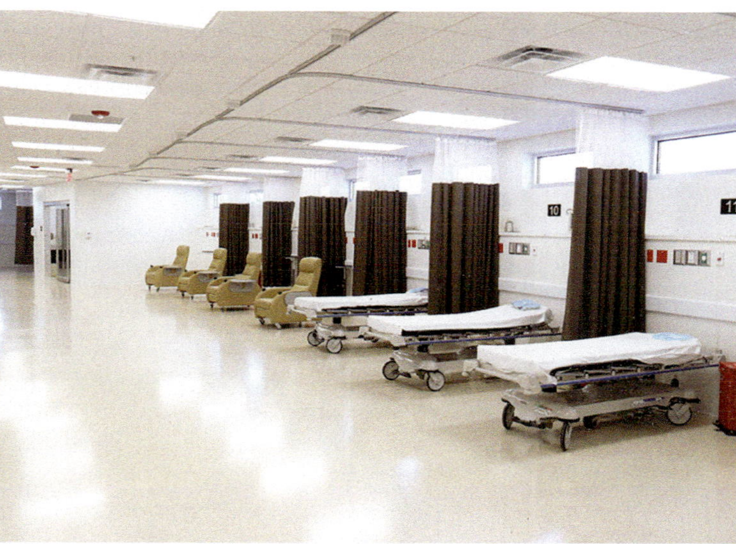

Fig. 6: Daycare unit.

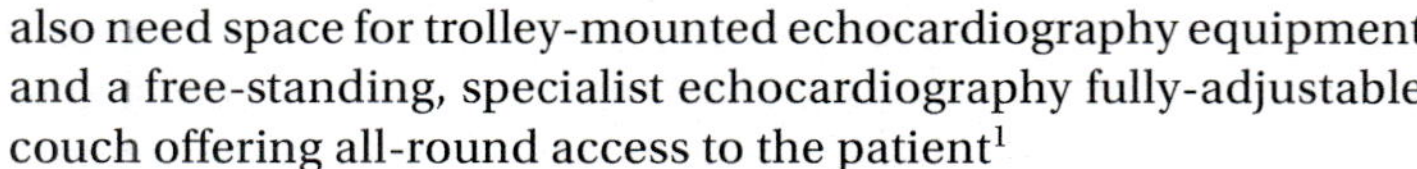

also need space for trolley-mounted echocardiography equipment and a free-standing, specialist echocardiography fully-adjustable couch offering all-round access to the patient[1]

- *Stress echocardiography room (Fig. 5)*: It will also need space for a treadmill or exercise bike and trolley-mounted 12-lead ECG monitor and recorder, sphygmomanometer and stands/pumps for administering drugs[1]
- *Transesophageal echocardiography rooms*: The couch should provide head-down tilt for use when sedating patients (to clear an airway in the event of the patient vomiting). A separate recovery bay, located in an adjacent space, will be required for recovery of sedated patients. Children undergoing transesophageal echocardiograms (TEEs) require a general anesthetic[1]
- *Interview room*: A separate interview room, close to the echocardiography rooms, will be required if fetal echocardiography is being carried out[1]
- *Tilt room*: It will need to contain trolley-mounted ECG equipment and beat-to-beat blood pressure monitoring and recording equipment (specialist tilt monitor), a free-standing, fully-adjustable tilting couch offering all-round access to the patient, and computer workstation for the cardiac physiologists.[1]
- *Rhythm analysis room*: This room should be equipped with relevant equipment for retrospective analysis of 24-hour ECG and BP data, and mechanical cooling will be required to suit the number of workstations. There should be links via modem and fax machines.[1]
- *Echocardiography reporting room*: A room for the retrospective reading and reporting of echocardiography data should be provided.
- *Vascular lab*: Diagnostic studies of the blood vessels are performed in a vascular lab to detect blood clots, calcium buildup, fatty deposits, and so forth. A vascular lab might be set up with two rooms, one for carotid artery studies of the neck and one for studies of the extremities. A third room would be an office for the sonographers.[1]
- *Implantable devices clinic room*: A room is required for analyzing and programming implantable devices that have already been inserted.

DAYCARE UNIT (FIGS. 6 AND 7)

A daycare unit is a place where patients are kept in the daytime and allows the patients to return home on the same day. In daycare center,

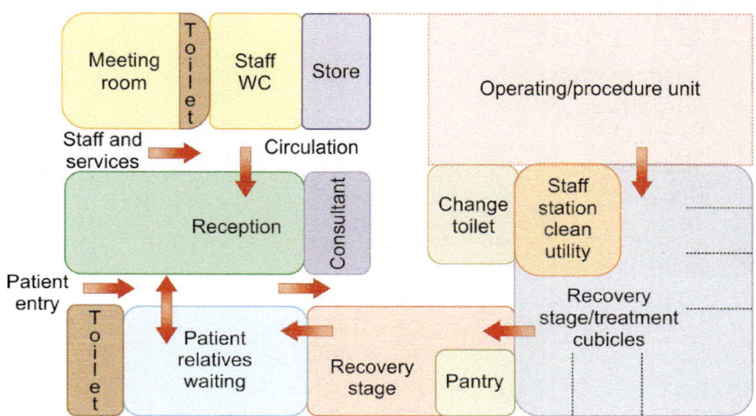

Fig. 7: Functional area of daycare.

operative procedures are performed or chemotherapy, if required, is administered. A daycare unit in a heart center has got a special importance because ambulatory patients of heart disease require frequent follow-up with supportive treatment for the adverse effect of treatment and operative procedure.

Key Planning and Design Parameters[2]

The facilities and standards of care should be comparable to those provided to inpatients. The waiting areas should be separate from recovery and procedure area. Patient bed spaces should be provided with suction, oxygen and nurse call facilities. All door widths should allow easy access for trolley bed/trolley transfer. The fittings and fixtures such as bed screens should ensure privacy and dignity to the patients. Arrangements should be made for about 10% of the patients to spend the night after the procedure/treatment under medical supervision. In daycare unit, dedicated and separate room for the storage, documentation and retrieval of clinical records should be planned. Floors and wall finishes should be seamless, impervious. Flooring should be non-slippery. The intersections of walls and floors should be coved in continuous materials. Joints, if any, should be thermo-sealed. General and individual offices should be provided for administrative and professional staff, which should be away from public and patient area. The daycare unit requires being contiguous with the catheter laboratories and minor cardiac procedures rooms. It should be nearby to cafetaria.[1]

INPATIENT AREA (FIGS. 8 AND 9)

A key element that should be addressed in all patient accommodation is that of privacy and dignity. Several benchmarks of good practice, focusing on the issue of respect for the individual so that:[1,12]

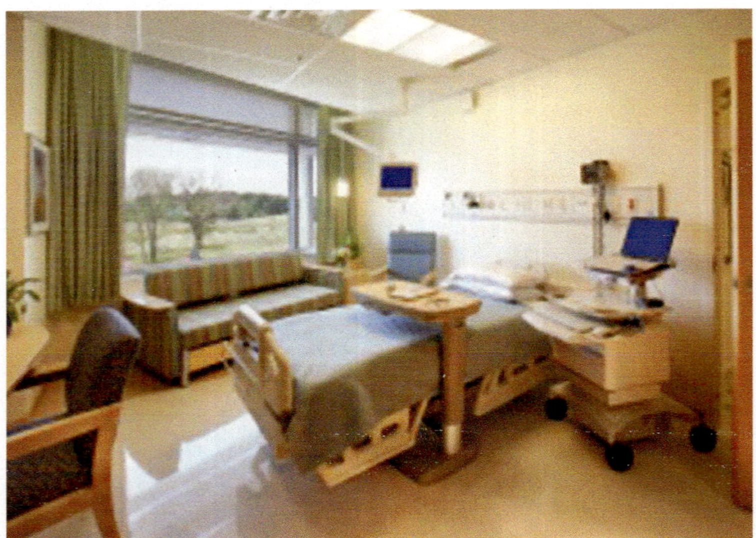

Fig. 8: Inpatient area.

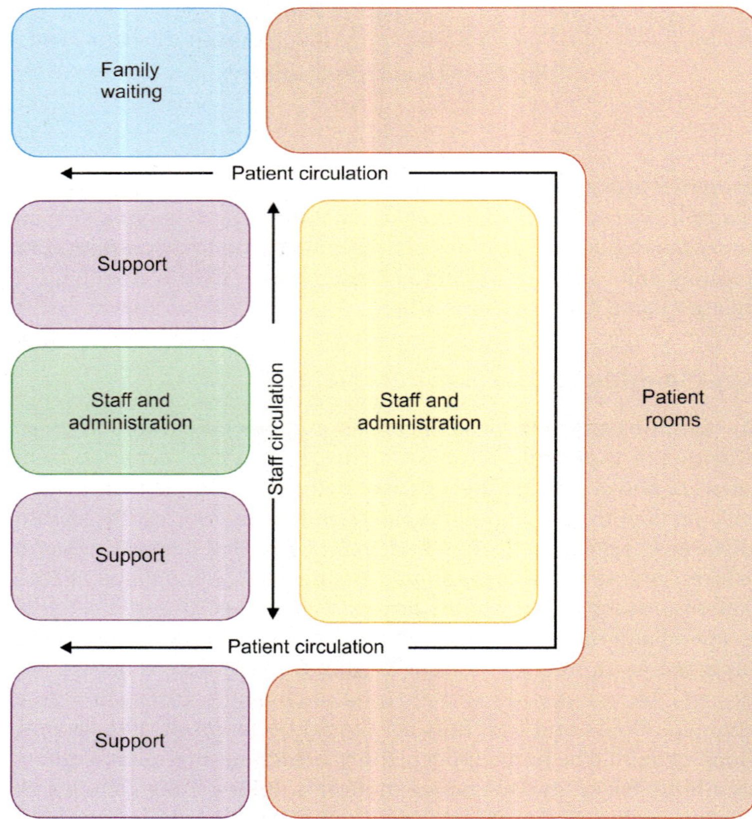

Fig 9: Functional diagram of inpatient area.

- Patients experience care in an environment that actively encompasses individual values, beliefs and personal relationships.
- Patients' personal space is actively promoted by all staff.
- Communication between patients takes place in a manner that respects their individuality.
- The care of patients actively promotes their privacy and dignity and respects their modesty, including gender segregation.
- Patients can access an area that safely provides privacy.
- Inpatient accommodation for cardiac patients does not differ from inpatient accommodation for other patient groups and *comprises surgical and medical wards*. There should be separate, dedicated cardiac wards for children, adolescents and adults.
- Accommodation for adult
  - Single bedrooms: The size of single rooms are 20 sqm.
  - Four bedded rooms: The size of rooms is 50 sqm.
  - *Space around the bed:* The minimum recommended clear space around the bed is now 3.0 m. This can be achieved within the new space allowances for single bedrooms and multibedded rooms.

En-suite sanitary facilities for single bedrooms: They are suitable for ambulant and semi-ambulant patients, the majority of independent wheelchair users, and patients requiring assistance from staff. For greatest flexibility of use, all sanitary facilities in inpatient areas should be accessible and manageable by people with physical or sensory disabilities with/without assistance.

Isolation suites: Single bedrooms provide effective isolation for many patients. In some cases, however, a greater degree of isolation may be required. It includes bedroom, en-suite sanitary facilities, and lobby. Single-bed rooms provide the most effective facility for isolating patients with a variety of infections, such as MRSA.

Dirty utility rooms: Ideally, a dirty utility room should serve no more than 15 beds. This reduces travel distances for staff, making better use of nursing time and reducing the risk of spillage and cross-contamination.

CARDIAC INTENSIVE CARE UNIT (FIG. 10)

The inter-society commission for heart disease resources has made following recommendations regarding cardiac surgery intensive care unit:[2,13]

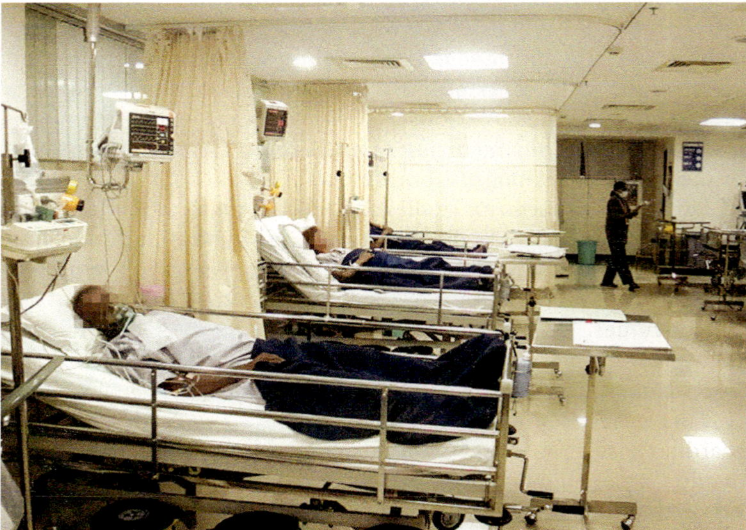

Fig. 10: Cardiac intensive care unit.

- This unit should be designated for the immediate postoperative care of cardiac surgery patients. It should be located within or immediately adjacent to the clean area. In general, the number of available beds should be approximately half the number of cardiac operations performed each week. A program conducting a minimum of 200 open heart operations a year with anticipated growth should plan for a four to six bed unit.
- Each bed should be in an individual cubicle measuring at least 15 sqm with no horizontal dimension less than 3.0 m. Metal and glass enclosures are satisfactory. It is desirable that wall on the one side of the room be of movable foldaway variety to allow for the enlargement of the room when needed in emergency.
- Direct observation of all the patients from a central nursing station should be possible. If larger units are planned then separate nursing stations should be established for each group of six beds. There should be approximately 10 sqm storage space for a four to six bed unit.
- A core laboratory equipped to determine blood gases and other stat tests should be designed within the intensive care unit. There should be interdepartmental communication system such as telephone, a hot line to serve emergency situations and an alarm capable of summoning appropriate personnel to assist in emergency. Cardiac surgery intensive care unit (CSICU) must have its own X-ray equipment.
- Each bed cubicle should be equipped with piped-in oxygen, a minimum of two independent suction outlets and three duplex electric outlets with equipotential grounding system. A sink with foot operative faucets should be available to each cubicle. Bed should be hydraulically or electrically or manually operated, relatively light weight, easily movable and readily adjustable to Trendelenburg, Fowler and other positions. The beds should be positioned to provide space for all necessary equipment and for personnel to deliver routine as well as emergency care.
- *Bed-boards* should be available at every bed for cardiac resuscitation. Each cubicle should have immediate access to a completely equipped cardiopulmonary emergency resuscitation cart including a defibrillator and a respirator in good working order. At least two transvenous catheter pacemakers with self-contained power source should be available at all times in 4–6 beds units with an increased number for larger units. If pediatric cardiac surgery is also being performed, then a separate cardiac surgery intensive care unit for pediatric patients is desirable.

INTERMEDIATE OR 'STEP-DOWN' AREA

An intermediate intensive care area for patients discharged from intensive care unit is highly desirable. This should be adjacent to or near the CSICU and specialized nursing care, cardiac monitoring and immediate resuscitation capabilities should be available. It should contain about the same number of beds as the intensive care unit.[2,13]

HIGH DEPENDENCY CARE AREAS

Coronary care units (CCUs) are required for the continuous monitoring of patients suffering from cardiac abnormalities or acute cardiac emergencies, such as acute myocardial infarction (AMI). A CCU may also accommodate patients not stable enough to return to a cardiac ward after an invasive procedure and/or patients requiring an initial assessment. CCUs will not normally accommodate patients requiring artificial respiration will be admitted on a temporary basis to a CCU.[1]

OPERATING THEATERS

Facilities for Cardiac Surgery

The cardiac operation theater suite should provide a safe operating environment for inpatients to undergo simple procedures, closed and open-heart cardiac and thoracic surgery, and heart/lung transplants including facility for teaching and research.[1]

Dimensions

All theaters in which cardiac work is carried out should be of a minimum area of 63 m^2, broadly rectangular and with a minimum dimension in any single direction of 7 m. They should be grouped in pairs, each capable of supporting the broad range of cardiac and cardiothoracic work undertaken.[1]

Occupancy[1,12]

- A lead and one or two support surgeons with a scrubbed practitioner and nonscrubbed 'runner'
- An anesthetist and anesthetist's assistant
- A monitoring technician.

When a coronary bypass operation is being undertaken, the above occupancy will be increased by a further surgeon; and a perfusionist to operate the heart bypass machine.

Components: Cardiac operation theaters need to be larger than standard operation theaters (OTs) to accommodate additional staff and equipment with additional perfusion preparation room. The recovery area does not need to be as large as for standard OT.[1,12]

Perfusion preparation room(s): It should be adjoining each theater for cleaning and setting up of perfusion (heart/lung) machines, separate for each theater, or shared between pairs of theaters. There should be at least three perfusion machines for each pair of theater (i.e. one per theater, plus one spare).[1,12]

Perfusion storage room: A storage space for disposable equipment is required, adjacent to the perfusion preparation room, large enough to enable storage of large quantities of disposable packs and volumes of fluids. It will require heavy-duty shelving.

Recovery area: A four-bed recovery room is recommended for a facility comprising four cardiac OTs[1] (this is less than those recommended for other OTs as large number of cardiac surgical patients go directly to CCUs rather than remaining in recovery).

Equipment store: A storage area for infusion pumps, echocardiography machines and mobile X-ray equipment is required. Facility for recharging and a shelved unit with spaced access to electrical plugs should also be provided.[1,12]

Surgical suite:[2,14-16] Medical research council has laid down minimum basic requirements for operating room suites for control of infection and for comfort. The operating room suite should be independent of the general traffic and air movement in the rest of hospital. The rooms of the operating suite should be so arranged that there is continuous progression from the entrance, through zones that increasingly approach sterility, to the operating and sterilizing room. People working within the suite should be able to move from one clean area to another without having to pass through unprotected or traffic areas. It should be possible to remove dirty materials from the suite without having to pass through a clean area.

The operating rooms should be divided into four zones:[16]

- Protective zone—which includes entrance lobby, recovery rooms and changing rooms.
- Clean zone—includes anesthesia rooms, scrub rooms and inner lobby.
- Sterile zone—includes operating rooms, sterilizing room and lay up room.
- Disposal zone—includes sink room.

The cardiac operating room should be large enough to comfortably contain the patient, the anesthesia machine, monitoring equipment, the perfusionists equipment including devices other than the pump oxygenator (such as IABP and cell saver devices), and the requisite nursing supplies and sterile area. The cardiac operating rooms should be 55–75 sqm in size, have adequate electric grounding, oxygen and vacuum supply, proper illumination and be capable of supporting and technical equipment utilized in cardiopulmonary bypass, including pump oxygenators, heat exchange equipment, cell saver, anesthetic apparatus and assist devices.[15]

Walls should be impervious. Suitable finishes include an epoxy resin type of paint and solid material sheet with welded joints. The walls, ceiling and floors should be light in color. Pale blue or green is acceptable as strong colors will distort the color rendering of light sources and should be avoided.

Corridors are better if not less than 3–4 m wide. Natural lighting from windows is not recommended for major operating rooms.

Special requirements of cardiac surgery operating room include:[1,2]

- A minimum of 90 amperes (optimum 120 amperes) of peak load current.
- Special plumbing installation for the pump-oxygenator if the pump is not self-contained. These should include hot, cold and waste water.
- Nine to twelve outlets, three on each of three or four walls.
- A capability of lighting two operating fields simultaneously.
- A capability of direct audio communication between cardiac operating room and the blood bank, the nursing supervisor's desk, the clinical and pathological laboratory and X-ray department is recommended.
- The ambient light recommended in cardiac operating room is 200–250 lux to be provided by LED lamps. At the operative site, the illumination recommended is 2500–5000 lux.

Storage space and pump room: A room should be designated in the clean area as a pump room in which the extracorporeal pump oxygenators, pump assist devices for intra-aortic balloon pump and all necessary equipment are stored, conditioned and maintained. It is desirable to have the pump room and the storage area within the surgical suite, preferably with both inside and outside access.[1]

Suction:[3] A minimum of three and preferably four separate sources of suction are recommended. One source should be available to the anesthetist at all times while two or three lines of suction are required by the operating team. All lines should be independent to obviate the consequences of central blockage.[1]

Anesthesia utility pedestal: Cardiac surgery requires more equipment than most other types of surgery so the floor tends to become cluttered with tubing's and power cords. To solve the problem of this vermicelli of tubing's anesthesia utility pedestal can be used. These pedestals may be ceiling-mounted or floor-mounted. These pedestals provide connection for oxygen, anesthetic gases, compressed air, three or four suctions, two or more shielded electric outlets, electrocautery units, telephone jacks, mounts and connections for the monitors.[1]

Blood gas laboratory: Blood gas results should be available early during cardiopulmonary bypass. Therefore, a core laboratory in the surgical suite is convenient for the rapid performance of blood gas, pH and electrolytes. Such a laboratory requires a space of 20 sqm and can service both the operative room and surgical intensive care unit.[1]

Ventilation requirements: Inter-society commission for heart disease resources has recommended following specifications for operating room air:[1]

- Air changes—at least 25 per hour
- Temperature—between 22 ± 2°C (optimum 60°F)
- Humidity 50 ± 5%
- High efficiency particulate filters for filtering of incoming air
- A higher pressure of air is required within the operating room than in the corridors of surgical suite. The exhaust vents should be unobstructed by furniture or personnel.

Heart/lung bypass machine room:[11] The heart lung machine is stored in the heart lung prep room adjacent to and directly accessible from the cardiac operating room. Particular attention should be given to the width of the doorway so the heart/lung machine will fit through it. Accessory supplies required for bypass procedures also are stored in the heart/lung prep room. The room is sufficiently large to allow breakdown, essential cleanup and storage of parts, and to accommodate at least two heart/lung machines, one of which provides back-up function in case of mechanical failure of the other machine. Clean bypass machines are transported to the cardiovascular operating room via the clean core. Soiled bypass machines are moved from the cardiovascular operating room to the heart lung prep room where they are cleaned.[17]

Pendant services: Two ceiling pendants for pipeline services should be designed; one for surgical team and one for anesthetist. Anesthetic pendant should be retractable and have limited lateral movement and provide a shelf for monitoring equipment. It should have oxygen, nitrous oxide, four bar pressure medical compressed air, medical vacuum, scavenging terminal outlets and at least four electric sockets.[18]

Piped gases in the OT: Automatic/semi-automatic fail safe manifold room to be designed. Two outlets for O_2 and suction and one for N_2O are a minimum in each OT. Pipeline supply system should be able to cut off from mainline if the problem occurs anywhere along the delivery hosing/tubing.[18] The schedule of accommodation is depicted in Table 2 and floor plans in Figure 8 to 15.

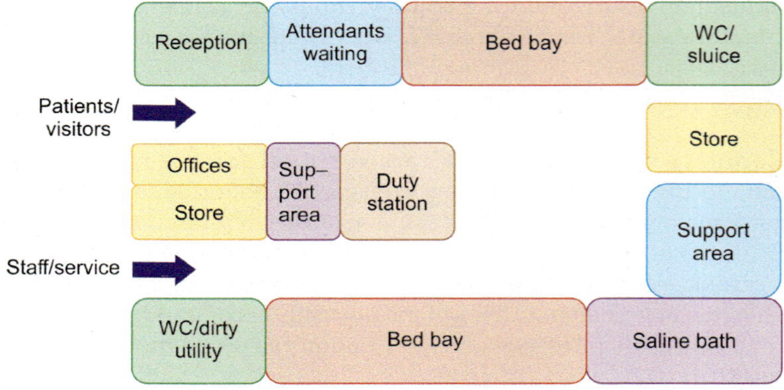

Fig. 11: Functional relations of ICU.

Table 2: Schedule of accommodation.[11,19-21]

Room/Space	Requirement	Area in sqm
Waiting area	Minimum NSF; provide an additional 55 NSF per each increment of two projected exam/treatment rooms greater than three 100 NSF provides for three standard seats, one wheelchair accessible seat and waiting space for one stretcher. Additional 55 NSF allocates 25 NSF for one accessible seat and 30 NSF for two standard seats	9.3
Sub-waiting	Minimum NSF; provide an additional 15 NSF per projected exam/treatment room greater than three	3.7
Reception	Minimum NSF; provide an additional 10 NSF per projected exam/treatment rooms greater than three	7.5
Consultation room	Provide one per cardiology suite	11.2
Exam room, cardiology	Divide the projected number of annual new cardiology exam clinic stops by minimum workload to generate one room; and the projected number of annual follow-up cardiology exam clinic stops by minimum workload to generate one room; provide one room for each whole increment	11.2
Catheter laboratories		
Cardiac catheterization laboratory	Divide the projected number of annual diagnostic cardiac catheterization clinic stops by minimum workload to generate one room; and the projected number of annual interventional cardiac catheterization clinic stops by minimum workload to generate one room; provide one room for each whole increment	55.8
Cubicle, patient prep/recovery	Provide two per cardiac catheterization laboratory suite	7.5
Nourishment station	Provide one per cardiac catheterization laboratory suite	5.6
Medication area	Provide one per cardiac catheterization laboratory suite	7.5
Nurse station	Minimum NSF; provide an additional 60 NSF per each whole increment of four patient prep/recovery cubicles greater than four	5.6
Scrub/gowning area	Provide one per every two cardiac catheterization laboratories	7.5
Control room	Provide one per every two cardiac catheterization laboratories	16.8
Viewing room	Provide one per every two cardiac catheterization laboratories	9.3
Storage, equipment	Minimum one; provide an additional one if the total number of cardiac catheterization laboratories is greater than two	12.6
Supply room, sterile	Provide one per every two cardiac catheterization laboratories	9.3
Cardiac catheter instrument room	Provide one per cardiac catheterization laboratory	9.3
Cardiac catheter system component room	Provide one per every two cardiac catheterization laboratories	12.5
Equipment cleanup room	Provide one per every two cardiac catheterization laboratories	9.3
Digital quality control area	Provide one per cardiac catheterization laboratory	16.8
Digital archival storage room-PACS	Minimum NSF; provide an additional 10 NSF per diagnostic room greater than four	13.1
Housekeeping aids closet	Provide one per cardiac catheterization laboratory	3.8
Counseling	One per catheterization laboratory	30
Electrophysiology		
Sub-waiting	Provide an additional 15 NSF per projected exam/treatment room greater than three	3.7
Tilt table testing room	Provide one per cardiology suite	16.8
Pacemaker ICD interrogation	Provide one per cardiology suite	11.2
Storage, pacemaker equipment	Provide one per cardiology suite	5.6
Procedure room, electrophysiology	Divide the projected number of annual electrophysiology clinic stops by minimum workload to generate one room. Provide one room for each whole increment	37.2
Control and observation room	Provide one per EP procedure room	13.1
Echocardiography area		
Resting ECG rooms	Divide the projected number of annual ECG clinic stops by minimum workload to generate one room; provide one room for each whole increment	11.2
Holter fitting rooms/cubicles	Provide one per cardiology suite	11.2
Holter monitor workroom	Minimum NSF; provide an additional 80 NSF per each EKG technician FTE position authorized greater than two	14.9
Echocardiography rooms	Divide the projected number of annual echocardiograph clinic stops by minimum workload to generate one room; provide one room for each whole increment	13.1
Cubicle, dressing, echocardiograph	Provide one per echocardiograph room	3.3
Stress echocardiography rooms	Provide one per cardiology suite	18.6
Stress testing treadmill	Divide the projected number of annual stress test clinic stops by minimum workload to generate one room; provide one room for each whole increment and if stress testing is authorized	23.3

Contd...

Contd...

Room/Space	Requirement	Area in sqm
Cubicle, dressing, stress testing treadmill	One per stress testing treadmill	3.3
Storage, echocardiograph supplies	Provide one per cardiology suite	7.5
Transesophageal echocardiography rooms	Provide one per cardiology suite and if transesophageal echocardiograph procedures are authorized; provide an additional TEE room if the projected number of TEE procedure clinic stops is minimum workload to generate one room or greater	20.5
TEE recovery bay	Provide one per TEE Room	7.5
TEE scope wash room	Provide one per cardiology suite and if transesophageal echocardiograph procedures are authorized	9.3
Echocardiography reporting room	Minimum NSF; provide an additional 80 NSF for each echocardiograph room greater than two. Minimum NSF provides area for two workstations	14.9
Nuclear medicine room	Provide one per cardiovascular laboratories	
Operating theaters 63 m^2 (55–75)		
Perfusion preparation room	Provide one per cardiovascular operation theater	
Perfusion storage room	Provide one per cardiovascular operation theater	
Recovery area	Provide one per cardiovascular operation theater	
Equipment store	Minimum one; provide an additional one if the total number of cardiac catheterization laboratories is greater than two	12.6
Storage space and pump room	Provide one per cardiovascular operation theater	
Blood gas laboratory	Provide one per cardiovascular operation theater	
Support areas		
Utility room, clean	Provide an additional 20 NSF if total number of exam/treatment rooms is seven or eight; provide an additional 60 NSF if total number of exam/treatment rooms is greater than eight; maximum 160 NSF	9.3
Utility room, soiled	Minimum NSF; provide an additional 20 NSF if total number of exam/treatment rooms is between sixteen and thirty; provide an additional 40 NSF if total number of exam/treatment rooms is greater than 30; maximum 120 NSF The soiled utility room provides an area for cleanup of equipment, utensils and for disposal of waste material	7.4
Storage, stretcher/wheelchair	Provide two per cardiovascular laboratories	5.6
Alcove, crash cart	Provide one per cardiovascular laboratories	1.9
Storage, equipment	Provide one per cardiovascular laboratories	11.2
Housekeeping aids closet	Provide one per cardiovascular laboratories	3.8
Staff and administrative areas		
Office, chief of cardiology	Provide one cardiovascular laboratories	14.0
Office, secretary and waiting	Provide one per cardiovascular laboratories	14.0
Office, physician	Provide one per physician	11.2
Office, nurse manager	Provide one per nurse manager	11.2
Cubicle, nurse technician	Provide one per nurse technician	7.5
Cubicle, administration	Provide one per administrative position authorized	7.5
Patient records	Provide one if handling and storage of patient records is authorized	7.5
Copy room	Provide one per cardiovascular laboratories. This space is used for copier/fax/mail distribution	7.5
Storage, forms/literature	Provide one per cardiovascular laboratories	7.5
Conference room	Provide one per cardiovascular laboratories	27.9
Lounge, staff	Minimum NSF; provide an additional 15 NSF per each FTE position authorized greater than five; maximum 210 NSF	7.5
Locker room, staff	Minimum NSF if total number of clerical FTE positions authorized is between five and thirteen; provide an additional 6 NSF per technician FTE position authorized greater than thirteen; provide locker space only for those FTEs without assigned office or cubicle space	7.5
Toilet, staff	Minimum one; provide an additional staff toilet for each increment of five FTE positions authorized greater than fifteen	4.7
Miscellaneous		
Toilet, public	One per cardiovascular laboratories	4.7
Toilet, patient w/shower	One per cardiovascular suite and if stress testing treadmill is authorized	6.6
Toilet, patient	One per cardiovascular laboratories	4.7

[NSF: net square feet (area of usable space for furnishing, equipment and personnel)]

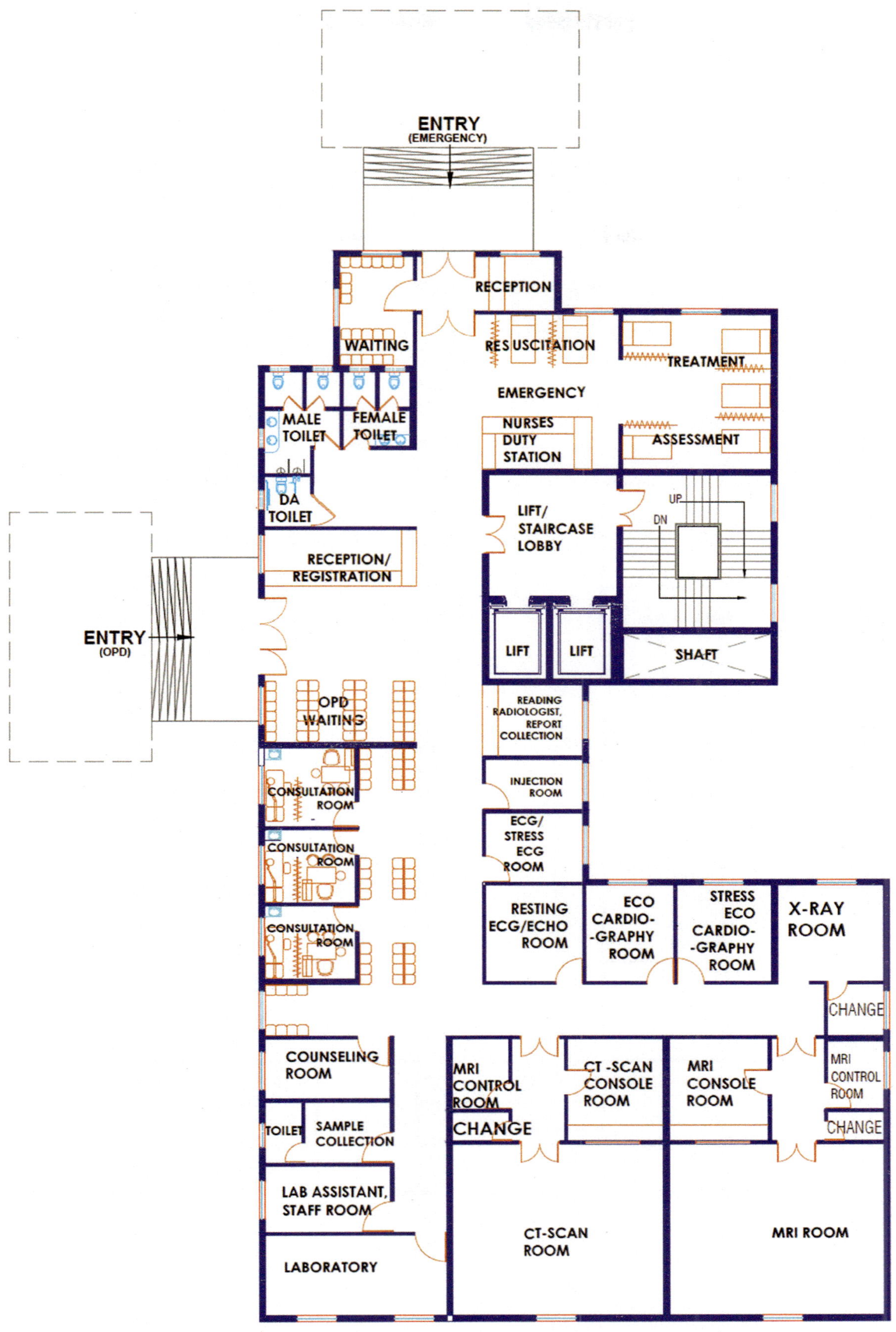

Fig. 12: Ground floor plan.
(DA: differently abled)

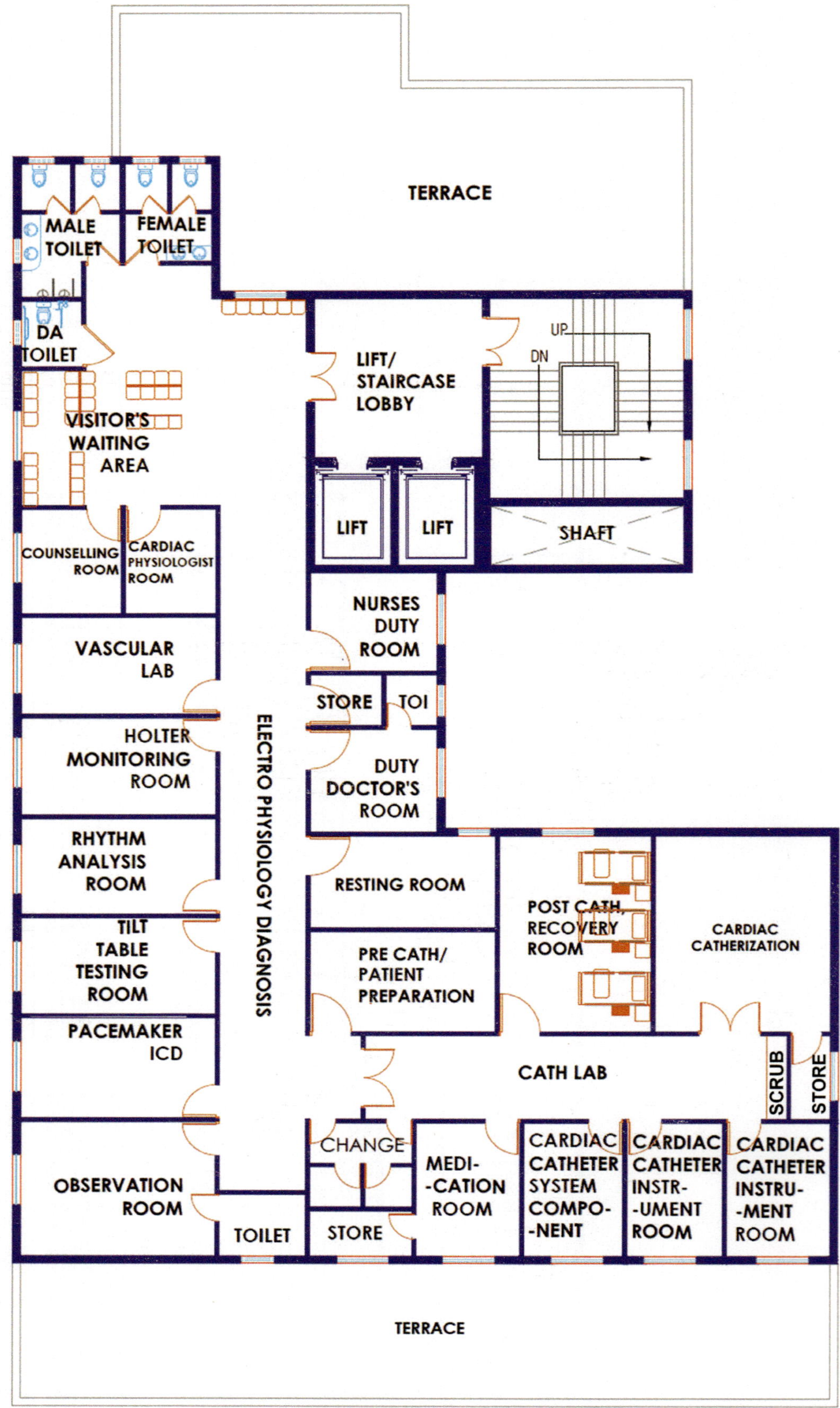

Fig. 13: First floor plan.
(DA: differently abled)

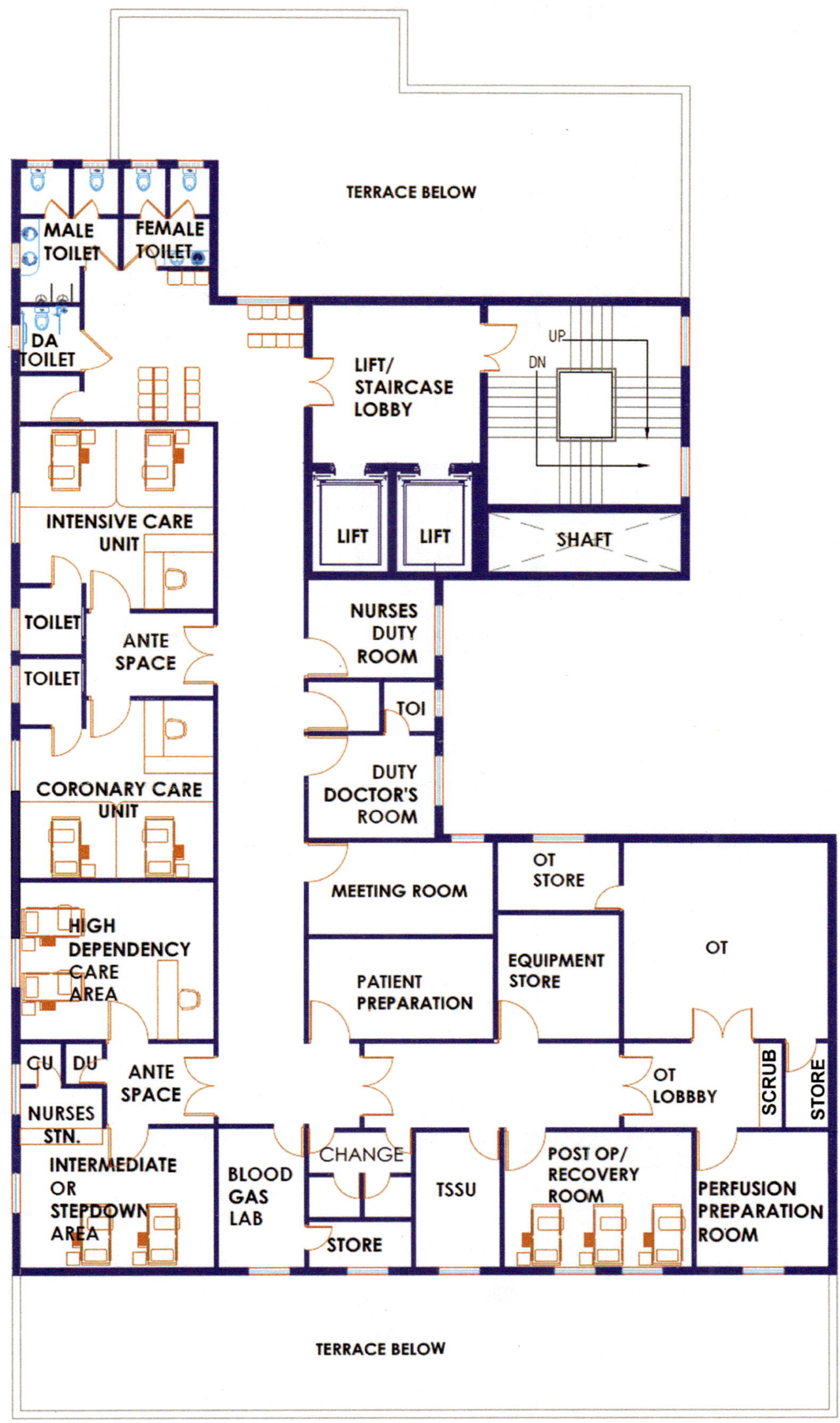

Fig. 14: Second floor plan.

(DA: differently abled; CU: clean utility; DU: dirty utility)

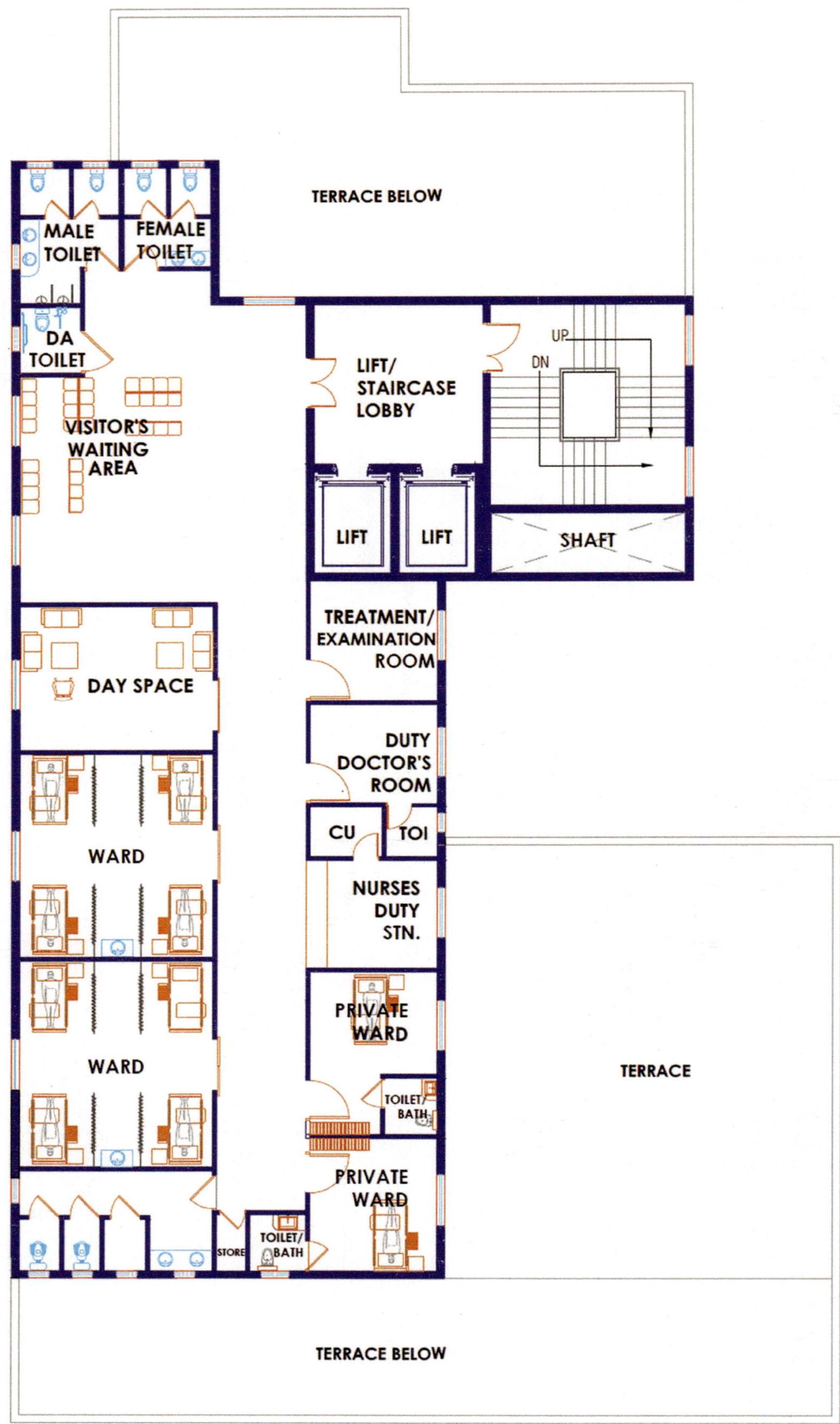

Fig. 15: Third floor plan.
(DA: differently abled)

CONCLUSION

Cardiothoracic and vascular center is a unique healthcare establishment, not because it pertains to a unique superspecialty, but because it caters to the needs of patients who need a unique care. Planning and designing should be done keeping this into consideration.

REFERENCES

1. www.hfs.scot.nhs.uk.
2. Scannell, J. "Optimal resources for cardiac surgery", The American Journal of Cardiology, 197511.
3. www. dph.state.il.us
4. www.rsconstruction.com
5. Popp RL, Fortuin NJ, Johnson ML, Kisslo JA Jr, Optimal resources for ultrasonic examination of heart. Circulation. 1982;65:423A-31.
6. Health Building Note 28. Facilities for cardiac services. 2006,pp. 19-21.
7. Pepine CJ, Allen HD, Bashore TM, Brinker JA, Cohn LH, Dillon JC, et al. ACC/AHA guidelines for cardiac catheterization and cardiac catheterization laboratories. Circulation. 1991;84:2213-47.
8. circ.ahajournals.org
9. HBN 28. Facilities for cardiac services; 2nd edn, 2006.
10. www.wbdg.org
11. "Practice of Medicine: Primary Care", Medical and Dental Space Planning, 2015.
12. www.dhsspsni.gov.uk
13. Scannel JG, Brown GE, Buckley JM, Ebert PA, Laufman H, Rackley CE, et al. Report of the Inter-Society Commission for Heart Disease Resources. Optimal resources for cardiac surgery: Guidelines for program planning and evaluation. Circulation. 1975;52:A 23-41.
14. "Design and Ventilation of Operating-room Suites for Control of Infection and for Comfort", The Lancet. 1962;1110.
15. Gupta SK, Kant S, Chandrashekhar R. Operating unit–planning essentials and design considerations. Journal of Academy of Hospital Administration. 2005;17:1-12.
16. Hambraeus, A.. "Protection of the patient in the operating suite", Journal of Hospital Infection, 1980.
17. www.cfm.va.gov.
18. www.ijaweb.org.

OTHER REFERENCES

- http://www.whc.int/cardiovascular_diseases/en
- Reddy KS. Cardiovascular diseases in India, World Health Stat Q. 1993;46:101.
- Singh RB, Sharma JP, Rastogi V, et al. Social class and coronary disease in rural population of north India. The Indian Social Class and Heart Survey. Eur Heart J. 1997;18:588.
- Working group on integrated prevention and control of cardiovascular diseases and diabetes (Kuala Lampur, Malaysia), 17–21 November, 1997.
- WHO. Technical Report. Serial No. 678;1982.
- Park JE. Park's Textbook of Preventive and Social Medicine, 19th edn. 2007. pp.303.
- Collis JL, D'Abreu AL, Clarke DB. Fundamental techniques in cardiac surgery. In: A practice of thoracic surgery, 3rd edn. Edward Arnold (publishers) Ltd; London. 1971.pp.291-2.
- Murray CJ, Lopez AD. The global burden of disease: A comprehensive assessment of mortality and disability from diseases, injuries, and risk factors in 1990 and projected to 2020. Cambridge, MA: Harvard University Press; 1996.
- Reddy KS. Cardiovascular disease in non-western countries. N Engl J Med. 2004;350:2438-40.
- O' Connor, Ramsay JG, Wynands JE, Kaplan JA. Anesthesia for myocardial revascularization. In: Kaplan JA, (Ed) Cardiac Anesthesia, 3rd edn. Sydney: WB Saunders. 1993.pp.587-613.

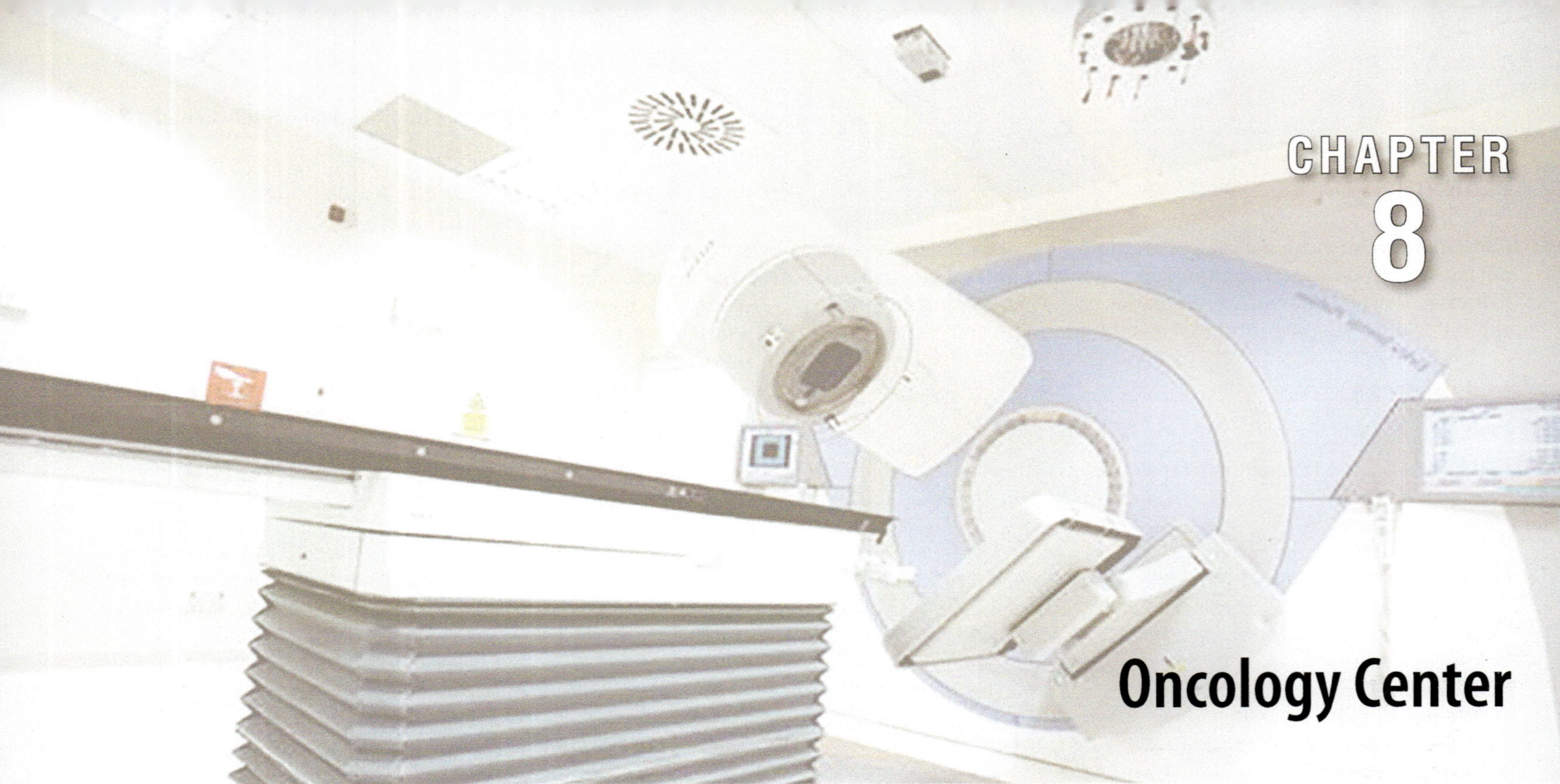

Oncology Center

AS Rana, Shakti Kumar Gupta, Sunil Kant, R Chandrashekhar

INTRODUCTION

Oncology center requires specific facility designing, because of complex nature of disease and complexity of treatment. Cancer patients require multidisciplinary treatment from medical oncology, surgical oncology and radiation oncology departments, etc. Besides this, diagnosis of disease requires special methods of investigations, to identify, to classify the type and severity of disease and spread of disease. Hence, to develop a cancer treatment (oncology) center special knowledge of disease process, diagnosis and treatment modalities is imperative and it requires the most appropriate physical space, equipment and trained manpower.

FUNCTION

Oncology center is expected to take comprehensive care of cancer patients like any other health organization in community which provides services of prevention, early diagnosis, treatment, disability limitation, and rehabilitation. Beside this education, training of different categories of health personnel, generation of data and research are important component of the organization. Cancer hospitals also provide palliative care and pain relief in the incurable and terminal cases.

KEY PLANNING AND DESIGN PARAMETERS

- Evidence-based design
- Healthy architecture
- Green architecture
- Intelligent building
- Ergonomically design building (Disabled friendly/physically handicapped)
- Barrier-free building
- Value-added services.
  - Embrace newer technology and innovation
  - Supportive patient and family friendly atmosphere
  - Operational efficiency
  - Design for future flexibility
  - Staff friendly
  - Minimize disruption during expansion construction.

Location and Building Planning

The location of the oncology center should have the following characteristics:

- Suitably/centrally located well connected with public transport.
- Provide safe and secure external and internal environment.
- Easy to locate, clearly visible from the approach road, with good directional signage from nearby major roads.
- Unhindered entrance, with visible, well-identified entrance, and a clear route from parking.
- Large enough to meet the present and projected demands.
- Enough space for parking.
- Place for night stay for visitors.
- Blending with culture and vernacular architecture.
- Provision for optimal utilization and recycling of natural resources.

Surgical and radiotherapy facilities are required hence

- Operation theater is to be planned in modular way with intraoperative radiotherapy measures.
- Gamma knife and cyber knife are advancement in radiation oncologist which requires amalgamation in onco-surgery.
- Radiotherapy is a modality of treatment which has to be planned as per Atomic Energy Regulatory Board (AERB) guidelines.[1]
- Disposal of radioactive waste is another necessity, which requires designing accordingly.

PLANNING CONSIDERATIONS

OPD Planning

Following design consideration should be taken into account:

- To be located at a place, which is readily approachable from main road and main entrance.
- Ambulance or any other patient vehicle should reach the alighting point
- Prevention of noise and pollution is to be considered in the planning.
- Outdoor garden and sufficient parking space to be provided.
- Patients with different degree of disability need special provisions in designing.
- Peak hour rush should be taken into consideration.
- It should be ensured that patient flow is in one direction, in a functional sequence and back flow of traffic must be regulated.
- Reception should be near the entrance, so that the first contact point is easily and conveniently reached.
- Privacy and dignity of the patient is to be maintained.
- Provision for expansion in future without hindrances in the routine work should be kept.
- All diagnostic facilities should be planned in such a way so that they are shared with inpatient department.
- Educational resources for patients and attendants should be displayed in waiting areas and lobbies.
- Functional areas should be designed in a way so as not to allow extraneous traffic. The flow of patients and visitors should be unilateral.
- Waiting areas and public spaces should be large enough to accommodate not only the patients but anticipated attendants.
- Subwaiting areas adjacent to various clinics, needs special consideration.
- Palliative and pain relief center/suite should be planned with OPD
- Natural light and good ventilation to be included in design.
- View of the outside from waiting areas to be considered in design.

Physical Facilities

The physical facilities to be planned are:

- Public area
- Clinical area includes consultation rooms, special procedures rooms, etc
- Administrative area
- Circulation area.

Public Area

Entrance

- Entrance should be easily accessible, with wide doors, ramps and steps.
- There should be a covered porch and sufficient space for parking ambulance or cars.
- The main entrance must have gentle sloping ramps with gradient of 15°–20°, steps and handrails should also be provided.
- All entrances must have provisions for geriatric and physically challenged persons.
- Entrance door should be double door with a width of 1.5 m, i.e. total width 3 m.
- Automatic opening doors fitted with sensors and dust catcher are important for keeping the OPD dust free.

Reception and Enquiry Desk Considerations

- Easily visible from front entrance and main waiting area.
- The height of the desk should be adapted to the need of the wheelchair patients.
- Each registration clerk requires 1.25 m length of reception counter with adequate drawers and shelves.
- An area of 6 sqm is recommended as minimum working space for each clerk, allowing for circulation behind the counter.
- Separate counters should be provided to ensure privacy of discussion between patients and reception staff.

Main Waiting Area

- It should be adjacent to consultation rooms.
- It should be larger than general hospital OPD area because cancer patients are generally accompanied by more than one attendant. Peak hours rush should be accommodated comfortably.
- Patients in wheelchair and trolleys require more space in waiting areas. Space recommended is 3.5–4 sqm area per patient.

Subwaiting Areas

- Recommended space is 0.8 sqm per patient for one-third of the average daily number of the patients attending OPD in one session. It should be shared between the various consultation rooms.
- A call system should be provided to direct the patients to appropriate rooms.
- Washrooms for male and female should be provided, one for each 200 users (patients and attendants). Space required is 12 sqm.
- Drinking water facility.

Value-added Service

- Coffee/tea and snack bar may be located near the waiting area
- Book and utility shop
- Telephone kiosks
- Prayer room.

Clinical Area

- Consulting rooms for surgery, obstetrics and gynecology, ENT, dental OPD and room for radiotherapist and medical oncologist.
- Number of OPD rooms depends on the workload, type of cancer prevalent in the community of that geographical area, and mandate of the hospital.
- Single consultation room with shared examination facility. It should accommodate doctor's chair, table, patients chair, patients trolley, or wheel chair, attendant's chairs, washbasin, examination couch and equipment for examination.
- For intercommunicating combined consulting and examination room, an area of 15 sqm is recommended for each room.
- For common examination room between two consulting room and more consulting rooms, size of each consulting room should be 12 sqm and size of examination room should be 9 sqm.
- Size should be little larger than the usual consulting room to provide the space for more number of attendants and trolleys/wheel chair, i.e. 15–20 sqm.
- Special equipment required in certain departments for examination needs separate space.

Counseling Rooms

- Counseling of the patients and their attendants regarding disease management.
- 20 sqm room should be planned to accommodate 10 people with comfortable sitting arrangement.

Ancillary Area in Clinical (Treatment) Area

Treatment, dressing and injection room should be planned. A waiting area for at least 20 people at a time to be planned. Usual norm is 0.6–0.8 sqm per patient.

Pharmacy and Store

- 3–4 drug distribution counters should be planned with a waiting area of 20 sqm for 20 people.
- A store area of 15–18 sqm attached to pharmacy counter should be planned. Cytotoxic drugs are hazardous and should be stored in locked and alarmed facilities. Cytotoxic drugs delivery and distribution is recommended not to use pneumatic tubes.

Procedure Room/Minor OT

- Minor OT of 40 sqm for small procedures like biopsy, FNAC, Pap smear, etc. should be planned.
- Includes shelves for storage of equipment and emergency drugs.
- A small 6–7 sqm anteroom for preparation with a bed should be planned.
- Injectable cytotoxic drugs for use in chemotherapy must be prepared in a dedicated pharmacy aseptic unit.

Auxiliary Area

- *Sample collection room*: It includes a central sample collection facility to collect urine, stool and blood. Blood collection room of 12–15 sqm with a couch, a chair with arm rest, technician chair, table with rack, drawer for keeping tubes, glass bulbs, requisition forms, etc. Routine examination facility should be attached to the OPD.
- A washroom and toilets separate for male and female to be provided of 12 sqm area each.

Medical Imaging Services

- It includes X-ray, ultrasonography, CT, MRI, and requires different sizes room with radiation safety measures
- Preparation room
- Common toilet
- Film processing room, and film storage room
- Radiologist room, computerized control station
- Report counter with office.

Blood Bank

These services are planned like in any other hospital. This needs space allocation in OPD block.

Health Education Facility, Medicosocial Services Facilities

These focuses on cancer related services and imparts education regarding the disease, preventive measures and availability of the treatment facilities. Space allocation should be done in the OPD area.

Administrative Areas

- Registration and information
- Cancer registry office and record room
- *Administrative office*: A room of 15–20 sqm for OPD administrator and assistant with computer facility
- Office for personnel section, requisitions, making reports and doing general correspondence
- Cash counter and accounts
- Housekeeping office
- Store for material
- Janitor closet for housekeeping and cleansing materials, size of 4 sqm to be planned
- Changing place and toilet of 10 sqm, for house keeping staff
- Storage area for OPD linen, general items and drugs to be created having 8 sqm space
- Nursing supervisors office
- Common room for nursing staff with attached toilets should be provided
- Beside these space required in OPD block to cater for.
  - Engineering services
  - Security services
  - Air handling units
  - Lifts/elevators
  - Ramps and stairs.

Table 1: HVAC requirements.

Parameters	*Specification*
Air pressure in relation to adjacent area	Positive
Minimum air changes	10
Relative humidity	45 ± 5%
Temperature °C	22 ± 2

Heating, Ventilation, and Air Conditions System (Table 1)

Refer Table 1.

Lighting

- Preferably natural light.
- Light of 300–500 lux, is recommended in examination room, corridors and facility light of 100 lux and waiting area of 200 lux.

KEY PLANNING AND DESIGN PARAMETERS[2]

The following are the main planning and design considerations:[2]

- Facilities and standards of care should be comparable to those provided to inpatients.
- Waiting areas should be separate from recovery and procedure area
- Patient bed spaces should be provided with suction, oxygen and nurse call facilities.
- All door widths should allow easy access for trolley bed/trolley transfer.
- Fittings and fixtures such as bed screens should ensure privacy and dignity to the patients.
- Arrangements should be made for about 10% of the patients to spend the night after the procedure/treatment under medical supervision.
- In daycare unit, dedicated and separate room for the storage, documentation and retrieval of clinical records should be planned
- Floors and wall finishes should be seamless, impervious. Flooring should be nonslippery.
- Intersections of walls and floors should be coved in continuous materials. Joints if any should be thermo-sealed.
- General and individual offices should be provided for administrative and professional staff, which should be away from public and patient area.

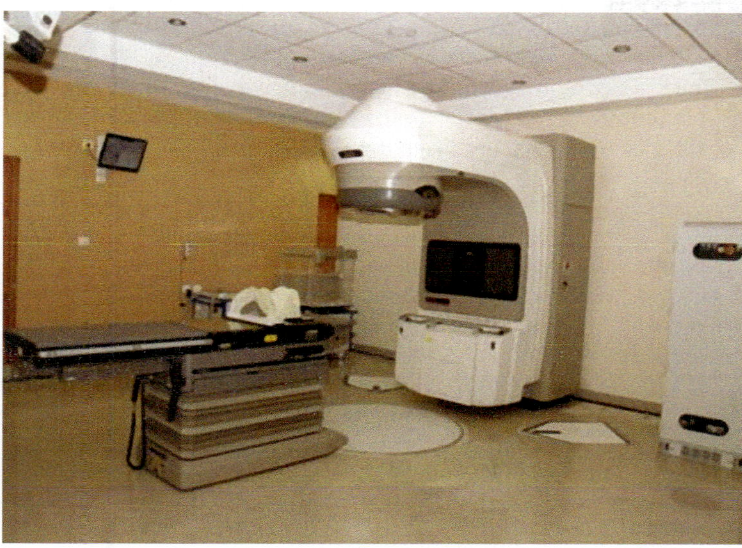

Fig. 1: Daycare treatment room.

Entry Area

- Wheelchair storage, reception and information counter should be planned
- Convenient access to waiting area and to public toilet facilities should be planned.

Treatment Rooms/Area (Fig. 1)

In a medical oncology daycare unit, treatment rooms/area should be provided for supervised administration of drugs. Facilities should be similar to preoperative holding or recovery area. Provision of dedicated chemotherapy facilities for children must be planned.

Preparation Room

Patients undergoing procedures, such as biopsy, endoscopy require space for preparation, equipment, bench and cupboards for sets of procedure, examination couch and screening (curtain) facility.

Recovery Areas

- For patients who have either undergone procedures with local anesthesia or *general anesthesia (GA)* but require further observations should be kept in recovery
- Changing facilities to be planned.

DAYCARE

Schedule of Accommodation of Daycare

Refer Table 2.

Table 2: Schedule of accommodation of daycare.

Room/Space	*Area in m²*
Space for 4 beds	28–30
Bays for hand washing	1
Bays for mobile equipment	4
Bays for trolley	2
Change cubicle for patients	2
Change cubicle for disabled patients	5
Clean utility	12
Dirty utility	10
Office	8
Operating room (minor)	36
Treatment room/area	9
Recovery area	
Patient holding	9
Recovery room	9
Staff station in recovery area	14
Store for equipment	9–20 sqm
Store for linen	2
Store for general items	9
Cleaners room	4
Toilet for patients with change facilities	4
Circulation area	35%
Staff and support areas	
Consultation room	12
Interview room	9
Waiting (depending on size of facility)	6–18 sqm
Toilets staff	2
Reception	10
Office work station	6
Office single person	9–12 sqm
Office shared by 2 persons	12
Shared areas	
Change room—staff	8–10 sqm
Disposal room	8
Meeting room	20
Parameters	Specification
Air pressure in ward	Positive
Minimum air changes ward and other area	8–10
Relative humidity	45 ± 5%
Temperature °C	22 ± 2
Pressure in OT	Positive
Minimum air changes OT	15
Filtration efficiency	HEPA filter
Light OT	1,00,000–1,40,000 lux
Light ward	300 lux
Doctors examination room	500 lux

PLANNING OF RADIODIAGNOSIS AND RADIOTHERAPY DEPARTMENT (FIG. 2)

Areas

There should be proper demarcation of work areas for each activity. Approximate space requirement should be proposed on the basis of the information available about the number of equipment, work load, available resources, and type of equipment planned.

Patient waiting area, reception, changing room and toilets should be planned.

Circulation area: 35% of the planned area of treatment area.

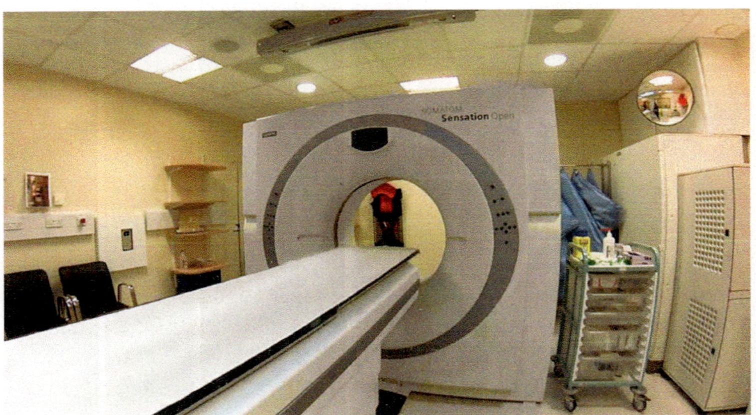

Fig. 2: Radiodiagnosis.

Administrative area: It includes record room, reporting area, conference room, staff room with toilets and library.

Technical area: It includes consultant room, equipment rooms, film and other stores.

Space for Patient Area

Subwaiting for patients with their attendants, and separate waiting area for patients on trolleys and wheelchair should be created. 1.3 sqm per patient norms are suggested but space requirement may increase due to attendants.

Circulation Area

The corridors should be 2.4 m wide to facilitate patient movement, including those on stretchers/wheelchairs.

Dressing room for staff and patients with toilets should be planned separately with good ventilation, lighting, mirror cloth hooks, closets, chairs and benches as per requirement.

Administrative Area

Offices of consultants, registration areas, rooms for technical staff with toilets, stores, maintenance staff of engineering.

Technical Area

Space for X-ray room facility:

- The size of X-ray rooms will depend upon the capacity and type of the equipment to be installed
- Approximately 40 sqm (length 6.7, width 5.8 m and height 3.3 m)
- Door opening 1.5 m
- A lead glass window or screen should be planned between X-ray machine and control panel
- It also requires cassette changing window
- Digital X-ray machine preferred.

Related Area in X-ray Department

Film auto processor area and film storage area:

Recommended protective shielding in X-ray department:[3]

- A standard poured concrete wall of about 12 cm is needed. The recommendation for wall thickness for radiation protection is based on a minimum X-ray room size. Calculate the desired thickness of material on the basis of total radiation exposure of 150 milli amperes minutes a week at 100 kV.
- Thickness would be required to provide a lead equivalent of 1 mm. If cinder blocks or bricks are used, a thickness of about 12–15 cm will be required depending upon the density of the material actually used, i.e

  (Thickness of concrete) × (2.35 g/cubic cm) =
  thickness × density (of similar material)[3]
- Within the X-ray room, two specific high-risk areas are: the wall behind chest stand which is protected by concrete wall thickness of 20 cm and the wall of the dark room, protected by 10 cm concrete thickness.
- If the X-ray unit is properly positioned, i.e. X-ray beam should not point at the wall of the dark room.
- The design should incorporate the shielding of control panel area. There should be a shield of 1 mm lead equivalent, at least 75 cm wide in front of the control panel and extending 50 cm on either side.
- It should be 2 m in height and should have a glass window with at least 1 mm lead equivalent (25 × 25 cm in size) situated in the central panel at the eye level, for visualization by operator. The patient should wear lead protective clothing.
- The windows should be provided at 1.5 m height from the floor for light and ventilation and persons restricted access within 1 m of window.

GUIDING PRINCIPLE FOR X-RAY ROOM LAYOUT

- *Location*: Ideally X-ray room should be located on ground floor and should be conveniently accessible from outpatient as well as in patient area.
- Functional needs are best served by locating X-ray room at the end of wing so that activities within the department are undisturbed by traffic to other parts of the center.
- Storage area, require approximately 2 sqm space.
- If digital X-ray facility is planned appropriate amendments will be required.

SCHEDULE OF ACCOMMODATION FOR MEDICAL IMAGING UNIT[2]

Digital Radiography and Fluoroscopy (Table 3)

Fluoroscopy Room

- *Dimension*: 6 × 3 m
- *Ceiling height*: 3 m
- *Attached toilet*: 4 sqm.

HVAC

Refer Table 4.

CT/MRI UNIT

CT Scanning

Functional Areas

The functional areas include the following:[2]

Table 3: Radiography and fluoroscopy room.

Room/Space	Area in m^2
General X-ray room	38–42
Film storage	25
Film processing (for daylight processing)	10–30
Dark room	8–10
Dirty utility	10
Clean utility	12
Reception	10
Reporting room	10–30
Store	10–15
Toilet for patient	4
Toilet for disabled persons	5
Computer processing area	50
Fluoroscopy preparation/storage	10
Fluoroscopy viewing	10
Fluoroscopy imaging	40
Patient change room	2
Hand washing	1
Staff and support areas	
Office single person (depending on staffing establishment)	9–12
Office (4 person shared)	20
Shared areas	
Staff room (depending on staffing establishment)	15–20
Toilet staff	2
Waiting (depending on patient load)	20–45
Meeting room	20–30

Table 4: HVAC.

Parameters	Specification
Air pressure in relation to adjacent area	Positive
Minimum air changes	10
Relative humidity	45 ± 5%
Temperature °C	22 ± 2

- *CT imaging room*: Area requirement is in the range of 38–42 sqm. The room should be located adjacent to the CT control room. There should be clinical scrub facilities adjacent to the room.
- *CT console room*: It accommodates the computer and other controls for the equipment. A viewing window permitting full view of the patient should be provided.
- The room should be located with direct access to the CT imaging room and ready access to film processing areas. Area requirement is 6–8 sqm.
- *CT computer room*: It provides area for the computer and generator modules associated with the CT scanning equipment and should be located adjacent to the CT scanning and console room. The area required is about 6 sqm.
- *Scrub up/Gowning area*: An area of about 6–8 sqm is required.
- *Patient holding areas*: A patient bay of approx 9 sqm is required for holding/recovery. Two bays per scanning room are recommended.
- *Patient toilet and change facilities*: An approximate area of 4 sqm is required. Other areas, which should be planned, include staff change and toilet facilities and storage. Circulation area of about 35% should be provided.

MAGNETIC RESONANCE IMAGING (FIG. 3)

Functional Areas (Table 5)[2]

MRI computer room: This is to accommodate the computer equipment. Recommended space is 40–50 sqm. The room should be located adjacent to the MRI scanning and console room.

MRI console room: This is required to accommodate the computer and other controls of the equipment. There should be a window to provide full view of the MRI room. A minimum space of 10 sqm is recommended. It should be located with direct access to the MRI scanning room.

MRI MACHINES

The other areas required along with the recommended space requirements are as follows:

Shared areas: If MRI is provided as a freestanding unit, following facilities will have to be provided as additional requirement.

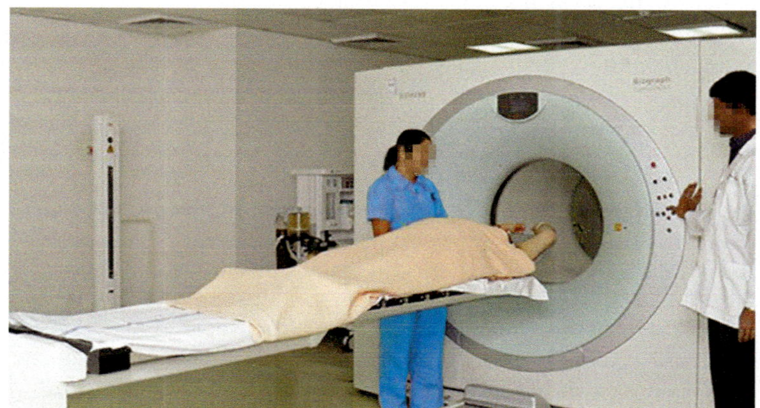

Fig. 3: Magnetic resonance imaging.

Table 5: MRI room.

Areas	Recommended space requirements in m^2
Patient bay	9
Office for single person (depending on staffing)	9
Hand washing bay (many may be required)	1
Anesthesia induction (optional)	15
Toilet for patients	4
MRI room	40–50
Console room	35
MRI computer room	10
Reception	10
Waiting	12
Film storage	8–12
Clean utility	12
Dirty utility	10
Linen bay	2
Trolley bay	3
Toilet for staff	4
Locker room for staff	6
Circulation space	35%

RADIATION PROTECTION[4]

If radiology rooms are isolated and built so that people cannot come within 1 m of its outside walls, no protection to walls is required. However, as this is not always possible, the walls of the rooms where radiographic machines are located have to be adequately reinforced.

Basis of Calculation of Wall Thickness

The unit of measurement used for this purpose is "mA second", which is the product of the current flowing through the X-ray tube and the duration of exposure.

- For a 100 mA machine, a wall thickness equivalent to 1 mm of lead is required
- 1 mm to lead thickness
  - = 12 cm of poured concrete
  - = 10 cm of sheet glass
  - = 5 mm of steel

- The appropriate wall thickness using different materials can be calculated using the following equation.

  Thickness of concrete × 2.35 g/cm^3 Thickness of other material × Density of other material

KEY PLANNING AND DESIGN PARAMETERS[2]

This facility is a part of radiodiagnosis, required by many clinical departments, should be located at a place where it can be easily accessible from OPD, in patient and at the same time radiation safety is required.

Special provision must be adhered to as per recommendations of regulatory authorities for storage and disposal of radioactive substances. Supporting spaces have to be planned such as:

- 'Hot' lab where radiopharmaceuticals are prepared having lead lined containers and refrigerators, exhaust radioisotope and approved system for radioactive waste collection and disposal.
- Dose room where patients are injected with radiopharmaceuticals.
- Flooring should meet load requirements for equipment.
- Floors and walls should be constructed of materials that are easily decontaminated in case of accidental radioactive spills.
- Walls should have provision of vents of radioactive gases as well as medical gases and vacuum.
- Provision for wiring, ducts or conduits should be made in floors, walls and ceilings.

PET Camera Room (Fig. 4)

A size of approximately 40 sqm is recommended. Ceiling height recommended is 3 m.

The following design parameters should be considered for the room:

- Room lighting should be controllable and glare-free.
- Floor should be antistatic.
- Floor should be structurally suited to bear the weight of the equipment, which may exceed 3,000 kg.
- Provision should be made for medical gases, medical air and suction.
- Visibility between camera and control rooms should be ensured.

PET Control Room (Fig. 5)

It provides for the computer and control for the positron emission tomography (PET) equipment. It should be of minimum of 10 sqm[2].

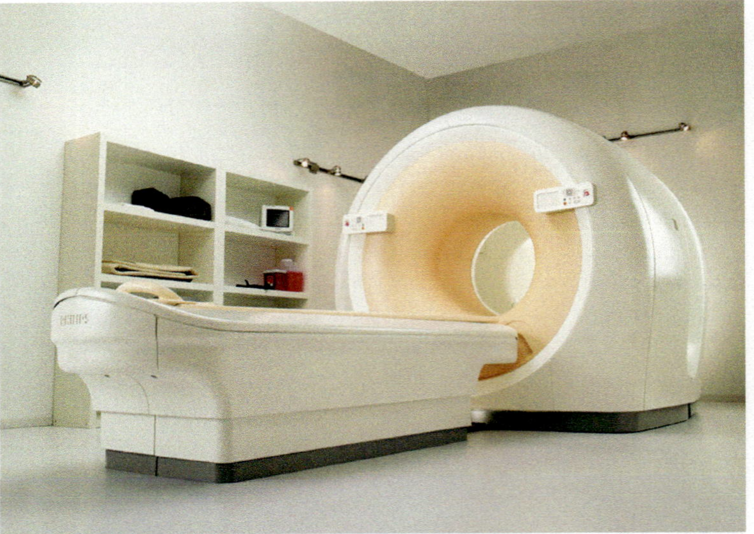

Fig. 4: Positron emission tomography scan.

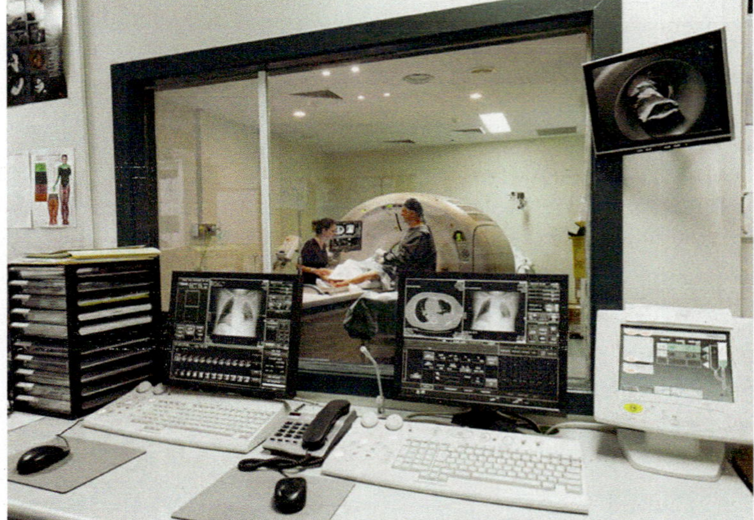

Fig. 5: Positron emission tomography scan control room.

Preparation Room

- It is required for preparing radiopharmaceuticals and injecting patients.
- It should have ready access to patient waiting areas and laboratories.
- It should be minimum 12 sqm and the room would require working benches and hand basin.
- A subwaiting area with chairs and provision for wheelchairs is required for patients who have received an injection of imaging agent and are awaiting the scanning procedure.
- The area requires radiation protection screening as the imaging agents emit a low level radiation.
- The toilet used by patients injected with radiopharmaceuticals should have a radiation shielding. The disposal is connected to delay tank before it is discharged to sewer line.

Waiting Areas

- A patient bay area is required for patients on beds/trolleys who have received an injection of imaging agent and are awaiting the scanning procedure.

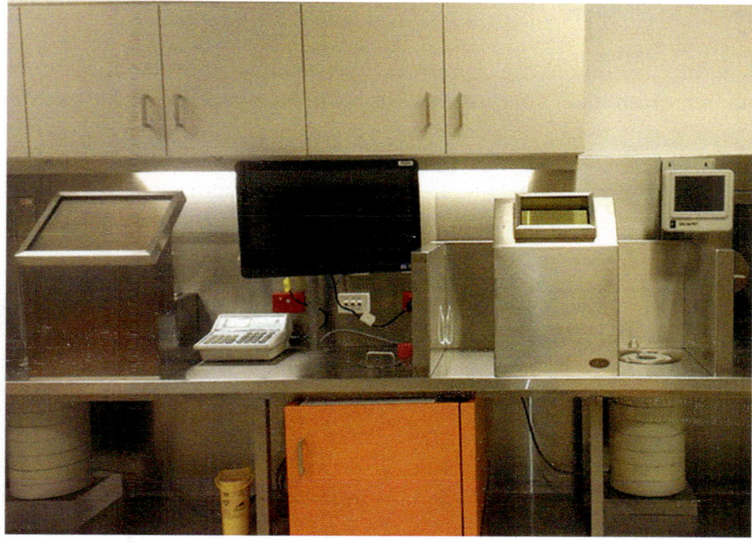

Fig. 6: Hot laboratory.

- Radiation protection screening will be required since the imaging agents emit radiation. Area recommended is 10–12 sqm.

Hot Laboratory (Fig. 6)

- It would require laboratory benches and also radiation protection. An area of 20 sqm is recommended.
- The storage and disposal from this room should be as per the recommendation of concerned statutory authority.

Quality Control Laboratory

It would require laboratory work stations, sink and radiation protection. An area of 10 sqm is recommended.

Disposal of Liquid Waste through Delay Tanks

The liquid radioactive waste (Effluent of patients admitted in isolation room) is disposed through special sanitary sewage system that connects the isolation room to the delay tank. The passage designed is to be smooth to prevent any logging in pipes. More water is poured with each flash to dilute the effluent. The effluent is stored in delay tank for a period of ten half-lives of the isotope having maximum half life. There are two delay tanks with sufficient capacity to hold the waste for more than 3 months. These tanks are used turn wise so as to allow maximum time for decay before discharge into normal sewage system. The delay tank is checked for radioactivity before final discharge.

KEY ISSUES

The following should be ensured:

- Radiation protection
- Sink and floor drain
- Dedicated three phase power supply
- Chilled water supply
- Compressed air supply
- Gas bottle storage
- Air conditioning with filtered exhaust system and negative pressure selective to the surrounding area. Structural requirements for weight bearing since weight of the cyclotron and ancillary equipment is 40,000 kg (40 tons).

Cyclotron Control Room (Fig. 7)

It is required for the user to control the operation of the cyclotron.

The room would require a minimum of 10 sqm. It should have direct access to the cyclotron room. The other areas required for PET are (Table 6).

HVAC

Same as MRI/CT scan.

SPECIFICATIONS FOR THE LAYOUT OF RADIOTHERAPY FACILITY

To establish a radiotherapy facility, the user institution must go through the regulatory requirements as mentioned in the Atomic Energy (Radiation Protection) Rules, 2004 and AERB Safety Codes (AERB/SC/MED-1 and 3). No regulatory clearance is issued for establishing the radiotherapy facility by AERB, unless the user complies with the

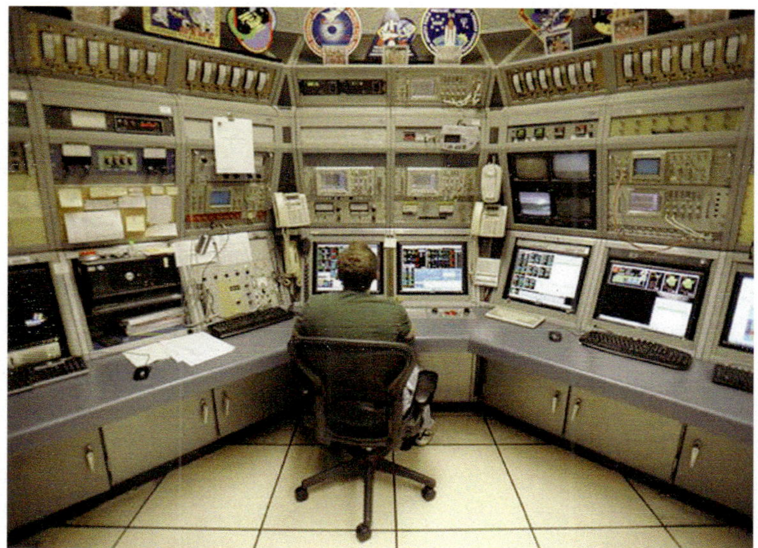

Fig. 7: Cyclotron control room.

Table 6: Positron emission tomography area.

Room area	*Recommended areas in m^2*
Anesthetic induction—room (optional)	15
Bay hand washing	02
Office single person (many may be required)	09
Circulation area	35%
Shared areas	
Clean utility	12
Dirty utility	10
Preparation room	12
Reception	10
Staff station	14
Store	12
Mobile equipment	04
Toilet for staff	02
Waiting (for non-injected patients and visitors)	15
X-ray imaging and reporting	12

regulatory requirements, specified in these documents. The first step to establish a radiotherapy facility is to submit the layout plan of the radiation installation and get it approved from AERB from radiation safety standpoint. It is advisable to take services of experienced radiation oncologists, medical physicists, the supplier of radiotherapy equipments and architects to prepare the layout plan of the radiotherapy facility. *The room layout plans (to scale 1:50) and the site layout plan (to scale 1:500) must be prepared and sent along with the filled in Performa AERB/RSD/RT/PLAN to the Head, Radiological safety Division, Atomic Energy Regulatory Board for approval.*[5]

Plan Approval

It is recommended to prepare the layout drawings (to scale) as per the standard layouts prepared by this Division and submitted to the *Head, Radiological Safety Division, AERB* for approval. The standard layouts are prepared based on typical workload for various facilities and for full occupancies around the installation from radiation safety standpoint. The standard layouts are advantageous as they allow structures to be built in future around the installations without any modification.

Site Selection

The location of the radiotherapy installation should be so chosen that it is away from unconnected facilities and is close to the related facilities such as Simulator Room, Mould Room, Patient Waiting Area, Treatment Planning System Room, Radiation Oncologist(s) Room, Medical Physicist(s) Room, etc.

Construction Material

The construction material to be used for radiotherapy room should be concrete of density 2.35 g/cc. However, where structural requirements so demand, RCC may be used. In case hematite concrete is used, the thicknesses may be reduced in inverse proportion to the ratio of the densities.

Viewing System

For observing the patient under treatment and the gantry movement from the control room (in case of teletherapy) appropriate viewing system must be provided. This can be achieved by providing closed circuit TV system (CCTV). In addition a backup arrangement must be made, which can be achieved by either having a spare CCTV or by using mirrors and an observation window of appropriate dimensions and at a convenient height from the floor must be provided in the door interlocked door for observing the patient conveniently from the operator's position.[3]

Conduit

A conduit of 5 cm diameter should be provided in the wall to enable cables of radiation measuring instruments to pass through from the control room to the treatment room. The conduit should be fixed in the specified wall at an angle between 20° and 45° to the horizontal. The lower end of the conduit should be located in the treatment room at a height between 15 cm and 20 cm from the inside finished floor level. Any conduit required in the maze wall can be parallel to the floor at a height of 15–20 cm from treatment floor level.[3,6]

Door Interlock

The door leading to the treatment room may be an ordinary wooden door of width 1500 mm. This door should be so interlinked to the control panel by electrical interlocks that the unit cannot be operated when the door is open. The door opening to control room, which is provided to keep the control panel as well as the treatment room secured, may be a collapsible grill door or any other type as per requirement.[3,6]

Air-conditioning

The treatment room should be air-conditioned. In case central air-conditioning is to be provided in the radiation therapy room, the ducts for central air conditioning should be taken along the wall of the entrance door and left at the desired location without making any opening on any wall. In case split air conditioners are to be provided in the radiation therapy room, conduits of minimum diameter consistent with the requirement and making an angle between 20° and 45° with the horizontal should be provided. The opening of these conduits in the treatment room should be at a height about 1.5 m from the floor of treatment room. The details may be finalized in consultation with AC Engineers. Although it is not common nowadays, if window air-conditioning is to be provided in the radiation therapy room, it must be provided on the secondary walls (not on the primary wall) in case of teletherapy installation. Moreover, the lower end of the openings should be located at a minimum height of 250 cm from the floor level outside and should further be covered with a baffle arrangement. The thickness of the baffle must not be less than 30 cm of concrete and width of the baffle and the length of its vertical portion should be such that 30-cm wide overlap is available all around the openings. The dimensions should be the minimum required for fixing the air-conditioners. The length may be decided in consultation with the firm installing the air conditioners and should be such as to permit efficient functioning of the air conditioners. In the case of accelerator installations special ventilation arrangements are required. It is desirable that the control room is also air-conditioned. Air conditioners for the control room may be located anywhere in its brick walls as per convenience. However, central air conditioning is recommended.[3]

Warning Lights

A red warning light should be provided above the interlocked door and should be so interlinked to the control panel that the light glows when the source is in the 'ON' position.[5]

Other Requirements

Electrical ducting requirements and also any pit, load specifications, conduit, etc., should be decided in consultation with the firm installing the unit, before commencement of the actual construction work.

Construction Restraints

It may be necessary for the installation of the unit that some portion of the wall or ceiling be constructed after bringing the crates carrying the unit into the treatment room. This may be decided in consultation with the firm installing the unit. It may also be ensured from the supplier of the unit before starting construction work that the maze/labyrinth provided in the drawing is adequate for the movement of the various components of the radiotherapy unit with or without crates.[3]

Associated Facility

Associated and supporting facilities of the radiation therapy department include simulator room, treatment planning system room and mould room doctors' room, physicists' room, examination room, etc. relative to the radiotherapy room. The institution must show all these facilities in the installation site plan.

Ramp

In case of Telecobalt installations, a ramp may be provided in close proximity to the teletherapy installation to facilitate easy movement of the crates carrying the unit to the teletherapy room. The ramp is also useful in future during source replacement operation, which is to be carried out once in every 5–7 years. For this work, a new cobalt-60 source is brought in a transport container weighing 2–3 tons. This container is to be unloaded from a truck and taken into the telecobalt room. The height and slope of the ramp should be so adjusted that the transport container can be unloaded with ease from the truck and transported into the teletherapy room on a suitable trolley.[3]

Beam Stopper

In certain instances, it is difficult to meet the shielding requirements of a teletherapy installation due to structural and space constraints. This situation may arise when (i) a teletherapy unit is to be installed in an existing room, (ii) a stationary telecobalt unit in an existing installation is to be replaced by a rotational telecobalt unit, or (iii) a telecobalt unit is to be replaced by an accelerator. Installing a teletherapy unit with a beam stopper can circumvent this difficulty. The beam stopper completely intercepts the primary beam and reduces its intensity approximately by a factor of 1000 and thereby decreases the shielding requirements for the primary barrier.[3]

Starting Construction Work

The institution should undertake no construction work unless the institution has duly obtained prior approval of AERB for the specific layout of the installation.

RADIOTHERAPY UNIT PLANNING

Spaces common to all activities include:[1,7]

- *A registration area*: An area should be designated for clerical staff to make bookings and register new patients, sign in patients under treatment and retrieve files for follow-up patients.
- Office space for physicians and physicists.
- *Laboratories*: a physics laboratory with cabinet space to store phantoms, ionization chambers, electrometers, cables and film should be available. If thermo-luminescent dosimetry (TLD) and film dosimetry are available, an area should be designed for these activities.
- A darkroom, the darkroom should be located conveniently near the simulator, external beam therapy and brachytherapy activity rooms.
- *A filing room*: a file storage area should be provided sufficient for long-term storage of documentation.
- Space to provide air conditioning for the entire facility; a minimum, air conditioning should be provided for the treatment rooms, planning room and the treatment control areas where computers are located.

PLANNING OF TELETHERAPY FACILITY OR EXTERNAL BEAM THERAPY (FIG. 8)

An External Beam Facility Requires

- Examination rooms
- Waiting areas
- Doctor's room
- Physicist's room
- Mould room
- Simulator room
- Treatment planning room
- Treatment room (bunker)
- Simulator room, treatment-planning room and treatment room should be designed in consultation with the manufacturer of the equipment[1]
- The requirements for power, air conditioning, monitoring ports and emergency system should be incorporated in the design.[8]

Site Selection

- An ideal site is such that it is away from unconnected facilities and is close to the related facility such as simulator room, treatment planning system room, mould room, doctor's room, physicist's room, examination room, patients waiting hall, etc.[3]
- For selected site approval should be obtained from AERB.
- The location of the teletherapy room should be such that it has open areas on two sides to avoid the radiation exposures to the members of the public and others not involved in radiation work.
- The installation should preferably be on the ground floor, or in the basement taking into account the load considerations vis-à-vis the weight of the teletherapy unit (app. 6 tons) and the weight of the transport flask (app. 2 tons) during each source replacement.
- Ground floor level at one end of the corridor or as an independent wing.

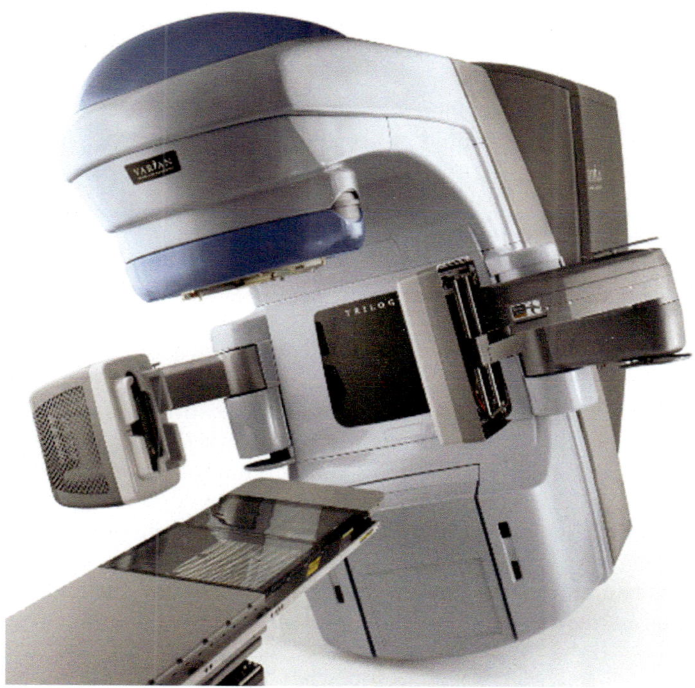

Fig. 8: External beam therapy.

- Installation of the unit in the basement should also be considered if it is cost-effective taking into account the other parameters, such as water seepage air conditioning requirements, etc.

Examination rooms: The examination rooms should be in close proximity to the treatment room and should include:[1]

- Standard table
- Gynecological examination table
- Head and neck examination chair
- Appropriate examination instruments and medical supplies.

Waiting Areas

- There should be separate waiting areas for patients attending clinical visits and those awaiting treatment. The clinical waiting area should have space for approximately eight patients for each physician.[12]
- The treatment waiting area should be adjacent to the treatment room with space for seating of about twelve people for each machine.[12]
- There should also be an area provided for stretcher patients. This area should be adjacent to the treatment area but preferably separated from the ambulatory patients. The area should be large enough to accommodate three stretchers.

Simulator Room[1,5]

- The shielding of the simulator room shall be designed according to the recommendations of AERB, paying due regard to the requirements of the BSS (Basic Safety Standards, an IAEA publication giving requirements for radiation safety) and the regulatory authority.
- The room should be large enough to accommodate the simulator, allowing the full range of motion of the treatment table.
- A means for securely mounting the patient positioning lasers to the wall at points appropriate for projection of lines through the isocenter should be included in the plans.
- A means for dimming the room lights should be considered in the design of the room.
- Adequate space should be planned for cabinetry; to store treatment devices and daily used quality assurance equipment.
- If the immobilization devices are to be fabricated in the simulator room, cabinet space to store supplies for their fabrication should be planned.
- A sink should be provided in this room.
- A viewing window should be provided for the control room.

EQUIPMENT FOR EXTERNAL BEAM RADIOTHERAPY (FIG. 9)

Area Requirements

The dimensions of the teletherapy room are dependent on:

- The unit specifications such as the size of the unit, the couch movement space required for rotation of the arm and servicing of the unit, easy maneuverability during source loading operation, etc. A typical plan for housing a cobalt rotational teletherapy unit (12,000 RHM) is shown in the drawing.
- The entry passage width should be decided by the easy movements of the crates carrying the unit during installation and transport flask containing the source during every source-loading operator.
- The easy maneuverability of the non-ambulatory patients.

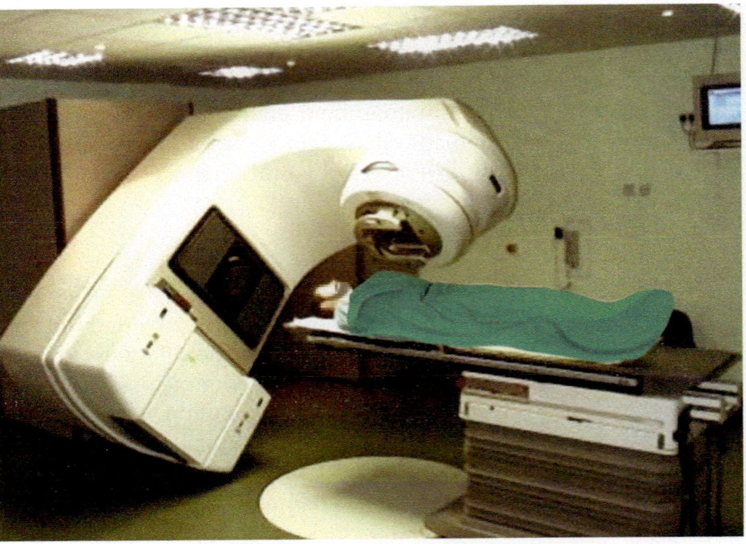

Fig. 9: External beam radiotherapy.

SPACE PLANNING FOR SIMULATOR COBALT 60 LINAC (FIG. 10)

Minimum size should be as follows:

- Simulator room—25 sqm
- Accelerator rooms—65 sqm
- Cobalt rooms—45 sqm.

Treatment Planning Room[1,8]

- The treatment planning room should be located in close proximity to the simulator room, although the two areas do not have to be adjacent.
- The room should be large enough to house the treatment-planning computer with its video monitor, a printer and plotter, a digitizer tablet and other required computer equipment.
- Space planning should be done for supplies of paper and pens or ink for the printer and plotter.
- An area designed to accommodate an L-shaped arrangement of the digitizer tablet and video monitor is frequently more desirable than a linear arrangement with the two devices side by side.
- Space for light boxes and a high intensity light for viewing CT scans and plane X-ray films should be planned.
- In larger centers, more than one computer video terminal should be planned.
- *Mould room*: Making immobilization, shielding and shaping devices for RT patients.
- Space should be planned for a mould room to fabricate custom designed blocks and compensators.
- Space for tools, a block cutter and counter-top workspace for pouring and mounting the blocks is required.
- Storage space for supplies of styrofoam, trays and shielding material for custom blocking is necessary. Adequate ventilation should be provided if shielding materials are melted in this area.
- If immobilization devices are fabricated in the mould room, space for a patient couch should be planned.

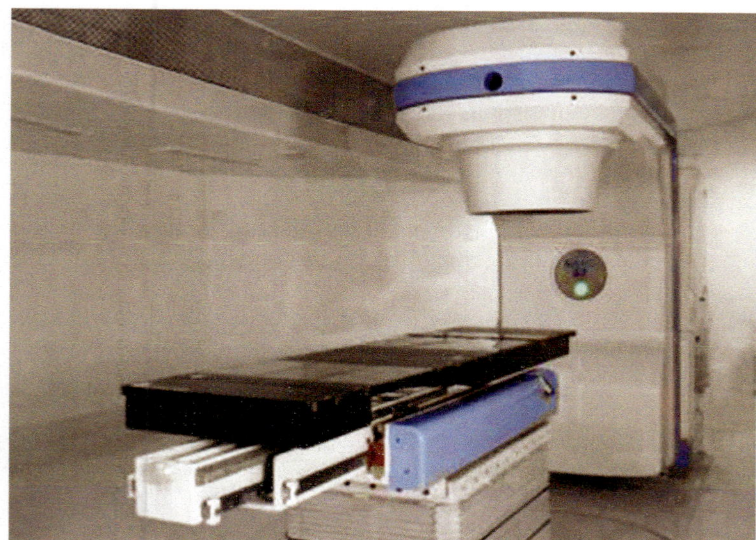

Fig. 10: Cobalt-60 linac.

- A sink with a refuse trap and churner should be fixed in this room, as plaster of Paris is frequently utilized.

TREATMENT ROOM OR EQUIPMENT ROOM

- The room should be large enough to accommodate the treatment machine, allowing the full range of motion of the treatment table. If total body irradiation (TBI) is planned, a larger treatment room is required.[7]
- A door interlock or other suitable means to prevent unauthorized access should be planned.[7]
- A sign should be posted at the entrance warning of the radiation hazard, in accordance with regulatory authority requirements.[10]
- For a 60-Co unit, an area radiation monitor safe against a power failure should be visible on entering the room.
- A means for dimming the room lights should be planned in the design of the room.[7]
- Adequate space should be planned for cabinetry, to store treatment devices, immobilization devices, blocks and daily used quality assurance equipment.[7]
- A means for secure mounting of patient positioning lasers to the wall at points appropriate for projection of lines through the isocenter should be included in the plans.[1,7]
- A heavy electrically operated door at the entrance to the room or an alternative to this is an appropriately designed extended corridor (called a maze) leading into the room should be planned.[7]
- At the entrance to the maze, a lightweight physical barrier or an optical barrier with appropriate interlocks should be erected. (The design of such a barrier should take into account the need to detect the passage of a child.) This has the advantage of allowing rapid access to the treatment room in the event of a power cut. However, the maze will take up additional space.[7]
- Space for a console immediately outside the treatment area overlooking the treatment room door should be planned. This console area should be large enough to accommodate not only the control console for the unit but also a source storage and preparation room, operating room, treatment planning room and patient room.

These facilities should not be too widely separated, in order to reduce distances over which patients and sources have to be transported. The relative proximity of these facilities can significantly influence procedure flow and efficiency.[7]

- Facility design should incorporate features to avoid transport in elevators of patients containing radioactive sources (separate elevators for materials).
- Sterilization facilities for applicators should be incorporated in the planning. The sterilization process should be appropriate to prevent damage of the applicators.

Teletherapy Unit[1]

- The teletherapy equipment should meet the specifications as per requirement and specified in the venders documents and clinical requirement.
- Consider very carefully whether the required clinical, technological and financial infrastructure is available to support the investment and maintenance.
- Orthovoltage equipment is found to be a cost-effective alternative to the use of electrons for surface and shallow lesions.

Shielding Calculations

The shielding thickness of the walls and ceiling arc computed using the parameters such as (i) the specification of the unit; (ii) work load *W* (*R*/*wk* at 1 m); (iii) use factor *U*; (iv) the occupancies around T; (iv) the material used for construction and its density the portions of the walls of the room facing the primary beam are considers as primary barrier and the remaining portions are taken as secondary barriers. *W* is assumed not to exceed 1.5 × 10 resque 5 *R*/*wk* at 1 m. *U* is taken as ¼ for primary beam and 1 for on position leakage radiations. The value of *T* is taken as 1 for fully occupied areas such as offices, laboratories, etc., 1/4 for partially occupied areas viz., corridors, restrooms elevators and 1/16 for occasionally occupied areas such as toilettes, stairways, open ground, etc. The thickness of protective barriers are arrived at by calculating reductions factor.

The allowable reduction factor of a protective barriers for primary barrier is given by

$$RF = W\,U\,T/p\,d\,sq \qquad (1)$$

where, p = maximum permissible exposure in R/week (0.04 R for radiation workers and 0.002 R for non-radiation workers).

d = distance in meters from the source to the point of interest.

W is expressed in R/wk at 1 m

Log_{10} *(RF)*: $\text{Log}_{10}\,(W\,U\,T)/(p\,d^2)$ = number of tenth values of CO-60 radiation.

Secondary Barrier for Leakage Radiation

The maximum "ON" position leakage radiation allowed from the housing of telecobalt unit at 1 m from the source, i.e. 0.1% of the primary dose at 1 m.

The allowable RF of secondary protective barrier is given by

$$RF = (0.1 \times 10^{-3}\,WUT)/(p \times d^2) \qquad (2)$$

Here $U = 1$, d = distance in meters from isocenter to the point of interest. Other factors are same as given in A.

Log_{10}(RF) of secondary barrier for leakage radiation will give number of tenth values of shielding material required.

Secondary Barrier for Scattered Radiation

Radiation is scattered from the patient in all directions. The amount of scattered radiation depends on the incident radiation dose on the scatterer, quality of radiation and angle of scattering. The ratio of scattered dose to incidence dose measured at 1 m distance from the scattered is called scattering coefficient and it is denoted as α. The value of α is given as function of the angle of scattered.

The allowable *RF* of secondary protective barrier is given by

$RF = \alpha\ W U T / p\ d^2$

$U = 1/4$ for scattering radiation with scattering angle less than 90°

$U = 1/2$ for 90° scattering radiation

Log_{10} (RF) of secondary barrier for scattered radiation will give number of tenth values of shielding material required.

When the difference between the shielding thickness as per B and C is less than 1 half values thickness for same secondary barrier then the shielding thickness of larger one is increased by 1 HVT to get secondary barrier thickness.

Width of Primary Radiation Area

Due to the divergence property of electromagnetic radiation, i.e. (both X-ray and Gamma-ray) size of the primary field increase as one goes away from the source. The width of the primary field falling on the primary protective barrier can be evaluated from the principle of similar triangle.

Width of the primary field = [(D × f/s) + 60] cm

Where D = the distance between source and primary wall given in meter

F = Maximum field size at SAD position given cm × cm

A = SAD of the unit given in meter

60 = The safe margin

A maze wall d is provided in the treatment room which helps in reducing the area of scatterer (i.e. portions of wall, ceiling and floor receiving the radiation scattered from the patient), thereby reducing the exposure at the door position.

Important Atomic Energy Regulatory Board Rules[5,7]

Radiotherapy follows the guidelines of ARRB very rigidly. Safety of the service provider is as important as of the patients. There are certain rules of AERB which need to be mentioned:

The 5 (n) "planning" means planning for the provision of appropriate

- Building layout
- Radiation shielding
- Protection equipment, and
- Operational procedures, to ensure adequate protection in course of handling radioactive material or radiation equipment and performing related operations in the proposed radiation installation; (o)"quality assurance tests" means conducted to ensure performance and reliability of the radiation equipment in accordance with the design specifications.

Planning of Radiation Installations[5]

- The location and planning of a radiation installation shall be such as to ensure adequate protection to the members of the staff, patients and the public.
- Appropriate measures to achieve this objective shall include the following measures, namely:
  - A radiation installation shall have integrated facilities at one location for the handling of radiation equipment and radioactive materials.
  - A radiation installation shall be located as far away as feasible from high occupancy areas, pediatric and maternity wards and other facilities of the institution that are not directly related to radiation and its use.
  - The layout of a radiation installation and safety equipment shall be so planned that all the radiation handling operations can be performed in a safe manner.

Commissioning of a Radiation Equipment or Radiation Installations (Tables 7 and 8)

Any radiation equipment or radiation installation shall be commissioned only after all aspects including design, planning, construction and operation have been duly approved by the competent authority.

PLANNING OF BRACHYTHERAPY FACILITY (FIG. 11)

Site Selection

A brachytherapy department should preferably be located in one corner or confined to one wing of the building in close proximity to the related radiotherapy and associated facilities. In the case of radiotherapy centers envisaging both teletherapy and brachytherapy facility, it is economical to locate the brachytherapy department above the teletherapy room so as to take advantage of the thicker ceiling of the teletherapy room.

General Layout

The minimum requirements for a brachytherapy department using manual systems are source storage and preparation room, minor surgery room (operating room), treatment planning room nurses station and wards for hospitalization of brachytherapy patients. However, a full-fledged brachytherapy department will have additional rooms for doctor and physicist, patient examination room, reception and records room, waiting hall, etc. These facilities should not be too widely separated in order to reduce distances over which the patient and sources have to be transported. The relative proximity of these facilities can significantly influence procedure flow and efficiency. Facility design should incorporate features to avoid elevator transport of patients containing radioactive sources.[1]

Table 7: Commissioning parameters.

	Primary barrier			Secondary barrier		
	Lead	*Barium concrete*	*Concrete*	*Lead*	*Barium concrete*	*Concrete*
100 kV	2.5 mm	0.75 inch	6.5 inch	1 mm	0.25 inch	3 inch
250 kV	12 mm	6.5 inch	20 inch	7 mm	3.5 inch	12 inch
4 MV	26 mm	38.6 inch	5 ft	15 cm	2 ft	2.5 ft

Table 8: Barrier thickness.

Endpoint energy (MV)[b]	Material	TVL1 (em)	TVL 0 (em)
4	Concrete	35	30
	Steel	9.9	9.9
	Lead	5.7	5.7
6	Concrete	37	33
	Steel	10	10
	Lead	5.7	5.7
10	Concrete	41	37
	Steel	11	11
	Lead	5.7	5.7
15	Concrete	44	41
	Steel	11	11
	Lead	5.7	5.7
18	Concrete	45	11
	Steel	11	11
	Lead	5.7	5.7
20	Concrete	46	44
	Steel	11	11
	Lead	5.7	5.7
25	Concrete	49	46
	Steel	11	11
	Lead	5.7	5.7
30	Concrete	51	49
	Steel	11	11
	Lead	5.7	5.7
CO-60	Concrete	21	21
	Steel	7.0	7.0
	Lead	4.0	4.0

[b]End point energy based on values from Coben (1972).

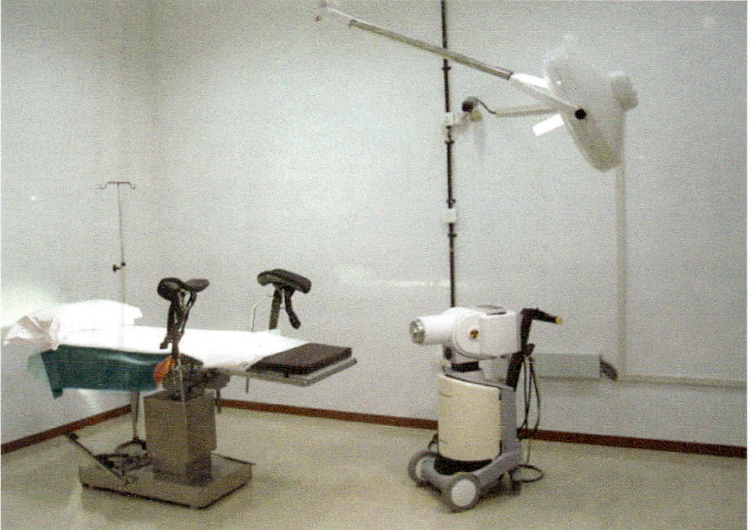

Fig. 11: Brachytherapy facility.

Shielding Requirements (Table 9)

In a brachytherapy department, wards alone require additional shielding for the walls, floor and ceiling. All other rooms do not normally require shielding. The planning of the wards will depend on (i) the type and strength of radionuclide used, (ii) number of beds, (iii) workload, (iv) the material used for construction and its density and (v) occupancy all around. In the case of a teletherapy installation, since the exposures are collimated, we have both primary and secondary protective barriers depending on whether a specific wall receives primary radiation or secondary radiation. However, while computing the shielding requirements for a brachytherapy ward, all the walls, ceiling and floor are considered as primary barriers since the exposures are panoramic, the attenuation by patient being assumed negligible. Hence, the computation of shielding requirements for a brachytherapy ward is similar to that of a primary protective barrier in the case of teletherapy room. The workload W is expressed in R/wk at 1 m and U is taken as 1. W is given by

$$W\,(R/wk \text{ at } 1 \text{ m}) = S \times \text{RHM} \times 40 \text{ h/week}$$

where S is source strength in curies.

Approximate half-value thickness and tenth-value thickness for heavily attenuated beam under-broad beam condition.

Table 9: Shielding parameters.

X-ray source	Half-value thickness (cm)		Tenth-value thickness (cm)	
	Lead	Concrete	Lead	Concrete
50 kV	0.005	0.4	0.018	1.3
100	0.025	1.6	0.084	–
0.5 MV	0.31	3.6	1.03	11.9
6	1.54	10.2	5.1	33.8
10 MV	1.69	11.7	5.6	38.6
20	1.63	13.7	5.4	45.7

Source Storage and Preparation Room[1,8]

- This room should be designed in accordance with the recommendations of AERB.
- It should be provided with a locked door to control access to the radioactive material.
- A sign should be posted on the door requirements.
- It should contain shielded storage for all sources and have facilities for receiving, preparing, calibrating and returning sources.
- An area radiation monitor should be visible on entering the room and while preparing the sources.
- Space for a workbench should be provided.
- A cabinet for the necessary instruments, equipment, treatment aid and the required documents should also be planned.
- Space for source transportation trolleys should be provided.
- Space for storage of radioactive material (sources) to allow decay to safe levels.

Operating Theater[1]

Cases require anesthesia for placement of applicators or catheters to contain the radiation sources, an operating room facility and recovery area should be planned.

An X-ray unit, preferably with fluoroscopic capabilities, is planned in the operating room because it enables the position of the applicator or catheters to be checked, and if necessary repositioned, before the patient leaves the operating suite.

Localization X-rays (orthogonal or stereo-shifted X-rays) required for dose calculation purposes should be planned with this unit. If no X-ray unit is in the operating room, these facility should be available elsewhere in the department.

Size of the operating room depends on the equipment planned, 45–55 sqm should be planned for the OT.

Treatment Planning Room

Treatment planning for LDR brachytherapy is usually performed on a general treatment planning system for teletherapy and brachytherapy using brachytherapy-planning software. Design elements of the treatment planning room could be obtained from AERB/DARP/RPAD.[1,8]

Patient Rooms[1,8]

- It is preferable to house each LDR brachytherapy patient in a separate room
- The rooms should be shielded according to the recommendations given by AERB/RPAD, paying due attention to the requirements of the BSS and the regulatory authority
- A sign should be posted on the door warning of the radiation hazard in accordance with the requirements of the regulatory authority
- A list with the maximum duration of daily visits by members of the general public should be posted on the door
- If several rooms are required, they should be adjacent to each other
- Nurses should attend the patient with special training in the care of radiation therapy patients
- A toilet for each room has added patient convenience but increases the risk of losing sources
- A bell connected to the nurses' station is essential as gynecological patients need to use bedpans and may not use even common toilets
- Storage for a bedside shield and emergency source container should also be provided.

REQUIREMENTS OF HIGH-DOSE-RATE THERAPY (FIG. 12)[8] AND TABLE 10

An high-dose-rate (HDR) brachytherapy facility requires:
- An operating theater
- A radiographic imaging system
- A treatment room
- A treatment planning area.

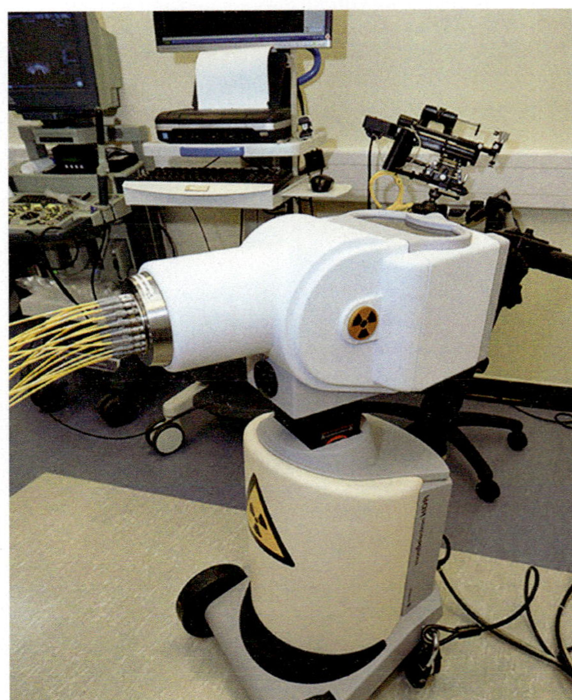

Fig. 12: High-dose-rate therapy.

Table 10: Requirements of high dose rate therapy.

Name of the space	*Allocated to person*	*Size of space*	*Number*
Chamber	Chief physicist	3.5 × 4 = 15 sqm	one
Chamber	Assistant physicist	15–16 sqm	one
Office	Steno-cum-clerk	12–15 sqm	one
Planning/conference room	Sitting for 6–8 persons	20–22 sqm	one

PALLIATIVE CARE UNIT PAIN CLINICS AND HOSPICE (FIG. 13)

Palliative care unit is requisite of the cancer hospital, because all cancers are not amenable to any type of treatment. Treatment in these units is done on short-term basis to relieve the patient on temporary basis.

SPACE PLANNING

Refer Table 11.

HVAC

Same as MRI/CT scan.

LIGHTING

Controlled light source is recommended in the treatment area. Other areas like conference room, treatment-planning rooms, Physicist room, and other chambers should be illuminated with 300 lux light. Corridors, toilets and stores, etc. required 100 Lux light. OT area needs 40,000–100,000 lux light.

Floor plans are depicted in Figures 14 and 15.

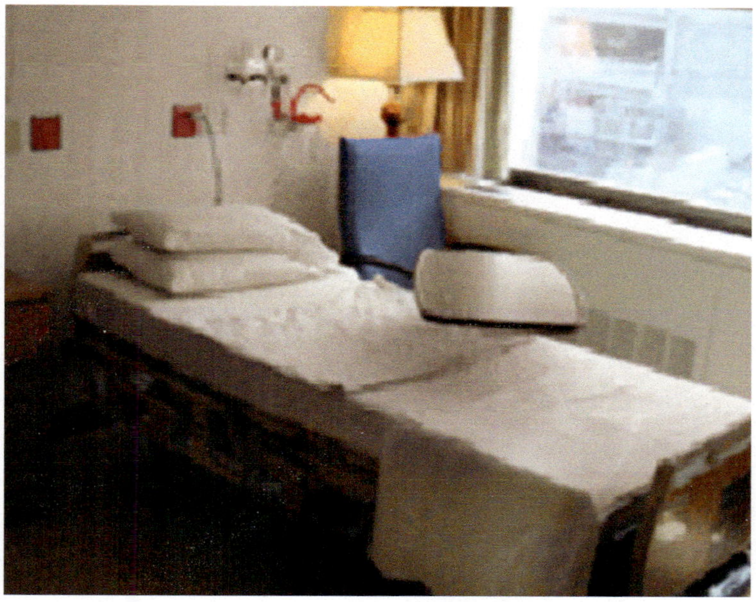

Fig. 13: Palliative care unit pain clinics and hospice.

Table 11: Palliative care unit.

Name of the area	*Space requirement in sqm*	*Remark*
Bed area	7–8/bed	
Treatment area	12–14	
Nursing station	6	
Changing room	9–10	
Store	6–8	
Facility for patients	8	2
Dirty utility	6	
Janitor closet	3–3.5	
Attendant room	6 sqm	
Pantry	9–10	
Trolly/wheelchair bay	6	
Waiting area	18–20	
Circulation area	35%	

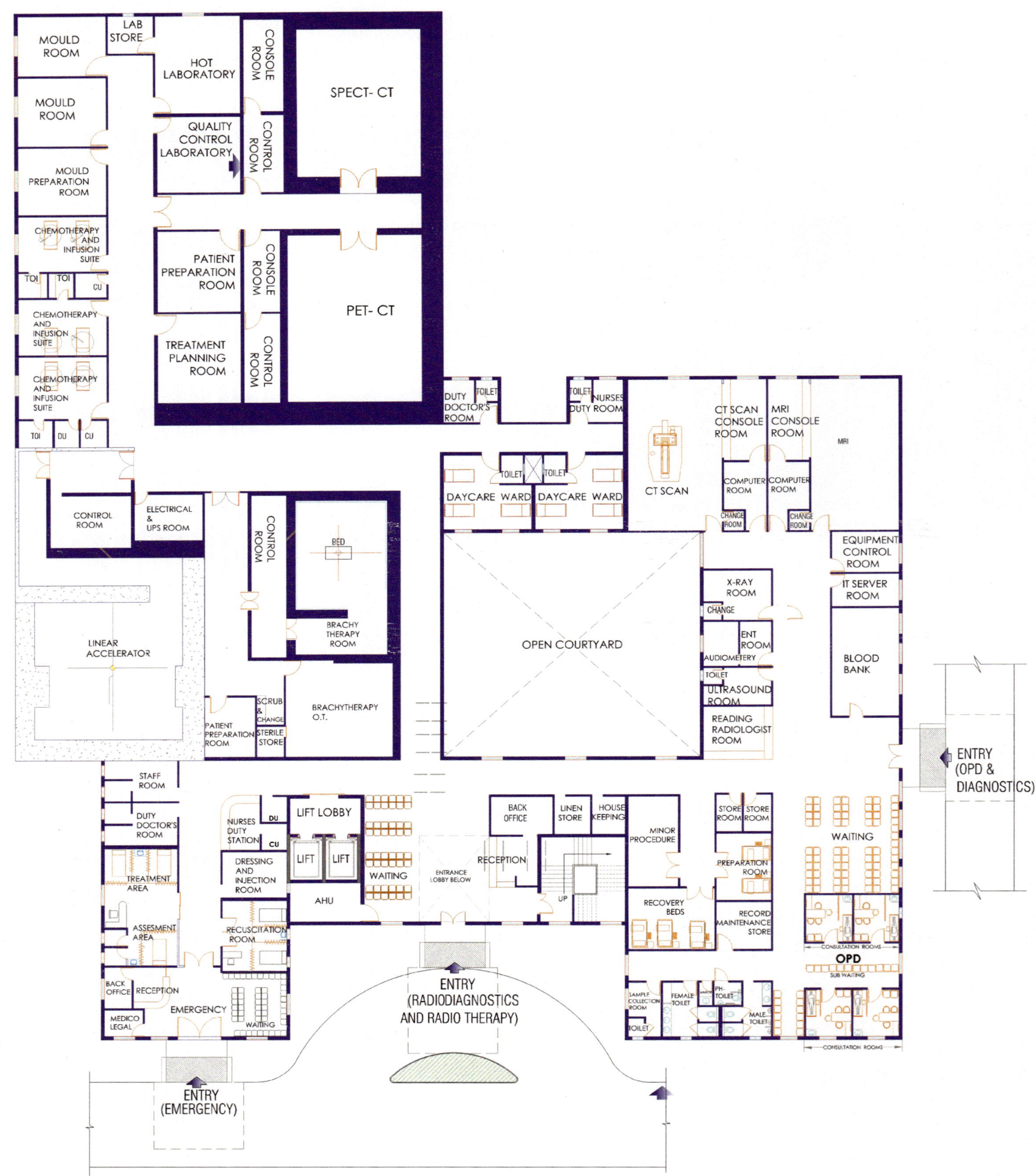

Fig. 14: Ground floor plan.

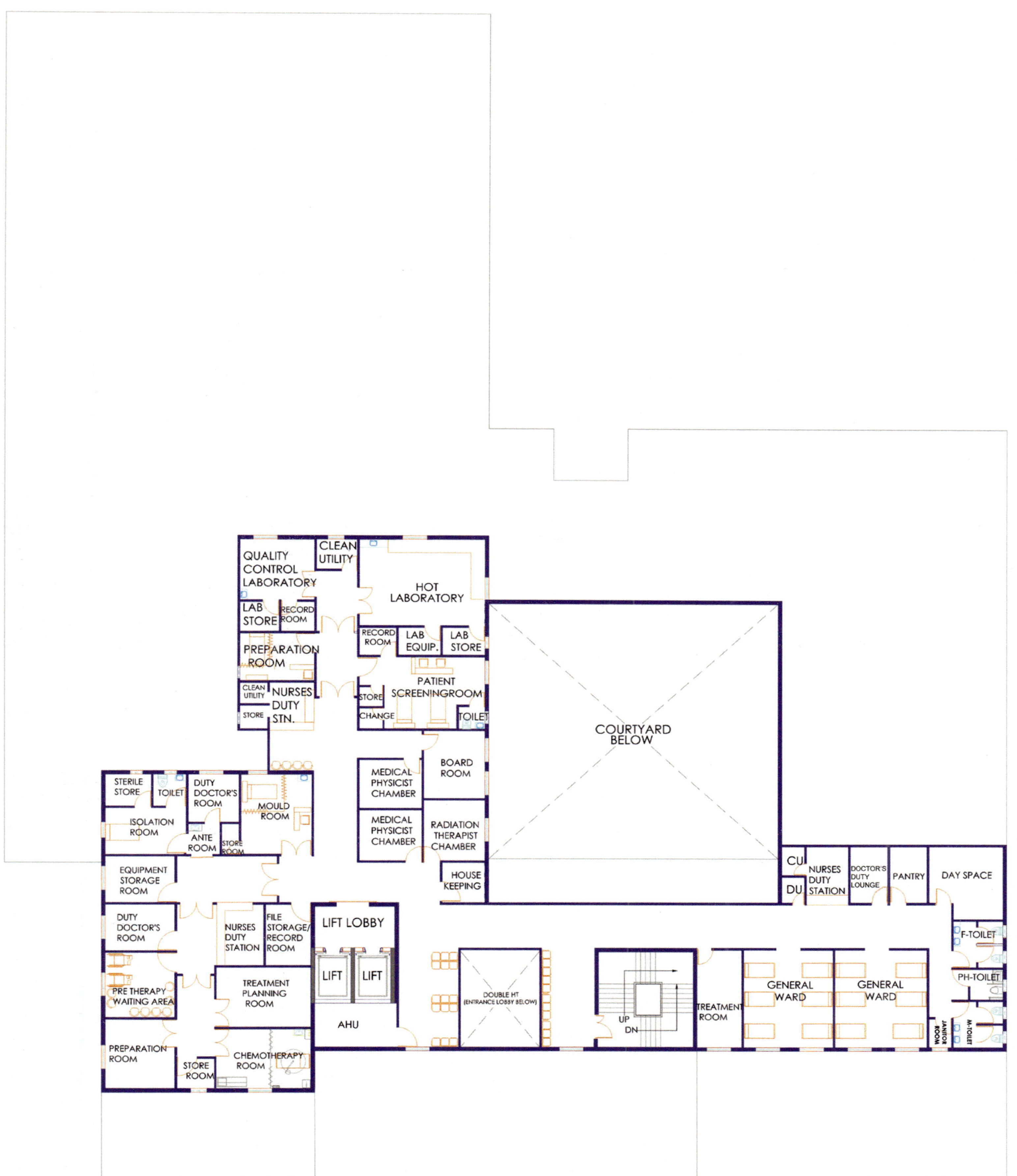

Fig. 15: First floor plan.

REFERENCES

1. www-pub.iaea.org
2. www.healthdesign.com.au
3. egyankosh.ac.in
4. www.scribd.com
5. www.aerb.gov.in
6. sgrdimsr.org
7. www.inca.gov.br
8. www.rpaz.co.zw

OTHER REFERENCES

- Advisory Committee on Radiological Safety (ACRS).
- AERB/RSD/RT/PLAN-Tech note-1-2006.
- AERB guidelineS, www.aerb.gov.in.
- Atomic Energy (Safe Disposal of Radioactive Wastes) Rules 1987, GSR 125, The Gazette of India, Part II, Section 3(I), February 28, 1987.111 111.
- Atomic Energy Act, 1962 (33 of 1962), September 15, 1962.
- GK Rath, BK Mohanti. The test book of radiation oncology"principles and practices. BI Churchill livingstone, 1st edn, 2000.
- Health Building Note 12 – OPD, Ministry of Health: London.
- Hospital Planning hand book, Rex Whitaker Allen, Illona Von Karolyl"–London, New York/Toronto.
- Iaea publications on clinical, medical physics, radiation protection, and safety aspects of radiotherapy.
- ICMR Annual report 2003–2004, ICMR 2005, and Jugal Kishore, National Health Programme of INDIA 6th Edition.
- International Atomic Energy Agency, Implementation of Microsource High Dose Rate (mHDR) Brachytherapy in Developing Countries, IAEA-TECDOC-1257, IAEA, Vienna, 2001.
- International Atomic Energy Agency, Mould Room Techniques for Teletherapy, Practical Radiation Technical Manual No. 4, IAEA, Vienna, 1999.
- International Atomic Energy Agency, Occupational Radiation Protection, IAEA Safety Standards Series No. RS-G-1.1, IAEA, Vienna, 1999.
- International Atomic Energy Agency, Organization and Implementation of a National Regulatory Infrastructure Governing Protection against Ionizing Radiation and the Safety of Radiation Sources, IAEA-TECDOC-1067, IAEA, Vienna, 1999.
- International Atomic Energy Agency, Radiological Protection for Medical Exposure to Ionizing Radiation, IAEA Safety Standards Series No. RS-G-1.5, IAEA, Vienna, 2000.
- International Basic Safety Standards for Protection Against Ionizing Radiation and for the Safety of Radiation Sources, Safety Series No. 115, IAEA, Vienna, 1996.
- International Basic Safety Standards for Protection against Ionizing Radiation and for the Safety of Radiation Sources, Safety Series No. 115, IAEA, Vienna, 1996.
- International Commission for Radiation Protection (ICRP), the National Commission for Radiation Protection (NCRP) in America, Regulatory and Safety functions of Atomic Energy in India.
- Radiation Protection Rules 1971, GSR 1061. The Gazette of India, Part II, Section 3(I), October 30, 1971.
- Recommendations of the International Commission on Radiological Protection, ICRP 60, 1991.
- RPAD, Radiological Physics and Advisory Division, (RP&AD) is providing advisory services to AERB.
- Sarin R. "Indian National Cancer Control Programme Setting sight on shifting targets " J Can Res Ther. 2005;1(4);240-8.
- Gupta S, Modern trends in Planning & Designing of Hospital, Jaypee Brothers Medical Publishers Pvt. Ltd, New Delhi.
- World Health Organization, Quality Assurance in Radiotherapy, WHO, Geneva, 1988.
- Health Building Note 02-01: Cancer Treatment Facilities. Dept of Health UK.

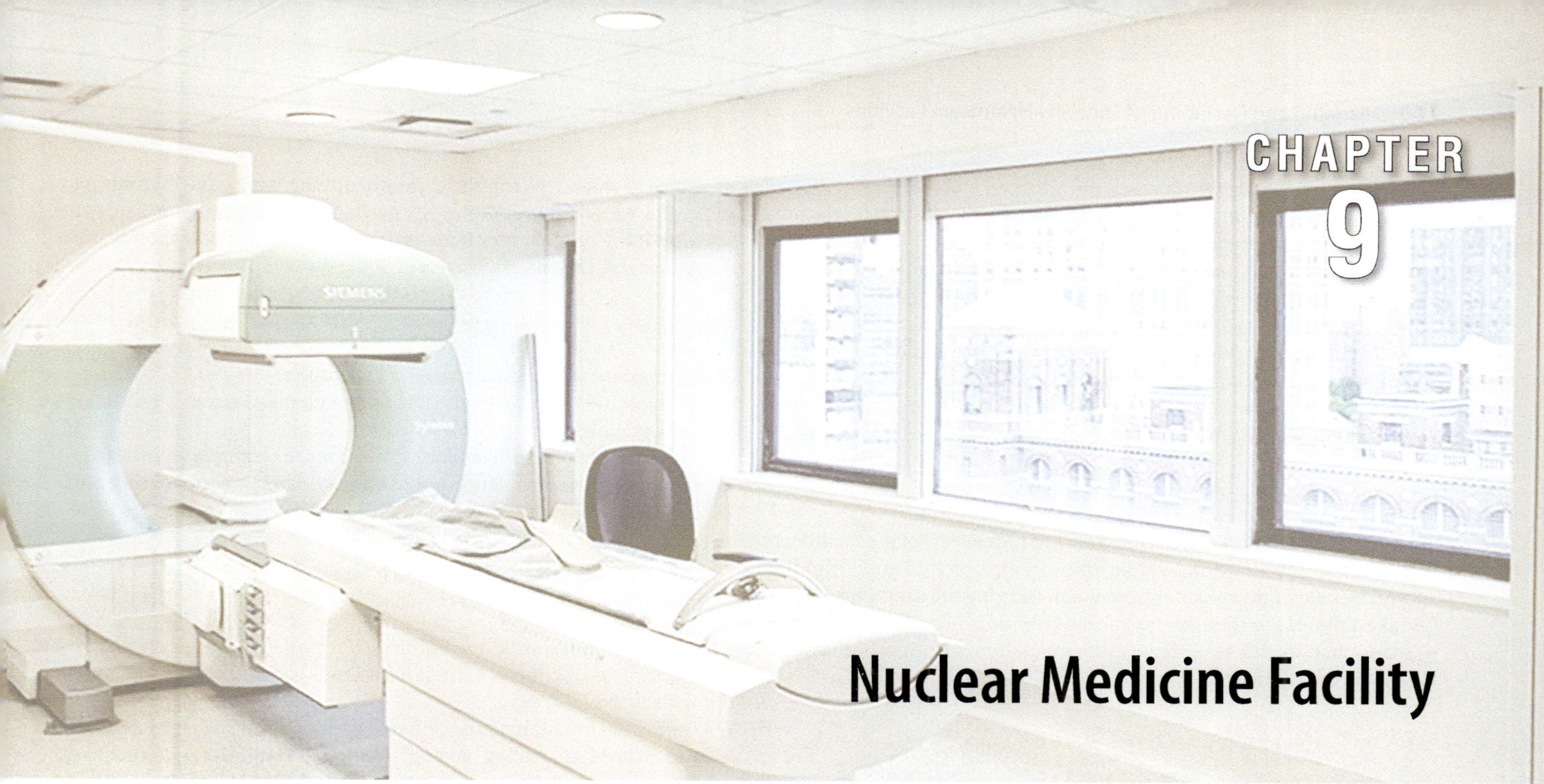

CHAPTER 9

Nuclear Medicine Facility

Neeraj Garg, Shakti Kumar Gupta, Sunil Kant, R Chandrashekhar

INTRODUCTION

Nuclear medicine specialists use safe, painless, and cost-effective techniques to image the body and treat disease. Nuclear medicine imaging is unique, because it provides doctors with information about both structure and function. It is a way to gather medical information that would otherwise be unavailable, require surgery, or necessitate more expensive diagnostic tests.

Nuclear medicine uses very small amounts of radioactive materials (radiopharmaceuticals) to diagnose and treat disease. In imaging, the radiopharmaceuticals are detected by special types of cameras that work with computers to provide very precise pictures about the area of the body being imaged. In treatment, the radiopharmaceuticals go directly to the organ being treated. The amount of radiation in a typical nuclear imaging procedure is comparable with that received during a diagnostic X-ray, and the amount received in a typical treatment procedure is kept within safe limits.[1]

FUNCTIONS OF FACILITY

Nuclear medicine is a safe, painless, and cost-effective way of gathering information that may otherwise be unavailable or require a more expensive and risky diagnostic test. One unique aspect of a nuclear medicine test is its extreme sensitivity to abnormalities in an organ's structure or function. As an integral part of patient care, nuclear medicine is used in the diagnosis, treatment, management and prevention of serious disease. Nuclear medicine imaging procedures often identify abnormalities very early in the progression of a disease long before some medical problems are apparent with other diagnostic tests. This early detection allows a disease to be treated early in its course when there may be a better prognosis.[2]

Although nuclear medicine is commonly used for diagnostic purposes, it also has valuable therapeutic applications such as treatment of hyperthyroidism, thyroid cancer, blood imbalances, and any bony pain from certain types of cancer.[2]

KEY PLANNING-LAYOUT PLAN APPROVAL

The user should submit to Atomic Energy Regulatory Board (AERB) two copies each of the proposed layout plan, site plan, and elevation drawing of the facility indicating the floor, nature of occupancy around, above and below, if any, has to be submitted in along with the application form AERB/RSD/NMF/SLA (downloadable from www.aerb.gov.in). On scrutinizing, the plans from radiologic safety point of view, necessary approval of facility is granted.[3]

Planning and Design Considerations

- Nuclear medicine facilities shall be located away from high patient and/or public occupancy areas and sources of intense radiation.[4]
- Active rooms, wards and areas of source storage and handling shall be marked with radiation symbol and legend denoting the identification of active area and presence of radiation hazard. Areas of high activity and contamination shall be demarcated by physical barriers. Active areas shall be arranged in increasing order of the activity with entrance from lowest active area.[4]
- Walls, floor and doors of the active areas shall have hard, washable, nonporous and leak-proof covering. Work surfaces shall be covered with nonporous and non-reactive material.[4]
- Plumbing shall provide direct flow of liquid effluents from active areas either directly to the delay tank or to the ultimate discharge point. Drain pipes and delay tank (for interim storage of high level radioactive waste) shall be leak-proof and corrosion-resistant.[4]
- Ventilation systems shall be of once-through type with unidirectional air flow from areas of lower activity to higher activity. The exhaust from fume hoods shall be let out directly into the open after filtering.[4]
- Radiation levels at the nurse station outside the wards shall not exceed 1 μSv/h.[4]
- The following radiation monitors shall be available in working condition and with recent calibration:[4]

- Portable beta-gamma area monitor(s).
- Contamination monitor(s) for personnel/area/surface/clothing
- Radioisotope calibrator.
- Calibration checked regularly and records maintained.

- Radiation levels around the in-house transport container should not exceed 1 μSv/h at 5 cm from the surface. Radiation symbol shall be permanently marked on its outer surface. Means shall be provided for securely locking the container.[4]
- The permanent shielding provided for radionuclide generator shall not be tampered with or removed.[4]

LOCATION

The unit should not act as a thoroughfare to other units of the healthcare facility. The floor loading weight of both equipment and shielding should be taken into consideration when locating the unit. Care should be taken to ensure that the location of the unit minimizes access by persons such as lost visitors, wandering patients from other units or those with criminal intent.[5]

LAYOUT AND FUNCTIONAL AREAS

The following rooms/spaces from the main functional zones of the unit:[5]

- Reception/administration
- Outpatient waiting
- Patient holding, observation and recovery area
- Treatment areas
- Clinical support areas
- Hot Lab/radioactive waste store (Fig. 1)
- Staff offices and amenities
- Teaching and research facilities in tertiary centers.

RECEPTION/ADMINISTRATION

Facilities will usually comprise:[5]

- Entry lobby and general public waiting
- Reception/enquiry desk
- Bookings office or alcove
- Administrative offices

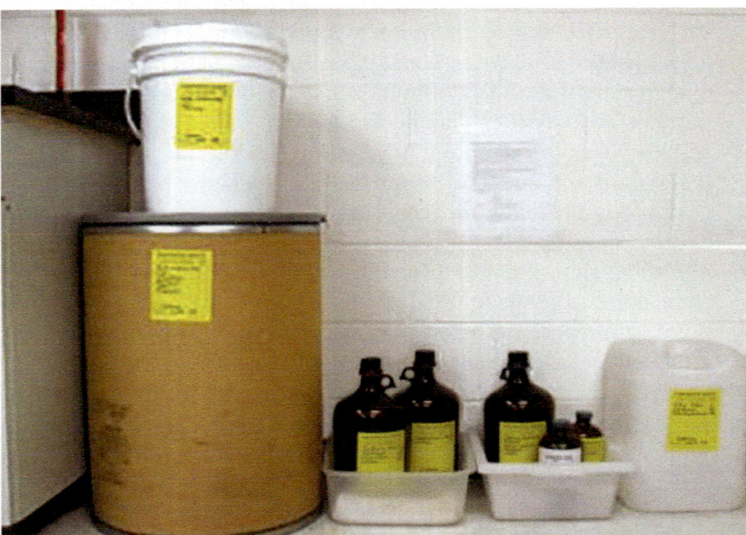

Fig. 1: Hot lab waste store.

- Clerical work area for filing, photocopying, and report typing
- Public toilets should be readily available but need not be inside the unit. If the nuclear medicine unit is part of a medical imaging unit, these facilities may be shared.

OUTPATIENT WAITING

The outpatient waiting area usually comprises:[5]

- Separate areas for dosed and undosed patients who may be ambulant or in wheelchairs.
- Access to toilets, shower and refreshments arranged so that dosed patients are not traveling across the undosed patient waiting area.
- Child play area, if required.

PATIENT HOLDING, OBSERVATION AND RECOVERY AREA

An area will be required for holding of inpatients, and recovery and observation as necessary of both inpatients and outpatients. It usually comprises the following:[5]

- Dedicated inpatient entry—direct is desirable if this can be achieved
- Curtained bed/trolley bays for holding, observation and recovery. The size of each bay and configuration of the overall space should permit both dosed and undosed patients to be held safely.
- A small staff base with hand basin.
- Ready access to dirty utility, linen trolley bay, sterile stock store.
- Resuscitation trolley—if only one, it is recommended to be parked in or near the stress testing room.

TREATMENT AREAS

All the following rooms are accessed by patients and require radiation shielding as advised by consultants:[5]

- Dosing/consult exam rooms—ideally adjacent to the dispensing hot lab
- Cardiac stress testing room
- Scanning room(s)
- Bone density room if provided.

CLINICAL SUPPORT AREAS

- Clinical support areas usually include the following areas. However, if collocated with a medical imaging unit, some areas listed may be shared:[5]
  - Viewing/reporting area
  - Dirty utility room
  - Disposal room
  - Equipment bays
  - Equipment and general stores
  - Sterile stock store or clean utility room
  - Print/server room.

HOT LAB/DISPENSARY AND RADIOACTIVE WASTE STORE

In the hot lab radioactive radiopharmaceuticals are stored, drawn up and prepared ready for administration to the patient. A lead screen will act as a barrier behind which dispensing occurs. Radioactive waste holding may also be incorporated into or adjacent to this space.[7,8]

STAFF OFFICES AND AMENITIES

Depending on the size and location of the unit and collocation with adjoining units, staff will need access to:[5]

- Staff room/beverage bay
- Meeting rooms and library
- Offices in accordance with staff establishment and teaching/research roles
- Toilets, showers and lockers.

Radioactive Iodine Sealed Bedroom

Some patients who receive radioactive I-131 treatment will require inpatient management within an especially shielded inpatient single bedroom. The physical location of the bed(s) will be dependent on the operational policy and service requirements for the facility. These rooms are usually associated with tertiary services, recognizing the role delineation/service capability profile of the facility.[5]

Parking

Patients and visitors will use the public parking facilities with access to drop-off areas and disabled parking. An identified parking area for vehicles delivering isotopes is essential. This should be in close proximity to the hot lab.

Patient Amenities

The following patient amenities should be available and, where possible, should be positioned so that dosed patients do not have to cross undosed waiting areas or public corridors to access these areas:[5]

- Toilets including access toilet
- Change cubicle/s and shower—for emergencies and post-stress testing hygiene.

PATIENT WAITING

Ideally, waiting areas should allow separation of dosed and undosed patients, particularly for patients undergoing cardiac scans who may wait for 45 minutes for uptake. It is preferable to separate dosed patients from people who accompanied them to the unit which may include young adults, pregnant women and children. Patients having a post-therapy I-131 scan should preferably be separated from patients having diagnostic scans.[2]

Disaster Planning

Each unit will have operational plans and policies detailing the response to a range of emergency situations both internal and external. Consider the ability to effect complete lock-down and issues such as the placement of emergency alarms, the need for uninterrupted or emergency power supply (UPS) to essential clinical equipment such as scanners, electronic sensor taps and services such as emergency lighting, telephones, duress alarm systems, servers and computers. Arrangements for management of spills and radioactive exposure should be in place. An emergency shower with eyewash station should be readily accessible to staff, patients and the public in case of contamination.[5]

WALLS

Walls should be washable and easily decontaminated in the event of a radioactive spill.

Finishes

Floor Finishes

Floor finishes and junctions should be impermeable and nonabsorbent in case of radiation spills.

FIXTURES, FITTINGS AND EQUIPMENT

General

High cost engineering areas which should receive careful consideration by design teams include:[5]

- Lighting and the impact of deep planning on lighting requirements
- Number of sanitary fittings and the potential for reducing these by strategic location
- Extent of the required emergency and uninterrupted power supply
- Extent of provision of emergency doors
- The need for and the cost benefit/implications of a pneumatic transport system
- Extent of provision of essential back-up systems (e.g. Dual generators, chillers, boilers and dual electrical circuits).

BUILDING SERVICE REQUIREMENTS

Construction

In constructing the unit, following issues needs to be addressed:[5]

- Ensure that new and existing floor structure and finishes are adequate to meet load requirements for equipment, shielding, patients, and personnel.
- Ensure that walls contain the necessary support systems for medical service panels.
- Provision should be made for cable trays, ducts or conduits in floors, walls, and ceilings as required for specialized equipment.
- Integrity of the shielding should not be compromised by ducts and penetrations.
- Ceiling height in the scanning rooms should be a minimum of 3 meters.
- Ceiling mounted equipment should have properly designed rigid support structures located above the finished ceiling.
- Tiled ceiling should be considered for ease of installation, service and remodeling.

ELECTRICAL SERVICES

A sufficient number of power outlets, both general and essential supply, including three phase outlets, are required for current and anticipated future needs. An emergency back-up system for the power supply should be available for high priority equipment and illumination.[5]

Provide uninterrupted power supply (UPS) to cameras, acquisition and workstations and servers to prevent data loss and/or damage during power surges or brownouts.[5]

HYDRAULIC SERVICES

When routing hydraulic services and air-conditioning ducts in ceiling spaces, avoid the space above gamma cameras as water leaks can cause significant damage.[5]

The need for delayed holding tanks to patient toilets in the unit will be dependent on the local water authority requirements and advice from the radiation safety officer.[5]

INFORMATION TECHNOLOGY AND COMMUNICATION SYSTEMS

The infrastructure for the following should be considered for the present and possible future expansion:[5]

- Wireless technology
- Voice/data systems
- Video conferencing capacity
- Duress call-fixed and personal (optional)
- CCTV monitoring systems of entry points, if considered necessary and in the scanning and uptake rooms
- Infrastructure for PACS, electronic records and imaging information management system
- Server room
- Patient/nurse and emergency call systems compatible with existing hospital systems.

MECHANICAL SERVICES

Additional cooling and ventilation will be required in scanning rooms and associated computer equipment rooms as the equipment is sensitive to excessive ambient heat. Avoid large temperature changes in scanning rooms (>4°C/h) because of the possibility of crystal fracture in gamma cameras. General air-conditioning needs to cool equipment but not to be blown over partially undressed patients.[5]

To maintain a high level of staff concentration and to minimize the possibility of accidents, the temperature of the unit should be maintained within a comfortable range not exceeding 25°C.[5]

Smoke detectors in treatment rooms should be sensitive to radiation, i.e. photoelectric.[5]

MEDICAL GASES

Oxygen, suction and medical air will be required in all scanning rooms, stress testing rooms and to patient bed bays.[5]

Nitrous oxide and scavenging will be required in rooms where general anesthesia may be administered, particularly in units where children are treated.

RADIATION SHIELDING

The principles of radiation safety and protection should be developed and integrated into the design and documentation of the unit from the earliest stages and it is important to brief design team comprehensively.[5]

LOCATION AND RELATIONSHIPS

Rooms are ideally provided in pairs with direct access between rooms so one nuclear medicine technologist can monitor two patients, if necessary. Ready access is required from dosing rooms and dosed patient waiting areas.[5]

CONSIDERATIONS[5]

- Floor structure should support the equipment weight.
- UPS power is required to the cameras and associated acquisition/processing workstation/s to prevent data loss and/or damage during power surges or brownouts.
- Individual room temperature and humidity control is required.
- Dimmable down lighting should be placed so that lights do not shine directly into the patient's eyes.
- Bed/trolley access is required plus space to park a bed or trolley and planning.
- It should be a body protected electrical area.

In addition to the camera/CT, fixtures, fittings and equipment will include:

- Collimator rack(s)—the collimator is a directional guide. The size and length of the collimator holes determine which gamma rays reach the detector in the camera. A range of collimators will be required. Collimator racks vary according to the model/level of gamma camera.
- ECG trigger and monitor for cardiac scans.
- CCTV camera (optional in SPECT/CT room).
- Protective lead clothing.
- Medical gases—oxygen, suction, medical air on service panel.
- Nurse and emergency call system.
- Power outlets on the medical services panel.
- Hand basin.
- Pat slide wall-mounted.
- Storage/prep bench and shelving.
- TV-fixed or portable (optional).
- Overhead power to avoid floor leads.

Computer data points near gamma camera unit as well as processing workstations. Scanning rooms also need to consider the space requirements for servicing equipment and machines which is frequently done *in situ* given the size of these machines. Machines may be pulled apart to provide access to internal workings thus occupying a larger space than when operational.[5]

CONTROL BAY

The control bay may be integral to the SPECT scanning room but should be separate area for SPECT/CT (as per CT imaging requirements).[5] It requires:

- A lead observation screen for the ordinary camera to shoulder height and for SPECT to full height
- A workbench
- Chair(s)
- Viewing monitors
- Bookshelves
- CCTV monitor if CCTV camera installed in SPECT/CT room.

POSITRON EMISSION TOMOGRAPHY-COMPUTED TOMOGRAPHY (PET CT) (FIG. 2)[5]

Major considerations for site planning: (Fig. 3)

- Space
- Power
- Floor loading concerns
- Radiation shielding

Typical shielding requirements[5]

- Walls will require 12 mm to 25 mm lead
- Doors will need 8 mm to 12 mm lead. For door with lead 8 mm, mechanical assist openers will be needed
- Viewing window must be leaded glass or acrylic to match surrounding walls.

DOSING/CONSULT/EXAM ROOM

Description and Function

This room is for patient consulting, examination and administration of isotopes.

Location and Relationships[5]

Ready access to scanning rooms and undosed patient waiting is required. Ideally, it should be located adjacent to the hot/dispensing lab.

Considerations[5]

- Radiation shielding as advised by consultants.
- Appropriate radioactive signage on access doors.
- Computerized dispensing system.
- Sharps bins and a bin for general radioactive waste which may be located under a bench in lead-shielded cupboards.
- Design of a preparation bench incorporating a stainless steel sink and a lead shielded cover behind which actual preparation occurs. The cover may be fixed or hinged.

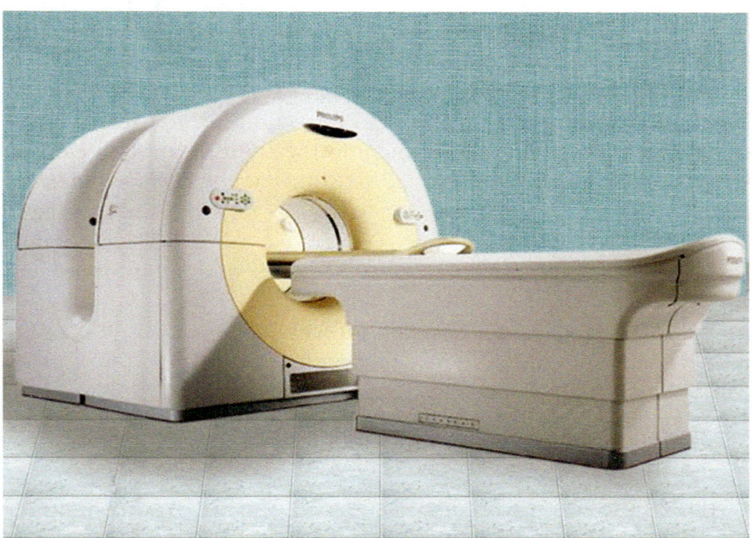

Fig. 2: PET camera.

- Sinks and basins with hands free taps for hand wash and decontamination.
- Fridges, freezers and storage cupboards for cold kits.
- Computer and label printer.
- Dose calibrator.

RADIOACTIVE WASTE HOLDING

Description and Function

A room for the temporary storage of radioactive material until it is fully decayed when it can be disposed of as per normal waste.[5]

Location and Relationships

Dual access to/from the unit is desirable but with external access, well-controlled.

Considerations

- Radiation shielding to be provided in accordance with advice from the radiation consultants.
- Bench for sharps bins.

BONE DENSITOMETRY ROOM (FIG. 4)

Location and Relationships

The room should be located at or near the unit entry to prevent patients coming into contact with dosed patients waiting scanning or having to pass in front of the scanning rooms. The scanner should be separated by distance or shielding from adjoining areas used by dosed patients. Check whether high radiation levels from nearby patients, e.g. I-131 or PET could interfere with data/image quality of BMD scans. Provide ready access to undosed patient waiting areas or alternatively these patients may use the general public waiting area.[5]

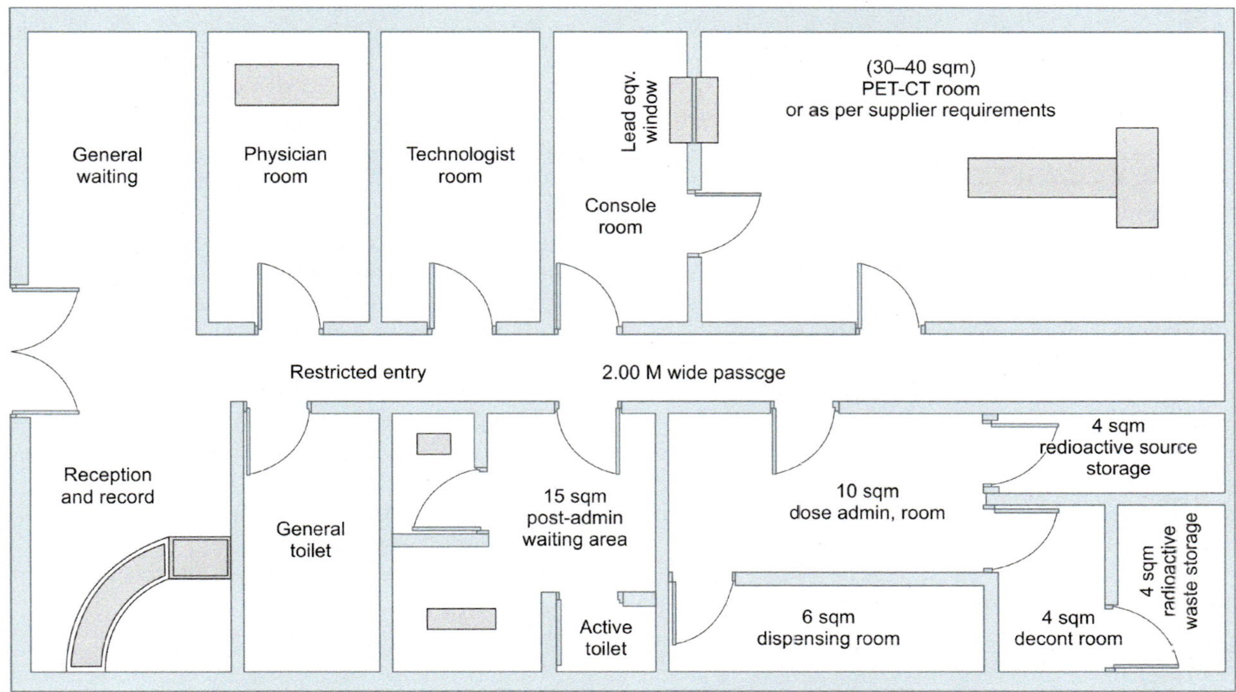

Fig. 3: Layout of PET CT.

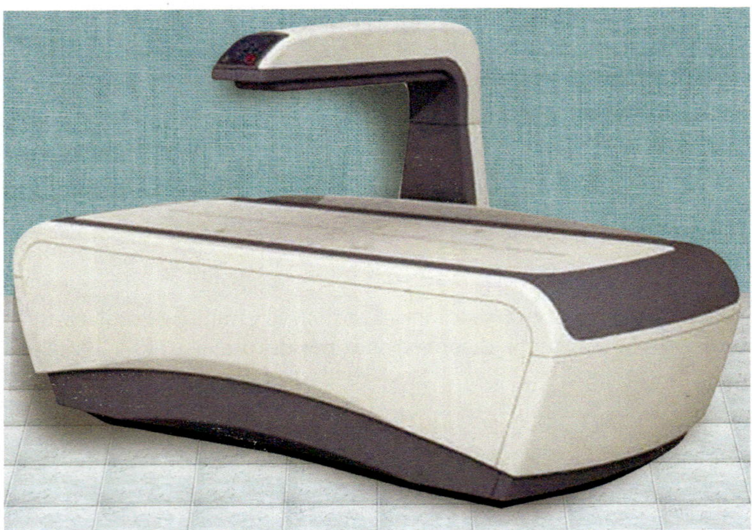

Fig. 4: Bone densitometry room.

Considerations[5]

- Bone densitometer machine—dual-energy X-ray absorptiometry-DXA or DEXA
- Computer workstation
- Office chair
- Visitor chair
- Shelving for gowns, positioning pillows, braces, etc.
- Hand basin
- Shielding as necessary.

Note: Modern machines have a very low radiation dose for the scans.

ENVIRONMENTAL CONSIDERATIONS

Natural Light

Natural light is desirable in all patient areas, the staff room, and controllable in reporting rooms. External windows provided in scanning and uptake rooms should be assessed by a radiation consultant for shielding requirements. In practice, it may be difficult to shield windows equal to wall shielding levels.[5]

Privacy

Visual and acoustic privacy is required in all consultation, examination rooms, and treatment spaces/scanning rooms. Patients on beds/trolleys should not have to pass through public circulation space in order to access treatment areas. Patients will also require privacy to discuss billing and private health related concerns.[5]

Signage

Visible warning signs are to be provided at every entry to a room where unsealed radioactive material is stored or used. Visible warning signs are also required to rooms with irradiating apparatus-bone densitometry, PET and SPECT/CT systems.[5]

SPACE STANDARDS AND COMPONENTS

Building Elements

Building elements include walls, floors, ceilings, doors, windows and corridors.

Doorways and turning circles should be sufficiently wide and high to permit the maneuvering of wheelchairs, trolleys and equipment without risk of damage or manual handling risks, and to allow ingress/egress of equipment for installation or removal.[5]

Ensure that floors are able to support the weight of equipment, and shielding, and that equipment is not located in vibration prone areas. Consider the need for shielding to floors or ceilings directly above, below or adjacent to the unit.[5]

Ensure that the allowances in some equipment specification manuals provide adequate space for complex transfers requirements such as patient from ICU bed to scanner.[5]

Doors and Doorways

Doorways should be sufficiently wide and high to permit movement of bariatric patients on large hospital beds, traction beds, wheelchairs, trolleys, equipment and accompanying staff escort without risk of damage or manual handling risks. Sliding doors may be appropriate, if provided, there is an area of wall of sufficient length.[5]

Provide the same level of shielding to vision panels in doors to treatment rooms and hot labs as to the adjoining walls. Doorways to scanning rooms should be flush to the floor for ease of camera installation and movement of equipment such as collimator carts.[5]

Radiation Shielding

Advice should be sought for each project from the radiation safety officer. Radiation shielding will be required to a number of areas within the unit.

These areas include but are not limited to the following:[5]

- Gamma camera rooms
- SPECT scanning room
- SPECT/CT scanning room
- PET/PETCT scanning room
- Dosed patient waiting area
- Reception and other rooms adjacent to dosed patient areas
- Consider the need for shielding to floors or ceilings directly above or below treatment rooms or hybrid SPECT/CT rooms.

Storage

Provide different storage areas to cater for clinical and nonclinical supplies and equipment. These include:[5]

- Storage in the scanning rooms to reduce manual handling issues associated with movement of heavy or bulky articles such as collimators and scanning phantoms.
- Equipment bays for mobile items such as portable TVs, wheelchairs, trolleys, lifters and ultrasound scanners. Equipment bay for technegas unit and argon cylinder(s). The *technegas unit* is bulky and sits on a trolley about 600 × 800 mm which can be wheeled to bedside or camera for patient to inhale technetium-99 (99mTC). When not in use, it needs parking space alongside a large cylinder of argon gas.
- General storage for smaller equipment items.
- Storage for office supplies.
- Storage for sterile stock and medical consumables.
- Storage for cleaning supplies.

Consider the impact of finishes, surfaces and fittings on safety. In particular, consider:[5]

- Slippery or wet floors.
- Protrusions or sharp edges.

Box 1: Key planning and design variables for nuclear medicine facility.[1-6]

- Prior approval of proposed layout plan, site plan, and elevation drawing of the facility from the AERB
- Nuclear medicine facilities should be located away from high patient and/or public occupancy areas and sources of intense radiation and appropriate segregation should be utilized
- Facility has to follow the principle of low active area to high active area, that is, entrance of the facility should have reception/general waiting area, and at the end hot laboratory cum radiopharmacy/radioactive waste storage is to be planned
- Pre-commissioning inspection of the facility by AERB official(s) to ensure that the construction of NM facility is as per the approved plan
- The radiopharmaceutical formulation should be prepared, handled, administered to the patients, and disposed of in a safe manner taking into account adequate radiation protection measures
- Any unusual event that has resulted or has the potential to result in overexposure to the workers or public should be reported to the AERB
- Active rooms, wards and areas of source storage and handling should be marked with radiation symbol and legend denoting the identification of active area and presence of radiation hazard
- Radioactive material should not be disposed off without prior approval of the competent authority
- Prior appointment of staff including Radiation Safety Officer
- Provisioning of personnel monitoring devices and protective equipments to radiation workers
- Provisioning of adequate shielding to avoid any radiation hazard. Walls will require 12 mm to 25 mm lead and doors will need 8 mm to 12 mm lead
- Expansion of the scanning rooms to allow for upgrades to the equipment which will require additional shielding, increased load bearing capabilities and services requirements
- Separate waiting areas for dosed and undosed patients
- Walls, floor and doors of the active areas should have hard, washable, nonporous and leak-proof covering. Work surfaces should be covered with nonporous and nonreactive material
- Ventilation system should be of once-through type with unidirectional air flow from areas of lower activity to higher activity
- Availability of radiation monitors in working condition and with recent calibration
- Easy, direct access for delivery of isotopes
- A separate toilet room for the exclusive use of injected patients with sign requesting patients to flush the toilet well should be displayed to ensure adequate dilution of excreted radioactive materials and minimize contamination
- Ensure that new and existing floor structure and finishes are adequate to meet load requirements for equipment, shielding, patients, and personnel.
- Integrity of the shielding should not be compromised by ducts and penetrations

- Stability and height of equipment or fittings.
- Fittings which should be well above floor level and/or waterproof.
- Adequate protection for workers against infection and any other hazards—particularly radiation exposure.
- Manual handling of technetium generators. The generators weigh up to 20 kg and a hoist may be required to transfer from transport package to benchtop and vice versa. The hoist should be capable of slow, accurate manipulation to avoid damage to the molybdenum (Mo-99) column within the generator shield.

Note: All the walls/partitions of the nuclear medicine laboratory should be made of 230 mm brick or 150 mm concrete. Fume hood to be installed; if required.

Decontamination room is optional. The active toilet may be used for personnel decontamination by providing a shower and wash basin.

Note: All the walls/partitions of the PET facility should be made of concrete only, the thickness of which will depend on the required workload and the area of the room, position of the bed and the occupancies all around. The ducting line of the fume hood should be shown in the plan.

Also, the plumbing and ducting line from the isolation ward to the delay tank is to be shown clearly.

Decontamination room is optional. The active toilet may be used for personnel decontamination by providing a shower and wash basin.

Facilities using Ge-68/Ga-68 generator will require a Hot lab of 12 sqm area.

Radioactive waste storage room for PET facility is optional. However, an alternative place has to be identified in the hot lab for storage of decayed Ge-68/Ga-68 generators.

Note: The capacity of the delay tank for a single patient should be 3,000 L each.

Key planning and design variables for nuclear medicine facility are summarized in Box 1.

CONCLUSION

In nuclear medicine facility, the radiopharmaceutical formulation should be prepared, handled, administered to the patients, and disposed of in a safe manner taking into account adequate radiation protection measures.[6] Radioisotopes should be stored, used, and transported safely and securely all the time. It ensures safe handling, physical security of radioactive materials, patient protection and management of radioactive wastes, and provide for detection of hazardous situations and initiation of prompt remedial measures to mitigate consequences.[3,4]

REFERENCES

1. www.limamemorial.org
2. nuclearmedicine.stanford.edu
3. www.ncbi.nlm.nih.gov
4. www.aerb.gov.in
5. healthfacilityguidelines.com.au
6. www.crcpd.org

OTHER REFERENCES

- AERB and Australian Guidelines for Nuclear Medicine Facility.
- Regulatory requirements for designing PET-CT facility in India. Ind J of Nucl Med. 2010

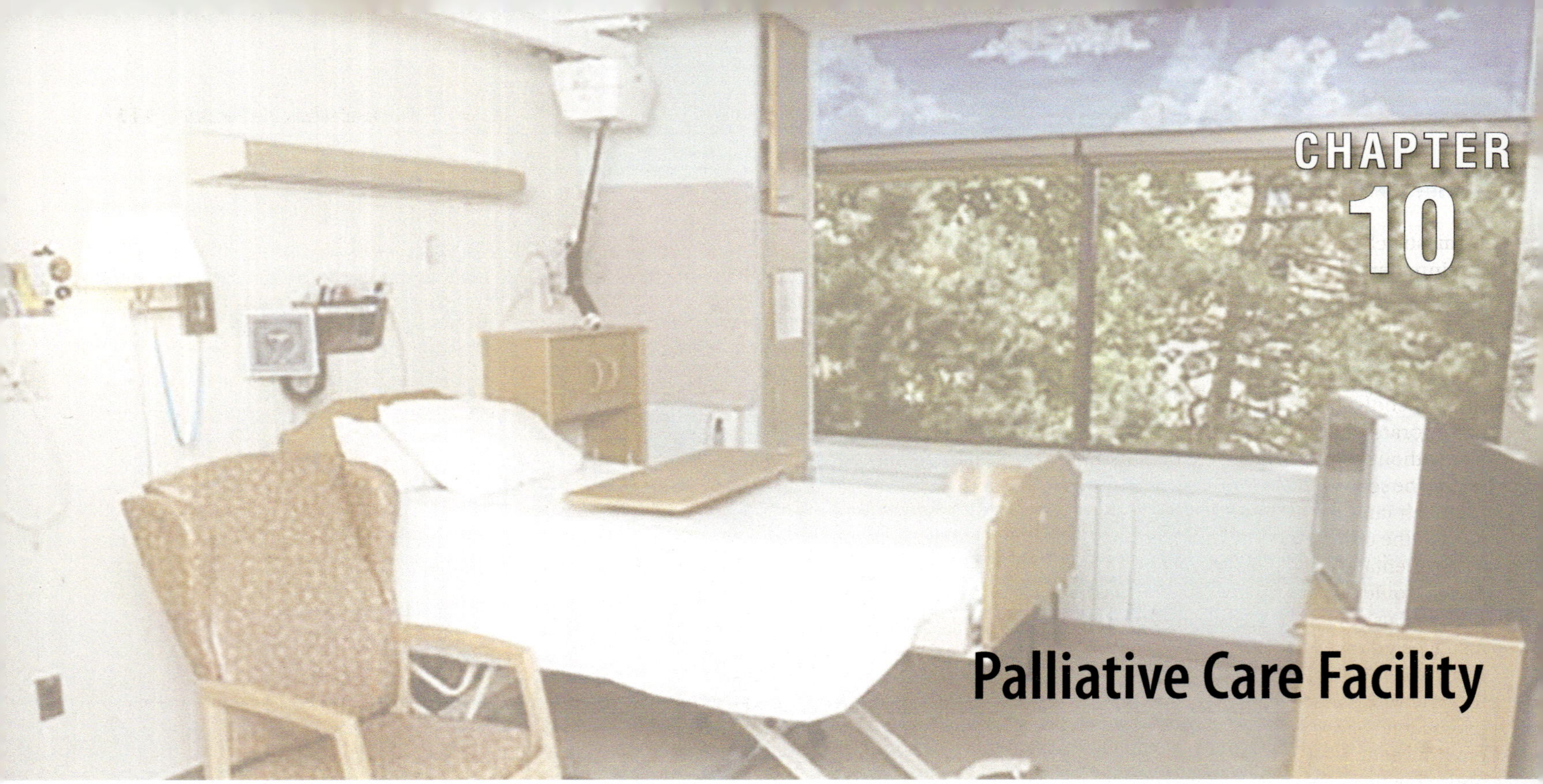

CHAPTER 10

Palliative Care Facility

Maneesh Rathee, Shakti Kumar Gupta, Sunil Kant, R Chandrashekhar

INTRODUCTION

Not every patient can be saved, but his illness can be eased by the way doctor respond to him, by emphasizing the need for effective symptom control, the care of patient and family as a unit and interdisciplinary team approach. Palliative care is medical care provided by an interdisciplinary team, including the professions of medicine, nursing, social work, chaplaincy, counseling, nursing assistants and other healthcare professionals, focused on the relief of suffering and support for the best possible quality of the life for patients facing serious life-threatening illness, and their families. It aims to identify and address and physical, psychological, spiritual and practical burdens of illness (Fig. 1).[1,2]

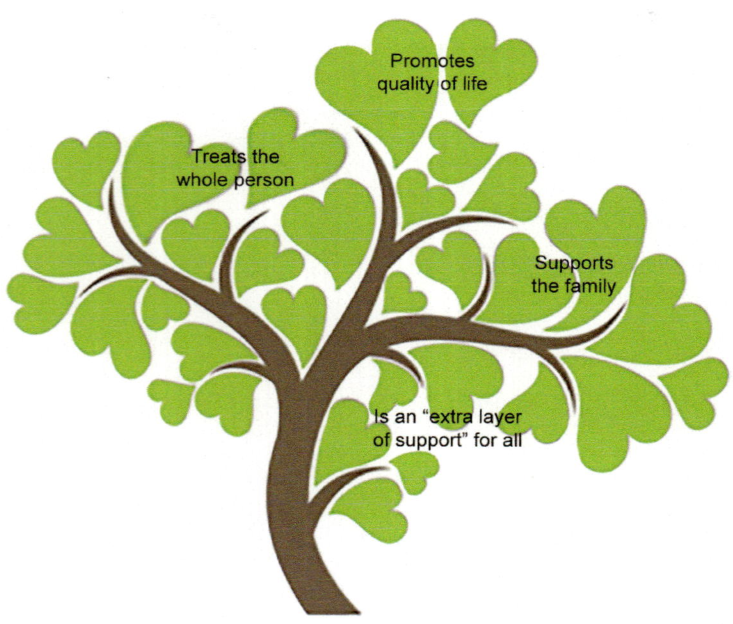

Fig. 1: Holistic approach to palliative care.

Functions of the Facility

The effort to integrate palliative care into all healthcare for debilitating and life-threatening illnesses should help to ensure that:[2]

- Pain and symptom control, psychosocial distress, spiritual issues and practical needs are addressed with patient and family throughout the continuum of care.[2]
- Patients and families obtain the information they need in an ongoing and understandable manner, in order to know their condition and treatment options. Their values and goals are elicited over time; the benefits and burdens of treatment are regularly reassessed; and the decision-making process about the care plan is sensitive to changes in the patient's condition.[2]
- Genuine coordination of care across settings is ensured through regular and high-quality communication between providers at times of transition or changing needs, and through effective continuity of care that utilizes the techniques of case management.[2]
- Both patient and family are prepared for the dying process and for death, when it is anticipated. Hospice options are explored, opportunities for personal growth are enhanced and bereavement support is available for the family.[2]

PLANNING CONSIDERATIONS

Site Selection

The palliative care facility should be located on the ground floor or adjacent to the tertiary care hospital. It is suggested that there should be close, collaborative, service and operational linkages between palliative care center and a tertiary care hospital facility specialty in the areas of pharmacy, radiology, and treatment interventions. Due considerations should be given to the road network and availability of public transport facility. The unit should harmonize with its environment, as far possible. The formal institutional appearance and environment should be avoided considering the complex emotions of the patients and their relatives.

General Principles of Design

Domestic character of the hospital should be created particularly for the inpatient areas. This should be achieved by careful attention to such considerations as quality of light, exploiting views, use of color selection of furniture and finishes. The physical accommodation for patients should be of interest and have a relaxed atmosphere, and consistent with the requirements of nursing care. A clear, legible and 'user-friendly' signage system (both internal and external) should be incorporated in the design. The circulation pattern should be simple and without criss-cross. The circulation route for OPD and IPD patients should be segregated. The environment should offer privacy to patients and their families. Sheltered outdoor spaces should be created in and around the unit for the utilization by patients, staff, and visitors, and to assist orientation. Patients should be provided with a view to the outside. There should be flexibility in the planning of defined areas to maximize potential use of the facilities and to meet possible future changes, with a suggested overall expansion factor of approximately 25–30%. This factor will require particular consideration for each project, and should identify those areas of the project considered most likely to require expansion. Careful consideration should be given to ensure a quiet environment, with a higher than normal level of sound containment and acoustic privacy, for patients and their families. This effect of noise can be reduced by locating noise generating rooms away from those requiring quietness, by isolating sound sources with sound containing partitions and doors, by absorbing sound with acoustic materials and by the incorporation of floor coverings, curtains, and other materials that do not reflect sound. Cultural aspects of the concerned region should also be accounted for. In view of the possibility of unpleasant odors in bedrooms, bathrooms, WC's, and day areas, the level of ventilation provided should be of a high standard. While recognizing this need for mechanical ventilation in particular areas, it is desirable that natural ventilation should be used wherever possible, and every effort should be made to avoid draughts. The fittings and finishes that are of low maintenance should be chosen. It is recommended to follow the principle of integrated design and universal access as some of the patients may have disabilities. All statutory requirements in design should be followed. Visual integration of artwork should be integrated in the complete design of palliative care center.

Planning

The building should be planned in such a manner that travel distances are reduced for the users.

- Long corridors should be kept to a minimum, to avoid any institutional activities, and should have natural light and views to the outside.
- Circulation spaces should be designed to accommodate appropriate activities, and should have natural light and views to the outside.
- Necessary space/room should be provided for moving and turning of wheelchairs/hospital beds throughout the design of the palliative care center.

Sitting Relationships

Core activities of patient care should be located close together centrally and supportive activities more peripherally. Patient's rooms should also have easy access to facilities for therapies, and should also be designed to deliver such services at bed side in case required.

Furniture and Finishes

The selection of furniture and fittings should take into account the following considerations:

- Performance (including clinical and infection control), appearance, durability, maintenance, flexibility in use, fire safety, cost, acoustics
- Ease of use for those with sensory or physical disability is of primary importance
- Beds of adjustable height to allow for nursing on the one hand, and independent transfer on the other should be provided.

External Design

External design of palliative care center should be of high quality with an open and welcoming character. Following aspects should be considered:

- It should not in any way reinforce the feelings of fear and anxiety to the patients.
- In addition to the normal activities and functions of the exterior of an acute care setting, such as access, parking, garden space, storage and so on, a palliative care center should have additional requirements for educational and other purposes.
- Car parking should be able to accommodate the vehicles for the patients, relatives, staff, religious teachers, consultants and home care team if same is functional.

Functional Areas: Inpatient Unit

A wide range of specialist services should be provided to patients and their families, including medical, nursing, paramedical, psychosocial and spiritual care:

- About 50% inpatient beds should be provided in single room with attached toilet for ease of nursing, treatment and need of relatives.
- Remaining beds may be arranged in cubicle of 4 bed rooms. Individual spaces should be created with the help of design elements and furniture items.
- Each bed space to be provided with natural light and outside views. Principles of evidence-based design to be followed
- Access to the ward should be directly from outside
- The width of any external door provided should be sufficient to allow the passage of a bed. Steps should be avoided, and a safe balcony, terrace or other paved area should be provided.
- Design of wards, and supporting operational policies, should allow for the greatest flexibility in terms of the gender mix of patients at any given time and facilitate the achievement of high standards of privacy and dignity for patients.

Single Bedrooms, with En Suite Water Closet and Shower Facilities

Single rooms should be grouped together. The size of the room should be 20 sqm.

- The size of a single bedroom should be enough to accommodate 1–2 relatives during day time and one at night time. The room should be provided with a wall mounted seat or sofa cum bed (single) which can function as pull down type extra bed during night. Room should have extra storage space for hospital linen.
- Each single room should have sufficient space around the bed to allow for the full range of high dependency nursing activities to take place, and for the safe use and positioning of equipment.

- It is recommended that one or two single bedrooms in each specialist unit should be equipped with electrically operated ceiling hoists, allowing for the transfer of patients from bed to a chair or to the en suite bathroom.
- It is recommended that patient's room should be provided with:
  - Attached toilet/bathroom with [Wash Hand Basins (WHB)—height adjustment possible if required]
  - Additional WHB in the room
  - Central gases
  - Natural lighting and ventilation
  - Artificial lighting for reading, therapeutic procedure and night dimmable light
  - Adjustable ventilation and air extractor system
  - Telephone
  - Television/DVD player
  - Controllable piped music
  - Facility for drinking water
  - Storage space
  - Bed side locker
  - Wardrobe and place for displaying personal items
  - Two nurse call bells strategically located
  - Bed pan.
- All bedrooms and bathrooms should be wheelchair accessible.
- A curtain should be provided inside the door of each single room, in order to maintain patient privacy. The basin should allow the patient to sit at it to wash. Taps are to be chosen that are suitable for patients with reduced dexterity. The vanity mirror should be fitted at a level that will allow it to be used from a standing or sitting position. It should be capable of being concealed when not wanted.
- The toilet bowl should be positioned to allow carers to give assistance from either or both sides, where planning permits. En suite layouts should be designed in such a way to facilitate left-hand or right-hand use, to ensure the availability of Water Closet (WC) facilities that permit lateral transfer in each direction.
- Taking account of the specific and particular needs of single rooms as noted above, it is recommended that in new developments they should be up to 20 sqm each in floor area, including the en suite bathroom. The provision of various individually sized rooms up to this limit may be appropriate.
- Projection system for creating suitable environment.

Four Bedrooms, En Suite

The recommended make for single room will also apply to 4 bedroom cubicle. Other salient points to be kept in mind are the following:
- Size of 4 bedded cubicles should be 60 sqm
- Separate accommodation should be provided away from the ward for relatives who wish to stay over with a patient.
- A small sitting area should be provided for the enjoyment of patients and visitors. This should preferably have natural light and a view to the outside.

Isolation Room

Each ward should have an isolation room. These isolation rooms should have following essential features:
- These rooms should have an ante-room or lobby with a WHB and a clothes rack for protective clothing.
- The isolation room should be provided with an air management system for the control of infection and negative pressure should be maintained.
- Isolation room should be provided with an additional area for lobby, containing gowning and utility area.

Nursing Station

It should be so positioned that the nurse(s) on duty can communicate easily with patients and have immediate and direct access to patients. It should allow for at least 2 people to work comfortably, (on a 24 hours basis) as well as providing space and support for ward staff. It should have provision for keeping controlled drugs in the form of lockers.

The following accommodation should be provided, for sharing between wards.
- Wheelchair and equipment store
- *A quiet room*: It should be provided for complementary therapies, including aromatherapy, acupuncture and music therapy.
- *Interview room*: This room should be provided for meetings between staff, patients and their families. The door should be wide enough to allow for the easy movement of a wheelchair, or on occasion, a bed. The room should be large enough to accommodate approximately 10 people and should have a non-clinical and comfortable character. The room will also be used to accommodate distressed families after a death. A telephone point should also be provided.
- *Store for patient's belongings*: A small room or cupboard space should be provided for the storage of personal effects and items belonging to deceased patients while awaiting their collection by the patient's family.

Other Inpatient Ward Accommodation

A range of other facilities and spaces should be provided in the ward or the specialized palliative care inpatient unit, like ward pantry and kitchenette, dirty utility and sluice room, clean utility room, linen store, cleaner's room, public toilets, staff toilets.

Activity room: To utilize the available skill of the patient for creative work/skill, they possess and can be put to use when they feel physically comfortable.

Pharmacy

The palliative care center should have an independent pharmacy.

Dietary Services

Following points should be considered for dietary services:
- Accommodation should be provided for the facility in the light of the policy of the center for provisioning of diet to the patients.
- In addition, a pantry should be provided for the need of relatives spending long hours with patients.

Rehabilitation Department

Facilities for various therapies (physiotherapy, occupational therapy, and speech therapy) should be provided close to one another, to facilitate speedy referrals, joint working, and the flexible use of departmental accommodation and to assist in multidisciplinary team approach. Each of above facility should have administrative and technical area which should be planned with due consideration of patient's dignity and privacy.

Spiritual Care/Yoga

Facilities should be provided in the inpatient unit, for suitably trained spiritual teacher to give spiritual care. This room should be capable of accommodating approximately 10–12 people on a daily basis, including wheelchair and bed access.

Mortuary

The facility should be provided for holding and viewing of remains, it should also have provision of suitable accommodation for relatives and a prayer room.

Medical Stores/Dispensary: The policies should be laid down for:
- Procurement of store
- Storage
- Distribution of stores
- Urgent issue of items
- Maintenance of equipment
- Controlled dangerous drugs.

Communications System: The palliative care center should have the following systems for intramural and extramural communication:
- Nurse call system
- Public address system with facility for zone paging
- Intercom telephone system for internal communication
- A telephone system for contact with external agencies. It also offers facility for the patients to make long distance calls directly from their room and has facility for remote metering. Public telephones are also required at convenient locations such as the visitors area
- Cellular phone system for staff on call duty
- Closed circuit television system for isolation rooms and for surveillance purposes.

Functional Relationship

Functional relationship of the components are given in Figure 2.

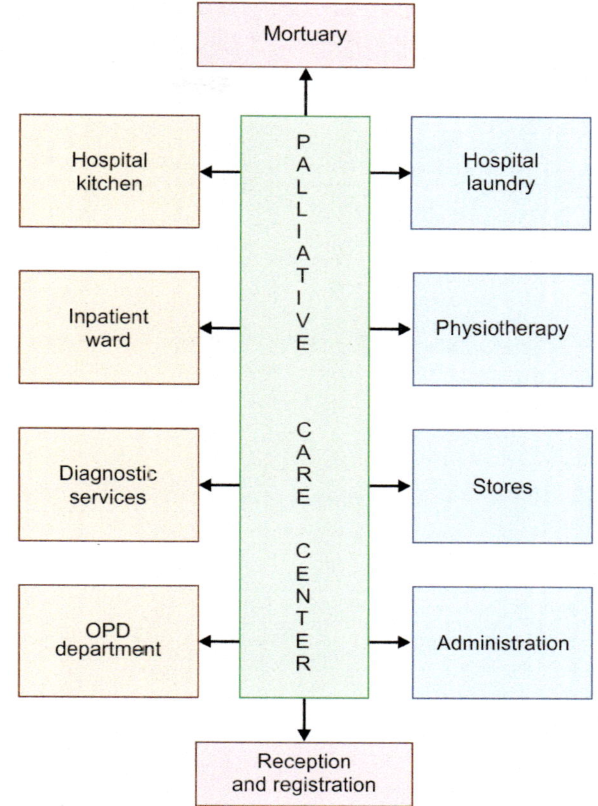

Fig. 2: Functional relationship.

SCHEDULE OF ACCOMMODATION

Schedule of accommodation for a 50 bedded palliative care center are given in Tables 1 to 7 and Figures 3 to 6.

A suggested functional layout of palliative care center is shown in Figures 3 and 4 and layout in Figures 5 and 6.

Table 1: Schedule of accommodation—OPD.

Sl. No.	Facility	Size (sqm)
1.	General waiting	24.0
2.	Public utilities	14.0
3.	Enquiry counter	10.0
4.	Admission discharge	10.0
5.	Cash counter	10.0
6.	Staff accommodation	12.0
7.	Chemist	12.0
8.	Gift book shop	10.0
9.	Ambulance station	10.0
10.	Exam/consultation (2)	15.0
11.	Sub-waiting	15.0
12.	Nurse's desk	12.00
13.	Sample collection	10.0
14.	Side laboratory	15.0
15.	Sub-waiting	18.0

Table 2: Schedule of accommodation diagnostic services.

Sl. No.	Facility	Size (sqm)
1.	*Imaging*	
2.	*Reception* • Enquiry/Registration • Queing track • Records • Sub-waiting	 12.0 12.0 10.0 15.0
3.	*General X-ray* • Radiography room • Control room • Change room • Sub-waiting	 28.0 7.0 7.0 15.0
4.	*Ultrasound* • Ultrasound room • Change room • Sub-waiting	 12.0 7.0 15.0
5.	*Support* • Dark room • Film/Chemical store • Reporting • Archive/Record	 12.0 10.0 15.0 10.0
6.	*Staff* • Consultant (1) • Residents • Technicians • Staff toilets	 12.0 12.0 12.0 7.0

Table 3: Schedule of accommodation—ICU.

Sl. No.	Facility	Size (sqm)
1.	*Patient care area*	
2.	*Nursing station* • Central console • Clean utility • Pantry • Store • Equipment park • Dirty utility • Janitor • Trolley park • Patient beds intensive care beds 4 • Patient conveniences • Relatives bay • Nurses duty • Doctors duty • Staff change	 20.0 7.0 7.0 10.0 10.0 7.0 3.0 10.0 42.0 7.0 12.0 12.0 12.0 7.0

Table 4: Schedule of accommodation—physiotherapy.

Sl. No.	Facility	Size (sqm)
	Therapies	
1.	Reception/record	12.0
2.	Electrotherapy	15.0
3.	Massage therapy	10.0
4.	Thermo therapy	10.0 each
5.	Gymnasium	30.0
6.	Traction	10.0
7.	Store	10.0
8.	Physiotherapist with attached toilet	15.0
9.	Sub-waiting with toilet	15.0

Table 5: Schedule of accommodation inpatient area.

Sl. No.	Facility	Size (sqm)	Remarks
1.	Single bedded rooms	15	
2.	Double bedded room	25.00	
3.	Multibedded rooms	42	4 beds
4.	Single isolation bedroom	15.00	
5.	Bay—mobile equipment	4.00	
6.	Bay—linen	2.00	
7.	Bay—hand washing	1.00	In addition to hand basins in bedrooms
8.	Bathrooms/toilets	3–5	Assisted bathroom facilities to be provided
9.	Toilet disabled	5.00	
10.	Treatment room	10–16	Wash hand basins, mechanical ventilation, compressed pipe medical gas
11.	Clean utility	10.00	
12.	Dirty utility	10.00	
13.	Nursing station	14	Have access to clean utility, treatment rooms and patient care areas
14.	Dining room	18.00–21.00	
15.	Interview room	12.00	May also be used for family overnight stays
16.	Meeting room small	12.00	Quiet sitting room, access to an outdoor area is desirable
17.	Office single person	9.00	Unit manager
18.	Office-3 person shared	16.00	Dependent on staffing establishment
19.	Pantry	8.00	Stainless sink, wash hand basins
20.	Store equipment	10.	
21.	Lounge patient	15.00	
22.	Circulation %	35%	
Shared areas			
1.	Bathroom	10.00	
2.	Cleaner's room	4.00	
3.	Disposal room	8.00	
4.	Meeting room	10.00	
5.	Multipurpose activities room	30.00	For inpatients and day patients
6.	Reception	10.00	
7.	Toilet staff	2.0	

Table 6: Schedule of accommodation—mortuary.

Sl. No.	Facility	Size (sqm)
1.	Autopsy	20.0
2.	Body store	10.0
3.	Body wash	10.0
4.	Staff accommodation	10.0
5.	Public utilities	3.0
6.	Sub-waiting	14.0

Table 7: Schedule of accommodation for 50 bedded palliative care center.

Sl. No.	Facility	Size (sqm)
1.	*Palliative care center administration*	
	• Medical superintendent	21.0
	• Secretarial staff	15.0
	• Sub-waiting	18.0
2.	*Nursing administration*	
	• Matron	14.0
	• Secretarial staff	15.0
	• Sub-waiting	12.0
3.	*General administration*	
	• Personnel office	14.0
	• Accounts office	18.0
	• Purchase office	18.0
	• Secretarial staff	15.0
	• Sub-waiting	12.0
4.	*Hospital information*	
	• Supervisor	10.50
	• Computer room	21.00
5.	*Security/fire*	
	• Supervisor	10.50
	• Secretarial staff	7.0

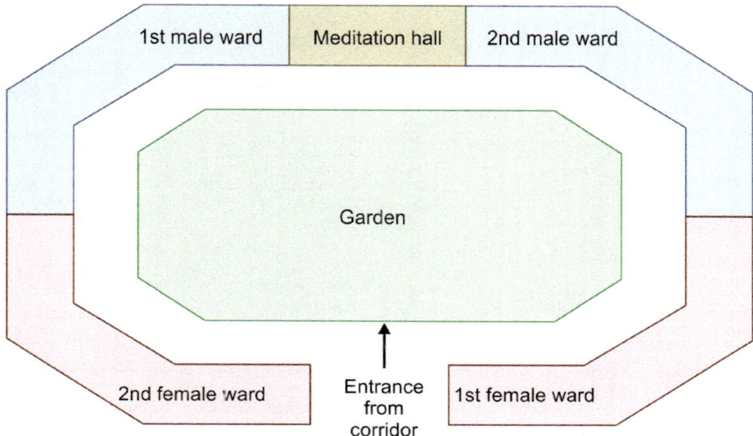

Fig. 4: Functional diagram of the inpatient areas on the first floor of the palliative care center.

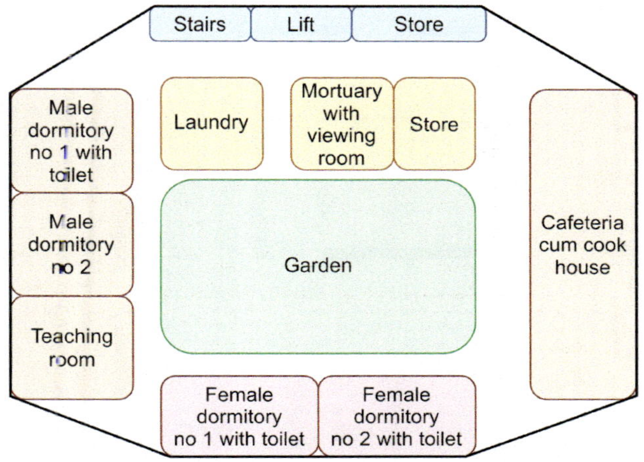

Fig. 3: Functional diagram ground floor of palliative care center.

CONCLUSION

Palliative care services aim to support patients of all ages with debilitating and life threatening illness, and their families, through the full course of the illness, regardless of its duration, until cure or until death, and through the bereavement period. Palliative care is delivered through skilled and interdisciplinary attention to pain and other distressing symptom; emotional, spiritual and practical support; assistance with complex medical decision-making; and coordination across the continuum of healthcare settings. The goal is to help the patient and family achieve the best possible quality of life in accordance with their values, needs and preferences.[2]

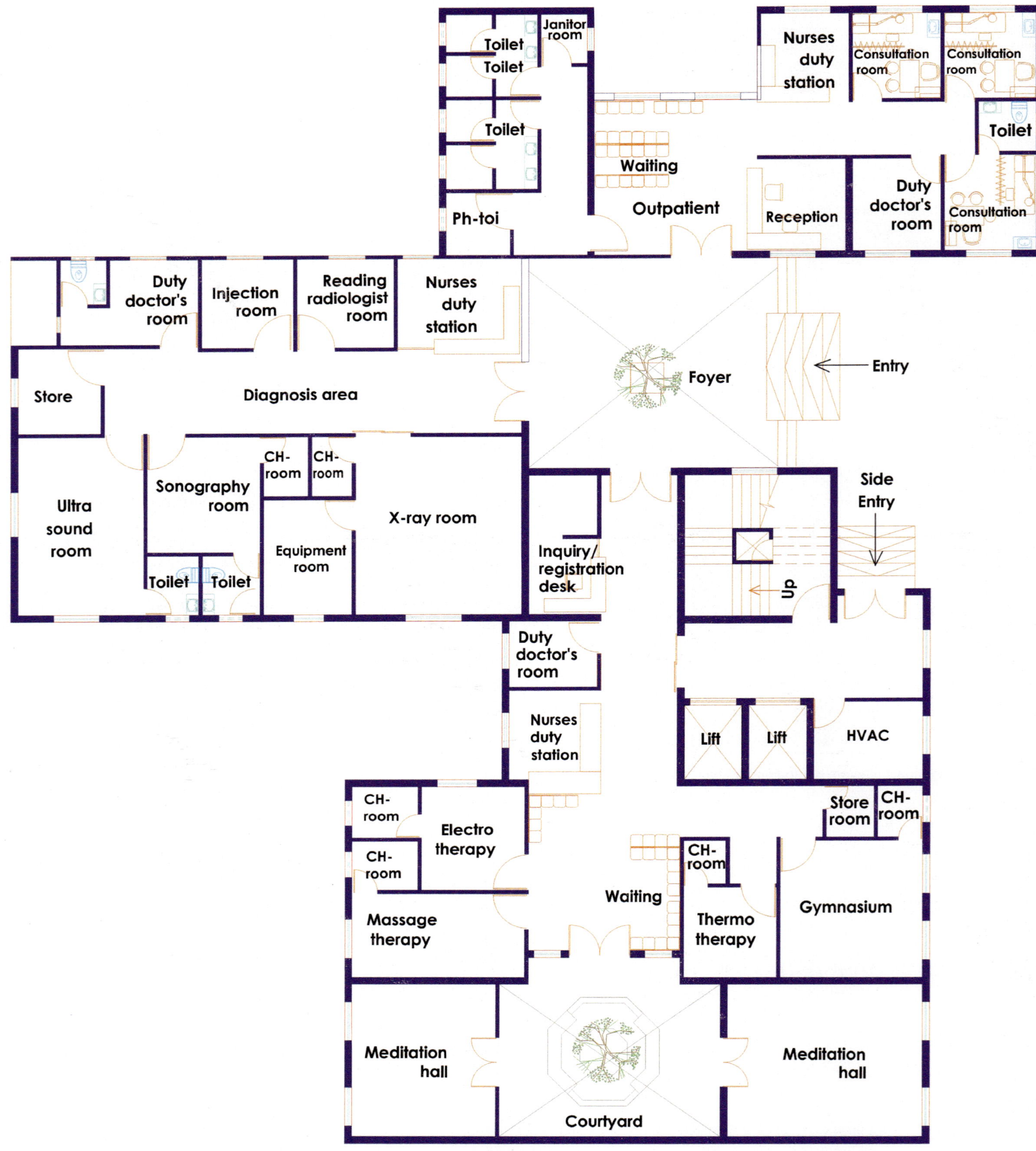

Fig. 5: Ground floor plan.

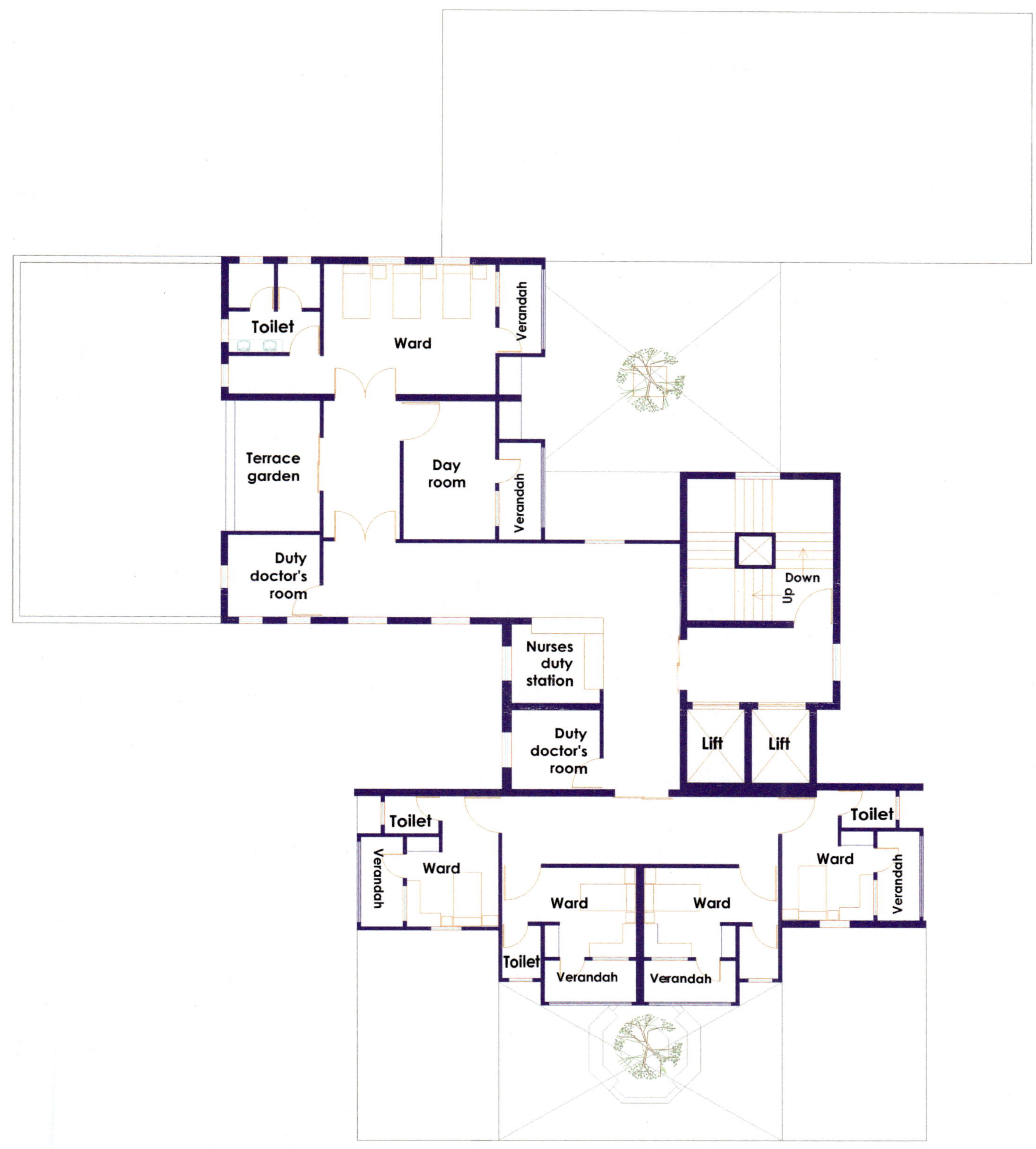

Fig. 6: First floor plan.

REFERENCES

1. arcweb.sos.state.or.us
2. growthhouse.typepad.com

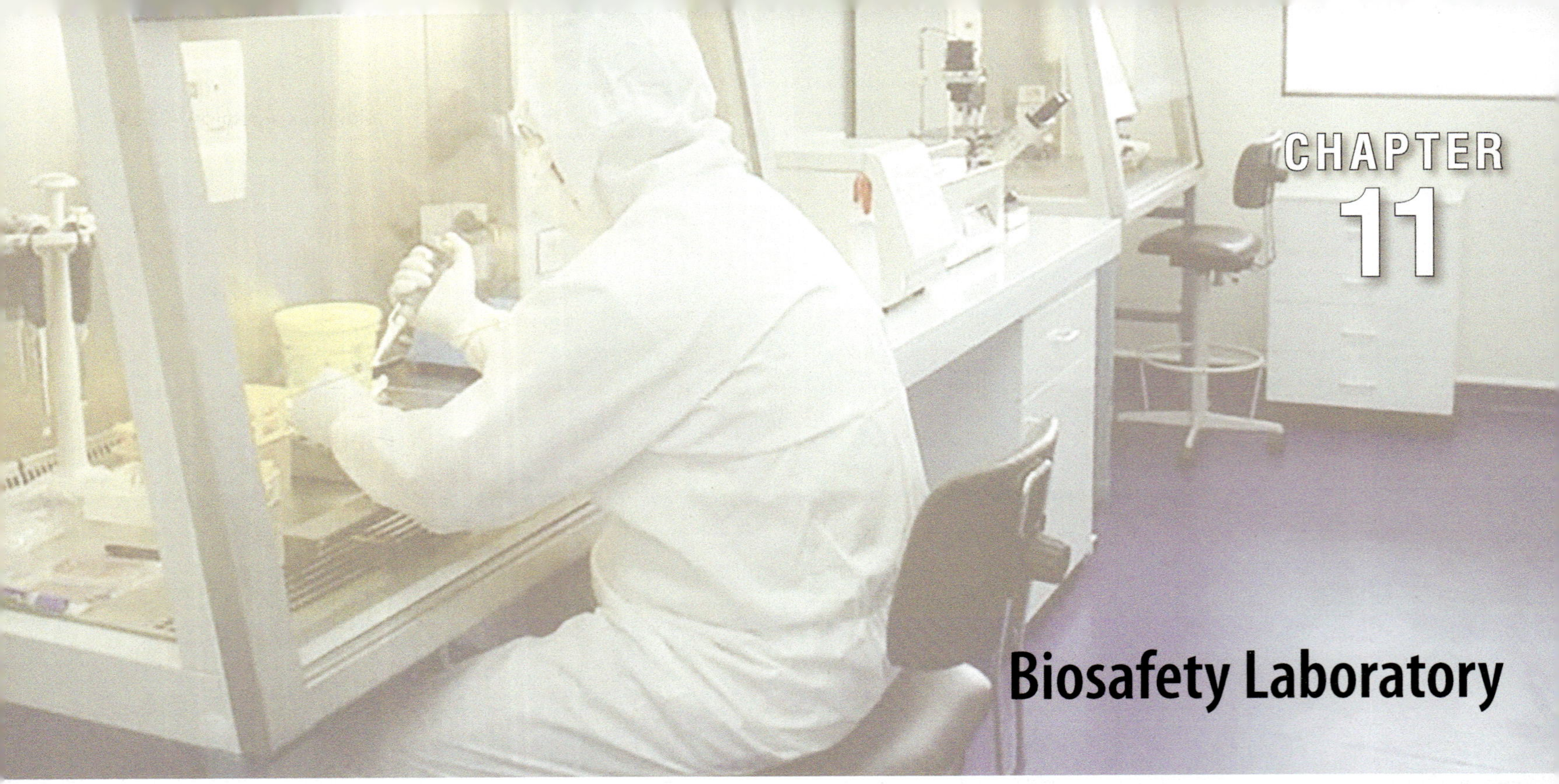

CHAPTER 11

Biosafety Laboratory

Dinesh Negi, Shakti Kumar Gupta, Sunil Kant, R Chandrashekhar

INTRODUCTION

To control epidemics and protect public health, medical researchers should be able to identify naturally occurring microbes at the earliest and develop appropriate diagnostic tests and vaccines for them. In combating bioterrorism, where deliberate release of a microbe into a community is done, in which it is not a current health concern identical scientific skills and strategies are required.[1,2]

The World Health Organization (WHO) has long recognized that safety and, in particular, biological safety are important international issues. It continues to provide international leadership in biosafety by addressing biological safety and security issues regarding risk assessment, safe use of recombinant DNA technology and transport of infectious materials. Recent world events have revealed new threats to public health through deliberate misuse and release of microbiological agents and toxins the protection of microbiological assets from theft, loss or diversion, which could lead to the inappropriate use of these agents to cause public health harm.[3-5]

FUNCTIONS OF FACILITY

The function of the facility is to impart research, training and patient care. These functions include:[6]

- Studying diseases naturally present in the environment.
- Understanding how pathogens cause disease.
- Developing new ways to detect and diagnose diseases.
- Aiding biomedical research and training.
- Producing new vaccines and treatments.
- Assisting national, state, and local public health efforts in the event of a bioterrorism emergency.

Biodefense is one of the stated purposes of the facility. This means that the facility will help to defend nation and the world against biological threats, both natural and man-made, by studying agents that already are or may become threats in the future.[6]

KEY PLANNING AND DESIGN PARAMETERS

There has been a considerable change in the design and construction of biomedical and microbiological laboratories. Advances in technology and knowledge have resulted in the establishment of high-containment laboratories which are highly sophisticated facilities, and which require specialized expertise to design, construct, operate, and maintain. Since these facilities are intended to contain dangerous microorganisms, usually in liquid or aerosol form, even minor structural defects—such as cracks in the wall, leaky pipes, or improper sealing around doors—could have serious consequences. Supporting infrastructure, such as drainage and waste treatment systems must also be secure. High-containment laboratories are expensive to build and maintain and any breach of security can result into a serious public health crisis.[7]

Figure 1 shows various barriers which should be considered while designing a biosafety laboratory. The barriers are classified in three categories:

Primary barriers: This consists of safety equipment and control practices.

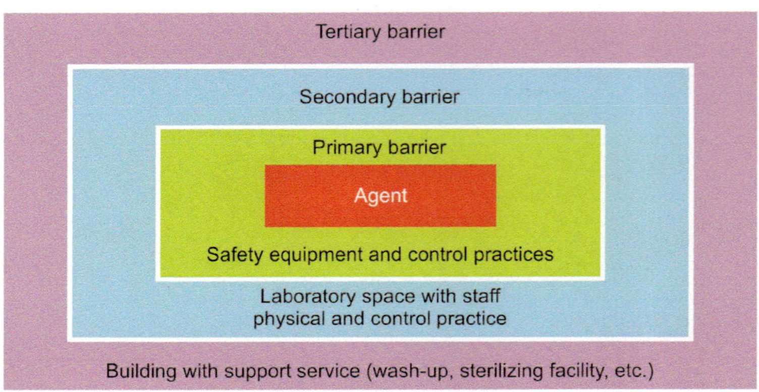

Fig. 1: Barriers in biosafety laboratory.

Secondary barriers: The laboratory space with staff and physical design with access control are included in this category.

Tertiary barriers: The building with support services provide tertiary barrier to the facility.

Depending upon the purpose of the laboratory various combination of the barriers are employed and accordingly the laboratories are designated levels from BSL-1 to BSL-4. Facilities, safety equipment and procedures in various BSL are shown in Table 1.

The features that distinguish a BSL-4 laboratory from lower level (BSL-1, 2, 3) microbiological laboratories are (Fig. 2):

- Provisions for access control.
- Safety measures for staff working in such laboratories
- Use of biosafety cabinets or fume hoods for all laboratory activities
- A specialized ventilation system ensuring directional airflow
- Exhaust of air after due contamination.

A BSL laboratory may be a single laboratory, a suite of laboratories or an entire building (Fig. 3). The primary objective of this type of facility is to provide the best possible physical containment of hazardous

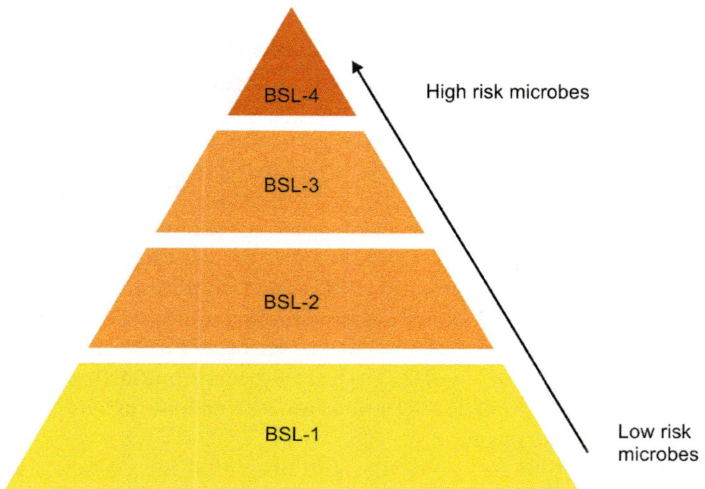

Fig. 2: The BSL levels and microbes risk.

Table 1: Facilities, safety equipment and procedures in venous BSLS.[8,9]

Biosafety level	*1*	*2*	*3*	*4*
Facilities	Standard well-designed experimental animal and laboratory facilities	*Level 1 plus*: Separate laboratory, room surfaces impervious and readily cleaned, biohazard sign	*Level 2 plus*: Controlled access double door entry and body shower, air pressure must be negative at all times, no recirculation, HEPA filtration, backup power	Level 3 plus: Specialized, secure, completely self-contained unit with specialized ventilation, fully monitored; airlock entry and exit
Safety equipment	Hand washing facilities, laboratory coats	*Level 1 plus*: Autoclave, HEPA filtered class I or II biological safety cabinet, personal protective equipment	*Level 2 plus:* Autoclave, HEPA filtered class II biological safety cabinet, personal protective equipment to include solid front laboratory clothing, head covers, dedicated footwear, and gloves, appropriate respiratory protection	*Level 3 plus*: Class III biological safety cabinets, positive pressure ventilated suits
Procedures	Basic safe laboratory practices	Use of personal protective equipment laboratory coat worn only in the laboratory, gloves, decontamination	Staff fully trained, written protocols; showers, wastes disposed of as contaminated, use of biological safety cabinets, personal protective devices	*Level 3 plus*: Access only to certified staff, rigorous sterilization/decontamination procedures

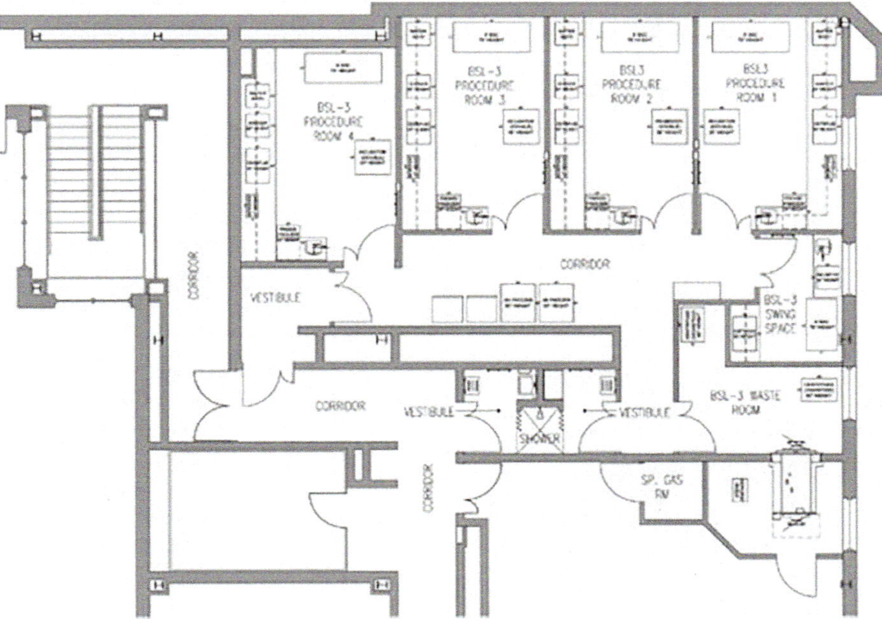

Fig. 3: Biosafety laboratory.

microorganisms or biological agents. All laboratory manipulations should be performed in a biosafety cabinet (BSC) or other enclosed equipment.

The biosafety cabinet is relied upon as the primary device in BSL laboratories for protecting products, personnel or the environment. In contrast are chemical fume hoods designed to provide only personnel protection.

The pressurized laboratory space serves as a secondary containment barrier. General exhaust air from the laboratory is often treated with high efficiency particulate air (HEPA) filters before it is exhausted outdoors. A dedicated exhaust system may be required, depending on the class/type of biosafety cabinet used. One other functional aspect of a BSL laboratory is the need for gaseous decontamination, essentially requiring a "tight" space. Penetrations must be capable of being sealed for fumigation purposes.

The ventilation system design and operation have a key role in biological containment facilities, a thorough understanding of the specialized requirements (HVAC) is necessary to safeguard researchers and other building occupants from potential exposure through inhalation.

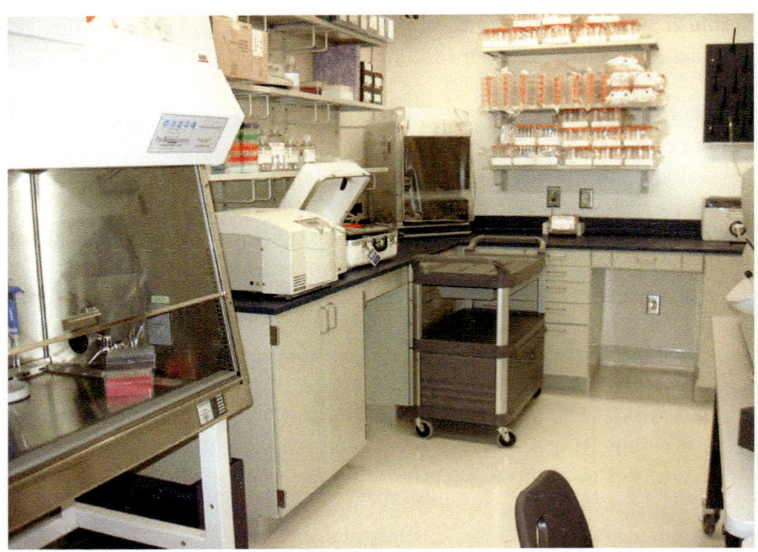

Fig. 5: Biosafety level 3.

Biosafety Level 1 (BSL-1)

The most basic level of containment is level one, which uses standard microbiological practices and no special primary or secondary barriers, other than a sink, for hand washing. The type of microorganisms present is not known to cause disease in healthy humans. Normally, this is the level at which water-testing, undergraduate and secondary educational training and teaching laboratories operate.

Biosafety Level 2 (BSL-2) (Fig. 4)

This level is applicable to clinical, diagnostic, teaching and other laboratories where moderate risk agents are present but not known to be transmissible by the aerosol route. The primary hazard to personnel is from exposures through the skin, mucous membrane exposure or ingestion. Procedures with aerosol or high splash potential must be conducted in primary containment equipment, such as a BSC (biosafety cabinet). Secondary barriers, such as hand washing sinks and decontamination facilities, must be available to reduce environmental contamination.

Biosafety Level 3 (BSL-3) (Fig. 5)

At this level, the risk of respiratory transmission causing serious and potentially lethal infections is present, and more emphasis is placed on primary and secondary barriers for protection. All laboratory manipulations should be performed in a BSC or other enclosed equipment. Secondary barriers include controlled access, often double-door entry through the use of an anteroom or airlock, and air movement that is directional and single-pass.

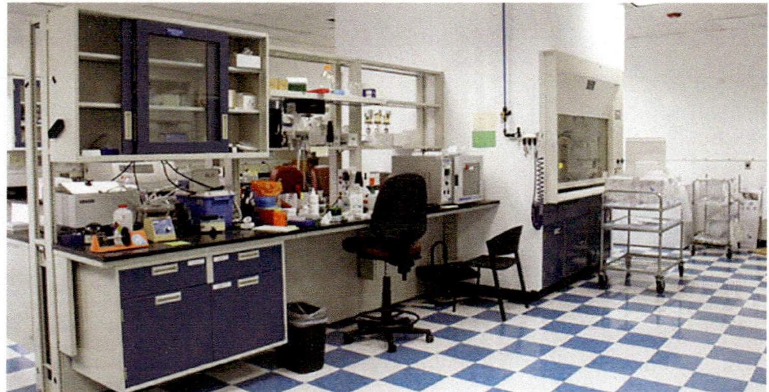

Fig. 4: Biosafety level 2.

Biosafety Level 4 (BSL-4)

At this level, dangerous and exotic agents pose a high individual risk of life-threatening diseases, which may be transmitted via the aerosol route and for which there is no available vaccine or therapy. All manipulations pose a high risk of exposure, not only to laboratory personnel, but also to the community and the environment. Work is conducted in a class III biosafety cabinet or in a full-body, air-supplied positive-pressure personnel suit. The facility is generally a separate building or a completely isolated zone. Complex ventilation and waste management systems are used to prevent the release of viable agents.[10,11]

The summary of biosafety level requirements are shown in Table 2 and containment levels in Table 3.

BSL-4 laboratory differs from BSL-3 laboratory in following ways:[12,13]

- Laboratory personnel receive specific and thorough training to handle extremely hazardous infectious agents. Their supervisor are competent scientists who are trained and experienced in working with these agents.
- Laboratory personnel understand the function of primary and secondary barriers and laboratory design features. They are trained in standard and special microbiological practices and the proper use of primary containment equipment.
- The laboratory director strictly controls access to the laboratory.
- The laboratory is in a controlled area within a building, completely isolated from all other areas of the building, or is in a separate building.
- All activities involving agent manipulation within the work area of the laboratory are conducted within a class III BSC, or within a class I or class II BSC used in conjunction with a one-piece, positive-pressure protective suit that is ventilated by a life-support system.
- The BSL-4 laboratory, or maximum containment laboratory, has special engineering and design features to prevent dissemination of microorganisms to the environment.

Table 2: Summary of biosafety level requirements.[12]

Sl. No.	Biosafety level	1	2	3	4
1.	Isolation of laboratory	No	No	Desirable	Yes
2.	Room sealable for decontamination	No	No	Yes	Yes
3.	Ventilation:				
	– Inward air flow	No	Desirable	Yes	Yes
	– Mechanical via building system	No	Desirable	Yes	No
	– Mechanical, independent	No	Desirable	Yes	Yes
	– HEPA filtered air exhaust	No	No	Desirable	Yes
4.	Double-door entry	No	No	Yes	Yes
5.	Airlock	No	No	No	Yes
6.	Airlock with shower	No	No	No	Yes
7.	Anteroom	No	No	Yes	No
8.	Anteroom with shower	No	No	Desirable	No
9.	Effluent treatment	No	No	Desirable	No
10.	Autoclave:				
	– On site	Yes	Yes	Yes	Yes
	– In laboratory room	No	No	Desirable	Yes
	– Double-ended	No	No	Desirable	Yes
11.	Biological safety cabinets:				
	– Class I	No	Optional	Yes	No
	– Class II	No	Desirable	Yes	Yes, in conjunction with suit laboratories
	– Class III	No	No	Desirable	Yes, in conjunction with cabinet laboratories

Table 3: Containment levels.[15]

Matrix x 1	Containment level 1	2	3	4	Laboratory location and access
1	●	●	●	●	Separated from public areas by door
2		●	●	●	Access limited to authorized personnel
3		●	●	●	Laboratory room doors to have appropriate signage (e.g. biohazard sign, containment level, contact information, entry requirements)
4	●	●	●	●	Size of door openings to allow passage of all anticipated equipment
5		●	●	●	Doors to the containment laboratory lockable (this does not apply to areas within the containment laboratory)
6			●	●	Doors to provide restricted access by installation of a controlled access system (e.g. card key) or equivalent
7			○	●	Electronic locking systems to be backed up with a physical key-lock system
8		○	●	●	Office areas to be located outside of containment laboratory. Paperwork stations for data collection can be within containment laboratory provided they are located away from laboratory work areas
9			●	●	Entry to laboratory to be provided via an anteroom
10			●		Anteroom door(s) located between the clean and dirty change rooms not to be opened simultaneously with either the containment laboratory door or the clean change entry door (Interlock, visual or audible alarms, or protocols are all acceptable means)
11				●	Anteroom door(s) located between the clean and dirty change rooms not to be opened simultaneously with either the containment laboratory door or the clean change entry door (interlock only)
12			●	●	Interlocked doors, if present, to have manual overrides for emergency exit
13			●	●	Entry to laboratory zone to be provided with clothing change areas separating personal and laboratory clothing dedicated to that zone (i.e. "clean" change area separated from "dirty" change area)
14			●	●	Exit from laboratory to be provided with a walk-through shower on the containment barrier (i.e. between "dirty" and "clean" change anterooms) (CL3 laboratories manipulating organisms, such as HIV, that are not infectious via inhalation, are not required to fulfill this criterion)
15				●	Entry to laboratory to be provided via anteroom with airtight doors (e.g. inflatable or compression seal); for laboratories using only a class III BSC biological safety cabinet line, airtight doors are not required
16				●	Entry to laboratory zone to be provided with a suit change area, a chemical shower on the containment barrier (i.e. between the laboratory and suit change area) and water shower on exit from the zone (i.e. between "dirty" and "clean" change areas); for laboratories using only a class III biological safety cabinet line, suit change area and chemical shower are not required
17			○	●	Containment laboratories to be located in close proximity to supporting mechanical services to limit the amount of potentially contaminated services
18			○	●	Containment laboratories to be located away from external building envelope walls
19			○	○	A laboratory support area to be provided adjacent to the containment facility for all supporting laboratory manipulations

Thus, BSL-4 laboratories are protected with primary, secondary, and tertiary barriers. Primary barriers include suits and gloves scientists wear and the biosafety cabinet. The biosafety cabinets have an integral HEPA filter in addition to two HEPA filters in the exhaust. Biosafety cabinets become another layer of protection and a place to capture organisms before they escape. Secondary barriers include airlocks, chemical showers, doors, walls, kill tanks, and sterilizers. Tertiary barriers include fences around complexes and security guards.[14,16]

Classification of Infective Microorganisms by Risk Group[5]

Risk group 1 (no or low individual and community risk): A microorganism that is unlikely to cause human or animal disease.

Risk group 2 (moderate individual risk, low community risk): A pathogen that can cause human or animal disease but is unlikely to be a serious hazard to laboratory workers, the community, livestock or the environment. Laboratory exposures may cause serious infection, but effective treatment and preventive measures are available and the risk of spread of infection is limited.

Risk group 3 (high individual risk, low community risk): A pathogen that usually causes serious human or animal disease but does not ordinarily spread from one infected individual to another. Effective treatment and preventive measures are available.

Risk group 4 (high individual and community risk): A pathogen that usually causes serious human or animal disease and that can be readily transmitted from one individual to another, directly or indirectly. Effective treatment and preventive measures are not usually available.

Biosafety Cabinets (Fig. 6)

The biosafety cabinets (BSC) is the primary containment barrier and all work involving infectious material must be conducted within it. The cabinets are designed to protect personnel, products and the environment from exposure to biohazards and cross-contamination. There are three classes of cabinets that may be used, depending on the level of protection desired. While all classes may be found in BSL spaces, class II cabinets are the most common and within this class, there are four types of cabinets. These types—known as A1, A2, B1 and B2—differ by their operating requirements, primarily in flow velocity and the percentage of air exhausted (Table 4).

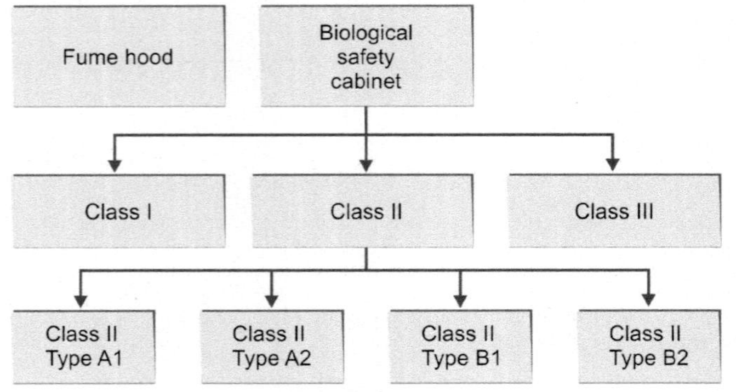

Fig. 6: Biosafety cabinets.

Table 4: Operating requirements of class II biological safety cabinets.[19]

Type	Inflow velocity	Exhaust amount	Exhaust through HEPA filter	Plenum pressure
A1	75 fpm (0.38 m/s)	30%	Optional	May be positive or negative
A2	100 fpm (0.5 m/s)	30%	Optional	Negative
B1	100 fpm (0.5 m/s)	70%	Yes	Negative
B2	100 fpm (0.5 m/s)	100%	Yes	Negative

Operation of Biosafety Cabinet

In class II cabinets, an internal blower draws airflow around the operator into the front opening and then into the front grille. At the same time, downward laminar flow of HEPA-filtered air minimizes the chance of product cross-contamination along the work surface of the cabinet. The downward moving air divides as it approaches the work surface, with the blower drawing part of the air to the front grille and the remainder toward the rear grille. Cabinet air exhaust is discharged through the rear plenum into the space between the supply and exhaust filters located at the top of the cabinet. The air passes through a certified exhaust HEPA filter, making it contaminant-free for either recirculation into the laboratory or extraction from the building.

Characteristics of Class II Biosafety Cabinets

- Leak-tight construction
- Requires two HEPA filters—supply and exhaust
- Airflow patterns
  - Clean (filtered) air flows down to the work surface
  - Downflow air splits 2–6 inch (5–15 cm) above the work surface
    - ◊ Some to rear of front grille
    - ◊ Some to rear of cabinet
- Intake air is drawn into the front of the front grille
- Air leaves work area and is HEPA filtered prior to being exhausted or recirculated in the cabinet.

Volumetric Offset versus Differential Pressurization Control

Maintaining correct room balances across cascaded pressurization zones can be complex from a ventilation control standpoint. Volumetric off set control, however, has proven to be a very effective method of achieving pressurization control in laboratories. Differential pressure control, controlling to a specific pressure, has historically been more difficult and less stable. The American National Standards Institute (ANSI) and the American Industrial Hygiene Association (AIHA) support the use of volumetric offset over differential pressurization for laboratory environments. "Specifying quantitative pressure differential is a poor basis for design...What is really desired is an offset air volume."[18]

"No specific pressure differential is required by the BMBL, and design basis varies widely between laboratories. The basis for determining the differential should be to create sufficient directional airflow to allow containment to occur during planned or unplanned breaches in the barrier."[5] A common differential used in BSL-3 laboratories is approximately 0.05 inch WC (12.45 Pa). As per Health Canada's *Laboratory Biosafety Guidelines*, "Directional inward airflow provided such that air will always flow toward areas of higher containment (e.g. ±25 Pa differential)."

Architectural Tightness (Figs. 7 and 8)

Due to the need for gaseous decontamination, BSL-3 laboratories must be designed as "tight" spaces. Air treatment systems for fumigation require that penetrations in walls, ceilings, and floors be sealed. For the ventilation system, accommodation must be made to seal the duct or reduce the airflow through the space, depending on the decontamination agent. Specifically, significantly reduced airflows or conventional shut-off devices may be required. For certain decontamination agents or other emergency conditions, bubble-tight dampers may be installed.

'Leak tight' is a term that may also be used in reference to the duct system, which is typically outside the containment barrier (room) and before any HEPA filtration or ultraviolet (UV) decontamination. In the event, the exhaust side becomes positively pressurized, the concern exists that potentially contaminated air may leak into surrounding areas. In this scenario, the definition of "leak tight" or "airtight" is based on a given loss of pressure over a stated time period.[16,17]

The *Handbook of Laboratory Safety* suggests a minimum of 6 air changes per hour (ACH) with a range from 10–20 air changes per hour for higher risk laboratories.[7] Designs for 10–12 air changes per hour for BSL-3 facilities appear to be common and this may be lowered to 6 ACH at night when the laboratory is unoccupied. The air change rate will likely be determined by equipment exhaust requirements.[19,20]

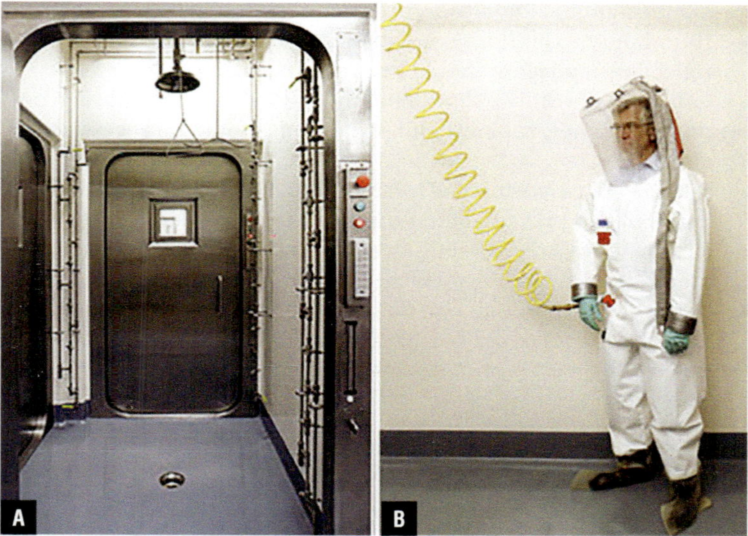

Figs. 7A and B: (A) Airlock entrance in laboratory's hot zone; (B) A biohazard suit.

High-efficiency Particulate Air Filtration

The biosafety cabinet incorporates a HEPA filter in its exhaust and/or supply system, additional filtering is optional in a BSL-3 laboratory, "The need for filtration should be reviewed with the appropriate safety officers."[8] However, the use of HEPA filtration on the room's general exhaust is considered a prudent practice in most cases. If the valve is

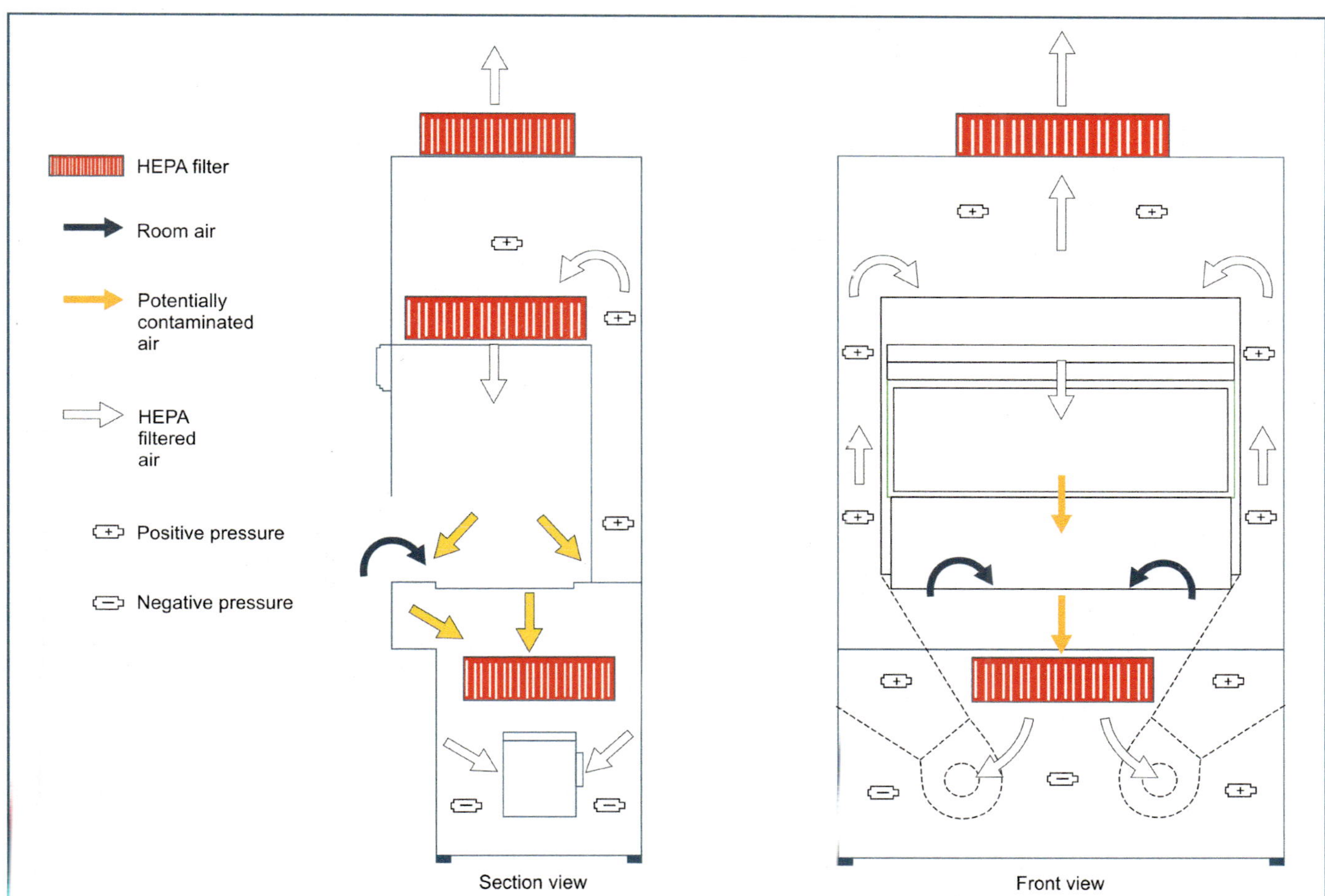

Fig. 8: Characteristics of all class II type B1 biosafety cabinet.

located outside of the containment perimeter, consideration should be given to isolation of valve casing leakage and HEPA filtration of pressure monitor lines, including valve pressure switches and pressure monitor sensors. "HEPA filter housings should have gas-tight isolation dampers; decontamination ports; and/or bag-in/bag-out (with appropriate decontamination procedures) capability. The HEPA filter housing should allow for leak testing of each filter and assembly. The filters and the housing should be certified at least annually."[11,21]

DESIGN REQUIREMENTS (FIGS. 9 AND 10)[5,18-20]

- The international biohazard warning symbol and sign must be displayed. On the doors of the rooms where microorganisms of risk group 2 or higher risk groups are handled.[22-24]
- Only authorized persons should be allowed to enter the laboratory working areas.
- Laboratory doors should be kept closed.
- Ample space must be provided for the safe conduct of laboratory work and for cleaning and maintenance.
- Walls, ceilings and floors should be smooth and the structure should be earthquake resistant and even in severe condition even the hair crack should not appear. The floor should be easy to clean, impermeable to liquids and resistant to the chemicals and disinfectants normally used in the laboratory. Floors should be slip-resistant.
- Bench tops should be impervious to water and resistant to disinfectants, acids, alkalis, organic solvents and moderate heat.
- Illumination should be adequate for all activities. Undesirable reflections and glare should be avoided.
- Laboratory furniture should be sturdy. Open spaces between and under benches, cabinets and equipment should be accessible for cleaning.
- Storage space must be adequate to hold supplies for immediate use and thus prevent clutter on bench tops. Additional long-term storage space, conveniently located outside the laboratory working areas, should also be provided.
- Space and facilities should be provided for the safe handling and storage of solvents, radioactive materials, compressed and liquefied gases.

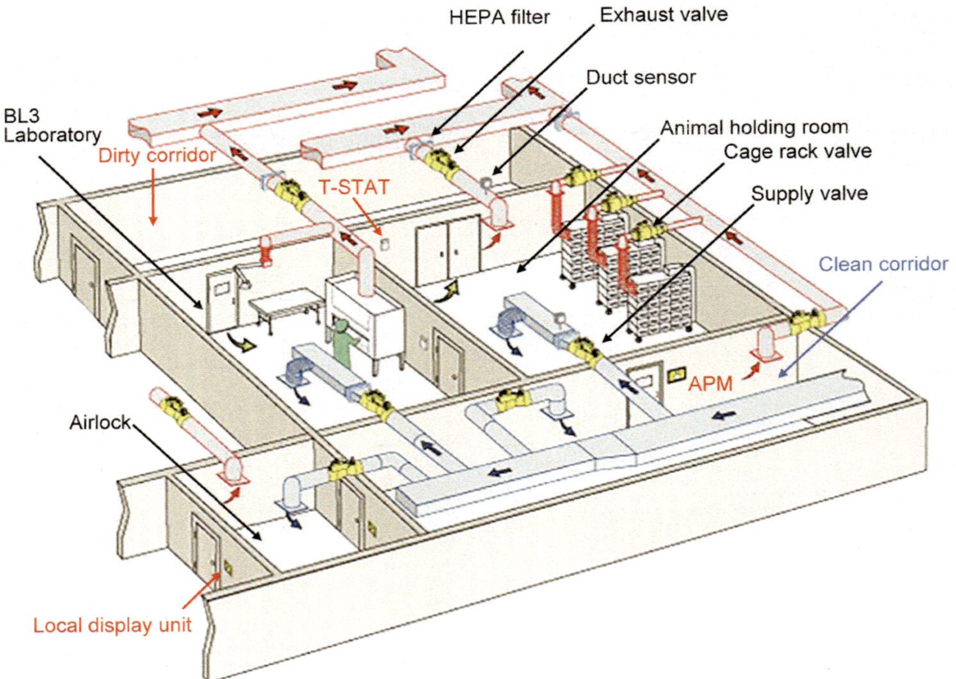

Fig. 9: HVAC biosafety laboratory.

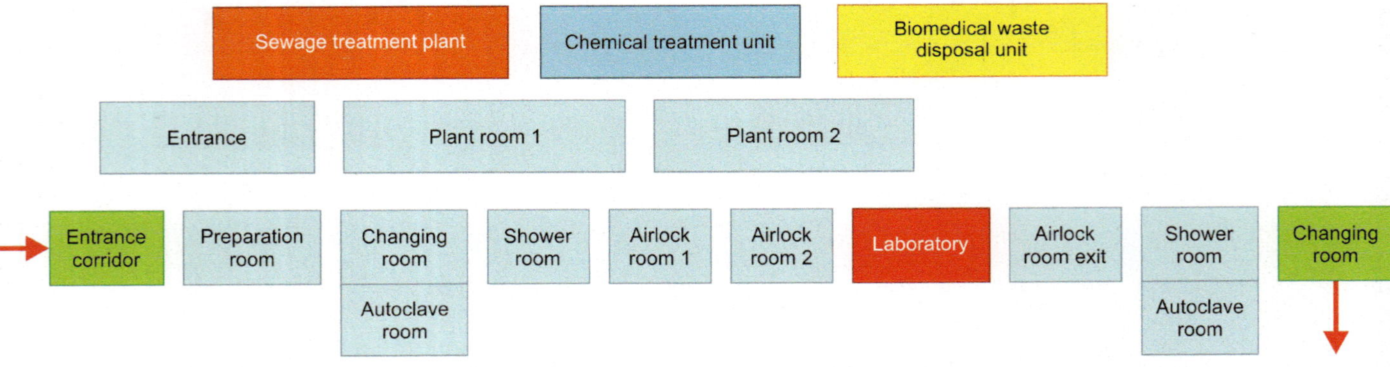

Fig. 10: Diagrammatic depictor of biosafety level.

- Facilities for storing outer garments and personal items should be provided outside the laboratory working areas.
- Facilities for eating and drinking and for rest should be provided outside the laboratory working areas.
- Hand washing basins, with running water if possible, should be provided in each laboratory room, preferably near the exit door.
- Doors should have vision panels, appropriate fire ratings, and preferably be self closing.
- At biosafety level 2, an autoclave or other means of decontamination should be available in appropriate proximity to the laboratory.
- Safety systems should cover fire, electrical emergencies, emergency shower and eyewash facilities.
- First-aid areas or rooms suitably equipped and readily accessible should be available.
- A dependable supply of good quality water is essential. There should be no cross connections between sources of laboratory and drinking-water supplies. An ant back-flow device should be fitted to protect the public water system.
- There should be a reliable and adequate electricity supply and emergency lighting to permit safe exit. A stand-by generator is desirable for the support of essential equipment, such as incubators, biological safety cabinets, freezers, etc., and for the ventilation.
- A line diagram is indicated in Figures 13 and 14.

SPECIAL REQUIREMENT FOR BSL-4 (FIG. 11)[5,25,26]

The features of a containment laboratory—biosafety level 3 also apply to a maximum containment laboratory—biosafety level 4 with the addition of the following:

Primary Containment

An efficient primary containment system must be in place, consisting of one or a combination of the following: *Class III cabinet laboratory*. Passage through a minimum of two doors prior to entering the rooms containing the Class III biological safety cabinet(s) (cabinet room) is required.

The biosafety cabinet provides the primary containment.

- A personnel shower with inner and outer changing rooms is necessary. Supplies and materials that are not brought into the cabinet room through the changing area are introduced through a double-door autoclave or fumigation chamber.
- Once the outer door is securely closed, staff inside the laboratory can open the inner door to retrieve the materials.
- The doors of the autoclave or fumigation chamber are interlocked in such a way that the outer door cannot open unless the autoclave has been operated through a sterilization cycle or the fumigation chamber has been decontaminated.
- A protective suit laboratory with self-contained breathing apparatus differs significantly in design and facility requirements from a biosafety level 4 laboratory with class III biological safety cabinets.
- The rooms in the protective suit laboratory are arranged so as to direct personnel through the changing and decontamination areas prior to entering areas where infectious materials are manipulated.
- A suit decontamination shower must be provided and used by personnel leaving the containment laboratory area. A separate personnel shower with inner and outer changing rooms is also provided.
- Personnel who enter the suit area are required to don a one-piece, positively pressurized, HEPA-filtered, supplied-air suit. Air to the suit must be provided by a system that has a 100% redundant capability with an independent source of air, for use in the event of an emergency.
- Entry into the suit laboratory is through an airlock fitted with airtight doors.
- An appropriate warning system for personnel working in the suit laboratory must be provided for use in the event of mechanical system or air failure.

Controlled Access

The maximum containment laboratory—biosafety level 4 must be located in a separate building or in a clearly delineated zone within a secure building.

Entry and exit of personnel and supplies must be through an airlock or pass-through system.

On entering, personnel must put on a complete change of clothing.

Before leaving, they should shower before putting on their personnel clothing.

Controlled Air System (Fig. 12)

- Negative pressure must be maintained in the facility.
- Both supply and exhaust air must be HEPA-filtered.

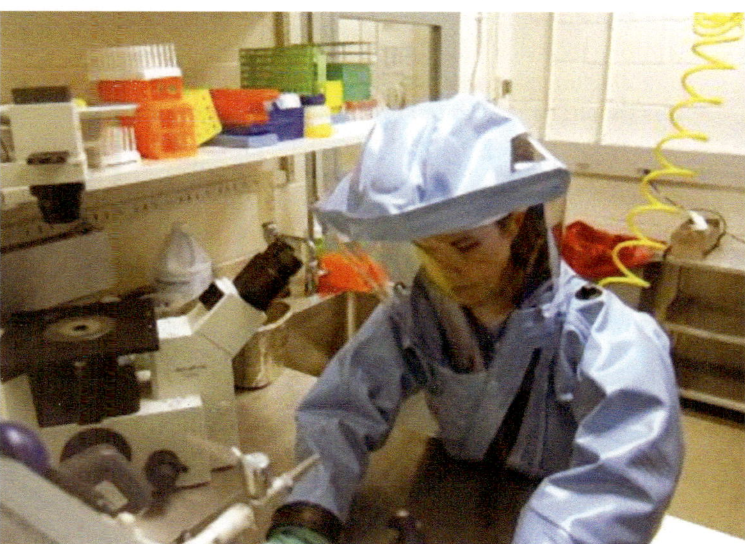

Fig. 11: Biosofety level 4.

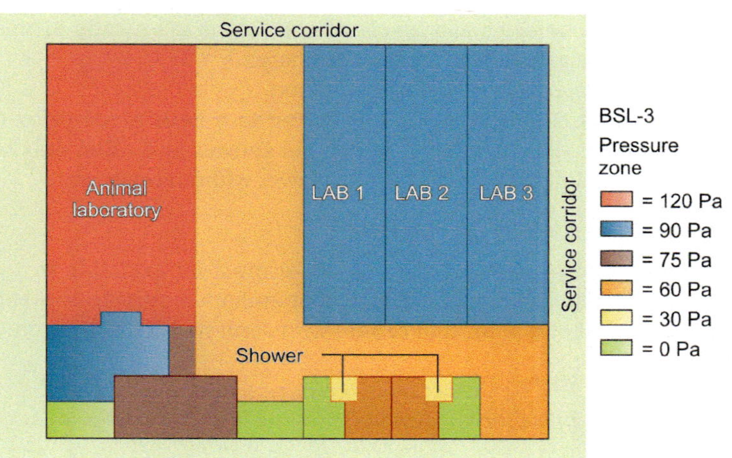

Fig. 12: Pressure zone.

- Supply air to the class III biological safety cabinet(s) may be drawn from within the room through a HEPA filter mounted on the cabinet or supplied directly through the supply air system.
- Exhaust air from the class III biological safety cabinet must pass through two HEPA filters prior to release outdoors.
- Cabinet must be operated at negative pressure to the surrounding laboratory at all times.
- A dedicated non-recirculating ventilating system for the cabinet laboratory is required.

Suit Laboratory

- Dedicated room air supply and exhaust systems are required.
- Supply and exhaust components of the ventilating system are balanced to provide directional airflow within the suit area from the area of least hazard to the area(s) of greatest potential hazard.
- Redundant exhaust fans are required to ensure that the facility remains under negative pressure at all times.
- Differential pressures within the suit laboratory and between the suit laboratory and adjacent areas must be monitored.
- Airflow in the supply and exhaust components of the ventilating system must be monitored, and an appropriate system of controls must be used to prevent pressurization of the suit laboratory.
- HEPA-filtered supply air must be provided to the suit area, decontamination shower and decontamination airlocks or chambers. Exhaust air from the suit laboratory must be passed through a series of two HEPA filters prior to release outdoors.
- Alternatively, after double HEPA filtration, exhaust air may be recirculated, but only within the suit laboratory.
- Under no circumstances should the exhaust air from the biosafety level 4 suit laboratory be recirculated to other areas.
- Extreme caution must be exercised if recirculation of air within the suit laboratory is elected.
- Consideration must be given to the types of research conducted, equipment, chemicals and other materials used in the suit laboratory, as well as animal species that may be involved in the research.
- HEPA filters need to be tested and certified annually.
- HEPA filter housings should be designed to allow for *in situ* decontamination of the filter prior to removal.
- Alternatively, the filter can be removed in a sealed, gas-tight primary container for subsequent decontamination and/or destruction by incineration.

Decontamination of Effluents

- All effluents from the suit area, decontamination chamber, decontamination shower, or class III biological safety cabinet must be decontaminated before final discharge.
- Heat treatment is the preferred method.
- Effluents may also require correction to a neutral pH prior to discharge. Water from the personnel shower and toilet may be discharged directly to the sanitary sewer without treatment.

Sterilization of Waste and Materials

A double-door, pass-through autoclave must be available in the laboratory area. Other methods of decontamination must be available for equipment and items that cannot withstand steam sterilization.

Airlock Entry Ports

Airlock entry ports for specimens, materials and animals must be provided.

Emergency Power

Emergency power and dedicated power supply line(s) must be provided.

Containment Drain

Containment drain(s) must be installed.

Support System

- Support system should be designed in such a manner that it is in close vicinity for a strict control.
- It should be fully secure and only authorized, trained persons should be allowed.
- There should be a detailed written approved protocol by biosafety officer in consultation with the maintenance in-charge.
- Design should allow the maintenance of the laboratory from outside without having to enter in the laboratory area.
- A fully well-designed power backup with clean uninterrupted power supply should be available.
- Laboratory should have self-explanatory signage's and instructions widely displaced at various appropriate place in and around the laboratory.
- Design should allow that even in the disaster situations the services are not affected.

Personal Protection[26]

- Laboratory coveralls, gowns or uniforms must be worn at all times for work in the laboratory.
- Appropriate gloves must be worn for all procedures that may involve direct or accidental contact with blood, body fluids and other potentially infectious materials or infected animals. After use, gloves should be removed aseptically and hands must then be washed.
- Personnel must wash their hands after handling infectious materials and animals, and before they leave the laboratory working areas.
- Safety glasses, face shields (visors) or other protective devices must be worn when it is necessary to protect the eyes and face from splashes, impacting objects and sources of artificial ultraviolet radiation.
- It is prohibited to wear protective laboratory clothing outside the laboratory, e.g. in canteens, coffee rooms, offices, libraries, staff rooms and toilets.
- Open-toed footwear must not be worn in laboratories.
- Eating, drinking, smoking, applying cosmetics and handling contact lenses should be prohibited in the laboratory working areas.
- Storing human foods or drinks anywhere in the laboratory working areas is prohibited.
- Protective laboratory clothing that has been used in the laboratory must not be stored in the same lockers or cupboards as street clothing.
- Children should not be authorized or allowed to enter laboratory working areas.

Training

Training is one of the most essential and pillar of the successful biosafety. All categories of staff should be trained and it should not be one time program. Ongoing training is a must. The floor plans are depicted in Figures 13 and 14.

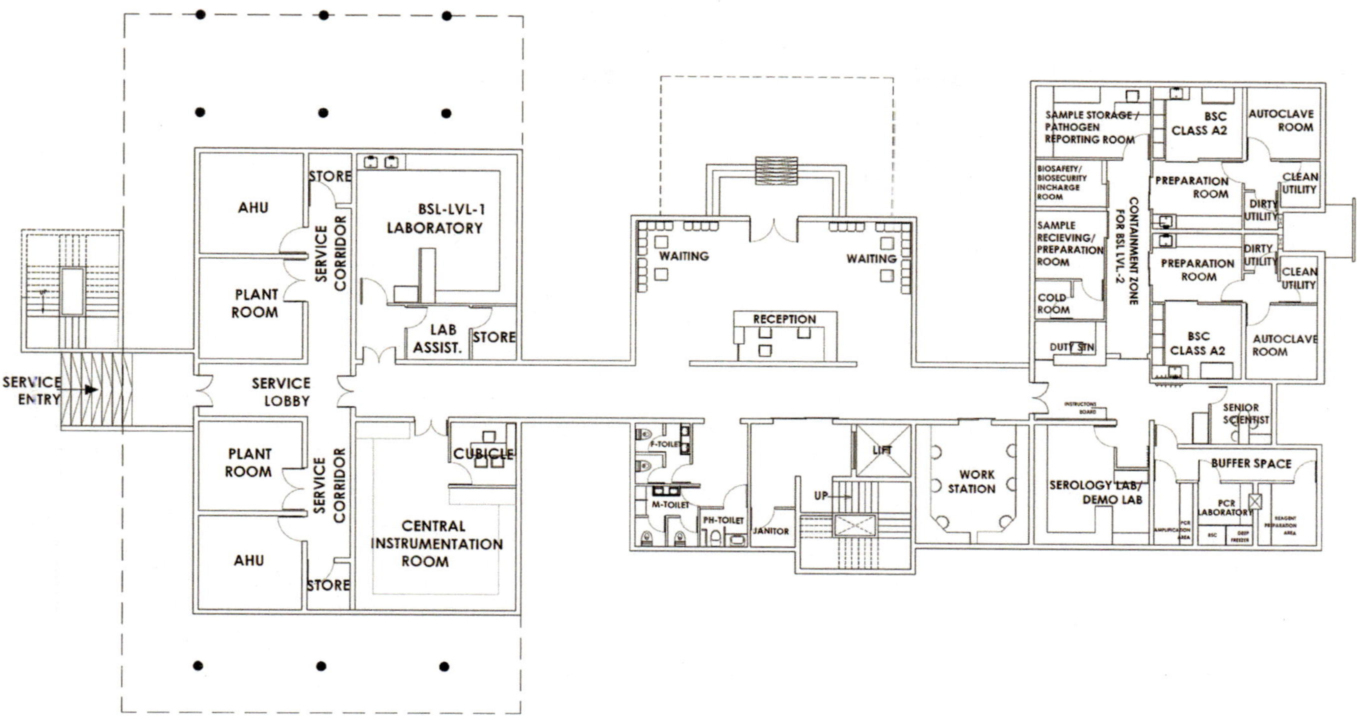

Fig. 13: Ground floor plan.

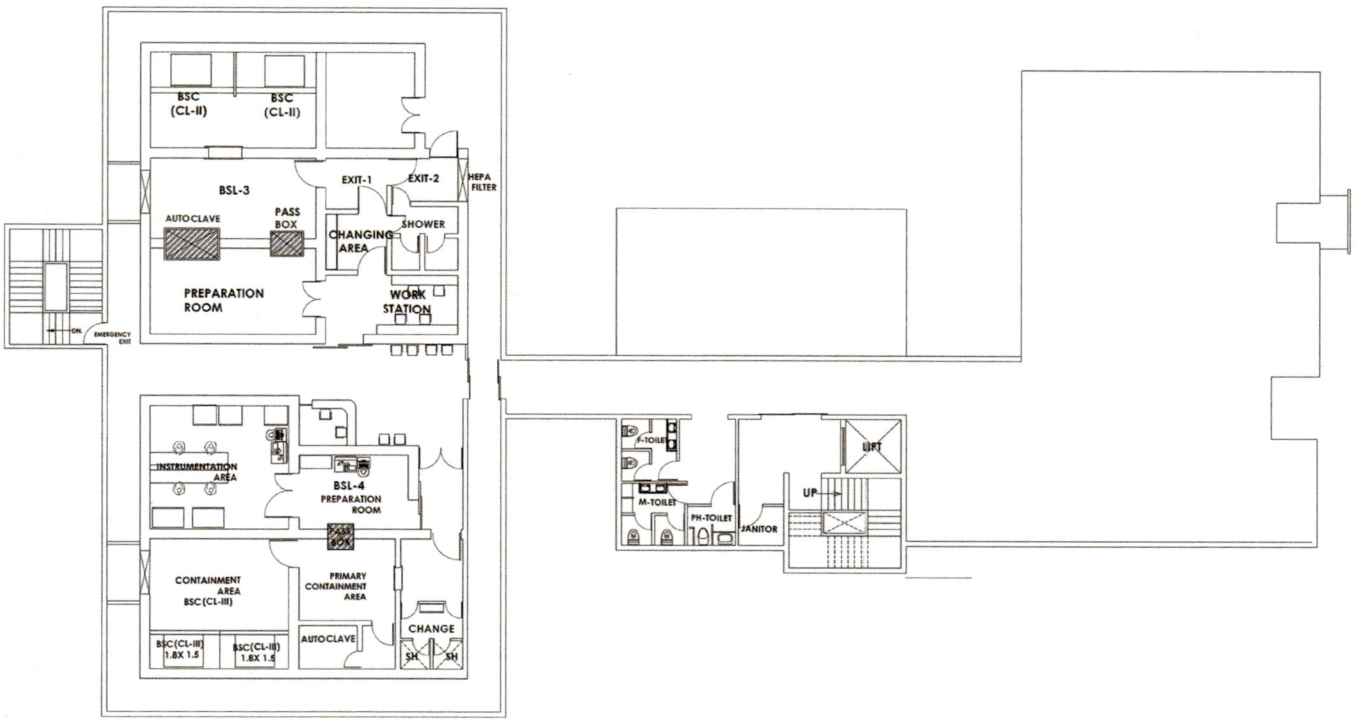

Fig. 14: First floor lab.

CONCLUSION

The design, construction and operations of biosafety laboratories are complex and need appropriate planning and design considerations. Safety of staff, visitors and community depends on these and should be accordingly addressed.

REFERENCES

1. "Need of lab biosafety. (Report)", Technology Times; Jan 26 2014
2. www.ocrwm.doe.gov
3. Laboratory biosafety manual, 3rd edition. World Health Organization; 2004.
4. www.wfcc.nig.ac.jp
5. ehs.kenyon.edu
6. dhc.ucdavis.edu
7. apps.searo.who.int
8. fens.sabanciuniv.edu
9. www.animalcare.mcgill.ca
10. www.animallab.com
11. ehs.mst.edu
12. www.staffsenate.lsu.edu
13. www.bordeninstitute.army.mil
14. talasthailand.org
15. www.phac-aspc.gc.ca
16. hpac.com
17. DiBerardinis. Laboratory Hoods and Other Exhaust Air Contaminant—Capture Facilities and Equipment, Guidelines for Laboratory Design Health Safety and Environmental Considerations; 2013.
18. newmaticengineering.com
19. www.nuclearsafety.gc.ca
20. Furr K. Laboratory Facilities—Design and Equipment. CRC Handbook of Laboratory Safety, 5th edition; 2000.
21. www.kcumb.edu
22. health.go.ug
23. qualityalchemist.com
24. www.tbcare1.org
25. The maximum containment laboratory—Biosafety Level 4.", Laboratory Biosafety Manual, Chapter 5 20040101.
26. scientificinternational.co.in

OTHER REFERENCES

- American Society of Heating, Refrigerating and Air-conditioning Engineers (ASHRAE) Inc.
- ASHRAE Handbook: 2007 HVAC Applications. Atlanta, GA: ASHRAE; 2007.
- Centers for Disease Control and Prevention (CDC) and National Institutes of Health (NIH).
- Biosafety in Microbiological and Biomedical Laboratories (BMBL), 5th edition. Washington.
- DC: U.S. Government Printing Office, 1999. Also available online at http://www.cdc.gov/od/ohs/biosfty/bmbl5/bmbl5toc.htm.
- Centers for Disease Control and Prevention (CDC), The Office of Health and Safety.
- Information System (Ohasis). Primary Containment for Biohazards, Section III. Available online at http://www.cdc.gov/od/ohs/biosfty/bsc/BSC2000sec3.htm.
- Crane, Jonathan T. Hot Zone Laboratories. ASHRAE Journal; 1999.pp.28-31.

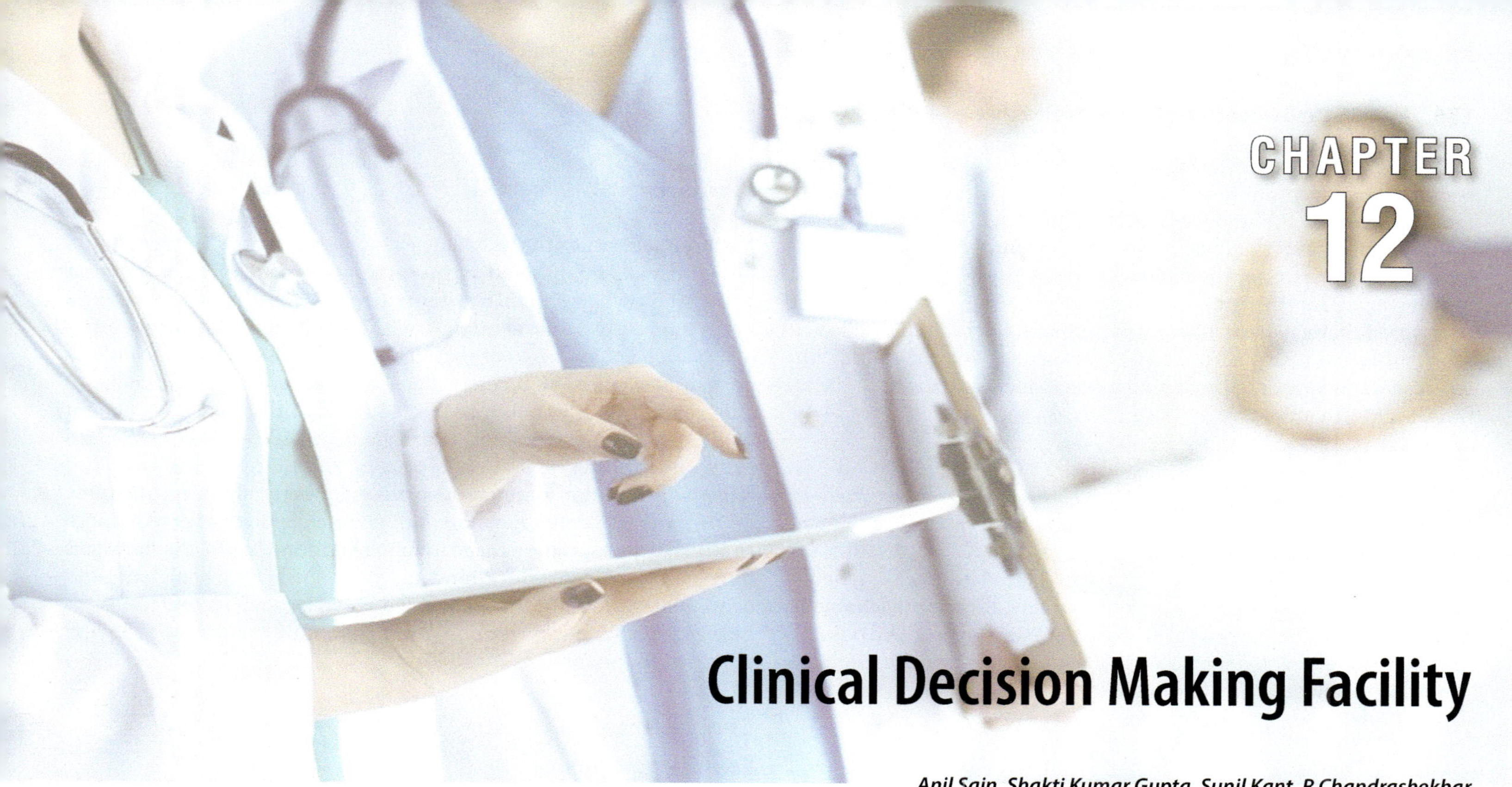

Clinical Decision Making Facility

Anil Sain, Shakti Kumar Gupta, Sunil Kant, R Chandrashekhar

INTRODUCTION

Clinical decision making is the process by which a clinician determines, which patient needs what kind of treatment and when.[1] The first choice of any person falling ill is, the General Practitioner, where he feels that he will be able to afford the cost of a reasonable consultation. At the same time, making a clinical decision becomes a challenging task for the General Practitioners who usually do not have an in-house adequate diagnostic support and end up referring their patients to other facilities thereby losing their own credibility and also subjecting the patients to further stress. This is the reason that a need was felt to develop a facility where a common man, when in need of medical attention, can come to a General Practitioner and expect to get satisfactory treatment for his ailments without having to shuttle between the doctor's clinic and diagnostic centers. At the same time, the General Practitioner is able to work with dignity and contribute effectively in healthcare delivery.

FUNCTIONS OF THE CLINICAL DECISION MAKING FACILITY

The "Clinical Decision Making" facility should ensure that the General Practitioners are able to make clinical decisions without the patients having to go to other facilities.

The facility should be managed by qualified and experienced General Practitioners having a support of in-house radiologist, laboratory and ECG facility. They should first try to arrive at a diagnosis with the help of these in-house diagnostic facilities. Medicines prescribed should be made available at the in-house pharmacy. If some injection is to be administered it should be done by the in-house staff nurse. Any dressing of the wound required should be done in the treatment room. In case the need is felt that the patient requires to be kept under observation for some time for example to give some I/V fluids, administer oxygen or nebulization, it should be done in the daycare room which may have two to three beds. The daycare room obviates the need for referring the patients to higher centers for small procedures as stated above.

In case, the General Practitioner is not able to make a decision, help of specialists should be sought in-house. This can be in two ways. Firstly, by having visiting specialists in the facility, and secondly, by using telemedicine technique. In case any major intervention is required as advised by the specialists, the patients should be guided to get those interventions done from an appropriate place as per their paying capacity, with the help of the "Information Portal", a strong management information system, maintained for this purpose. An exhaustive database of referral centers in the city providing specialized interventions should be maintained. A list of specialists and superspecialists performing various procedures in their respective fields should be maintained. The cost of treatment available at various centers along with information about various value-added services available at different centers should be available at this facility. Official at the "Information Portal" should help the patient in getting the appointment in that particular facility. Thus, decision making should be possible under one roof, saving time, money and other resources.

Another value-added facility should be a network with the referral hospitals to provide vehicles to take the patients to the specialists at the appointed time and drop them back to their residence. In case a follow-up is required after a procedure/intervention, it should be done at this facility, by the physicians of the facility in consultation with the specialists on phone or via telemedicine.

In this facility, the entire team should be available during daytime and a General Practitioner should be available round the clock. At night, the General Practitioner should be assisted by a nursing attendant to attend and guide the patients. If possible the doctor on duty should solve the patient's problem in-house or guide him to a suitable facility. Electronically maintained records for the follow-up patients will be of great help. Security should be available round the clock and also an ambulance with driver should be available to escort the patient to the required facility.

All care should be taken by a dedicated team of personnel to see that a patient/visitor coming to the facility feels relaxed and comfortable. There should be provision for playing music from a central place and should create a soothing atmosphere for the visitors. At times, it is inconvenient for the patient to attend the clinic, especially for the postoperative or very old patients. Arrangement should also be made for domiciliary visits for the patients if desired.

Convenience of the patient should be of prime importance. It should be assured that a patient, already in problem due to his disease is no more subjected to any sort of anxiety or harassment due to difficulty in decision making or approaching the right facility at the appropriate time, for his treatment.

KEY PLANNING AND DESIGN PARAMETERS

Location

The facility should be located in a central place within easy reach of the population it is catering for. It should be easily approachable by public and private transport at all hours. Since, it may not be possible to have a large area for such a facility in such a central location, it is proposed to have a facility designed in two floors. However, variations can be done as per space available.

Design Features

Facility should be so designed that it is easily accessible to patients with different degrees of disability. The patients entering the facility should find the environment friendly and welcoming and their dignity and privacy should be maintained. There should be sufficient waiting areas, recommendation being 0.8 sqm per patient, for one-third of the average daily load.[2] The design should allow natural light and good ventilation and should provide good view of outside. There should be scope for future expansion.

The facility should have the following physical areas:[3]

- Public areas
- Clinical areas
- Administrative areas
- Ancillary areas.

Public Areas

Entrance

The entrance of the facility should be so designed that it is user-friendly for the handicapped and it should be possible to wheel in the patients (Fig. 1). The floor should be skid free and the entrance should have a double door with a width of 1500 mm to facilitate passage of stretchers and wheelchairs.

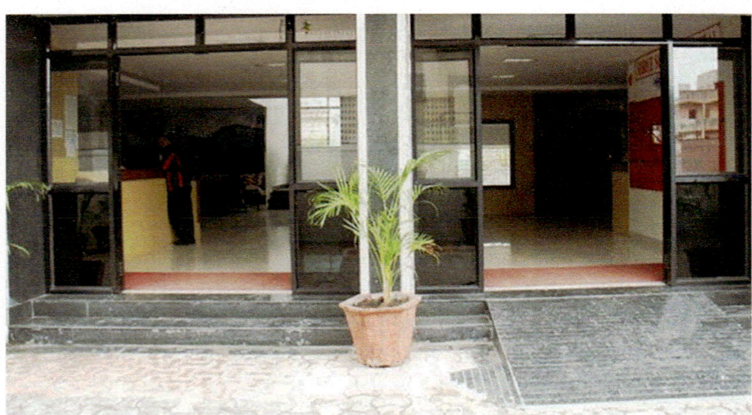

Fig. 1: User-friendly entrance.

Reception and Waiting Area

As the patient enters the building he reaches the foyer. This area should be esthetically maintained as this is going to give the first impression of the facility. This should be the area from where the patient is going to be guided to various other areas. There should be a reception desk which should be so designed that it affords some privacy to the patient talking to the receptionist. Adequate waiting space (Fig. 2) with seating facility should be planned according to the peak patient load expected and care should be taken to provide for adequate space for public utilities separately for males and females. The cash and registration counter should not be placed directly adjacent to the flow of the patients so that movement of people is not obstructed. There should be appropriate signage, public telephone booth, display racks for promotional and educational material, space for wheelchairs and drinking water facility. Value-added services such as machines for beverages and snacks, mobile phone charging facility, etc. may be provided in the foyer.

Clinical Areas

Consultation Room

Room of area about 12 sqm is adequate for a consultation and examination. This also includes space for examination tables, a wash basin, instruments trolley, an X-ray viewing screen, desk and chair for doctor as well as chairs for the patients/visitors. Rooms for the specialists should be provided with extra fitments/furnishings as per requirement of the particular specialist, in addition to the above.

Treatment cum ECG Room

The treatment cum ECG room should be provided with a patient's couch to perform some small procedures like dressing of a wound, incision and drainage of an abscess, suture removal, ECG, etc. Storage space for the material and equipment required should be provided as also provision for a wash basin.

Daycare Area

There should be daycare beds for patients requiring observation for short period, for example, patients of dehydration requiring only I/V fluids, asthma patients requiring nebulization, etc. A nursing counter and attached washrooms should be provided.

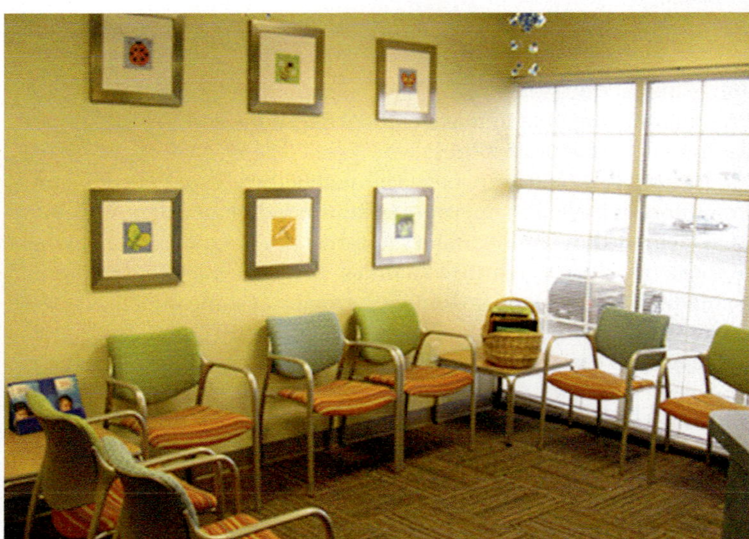

Fig. 2: Waiting spaces.

Administrative Area

Administrator's Office

In administrator's room, apart from the routine furnishings for the administrator and the visitors, there should be provision for installation of the monitoring screen of the CCTV system so that the administrator can observe the activities of the vital areas of the facility, sitting in his room, and can make a random check of the functioning of the officials. A separate adjacent room should be provided for the office of the administrator. There should also be a provision for an attached toilet.

Store

A store is essential from where all the supplies are made available. It is planned on the first floor of the facility in proximity to the ancillary facilities and daycare area to which it caters to, most of the times.

Ancillary Facilities

Laboratory

Apart from the working stations the laboratory should include sample collection area for urine, stool and blood. A washroom and toilets, separately for males and females should be provided.

Imaging Area

X-ray room (Fig. 3) should have separate washroom and cubicles for changing clothes for the patient apart from film processing and actual working area. Similarly, ultrasound room (Fig. 4) should also have a separate washroom.

Pharmacy

The in-house pharmacy should be so located on the ground floor that patients can take the required medicines without obstructing the movements in the facility. For this, if required pharmacy counter can be opened in the outer wall of the room instead of the interior wall.

Physiotherapy Unit

A physiotherapy unit (Fig. 5) is also planned in the facility for the convenience of orthopedic and postoperative patients. Gadgets/equipment required for various types of mobilization exercises should be available and interiors should be designed accordingly.

Special Equipment and Space Requirement

The unique feature of the facility would be its information portal. It should house two facilitators having completely independent computer units with a display screen on the wall for each. The patients seeking help should be detailed about the facilities available in the city for their specialized treatment and would also be shown video recordings on the wall panel, about the features of the various specialized centers available for treatment. Suitable electrical and cable connections would be needed and also place for the patients to sit and watch the clippings.

Along with this, there should be a provision for tele-linking with other secondary and tertiary care centers so that on-line opinion of specialists can be sought whenever required.

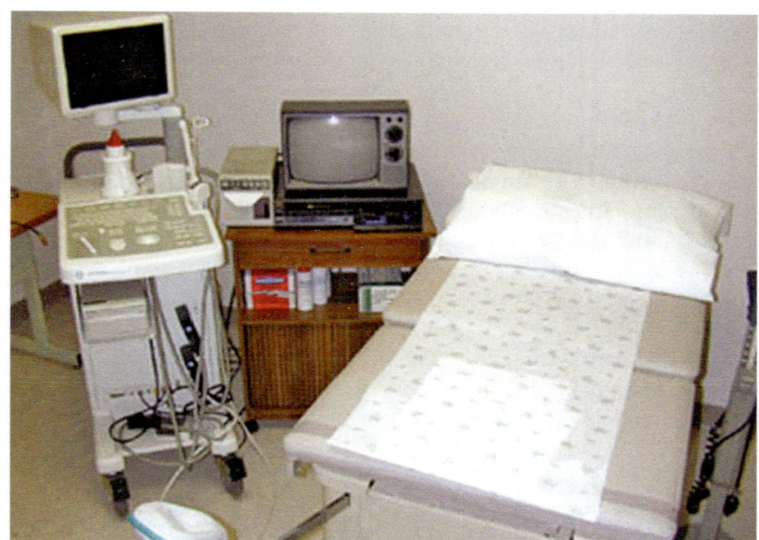

Fig. 4: Ultrasound room.

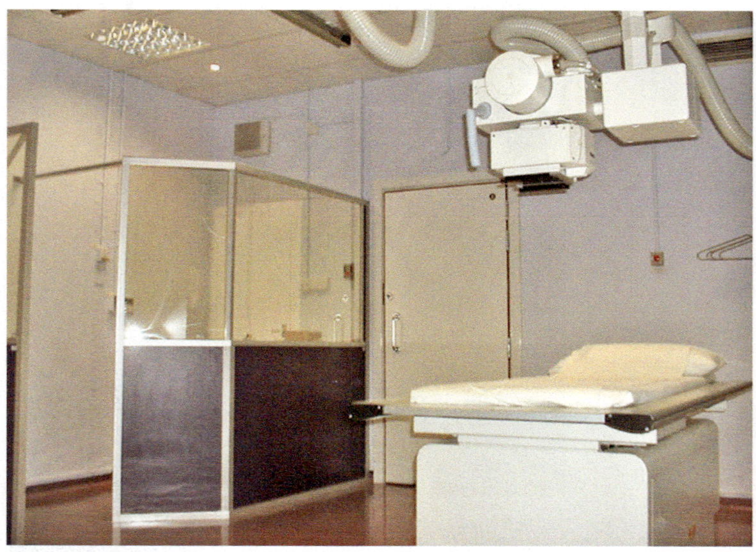

Fig. 3: X-ray room.

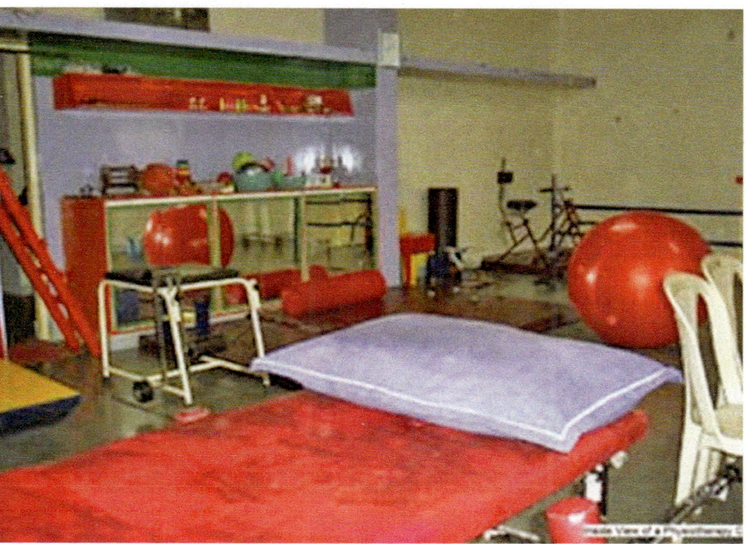

Fig. 5: Physiotherapy unit.

LAYOUT

Board Room

A board room (Fig. 6) should be planned in the facility which may be used for sharing knowledge between the health professionals as well as for educating patients. Apart from ample and comfortable seating it should be equipped with all audio-visual aids required for effective communication.

Cafeteria

A cafeteria should also be planned to meet the food and beverage requirements of staff and patients. It should serve healthy and hygienic food.

Hospital Attendants' Room

A room should be provided for the hospital attendants where they may change into their uniforms and may have refreshments or refresh themselves. It should have cupboards to keep their belongings. This room should also have a panel for the call bell so that they may know where they are required and may reach there immediately.

Janitors Closet

A closet (Fig. 7) should be provided at an appropriate place to house the Janitor's equipment and materials. It should have proper air exhaust to get rid of moisture and keep all the articles away from the public view so as not to disturb the esthetics of the facility.

Vertical Movement

A ramp with non-skid flooring should be provided with suitable railings, apart from a lift and staircase for easy movement of patients on wheelchairs/trolleys in case of power failure or any other exigency.

Circulation Area

Area should be available as circulation space. This includes area corridors, ramps and staircase.

Atrium

A central atrium should be planned with rooms all around it. There should be corridors in front of the rooms providing sufficient sub-waiting area for seating the patients and space for moving about. The atrium should be open to sky and provide adequate lighting and ventilation in the facility. Esthetics of the facility may be augmented by placing water fountains and decorative plants in the atrium.

Eco-friendly Facility (Fig. 8)

Measures must be taken to provide for rain water harvesting. There should be provision for installing solar panels on the roof to use the eco-friendly solar power as it is going to be a statutory requirement for the buildings of the future. Also a room should be provided for housing

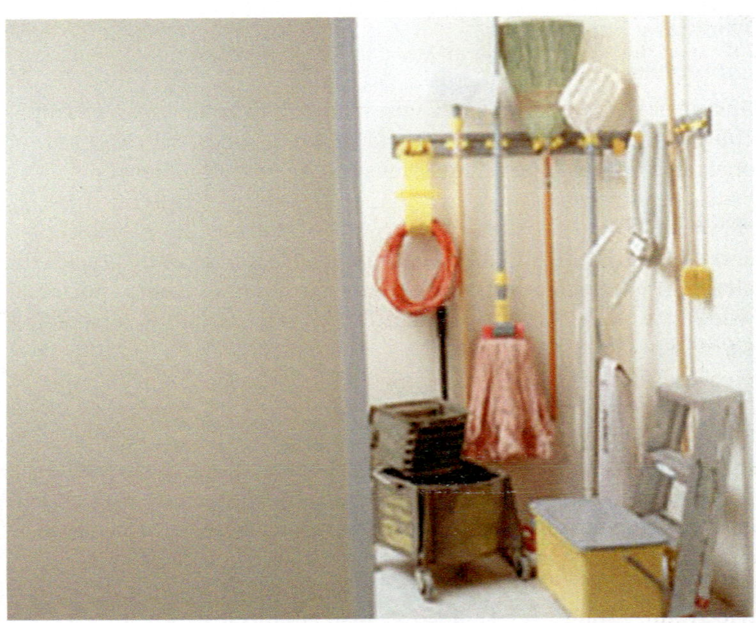

Fig. 7: Janitors closet.

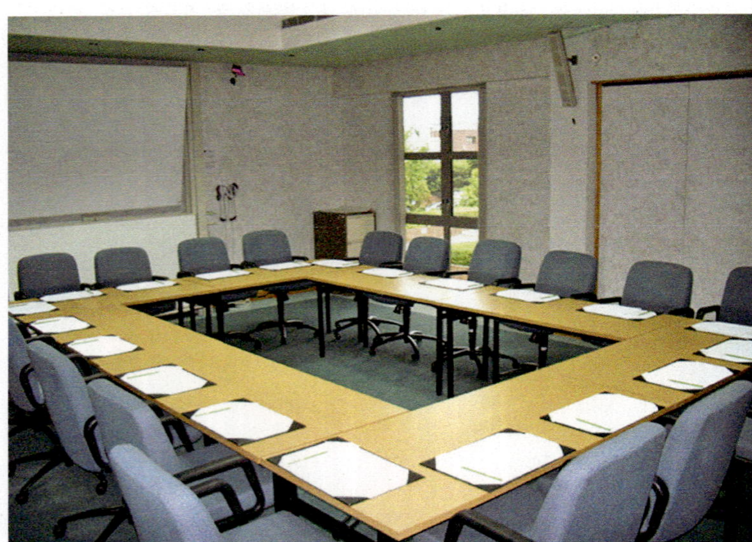

Fig. 6: Board room.

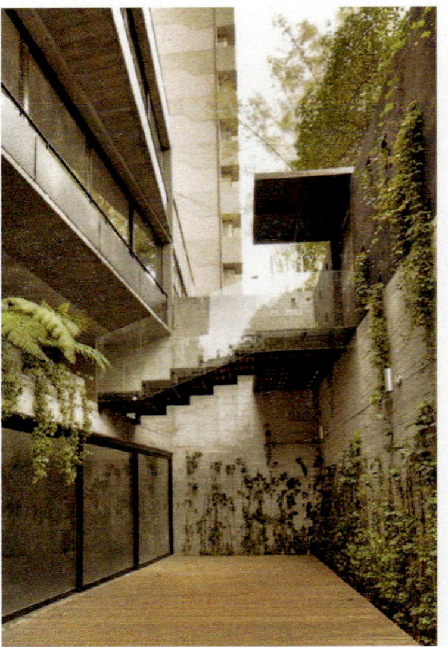

Fig. 8: Eco-friendly facility.

the batteries to be charged by the solar panels installed at the top of the building.

Open Area

The facility should be so built that it has open area surrounding the building with ample greenery. It should provide necessary light and ventilation from all sides and a good view of the outside. It should also provide sufficient parking space for the vehicles of the visitors and the vehicles/ambulance of the facility. A guard room should be provided near the entrance and there should be a provision for a room for the drivers.

Biomedical Waste Management

Bins should be installed at strategic locations for proper segregation and disposal of the waste generated in the facility. Adequate information should be given with the help of signboards alongside the bins for the same. Outsourcing may be done with the waste management agencies for collection and disposal of the waste.

HVAC—Heating, Ventilation, and Air-conditioning

The building should be planned in such a way that corridors and other open areas are well ventilated and lighted. The central atrium should provide the necessary light and ventilation and the facility is open on all sides. Centralized air-conditioning should be provided in the rooms and ducting should be done accordingly to cover all the areas where air-conditioning is required.

Signage

Measures care should be taken for appropriate and effective signage. A literate person should be able to reach the desired place on his own, following the signage and there should be no confusion or need to seek guidance. In the very first place, there should be an attractive and legible bilingual sign board outside the facility. From the main entrance, the visitor should be guided to the reception. At the, there should be explicit sign board depicting the layout plan of the floors showing what all facilities are available and where all they are located. Each room should be numbered and effective arrow signs should be able to lead the visitor to the desired place. A receptionist should also be available to the visitors. The mission statement of the facility should be clearly spelt out and written on a board hanged at a convenient place in the reception area. All sign boards should be bilingual with graphic representation wherever possible. The place where patients are required to wait should be provided with display panels showing when the patient sitting outside is likely to get his turn.

Schedule of Accommodation[2-5]

A suggested schedule of accommodation is shown in Table 1 and line diagrams in Figures 9 and 10.

Table 1: Schedule of accommodation.

Sl. No.	Facility	Area (sqm)
1.	Reception	8
2.	Registration and cash counter	8
3.	Waiting area	15
4.	Consultant rooms (4 nos)	12
5.	Treatment-cum-ECG room	15
6.	Physiotherapy room	20
7.	Pharmacy	15
8.	X-ray room	20
9.	Office	12
10.	Washrooms 2 Nos (patient and staff)	12 each
11.	Room for housing batteries/generator	5
12.	Specialist room (3 nos)	12 each
13.	Cafeteria	20
14.	Ultrasound	12
15.	Laboratory	28
16.	Committee room	20
17.	Radiologist's chamber	12
18.	Administrator's room	12
19.	Daycare ward	25
20.	Store	24
21.	Doctors' duty room	10
22.	Nurses' duty room	10
23.	Circulation area	30% approx

The ground floor should lead to the first floor via a gradually graded ramp and also there should be a provision for a lift and a staircase.

Planning for the areas, as above, a covered *area of 600 sqm* should be sufficient, if the whole facility is planned on two floors altogether. With the open space required for the parking, provision for green area and rain water harvesting facility area comes to *2400 sqm*. The floor plans are shown in Figures 9 and 10. However, the plan may vary as per the availability of space and accordingly vertical expansion can be thought of.

CONCLUSION

The facility planned can be operationalized in both government and private setup. The facility has been proposed with the idea of providing carefree health services to the public. People may be able to get the best treatment at a price they can afford under one roof.

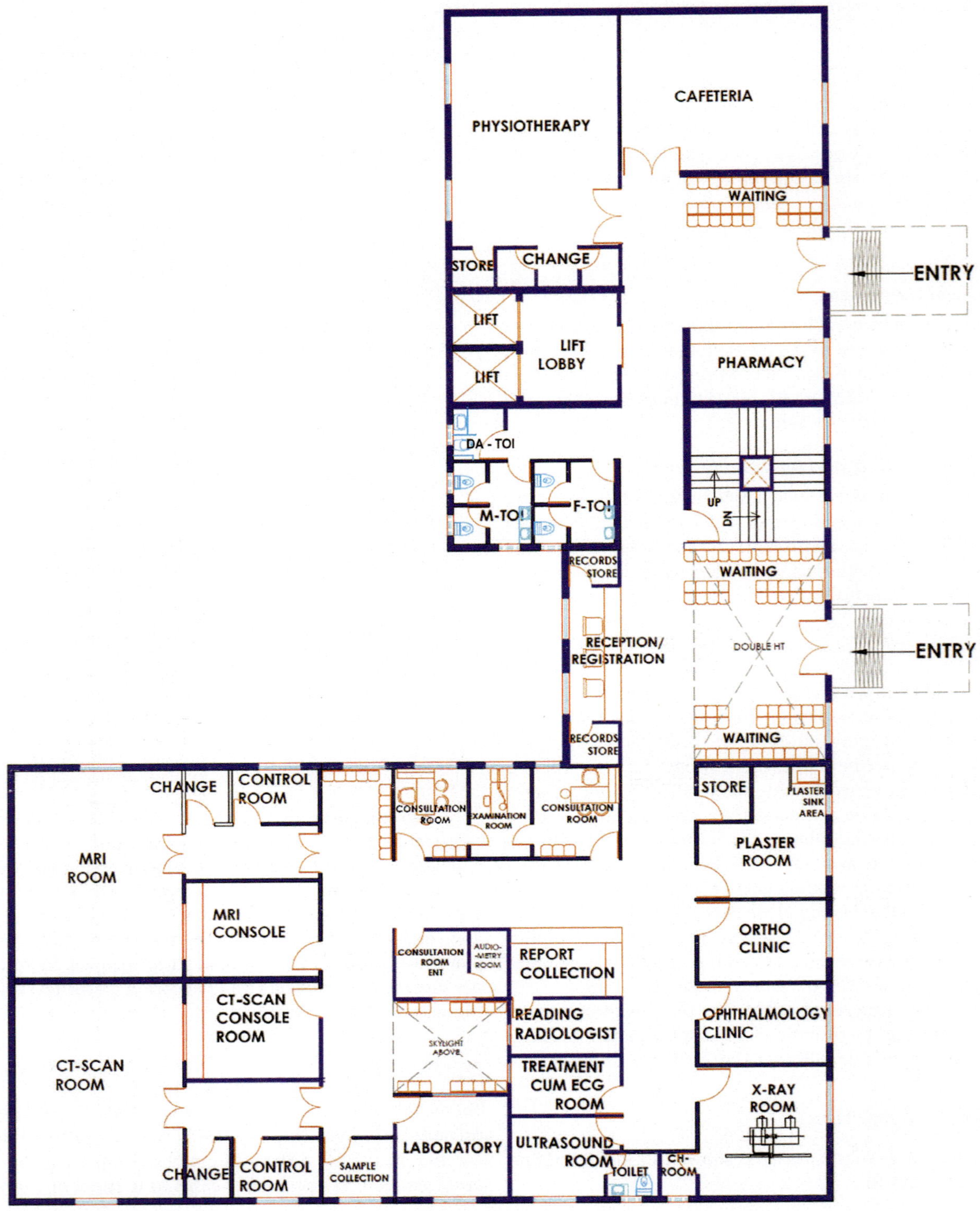

Fig. 9: Ground floor plan.
(DA: differently abled)

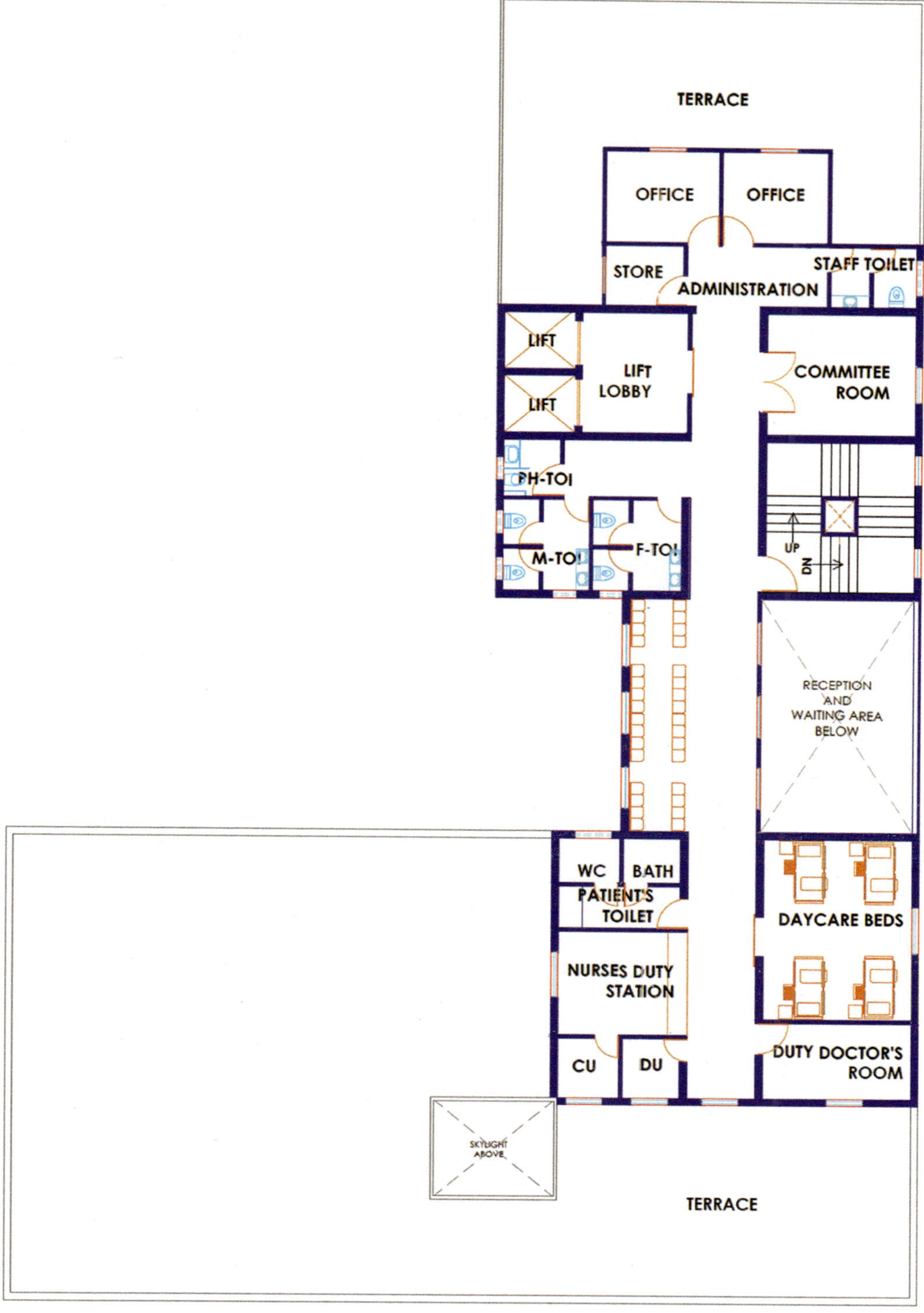

Fig. 10: First floor plan.

REFERENCES

1. Goldberg C. A practical guide to clinical medicine: A comprehensive physical examination and clinical education site for medical students and other health care professionals. 2008. Available from *URL:https://meded.ucsd.edu/clinicalmed/thinking.htm*
2. Gupta SK, Kant S, Chandrashekhar R, Satpathy S. Modern trends in planning and designing of hospitals: principles and practice. Jaypee Brothers Medical Publishers Pvt. Ltd, New Delhi; 2007.
3. Francis CM, D'Souza MC. Hospital administration, 3rd edn. Jaypee Brothers Medical Publishers Pvt. Ltd, New Delhi; 2004.
4. Davies RL, Macauly HMC. Hospital planning and administration. Jaypee Brothers Medical Publishers Pvt. Ltd, New Delhi; 1995.
5. Kunders GD. Hospitals: facilities planning and management. Tata McGraw-Hill Publishing Company Limited, New Delhi; 2005.

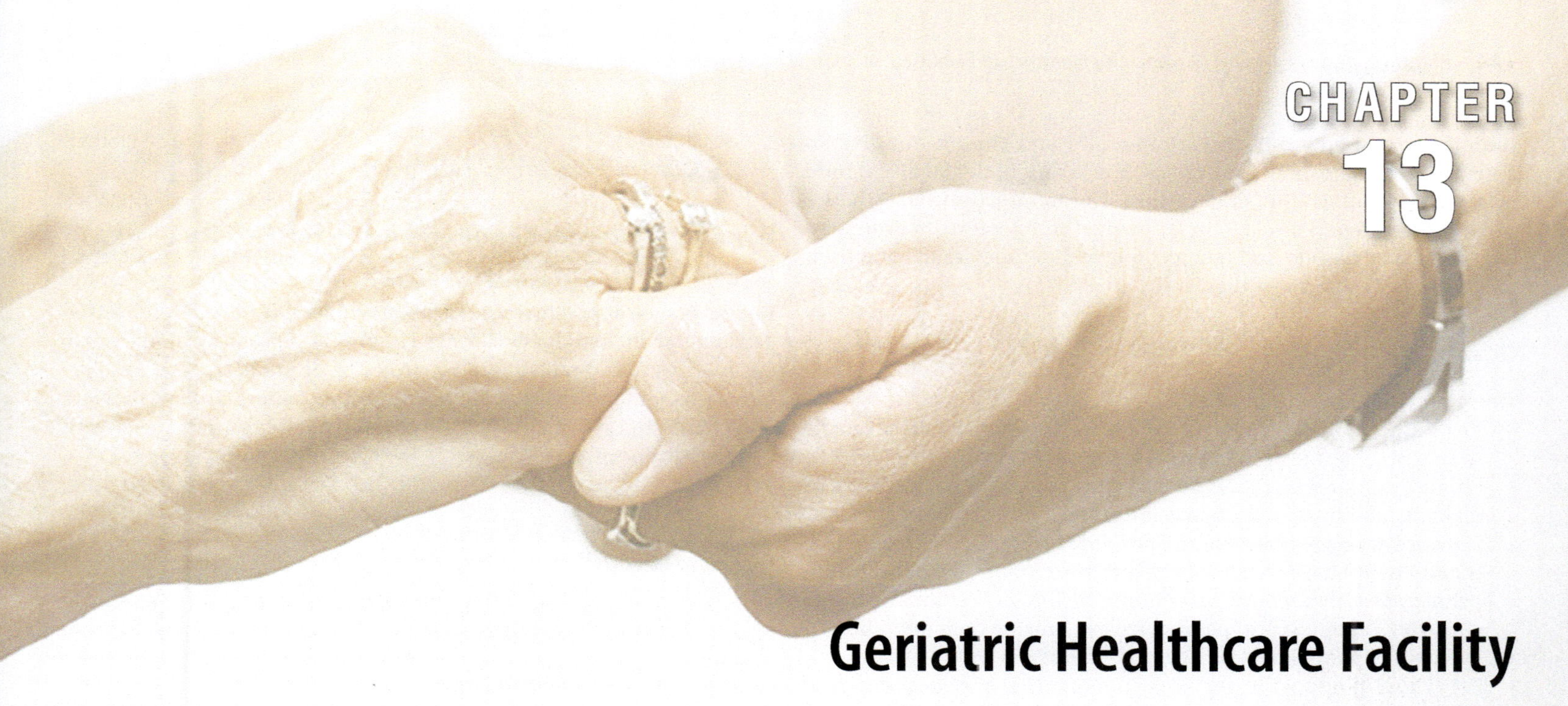

Geriatric Healthcare Facility

Jitender Mehta, S Satpathy, Shakti Kumar Gupta, Sunil Kant, R Chandrashekhar

INTRODUCTION

As one ages into the senior years, vision, mobility, hearing, cognition, perceptual ability, general physical ability and endurance commonly declines. Superimposed upon this normal aging process will be a variety of chronic and acute medical conditions and symptoms that increase in frequency with age, further reducing the senior's functional ability.[1]

The French physician Charcot (1881) was the first to advocate for a specialty of geriatric medicine in his lecture series on medicine of old age, which were translated and published in English in 1881.[2,3] These aroused scientific interest in the field.

As the value of geriatric services became established, geriatricians became more involved in the acute care of patients in general hospitals. Later, the concept of a close clinical relationship between geriatrics and orthopedics was instituted in Hastings.[4,5] The first chair of geriatric medicine was established in Glasgow in 1965.[2,6]

Global scenario[7-9]

One out of every ten persons is now 60 years or above; by 2050, one out of five will be 60 years or older; and by 2150, one out of three persons will be 60 years or older with the current trends.

The older population itself is aging.

The oldest old (80 years or older) is the fastest growing segment of the older population.

They currently make up 13% of the 60+ age group and will grow to 20% by 2050.

The number of centenarians (aged 100 years or older) is projected to increase 14-fold from approximately 2,65,000 in 2005 to 3.7 million by 2050.

Indian scenario

The growth in the aging population in India has been faster than in other developing countries. In 1947, when India became independent of British rule, life expectancy wavered around 32 years.[10]

The life expectancy has nearly doubled to 63 years in 2000 with the projected increase to 74 years by 2045–2050.[1]

The issue of the aging of populations, with its vast implications both for overall development at the national level and for the welfare and safety of older individuals, is therefore one which will concern all countries in the relatively near future; it already affects some of the more developed regions of the world.[11] The current demographic revolution is predicted to continue well into the coming centuries.[12]

NEED FOR THE FACILITY

Elderly people are highly prone to mental and physical morbidities due to aging of the brain, problems associated with physical health, cerebral pathology, socioeconomic factors such as breakdown of the family support systems, and decrease in economic independence. The mental disorders that are frequently encountered include dementia and mood disorders. Other disorders include neurotic and personality disorders, drug and alcohol abuse, delirium and mental psychosis.[13-15]

The rapid urbanization and societal modernization has brought in its wake a breakdown in family values and the framework of family support, economic insecurity, social isolation, and elderly abuse leading to a host of psychological illnesses.[16] The socioeconomic problems of the elderly are aggravated by factors such as the lack of social security and inadequate facilities for healthcare, rehabilitation and recreation. A vicious cycle is thus created.

With these social, epidemiological and demographic trends coming together, India is expected to follow the situation in the West where demand for long-term care is growing and main reasons for a need of a protective geriatric care facility in India are evident from these facts as the facilities and infrastructure existing in India are meager and inadequate.

KEY PLANNING AND DESIGN PARAMETERS OF THE FACILITY

In spite being highly technical and scientific facility, the center should be like a home in looks and appearances, with all the technicalities seemlessly embedded in the architecture and should not give an appearance of a hospital for the sick. The layout of the facility should be more horizontal rather than vertical. The architecture and esthetics of the facility should have elements of local architecture incorporated to give an accustomed and comfortable feel to the patients and their relatives. Design to create dignity.

Goals

The facility should:

- Provide a quality residential aged care health system for those unable to remain at home or in the care of friends or relatives.
- Should be affordable, accessible, flexible and equitable. Recognizes diversity and promotes choice and respect for users and workers.
- Provides access to planned, and properly resourced and integrated, quality healthcare. Integrates health promotion and prevention, primary healthcare and community health, subacute and acute care, rehabilitation and palliative care. Provides rehabilitation to ensure best functional and cognitive status.
- Provision of adequate services such as OPD services, daycare, residential care, respite care and hospice beds, especially for the very frail, with an environment which caters to the specific needs associated with people with cognitive impairments, with the services set up to cater for the increasing numbers of 'frail older' people with acute illness and complex care needs.[17-19]

The Safe Design Process Steps

The safe design process is a collaborative risk management process implemented at the design stage of a product. Such processes can only be effective if the parties to the design, development and ownership of a product adopt the safe design process as a responsibility and documented procedure in their everyday business strategy.[16,20]
Steps in the process are:[20]

- The product owner initiates the safe design process through the procurement process.
- Identify and assemble a risk management team.
- Set out the context for the review.
- Collate information about risks associated with all stages of the product's life cycle.
- Review the design to identify health and safety risks and redesign options to eliminate or minimize the identified risks.
- Establish a residual risk register and record details of risks not eliminated.
- Use the residual risk register to inform life cycle stages of risk applicable to each life cycle stage.
- Review the process and product to update the register and inform the designer.

Objective Design Considerations

These designs should be targeted at three prime groups/areas:[20]

- Direct care workers who handle patients/residents
- Managers and designers and
- For the design and layout of the main patient/resident handling areas within hospitals and aged care facilities, including:[20]
  - Bedrooms
  - Bathrooms/en suites
  - Dining/lounge and recreational rooms (aged care)
  - Areas with specific function corridors
  - Reception
  - Exteriors
  - Other relevant areas, e.g. equipment/aids storage.

Common/External Requirements in the Facility

External Works

Buildings such as psychiatric and geriatric units require secure, enclosed gardens for the occupants. These should be pleasantly landscaped, easily supervised and without hazards. The orientation of these areas as regards sunlight, privacy, etc. are important factors. The site network and circulation system must allow covered outside entrance way with drive-up drop-off area.[21]

Outdoor Areas Design

Flow and Layout[19]

- Variety of accessible and inaccessible landscape areas
- Consideration of therapeutic and sensory plantings/ raised garden beds
- Screening and shelter/activity areas
- Minimum access widths for paths around buildings, passing spots, materials.

Furniture and Fixtures[19]

- Perimeter fencing—security and design
- Water features—safety features and management
- Outdoor chairs and tables—heights and ergonomics
- Garden ornaments and lighting
- Garden equipment.

Considerations of Use

Equipment—a variety of equipment may be used in development and maintenance of this.

Potential Hazards/Risks[19]

Slippery/wet paths; space restrictions; inadequate shelter; inadequate light; poorly secured; uneven surfaces, poorly lit.

Security

The security of patients, visitors and staff must be a balanced approach against the needs of ease and access and egress to the facilities and should include the following security concepts:[21]

- The design principles of the developments should take into account the latest security initiatives as well as general design techniques.[21]
- Clear delineation between public and controlled areas, and avoidance of unobserved areas and hiding places.[21]
- The use of the healthcare buildings and parts as may be required at different times of the day.
- Security design should be subtle and include natural barriers, access control points.[21]

Safety and Environmental Systems

- Fire protection system—exits, doors, equipment, fire rating requirements for building and introduced materials, compartmentalization.[16,20]
- Electrical/network system—light switches, plug outlets, cabling, lifts as per specifications.[16,20]
- Climate regulation system—heating, cooling, water temperature/ flow rates.

- Water reticulation, pipe work and control of backflow[20]
- Materials selection—low emissions, fire rating.

Infection Control Considerations

- As per biomedical waste management and handling rules 2016 the clinical waste is to be treated appropriately, contained and transported carefully. Arrangements for collection impact on design and the location, size and infrastructure of the aged care facility.[20]
- Waste disposal facilities—clear access to waste disposal facilities, including sluices, section for storage of clean items should be carefully defined and protected from vapors, splashing or aerosols during procedures, hand washing, equipment washing, ultrasonic cleaning and reprocessing.[20]
- Clinical hand basins—in all areas which resident treatment may occur with hot and cold water, nontouch taps, supplies of liquid hand wash, and disposable paper towels. Taps should have anti splash devices.[20]
- Work areas—adequate lighting, good ventilation and suitable receptacles (container) for the disposal of waste, easy access to equipment and safe storage for equipment not in use. Adequate bench space, at least one stainless steel sink or trough deep enough to accommodate instruments and other equipment requiring cleaning (double sinks are preferred), space for ultrasonic cleaners.[20]

Lighting

Seniors require 30% more light for equivalent vision, and up to 5 times brighter light in areas for reading and task completion:[1,22]

- Ensure no glare and light to be used are LED
- Cove lighting should be considered wherever possible; Cove lighting is a form of indirect lighting built into ledges, recesses, or valences in a ceiling or high on the walls of a room. It may be used as primary lighting, or for esthetic accent. Cove lighting is valued because it hides the fixtures, and because it provides a very even, warm light.
  - Direct illumination on vertical surfaces.
  - No highly polished surfaces.
- Avoid pooled lighting and shadows (sconces, i.e. a decorative wall bracket for holding candles or lights, table lamps)
- Provide night lighting in patient washrooms, and foot light in room
- Ensure focused light on signs and other way finding cues
- Ensure consistent levels of brightness in adjacent areas
- Create gradual changes of light levels when coming in from outdoors.[22-25]
- Remote audio controlled highting system should be used.[29]

Noise/Sound

High noise levels can lead to anxiety, confusion and fatigue from over stimulation and difficulty hearing that which is spoken to the senior. Background noise can create misinterpretations of what is happening in the environment.

- Reduce the use of the public address system as much as possible and turn off in patient bedrooms.[1]
- Combine a visual display that scrolls slowly to inform patients in a waiting area.
- Reduce background ambient noise (e.g. ventilation systems, radio).
- Have hearing amplifiers available in all patient contact areas.
- Reduce the number of hard surfaces and "echoes"[1]
- Use quality acoustical ceiling and wall products
- Consider heating and ventilation structure to reduce noise when installing.[1]

Décor

- Use colors at the warm end of the spectrum (blue tones are difficult to see)[1]
- Pastels and low contrast colors are difficult to see and define
- Use color to define functional areas (i.e. yellow hallway, green rooms, amber activity room)
- Use color contrast to highlight areas such as doors to assist way finding.

Catering

The facilities need catering both for staff and clients/patients. A central kitchen facility with satellite areas in each of the units will be a requirement. Either a central staff restaurant or individual units in some of the facilities will be a necessity. If a central kitchen is not provided, individual kitchens will be needed in many of the units.[21]

Nutrition

Following is the nutritional considerations in the geriatric set-up:

- *Goal:* To maintain or improve nutritional intake at meals and provide a quality mealtime experience that fosters dignity and pleasure in eating, as well as respecting cultural and personal preferences, for as long as possible.[26]

Guiding Principles[26]

- The adequate intake of nutrients is necessary to maintain physical and emotional health.
- The quality of mealtime is an indicator of quality of life and care of an individual.
- Mealtime is an opportunity not only to ingest nutrients but also to maintain critical social aspects of life.
- The social components of meals should be observed, including mealtime rituals, cultural norms and food preferences.
- Persons should be encouraged and assisted to self-feed for as long as possible.
- Persons dependent in eating should be assisted with dignity.

Furniture[1]

- Tables
  - Sturdy 4 legged
  - Rounded corners
  - Edges defined with contrasting color borders
  - Matte tabletop
  - Contrast table settings to assist with depth perception.
- Beds
  - Electric adjustable height to 18 inch low
  - Controller with "simple" technology and large easily identified buttons
  - Pressure relieving mattress
  - Avoid side railings that fold down to the floor.
- Bedside tables
  - On glides instead of wheels
  - Lever handles for easy glide drawers.
- Chairs
  - Seat: 18–19 inch high, 18–20 inch deep with firm cushion
  - Arms extended to front chair edge, 10 inch above seat height
  - Lumbar support
  - Nonslip easily cleaned fabric

- Clearance under front of seat to allow feet under front edge
- Stable/tip-free
- Minimal back recline and backwards seat tilt
- Chair legs able to be fit with blocks to further raise seat height.

Electrical and Fittings

- There are a number of items of fittings and fixtures found in acute and aged care facilities, some of which are necessary in the delivery of medical services (e.g. oxygen, gas, suction, IV and blood pressure machines) and other items (e.g. bedside tables, fixed shower screens, privacy curtains, etc.). These fixtures can impede staff when handling patients/residents. Choosing appropriate movable fittings, such as bedside tables, can contribute to better access and therefore to safer handling procedures. This also includes appropriate adjustable beds (electronic/hydraulic) and special lounge chairs that can assist in reducing staff injuries.[27]
- There should be enough electrical outlets for all personal and agency equipment, and they need to be located so as to minimize cords trailing across circulation areas, which can cause tripping hazards or impede movement of wheeled equipment.[19,28]
- The appropriate location of electrical and mechanical fittings (e.g. air-conditioners, ducted vacuum systems) can also have an impact on staff handling procedures and prevention of staff injuries.[19,28]

Specific Spatial Requirements Inside the Building

Waiting Areas

Guidelines of waiting area are depicted in Table 1.

Common Rooms Design (Fig. 1)[20]

Function: Multipurpose room for activities, relaxation.

Workflow and Layout

- Allowance for lounge chairs/recliners and tables sufficient for number of residents
- Separation of activities—passive/active

Table 1: Guidelines of waiting areas.[21]

Objectives of waiting area	*Guidelines*
Size and function	
• To provide an easily recognizable and welcoming entrance for the use of the public visitors, residents and staff	• Indicative size–30 sqm including waiting area • Entry may be through a front porch, hall lobby or foyer space
• To incorporate a waiting area	• The waiting area should allow space for wheel chair access particularly at the reception counter
• To provide a sense of place to assist visitors to familiarize themselves	• Provide room for family groups to pause near the entry door within easy sight of way-finding cues • Provide one entry point only and security • Design for access and mobility for frail, disabled and ambulatory persons
Location	
• To be the point of arrival and departure from the building	• The entrance should be given protection from the elements with a covered porch overhang to the Kerb edge • Provide direct uninhibited access to the reception area from the door • Provide direct access to public telephone and toilets for visitors
• To provide clean dry access for ambulatory or disabled persons • To enable screening of people coming and going	• Locate close to street pedestrian access and onsite parking • Visual access to main circulation corridor, reception, office and meeting room • Locate adjacent to the major circulation routes within the facility
Colors	
• To provide an easily recognizable entrance with a welcoming and caring atmosphere	• Provide welcoming bright colors and a domestic feel to the room
Signage	
• To enable easily read directional signage so visitors can orientate themselves and find their way throughout the facility without staff assistance	• Map "You are Here" or directory board at the hallway to the home • Directions to toilets and to telephone • Clear identification of the reception counter within line of sight from entrance door • Tactile signage • Letter size large enough and in contrast colors
Floors and floor finishes	
• To intercept grit, mud, water, organic matter and the like and resist heavy wear at the entrance • To be easily cleaned	• Adopt a nonslip surface just inside the door and a hard wearing floor covering to the remainder of the room
	• Mats at the entrance are to be feather edged and edge restrained so as not to create a tripping hazard. Mat wells are not to be used • Avoid steps and changes in color of adjacent materials in paths of travel because this can be perceived as a step by frail, disabled or ambulatory persons • Surfaces are to be arranged to reduce slip or trip hazards
Ceilings	
• To provide a light, reflective monolithic ceiling at a height that is in scale with the space • To be non-institutional in appearance	• Adopt set and painted plasterboard as a standard • Minimum height of ceiling is to be 2400 mm high • Where ceiling fans are to be used, ceilings are to be a minimum of 3000 mm high or 2700 mm to the underside of fan blades • Careful symmetrical arrangement of service penetrations

Contd...

Contd...

Objectives of waiting area	*Guidelines*
Walls	
• To provide visual and acoustic privacy between the entry and the other rooms/spaces • To provide finishes relevant to residential/domestic environments within the area	• Adopt 12 mm set and painted plasterboard as a standard • Provide wall protection to all areas which are subject to mechanical damage from chairs and the like by using 12 mm set and painted fiber cement dry wall sheeting to a height of 900 mm, or install a chair rail • Provide handrails that have a domestic character and feel
Doors and windows	
• To provide hands free entrance and controlled exit • To allow natural light, ventilation and a pleasant outlook	• Provide automatic opening, sliding glazed doors to front entry • All door openings are to be a clear minimum of 920 mm wide • Domestic scale clear glass windows with sills at chair-rail height • Openable windows will require insect screens
Lighting and fans	
• To achieve well lit floor surfaces in paths of travel and adequate light for reading in waiting areas	• Provide non-institutional light fittings centered over walkways • Use lighting to help provide a warm and welcoming ambience • Consider the use of table lamps as decorative elements and to de-institutionalize the space and provide task lighting for reading • If used, place ceiling fans in a manner to avoid ceiling fan flicker
Communications and data	
• To provide after hours communication and security from front door	• Consider provision of intercom, CCTV and night bell outside the entry doors
• To enable residents and visitors to access telephones	• Provide a keypad door opener at the front door with indicators in the reception area so that access through the doors can be visually monitored by reception staff • Provide for a public telephone either in or nearby the waiting area
Power	
• To provide sufficient individual power outlets so that there is no requirement for extension cords or double adaptors	• Provide power outlets for table lamps • In some cases, power may be required for snack dispensers, water coolers or coffee dispensers • Confirm the individual requirements of the user groups during project definition plan phase
Switching and controls	
• To ensure staff control and 24 h illumination	• Switching is to be in the adjacent reception area • Provide capability to automatically reduce light levels late at night and in daylight h
Ventilation/climate control	
• To provide a comfortable environment as per the local conditions, for the elderly and visitors who may wait there	• Where air conditioning is provided use individual room thermostat and control • Design for irregular numbers of people during the day • Provide insect screened natural ventilation as an alternative to mechanical ventilation
Loose and soft furniture	
• To emulate a "living room" atmosphere with robust, comfortable and furniture which can be easily cleaned with a domestic feel • To provide safe, comfortable furniture that is both attractive and suitable for use by elderly persons	• Typical furniture within this area will include comfortable seats, coffee table (carefully placed) with seating for up to six people • Use warm materials and textures and decorate similar to a residential entrance/living area • Avoid sharp corners. Side tables 720 mm high with rounded corners • Consider incontinence resistant fabrics for chairs. Chairs should generally have arms positioned directly over legs for maximum stability • Place furniture clear of the walkway between entrance door and main passage/reception allowing ample space for elderly persons using wheelchairs or walking frames • Expert consultants experienced in the requirements of furniture for the elderly should be engaged to assist in selections

- Television visual comfort and screen size/positioning
- Ease of movement
- Access and storage for wheelchairs and walking frames.

Furniture and Equipment

- Lounge chairs/recliners and tables
- Display cupboards/sideboards
- Storage cupboards
- Audio-visual.

Considerations of Use

Carriers—assisting with transfers and personal care
Change of use—rooms may be used for other purposes
Equipment—a variety of equipment may be used in this area.

Potential Hazards/Risks

Slippery/wet floors; space restrictions; inadequate ventilation; sharp edges; tripping; light pooling; visual problems, e.g. patterns/contrast.

Hallways

Salient features are:[1]

- Clear, unimpeded pathways wide enough for wheelchair/walker and caregiver in each direction (larger than minimum wheelchair access standard).
- Avoid shiny surface with glare
- Avoid long hallways without visual interruption
- Seating areas at regular intervals along long hallway

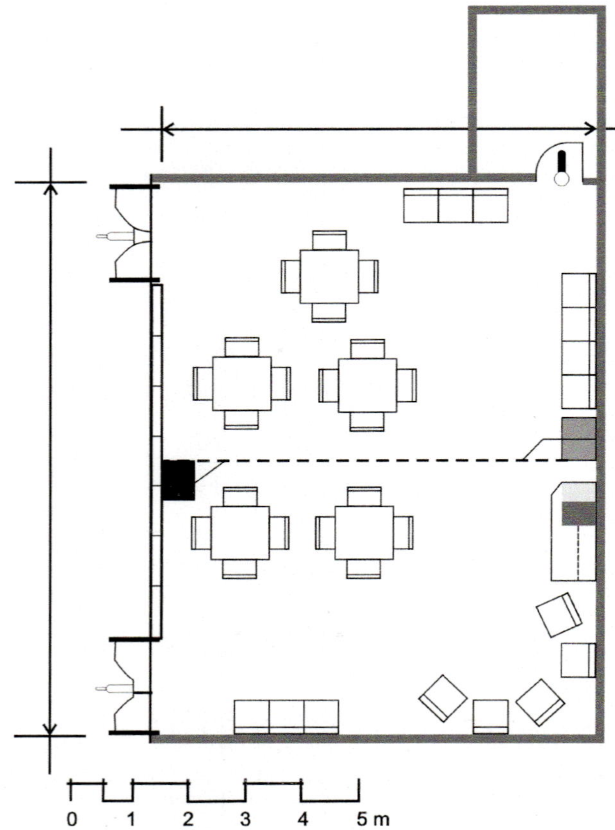

Fig. 1: Common room design.

- Hand railings in hallways to assist walking (1.5 inch diameter with 2 inch hand clearance—"easy grip" rounded style)
- Handrails extend beyond top and bottom landings.

Steps

- Conventional (6-inch risers; 12-inch treads) that will be expected
- Highlight step edge with contrast color (yellow).

Ramps

- Avoid if possible
- If required 5–8% slope of the area traveled
- Rest area every 30 ft
- Mark top and bottom with yellow strip.

Shock Absorbent Flooring

Table 2 shows the shock absorbent flooring.

Bedrooms[1]

- Visibly distinctive doorways and bed area
- Direct sight line to washroom from bed
- Call bells
  - Remote voice activated is ideal
  - Fixed to bed side
  - Large easily activated button.

Table 2: Shock Absorbent flooring in various areas.

Room	Facility	Floor finish
Bedrooms	Acute aged care rehabilitation	Cushioned vinyl or Wooden
Bathrooms/En suites	All	Nonslip vinyl or epoxy
Corridors	Acute aged care/Rehabilitation	Vinyl
Dining rooms	All	Vinyl

- Telephone
  - Black phone with large white push buttons with contrasting buttons/letters
  - Located within easy reach of the bed
  - Volume control
  - Suitable for use with hearing aids.
  - Mobile phone with special inbuilt features for aged.

BEDROOM DESIGN[20]

Function: Provision of bed, personal affects/furniture.

Workflow and Layout

- Required clear space on both sides, and end of the bed
- Storage of wheelchairs/walking frames, television/entertainment equipment/computer
- Access to the en suite/bathroom.

Furniture/Equipment

- Beds (variable widths) and wardrobes (built in/free standing)
- Side tables and chairs—ergonomic requirements
- Display cabinets, built in furniture
- Lifting machine at foot end of bed
- Medical equipment (e.g. Nebulizer).

Considerations of use

- Carriers—assisting with transfers and personal care
- Aging in place—provision for increasing dependencies of the inmates.
- Change of use—rooms may be used for other purposes
- Equipment—a variety of equipment may be used in the rooms so the space requirements should be anticipated.

Potential Hazards/Risks

Space restrictions; tripping points; non-electric beds; manual handling; uneven floors; sharp edges on furniture; poor levels of lighting/external glare; protruding bed controls; clutter, lack of adequate storage.

En Suites and Assisted Toilets[20]

Function: independent or assisted ablutions (Figs. 2 to 9).

En Suites and Toilets Design[20]

Workflow and Layout

- Toilet ideally located opposite door
- Minimum access space around the toilet for maneuverability for carers, person and equipment.
- Wheelchair and walking frame storage/access to basin.

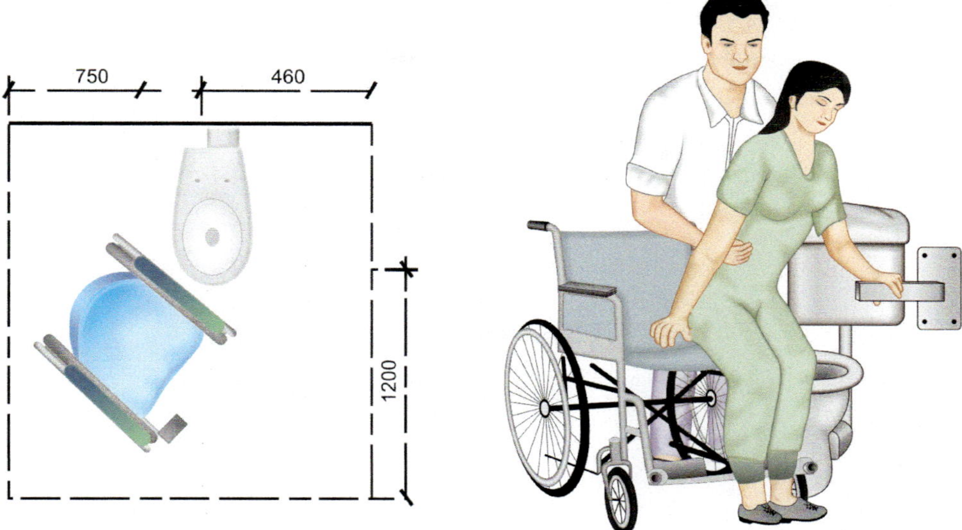

Fig. 2: The functional area for a wheelchair bound patient/resident who requires assistance in a side transfer.[20,24]

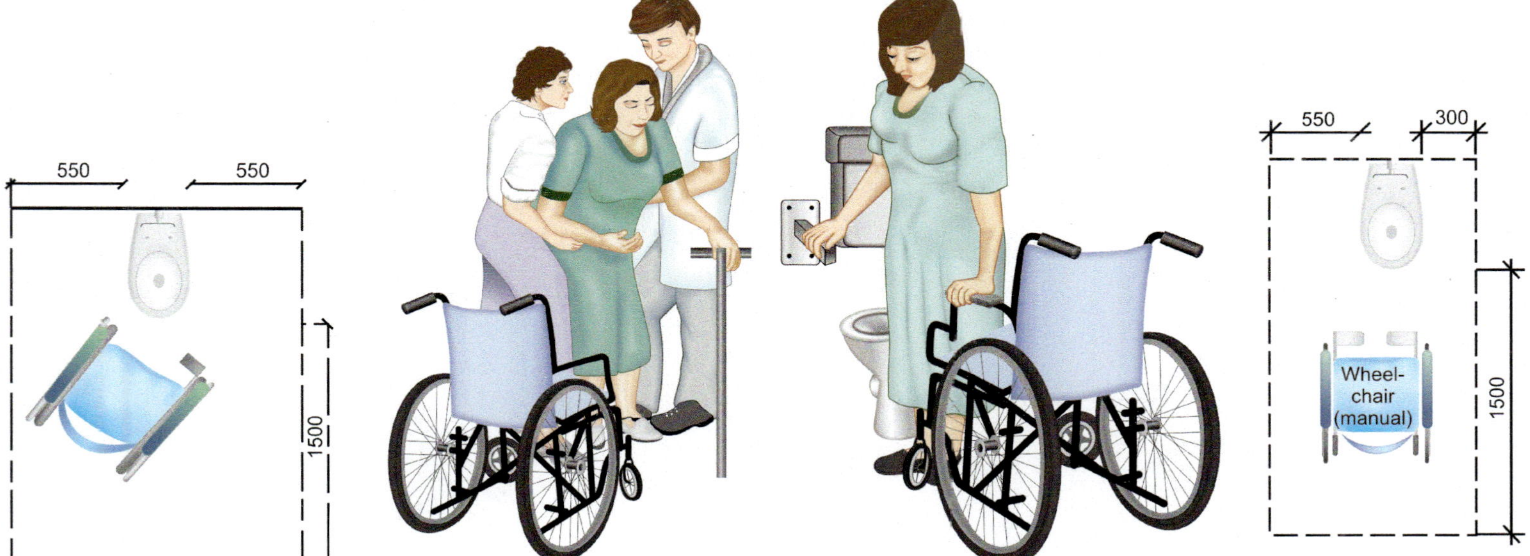

Fig. 3: The functional area for a patient/resident who can stand on both legs. This transfer requires the option of two staff assisting by standing either side. The wheelchair is placed as shown in the diagram. This is also sufficient space for a patient to transfer with the help of a swivel board/turntable.[20]

Fig. 4: The functional area needed by an independent wheelchair person—frontal transfer.[24]

Sanitary Ware/Equipment[20]

- Minimum specifications and access space apply
- Support arms on both sides of the toilet
- Ease of use of taps.

Considerations of Use[20]

- Carers/family—assisting with transfers and personal care
- Equipment—a variety of equipment may be used.

Potential Hazards/Risks

Slippery/wet floors; space restrictions; poor lighting inadequate ventilation; personal emergency—door locked; light pooling; visual problems, e.g. patterns/contrast.[20]

En suites and assisted toilets are often planned for the movement of independent patients/residents with disabilities. Detailed consideration in allowing for staff assistance is often overlooked however, for example, the situation of two staff assisting in the transfer of a patient/resident and the use of mobile lifting machines.[20]

The Figures 8 and 9 show the spatial requirements for manual handling around individual fixtures.

Toilet Transfers

Note that these diagrams exclude hand basins and showers, as they will be provided outside the minimum spatial zone required for toilet transfers.[20]

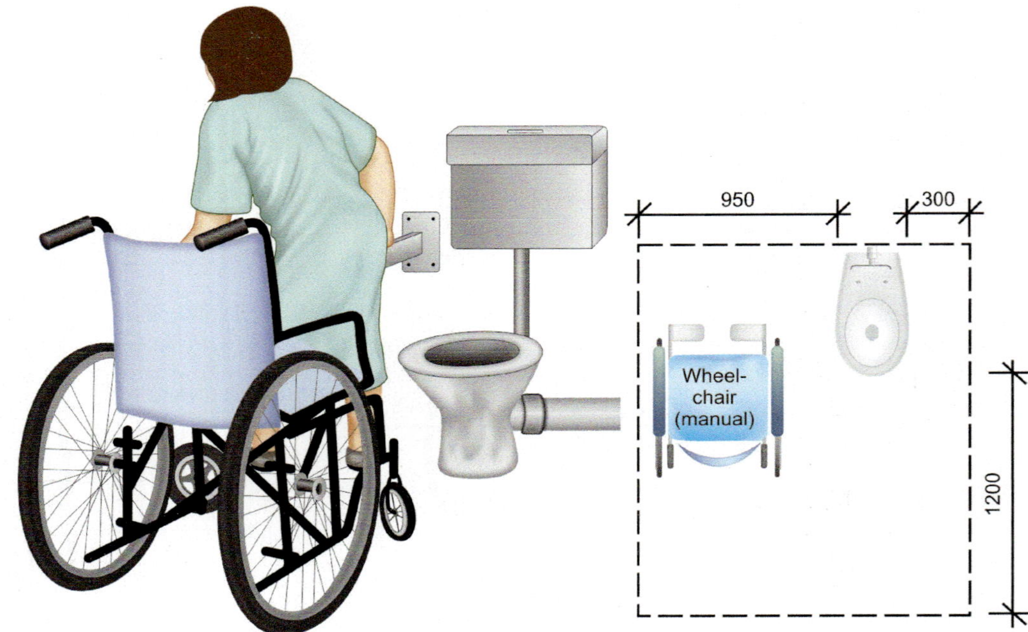

Fig. 5: The functional area needed by an independent wheelchair person—side transfer.[24]

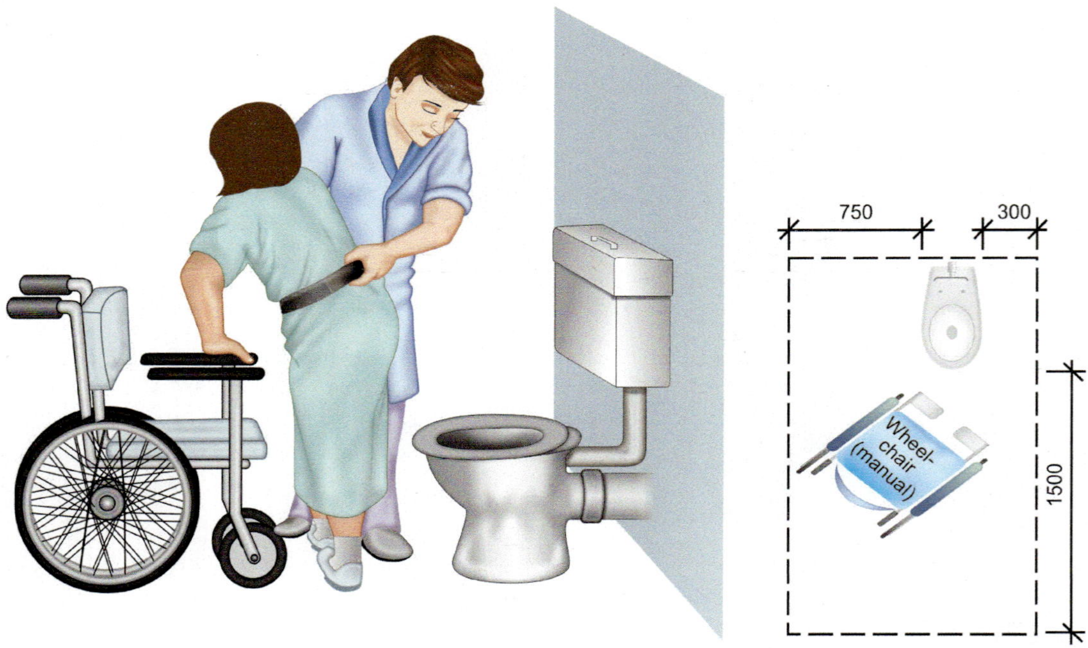

Fig. 6: The functional area for a wheelchair bound patient/resident, who can stand on one leg, required assistance by one staff with frontal transfer. The wheelchair is placed as indicated in the figure.[24]

The functional area for a wheelchair bound patient/resident, who can stand on one leg, requires assistance by one staff with frontal transfer. The wheelchair is placed as indicated in the Figure 6.[20]

Design for Daycare

Historically, the advent of nursing homes created a hospital-like environment where the elderly who could not care for themselves for medical reasons could be cared for (Diaz Moore, 2005). However, it became clear that nursing homes were not always a suitable environment for the elderly. A continuum of care including assisted living and adult daycare centers emerged to provide support and help in preventing or delaying the placement of the elderly, particularly those with dementia, in an institutional typesetting by providing a supportive environment and respite for the family caregiver.[28,29]

Automated distribution system general environmental concepts that are important to implement in a daycare center, especially for the clients with cognitive impairments, to maximize its therapeutic capabilities are broadly as follows:

Services that afford independence, autonomy and control by being adaptable to the users.

- Spaces that afford meaningful and culturally appropriate activity.
- Interior and exterior detailing that is familiar and non-threatening.
- Spaces, access points, pathways and services that use appropriate modes (light, color, pictorial, verbal, tactile) for presentation of essential information to assist appropriate task completion (i.e. cueing stimuli).

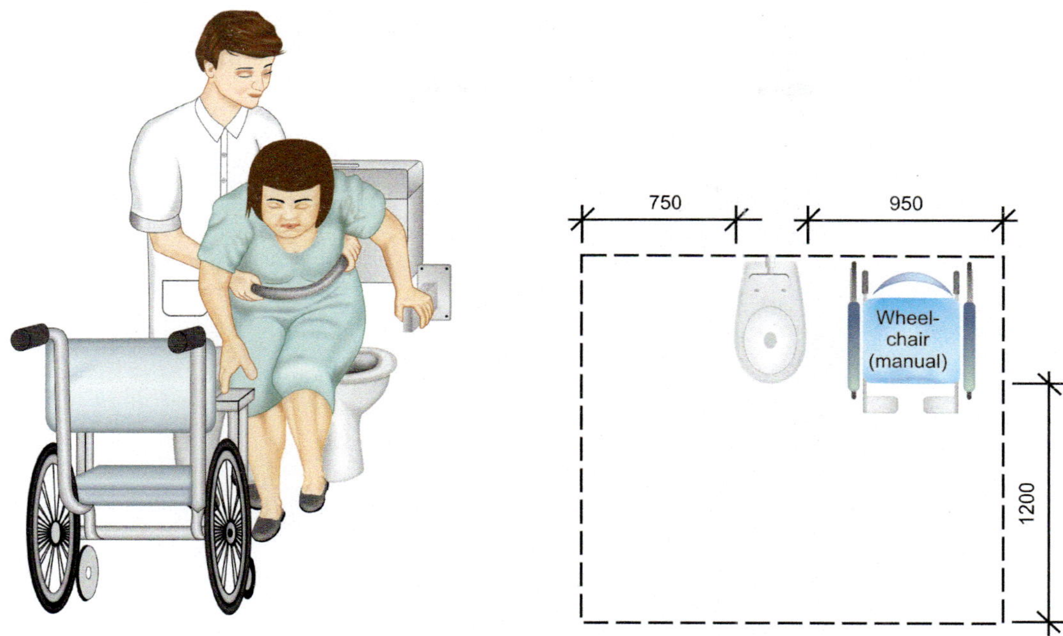

Fig. 7: The functional area for a wheelchair bound patient/resident—side transfer.[24]

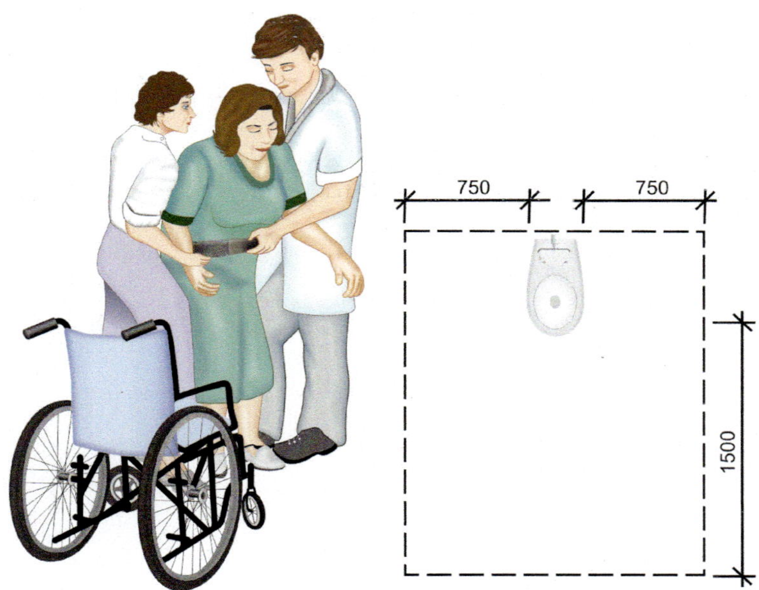

Fig. 8: The functional area for a patient/resident who can stand on both legs. This transfer requires the option of two staff assisting by standing either side. The wheelchair is placed as shown in the diagram. This is also sufficient space for a patient to transfer with the help of a swivel board/turntable.[20,24]

- Spaces, access points, pathways and services that eliminate unnecessary complexity and reduce extraneous sensory stimuli.
- Spaces, access points and pathways services that reduce agitation and opportunities for meaningless wandering.
- Spaces, access points, pathways and services that afford approach, reach, manipulation, and use regardless of user's limitations (i.e. highly negotiable).
- Spaces, access points, pathways and services that are tolerant of user related error (i.e. safe and secure).
- Spaces, access points, pathways and services that meet the needs of staff.

The guidelines of the National Building Codes, elements of an earthquake resistant buildings, green buildings, water harvesting also have to be kept in mind since the inception of the plan (Figs. 10 and 11).

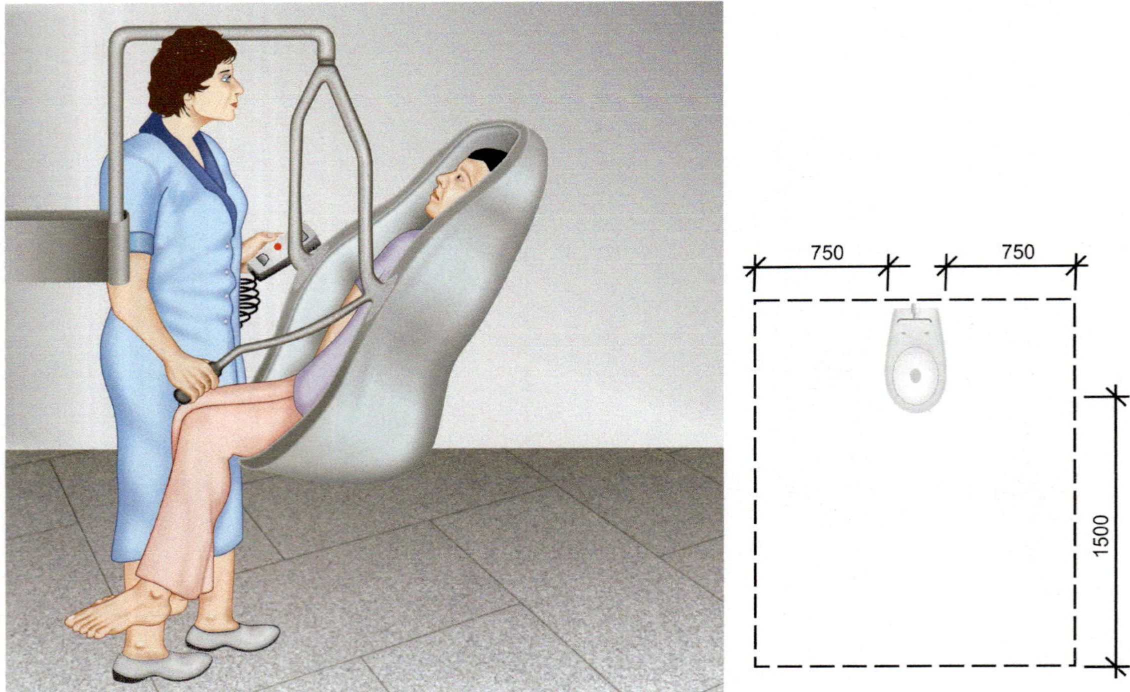

Fig. 9: The functional area needed for a patient/resident in a lifting machine and with assistance of one or two staff on either side. The transfer to the lifting machine has been done outside this area.[20]

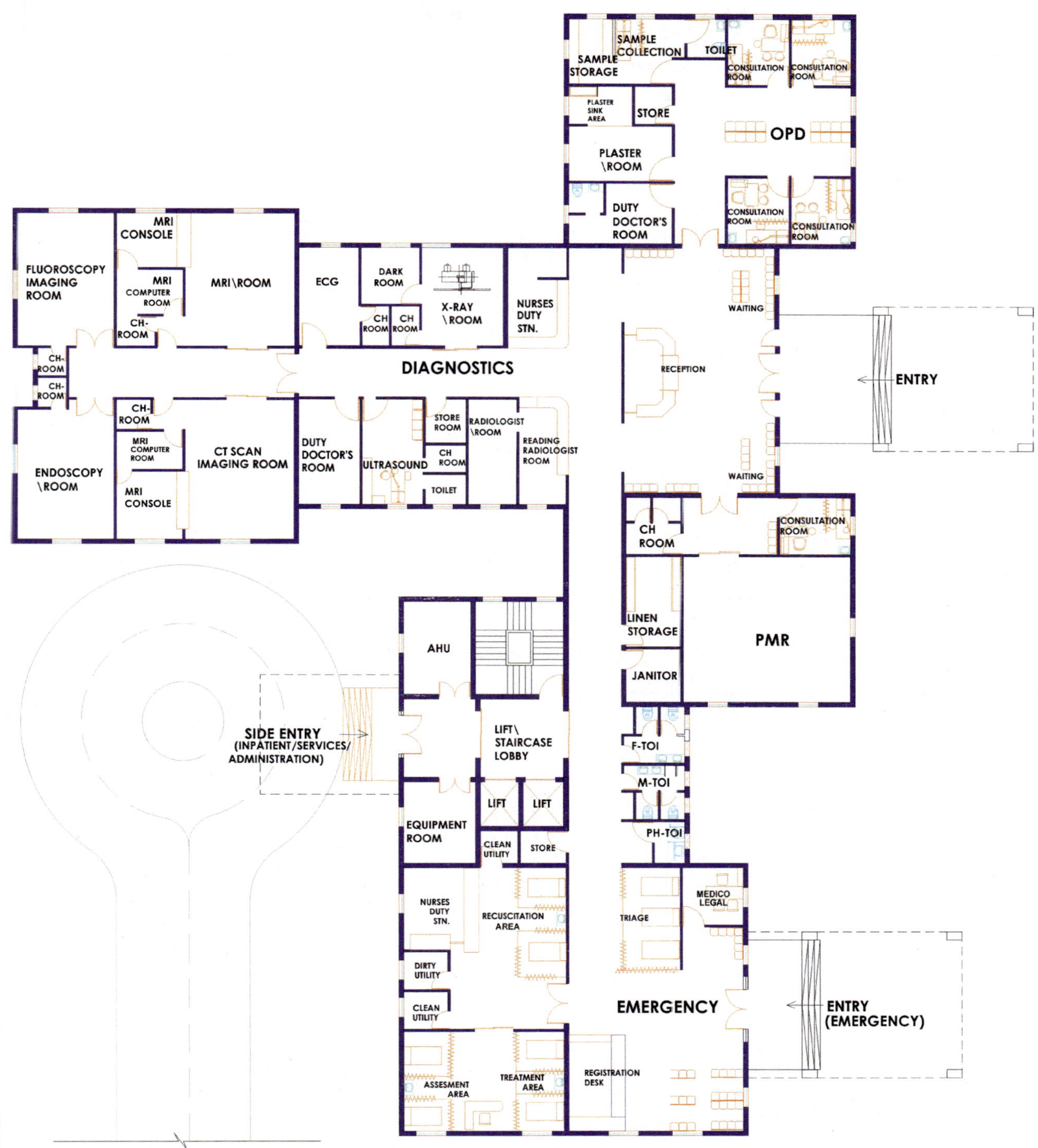

Fig. 10: Ground floor plan.

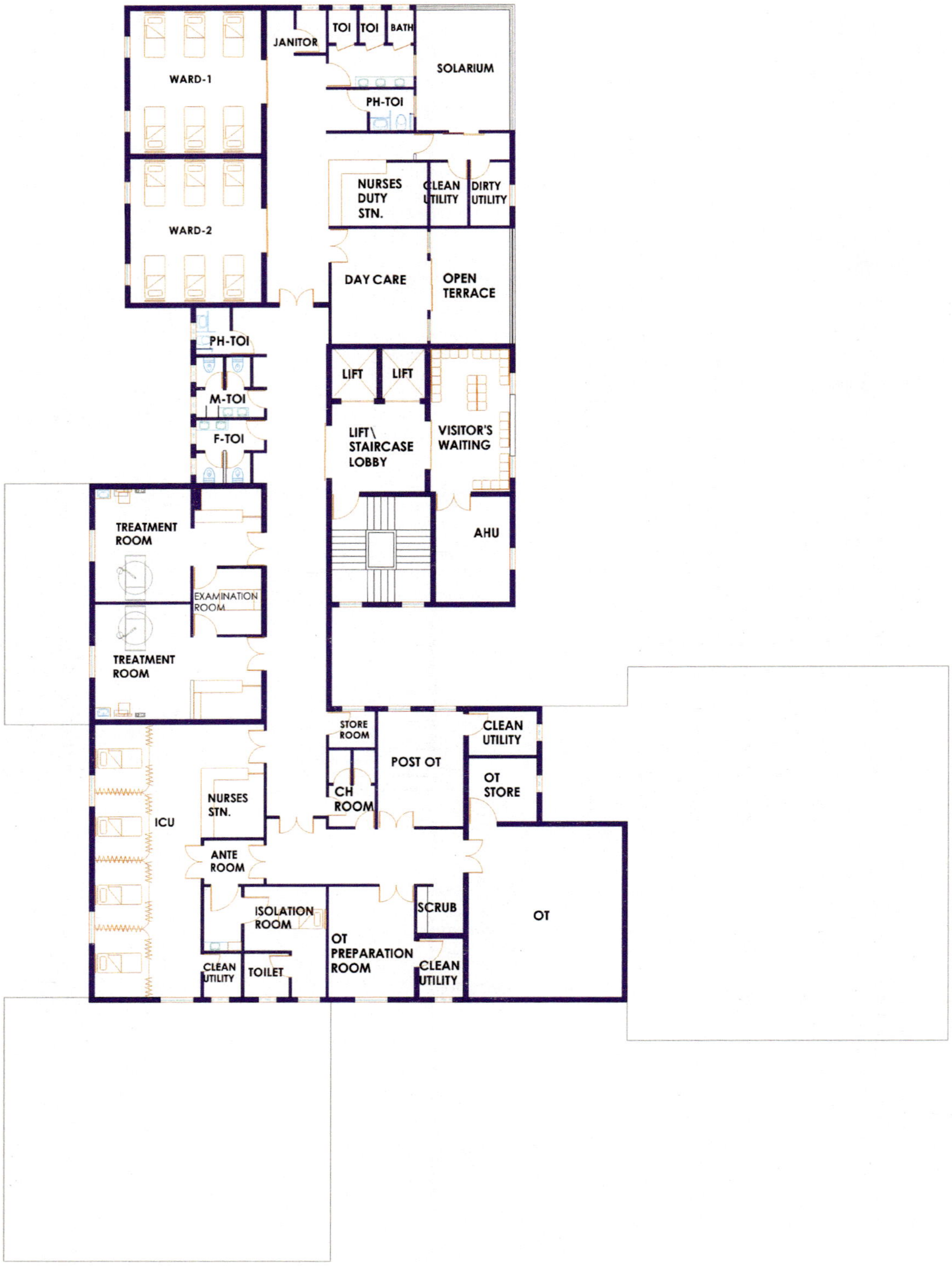

Fig. 11: First floor plan.

CONCLUSION

Over the past decades, India's health program and policies have been focusing on issues like population stabilization, maternal and child health, and disease control. However, current statistics for the elderly in India gives a prelude to a new set of medical, social, and economic problems that could arise. There is a need to highlight the medical and socioeconomic problems that are being faced by the elderly people in India, and strategies for bringing about an improvement in their quality of life also need to be explored.[3] In view of these parameters Government of India launched "National Programme for Healthcare of Elderly (NPHCE)", free specilized healthcare facility exclusively for elderly people through the State health delivery system.

The role of geriatric healthcare facility in society is multifold. With the increased longevity of life, there will be requirement of geriatric healthcare facility in large number in India. A complete, well-planned geriatric health facility will provide:[30]

- Linking between aging and societal development by treating aging as an opportunity for development
- Establishing sustainable system of social protection to guard against poverty in old age.
- Meeting the growing demand for accessible and quality healthcare, including long-term care for the elderly.
- Creating age-friendly environments and working with the government and other national and international organization for promotion of elders' well-being and health.

REFERENCES

1. www.rgpeo.com
2. www.rgpc.ca
3. Charcot JM, Hunt LH, Loomis AL Clinical lectures on the diseases of old age. New York: William Wood, 1881.
4. Devas MB. Geriatric orthopaedics Bri. Med. J. 1974;1(5900):190-2.
5. Irvine RE Geriatric orthopaedics in Hastings: The collaborative management of elderly women with fractured neck of the femur. Advanced Geriatric Medicine, 1983;pp.130-6.
6. Wykes L, Sir Anderson WF. British Geriatrics Society.September, 1-3. Retrieved May 13, 2018 from http://www.bgsnet.org.uk/pdf/Sept2001.pdf.
7. http://www.un.org/esa/population/meetings/EGMPopAge/EGMPopAge_21_RHuber.pdf
8. www.a4m.com
9. www.jiag.org
10. Johnson CS. Ageing and healthy life expectancy: Will the extended years be spent in good or poor health? J Indian Acad Geriatr, 2008;4:64-7.
11. www.un-documents.net
12. www.un.org
13. www.ncbi.nlm.nih.gov
14. Khandelwal SK. Mental health of older people. In: Dey AB, (Ed). Ageing in India. Situational analysis and planning for the future.Rakmo Press, New Delhi; 2003.
15. www.ijcm.org.in
16. Jamuna D, Reddy LK. The impact of age and length of widowhood on the self concept of elderly widows.Indian J Gerontol. 1997;7:91–5.
17. http://www.aag.asn.au/filelib/AHMAC_and_beyond.pdf
18. www.agedcareassociation.com.au
19. aag.asn.au
20. www.safework.sa.gov.au
21. www.ggda.ie
22. www.light.com
23. www.expresshealthcaremgmt.com
24. bralpowerassociate.blogspot.com
25. www.lightingassociates.org
26. www.consultgerirn.org
27. Work Cover Authority, Victorian. "Designing Workplaces for Safer Handling of Patients/Residents", Back Injury Among Healthcare Workers Causes Solutions and Impacts, 2003.
28. safework.sa.gov.au
29. Medical and Social Adult Day Service Programs: A Comparison of Characteristics, Dementia Clients, and their Family Caregivers. Research on Aging. 2001;23: 473-98.
30. www.johsonmedical.com

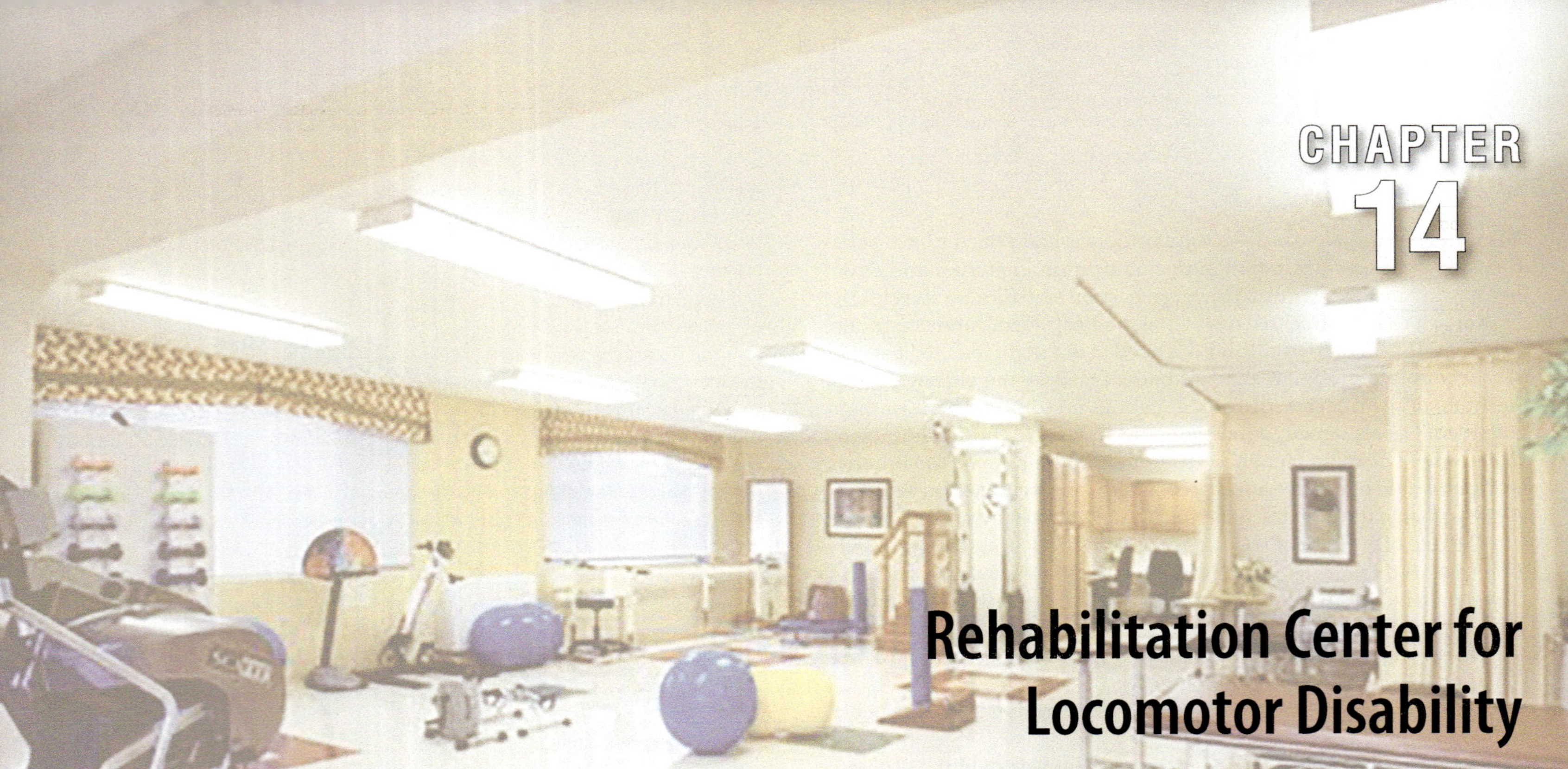

Rehabilitation Center for Locomotor Disability

Jitesh V, Shakti Kumar Gupta, Sunil Kant, R Chandrashekhar

INTRODUCTION

There is no universally agreed definition of disability. In the World Health Organization (WHO) report, disability is understood to be primarily a social phenomenon. It is society that disables people who have impairments, by failing to recognize and accommodate differences, and through the attitudinal, environmental and institutional barriers that it erects against people with impairments. Disability thus arises from a complex interaction between health conditions and the context in which they exist. The International Classification of Functioning, Disability and Health, (ICF), is WHO's framework for measuring health and disability at both individual and population levels.[1]

The International Classification of Functioning, Disability and Health, known more commonly as ICF, are a classification of health and health-related domains. These domains are classified from body, individual and societal perspectives by means of two lists: a list of body functions and structure, and a list of domains of activity and since an individual's functioning and disability occurs in a context, the ICF also includes a list of environmental factors.[2]

In India, the persons with disabilities (equal opportunities, protection of rights and full participation) Act 1995 define disability as one or more of the following: blindness, low vision, leprosy cured, hearing impairment, locomotor disability, mental retardation and mental illness. It says that to be considered disabled, a person must suffer from not less than 40% of any disability, as certified by a medical authority.[1]

FUNCTIONS OF THE CENTER

These should include:

- Rehabilitation
  - Assessment
  - Corrective surgery
  - Orthotics/implements/devices/equipment
  - Rehabilitation
  - Education
  - Vocational training
  - Community integration.
- Research
  - Data collection and compilation
  - Experimentation and innovation.
- Human resources development
  - Education
  - Research
  - Telemedicine.

PLANNING AND DESIGN CONSIDERATIONS

The following form the basis of the planning premises:

- *Continuum of care:* The needs of rehabilitation begin with the onset of any illness and continue beyond the acute phase and more. The need for the rehabilitation center to be co-located with hospital, therefore, needs to be considered.
- *Comprehensive care:* To provide comprehensive care in terms of multispecialty, multisectoral, multimodal intervention, needed in case of a rehabilitation patient, the departments should be planned in detail at the outset to avoid fragmentation and lack of coordination.
- *Completeness of care:* The completeness in terms of rehabilitation services must take into account the involvement of the caretakers of the person with disability through the process of rehabilitation along with the varied professionals involved.
- *Community-based care:* Recent evidence point to the need for community involvement in the rehabilitation process and inclusion of people with disability in all walks of life. To this end community awareness and participation should be considered in the setting up of a rehabilitation center.
- Evidence-based medicine suggest certain philosophies to be followed in patient care facility planning in general

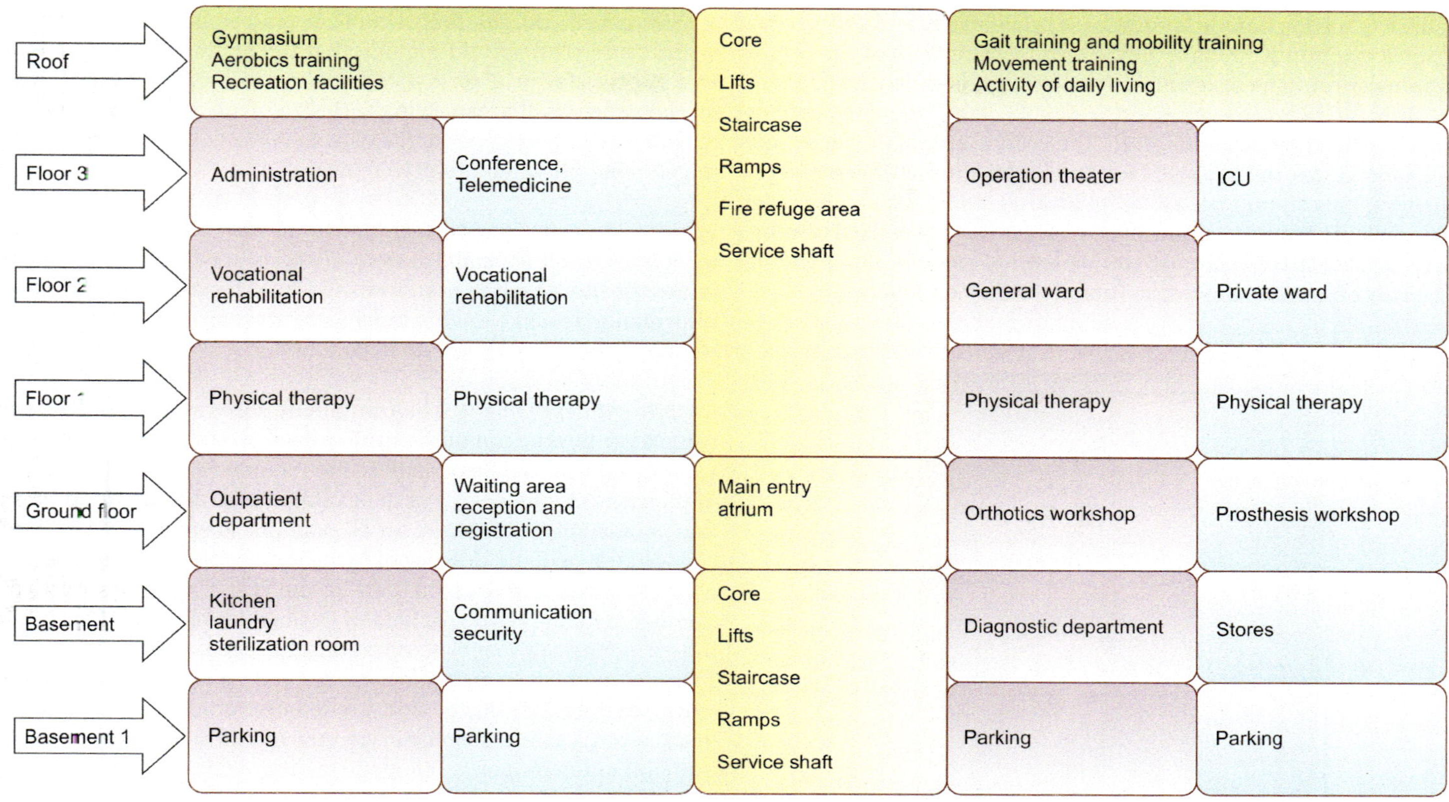

Fig. 1: Stack diagram.

- Patients have the right to appropriate communication in a warm, caring environment.
- Patients, their families, and the professional staff play unique and vital roles in the healthcare team.
- Patient is not an isolated unit but a member of a family, community, and culture.
- Patient is an individual with rights, responsibilities, and choices regarding his/her lifestyle and health.
- A supportive, friendly, and caring environment is an essential component of providing high-quality healthcare.
- The physical environment is vital to the healing process and should be designed to promote healing and learning, as well as patient and family participation in care.

Stack diagram is shown in Figure 1.

FACILITIES

The recommended specialties are:

- *Outpatient:* The interface with the community.
- *Inpatient:* Limited to the admission of the person requiring corrective surgery or for comprehensive assessment.
- *Rehabilitation services:* Will form the fulcrum of the establishment.
- *Vocational training:* The complete spectrum of the vocation training may not be feasible in the same establishment however; it should include work simulation and work assessment and prevocational training.
- *Community integration:* The care takers orientation and education, considering the home family as the fundamental unit of the community is to be catered for. The smooth transition of the patient from the rehabilitation to the home and the community should be addressed.
- Support services.

Location and access of rehabilitation center: It should be such that the facility should be easily accessible to the clientele as well as the staff and there should be easy access to the services of the hospital, in addition, the patient in the hospital would need to be assessed and planned for continued rehabilitation program.

Reception: It will form the interface of the facility with the community and therefore needs careful considerations of the under mentioned areas for the benefit and impression of the visitors. Reception and assistance should cater for the needs of wheelchair bound patients, which would entail a lower desk height, in addition to ensuring the privacy of the interaction. A reception desk with a low counter top is welcoming to all patients. Desk-height writing surfaces with knee space for use by wheelchair users and others who cannot stand while transacting business.[3]

Parking area should be accessible and must have mobility assistance for patient to move from the parking to the facility.

Security aspect for the parking area must be kept in mind during the planning stage including the surveillance camera and structural features like boom barriers and access control.

Signposting should be clear and keeping the user profile in consideration. The visitors will have multiple disabilities and therefore should be factored in the design consideration. The provision of wheel chair or assistive devices for mobility of patients within the facility should be catered for.

Ramps and patient lifts: The design of the ramps and patients lifts need to be catered for.

Ramped approach (Fig. 2): Ramp should be furnished with non-slip material to enter the building. Minimum width or ramp should be 1800 mm with maximum gradient 1:12, length of ramp should not exceed 9.0 M having double handrail at a might of 800 and 900 mm on both sides extending 300 mm. Beyond top and bottom of the ramp. Minimum gap from the adjacent wall to the handrail should be 50 mm.[4]

Motivation hall/library/waiting hall: The waiting area at the reception wing should form the major place for social interaction between the visitors. This should have seating arrangements which allow for considerable flexibility in terms of not having too many fixed seating facility, and has spaces adequate for wheelchair bound or patient on other forms of assistive devices to interact with each other.

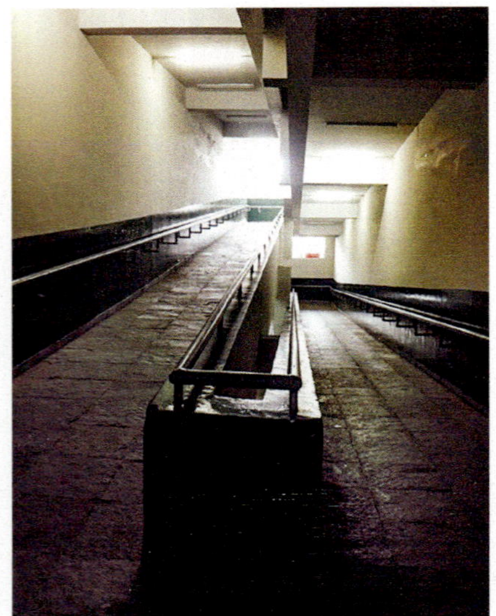

Fig. 2: Ramped approach.

Restrooms and facilities should be catering to the needs of the visitors and plan should include that the facility if barrier free and easily accessible to all forms of the visitors using the facility. The need for the patients with respect to the design of the toilet must be catered to with the turning radius of the wheelchair accounted (Fig. 3) for and the grab bar provided at suitable height.

Value-added services: A cafeteria would be a value addition in the reception area, the establishment of shops in which items produced in the vocational rehabilitation wing would form a motivating factor. Information kiosks, vending machines, toy rooms, gift shop, and play rooms are facilities which are desirable.

Outpatient department: The outpatient department forms the first step in the interaction of the professional with the patient. The sub-waiting area should be considered to include for both the categories of the visitors. The design of the examination rooms should be such that accessibility is ensured for all patients, keeping in view that the consultation will include not only the patient but the family member who will be an active participant in the rehabilitation process. The number of rooms will be decided by the load factor calculated based on the incidence, approach, acceptability and accessibility of the facility. There should be corridors which are wide enough for at least two wheelchairs to pass side by side. Conference room/cross consultation/board room is a must keeping in view the multidisciplinary approach in a rehabilitation program. Telemedicine should be planned to be set-up in the outpatient wing to cater for long distance learning as well as outreach program. Library is desirable in the outpatient department.

Inpatient department: The average length of stay varies rather remarkably in the inpatient wing of any rehabilitation facility. The number of the

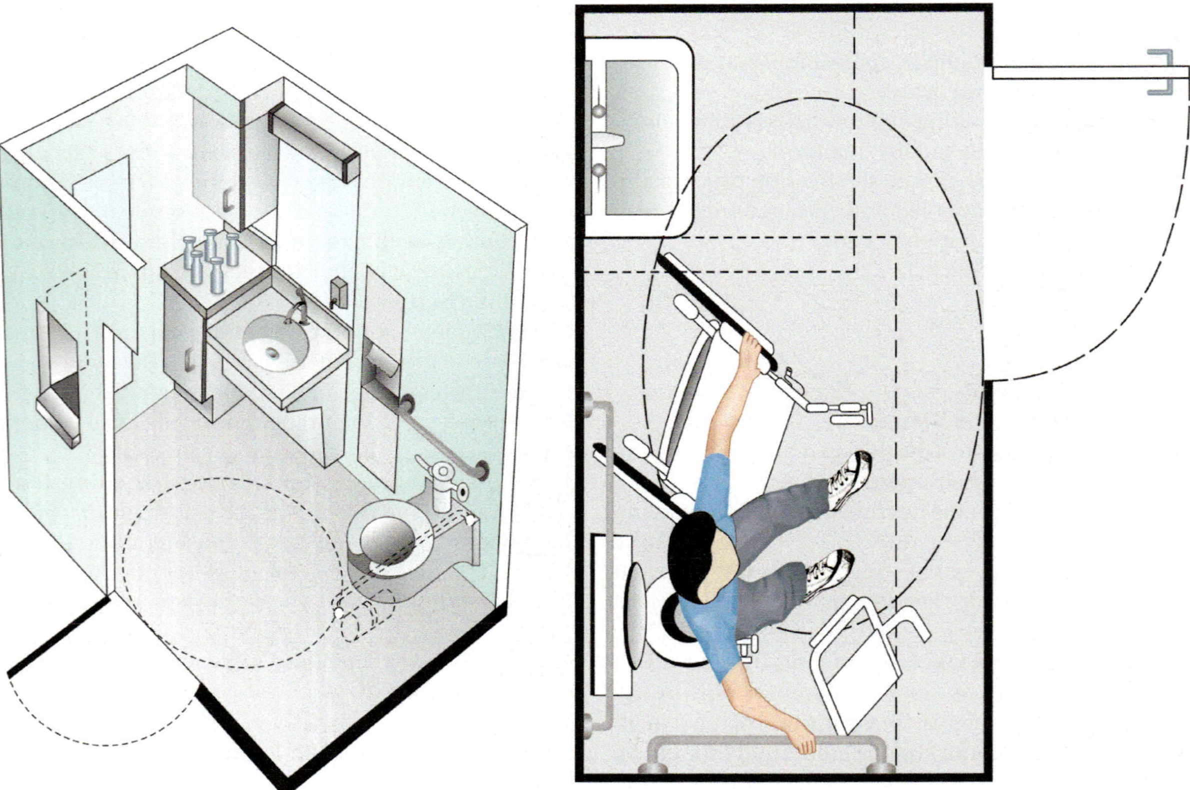

Fig. 3: Toilets should allow wheelchair movements.

beds, the size of each room, and the number of beds in each section will be based on the number of the patients, the type of the patient, the accompanying family members, need for privacy, and space for keeping assistive appliances within accessible limits, will form the design considerations of the inpatient wing. About 100% accessible rooms and facility is to be designed for the inpatient wing.

Operation suite: An operation suite for corrective surgeries, arthroscopy, minimally invasive surgeries, and rehabilitation specific surgeries needs to be catered for. An integrated modular OT needs to be planned and incorporated.

Intensive care unit (Fig. 4): An appropriate unit with requisite ancillary facilities should be planned in the inpatient wing.

Diagnostic wing: The diagnostic wing of the Rehabilitation Center is primarily focusing on the imaging services, and it is to be considered that comprehensive care for rehabilitation would require the full complement of the diagnostic facility.

Radiology: Imaging services has a major role to play in the rehabilitation center and the provision of and X-ray facility, a computed tomography (CT) scan, magnetic resonance imaging (MRI), bone densitometry need to be considered. A standalone dedicated facility for the rehabilitation center is fraught with the chance of underutilization and therefore, outsourcing of the facility might be considered. It is emphasized that the special nature of the patient visiting the rehabilitation center necessitates that the planning of such facility include barrier free and universal design principles.

Specialized investigations: Rooms for special investigations should be planned in a manner to incorporate special equipment, and the special needs of the patients attending this facility.

Support services: The need and the schedule for the under mentioned services should be considered during the planning phase and may be outsourced without compromising on the core competencies of the center depending on the scale of the establishment.

Kitchen: The kitchen services should be planned as per the specific requirements of the needs of the patients, daily store unloading access, stores of various natures including refrigeration, the work area to be impervious and easily cleanable, the need for heating appliances and water requirements for cooking and cleaning.

Cafeteria: A common cafeteria at the waiting hall catering for patient and staff should be planned and incorporated in the planning phase. The space requirements and the furniture and fixtures should be designed for the use of the disabled population visiting the center.

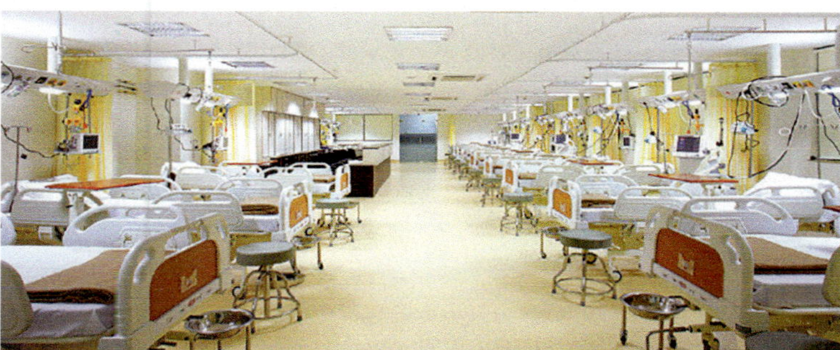

Fig. 4: Intensive care unit.

Laundry: The laundry for the center need to be planned and should cater for the load of the center in terms of the wash load from inpatient, OT, outpatient, rehabilitation and gymnasium.

Manifold: To cater for the surgeries primarily, a manifold need to be planned.

Communications, networking and IT: Special attention to the ergonomic design for use by the physically should be considered. The under mentioned components of the communications system need special attention at the planning stage.

- Telephones
- Public address system paging
- Mobile phones
- Television and entertainment system.

Security: Security of the facility should be comprehensively covered after the analysis of risk and the need of the special category of the patients in the facility. The following facets should be considered:

- *Infrastructure:* Including the perimeter wall, barriers, check post, observation posts and lighting.
- *Technology:* To include the webcam surveillance, network and access control.
- *Fire safety:* It should be considered comprehensively to include fire detection, alarm and evacuation systems.
- Administration and control areas should be catered for.

Housekeeping and biomedical waste management: It is preferable to incorporate the requirements of in-house/outsourcing at the planning stage.

REHABILITATION DEPARTMENT

- Prosthetics and orthotics department, scheme (Figs. 5 to 18)
- Physical therapy department scheme (Fig. 6)
- Physical therapy wing scheme (Fig. 7).

The rehabilitation wing forms the main focus of the center where the patient is expected to spend considerable time. The following modalities of physical therapy need to be provided for in the center for comprehensive care.

Hydrotherapy (Fig. 8): Involves the use of water in the physical therapy of disabled person. The equipment used includes:

- Whirlpools
- Jacuzzi
- Hubbard's Tank
- Pools of various sizes
- Cryotherapy.

Keeping in view the requirement of water and equipment specifically using water in controlled temperature, the design consideration should include nonslippery floor surface, easily cleanable surfaces; consideration for the electric power requirements should be catered for.

Heat and cold therapy: The use of various equipment to deliver temperature to various body parts as part of therapy. The equipment includes:

- Wax bath (Fig. 9)
- Moist heat therapy units (Fig. 10)
- Heat and cold packs (Fig. 11)
- Contrast bath (Fig. 12)
- Infrared light (Fig. 13)

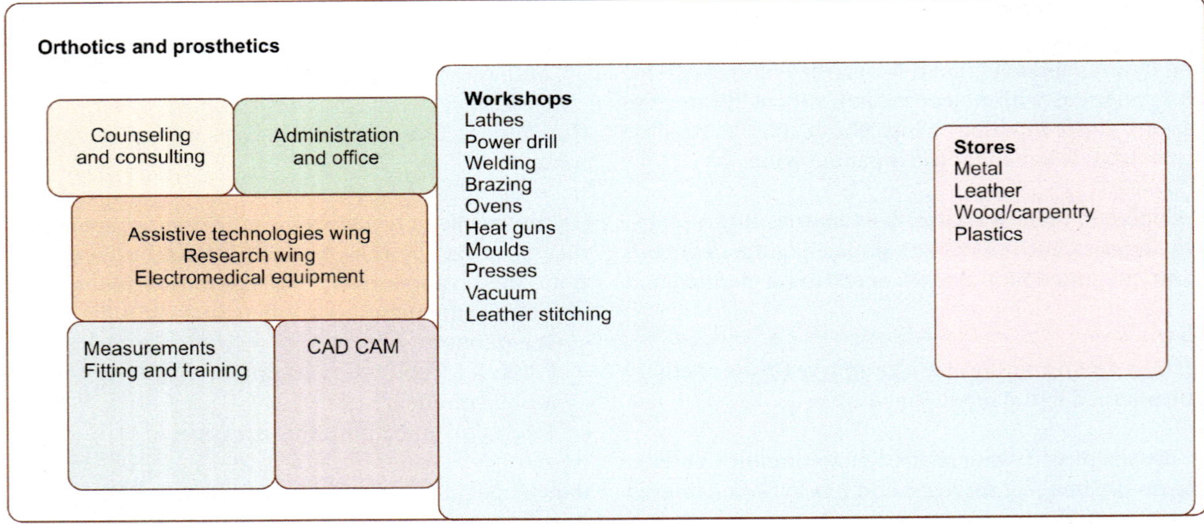

Fig. 5: Orthotics and prosthetics departments.

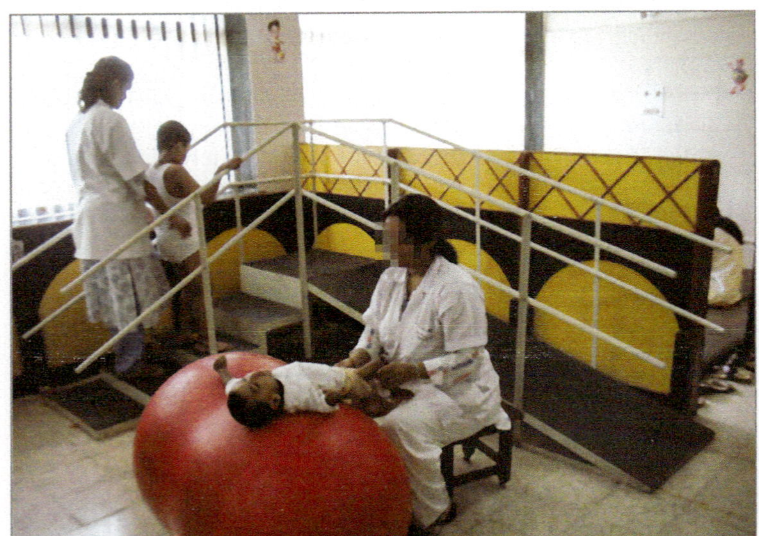

Fig. 6: Physical therapy department.

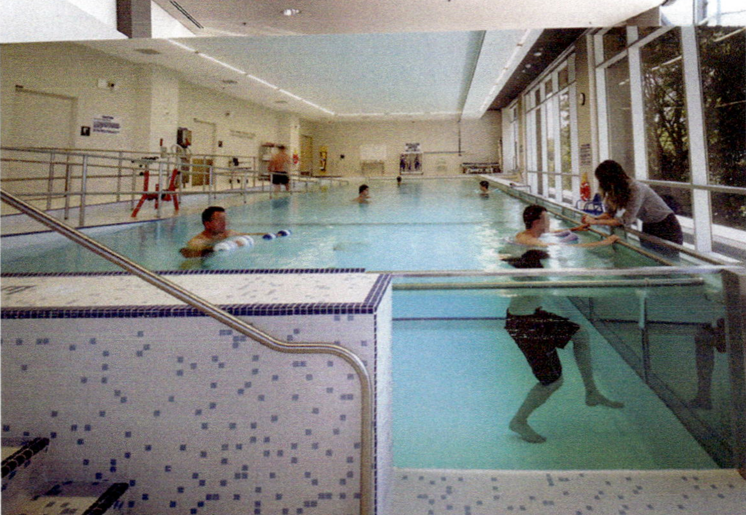

Fig. 8: Hydrotherapy.

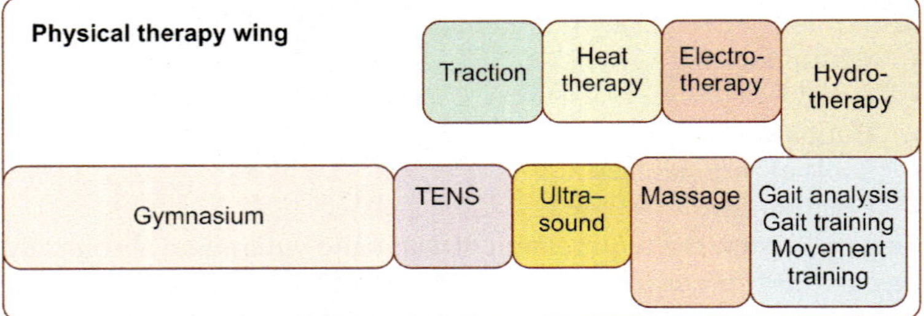

Fig. 7: Physical therapy wing.

- Ultraviolet lamp (Fig. 14)
- Short wave diathermy machines (Fig. 15).

Other equipment includes:

- Muscle stimulators (Fig. 16)
- Interferential therapy unit
- Ultrasound therapy unit

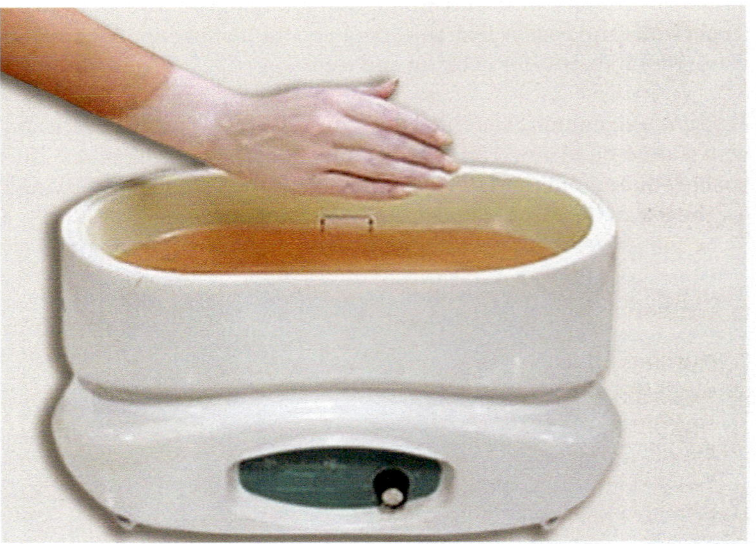

Fig. 9: Wax bath.

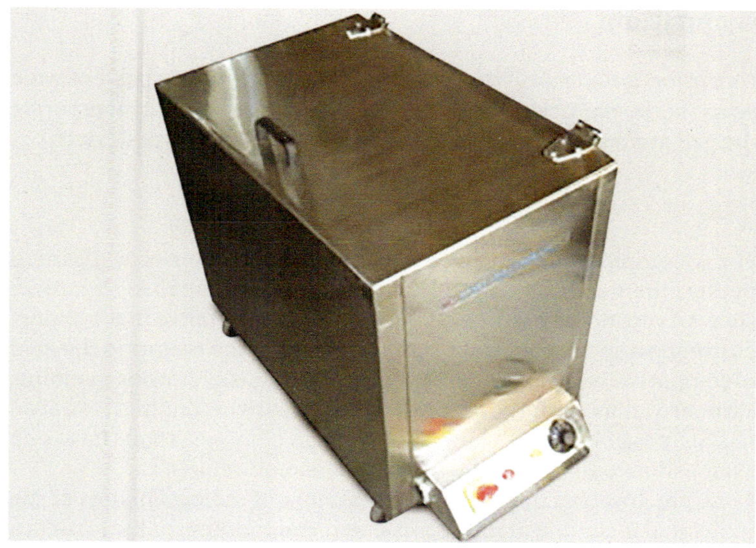

Fig. 10: Moist heat therapy units.

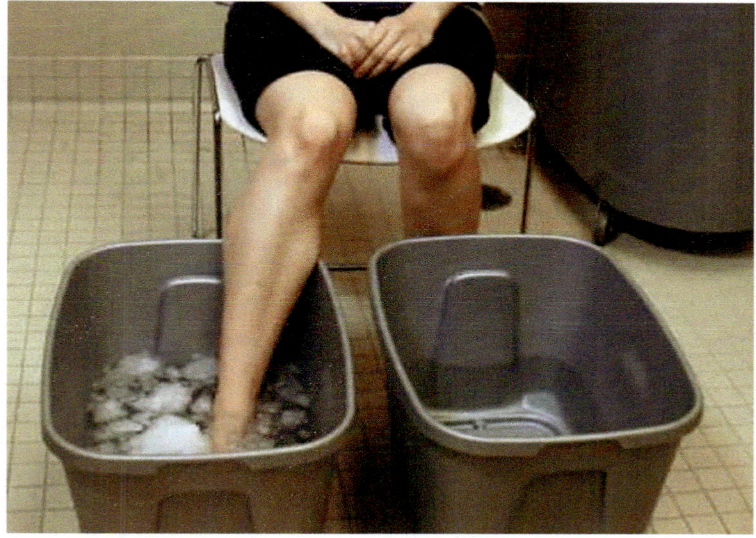

Fig. 11: Heat and cold packs.

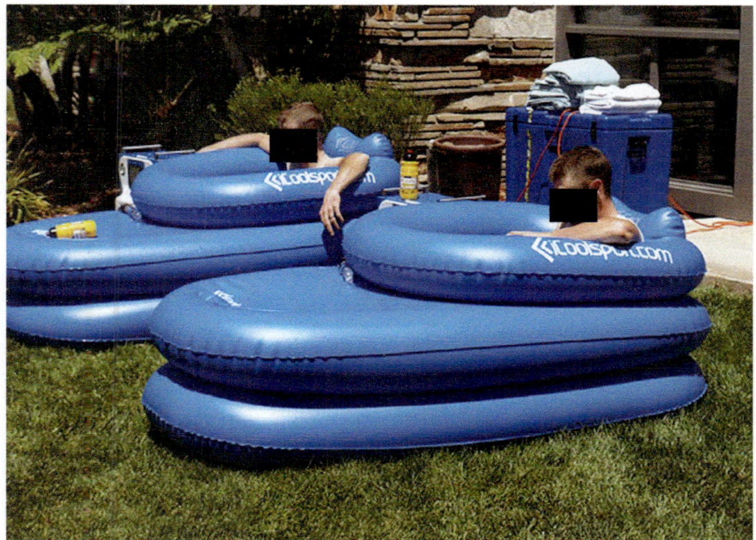

Fig. 12: Contrast bath.

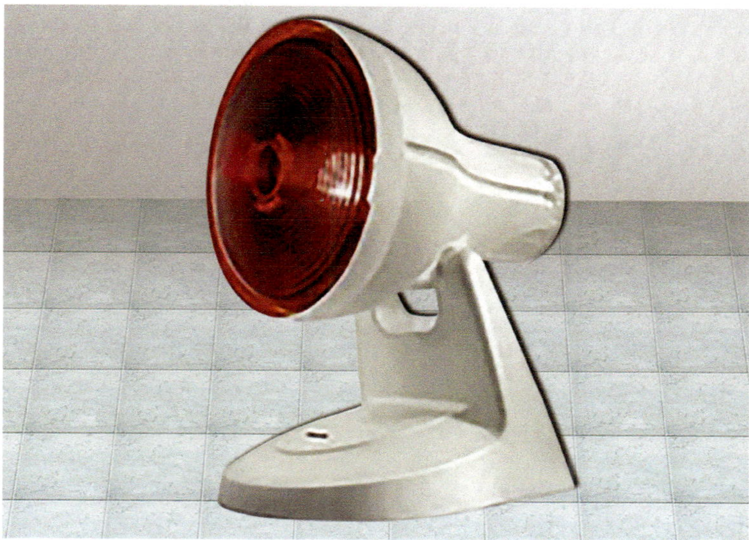

Fig. 13: Infrared light.

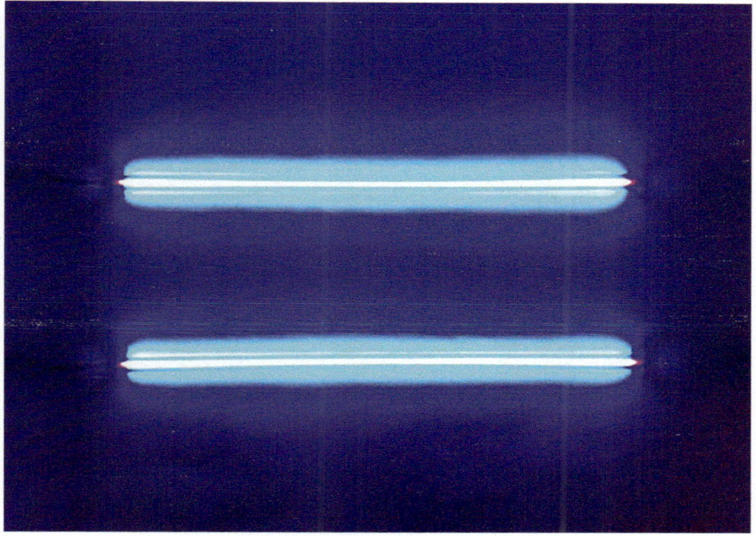

Fig. 14: Ultraviolet lamp.

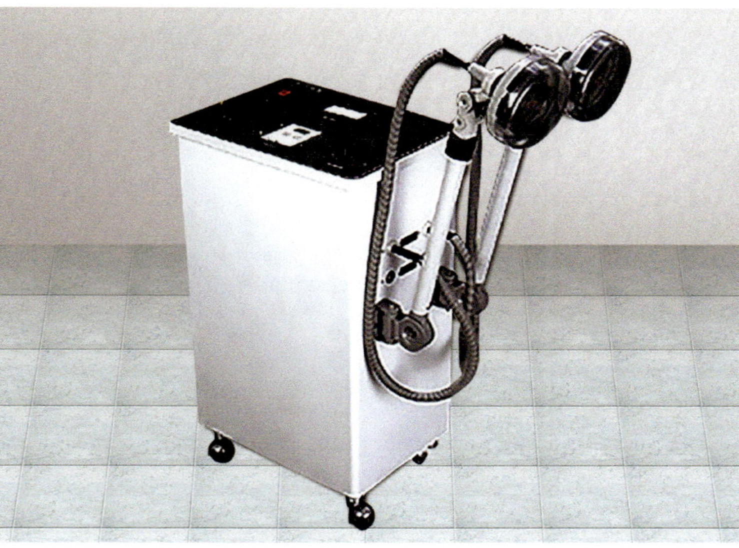

Fig. 15: Short wave diathermy machines.

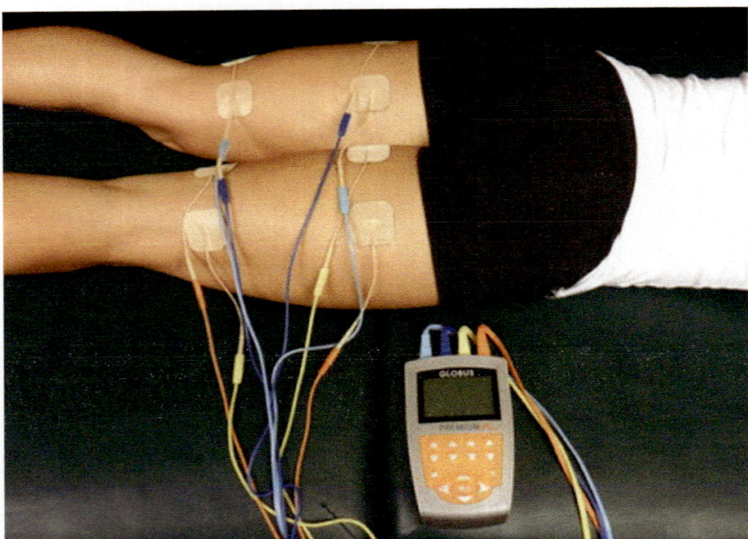

Fig. 16: Muscle stimulators.

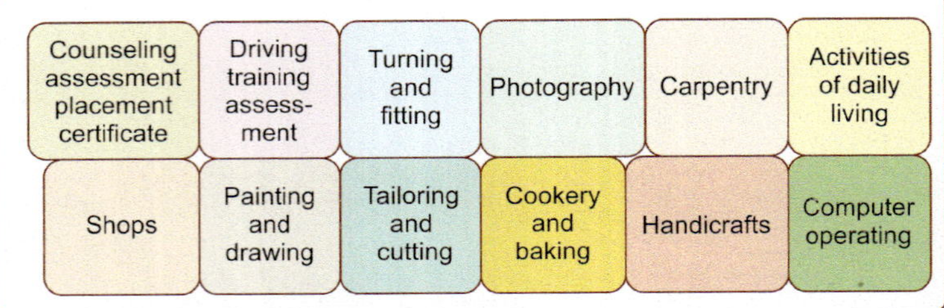

Fig. 17: Vocational training center.

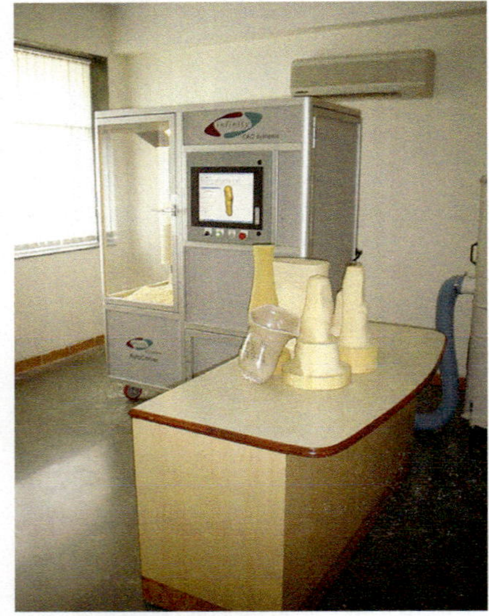

Fig. 18: Orthotics camera (CAD CAM).

- Transcutaneous nerve stimulator
- Iontophoresis.

Massage forms an important aspect of the therapy and the massage room with adequate privacy and appropriate tables need to be catered for.

Traction: The traction, otherwise known as "spinal decompression therapy", addresses the functional and mechanical aspects of discogenic pain and has been used by physiotherapists for years (Fig. 17).[5]

Gymnasium

Gait training and movement training: Gait training encompasses a wide scope of the physical rehabilitation program. This would incorporate the gait analysis, exercises and gait training with assistive devices.

VOCATIONAL TRAINING DEPARTMENT

For a complete and comprehensive rehabilitation of a disabled person the need for vocational training is inescapable. Figure 19 shows a vocational training department. It is imperative that training, customized and special training be imparted to the visitors in the field of computers, handicrafts, tailoring, dietetics, music, drawing/painting, carpentry, photography, turning and fitting, driver training. However, it is not possible for the complete spectrum of the vocations be at one establishment in view of the innumerable requirements.

A pre-vocation training and assessment of the capabilities of the individual including driving assessment and training for the same is a necessity.

Activities of daily living: There are two groups of daily living activities. These are referred to as the activities of daily living (ADL) and the instrumental ADL. The ADL are basic, routine tasks, such as bathing, dressing, eating and using the toilet, which most people are able to perform on a daily basis without assistance.[6]

There should be facilities that measure ADL for individuals and facilities should also have programs that teach and mentor individuals who are losing the ability to perform ADL. There are also devices and gadgets that are built to help people perform ADL. Some of these devices include: wheelchairs, walking sticks, long-handled brushes, special cups and bowls, bath seats, reachers to help with dressing, etc.

A counseling/testing/guidance cell/placement cell would add value to the establishment and must be incorporated in the planning stage.

The concept of combination of vertical and horizontal layout of the facility should be contemplated. This allows for more flexibility and expansion at a later date. This design concept will also be exemplary of universal design principles.

The universal design concept should be applied not only for the ease of the visitors but to serve as an exemplary model for others to emulate and apply in everyday living.

The schedule of accomodation for the center is depicted in Table 1.

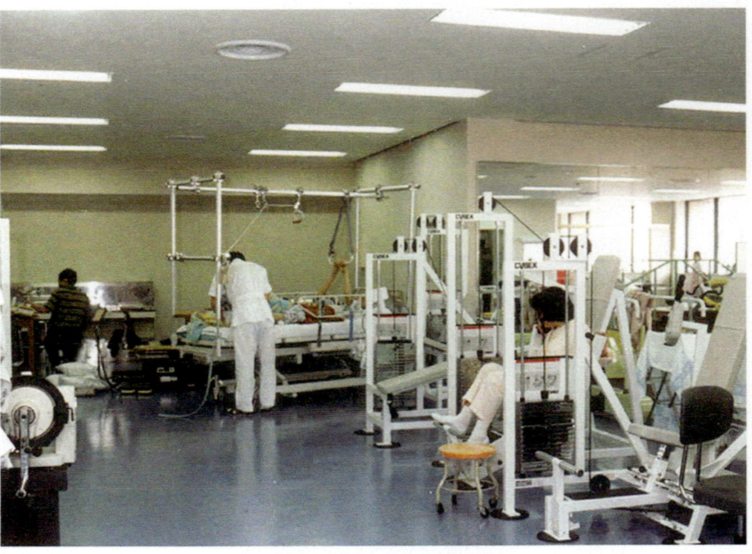

Fig. 19: Physiotherapy.

Table 1: Schedule of accommodation.

Room/Space	*Area in sqm*
Common parameters	
Toilets	5
Bathroom cum toilet	15
Outpatient department	
Reception	10
Waiting area	50
Consultation room	12
Examination room	12
Treatment room	15
Staff room	15
Store room	8
Meeting room	16
Inpatient area	
Bed area	7
Intensive case unit (ICU) bed area	20
Single bedroom	12
Multi-bedroom	50
Operation theater (integrated)	54
Diagnostic	
Reception	15
Collection center	12
Hematology	30
Microbiology	30
Biochemistry	30
Radioimaging	200
Special diagnostics	80
Support services	
Laundry	*
Kitchen	*
Central sterile supply department (CSSD)	*
Communication	*
Security	*
Workshops	
Reception	10
Measurement and fitting	15
Store	60
Administrative/staff area	20
Workshop	75
CAD-CAM	15
Physical therapy department	
Reception	10
Heat therapy	15
Hydrotherapy	60[@]
Traction	15
Ultrasound	15
Gymnasium	300
Playfields/recreation	100
Movement training	100
Activities of daily living	100
Vocational training	
Reception, administration	25
Placement cell, counseling room	15
Workshops, each	25[$]
Simulator, driving	15

Cont'd...

Cont'd...

*Should be demand based, outsourcing to be considered keeping the financial implications.
[@]Swimming pool is an option to be considered.
[$]Depending on the scope and type.

CONCLUSION

The concepts and technology for assisting the disabled are evolving. The planning and design needs to be inclusive comprehensive, futuristic aimed to facilitate a holistic rehabilitative program. Community integrated and targeted policies and practices for the rehabilitation of the disabled must be considered. A sample line plan drawing is shown in Figure 20.

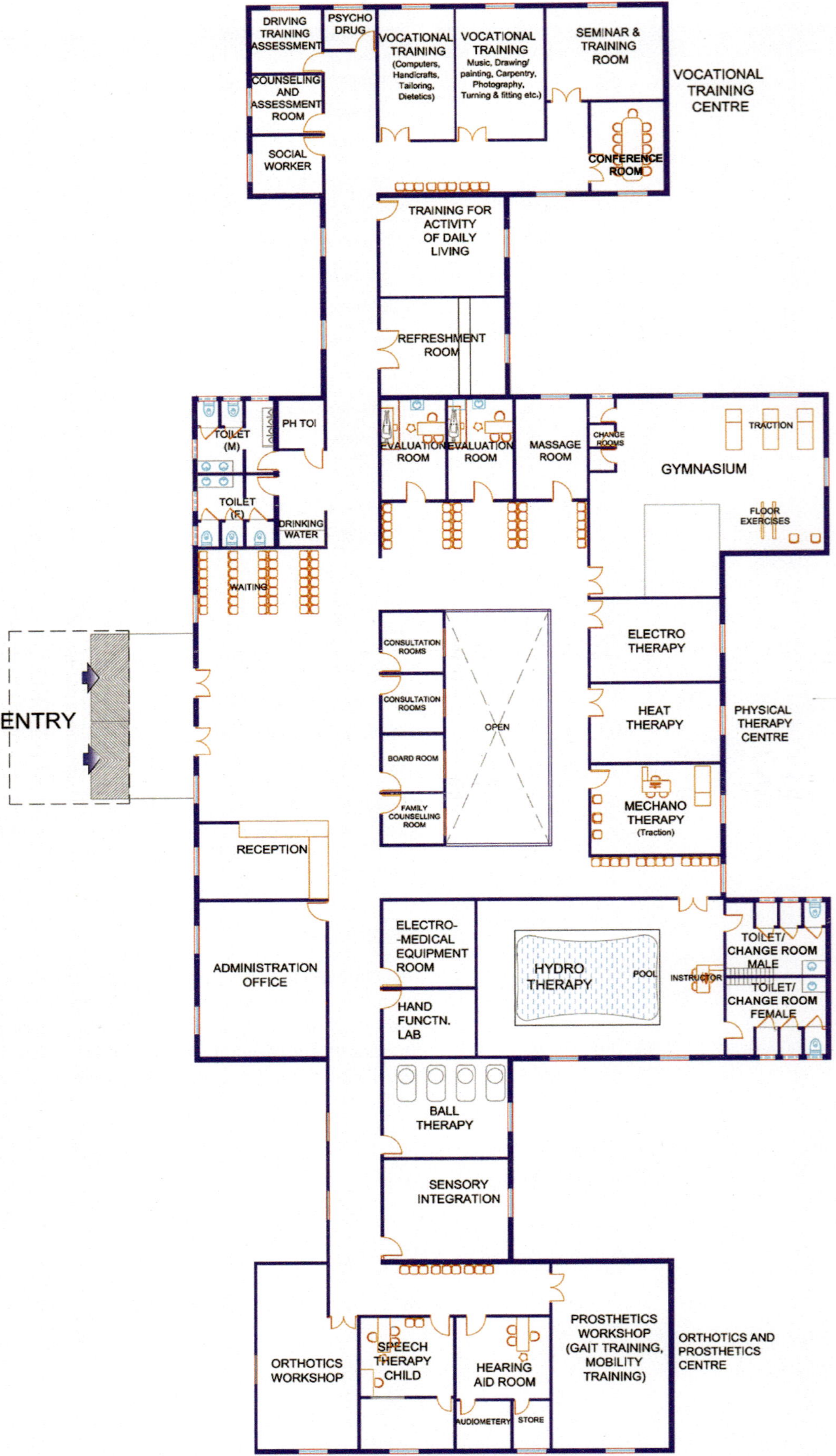

Fig. 20: Plan for rehab centre for locomotor disability.

REFERENCES

1. www.addc.org.au
2. ushik.ahrq.gov
3. www.fpg.unc.edu
4. http://disabilityaffairs.gov.in/
5. www.orthoneurospine.com
6. purehomecareservices.com

OTHER REFERENCES

- Gupta S, Kant S, Chandrashekhar R. Modern trends in planning and designing of hospitals. Jaypee Publishers Delhi 2007.
- World Health Organization. World report on disability, 2011.
- World Health Organization. Disability and Rehabilitation WHO Action Plan 2006–2011. 2011;1–7.
- Department of Veterans Affairs. Barrier free design guide. 2011.
- Ministry of Social Justice and Empowerment. National Policy for Persons with Disabilities.
- The World Bank. People with disabilities in India: from commitments to outcomes. 2007.
- United Spinal Association. Fire safety for wheelchair users at work and at home: safety manual.
- Department of Veterans Affairs. Polytrauma rehabilitation center, 2008.
- CPWD. Guidelines and space standards for barrier freebuilt environment for the disabled and elderly persons, 1998.
- Malkin J. Medical and dental space planning: a comprehensive guide to design, equipment, and clinical procedures, 3rd edn, 2002.
- Ministry of Social Justice and Empowerment. The rights of persons with disabilities bill, 2011.

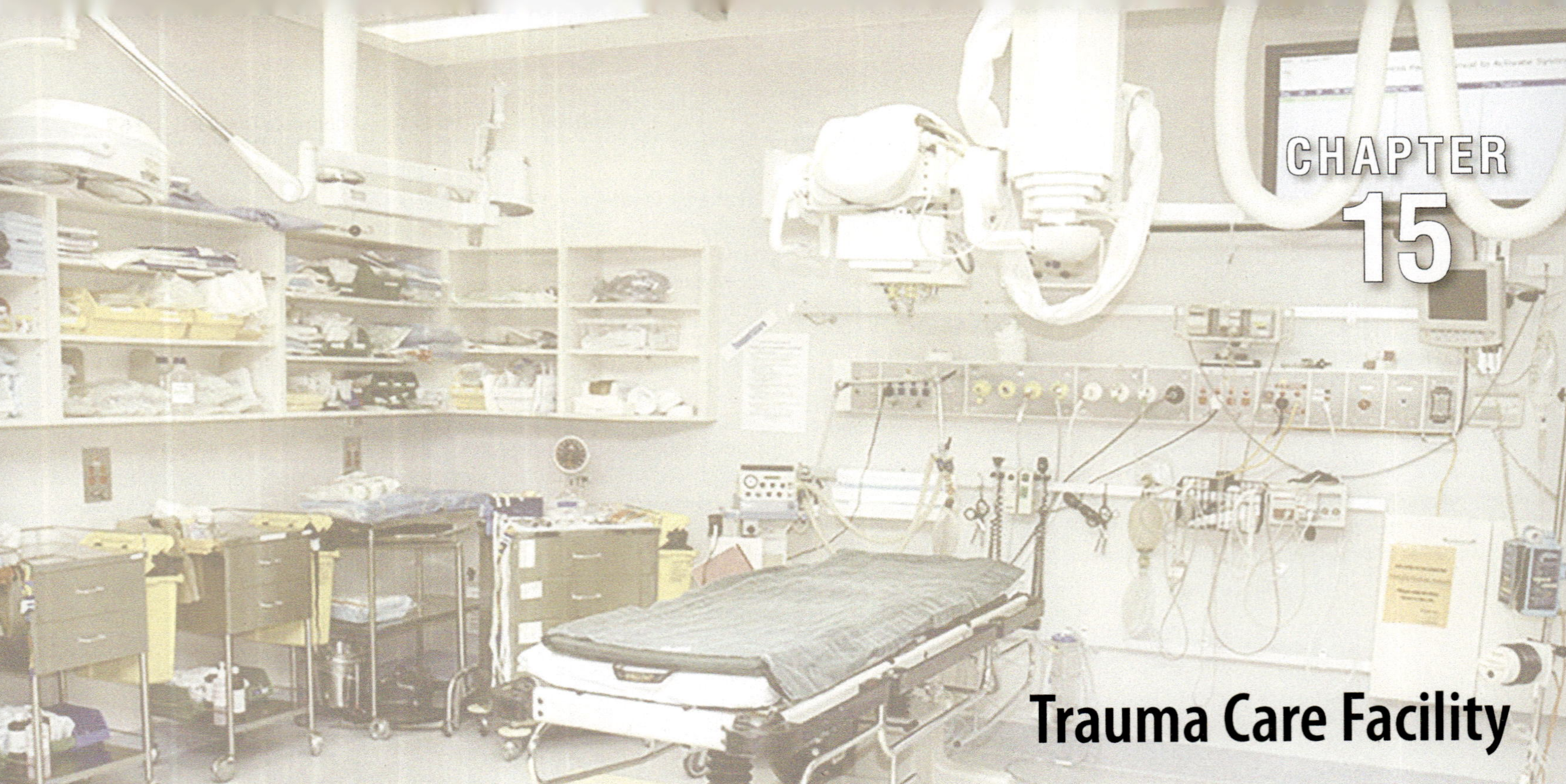

CHAPTER 15

Trauma Care Facility

Angel Rajan Singh, IB Singh, Shakti Kumar Gupta, Sunil Kant, R Chandrashekhar

INTRODUCTION

A *Trauma Care Facility* often referred to as *'Trauma Center'* is a healthcare institution that has the resources and capabilities necessary to provide trauma services at a particular level to injured patients.[1] Trauma center designation criteria set strict requirements for staffing, specialist availability, response times, training, quality improvement and community education. This facility verification and designation is an important foundation for the success of an inclusive trauma system.[2]

American College of Surgeons Committee on Trauma (ACSCOT) has classified trauma care facilities into four levels.[1,2]

Level I

- Usually serves as the lead institution in a trauma system.
- Manages a large number of severely injured patients with 24-hour availability of in-house surgeon and all related superspecialties like emergency medicine, general surgery, orthopedics, neurosurgery, cardiothoracic surgery, vascular surgery, etc.
- Provides community leadership in trauma research, education, and prevention.
- Admits >1,200 patients or 240 severely injured patients annually.

Level II

- Supplements the function of a Level I center in population-dense areas.
- Serves as the lead trauma facility in less population-dense areas.
- Provides full range of trauma care with 24-hour availability of in-house surgeon; superspecialties are available on call within 30 minutes.
- Coordinates outreach programs to incorporate smaller regional institutions.

Level III

- Capable of initial patient management.
- Surgeons must respond promptly and transfer agreements should be in place to facilitate transfers to Level I or Level II centers.
- Provides injury prevention, outreach activities, and education programs for nurses, physicians, and allied healthcare workers.

Level IV

- Located in a rural environment.
- Supplements care within a larger trauma system.
- Requires 24-hour coverage by a physician.
- Most patients require transfer to a higher level trauma center.

PLANNING PREMISES AND DESIGN CONSIDERATIONS

A trauma care facility can be a specialized area within a hospital building, a separate building adjunct to an existing hospital or a standalone facility self sufficient in all aspects. The core areas in all these three types remain consistently the same as detailed below, the difference being primarily in the scope of support facilities that needs to be planned for. A workflow diagram in this facility is shown in Figure 1 and line plans in Figures 2 and 3.[2]

CORE AREAS IN A TRAUMA CARE FACILITY

Patient Access[2]

- Ambulance entrance
- Walking entrance
- Decontamination area
- Helipad access.

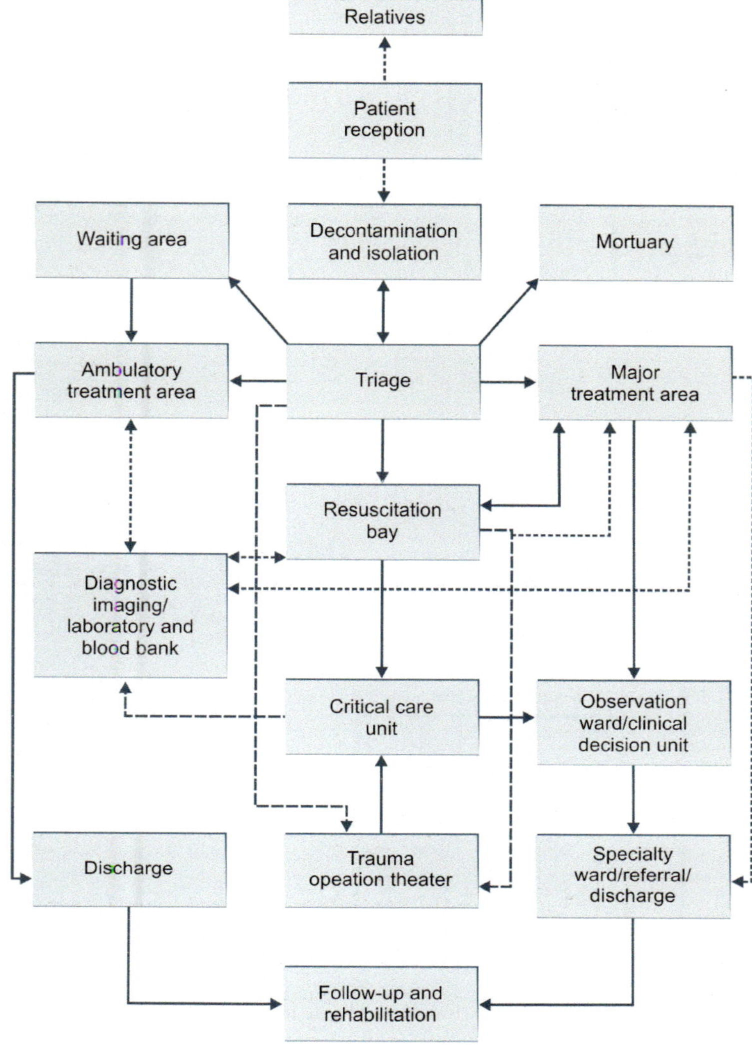

Fig. 1: Workflow in a trauma care facility.

Patient Care Areas[2]

- Triage and reception area
- Resuscitation area
- Treatment area
- Ambulatory care area
- Waiting area
- Observation ward/clinical decision unit
- Isolation rooms.

SUPPORT FACILITIES

Clinical Support Services[2]

- Laboratory services
- Radiology
- Blood bank
- Pharmacy
- Communications
- Central sterile supply department (CSSD)
- Manifold
- Security
- Mass casualty incident/disaster stores.

Facilities for Patients Relatives[2]

- Waiting area
- Communication room
- Toilets
- Prayer room
- Refreshment area.

Staff Facilities[2]

- Staff changing rooms
- Staff shower and toilets
- Staff dining area.

Office Accommodation[2]

- Administrative support
- Multi-person offices
- Individual offices.

Education and Training Facilities[2]

- Seminar room
- Library/computer access
- Storage area.

GUIDING PRINCIPLES

Important characteristics of a trauma care facility which influence the planning and designing process are as follows:

- High levels of activity
- High patient turnover
- Large multidisciplinary workforce
- Infection control requirements
- Access issues
- Interface with prehospital services
- Multiple interactions with in-hospital specialties/transfers
- Communications issues
- Major incident capacity
- Possibility of aggression/assault—security issues.

LOCATION[3]

The difference between life and death for severely injured people often depends upon the amount of time it takes to get them to a trauma center. The siting of trauma centers, however, is more complex than just maps of land area coverage showing ringed bands around each hospital. The speed and location of helicopters and ambulances, the number and location of trauma centers in a region, and the spatial relationships between these resources need to be considered.

Researchers from the University of Pennsylvania and Johns Hopkins University have developed the Web-based Trauma Resource Allocation Model for Ambulances and Hospitals (TRAMAH), a mathematical optimization model that uses population and access to existing trauma centers based on geographic relationships to ambulances and helicopters to simulate the effects of newly-sited trauma centers.

A similar model based on Indian variables could be used to decide on the geographic location of a trauma center in a specific area.

Further when a trauma center is built within an existing hospital premises, it should be located adjacent to the existing emergency department with common entry, registration point and triage areas.[2]

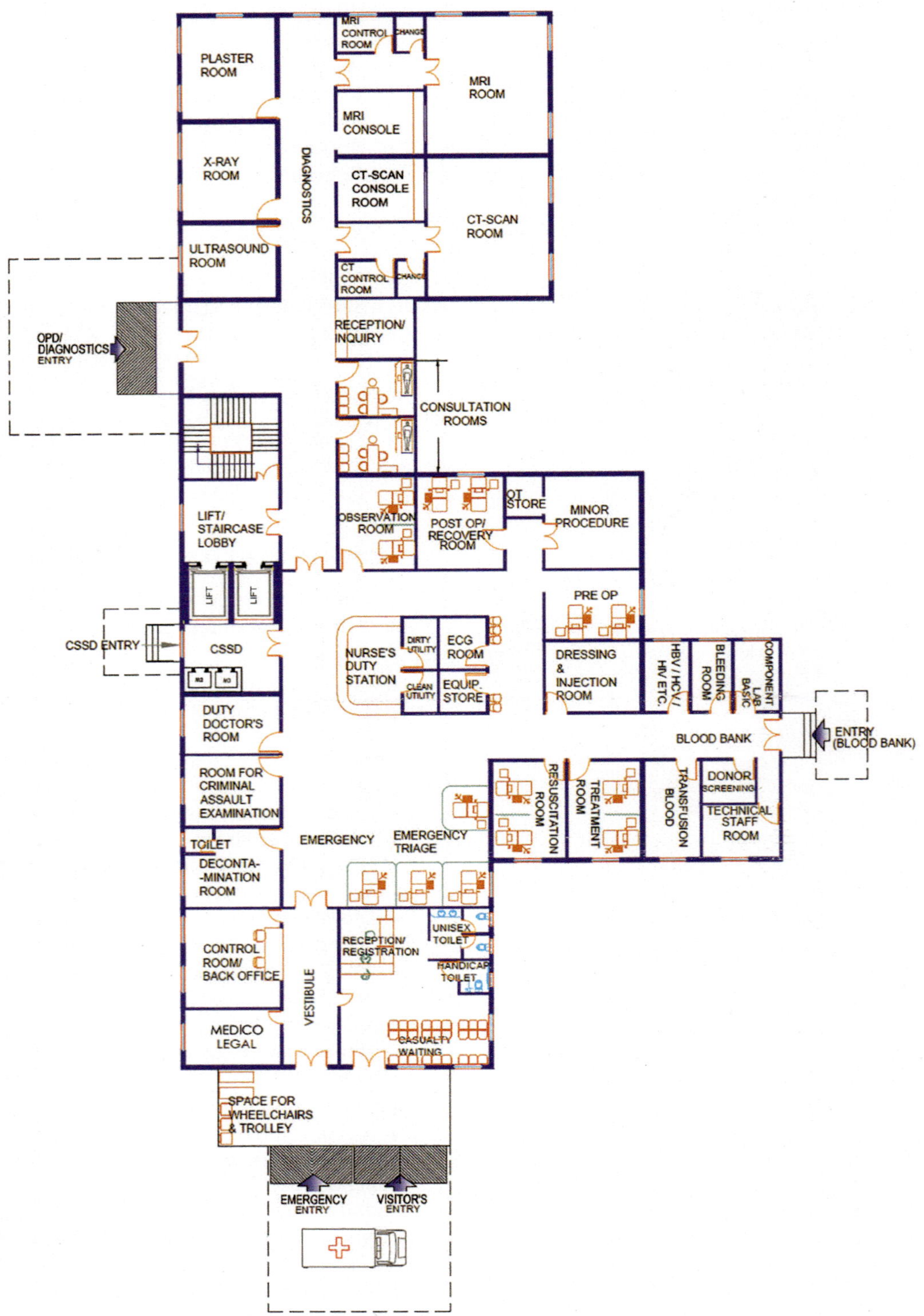

Fig. 2: Ground floor plan.

This will allow patients whose needs are best met in an area other than the trauma care facility to be redirected, depending on their clinical condition and local operational policies.

Conjoint triage ensures that patients who require resuscitation have the quickest route to the care they need, rather than being subsequently redirected from another access point or clinical area.[2]

This also enables provision of two *key connectivities* between the two facilities, namely the sterile connectivity and diagnostic connectivity.[2]

Sterile connectivity: It is a sterile corridor between the operating rooms (ORs) situated on the same floor in the two buildings. This helps the operating rooms staff and surgeons to travel between both ORs seamlessly.[2]

Diagnostic connectivity: This represents a corridor between two buildings at the level of laboratory and radiological services; which helps in sharing the diagnostic facilities between both facilities thereby enabling optimal utilization of the resources.[2]

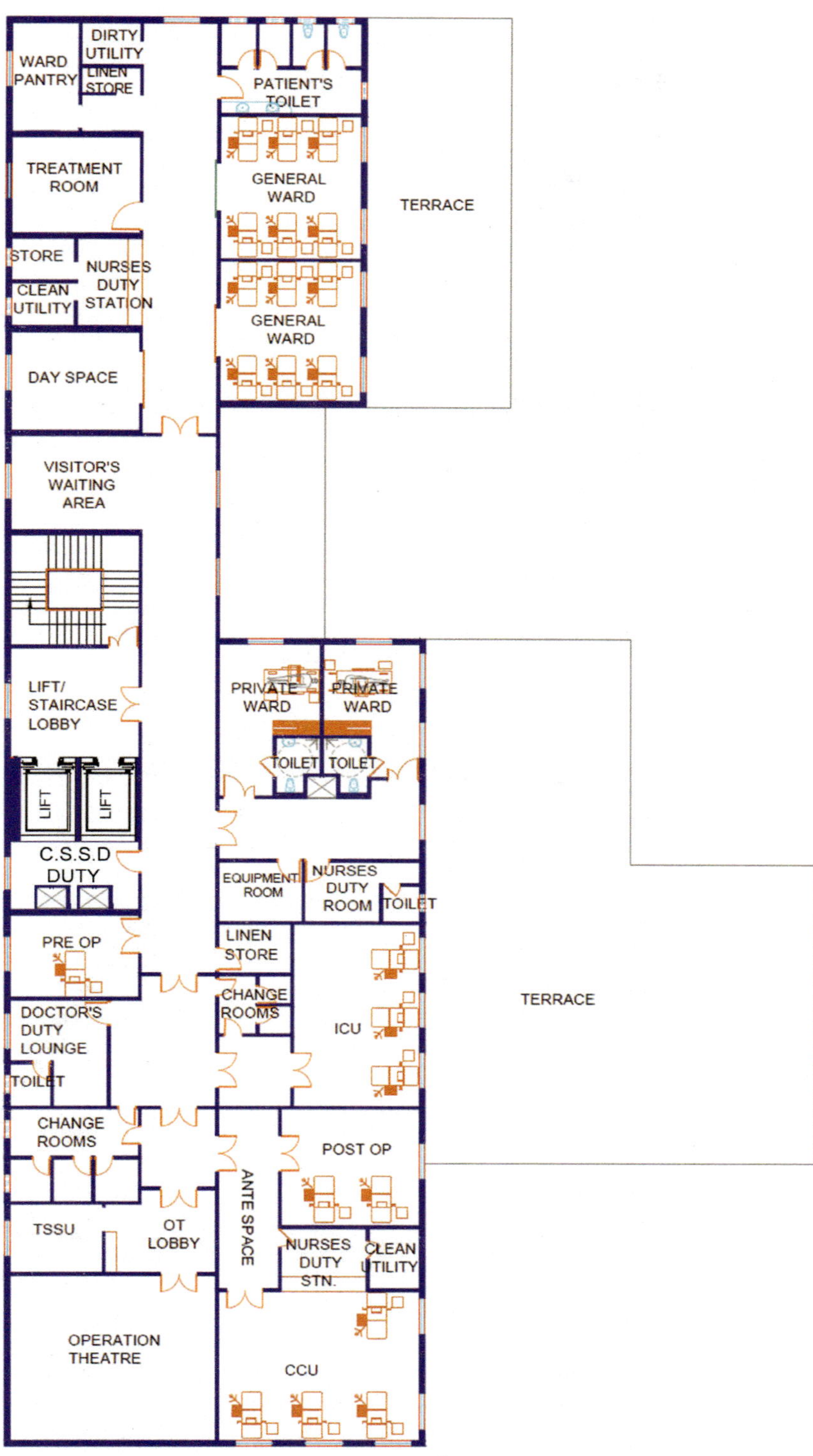

Fig. 3: First floor.

FACILITY ACCESS

There should be separate entrances to the trauma care facility for walking and ambulance patients. These entrances must never be used as general entrances to the hospital or as thorough fares for staff and other patients moving within the hospital, as this has a detrimental effect on patient care and privacy and potentially compromises patient and staff safety.[4]

There should be provision of adequate parking commensurate with the facility's requirements. Provision of Valet parking for patients who directly drive in should preferably be made.

Ambulance Access (Fig. 4)

As trauma care facility will often cater to incidents in which multiple casualties are expected, appropriate provision for a number of

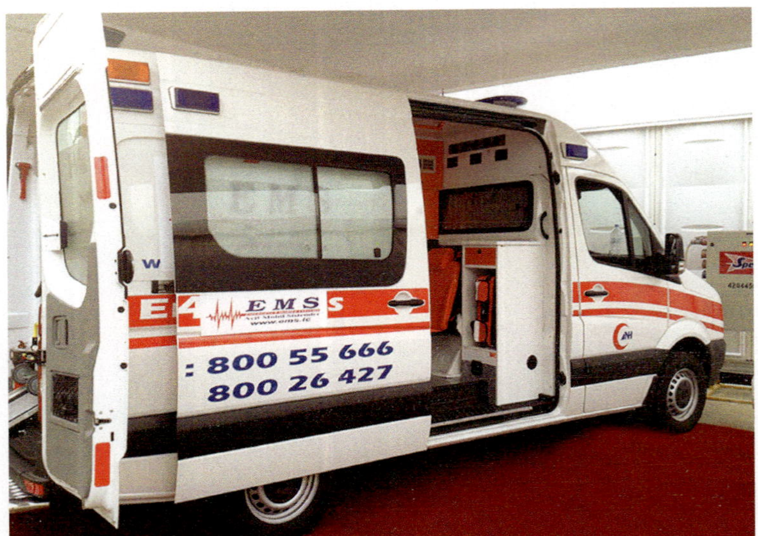

Fig. 4: Ambulance access.

ambulances to park close to the facility entrance and allow for safe patient disembarkation is required.[4]

The ambulance entrance should be close to the resuscitation room to minimize the interval between the ambulance and the resuscitation facilities. The route to arrive at a resuscitation bay should be direct and minimize the number of corners ambulance personnel have to push trolley-based patients around. It should also be private.[4]

There should be a canopy to keep patients dry while disembarking. The entrance should be well illuminated with an automated mechanism rapidly opening the outer door. Rapid access by emergency personnel must be achieved without compromising department security.[4]

The ambulance access area should be designed in conjunction with the ambulance service and facilitate appropriate turning circles, etc. Considerations will include ambulance design and engineering issues, requirements for the urgent and discrete cleaning of ambulances; major incident planning and facilities for storage of trolleys, wheelchairs and stretchers. Security personnel must be deployed on a 24/7 basis to ensure that all access routes remain clear.[4]

A route to segregate relatives arriving with ambulance patients to register patients or to be directed to an appropriate waiting area should be planned. Security personnel should control this area to maintain a car-free ambulance bay.[4]

Helipad Access

There are three principal options for siting a helipad:[3,5,6]

- At ground level
- On a rooftop
- On a low structure or mound near to the facility.

All options require airways clear of obstacles, such as trees and buildings, which helicopters will use when approaching and departing, as well as a clear space for the helipad and its immediate surrounds. These criteria can be difficult to achieve, particularly at ground level in congested areas and on small hospital estates, and may compromise a hospital's future development plans.[5-7]

Helipads built on rooftops (ideally above the facility to ensure a short transit for the patient) are the most effective from the aviation and strategic planning perspectives: they largely remove any constraints on future building plans, they provide the greatest choice of obstacle-free helicopter airways, and they reduce the environmental impact on the hospital and its neighbors.[3,5,6]

Ground-level helipads do not have these advantages but are cheaper to build and operate. The third option, building a helipad on a mound or low elevation structure above a car park or other occupied area, has some of the benefits on a roof-top site but costs less to construct and operate.[3,5,6]

Civil aviation guidelines regarding requirements for heliports laid down by Director General of Civil Aviation (DGCA), India cover all aspects of heliport planning, infrastructure including taxiways, aprons, markings, aeronautical lightings, emergency services, maintenance standards, physical characteristics, obstacle limitation surfaces to be provided for, etc. and should be diligently followed at the initial planning stage itself.

DECONTAMINATION AREA

Decontamination facilities may involve use of external facilities, such as inflatable units, or internal decontamination may be an option. Water drainage and ventilation of this area requires specific engineering specification and will need to be separate from the main hospital systems.

PATIENT CARE AREAS

Triage and Reception Area[2,4]

Triage is the sorting of patients for prioritization according to clinical acuity. Triage may occur before or instantaneously upon patient arrival (prehospital notification), within minutes of arrival, at the bedside or in a designated area. The triage/assessment area may include a designated area for ambulance patients and an area for ambulant patients. Patient movement between triage/assessment and the following areas should be considered—reception, waiting area, resuscitation, treatment and ambulatory care, patient toilets and diagnostic imaging.

Each triage/assessment cubicle should have the following:

- Service/examination panel
- Examination light
- Desk
- Chair on wheels
- Patient chair
- Trolley
- Computer console with nearby printer access
- Equipment for physiological measurement (e.g. to check vital signs, oxygen saturation, temperature, near-patient blood sugar testing), examination equipment, etc.
- Sharps containers
- Foot stool
- Waste bins
- Handwashing facilities
- Storage for wound dressings, etc.
- Access to paper-based documentation, if used.

Each *triage/assessment space* should be of not less than 16 sqm in size and should be trolley and wheelchair accessible. The minimum *combined Reception and Triage area* must be 1.8 sqm/1000 patient attendances per annum. There should be a minimum allocation of one triage/assessment cubicle per 10,000 annual attendances.[2,7,8]

The IT developments [e.g. faxing of electrocardiographs (ECGs), shared hospital and prehospital IT systems] may determine the need for additional space for prehospital services within the triage-cum-reception area.

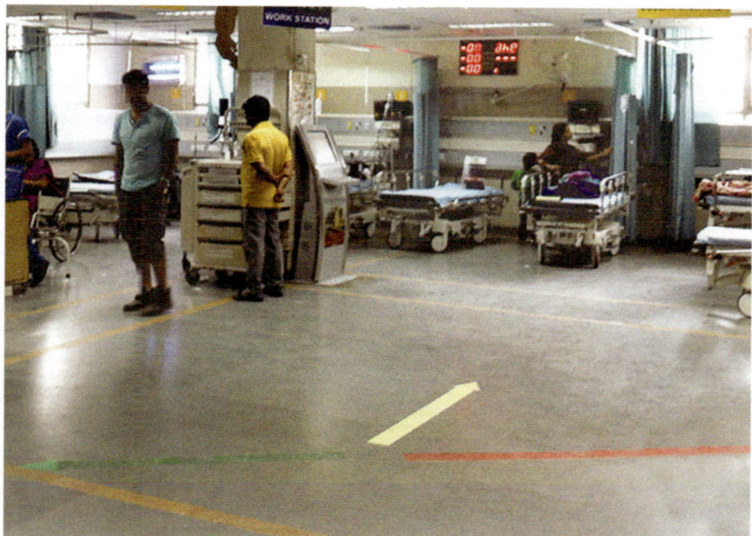

Fig. 5: Trauma resuscitation area.

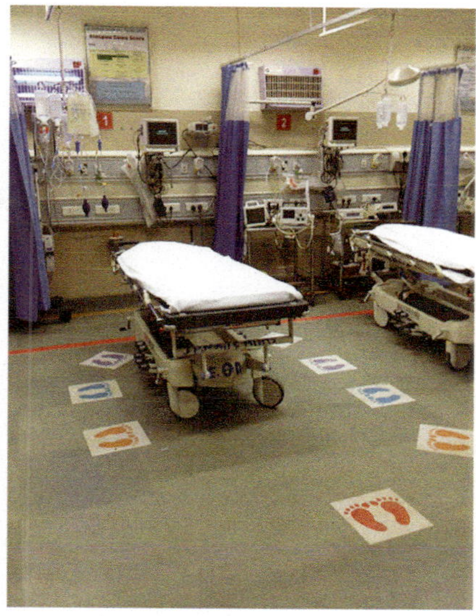

Fig. 6: Resuscitation trolley.

Trauma Resuscitation Area (Red Area) (Fig. 5)

The size of the trauma resuscitation area largely depends on the volume and acuity of trauma managed by the facility.[6]

Whenever possible, the trauma resuscitation area should be adjacent but physically separate from the remaining facility. Distinct entrances and exits for the trauma patient from the remainder of the facility are considered ideal. Access to nonmedical and any nonessential personnel should be limited. At the same time, convenient access to the radiology suite, operating room, and intensive care unit should be considered. If possible, a radiologic suite with access to plain radiography and computed tomography should be contiguous to or located close to the area.[6]

Radiation protection must be incorporated in the design including wall lining and staff and patient protection during portable X-ray. Sufficient room lighting and an overhead operating room light for each trauma stretcher are imperative and fixtures should not impede movement around the patient. To permit unimpeded circumferential access to the patient, monitoring equipment, suction, and gases should be mounted above the patient on fixed columns or movable overhead booms; the floors should be free of fixed hardware to avoid tripping. The ceiling mounts should be higher than the height of tall members.[2,9]

Trauma Resuscitation Area (Thumb Rules)[2,4,10]

For an average case-mix of 20,000 patients per year, a trauma center should have a minimum of two resuscitation bays with one additional bay per 10,000 patients per year.

There should be a minimum of 25 sqm per resuscitation bay excluding storage space. An additional one quarter to one third of this figure should be allowed for storage.

Each resuscitation area patient space must (Fig. 6):[4]

- Have sufficient space to ensure 360 degree access to the patient on an appropriate high specification resuscitation trolley.
- Have a high-specification patient trolley suitable for portable X-ray acquisition.
- Have full individual physiological monitoring, including ECG, NIBP, oxygen saturation, core temperature, invasive monitoring, end-tidal CO_2 monitoring, etc.
- Should have one ventilator for each resuscitation bay.
- Be fitted with three oxygen outlets.
- Be fitted with wall mounted suction.
- Have resuscitation equipment in each space for intubation, defibrillation with external pacing capabilities, cannulation, etc.
- Have an appropriate service panel with a minimum of 12 electrical sockets and four category 5 sockets.
- Have equipment or an overhead rail to hang IV fluids.
- Have handwashing facilities.
- Have a clock with timing facilities.
- Have an operating theater quality light.
- Includes a wall mounted ophthalmoscope/otoscope.
- Have overhead X-ray gantry or alternative immediately accessible imaging system.
- *Clinical waste facilities*: Sharps and clinical waste.
- A dedicated computer terminal with access to laboratory and diagnostic imaging results and the ability to request clinical investigations.

Within the resuscitation area, there should be access to:

- Resuscitation equipment sets for advanced airway management including surgical airway, emergency surgical procedures, urinary catheterization, central-line placement, etc.
- Two transport monitors for patient transfer to imaging and other clinical facilities.
- Two transport ventilators for patient transfer to imaging and other clinical facilities.
- Facilities for noninvasive ventilation.
- At least two twin diagnostic imaging monitors.
- A standard anesthetic machine.
- Medical air, nitrous oxide.
- Emergency ultrasound.
- Hands-free telephone.
- A locked cupboard for controlled drugs.
- Facilities for warming of resuscitation fluids.
- Equipment to warm patients and the ability to create an appropriately warm environment for the assessment of patients with major burns
- A rapid infusion device and other infusion pumps.
- Area for patient documentation/note-keeping/IT system access.
- Sterile procedure preparation area.
- Access to blood bank for urgent transfusion.

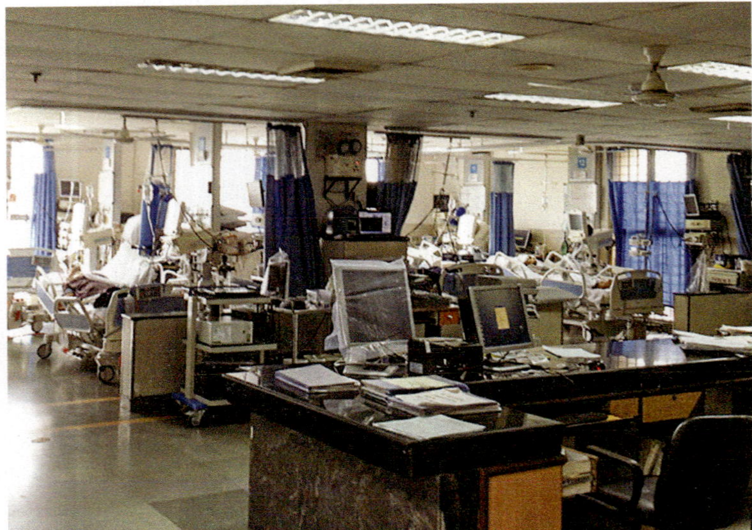

Fig. 7: Treatment areas.

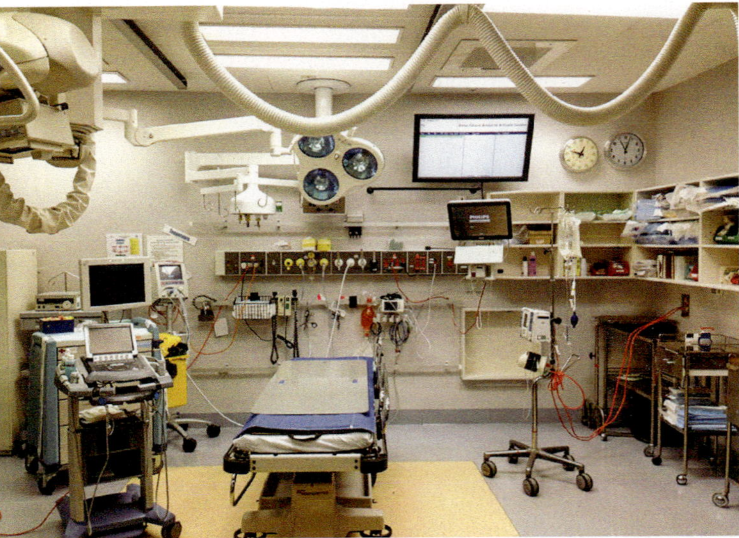

Fig. 8: Special function treatment rooms.

- Resuscitation equipment storage with re-charging capabilities
- Adequate worktop space for PCs, monitors, documentation, etc.

Combined Trauma Treatment and Imaging Room

The combined trauma imaging and treatment area is best viable in a multi-bay environment design and allows for the treatment and imaging of a minimum of four patients.

In a multi-bay environment, the individual spaces should be divided by half-length partition walls or mobile X-ray shielded lead screens. These walls/screens should be at least 2,500 mm high and 4,000 mm wide and should a high degree of construction radiation protection of approximately 2.5 mm of lead equivalent at energies of 150 kV. This level of protection will also allow the clinical trauma team to make use of mobile CT scanners which are fast catching up. Space should be left at the end of screens/walls to allow staff to move easily between bays.[11]

Treatment Areas (Fig. 7)

The optimal number of treatment cubicles will depend on the factors outlined in relation to the overall size of the ED. Estimating the number of treatment cubicles required will involve careful consideration of the volume and scope of services provided.[4]

The total number of treatment areas should be at least 1/1100 yearly attendances or 1/400 yearly admissions, whichever is greater in number. At least 50% of treatment cubicles should have centrally monitored physiological monitoring. Special function treatment areas are not considered in the calculation for treatment area cubicle numbers. All treatment area cubicles should be 16 sqm in size and should be directly observable from the staff duty base.[4,10]

Each treatment area should have:[4]

- Two oxygen outlets
- Wall mounted suction
- A service panel with a minimum of 10 electrical sockets and four category 5 sockets
- A patient trolley
- Swivel chair/stool
- Handwashing facilities
- Patient documentation equipment (writing boards/desk)
- Computer terminal and diagnostic image viewing facilities
- A surgical light
- ENT and ophthalmic examination panel
- Access to dressings and wound care equipment
- Clinical waste disposal bins.

Special Function Treatment Rooms (Fig. 8)

These include:

- Plaster room
- Dental examination room
- Designated room for ENT examination
- Ophthalmology assessment room with black-out capability
- Procedure room with operating theater standard lighting for suturing and wound care (minor OT).

These rooms should be located in close proximity of the major treatment areas and should be adequately equipped to perform the desired procedure.

Single/Isolation Rooms (Negative Pressure Rooms)

Isolation rooms are also advocated for the routine accommodation of patients who are potentially infected. These rooms should be located close to the entry/triage area so that patients can be transferred directly from the ambulance or triage and assessed therein without infecting the remaining facility.[4]

These rooms should have independent negative pressure ventilation and exit high efficiency particulate air (HEPA) filters may be used, if desirable. These rooms should preferably be located close to the outer walls to facilitate ventilation requirements.

TRAUMA OPERATING ROOM

Ideally, the trauma operating rooms (ORs) should be located nearby or adjacent to the resuscitation suite to minimize transportation time for an unstable trauma patient. On the basis of functional program and the schematic design, the size of the OR and the layout of the surgical suite should be established. An OR size between 600 sqft and 750 sqft can accommodate most surgical procedures that utilize management information system (MIS) equipment, a robotic arm, or portable imaging equipment. If considering fixed imaging equipment in the OR, room sizing requires specific planning in the context of the modality and type of procedures to be performed.[2]

HVAC System in Trauma Operating Room

The American Institute of Architects (AIA) guidelines recommend a minimum of 15 ACH (air changes per hour) with a relative humidity range of 45 ± 5% and a design temperature between 22°C and 25°C.[12]

To maintain an environment free of impurities, a design involving use of prefilters at the air handlers followed by high efficiency particulate air filters located above the diffusers through which the air enters the OR is recommended. The pre-filters may include charcoal filters to remove environmental contaminants. The diffuser panels in the ceiling should be located above the predominant position of the OR table (patient) to provide maximum benefit of the vertical downdraft air curtain effect. Return air should be located near the floor level as far from each other as possible.[2]

Lighting Requirements in a Trauma Operating Room

Trauma ORs are required to have general lighting as well as surgical lighting units located above the OR table. Surgical lights are preferably mounted on articulating arms, which provide a wide range of motion for positioning during various surgical procedures.[2]

The ability to dim the general room lighting should be available at the circulating nurse station. To enhance viewing of flat panel displays, consideration should be given to installation of a dimmable green down light.

Interior Finishes in a Trauma Operating Room

The AIA guidelines require the installation of a monolithic and joint-free (seamless) floor. The floor should be nonporous, slip-resistant in wet and dry conditions, handle frequent hard cleaning, and capable of handling heavy rolling loads.[12]

Wall finishes are required to be impermeable to fluids, free of fissures, open joints, or crevices that may retain dirt particles, and washable.

Ceilings are required to be monolithic, scrubbable, and capable of withstanding chemicals. Cracks or perforations are not allowed.[2]

All floor, wall, and ceiling-mounted fixtures and access panels are required to be sealed to prevent entry of dust and contaminants in the OR.

Systems Integration in the Trauma Operating Room (Fig. 9)

There are several design issues to consider when planning for MIS in the OR. Accommodating the equipment required for an MIS case requires more space and preparation and can take significant additional time. Considering the ergonomic configuration around the operating table (the position of the OR table, the height and position of the video displays, and the location of physiologic monitors) is important to provide relief from muscle fatigue and visual feedback to all members of the surgical team.

The additional equipment involved in MIS and the society of vascular surgery (SVS) places greater energy demands on electrical systems and greater heat loads for HVAC (heating, ventilation, and air-conditioning) systems to accommodate. Room setup, access and circulation around the OR table, and maintaining a hazard-free environment are also issues to address during design.

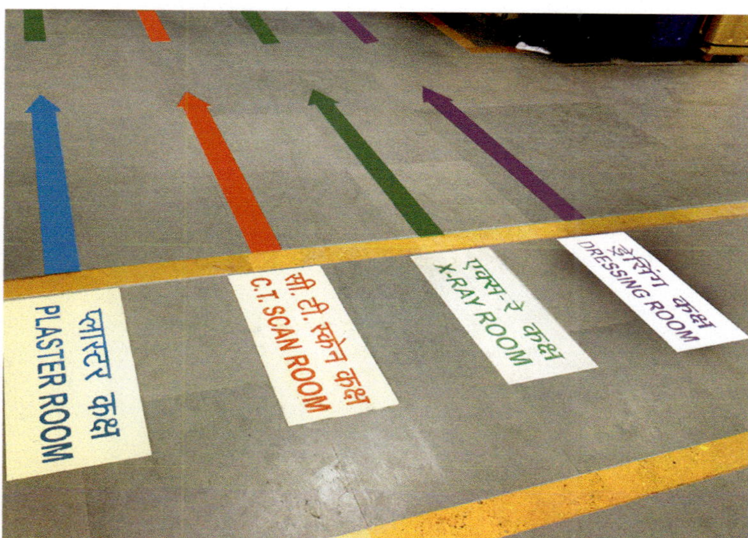

Fig. 9: Systems integration in the trauma operating room.

Imaging Systems in a Trauma Operating Room

The addition of fixed imaging equipment in the OR environment increases the size and complexity of the space. Building structure, OR size, as well as floor and ceiling loading require careful consideration.

Robotic Systems in the Trauma Operating Room

In planning for the use of robotic systems, consideration must be given to the size, structure, and utility capacity (power, telecommunication) of the OR. In addition, the OR layout needs to consider location and workflow of people, supplies, instruments, and equipment, along with the robot and associated systems.

Digital Information Management and Controls in a Trauma Operating Room (Figs. 10A and B)

An area of innovation in trauma ORs is the development of integrated OR, which makes it quicker and easier to set up and manage the OR environment. A single user interface connected to the MIS equipment, flat panel displays, OR lighting, HVAC, and medical equipment offers the circulating nurse the ability to rapidly set up and change the status of the OR environment.

Creating a digital information management and controls environment involves making significant infrastructure investments in the structured cabling system along with planning and integration of several elements, such as the MIS, SVS, integrated operating room (IOR), OR case management system, patient tracking system, medical devices with status information and control interfaces, and building automation system.

Conduit and cable tray systems to accommodate all potential information sources and destinations, large telecommunication equipment management rooms, increased HVAC capacity to handle additional heat loads, and location of the circulating nurse are key areas of consideration in the design of OR.

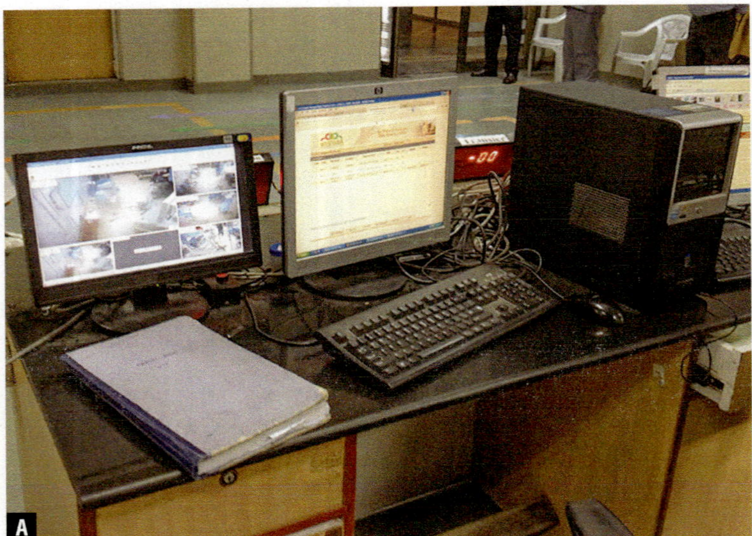

A

TIVE--TOWARDS SAFETY,EMERGENCY DEP

12:22 PM PAGE 3

TC-NO	NAME	BED NO	GCS SCORE	DIAGNOSIS	MLC-STATUS	CALL SENT TO	INVESTIGATION REQUIRED	WAITING-FOR	STATUS
384118	GURU DEV	10	15	HI,SFI	NON-MLC	SURGERY		REVIEW BY SPECIALIST	STABLE
384121	SAINATW IYER	13	15	MI	NON-MLC	ORTHO	X-RAY	REVIEW BY SPECIALIST	STABLE
384122	DONALISA KOMAL	14	15		NON-MLC			REVIEW BY SPECIALIST	STABLE
384124	MOHIT	15	15		NON-MLC			REVIEW BY SPECIALIST	STABLE
384128	VIJAY PAL NAGAR	16	15		NON-MLC			REVIEW BY SPECIALIST	STABLE
384129	MALLESHWARI	17	15		NON-MLC			REVIEW BY SPECIALIST	STABLE
384130	SATENDRA	18	15		MLC			REVIEW BY SPECIALIST	STABLE

Abbreviations: HI=Head Injury, SI=Spinal Injury,THI=Thoracic Injury,SFI=Superficial Injury,PF=Pelvic Fracture,ABDI=Abdominal Injury, LBI=Long Bone Injury,MI=Musculoskeletal Injury,A=Airway

B

Figs. 10A and B: Digital information management and controls.

Major Incident/Disaster Planning in a Trauma Care Facility

The major issues in the design of a trauma care facility are related to disaster preparedness. Four central themes in this regard are:

- Surge capacity
- Flexibility
- Information access
- Security.

Treatment areas must be rapidly converted into trauma resuscitation areas capable of providing the same level of patient care available in the trauma resuscitation area. Plans should be established to quickly convert space adjacent to the trauma resuscitation area into triage space and patient treatment areas. Nonclinical space (e.g. waiting rooms), parking garages, and parking lots can be converted into expanded triage or treatment areas.

Part of the expansion plan must include provisions for communication, materials management, and information technology. In addition, space and equipment for decontamination must be included in the surge capacity plan.

Surge capacity also applies to information systems; an adequate plan should be in place to make essential patient information available to providers in all of the areas that have been converted to clinical workspace. Security, a prominent issue in many trauma centers, becomes a larger issue during a disaster response. To protect patients and healthcare providers, the trauma care facility must have the ability to enact a total lockdown. Access to the clinical areas from inside and outside the facility must be strictly controlled. Establishing a security perimeter, such that access to the facility grounds is also limited is an additional consideration.

CONCLUSION

A trauma care facility is much more than mortar and bricks. Its all about appropriate resources both in the form of manpower and equipment supported by a suitable infrastructure.

Trauma care facilities like fire departments and police services are required to be available 24 hours a day, 7 days a week. This level of commitment by them and the reciprocal expectation from the community, force trauma centers to make considerable investments in readiness. This cost of readiness is expended regardless of the patient volume or paying capacity. Thus trauma care facilities have a large component of costs that are not factored in traditional budgeting mechanisms within health systems.[13]

Trauma care facility based care not only saves lives, it is a cost-effective way of treating major trauma. The costs per quality-adjusted life-year (QALY) gained themselves fund for a trauma care facility.[2]

To summarize, it is essential that while planning for a trauma care facility, a holistic approach for resource planning in the form of infrastructure, equipment, manpower and financial resources is taken.

REFERENCES

1. http://www.azhha.org/member_and_media_resources/documents/Bkgndr-Trauma.pdf
2. dghs.gov.in
4. www.iaem.ie
3. nahfo.org
5. dgca.nic.in
6. www.wales.nhs.uk
7. www.azhha.org
8. Huntington Memorial Hospital Receives Prestigious Level II Trauma Center Verification from the Ameri. Medical Devices and Surgical Technology Week; Feb 8 2015.
9. medcaretips.com
10. MacKenzie, et al. The Value of Trauma Center Care. The Journal of Trauma Injury Infection and Critical Care. 2010;69:1-10.
11. www.gov.uk
12. Guidelines for Design and Construction of Hospital and Healthcare Facilities. American Institute of Architects 1997.
13. www.ncbi.nlm.nih.gov

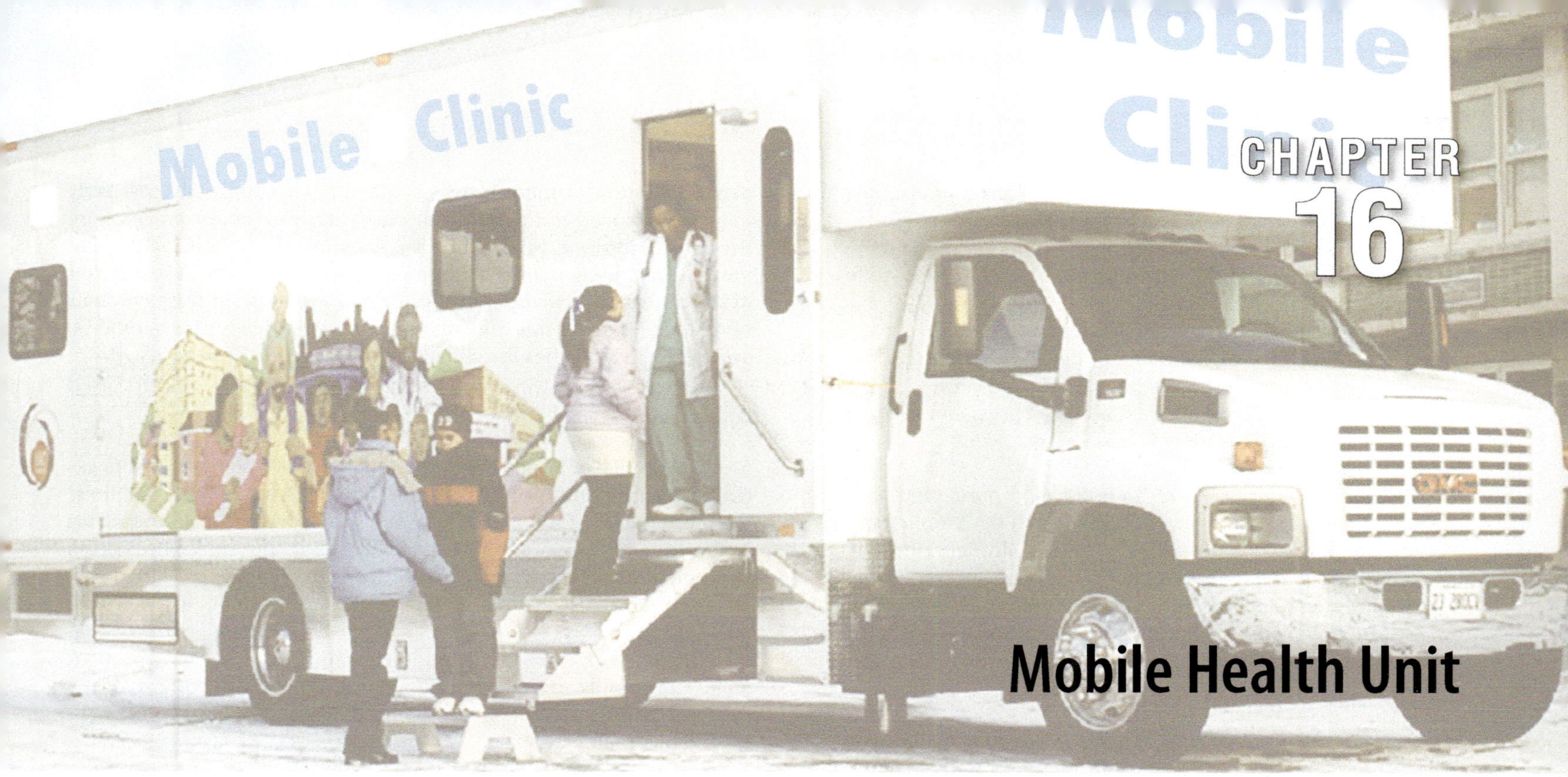

Mobile Health Unit

Saroj Kumar Patnaik, Shakti Kumar Gupta, Sunil Kant, R Chandrashekhar

INTRODUCTION

Mobile medical units have been envisaged to provide preventive, promotive and curative healthcare in inaccessible areas and difficult terrains, which are underserved or underserved areas under usual circumstances. Factors that negatively influence the existing public health system and call for the exigency are—Distance of the remote villages from public health institutions, geographical barriers to reach the pockets, lack of mobility support for field visit by the staff assigned to do the job, lack of medicines/equipment/manpower.[1]

Mobile Health Units (MHUs) also provide healthcare in unstable situations, such as armed conflicts, where fixed services cannot function for reasons of security. They are, however, a controversial way of providing healthcare, because of their cost, their irregular service provision and their logistical complexities.[2,3]

HISTORY OF MOBILE HEALTH UNIT

The structured MHU initially started as Mobile Army Surgical Hospital (MASH).

The MASH unit was conceived by Michael E DeBakey and other surgical consultants as the *Mobile Auxiliary Surgical Hospital.* It was an alternative to the system of portable surgical hospitals, field hospitals, and general hospitals used during World War II. It was designed to get experienced personnel closer to the front, so that the wounded could be treated sooner and with greater success. This proved to be highly successful; it was noted that during the Korean War, a seriously wounded soldier that made it to a MASH unit alive had a 97% chance of survival once he received treatment.

Worldwide, the last MASH unit was deactivated on October 16, 2006. The 212th MASH—based in Miesau Ammo Depot, Germany—was the first US Army hospital established in Iraq in 2003, supporting coalition forces during Operation Iraqi Freedom. The 212th MASH's last deployment was to Pakistan to support the 2005 Kashmir earthquake relief operations. Its equipment was donated to Pakistan.[4]

Over the past 50 years, the geographic areas in which MHUs have been used and the services delivered in this manner have changed dramatically. The MHU delivery concept originated in the 1940s. In the 1950s and 1960s, MHUs were popular in both domestic and overseas markets. It is used to deliver care to a convenient site for select consumers, such as the elderly, pregnant women, school children, and groups at recreational events and at work. Sound as these goals may seem, the purchase of a MHU usually is quite costly and in many instance does not live up to providers preconceived expectations. Questions relate to cost-benefit, cost-effectiveness, quality, and outcomes consistently confront stakeholders Accompanying the expansion of healthcare systems is the emphasis on offering a continuum of cost-effective care to consumers—even those living in outlying catchment areas. In some MHU can be a viable strategy for offering an array of services, including primary, secondary, tertiary, and specialized care to consumers living and working in diverse settings. However, the mobile model is not the answer in every situation.[5,6]

To encourage attendance at MHUs, the first services offered should be those of greatest interest to the population (e.g. vaccination as part of a planning program, the distribution of condoms in clinics dealing with sexually transmitted diseases or HIV/AIDS). The practice of tagging on service onto a vertical program is well established, and is described in WHO's sustainable outreach programs.[3,7]

SETTING OF THE MOBILE EMERGENCY FIELD HOSPITAL

Geographical and strategic siting is the responsibility of the administrative officer of local government in consultation with the medical authorities to the team. The choice of the site is influenced by:

- Accessibility, especially by road transport, of the areas, the mobile hospital is to cover.
- General communications and road communications, which can be, used as routes of general supply.
- Functional—the actual site is chosen for its advantages in helping the unit in its function of receiving, treating and evacuating the

sick and wounded. Various local conditions and circumstances are desirable:

- Central position in relation to the units served and proximity an airfield. Preferably, the unit should not be more than a mile distant from an airfield.
- Good roads in the immediate neighborhood.
- Adequate shelter, available either in building or afforded by natural objects, such as cliffs, woods and slopes
- Suitable soil for erection of tents and provision of drainage.
- Adequate water supply.
- Proximity to railhead.

All these circumstances change in order of importance according to the nature and terrain of the country in which the Mobile Emergency Medical Hospital is operating. Ideally, the Mobile Field Hospital should be sited centrally in relating to the affected areas. The unit should be deployed in the field such as at Health *Melas*, Mobile Camps to find out the functional efficacy during normal time at least once in a year.[8]

LAYOUT OF THE UNIT (FIGS. 1A TO E)

The senior most doctor, in-charge of the unit and his staff must keep the relative importance of the medical and domestic requirements in mind in planning the layout of the limit. The choice between accommodation in buildings or in tents or container model cannot be foreseen and therefore only the requirements are considered here. Priority must be given to medical needs; if buildings are available, they are required for operating theater, wards, X-ray apparatus, laboratory and stores, particularly of linen, blankets, clothing and dressing. These needs in order of priority.

Wards for surgical and medical divisions, officers, the special treatment center and infectious diseases; they may occupy buildings or large expanding hospital tents or container models.

- Operating theater and resuscitation room with the sterilizing room; they should be next to the surgical ward and may occupy a building or tents.
- Laboratory, X-ray, dispensary and medical equipment, including linen, blankets and clothing, in building, tents or vehicle as available.
- Doctor's room, reception may occupy buildings, adjacent ridge tents or vehicles with lean to tents on each side.
- The generators may be placed so that it may serve the theater, the wards, and the cookhouse and mess tent with greatest economy of cable.
- The water reservoir should be near the cookhouse, reserve water being held in bin/collapsible container, tanks or water cart itself at convenient sites in the camp.
- Toilets placed at sited selected to the leeward of the respective lines, which they serve.
- Refuse incinerator or pit placed to the leeward of the whole camp on lower ground, if possible.
- Laundering and disinfestations plant, it should occupy a ridge tent as near as possible to water supply.
- Sleeping sites.

SUPPLY CHAIN MANAGEMENT

General

The chief supplies, equipment is from the place of origin. Subsequent supplies should be from Medical Stores nearest to the site of disaster. Knowledge of the methods and routes of supply is the responsibility of the doctor incharge of the unit, local administrative officers who must obtain this knowledge as soon as possible after arrival in the area of operation. The main items are water, ration, petrol/fuel, sanitary, drugs, disposable surgical/medical items. Difficulties in supply are most likely to be experienced at the beginning particularly in remote areas where the communication is poor/or disconnected. The doctor incharge of the team and his man must make themselves responsible for collection of store due to them without waiting for stores to be delivered at their doorsteps. To avoid this difficulty one member of the team should be appointed to look after the collection of stores.

Water

Mobile Hospital of 50 beds requires about 20 L of water a head daily as comfortable minimum, but in times of shortage, it is possible to continue for some time on as little as 8 L a head daily. Water tenders must be available to draw the necessary supply from water point and water purification equipment must be an integral part of every mobile medical unit.

Ration

The initial supply should be obtained from the place of origin for the patients as well as the medical personnel. Subsequent replenishment should be obtained locally.

Petrol/Fuel

These supplies are usually available from the nearest supply depot. The team should carry some quantity of fuels for the Generators and for the ambulance at the time of departure.

Medical Equipment

It is particularly important to ensure that the initial medical equipment to scale, as well as replenishment is received. For this purpose, the team leader should make arrangements to check all medical gadgets on formation of the unit and arrange for any deficiencies to be made good before the unit proceeds to the area of operations.

Communication

Mobile telephone at least five should be available to have direct contact with the officials or the Central and State Health and other administrative official in order to brief them on the situation and seek any direction.

PLANNING AND DESIGNING PARAMETERS OF 50-BEDDED CONTAINERIZED MHU

This module comprises of basic OPD, operation theater module including diagnostics and in addition will have dental unit, ward unit, ancillary units (kitchen, laundry, additional toilet complex, stores, additional power and water supply), living accommodation and administrative unit.

The 50-bed mobile hospital module will comprise of the following facilities:

- Reception
- OT module
- Wards
- Dental
- Medical and hospital stores
- Laundry
- Kitchen
- Toilet complex
- Office complex
- Residential accommodation complex.

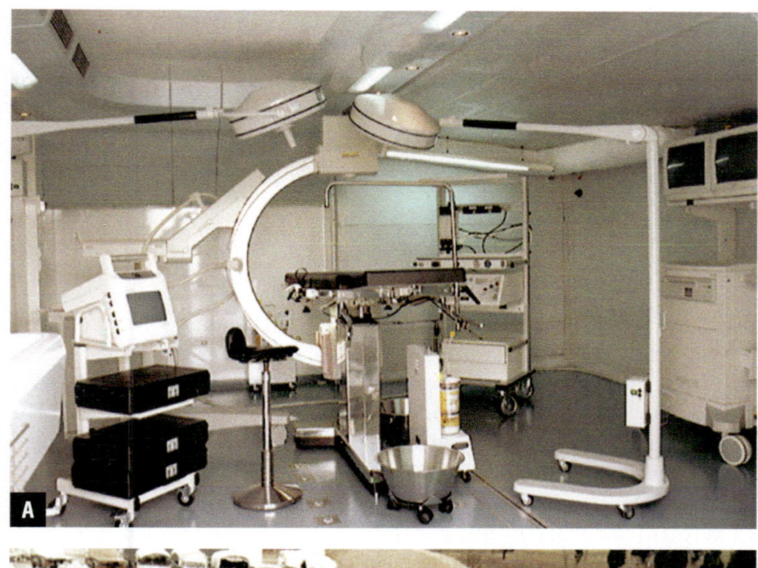

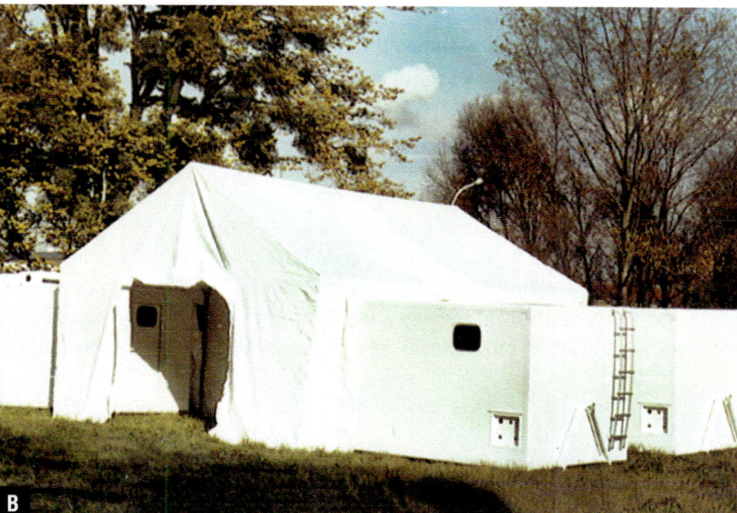

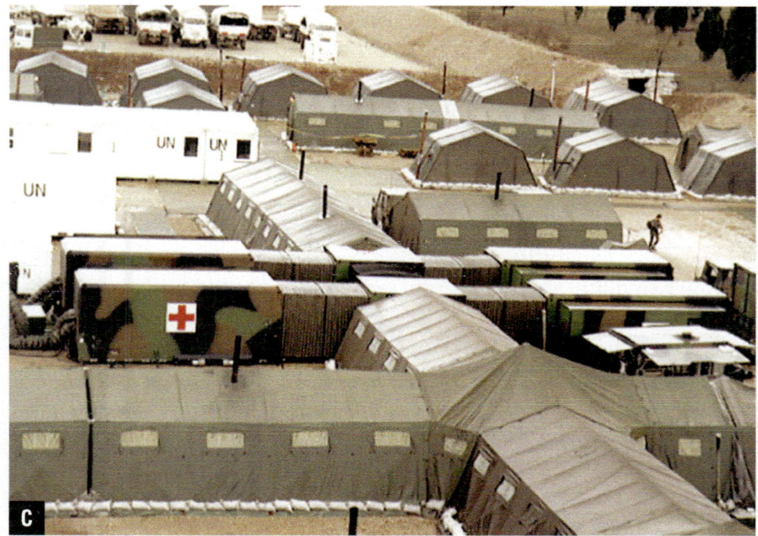

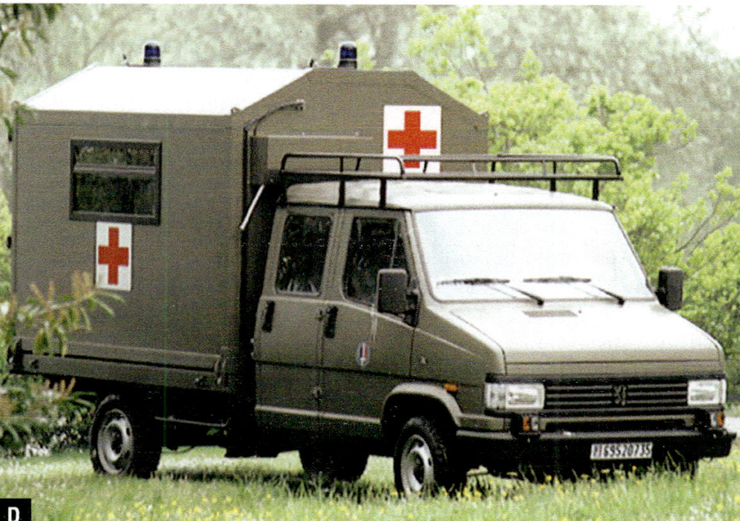

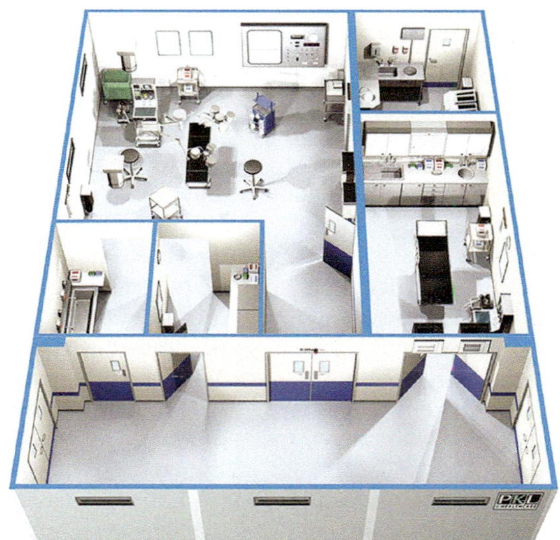

Figs. 1A to E: Layout of mobile hospital.

Containers/Tents needed to deploy a 50-bed mobile hospital:

- Reception modul : 1 × expandable container
- OT module : 7 × standard/expandable containers and 1 × inflatable tent
- Dental : 1 × standard container
- Wards : 3 × inflatable tent
- Medical stores : 1 × standard container
- Hospital stores : 2 × standard containers
- Hospital laundry : 1 × standard container

CONFIGURATION

Configuration for 50-bed mobile medical treatment facility:

- Expandable containers (1:3) : 03
- Expandable container (1:2) : 01
- Standard containers : 16
- Inflatable tents : 09

  Total containers : 20

Deployment: The mobile medical treatment facility will be fully deployed and functional within 30 minutes for primary consultation room and 4–6 hours for the 50 bed mobile treatment facility (Figs. 2A to E).

Dental Unit

This unit will be utilized for a single chair dental clinic. It will be based on a single, fixed volume ISO specified 6 m container. The sides and ceiling should be made of sandwich aluminum panels. All internal corners to be rounded off for easy cleaning. Suitable high-grade insulation material should be provided in between outer and inner paneling to withstand extreme climatic condition ranging between –10°C + 50°C. The floor should be covered with heavy duty vinyl flooring of high quality without joints. There should be suitable drain hole for easy washing of floor with facility to close the hole when not in use. There should be adequate number of windows with fixed double layer glass with sun protection film. Provisions of opaque blinds should be made for use under blackout conditions. Door should have automatic hydraulic door closing system. The container should be fitted with inherent lifting device (hydraulic/manual jacks) to facilitate easy loading/unloading of container from the prime mover without the help of crane or fork lift.

Fittings

- *HVAC (Heating, ventilation and air conditioning) system*: It will consist of AC to ensure ambient temperature of 20–25°C under extreme climatic conditions with temperature variation of –10°C to +50°C. It should also have heating facility for use during winters. Noise and vibration levels should be low.
- *Air circulation (Fan)*: Four wall mounted oscillating fans to be provided of 45 cm diameter in the container. The fans should be fitted with electronic regulators.
- *Illumination*: The following should be provided:
  - *Internal illumination*: Flush mounted light fitments with LED to ensure brightly lit interiors.
  - *External illumination*: Waterproof electric light fitments, one above each door for providing external illumination at entry and exit doors.
  - *Power points*: Multi-pin 15/5 Amp power points should be provided for all electromedical equipment. In additions four power points for X-ray compartment and six power points for laboratory compartment to be provided.
  - *Water supply*: The container will be provided integral water supply of minimum 50 L with facility for running hot and cold water.
  - *Storage cabinets*: There should be a provision for lockable wall mounted storage cabinets to store dental equipment and consumables.
- *Equipment and furniture*: The container for the dental unit will be fitted with the following equipment:
  - Pantographic, electrically operated physiological compact dental chair and unit with complete attachments : 01
  - Tabletop autoclave : 01
  - Dental X-ray unit with RVG : 01
  - Water distiller : 01
  - Basic dental instruments kit : 01
  - Ultraviolet storage cabinet : 01
  - Laptop computer with latest technology update with software

Ward Unit

Ward unit will be based on fully integrated, self-inflating, self-supporting double-layered airbeam tents/shelters. It should be possible to erect the shelter at the site, using not more than three persons and have it fully functional within twenty minutes. Each shelter should be capable of laying out 10 beds of size 180 cm (L) × 75 cm (W) × 70 cm (H). There should be a minimum distance of 75 cm between two beds when laid out. Each shelter should have the following characteristics:

- Should be designed for maximum interoperability and interconnectivity that incudes hard to soft and soft to soft connections.
- It should have the capability to provide space for pharmacy within the patient ward utilizing preinstalled lockable cabinets for medical supplies/store for 72 hours.
- Be capable of operations using standard generators/commercial power source
- Have the capability to provide an integrated filtration system for dust and sand in all areas with provision for NBC filters.
- Have the capability to provide integrated environmental control that can maintain the internal temperature in the range of 20–25°C with outside ambient temperature of –10°C to +50°C.
- It should have an interior noise level less that 60 dB during normal operations.
- It should have capability to provide an integrated floor system that is non-conductive, non-skid and easy to clear with minimal vibrational movement when walking over the floor.
- It should have the capability of an integrated solar shield to facilitate thermal efficiency.
- It should be composed of materials that are durable, rugged and support life cycle of 20 years.
- It should have the capability to be adoptable to all terrain types, altitudes, and climate and weather conditions from –10°C to +50°C.
- It should be able to operate in 5–100% relative humidity.
- It should be capable of operation under normal environmental conditions and hazards, such as, but not limited to shock, corrosion, vibration, dust, smoke, fungus and lightening. It should be corrosion resistant and the design and construction should limit contact between dissimilar metals to prevent galvanic corrosion. It should not support the growth of fungi.
- It should be capable of operation in sustained winds of 60–80 km/h with gusts of up to 100 km/h.
- It should inhibit snow accumulation and remain fully operational under heavy snow load. It should not be degraded by snow, freezing rain or ice removal procedures.
- It should prevent accumulation of rainfall and withstand, without leak, heavy rainfall in moderate steady winds.
- It should be repairable under field conditions after sustaining small arms and splinter damage.
- It should have the capability to provide collective protection under NBC conditions. It should have an option for integrated NBC soft wall shelter liner and integrated NBC filtration system.
- It should be compatible with standard camouflage techniques. It should have removable red crosses with white background (Figs. 3A to C).

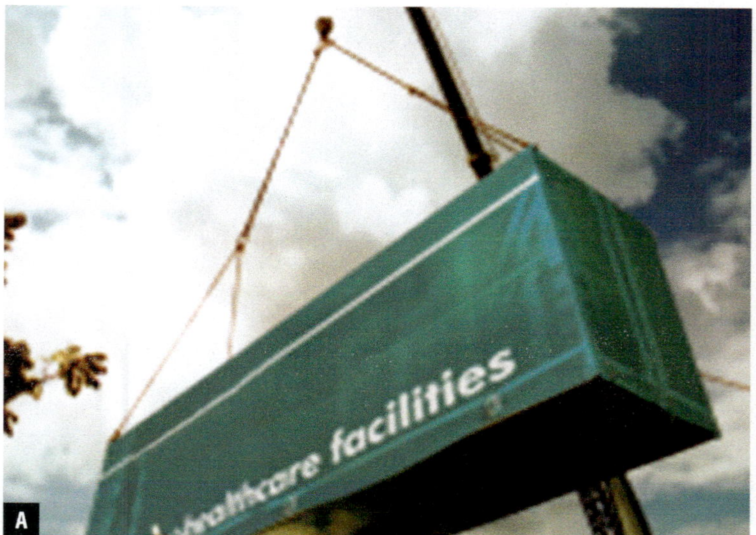

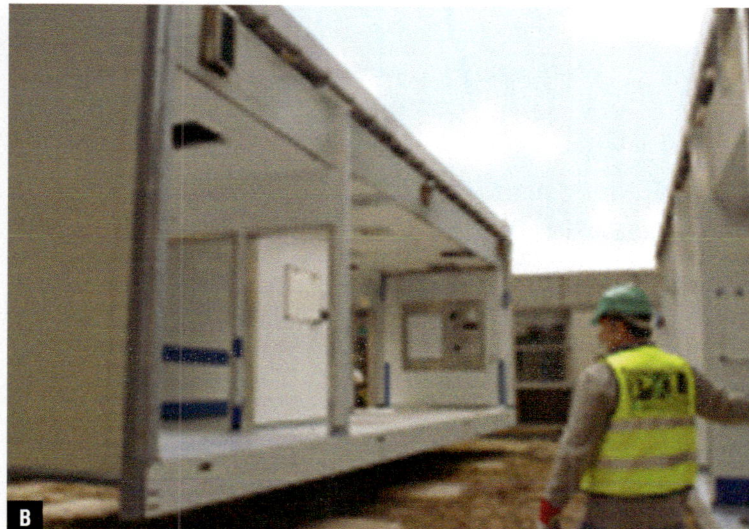

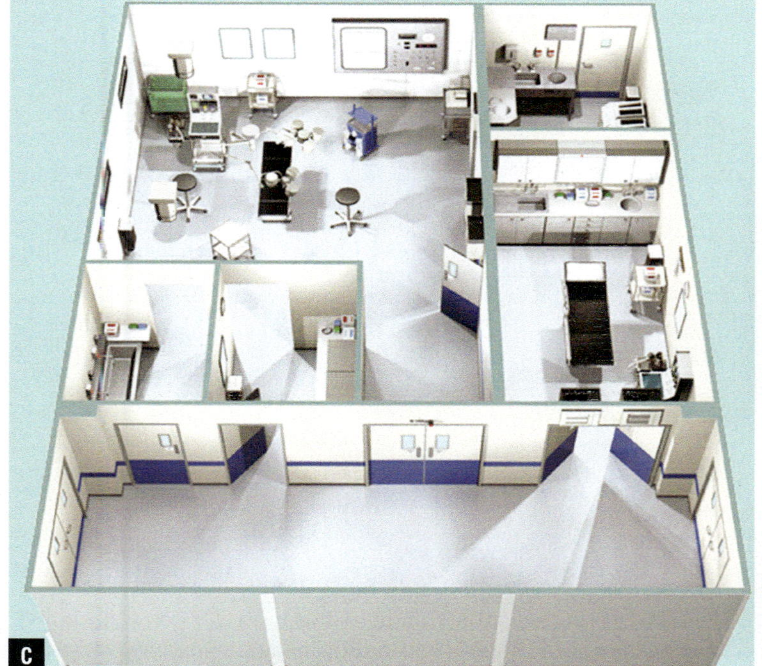

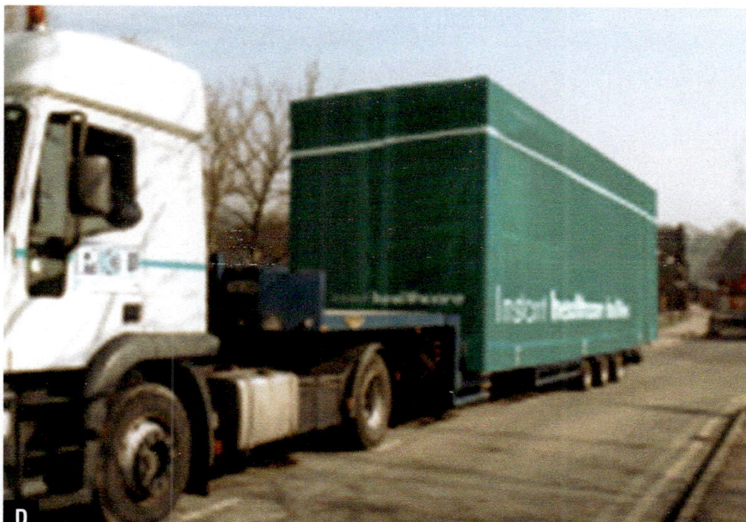

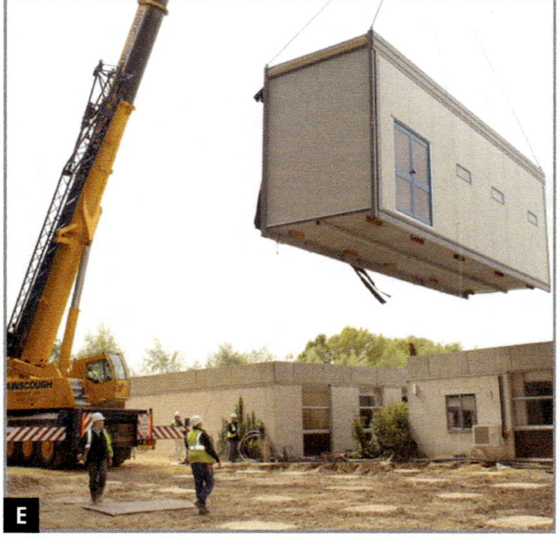

Figs. 2A to E: Containers for Mobile Health Unit.

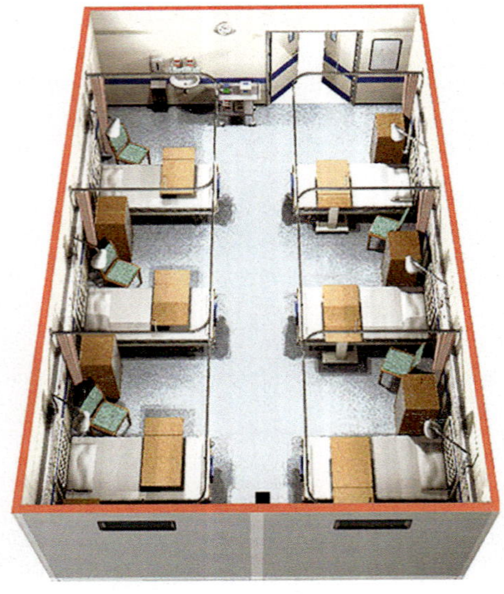
A

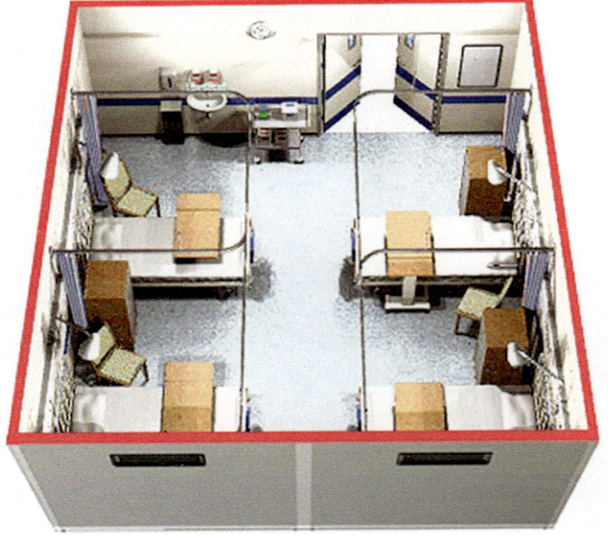
B

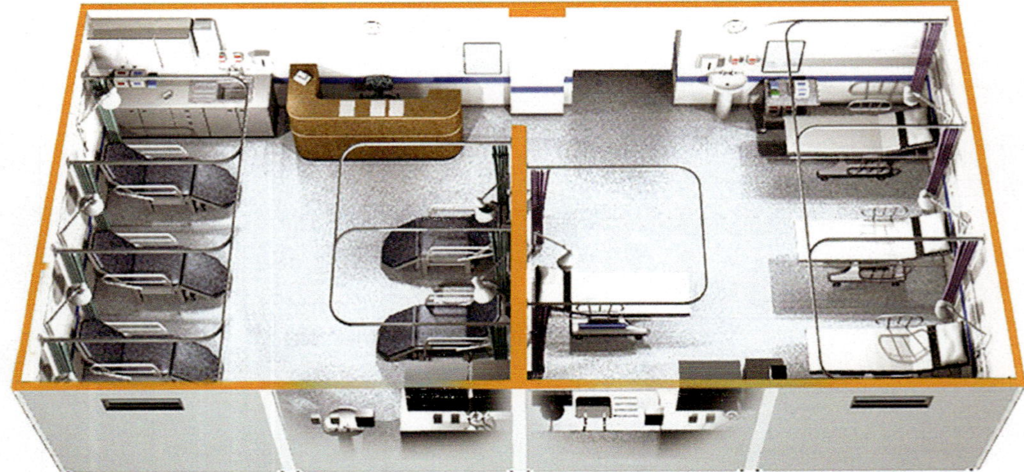
C

Figs. 3A to C: Various mobile wards.

Fittings

- *HVAC system:*
  - The ward shelter should have integrated environmental unit to maintain the inside temperature between 20–25°C centigrade under extreme climatic conditions (temperature variation -10°C to +50°C).
  - It should have optional facility to provide an integrated filtration system for dust, sand and bacteriological and chemical warfare agents.
- *Illumination*: The shelter should be fitted with integrated lighting of LED type to provide sufficient illumination inside the shelter.
- *Power points*: There should be a provision of minimum of six 15/5 Amp multi-pin power points between two beds. All cables/ electric wiring should be integrated within the shelter.

Furniture

Following medical furniture will be required for each ward shelter:

- *Beds 10:* Each bed should have dimensions of 75 cm (W) × 180 cm (L) and 70 cm (H). It should be foldable. Each bed to be provided with mattress of 05 cm thickness of high density foam covered with waterproof and stain-resistant material. Each bed should be fitted with two IV stands.
- *Bedside table-10*: Table should be folding type with two shelves. Dimensions of each table should be 45 cm (L) × 30 (W) × 90 cm (H).
- *Table for nursing station-01:* It should be foldable type with collapsible legs of dimensions 90 cm (W) × 120 cm (L) × 90 cm (H).
- Revolving chair : 01
- Patient stool : 01
- Camp chair (folding) : 06
- Wall clock : 01
- Racks for storing essential medicines with four shelves each : 02
- Washbasin with running hot and cold water
- Patient screen hospital (folding) : 04

Medical Stores

The medical stores for the hospital will be carried in a standard, fixed volume IOS specified 20 ft container. The walls and ceiling will be made of sandwich aluminum panels. There should be suitable insulating material filled between the outer and inner paneling to provide insulation under extreme climate conditions with temperature variation between -10°C to +50°C. All inner corners to be rounded off for easy cleaning. There should be provision of a drain hole in the floor. The floor should be covered with heavy duty vinyl flooring without joints. The container should be fitted with inherent-lifting device (hydraulic/manual jacks) to facilitate easy loading/unloading of container from the prime mover without the help of crane or fork lift.

Fittings

- *Heating, ventilation and air conditioning system*: It will consist of air conditioning to ensure ambient temperature of 20–25°C under extreme climatic conditions with temperature variation of –10°C to +50°C.
- *Illumination*: The following should be provided:
  - *Internal illumination:* Flush mounted light fitments with LED to be provided inside the container to have brightly lit interiors.
  - *External illumination*: Waterproof electric light fitments, one above each door for providing external illumination at entry and exit doors.
- *Power point*: 06 Multi-pin 15/5 Amp power points to be provided
- Hand wash facility with running hot and cold water and water storage, if 100 L to be provided.

Furniture

The following furniture should be provided:

- Folding table of size 60 cm (W) × 90 cm (L) × 90 cm (H) : 01
- Revolving chair : 01
- Frost-free refrigerator of 250 L capacity : 02
- *Storage cabinet:* The container should be equipped with lockable storage cabinets along all walls and in a free-standing row along the center of the container. The cabinets shall extend to ceiling height and have adjustable shelves for storage of items of different size. The shelves should have a minimum depth of 45 cm.

Information Technology Stores

There should be provision of one computer of latest technology with LCD monitor, laser printer and UPS (The specifications will be finalized at the time of tendering). There should be facility for intercom between different modules, satellite phone link, internet access and provision for telemedicine. There must be provision of integrated LAN between all modules for data and information exchange.

Miscellaneous Points

Joining Module (Fig. 4)

There will be a provision of providing covered connections between various modules so that the mobile hospital is laid out as integrated unit. It should be possible to move between various wards and department without leaving the hospital environment. The joining modules should be flexible and provide all weather protections with integrated flooring. They should be able to connect equally with both elements of the hospital, that is, both hard-walled containers and soft-walled inflatable tents/shelters. The module will have integrated lighting and have capability of being joined together to form corridors whenever required. It should have the capability to join two, containers/tent on different levels due to uneven ground.

There will be a provision to load/upload patients from ambulance vehicles in bad weather conditions like rain, snow, etc. A place for visitors/attendants should be available. These can be provided by using inflatable tents.

Container Loading and Unloading System (Figs. 5A to C)

All containers should be fitted with inherent lifting device (hydraulic/manual jacks) to facilitate easy loading/unloading of container from the prime mover without the help of crane or fork lift. However, a crane or any other suitable device/hook system should be provided for loading and unloading the containers from/to the prime movers when the built in jacks cannot be used for loading the containers on other means of transport like train, ship, etc. This container handling system should be able to be carried on the prime mover and have the same cross country mobility as the rest of the containers.

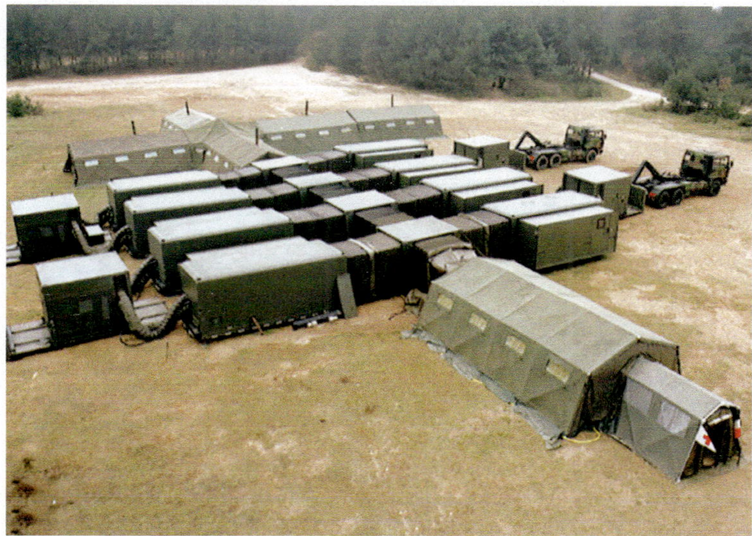

Fig. 4: Joining module of mobile hospital.

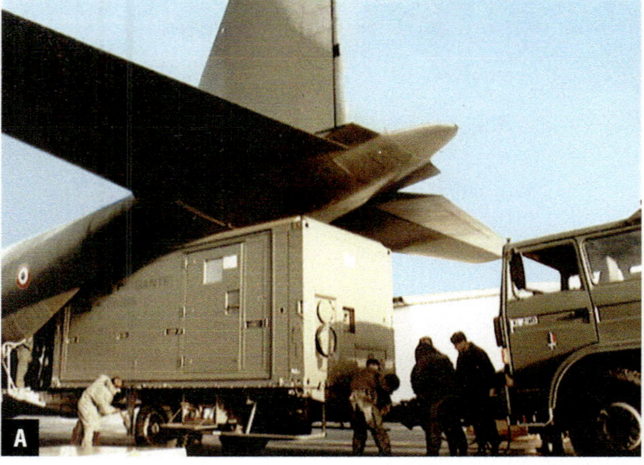

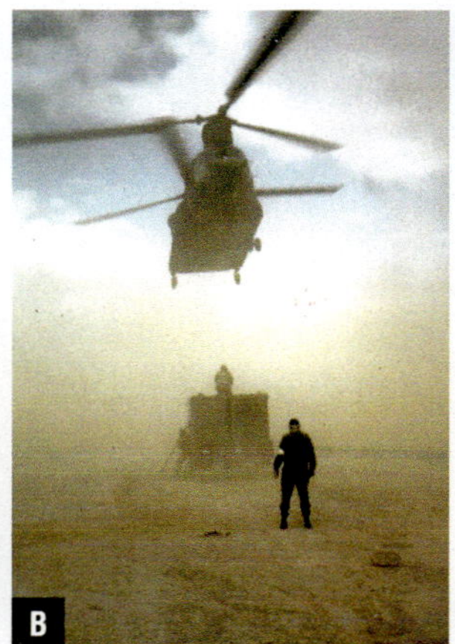

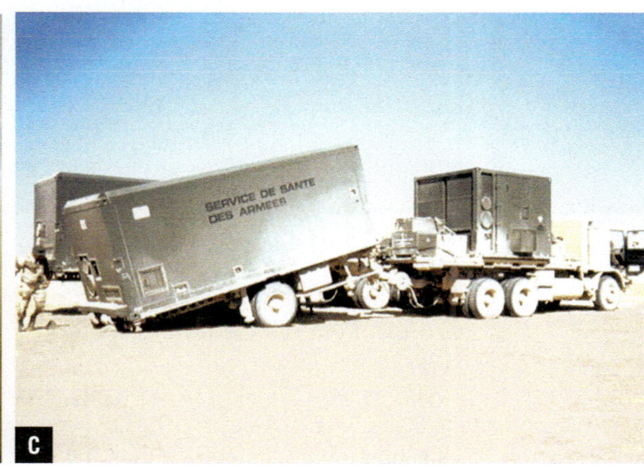

Figs. 5A to C: Container loading and unloading.

MOBILE HEALTH SYSTEMS

Mobile Hospital

Mobility

The 6.0 m ISO container concept gives high mobility by road, rail, sea and air.

Modularity (Figs. 6A to D)

The modular design allows changes in the capacity of the reception and treatment wards and in the type of medical facilities depending on the requirements of the mission.

Technical Core

A technical core of the same standard as a normal hospital.

MOBILE CLINIC SYSTEM (FIGS. 7A TO F)

The construction and basic fittings of the units are identical whatever their specialization, thereby simplifying training, logistic support and maintenance. Various specialized units are depicted in Figs. 7 and 8).

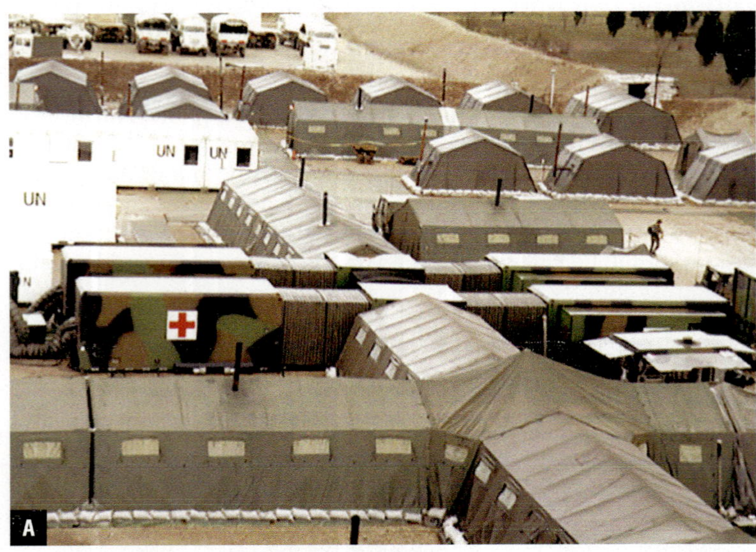

A
French hospital in Bosnia

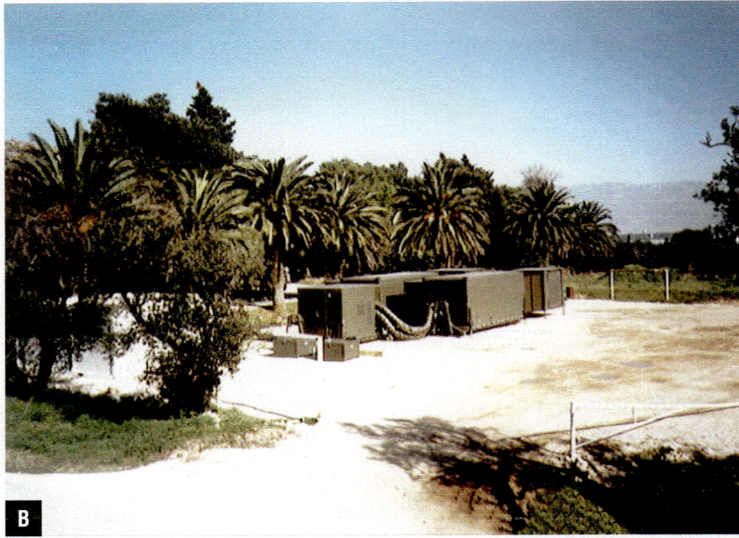
B
British hospital in Croatia

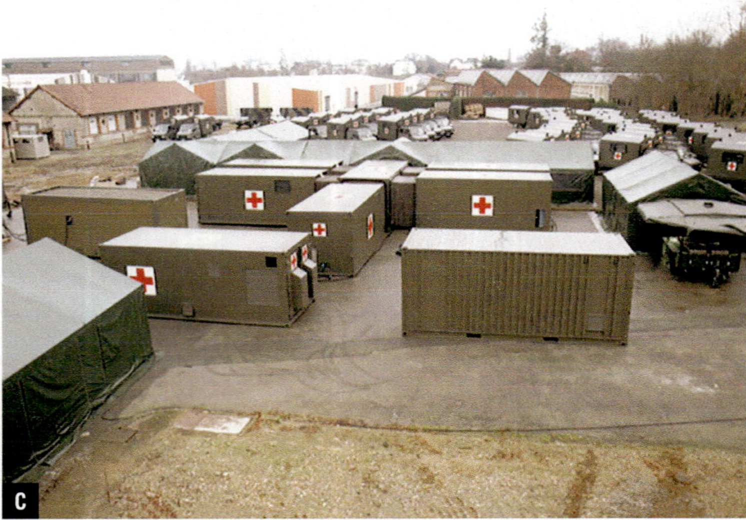
C
French hospital in Bosnia

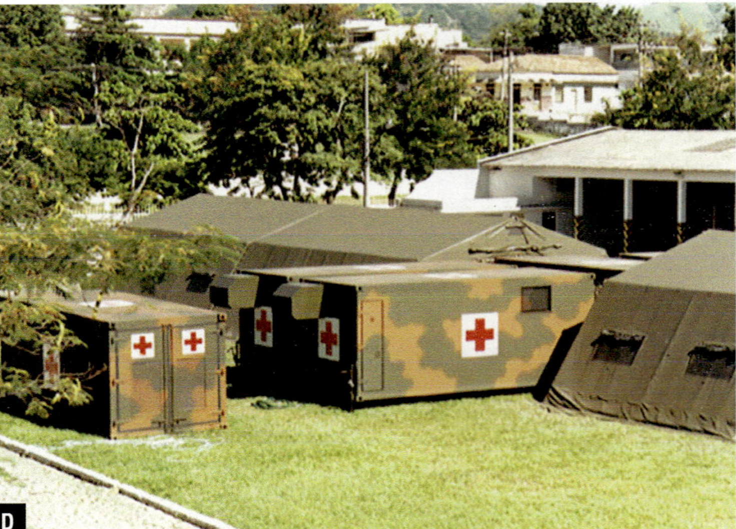
D
Brazilian hospital

Figs. 6A to D: Modularity.

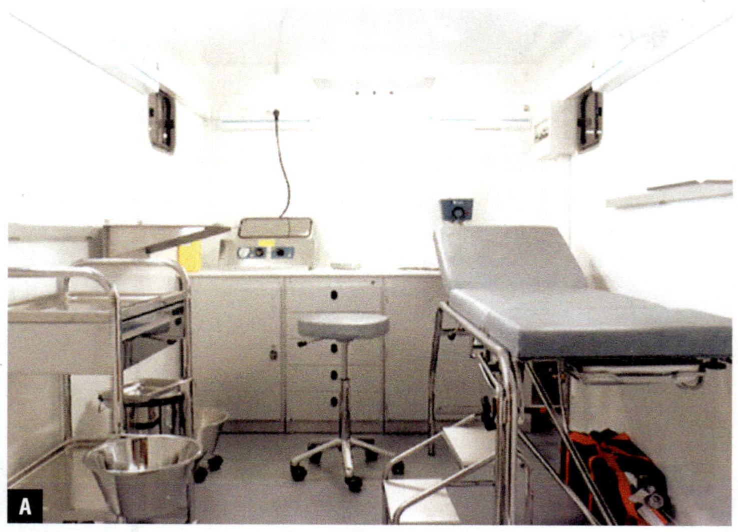
A
General medicine

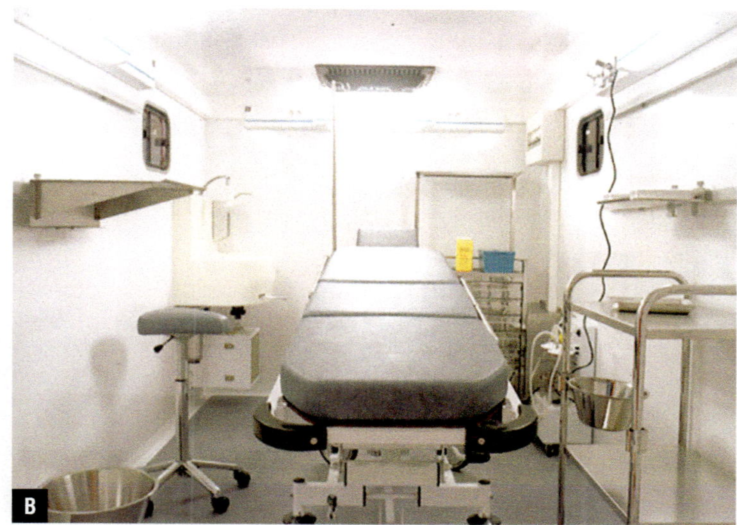
B
Minor surgery

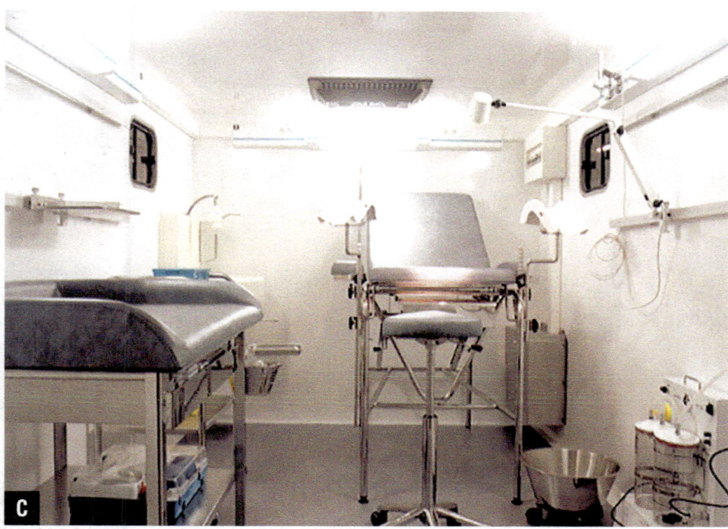
C
Gynecology

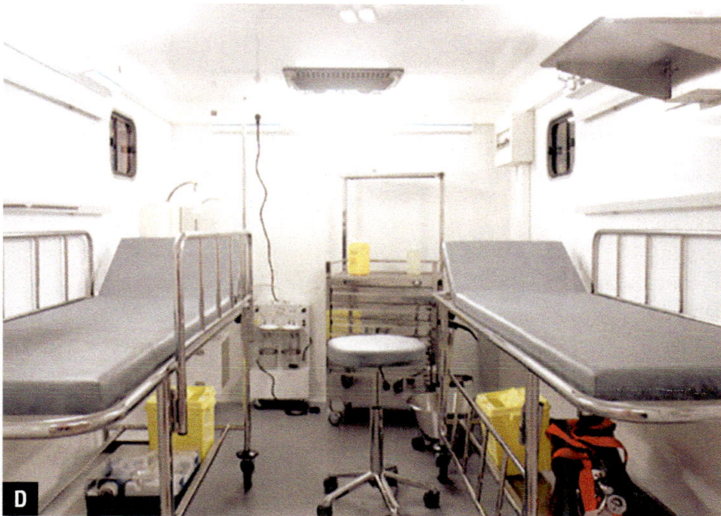
D
Intensive care

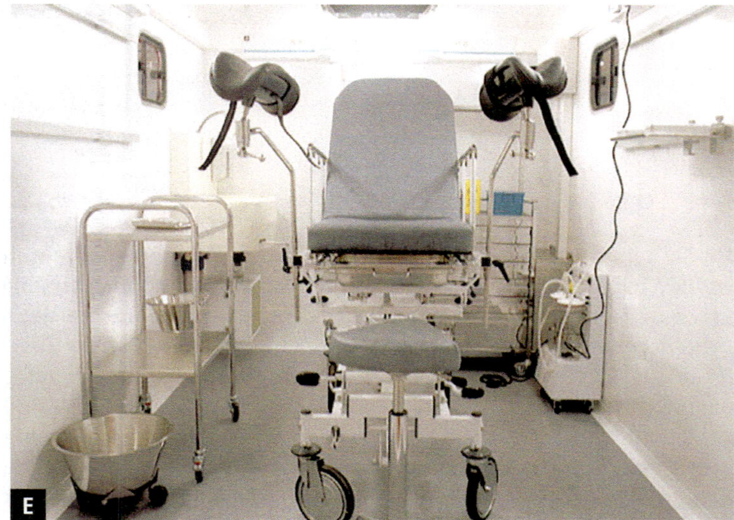
E
Obstetrics

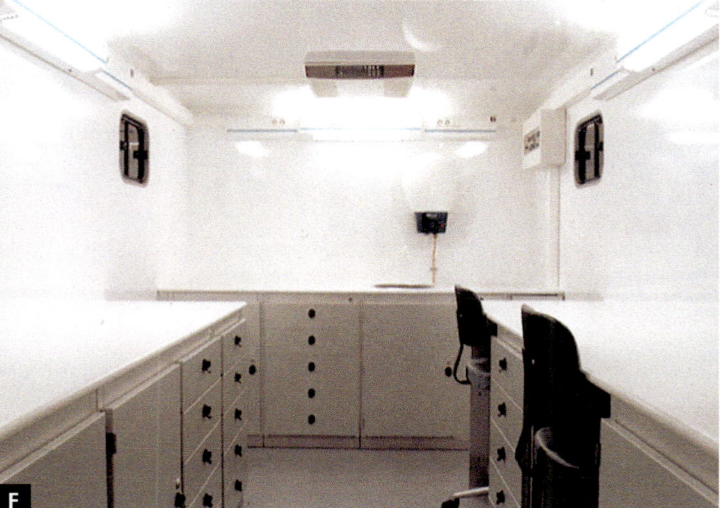
F
Laboratory

Figs. 7A to F: Specialized units.

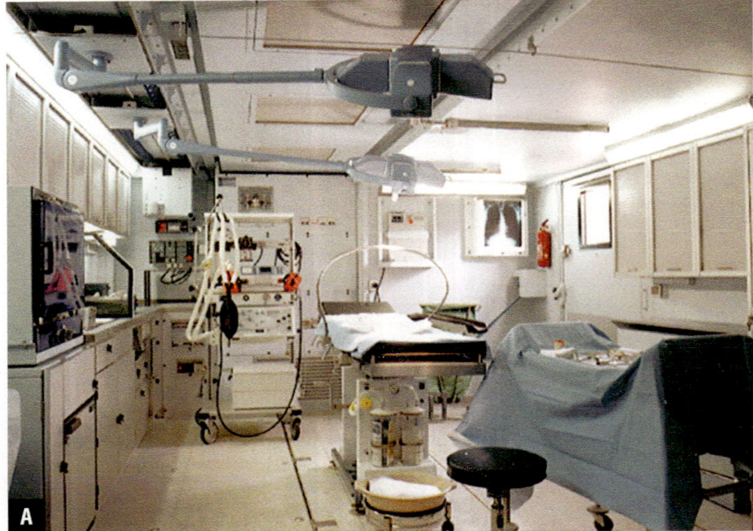

Surgical module

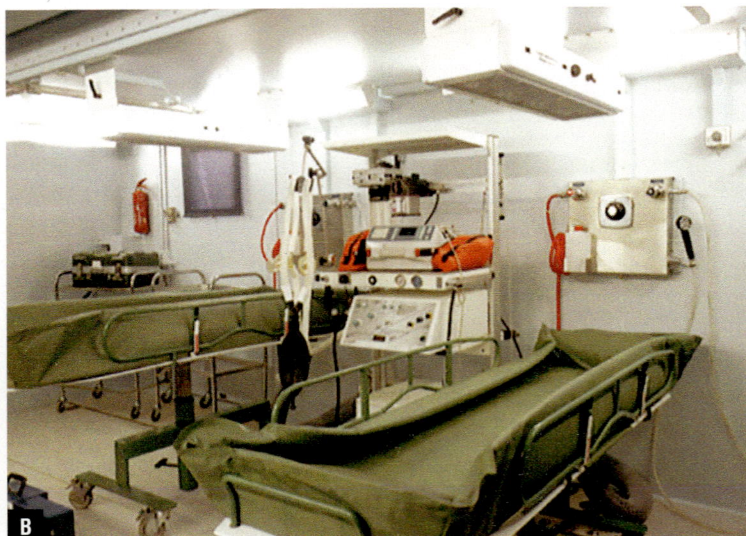

Burn module

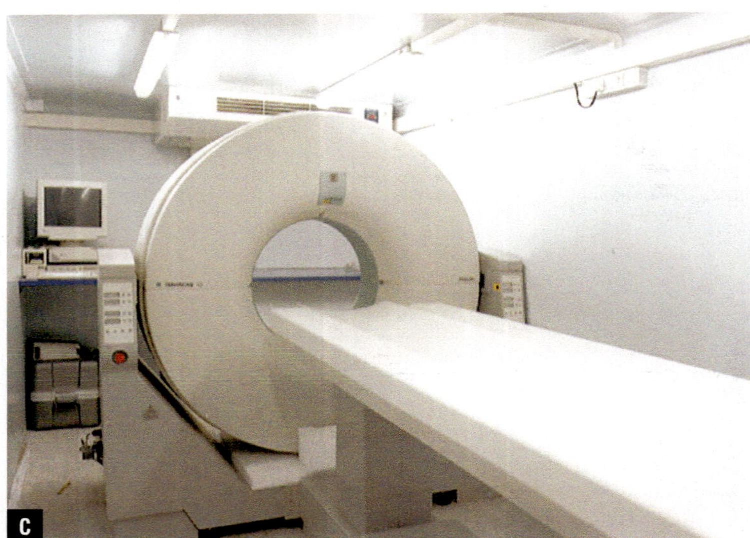

Scanner module

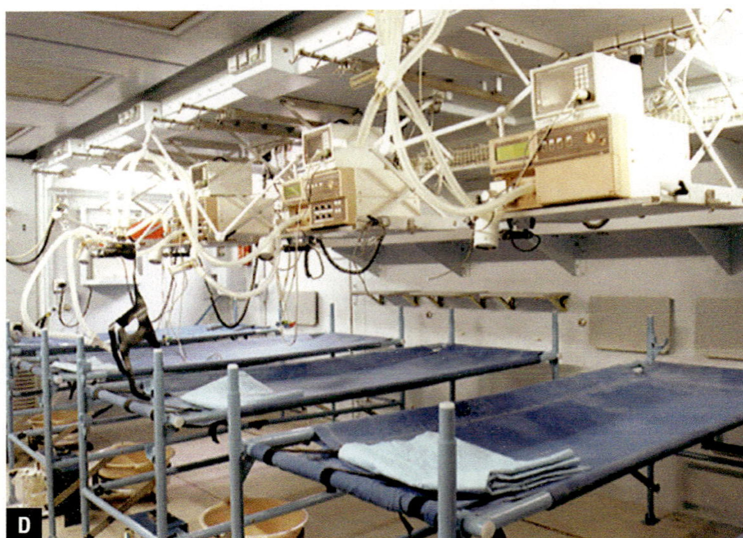

Intensive care module

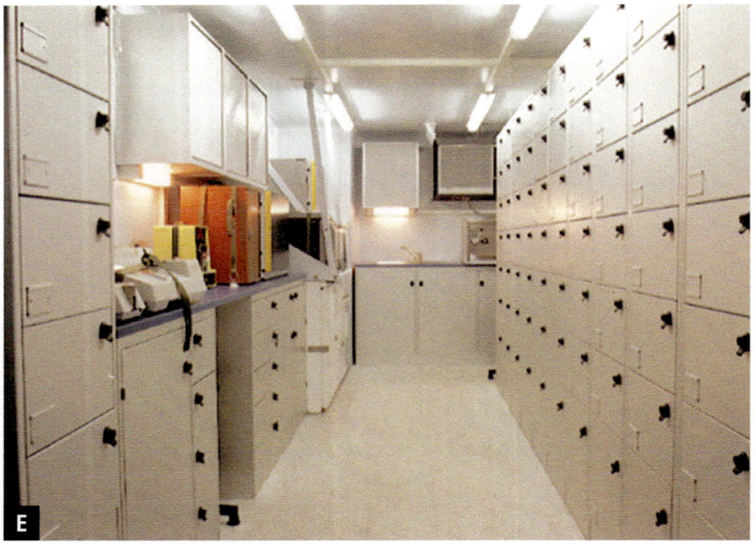

Laboratory module

Figs. 8A to E: Clinical System: Different modules.

CONCLUSION

Mobile health units have their uses, but they must be considered carefully, in emergency situations and areas affected by conflict, mobile units may be the only way to provide a selection of priority services to the population. Setting up mobile health services is never easy, and several factors need to be taken into account the possible modes of action, their role in the healthcare system, whether they respond to the priority needs as assessed, whether resources are available to implement these services, and whether this is and appropriate strategy. The services provided must be chosen carefully, in order to respond to health priorities. MHUs have a number of drawbacks (Communication, logistics, scheduling problems), and these must be considered. Nonetheless mobile health units can be a suitable option for outreach programs, and to bridge the mismatch between demand and supply of healthcare delivery system.[2,3]

REFERENCES

1. www.nrhmorissa.gov.in
2. www.odihpn.org
3. www.reliefweb.int
4. en.wikipedia
5. Deborah MS, Angeline B, Janice P, Eizabeth S. The Journal of nursing administration (Joxia). 1999; 29(2), pp 34-41, Copyright: © 1999 Lippincott Williams and Wilkins, Inc. Publication Type: (Articles) ISSN: 0002-0443 Accession: 00005110-199902000-00009 [Articles] Factors to Consider When buying a mobile health unit moulavi.
6. Moulavi D, Angelus B. Factors to Consider When Buying a Mobile Health Unit, "JONA Feb. 1999;29(2):34-41.
7. Mobile Health Units in emergency operations; Methodological approach. Stephane Du Mortier and Rudi Coninx, Number 60 June, 2007.
8. Chandrasekhar R. Report Emergency Mobile Field Hospital vide Director (EMR)'s letter No. D. 302020/6/2001—EMR, dated 8th May, 2001.

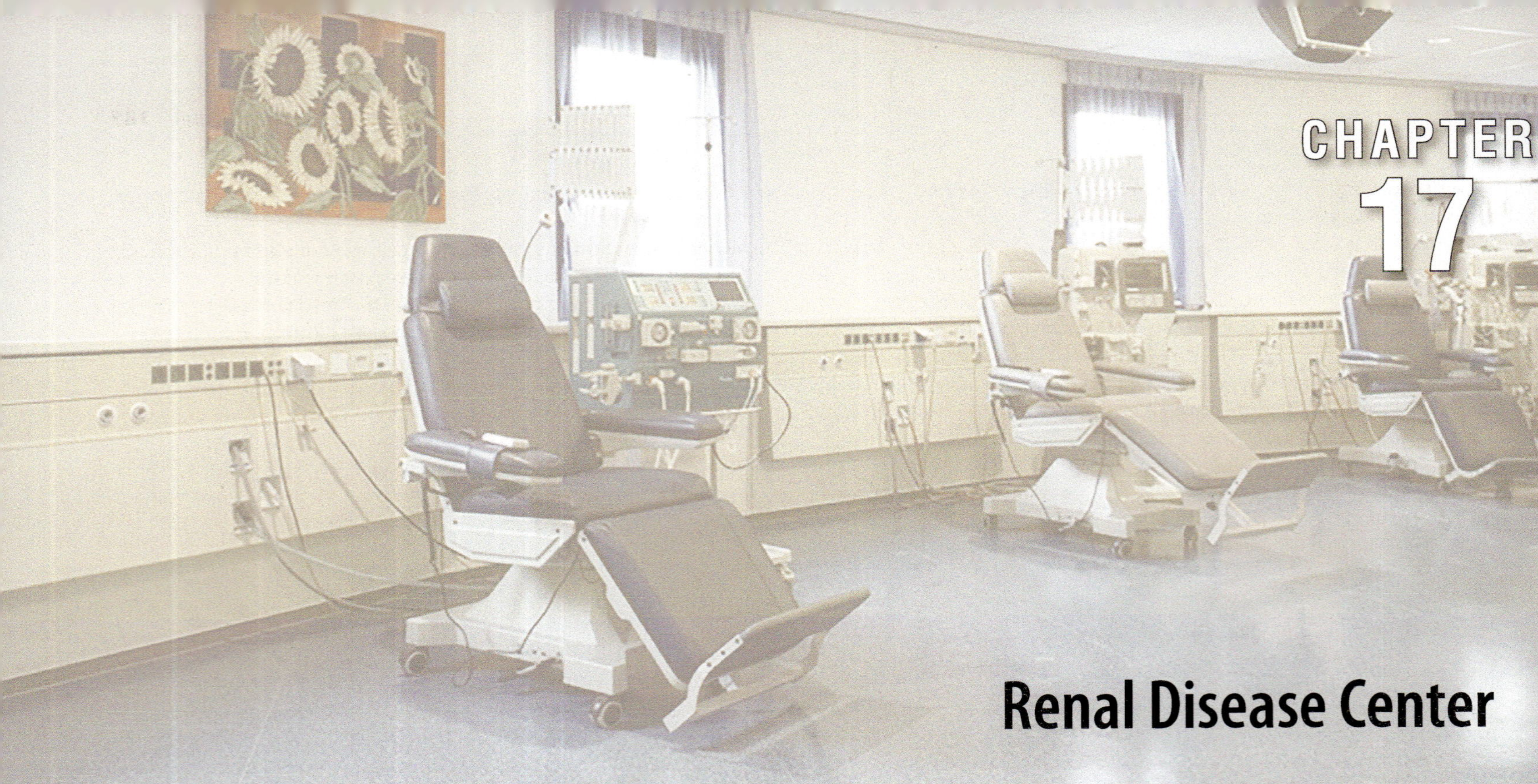

Renal Disease Center

Priti Goel, Shakti Kumar Gupta, Sunil Kant, R Chandrashekhar

INTRODUCTION

The prevalence of chronic renal failure is high and for effective management of end-stage renal disease, it is essential to have facilities of a renal disease center.

FUNCTIONS[1]

The function of the main renal unit is to provide a continuum of care for adult patients suffering from renal disease at all points on this continuum. Patients attending a main renal unit might arrive there through the following:

- Referral from primary care
- Referral from nonrenal secondary care
- Referral from renal secondary care
- Referral from acute care services (A and E departments)
- Self-referral by established renal patients.

In addition to the provision of dialysis facilities (i.e. both hemodialysis and peritoneal dialysis), it also has:

- A renal transplant facility
- A renal ward for the care of acutely and chronically ill renal patients;
- An outpatient facility
- An administration facility
- A technical services area.

Patients and/or assistants may attend the main renal unit for home hemodialysis training to learn how to undertake independent hemodialysis in their homes. All renal patients attending the renal unit should be given a welcoming, calming and attractive environment.

GENERAL DESIGN CONSIDERATIONS OF A RENAL UNIT[1,2]

Access to Main Renal Unit

As the main renal unit uses a considerable amount of consumables and needs to dispose of-large volumes of clinical and nonclinical waste daily, it should ideally be situated on the ground floor.

Entrance

It should have a separate dedicated entrance for patients and their assistants and staff.

This entrance should be wide enough to allow access by disabled patients in wheelchairs or using walking aids, and should be able to comfortably accommodate a peak of patient/staff flows at dialysis-shift and working-shift changeovers.[1]

There also needs access to the hospital large enough to permit the patients to come to the unit on a bed. This link needs to be a covered "corridor".

There should also be an entrance to the ward and administration area which allows the medical staff an access without them having to go through patient waiting areas, such as those in outpatients or the hemodialysis area.[1]

Patients attending the main renal unit are likely to arrive at the unit by a variety of means—Public transport, taxi, ambulance, own transport, and assistants transport. To facilitate patient access, therefore, the entrance to the main renal unit should, where possible, be located near public transport routes.[1]

It is also important to provide dropping-off points for ambulances, taxis and assistants transport. The dropping-off point for ambulances should be large enough to accommodate several ambulances, as the ambulance staff may have to leave their vehicles there while taking patients to their destination within the main renal unit.[1]

The entrance to the unit should be covered so that patients transferring from a vehicle into the unit are not exposed to the weather. Other facilities provided should include:[1]

- Diapers-changing and baby/infant-feeding facilities
- Buggy/pushchair parking
- Public telephones
- Refreshment facilities.

Car Parking

Car parking spaces should be provided immediately adjacent to the unit and as near to the entrance of the dialysis area as possible. It is recommended that there is at least one dedicated parking space for every three dialysis stations.[1]

Project teams should bear in mind that, as the age of dialysis patients is likely to increase; thought should be given to the future needs for 'differently able' car parking spaces. Local practices might also require nearby a dedicated parking for community-based staff, a such as technicians for home hemodialysis and home-visiting nursing staff, which may have to carry heavy or bulky supplies or equipment between the main renal unit and their vehicles.[1]

Signage

There should be on-road and plated signage indicating that the drop-off bay, ambulance bay and delivery bay are for the main renal unit's exclusive use. The car parking spaces should be clearly marked to indicate that they are for the exclusive use of patients visiting the main renal unit. Accordingly, it is recommended that the 'differently able car parking' bays are also marked to indicate that they are for the exclusive use of differently able renal patients.[1]

There should also be signposting from the main renal unit to the main hospital, and especially those departments within the main hospital which are of particular relevance to renal patients: Radiology, cardiology and urology.[1]

Infection Control

The primary measures for prevention of BBV (blood-borne viral) transmission are:[3]

- All staff should cover cuts and abrasions with waterproof dressings
- Staff should wear protective clothing (gloves, aprons, and facial protection) whenever there is a risk of exposure to blood or body fluids.
- Staff should change gloves and aprons and decontaminate their hands in between attending to different patients, or different caring activities for the same patient.
- All exposed surfaces in and adjacent to each patient's treatment station should be washed with neutral detergent and hot water and thoroughly dried in between patient treatments; where there is visible blood, disinfection should be carried out.
- Care should be taken to avoid injury with sharp instruments
- Multi-use vials should only be used for individual patients
- Adequate treatment space and staffing should be provided to ensure safe working practices.

Information Technology

The project team should plan for the future and consider for allowing:[1]

- Computer monitoring of the dialysis-machine data
- Computerised transfer of patient information from the initial monitoring area to the dialysis machine, for example by electronic "key".
- Bed-head and dialysis-station access for staff to the renal data system, where telemetry might be a good idea.
- Integration of handheld devices with the system
- Provision of an internet connection at each dialysis station and bed-head for patients.

SPECIFIC FUNCTIONAL AND DESIGN REQUIREMENTS OF A RENAL UNIT[1]

Renal Outpatient Department

Location

Ideally, renal outpatient department should be located at the fringe of the main renal unit and be on the ground floor. It should be immediately adjacent to the patient dialysis (PD) area and the renal ward.[1]

The outpatient area should have covered links with other hospital departments, particularly radiology, cardiology, intensive care and urology. Access to adjacent areas that lead to the renal outpatient area should be fitted with disabled access facilities. The functional relationship is shown in Figure 1.

Reception/Waiting Area

Reception Office

Secretarial and other administrative staff is based in this office. Duties of administrative staff may include management of the patient appointment system, management of patient transport systems, general correspondence, and liaison with other parts of the healthcare system, preparation of reports and analysis of statistics.[1]

Waiting/refreshment Area

A waiting area should offer a comfortable and relaxing environment. There should be space for patients in wheelchairs to continue sitting in their wheelchairs while waiting, and for people using walking aids. There should also be a children's play area. A supply of general reading material should be available. There should be a next-patient call system to alert waiting patients when their appointment time has arrived. This

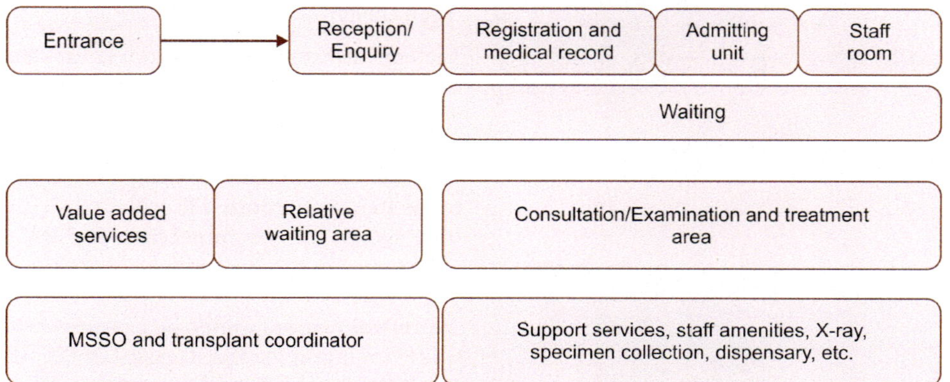

Fig. 1: Functional relationship of outpatient department.
(MSSO: medical social service officer)

could take the form of both an audible and a visual display system. A vending machine for hot and cold drinks is an option. A public telephone with an acoustic hood should be provided in accordance with hospital policy. A free phone for taxis should also be considered.[1]

Washroom for Patients and Escorts

Separate male and female washroom should be provided close to the waiting area for use by all the patients and assistants.

Examination/Treatment Room

Treatment Room

One or more treatment rooms will be needed for examining, assessing and treating patients. Patients may arrive in a wheelchair, on a stretcher trolley or in a bed. There should be enough room for one patient and three other people. Data points should be provided for picture archive and communication systems (PACS). A worktop is required where sterile packs, lotions and drugs for immediate use are stored and prepared for use, and where dressing/instrument trolleys can be prepared for use and/or held. An emergency call point and clinical wash-hand facilities are also required. The room should be sound-attenuated. Natural light is preferred but not essential. The treatment room should have easy access to both the clean utility and the dirty utility, and have enough space available for the disposal of clinical and nonclinical waste bins.[1]

Combined Consulting/examination Room(s)

The main renal unit houses various disciplines. Each discipline will need space to hold its own clinics (although not necessarily separate space). Therefore, the number of consulting/examination rooms that need to be provided for this purpose should be based on the size of the patient population, the number of clinics and consultants, and the number of services provided in other units.[1]

Venepuncture/Phlebotomy (Fig. 2)

This area will be used for taking and testing of blood specimens.

MSSO Room/Interview/Counseling Room

A Medical Social Service Officer (MSSO) room should be provided where patients and relatives can be interviewed in a relaxed environment that ensures that their privacy and dignity are maintained. Acoustic privacy is important. Semi-easy chairs and a desk space for one person should be provided.[1]

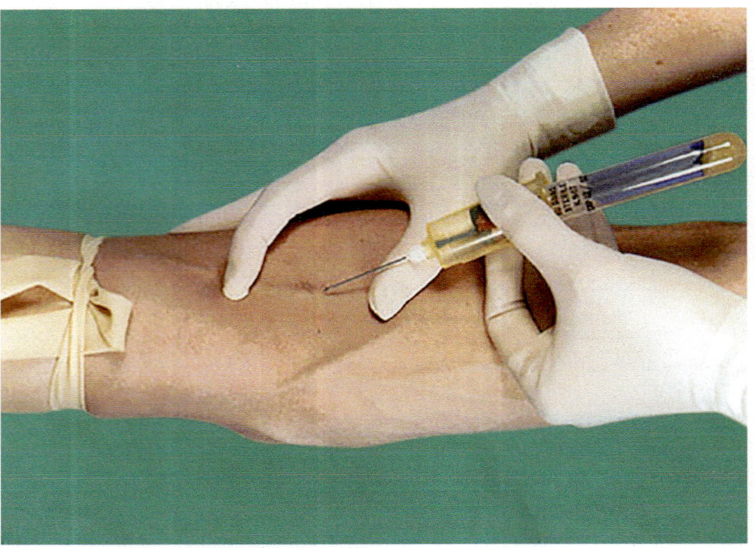

Fig. 2: Venepuncture/phlebotomy.

Office Accommodation

Nurse Manager's Office

This office is the administrative base for the renal outpatients area. It should be sufficiently private for confidential discussions among staff. The office should accommodate a workstation with computer and keyboard, seating for up to three other people, and storage for books and files.[1]

Support/Utility Services

Staff Restroom

Provision of rest-room facilities where staff can relax and take beverages and snacks, can be shared with other departments within the main renal unit. However, local considerations, including the length of clinics, may mean that such facilities should be included. Pantry facilities for staff may be needed if staff cannot easily use other renal-unit or hospital facilities for consuming or preparing food and beverages.[1]

Staff Change/locker Room

Separate male and female staff change/locker rooms should be provided where staff can change into a uniform and store outdoor clothing and other personal items.[1]

Personal full-length lockers for the secure storage of garments, footwear and small personal belongings are required. The number of lockers provided should be arrived at following consultation with staff, bearing in mind any likely future expansion of the unit, and included in the design brief. Separate male and female showers should be provided en-suite. The staff change/locker room door should be lockable.[1]

Staff Sanitary Facilities

Gender-specific sanitary facilities, including Western commode (WC) with wash-hand basins and a WC accessible to the disabled, should be located adjacent to the staff change/locker room.[1]

Patients' Sanitary Facilities

Separate male and female sanitary facilities, including WC with wash-hand basins, should be provided.[1]

General Storage Area

A back-up store specifically for sterile supplies such as bulk dressing packs, syringes and needles, will be required to supplement supplies held in the clean utility room and working supplies held in individual spaces within the department.[1]

Clean Utility

A clean utility room is required for storing and preparing drugs, medicines and lotions, and for holding a working supply of clean and sterile supplies. A controlled drugs cupboard—attached to a load-bearing wall and alarm—may be located here. A refrigerator will be required to store specific drugs. The clean utility should be adjacent to the treatment room. Clinical wash-hand facilities are required. The floor should have an impervious finish.[1]

Dirty Utility

A dirty utility room should be provided, where items of equipment may be cleaned and for the disposal of liquid and solid waste. The room should be fitted with a sluice sink, a sink-unit with drainer, a wash-hand basin, a work surface, cupboards and shelves (Fig. 3). Bedpan disposal

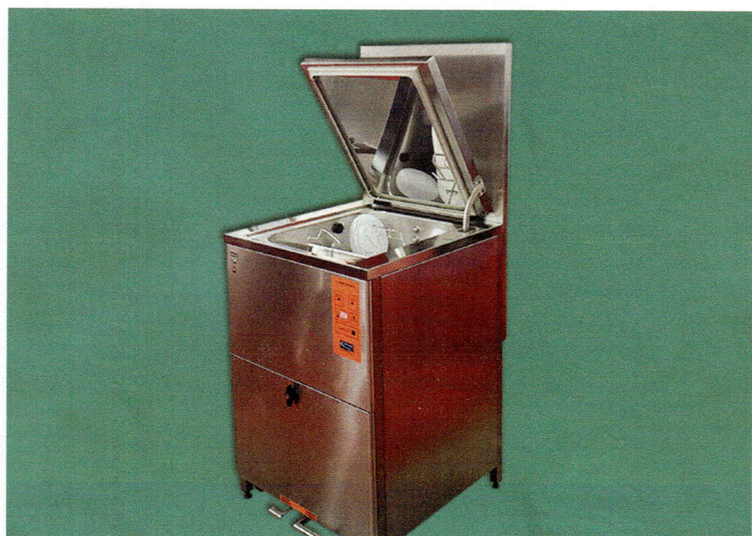

Fig. 3: Dirty utility—Bedpan sanitizer.

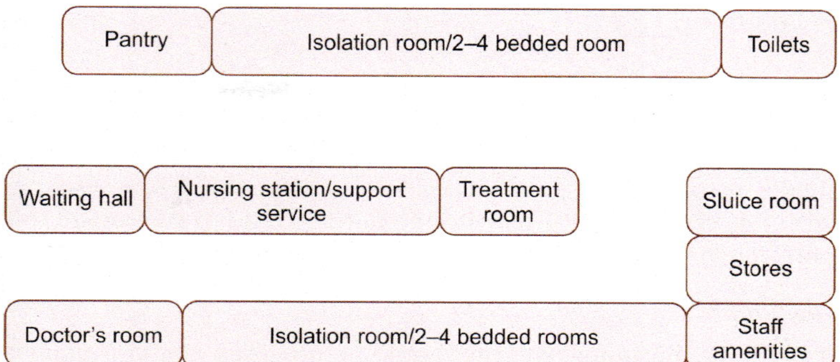

Fig. 4: Functional relationships of inpatient area.

facilities are required. Space should be available to park trolleys and for temporarily holding bags of soiled linen, etc. Pedal-operated sack-stands are also required. The floor should have an impervious finish. A secure collection area for clinical waste and nonclinical waste should be provided. There should also be separate external access for clinical waste bins.[1]

Disposal Room

The disposal room is the temporary storage point for all items of supplies and equipment which have to be removed for cleaning, reprocessing or disposal, for example linen, waste disposal and sharps. The room should allow for cleaning of any spillage from the clinical waste bags. The floor should have an impervious finish.[1]

Cleaners' Room

This could be shared with those available in other functional areas of the main renal unit. Space and facilities must be sufficient for parking and maneuvering cleaning machines and a cleaners' trolley, cleansing of cleaning equipment, and disposal of fluids and used cleaning materials. Hand washing facilities are also required. Shelving and vertical storage should not encroach on the working space or restrict access to the cleaners' sink.[1]

Electrical Distribution Cupboard

An electrical distribution cupboard, with lockable doors, housing the main isolators and distribution fuse switchgear should be:[1]

- Accessible directly from a circulation area (access space may be part of the circulation area).
- Sited away from water services
- Lockable.

FUNCTIONAL AREAS

Inpatient Accommodation

The functional relationships are shown in Figure 4.

Bed Spaces

There should be enough space in each bay or room for appropriate weighing equipment to be brought to the bedside or into the bay before a dialysis session. There should also be enough space to use a hoist, as there will be a greater number of wheelchair users in the main renal unit.[1]

Bed Provision

The total number of beds on the ward will need to be arrived at through local consultations, with assessment of current and projected demand.[1]

Bed-head Services

Every bed-head should have a nurse call button which can be reached by patients, and an emergency call button for staff. A communication and entertainment system with individual TV, radio, video and stereo headphone systems,[1] and a telephone handset that allows patients to both make and receive calls, should be provided.[1]

Televisions may be suspended from the ceiling, mounted on walls, placed on mobile units or, if flat-screen, secured to a swing-out arm for each patient. To avoid disturbance to other patients, sound outputs from radios, televisions and other auditory equipment should be through headphones only.[1]

Consideration should also be given to providing patients with laptop-computer access to the internet through a data-point or wireless connection. Each bed head should have outlets for medical gases and vacuum, and (where required) be plumbed for dialysis-standard water, and have drainage outlet points.[1]

Isolation Room(s)

Where an isolation room is provided in the renal ward, a negative air-pressure facility may be needed. The room should be accessible from the main renal ward and have a window through which the patients and staff can see one another. The door to the isolation room should be kept closed as much as possible so that the required direction of air movement is minimally disturbed. An emergency call button is needed in each isolation room. An en-suite shower and WC should be provided within the isolation room.[1]

Staff Base

The staff base/bases should be located so that staff sitting at the base can observe the patients in the bed bays/rooms under their care. Staff bases should not, however, be a source of disturbance to patients. The likely numbers of nursing staff, the choice and location of monitoring and computing equipment, storage policies and requirements for notes (with due regard to patient confidentiality), forms and other stationery must be considered. Work-surface provision should cater flexibly for differing and evolving configurations of computers and monitors. All staff bases should have terminals for ward and hospital communication systems, including computer, telephones, call systems and alarms, and at least one should have a fax terminal.[1]

Waiting Area

A waiting area should offer a comfortable and relaxing environment, with domestic-type finishes and furnishings. Different types of seating are required, and should include those suitable for older people. There should be space for patients in wheelchairs and for people using walking aids. Refreshment facilities offering hot and cold drinks should be provided.[1]

Day Room

A small day room for patients should be provided. Patients can sit and rest here after meals, watch television and listen to the radio. A bookcase with various reading materials should be provided, along with an occasional table. The day room should be accessible, with a variety of seating heights to help ambulant disabled people.[1]

Minor Operations Room(s)

Depending on the size of the ward and local policies and practices, a minor procedures room will be needed in which medical and nursing staff can perform minor diagnostic and treatment procedures requiring a clinical environment.[1]

Treatment Room

Same as outpatient.

Offices/Other Accommodation

Ward Sister's Office

This is the administration base for the ward sister. It should be sufficiently private for confidential discussions among the staff. The office should have a workstation with computer and keyboard, printer, photocopier, fax, seating for up to three other people, and storage for books and files. There should be space for a secure, controlled drugs cabinet to be installed on a load-bearing wall. This office should be near the staff base.[1]

Doctor's Office

A doctor's office should be provided in which medical staff can hold confidential discussions, make telephone calls and write up medical notes. It should be near the staff base.[1]

Support/Utility Services

Resuscitation Trolley Bay

A resuscitation trolley bay, with space for parking a resuscitation trolley (with defibrillator), a mobile suction unit and a cylinder of oxygen on a trolley, should be located with easy access to all spaces used by the patients.[1]

Clean Utility

Same as outpatient.

Dirty Utility

Same as outpatient.

Staff Restroom

Same as outpatient.

Staff Pantry

Pantry facilities are needed for the safe handling of food including the preparation of beverages and light snacks, for washing and storing crockery and cutlery, for storing a limited quantity of dry goods, and for the refrigerated storage of milk, etc. Equipment should include a stainless-steel sink and drainer, an electric water boiler, a microwave oven, a worktop with cupboards and a wash-hand basin.[1]

Equipment Store

Depending on the adjacency of the renal ward, this facility could be optional. If provided, this store should be large with plenty of racking. The exact size of the store will depend upon how frequently supplies are delivered. There should be provision for a bottled gas rack within this room. The store will require lockable and alarmed double doors.[1]

Fluid Store

A storeroom for bulk liquid deliveries should be considered. This room is optional accommodation.

General Storage Area

Same as outpatient.

Electrical Distribution Cupboard

Same as outpatient.

Peritoneal Dialysis

Location

Ideally, the peritoneal dialysis (PD) area should be located between renal out-patients and the renal ward or immediately adjacent to the two. The PD area should have signposted links with other hospital departments, particularly radiology, cardiology and urology.[1]

Functional Areas

Washroom for Patients and Escorts

Same as outpatient.

Wheelchair Storage Area

It may be possible for patients to take wheelchairs into the consultation or teaching/dialysis rooms but, if not, a wheelchair storage area should be included for patients who, while undergoing a consultation or dialysis/teaching session, have to leave their chairs.[1]

Training Room

This room is used to teach the patients how to perform their own peritoneal dialysis safely and adequately, and to provide advice and education for patients and their families, enabling them to make best use of this treatment. The room should be well-lit and ventilated. Space must be allowed for fluid-bag warmers and for carrying out fluid exchanges. The room should be able to accommodate three patients/assistants and a PD nurse. An examination couch should also be provided. Patients should also have access to mobile or wheelchair scales. A whiteboard and video/TV should be provided. A general wash-hand basin and clinical wash-hand basin should be supplied.[1]

PD Treatment Area

Each dialysis/teaching bay should be equipped with an emergency call button. Project teams should consider providing computer outlets and/or telephone points in each bay. There should be enough space within a bay to accommodate a nurse, a patient and an escort. Clinical wash-hand facilities are required, as well as a separate sink for the disposal of saline solution and other waste products. The floor should have an impervious finish—such as vinyl with welded joints and coved skirting—as the risk of spillage of body fluids and other contaminants is high.[1]

Consulting/Examination Room(s)

One or more combined consulting/examination rooms will be needed depending on the number of patients the PD area is likely to deal with at any one time.[1]

Treatment/Procedures Room (Fig. 5)

A treatment/procedures room may be needed for medical and nursing staff to perform minor diagnostic and treatment procedures which require a clinical environment; for example, line changes for continuous ambulatory peritoneal dialysis (CAPD) patients. The level of asepsis required will depend on the treatments/procedures proposed. An examination light should be provided. A clinical wash-hand basin is also required. An emergency call system for the staff and a nurse-call system for the patient should be provided within this room.[1]

Sister's Office

Same as outpatient.

Clean Utility

Same as outpatient.

Dirty Utility

Same as outpatient.

Fluid Store

This store should be large, with plenty of racking, as dialysis fluid is consumed in high quantities. The store may need double doors to the outside of the building for receiving delivered goods. Alternatively, bulk delivery of fluids might go to a store shared with other parts of the main renal unit and then be redistributed to the PD area internally. Dialysis fluids need to be moved around on trolleys and pallets; there should be enough space within the PD area and in connecting corridors between the PD area and other parts of the main renal unit for this to be done safely and easily.[1]

General Storage Area

Same as outpatient.

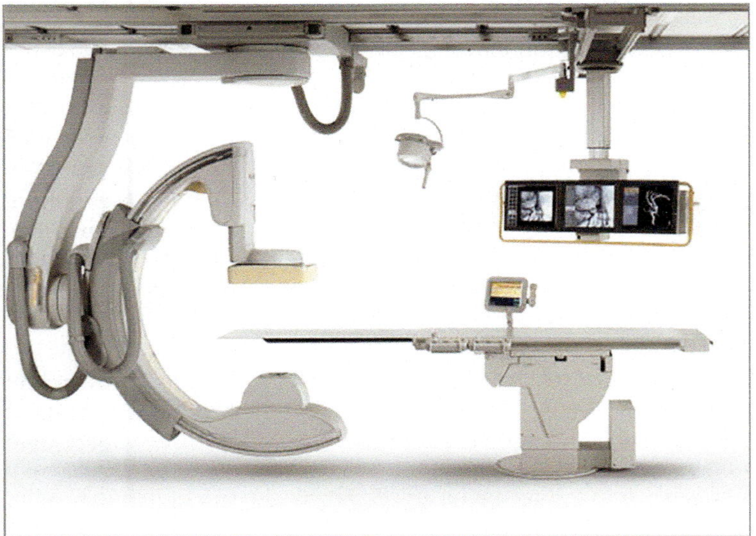

Fig. 5: Procedures room.

Hemodialysis Area

Location

Ideally, facilities for hemodialysis should be located at the fringe of the main renal unit and be on the ground floor. The hemodialysis area should be adjacent to the other areas within the main renal unit (peritoneal dialysis, renal outpatients, renal administration, renal ward, renal transplant, and renal technical services). The hemodialysis area should have covered bed-accessible links with other hospital departments, particularly radiology, cardiology, urology, diabetology and general wards.[1]

Functional Areas

Reception Office

An office is required at the entrance to the unit and adjacent to the waiting area for receiving and registering patients upon arrival and to provide the administrative and communication center of the unit. It must be possible for patients, escorts and staff to communicate easily. It is important to ensure that the reception office is accessible to people in wheelchairs and that counters or reception desks are suitable for patients in wheelchairs to be able to communicate with the staff at computer terminals. Consideration should be given to routing all telephone calls to and from the unit through the reception office.[1]

Waiting/Refreshment Area

A waiting area should offer different types of seating and should include those suitable for older people. The layout should be informal. There should be space for patients in wheelchairs and for people using walking aids. The waiting area is an important social space. The provision of notice boards and posters, low-level background music, a TV/video system, facilities for personal entertainment, and internet connections for patients using their own laptop computers can be made. A supply of reading material should be available. Refreshment facilities, public telephone with an acoustic hood, should be provided.[1]

Patient Changing Area/Locker Room

Separate male and female patient change/locker rooms should be provided where patients can change into comfortable clothing before dialysis and can store their outdoor clothing and other personal items while they are on the machines.[1]

Patients' Sanitary Facilities

Separate male and female sanitary facilities, including WCs with wash-hand basins, should be located adjacent to the patient changing/locker room. Patient sanitary facilities should include an accessible toilet, and baby changing facilities. Patients need to provide urine samples; thus, this area requires good ventilation.[1]

Wheelchair Storage Area

A wheelchair storage area should be included for patients who, while being dialyzed, have to leave their chairs.

Treatment Area

Patient-monitoring Area (Fig. 6)

This space is used to monitor and record patients' weight, blood pressure and general health before each dialysis treatment. Data may be recorded either on computer or on paper, depending on local policy. Facilities required include: chair weighing scales and wheelchair weighing scales, a desk and chair, storage for blood pressure equipment.[1]

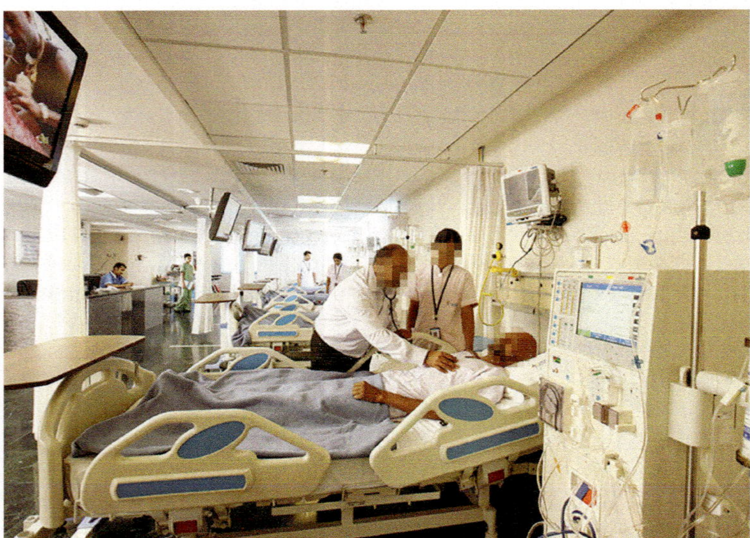

Fig. 6: Monitoring the patients.

Multifaith/Quiet Room

This room will be used as a quiet room for worship, meditation, reflection and counseling. Accessories of worship vary in accordance with denomination or faith, and, therefore, suitable storage cupboards should be provided. Appropriate washing facilities should be provided.[1]

Dialysis Area

The dialysis area should consist of dialysis stations in increments of three. Sufficient space must be allowed for the chair to be fully reclined, and for nurses to carry out procedures. Treatment stations will need to be arranged so that the patients can be attached to the machine either by arm or by cannulae in their neck or groin. If beds are to be used instead of reclining chairs, floor areas for each station will need to be reviewed, as area allowance is slightly larger for bed provision. One emergency call button (with an audible and visual alarm) per station should be provided.[1]

Facilities are required at the station for the storage of frequently used medical items, and for patients to carry out seated activities, including watching television, while undergoing dialysis. Storage shelves should be located so that items can be seen and reached easily by staff and patients. A mobile table may also be used by the patients for storing books, newspapers and other personal belongings, and by staff for recording the patient's notes.[1]

There should be at least one wash-hand basin between two stations. The basin should be located as near to the station as possible without causing risk of splashing and cross-infection. At each station, there needs to be:[1]

- An alcohol hand-rub dispenser
- A wall-mounted soap dispenser
- A towel dispenser
- A clinical and nonclinical waste bin
- A sharps container.

The floor should be slip-resistant, easily cleanable, and have an impervious finish with coved skirting, as the risk of spillage of body fluids and other contaminants is high.

Adequate adjustable lighting should be installed on walls and ceilings for use by staff carrying out procedures and by patients for reading, writing, etc. Lighting controls should be within easy reach of patients and staff. Consideration should be given to the provision of a communication and entertainment system with individual TV, radio, video and stereo headphone systems, and a telephone handset that allows the patients to both make and receive calls. Televisions may be suspended from the ceiling, mounted on walls, placed on mobile units or, if flat-screen, on a swing-out arm for each patient. To avoid disturbance to other patients, sound outputs from radios, televisions and other auditory equipment should be via headphones only. Consideration should also be given to providing access to the internet through a data point or wireless connection for patients who have laptop computers.[1]

The provision of medical gases, including oxygen, medical air and vacuum, at each station, is for local consideration.

Isolation Room

Same as inpatient.

Staff Base

Same as inpatient.

Resuscitation Trolley Bay

Same as inpatient.

Consulting/Examination Room

One or more combined consulting/examination rooms will be needed for consultation and examination. The room should be large enough to accommodate a doctor, a nurse, a patient (who may be in a wheelchair), and an escort/carer. Clinical wash-hand facilities are required. A telephone may also be required.[1]

Treatment/Procedures Room

Same as peritoneal dialysis area.

Training Room

This room is used for the general education of patients and their escorts.

Technical Services Manager's Office

Office space should be provided for the manager of the renal unit's technical services, as it is inappropriate to carry out managerial functions within the general working/maintenance area, and there is also a need for privacy. It should accommodate a workstation with computer and keyboard, seating for up to three other people, and storage for books and files.[1]

Support/Utility Area

Water-treatment Plant Room

For hemodiafiltration, the water quality must achieve ultrapure standards. To achieve ultrapure water standards "double-pass reverse osmosis (RO)" may be required, and this will have an effect on the space allocated to the water treatment room. It is important that the plant be close to the dialysis area (although not adjacent to it because of noise considerations) as this will shorten the distance covered by the distribution ring. There should be sufficient space to accommodate a maximum of two people to monitor, adjust service and repair the water treatment plant. The plant room should be sized to accommodate the plant and storage of chemicals. Areas within the plant room providing bulk storage of any corrosive liquids should be suitably sealed and bonded. The plant room floor should be sloped to a drain and treated with a chemical-resistant sealant, and the door accesses should have a lip and ramp to prevent water seeping to the rest of the unit in the event of a large water leak. The floor should also be "bunded" to contain any major water leakage. The door should be lockable for security.

The plant room should be adequately lit and ventilated. Mechanical ventilation may be necessary if the heat gain from the water treatment plant cannot be controlled by natural ventilation. The water treatment plant room should not house any other equipment other than that which is specific to its function.[1]

Clean Utility

Same as outpatient.

Dirty Utility

Same as outpatient.

Staff Restroom

Same as out patient.

Pantries: Patients and Staff

Same as inpatient.

Staff Change/Locker Room

Same as outpatient.

Staff Sanitary Facilities

Same as outpatient.

Equipment Store

Same as inpatient.

Fluid Store

A storeroom for "bulk fluid" deliveries should be considered. This is a different way of providing dialysis fluid and requires one or more tanks to be installed for storing the fluid. The size of this room will depend on the number of stations and the frequency of delivery. This room is optional accommodation as not every unit will use this system.[1]

Linen Storage

There must be segregation of clean and dirty linen. Dirty linen should be temporarily held in the disposal room. There should be sufficient space within the clean linen store for the storage of towels, pillows, blankets, etc. and access for linen trolleys to be loaded/unloaded.[1]

General Storage Area

Same as out patient.

Electrical Distribution Cupboard

Same as outpatient.

Home Hemodialysis Training Room

Location

It should have its own separate area—training should not take place where other patients are dialyzing. Ideally, it should be adjacent to the renal outpatients and hemodialysis area.[1]

This unit can share the reception/waiting area with the hemodialysis unit.

Renal Transplant Operation Theater

The minimum total number of operating rooms for the center must be:

- Organ retrieval : 1
- Kidney transplant: 2- Cadaver, 2- Live

At least, 2 operating suites for 20 beds must be dedicated for only kidney transplant procedures, if it is a part of multispecialty/tertiary care hospital.

Functional Areas[4,5]

Planning Parameters

An operating unit design with a sterile core must provide for no cross-traffic of staff and supplies from the decontaminated/soiled areas to the sterile/clean areas. The use of facilities outside the operating room for soiled decontaminated processing and clean assembly and sterile processing should be designed to move the flow of goods and personnel without compromising universal precautions or aseptic techniques in both departments.

Location

The operating unit should be located and arranged to prevent nonrelated traffic through the suite. As per the planning of this center, the operating room is preferably located on the last floor of the center.

Operating Suite (Fig. 7)

Preference of modular theater for procedure area which consists of prefabricated units for operating suites complete with integrated mechanical and electrical service including air-conditioning should be utilized. In addition, the operating room must integrate with the telemedicine department of the center.

- It must be prefabricated jointless operation theater with all structural steel sections of grade 43 to BS 4360 or equivalent Indian standard.
- The floor should be of the type that does not promote bacteriological growth and the finish should be 2 mm static conductive PVC tiles, laid on a semiconductive adhesive base. The floor finish should be smooth, nonslip impervious material, seamless, welded and washable and terminate at the room perimeter passing over a concealed cover former and continuing up the wall for 100 mm. The doors of the OT must be 2100 mm in height and 1500 mm in width for patient entry and 2100 mm in height and 1000 mm in width for staff's entry. All the doors should be hermetically sealed to maintain sterility and correct air pressure. The edges should get sealed in closed position. All doors should be able to be operated manually in the event of power failure.

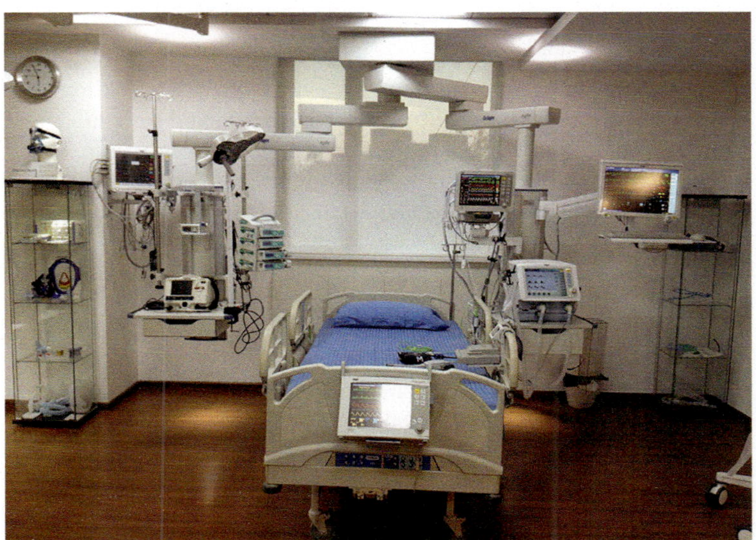

Fig. 7: Operating suite.

- The ceiling must be impervious, sound proof and seamless and its height must be 3.0 m. The ceiling should provide optimum air distribution over the patient area, integrated with shadowless lighting. The ceiling should be constructed with a plenum box supplied with central air-conditioning system. HEPA filters mounted on the exit from the supply ducting. It should include integral lighting and composite air/light diffuser. The laminar flow ceiling should have illumination across its total area.
- The lighting should be evenly distributed throughout the room. General illumination is furnished by ceiling lights. To minimize eye fatigue, the ratio of intensity of general room lighting to that at the surgical suite should not exceed 1:5, preferably 1:3. It should be sufficient to provide an illumination level of 1500 lux at the wound site and should be dimmable down to 3% of full lighting, without flicker. It is a combination of one major and one satellite light-head with intensity of about 1,10,000 for major and 1,00,000 for satellite light-head with individual intensity control arrangements for each light-head. The color temperature is 3300 K and color rendering index is 95 Ra. Shadow reduction is to be achieved by prismatic optical system.
- *The panels:* All controls within the theater should be located on a membrane control panel mounted in the theater wall. It must consist of time elapse clock, standard clock, temperature and humidity indicators, temperature and humidity set points adjust, plenum lighting controls, and medical gas alarms.
- *Medical gases:* Main storage of medical gases must be outside the facility and reticulated internally to gas outlets. Provisions shall be made for additional separate storage of reserve gas cylinders necessary to complete at least one-day's procedures.
- *Others:* Writing board, equipment storage unit, pressure stabilizer and surgical scrub system.

Reception Area

To receive patients to the unit, with general overseeing of day-to-day operations, control of entry and exit from the unit and completion of general administrative tasks.

Holding Area

This area must be located away from the operation theater complex and preferably it can be located in the ward floor area. The area should be 7.5 sqm and should have a clearance of 1.22 m which can hold a trolley/bed for the patient.

Patient Transfer Area

There must be an earmarked route for patient from the holding area and the operating theater and this can also be used for transfer of patients from different areas of the hospital to operating room. It will be convenient to have a separate route/corridor for the transfer of patients from all areas of the hospital to operating theater.

Storage

Adequate equipment store room(s) for equipment and supplies used in the operating unit should be provided. Equipment stores should be provided at the minimum rate of 10 sqm per operating room. Store rooms are best designed in an elongated rectangular form to allow easy access to all items. Storage bays should be provided for equipment such as portable X-ray machine, stretchers, warming devices and auxiliary lamps. Storage bays should be provided at the minimum rate of 5 sqm per operating room and minimum dimension of 0.8 m (1 m preferred). These areas should be out of corridors and traffic. This can be satisfied by recessing the bay with the corridor width. Adequate storage facility must be provided in the theater in the form of adjustable open shelving systems.

Equipment Room

An area for testing operating equipment also requires consideration in the planning stage of on-site facility needs. Part of the operating unit general store may be used for this function, or a dedicated room for this purpose may be necessary. Sometimes, it is referred to as the biomedical engineering room.

Recovery Area

It must have medication station, hand washing station, nurse station, and storage space for stretchers, supplies and equipment. The area should be 7.5 sqm and should have a clearance of 1.22 m to accommodate a trolley/bed. Administrative and staff area includes change rooms, staff rooms, offices and administrative space for clinical staff.

Change Rooms

Appropriate change rooms should be provided for male and female personnel (nurse, doctors and technicians) working within the operating unit. The change rooms should contain adequate lockers, showers, toilets, hand basins and space for donning surgical attire and booting. These staff rooms should be arranged to encourage a one-way traffic pattern so that personnel entering from outside the surgical suite can change and move directly into the operating unit and the entry must be from nonsterile area with proper infection control measures. The change room entrance door should be provided with locks or electronic access devices to prevent the entry of unauthorized persons into the operating unit.

Coffee Room/Lounge

It should be provided within the unit for staff to relax and prepare beverages. Inclusion of a window to the outside is desirable. Staff room may be made separately for various categories of staff, such as doctors, nurses, paramedical staff, etc. The air-conditioning of this area must be segregated by proper compartmentalization and connected to exhaust system.

Sterilizing Facilities

Sterilizing facilities with high-speed sterilizers or other sterilizing equipment for immediate or emergency use must be grouped to several operating rooms for convenient and efficient use. A workspace and hand washing facility should be included in this area. The facilities for processing and sterilizing reusable instruments may be located in other area of hospital unit such as central sterile supply department (CSSD).

Infection Control

A room must be provided for an infection control nurse with a table and chair along with required stationery and also for taking samples for testing. A clinical hand wash basin should be provided within the room. The room must be of 9 sqm.

Preparation/Lay-up Room

This is the room in the operating unit where clean or sterile materials are held and arranged prior to use during the operation.

Toilets

Toilets should be provided at the minimum ratio of one per operating room but no fewer than two. Showers should be provided at the minimum ratio of one per two operating rooms but no fewer than two. The toilets and showers are to be divided equally between male and female change rooms. It must be located in the nonsterile zone of the theater.

Security and Fire

The fire detection system should comprise smoke detectors and heat detectors located at strategic locations in the OT and connected to a fire alarm panel at a convenient location.

Clean Utility Room

The room may also provide storage for dangerous drugs. The clean utility should be a minimum of 12 sqm or 14 sqm when access is required from two sides of the room.

Dirty Utility Room

It may be combined with a disposal room for space efficiency. It should be a minimum of 10 sqm or 12 sqm when access is required from two sides of the room. If combined with disposal room, the combined room should be of 14 sqm.

Equipment and Special Fluids

The operation theater must be fully equipped with basic equipment such as anesthetic machines, cell shaver, rapid infuser, diathermy, venovenous bypass machine, central line catheters, cell separator, irradiators, flow cytometry, arterial blood gas (ABG) machine with lactate test, thromboelastography, AR gun, intraoperative USG machine, Doppler, cardiac monitor, patient-warming devices, refrigerator, deep freezes and special perfusion/preservative fluids such as Renogram for kidney transplant. An ice machine and cold-storage facilities should be provided for storage, transportation of organs, for treatment and patient use. These equipment must be provided with a room of 15 sqm with good lighting and storage shelves can be retrieved easily whenever required.

Operating Table

The OT table must be an electrohydraulic, operated on high storage capacity batteries and also must work on 220/240 V AC single-phase power supply; it must be disinfectant-resistant, radiolucent table top, with no crevices for ingress of liquids so as to enable proper infection control.

Intensive Care Unit[3]

Location

The intensive care unit of the center must be located in close proximity to the operation theaters which is easily accessible with lifts and ramps for doctors, staff, patients and visitors.

Functional Areas

Reception

The reception in the ICU acts as enquiry office, clerical office as well as center for coordination. It is to be provided with means of communication and separate work force for staffing it on 24 × 7 basis. Attached with the ICU is also a small waiting area where the attendants of critically ill patients can stay. It should be provided with reclining chairs and basic amenities of water, toilets and a television. The waiting area is important, as the attendants cannot be with the patient in the ICU. In India, usually one attendant is permitted with each patient, therefore, the waiting area should have appropriate space at the ratio of 1:1 to the number of beds in the ICU.

Patient Care Area

The following considerations are important for the patient care area in the ICU. Each bed should have adequate circulation space for 360° access to the patient. Space between the beds to be wide enough to accommodate large size trolleys typically required for dressing and movements for equipment, such as X-ray. Each bed should be clearly visible from the doctors/nurses duty station. Each bed must have dedicated equipment such as monitors, ventilators, etc. with manifold outlets and brackets for positioning and monitoring equipment. Distress call system should be installed on every bed. At least 15 sqm floor area for single-bed accommodation exclusive of service areas and at least 22 sqm floor area for multiple bed accommodation is recommended. The beds can be segregated for donor and recipients. Few beds must be earmarked for brain-dead patients who are potential donors.

Nursing Station

The nursing station in the patient area is to be on a raised platform for unhindered visibility. A common station for doctors and nurses can be made with separate tables for both. The station must have spaces for central monitoring system, clinical records, storage for frequently used medicines, consumables, equipment and an attached treatment bay. This bay is for housing various trolleys and resuscitation equipment. Monitoring equipment of each ICU bed must be independent in terms of equipment such as ventilator, cardiac monitor, medical gases, BP apparatus etc. Monitoring can also be made centralized where the parameters to be monitored are available at the nurse duty station in real-time mode. Mounting brackets for monitoring equipment should be sturdy and durable. It can be safely assumed that number of equipment will steadily increase over time.

Electrical Panels

Each bed must have at least 8 electrical points: Ventilator-1, two infusion pumps-3, multisign monitor-1, defibrillator-1, reserve-2. All the points in the panel must have 100% power backup, however, at least 4 points should be power backed up, i.e. always powered. The points should be composite type, i.e. should be able to take both 5 Amp and 15 Amp plugs. If all points do not have power backup, then the backed up points should be colored differently so that they are easily identifiable. All the plug points must be properly earthed.

Bed-head Panel

It should comprise outlets as follows—Two oxygen outlets, two vacuum outlets, one compressed air at 4 bars, one 9 W reading light, eight multipin 15 Amp, switch socket outlet combine (four to be backed up), one arm 1 Amp-60 W with adapter holder for vacuum collection jar, one infusion pump rail mount pole with adapter, two spare spaces, one nurse call switch (with wired remote).

Allied and Support Services

They include utility rooms, store rooms, linen, disposable room, cleaners room, pantry, staff amenities areas. These should be out of traffic paths but conveniently located outside the patient care area and should have independent access.

Equipment Room

Mobile equipment such as CPR trolleys and mobile X-ray units that are located within the ICU should require storage areas that are out of traffic paths but conveniently located for easy access by staff. Consideration should be given to the ever-increasing amount of equipment used.

Communication

The ICU should have communication facilities for communication with hospital staff, lab, blood bank and other key hospital departments. In addition to a standard telephone service, there should be a mechanism for emergency internal and external communications when normal systems fail such as mobile/paging. Plasma screen and telecom in areas linked up with ICU, so that entry to ICU is restricted and relatives can see their patients in waiting area, which not only prevents infection, but also prevents overcrowding and security problems of the area.

Hand Wash Facilities

Hand washing facilities should be provided conveniently to the staff station and patient and patient bed areas. A minimum of one hand wash unit per two beds is required though one such unit per bed is preferable. Along with this, there must also be alcohol-based hand rub disinfectants placed near each bed and in the areas easily accessible by the staff and attendants.

Circulation Space

When an open plan arrangement is provided, a circulation space of 2.4 sqm minimum clear widths should be provided beyond dedicated cubicle space. Separate cubicles and isolation rooms should be minimum 15 m^2. All doors and openings should be minimum 1.8 m wide to permit transit of heavy equipment, patient beds and trolleys. These should permit hassle-free movement and easy maneuverability.

Medical Imaging Services [2,3]

The diagnostic radiology services should consist of X-ray, fluoroscopy, ultrasonography, MRI scan and renal angiography.

Planning Considerations

- Easy access for the patients
- Adequate subwaiting area and having washrooms in close proximity
- Efficient record keeping preferably using picture archiving and communication system (PACS).

Design Considerations

- Flexibility in design to cater for future expansion in view of rapid advancements in technology
- Wide entrance and wide doors for the movement of trolleys and equipment
- Safety features as X-ray room is part of the complex. The design and construction of the X-ray room must cater to the guidelines issued by the Atomic Energy Regulatory Board (AERB) and Bhabha Atomic Research Center (BARC), such as thickness of the wall, lead lining and measurement of exposure to the staff, etc.

Location

Radiology services should ideally be located on ground floor and conveniently accessible to inpatient, outpatient and accident and emergency department.

X-ray Room

Optimum size of X-ray room 5.5 × 6 × 3 m^3 height is recommended. A control booth adequate radiation exposure protection should be located in the room. It is recommended that 2–4 well-lit and ventilated cubicles for each X-ray machine should be provided. For each X-ray room, two toilets should be provided.

Fluoroscopy Room

In fluoroscopy, radiopaque media is introduced into the body to create images of tissues that would not otherwise show up well on the X-ray. The room is recommended to be of 4.5 × 6 × 3 m height. The room should have an attached toilet. Intravenous pyelography is done in fluoroscopy room.

Ultrasound Room (Fig. 8)

Renal sonography is utilized to demonstrate soft tissue structures and to study physiological movements. The room should be minimum of 12 sqm. It should be located with access to patient toilet facilities from within the room. Facility for patient reception, registration and subwaiting should be provided based on the workload.

MRI Room

Magnetic resonance imaging (MRI) services may be provided as part of the medical imaging or as a free standing unit. It should be located with ready access to the emergency unit, operating unit and critical care area. Ground floor is the preferred location for an MRI unit.

Functional Areas

MRI computer room: It is required to accommodate the computer equipment. Recommended space is 35 sqm. It should be located adjacent to MRI scanning and console room.

MRI console room: It is required to accommodate the computer and other controls of the equipment. There should be a window to provide full view of the MRI room. A minimum space of 8 sqm is recommended.

Location: This provides the area and equipment for MRI scanning procedures. It should be located with direct access to console room. Magnetic and radiofrequency shieldings are required.

Schedule of accommodation of areas is shown in Table 1.

Renal Angiography

The angiography may be located within the medical imaging unit and it provides facilities for diagnostic X-ray investigation of renal blood vessels.

Functional Areas

Angiography room: It provides an area and equipment for angiography examination. The minimum space recommended is 40 sqm. A scrub suite for staff should be located outside the staff entry to the angiography room.

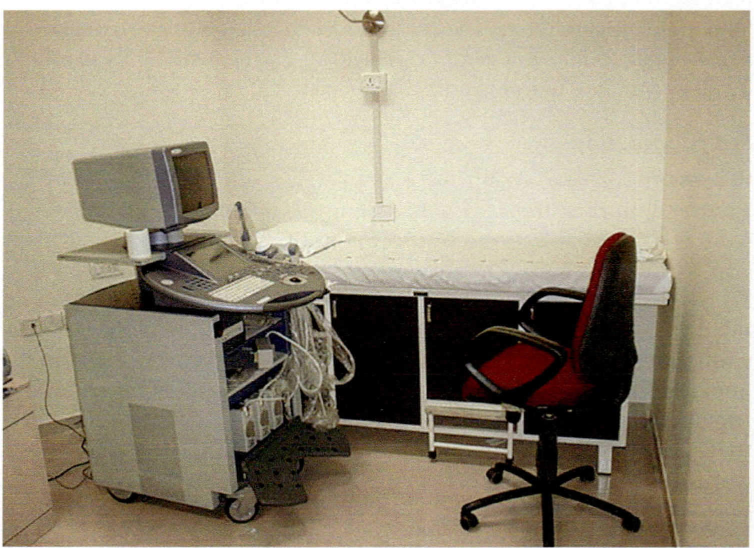

Fig. 8: Ultrasound room.

Table 1: Schedule of accommodation.

Areas	Recommended space requirements in sqm
Patient bay	9
Office for single person	9
Hand washing bay	1
Anesthesia induction	15
Toilets for patients	4
Change room for staff	8
Office for single person	9
Scrub up and gowning	8
Store	6–9
Toilets: Patient/staff	4/2

Control room: It provides for remote operation of the angiography equipment. A viewing window to permit full view of the patient should be provided. A space of 8 sqm is recommended.

Computer equipment room: A space of 6 sqm is recommended.

Laboratory Services

The laboratory of the center can be divided into two main categories:
- Routine laboratory
- Human leukocyte antigen (HLA) laboratory.

Routine Laboratory (Fig. 9)

- Biochemistry
- Hematology
- Microbiology
- Histopathology.

The lab must be provided with modules with each workstation consists of space for equipment such as microscope, incubator, centrifuge, etc.

Each workstation must be provided with below and overhead cabinets. The workstation should be equipped with vacuum, gas, electrical services, sinks and water. A revolving adjustable stool/chair must be provided along with each workstation. Adequate storage facilities for reagents, standards supplies, stained specimen microscopic slides and separate for chemicals and flammable liquids. The floor must be made of moisture-resistant tiles such as quarry or vitreous. The junctions of walls must be rounded and washable. The room must be provided with proper air-conditioning system, so that the windows can be closed, but important is to ensure that the air circulation from the lab is not connected in any way with that of the remaining parts of the hospital.

Human Leukocyte Antigen (HLA) Laboratory

The room must be spacious with stainless steel topped tables along with revolving stools. The overall space requirement is 2 rooms of 20 sqm with UV light, fumigation facility and positive pressure air-conditioning and lighting of 300 lux. Also at the entrance of the HLA lab, a change room for the staff before going inside the room with two entry doors to be provided (one for the entry of staff after changing which is fitted with automatic air shower for cleaning and maintenance only). A wash-basin at the entry of the lab is mandatory.

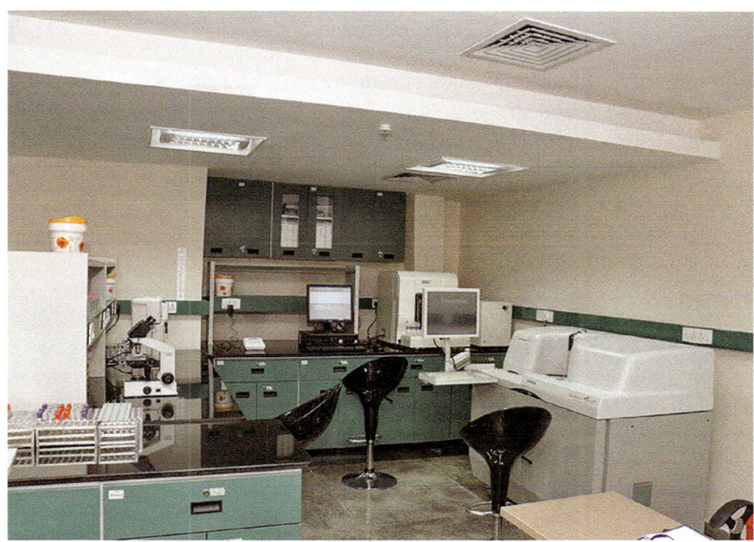

Fig. 9: Routine laboratory.

Renal Administration

Location[1]

Ideally, the administration area should be located so as to be easily accessible from all other areas of the unit. It should have a dedicated entrance off the renal ward, which should be appropriately signage to discourage patients, visitors, assistants from entering.

The administration area is essentially a suite of offices and should be appropriately equipped.

As the administration office is likely to be immediately adjacent to the renal ward, administration staff should be able to share this area's restroom facilities, staff change/locker facilities and staff sanitary facilities.

If not conveniently located elsewhere, the following facilities should be provided:
- A cleaner's room
- An electrical switch cupboard
- A general storage area
- Disposal facilities.

Office Accommodation

All offices should be sufficiently private for confidential discussions among staff. They should be able to accommodate a workstation with computer and keyboard, printer, fax and seating for up to three other people, and storage for books and files. A photocopier bay should also be provided.[1]

Office space should be provided for:[1]
- Renal services manager (this office is the administrative base for the renal unit)
- Nurse and medical consultants
- Medical secretaries
- Junior medical staff
- Dietitians
- Renal social workers
- Renal counselors
- Pharmacists
- Specialist nurses

- Research staff
- Professional development
- General administration (this could be either a suite of rooms, single open-plan office space, or a mix of the two)
- Home administration team
- Community staff
- Matron
- IT manager.

Engineering Services in Renal Unit

Flexibility of Design

In the light of the projected increase in demand for renal services, engineering services should be designed to accommodate future expansion.

Ventilation

Ventilation proposed must continue to be entirely compatible with the primary objective of maintaining infection control in the main renal unit. The main renal unit should use 100% fresh-air, low-velocity ventilation systems, where it is viable to do so, heat should be reclaimed from all extract systems using either recuperators or heat-recovery air-to-water coils. Cooling should be considered for the dialysis/treatment areas and isolation room(s) to achieve good comfort levels. Vents should not be positioned directly above patient-occupied areas, that is, directly over beds or chair positions. Grilles and diffusers should be located to provide even air.[1]

Water Services for Hemodialysis

The plant room should be located as near as possible to the renal unit in order to reduce pipe runs. Plant should be in a separate area to hot water/heating services.

New equipment should be capable of producing ultrapure dialysis fluid (bacterial counts <0.1 CFU/mL, and endotoxin <0.03 EU/mL). Ideally, this should be achieved using ultrapure water; however, water that meets the minimum standards can be used together with point-of-use filtration on the dialysis fluid. A routine testing procedure for water to be used in dialysis should form part of the renal unit's policy.[1]

Water Supply and Pipework

- The pipework should be constructed from rigid acrylnitrile butadiene styrene (ABS), food-quality cross-linked polyethylene (PEX) tubing, hardwearing polyvinyl chloride (PVC) or stainless steel, depending on the disinfection process to be used
- The pipework should be capable of being cleaned and/or disinfected by either chemical or heat treatment to maintain hygiene
- PEX can support both chemical and heat treatment
- It will be possible to use only chemical decontamination with ABS and PVC pipework (not heat)
- All treated water connections to dialysis machines should be of the dead-free-space design or have an automated facility to disinfect the tubing connecting to the dialysis machine on a regular basis.

Flexible hoses connecting the dialysis machine to the water supply and drainage outlet points should be provided with quick-release couplings. To avoid the risk of accidentally dislodging the drainage hoses from dialysis machines, it is recommended that the quick-release coupling be of a different size to the water-supply coupling to avoid confusion and cross-connection.[1]

Water Treatment Plant

The water treatment plant conditions should be monitored by the BMS and a plant status alarm panel providing visual or audible signals. The plant conditions should be capable of being transmitted to remote alarm panels.[1]

The water treatment plant should provide for total redundancy with dual softeners, circulating pumps, RO equipment and carbon filters. Carbon filters should be selected to achieve sufficient contact time to remove all chlorine and chloramines.[1]

Maintenance

With regard to the protection of the RO water treatment plant, devices for the control and safe isolation of engineering services should be in a separate secured room.[1]

Internal Drainage

Drainage pipework materials should be suitable for high-temperature waste at the time of automatic cleaning and disinfection (and also a range of disinfecting chemicals). It is possible that a protein-type residue will build up in the dialysis (solution) drainage pipework. It is, therefore, recommended that the pipework gradient from the discharge outlet point to the drainage system be greater than the usual 1 in 50.[1]

Acoustics

Efforts to ensure auditory privacy should not compromise patient safety during dialysis treatment (by interfering with clinical observation) and should not result in any requirement to increase nursing staffing levels.[1]

Electrical Installation

The electrical supply connections to electromedical equipment should comply with standard norms to avoid corruption of input data; some equipment may require automatic disconnection, with manual reset, following mains failure.[1]

Electrical Interference

Care should be taken to avoid mains-borne interference, harmonics and electrical radiofrequency interference affecting computers and other electronic equipment used in the main renal unit.[1]

IT and Telephone Wiring Systems

In addition to the monitoring of dialysis equipment and providing staff access to this data, the IT system should offer telemetry links to other areas within the main renal unit and to other hospital services.[1]

HEATING, VENTILATION AND AIR-CONDITIONING

The requirements of heating, ventilation and air-conditioning (HVAC) are listed at Table 2.

Table 2: HVAC in various areas.

Area	Air pressure	Air changes per hour	Relative humidity (%)	Temperature (°C)
Outpatient	Normal pressure	8–10	Normal filters	24+2
Renal ward	Positive	6–8	45+5	22+2
Treatment room (ward)	Positive	6–8	45+5	22+2
Pantry (ward)	Negative	10	45+5	22+2
Corridor	Negative	6	45+5	22+2
Disposal room (ward)	Negative	10	45+5	22+2
Dialysis area	Positive	6–8	45+5	22+2
Renal operating suite	Positive	20	45+5	22+2
OT preparation room	Positive	15	45+5	22+2
Recovery room	Positive	6–8	45+5	22+2
Corridor (OT)	Negative	6	45+5	22+2
Disposal room (OT)	Negative	10	45+5	22+2
TSSU	Negative	10	45+5	22+2
Radiology and lab services	Negative except in biochemistry and HLA lab	6–8	45+5	22+2

(HVAC: heating ventilation and air-condition; OT: operation theater; TSSU: theater sterile supply unit; HLA: human leukocyte antigen)

Technical Service Area of Main Renal Unit

Maintenance Room

Equipment storeroom: A separate equipment storeroom will be needed to store spare and isolated dialysis machines (the maintenance room itself should not be used to store any spare machines). A treated water supply, power and drainage facilities are required.[1]

The technical services area should have a treated water supply and drainage facilities maintenance room showing work bench and sink for cleaning of components and disposal of nontoxic fluids.[1]

Lighting

The lighting requirements are listed at Table 3.

The floor plans are listed at Figures 10 to 12.

Table 3: Lighting in various areas.

Area	Intensity
Renal outpatient:	
• Patient area	300–500 lux
• Corridor and waiting area	200 lux
Renal ward	
• Nursing station	500 lux
• Corridor	200 lux
• Support area	200 lux
Hemodialysis area	500 lux
Renal Tx. OT—General illumination	1500 lux
Renal ICU:	
• Clinical observation	500 lux
• Patient care area	300 lux
• Corridor	200 lux
Lab and radioimaging services	500 lux
Blood storage and issue unit	200 lux
CSSD and dietary	
Renal administration	

(CSSD: central sterile supply department; OT: operation theater)

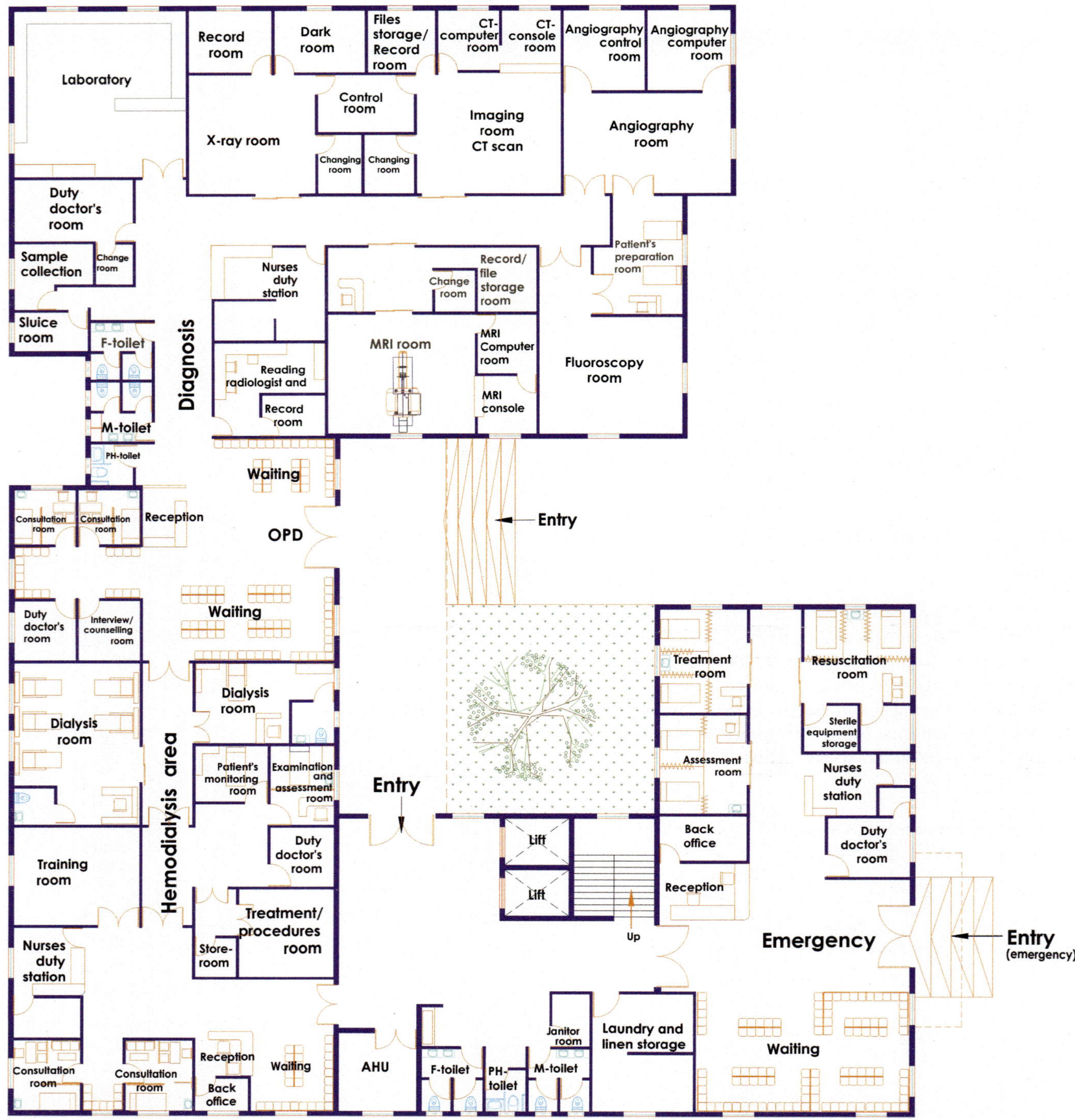

Fig. 10: Ground floor plan.

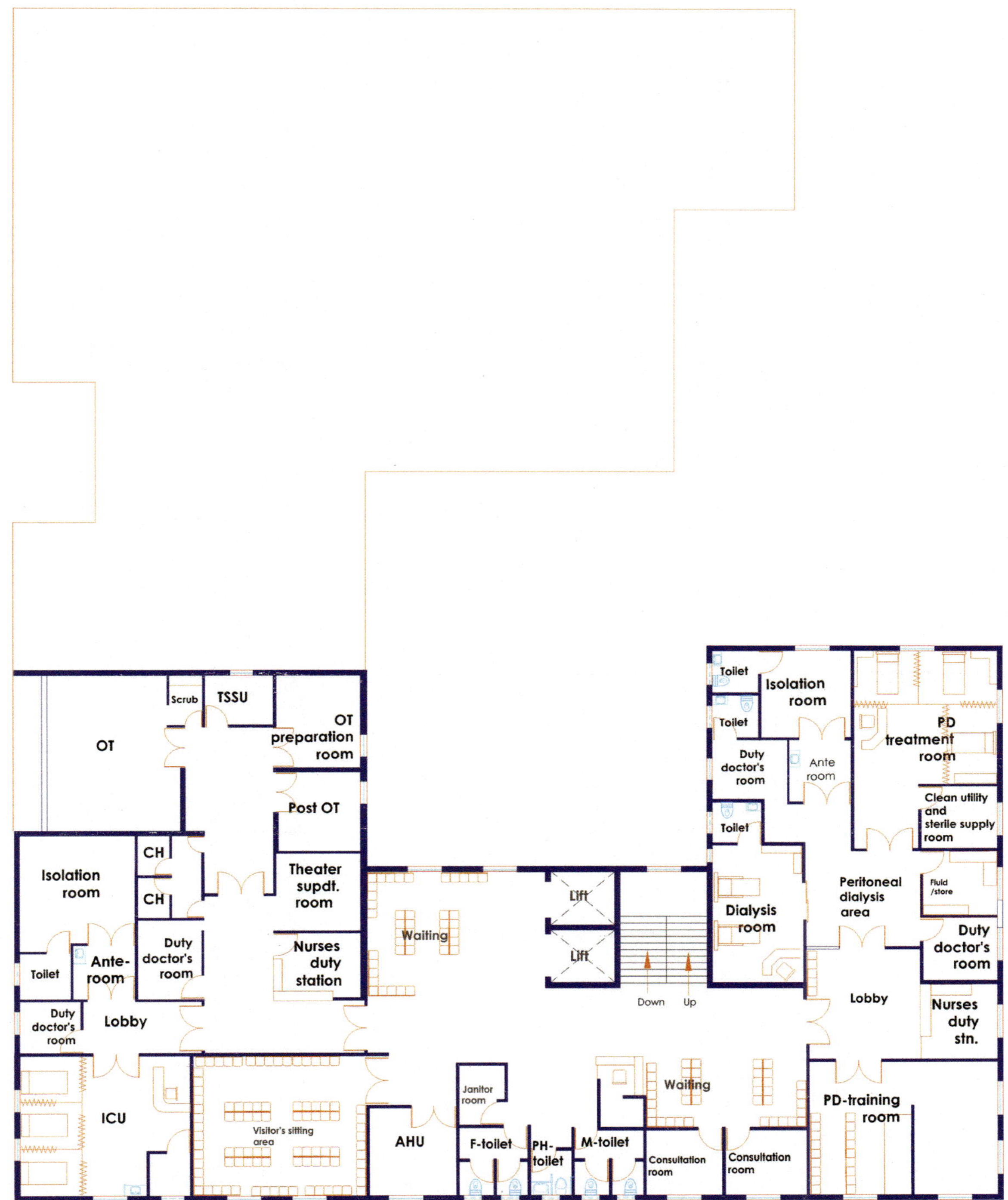

Fig. 11: First floor plan.

(AHU: air-handling unit; ICU: intensive care unit; PD: peritoneal dialysis; TSSU: theater sterile supply unit; OT: operation theater)

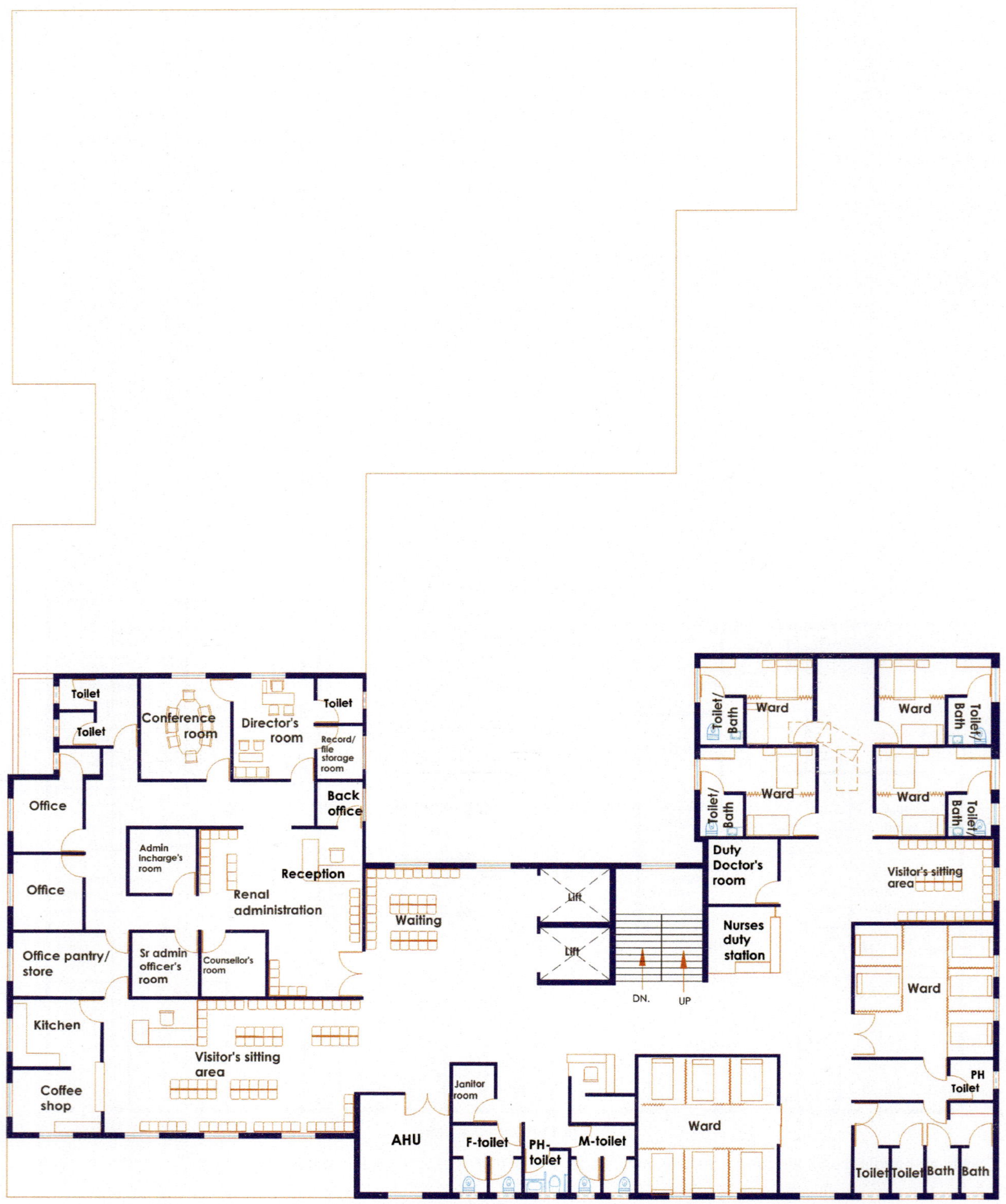

Fig. 12: Second floor plan.

REFERENCES

1. www.gov.uk
2. www.publications.doh.gov.uk
3. www.hivscotland.com
4. www.healthdesign.com.au
5. www.statehealthsocietybihar.org

OTHER REFERENCES

- Dash SC, Agarwal SK. Incidence of chronic kidney disease in India. Nephrol Dial Transplant. 2006;21(1):232-3; doi:10.1093/ndt/gfi094.
- Gupta SK, Kant S. Modern concepts of planning and designing. Jaypee Brothers Medical Publishers, 2007.
- http://www.mediescapes.com/dialysis_and_kidney_transplant.html
- http://www.spaceforhealth.nhs.uk/articles/general-service-considerations.
- Klahr S, Miller S. Acute oliguria. N Engl J Med. 1998;338(10): 671-5. doi:10.1056/NEJM199803053381007. PMID 9486997. http://content.nejm.org/cgi/content/full/338/10/671.
- MedicineNet, Inc. (2008-07-03). "Hyperkalemia". Available from: http://www.medicinenet.com/hyperkalemia/page4.htm. Accused May, 2009.
- Perneger TV, Whelton PK, Klag MJ. Risk of kidney failure associated with the use of acetaminophen, aspirin, and nonsteroidal anti-inflammatory drugs. N Engl J Med. 331(25):1675-9. PMID 7969358.
- Sakhuja V, Sud K. End-stage renal disease in India and Pakistan: Burden of disease and management issues". Kidney International 2003;63, S115–S118; doi: 10.1046/j.1523-1755.63.s83.24.x
- Your Kidneys and How They Work—How do kidneys fail? National Kidney and Urologic Diseases Information Clearing House. (NIDDK). NIH Publication No. 07–3195. August 2007.

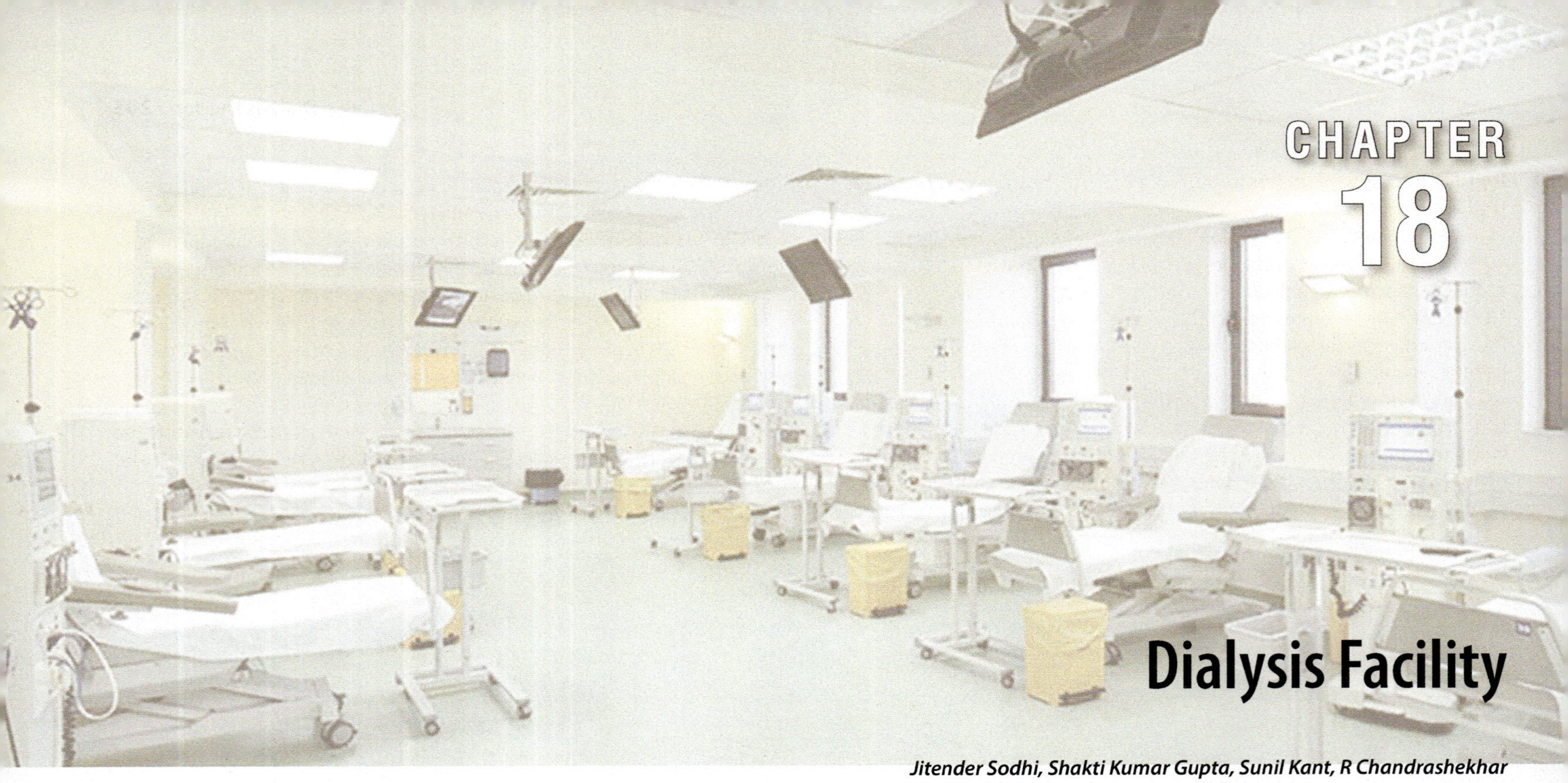

CHAPTER 18

Dialysis Facility

Jitender Sodhi, Shakti Kumar Gupta, Sunil Kant, R Chandrashekhar

INTRODUCTION

History

Dialysis was first described by Thomas Graham in 1854.[1] He prepared a bell-shaped vessel shown below (Fig. 1).

The wide open end of the bell was covered by a membrane created from an ox-bladder. He filled the bell-shaped vessel with urine and suspended it inside a larger container, filled with distilled water. After several hours, the bell-shaped vessel was removed. The larger container was heated so that the fluid inside boiled to dryness. Graham showed that the residue in the larger container consisted mainly of sodium chloride and urea, the principal components of urine. This proved that urea had passed through the membrane. Graham termed this process dialysis and proposed, together with Richard Bright, that this would form the basis of a treatment for renal failure. They predicted that it would take around 60 years to develop the process sufficiently to be used in the patients.[1,2]

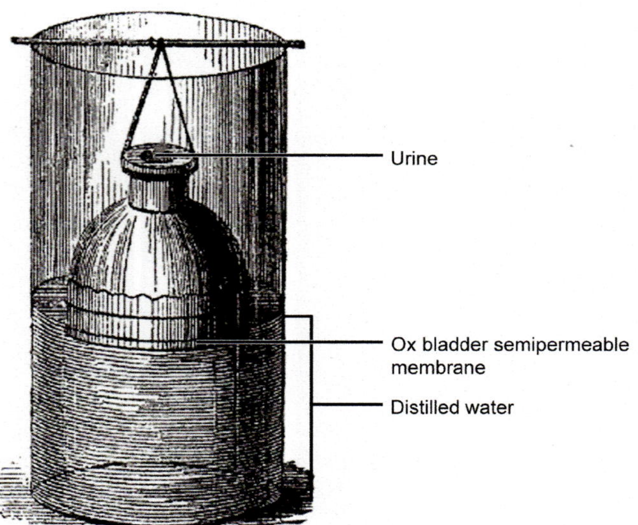

Fig. 1: Graham prepared a bell-shaped vessel.

Source: Based on Graham T philos trans R Soc Lond 1854;144:117-128.

The development of what eventually became a functional hemodialyzer was the cumulative effort of several membrane pioneers. Collodion membranes provided the first low-flux dialyzers. Fick was perhaps the first to use collodion membranes to selectively separate small molecular weight solutes (MW <5000) from blood through the process of diffusion.[3] This was shortly followed by the preparation of collodion tubes and the manufacturing process to control pore size and water permeability.[1,2]

While significant research with artificial membranes, including dialysis of animal blood against saline solution[3,4] and further characterization of membrane function and structure[3,5] was conducted between 1880 and 1913, it was not until 1914 that Abel et al. developed and tested the first efficient dialysis system at Johns Hopkins University School of Medicine. Their "vivi-diffusion" apparatus consisted of a filtering device made of cellulose trinitrate (collodion) tubes and an attached burette containing hirudin solution obtained from leech heads used as anticoagulant. That same year, Hess and McGuigan recommended high blood flows to avoid clotting or need for anticoagulation.[1,2]

The first human hemodialysis was performed in a uremic patient by Haas in 1924 at the University of Giessen in Germany. He used a tubular device made of collodion, cannulation of the radial and carotid arteries and the portal vein and hirudin for anticoagulation. Later that year he added a blood pump. In 1937, the first flat hemodialysis membrane made of cellophane was produced.[1,2]

A new phase in clinical hemodialysis started with the introduction of the Quinton and Scribner AV shunt in 1960. They used silastic tubes fitted with Teflon tips into the radial artery and cephalic vein in the wrist or the posterior tibial artery and saphenous vein at the angle as an arteriovenous shunt. The two tubes ended in expanded couplings to facilitate connection. This shunt provided for the first time continuous circulation of the blood when the patient was not attached to the machine, effectively eliminating clotting and provided ready access for repeated long-term hemodialysis, opening the door to chronic renal replacement therapy.[1,2]

The next significant advance in vascular access occurred in the 1960s when Cimino and Brescia first described their native arteriovenous fistula for chronic vascular access. These fistulas are generally created by an end-to-side vein-to-artery anastomosis. A mature native A-V fistula is by far the safest and longest lasting vascular access for hemodialysis.[1,2]

The major developments over the past four decades related to improvements in membrane biocompatibility and dialyzer design, volumetric control, sophisticated monitoring systems that provide online clearances, isothermal dialysis, high-flux membranes and convective modalities, such as hemofiltration and hemodiafiltration.[1,6]

DEFINITIONS

Dialysis (Fig. 2)

A type of renal replacement therapy which is used to provide an artificial replacement for lost kidney functions. There are two main forms of dialysis, hemodialysis and peritoneal dialysis, both of which are life-support treatments; but dialysis does not treat kidney diseases. Dialysis may be used for very sick patients who have recently lost kidney functions (acute renal failure) or for stable patients who have permanently lost kidney functions (chronic or end-stage renal failure).[1]

Dialysate

A solution of water and chemicals used in dialysate is provided in both single-patient and multiple-patient mixtures as determined by the medical staff (Fig. 3).[1]

Dialysis Center

A highly specialized program which provides facilities for the treatment of patients with irreversible renal insufficiencies. Treatment procedures require professional supervision by staff experienced in renal pathophysiology. The dialysis center may serve either or both inpatients and outpatients, depending upon the medical facility type, and may provide self-dialysis training for peritoneal dialysis in addition to on-site assisted dialysis, i.e. hemodialysis. The dialysis center administers both single-patient and multipatient hemodialysis systems (Fig. 2).[1]

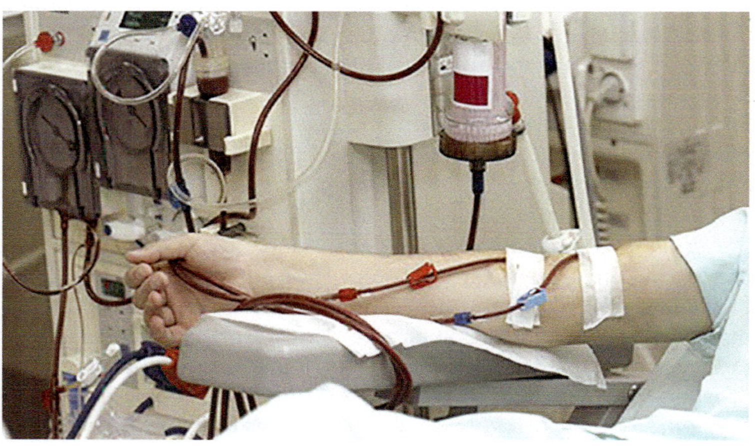

Fig. 2: Hemodialysis.

Hemodialysis

It is the form of dialysis typically conducted in a dialysis center. Hemodialysis relies on convective transport of a dialysate and utilizes counter-current flow, where the dialysate is flowing in the opposite direction to blood flow in an extracorporeal circuit (Figs. 4 and 5).[6]

Peritoneal Dialysis

Peritoneal dialysis (PD) is a treatment for patients with severe chronic kidney disease. The process uses the patient's peritoneum in the abdomen as a membrane across which fluids and dissolved substances (electrolytes, urea, glucose, albumin and other small molecules) are exchanged from the blood (Fig. 6).

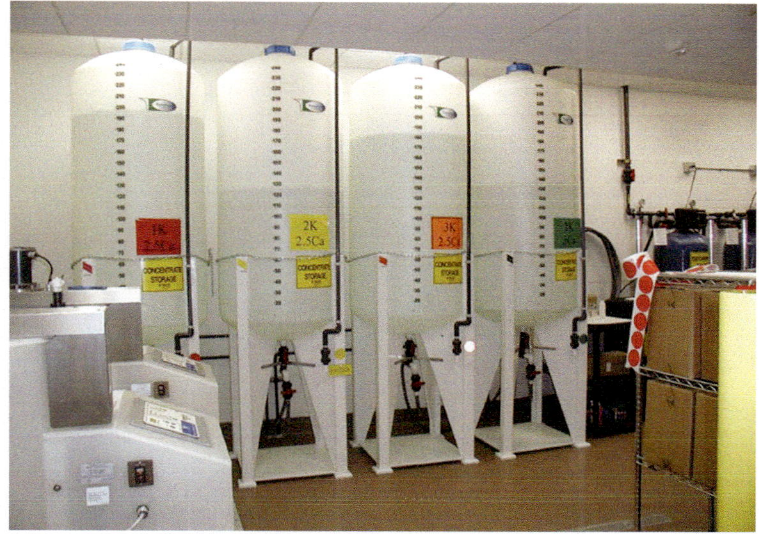

Fig. 3: Central dialysate.

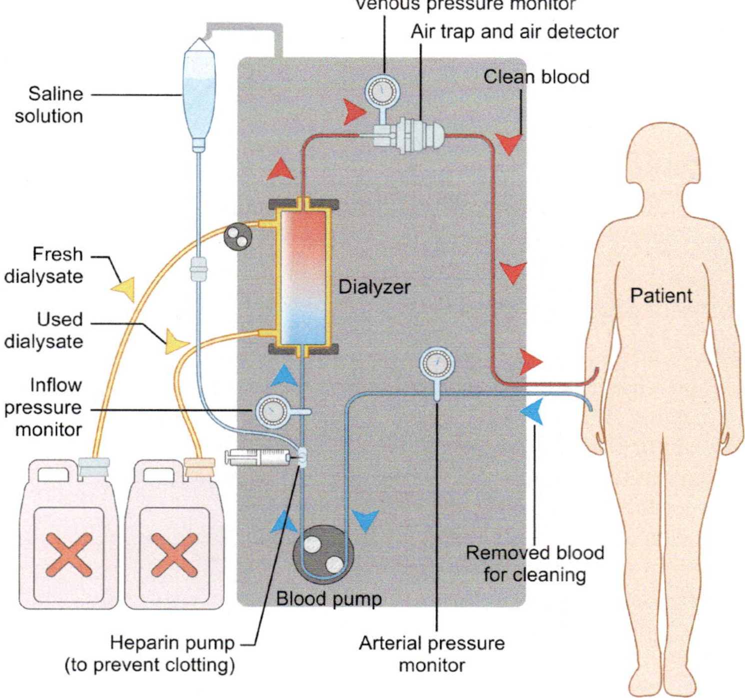

Fig. 4: Dialysis center (Schematic diagram of hemodialysis circuit).

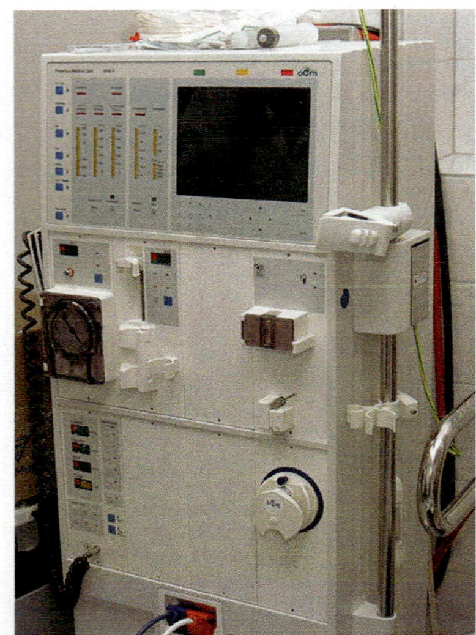

Fig. 5: Hemodialysis machine.

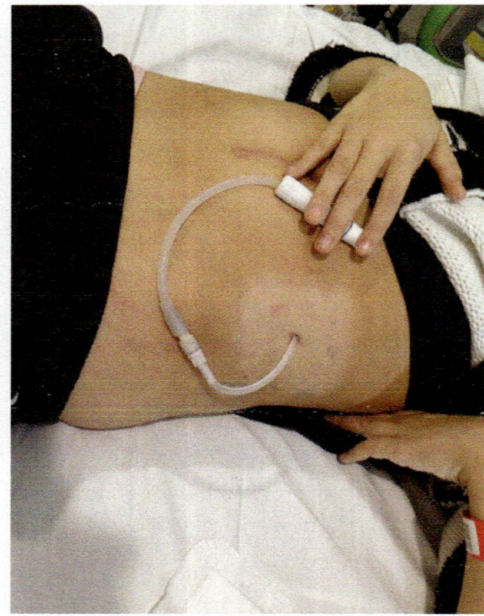

Fig. 6: Peritoneal dialysis.

Pathophysiology

The study of the disturbance of normal mechanical, physical, and biochemical functions which a disease causes or which causes a disease.[1]

Water Treatment (Fig. 7)

Dialysis water treatment implies various levels of pre-treatment and a final purification module prior to distribution of purified water through a hydraulic circuit.[1]

- *Deionization (DI) water*: Water which has been treated to remove contaminants. This system removes most mineral deposits, but microbial contaminants may remain.[1]
- *Feed water*: The untreated, potable water available throughout the facility through its water supply system.
- *Permeate water*: Fully treated purified water, stored in a tank, which is used in the preparation of dialysate.[1]
- *Pretreated water*: Partially treated water, sometimes available as feed water, which has had substantial reduction of mineral and/or microbial particles.[1]

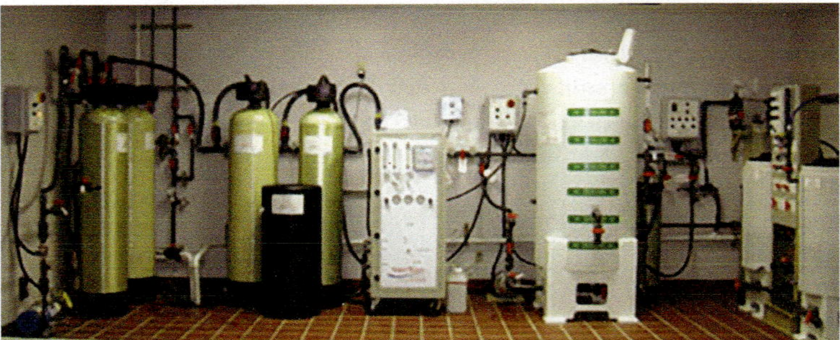

Fig. 7: Water treatment.

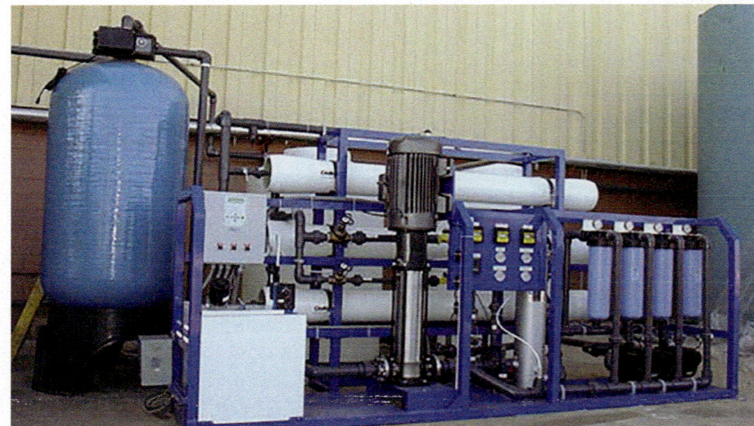

Fig. 8: Reverse osmosis plant.

- *Reverse osmosis (RO) water*: Usually, the final purification module in the treatment system, RO-based treatment modules produce water of optimal chemical and microbial quality (Fig. 8).[1]

Workload

Workload is the anticipated number of procedures or suite stops-that is processed through a department/service area. The total workload applied to departmental operational assumptions will determine overall room requirements by modality.[1]

GLOBAL BURDEN OF CHRONIC KIDNEY DISEASE

The number of patients with chronic kidney disease (CKD) worldwide is rising markedly. However, the absence of kidney registries in most of the low- and middle-income countries has made it difficult to ascertain the true burden of CKD in these countries. The global increase in the incidence and prevalence of CKD is being driven by the global increase in the prevalence of diabetes mellitus, hypertension, obesity, and aging. Most patients in low- and middle-income countries die because they cannot access renal replacement therapy because of the exorbitant cost. Community surveys have shown that the number of people with end-stage kidney disease is just the tip of the "CKD iceberg." The preventive strategies to stem the tide of CKD should involve educating the population on how to prevent renal disease; identifying those at risk of developing CKD; raising the awareness of the general public, policy makers, and healthcare workers; modifying the lifestyle of susceptible individuals; detecting early stage of CKD; arresting or hindering the progression of disease; and creating facilities for global assistance.[1,4]

Dialysis center is a highly specialized which provides facilities for the treatment of patients with irreversible renal insufficiencies. Treatment procedures require professional supervision by staff experienced in renal pathophysiology. The dialysis center may serve either or both inpatients and outpatients, depending upon the medical facility type, and may provide self-dialysis training for peritoneal dialysis in addition to on-site assisted dialysis, i.e. hemodialysis. The dialysis center administers both single-patient and multipatient hemodialysis systems.[1,4]

FUNCTION

An increase in the number of patients with diabetes and hypertension combined with poverty has led to an upsurge of patients with CKD. The mean age of patients with ESRD in India is between 32 years and 42 years, compared with 60 and 63 years in developed countries. Although the alternative option of renal transplantation for the treatment of ESRD is well-developed in India, it is severely hampered due to a lack of donors and the absence of a strong deceased donor program. Therefore, even patients who can afford transplantation have to opt for dialysis as the only possible treatment.[5]

Less than 10 percent of the total patients requiring dialysis are able to avail the facility, while only half of them are able to afford it on long-term basis—due to cost, time and logistical factors. Most dialysis units are privately run and the cost of dialysis beyond the means of most Indians.[5]

KEY PLANNING AND DESIGN PARAMETERS

The dictum of 'form follows function' is of prime importance in any planning premise. It is essential, therefore, to understand the following design considerations:

- The nurse station(s) must have a clear visual line of observation of each patient station and each patient toilet room entrance. Each nurse station should observe no more than ten patient stations; and, when multiple nurse stations are required, they should be arranged as each to observe as equal a share of the dialysis stations as possible.[1]
- Dialysis patients are highly susceptible to infections. The dialysis center should be located in an area which prevents cross-flow by other patients and staff; strategically placed and accessible handwashing stations throughout the patient treatment areas; and each dialysate return receptacle on the wall, centered at each patient station, and at a height such that it is easily accessible to clean repeatedly each day.[1]
- A minimum of 4 ft - 0 inch (1.22 m) clearance between beds or chairs and a headwall at each dialysis station at least 10 ft - 9 inch (3.28 m) wide should be provided.
- The dialysis station should not be less than 6 sqm to accommodate a bed or chair, the dialysis equipment and emergency equipment of needed.[7]
- The height of the dialysate receptacle should be coordinated with the equipment and the preceding parameter to inhibit an excessively long dialysate return hose; and any architectural systems used to conceal the gravity drain must be easily removable such as not to impede decontamination or modifications.[7]
- Dialysis patients are highly sensitive to and adversely affected by unsteady ranges of temperature, pressure, and humidity. Environmental systems must provide stable, consistent conditions.
- If the dialysis center biochemistry laboratory is authorized, patient toilets should be provided adjacent to the lab, and a pass-through into the lab should be provided.
- Patient confidentiality must be maintained when providing personal information to interview clerks and/or other staff. The physical design of the space should not encumber this requirement.[6]
- Staff areas should be located convenient to staff and separate from patient areas, and patient and staff circulations should be segregated. Since the dialysis center operates 24 hours a day/365 days a year, its staff lounge, staff lockers, staff toilets, and staff showers should not be collocated with those of adjacent departments unless they are in close proximity and always accessible to the dialysis center staff.[6]
- Dialysis equipment may connect directly into patient data information systems to input recordings of the treatment process. The designer must coordinate the interface of the equipment and the information system.
- Separate hemodialysis area should be designated solely for use of Hepatitis B patients for HCV-infected patients and isolation facilities may be required.

Facility Planning

What makes the design of a dialysis facility distinct is that patients spend 3–4 hours, 3–5 times a week in the clinic undergoing treatment. People of all ages with different degrees of kidney failure undergo dialysis. A warm, homelike, and flexible environment is a key part of the design philosophy, for both patients and staff.[8]

Space Criteria

Space planning criteria have been developed on the basis of an understanding of the activities involved in the functional areas of the dialysis center and its relationship with other services of a medical facility. These criteria are predicted upon established and/or anticipated best practice standards.

These criteria are subject to modification relative to development in the equipment, medical practice, vendor requirements, and subsequent planning and design.

Dialysis center capacity per year should be based on:[1]

$$\frac{\text{Operating days per year} \times \text{Hours of operation per day}}{\text{Minutes per clinic stop / 60 minutes}} = \text{Number of annual clinic annual clinic stops}$$

The schedule of accommodation is shown in Table 1.

Occupancy Rate

The number of patients that should be taken into account is an assumed occupancy rate. Occupancy rates of 85–90% are typically considered cost-effective. Most facilities will be hard-pressed to run at more than 95% of capacity annually because of cancellations, illness, staff shortages, and power outages.[8]

Although the general planning model for dialysis facilities for tertiary care hospital assumes 365 operating days per year and 24 hours of operation per day to support inpatient programs, the impact of this within the dialysis center will be on staffing, supplies, storage, and equipment processing rather than on the number of dialysis stations.[1]

The basic room efficiency factors for dialysis stations are 90% use during the peak hours of operation, including the time between patient use when staff members are preparing the space, and 80% use during

Table 1: Schedule of accommodation.

Room/ Space	*Area (sqm)*
Reception Areas	
Reception	7.5
Waiting	18.6
Toilet, Public	4.7
Patient Areas	
Renal dialysis, Bed station, Private	14.0
Renal dialysis, Chair station, Cubicle	7.5
Exam/Treatment Room	11.2
Support Areas for Patients	
Toilet, Patient	4.7
Toilet, Patient, Private	4.7
Toilet, Patient, Isolation	4.7
Locker room, Patient	4.7
General Support Areas and Facilities	
Utility room, Soiled	7.5
Utility room, Clean	9.3
Storage, Clean supply	7.5
Storage, Sterile supply	7.5
Storage, Clean linen	3.8
Storage, Equipment	9.3
Medication preparation	10.3
Alcove, Crash cart	1.9
Dialysate preparation room	14.0
Water treatment room	18.6
Alcove, Wheelchair/Stretcher	37.2
Housekeeping aids closet- HAC	37.2
Staff and Administrative Areas	
Nurse station	10.3
Office, Physician	11.2
Office, PA/Resident/Intern	11.2
Room, ANS/Sister-in-Charge	11.2
Cubicle, Dialysis support technician	2.8
Conference room	29.9
Facilities for Staff	
Lounge, Staff	7.5
Locker room, Staff	7.5
Toilet, Staff	4.7

the off-peak hours of operation. Using 85% as the mean which indicates that, on average for each inpatient dialysis station through the course of all operating hours, a dialysis station is prepared and ready for use but unoccupied 15% of the available time.[7]

This is the basis for determining a system-wide design standard for calculating the number of dialysis stations required.[7]

Example:[7] Assume the operating averages for dialysis centers are 6 days a week and 10 hours a day. Also assume each dialysis station uses averages 300 minutes (5 hours) per clinic stop, including clean-up and set-up: 6 operating days per week × 52 weeks per year = 312 operating days per year.

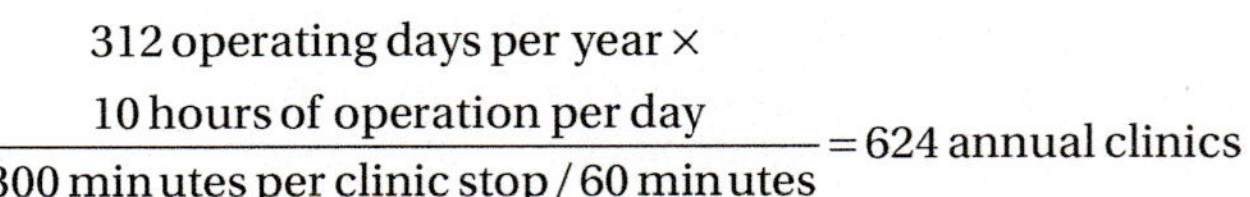

$$\frac{312 \text{ operating days per year} \times 10 \text{ hours of operation per day}}{300 \text{ minutes per clinic stop} / 60 \text{ minutes}} = 624 \text{ annual clinics}$$

This yields a maximum capacity of 624 clinic stops per year per dialysis station, assuming 100% utilization. However, 100% utilization is not realistic to achieve; thus, it is not realistic as a design standard. Apply the room efficiency factor as follows:[1]

624 × 85% = 530 annual clinic stops.

The number of annual clinic stops per dialysis station will be used as a criteria parameter to calculate the number of dialysis stations (Table 2).

Spatial Needs

Once the number of patients and a reasonable occupancy rate are defined, a space program is outlined to determine spatial needs; indicating patient and staff areas, support spaces, business offices, mechanical systems, and any other patient care spaces that are part of the facility's goals and objectives. The space program is usually a written list of rooms, room sizes, functions, equipment, and utility needs within each room, many of which are defined by code. Diagrams are also part of a space program to help define the general layout of the facility and to determine the circulation of patients, staff, and supplies.[8]

Reception Areas

- Reception—80 NSF (7.5 NSM) (Fig. 9)
- Waiting—200 NSF (18.6 NSM) (Fig. 10)
- Toilet, Public—50 NSF (4.7 NSM)
  (NSF, net square foot; NSM, net square meter).

Table 2: Workload parameter calculation.[1]

Dialysis center	*Average length of clinic stop (minutes)*	*Utilization rate*	*Minimum workload to generate one dialysis station*
Dialysis station	300	85%	530

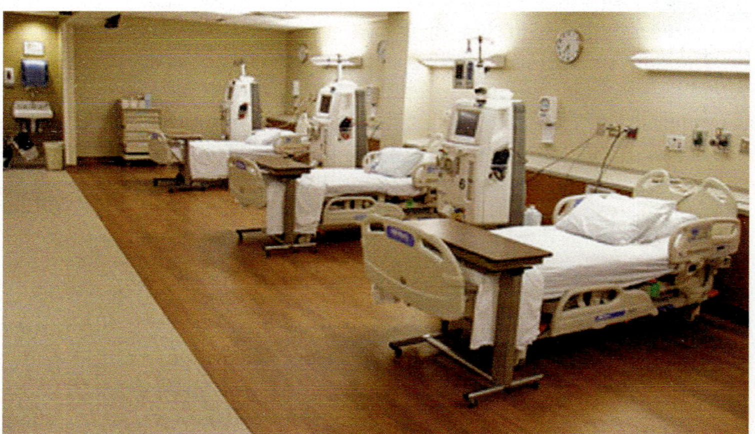

Fig. 9: Dialysis bed station.

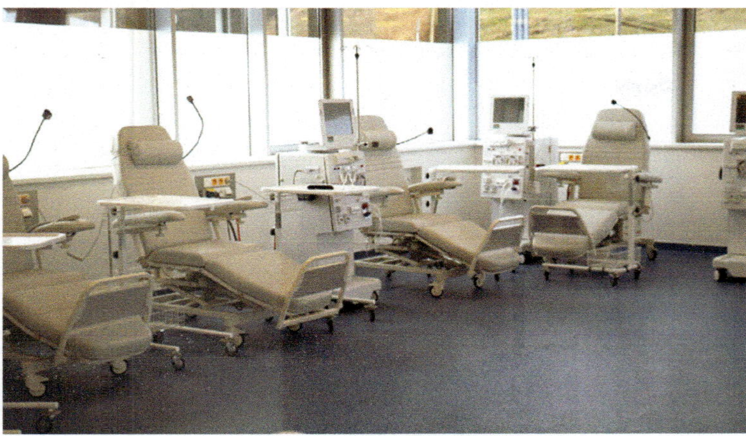

Fig. 10: Chair station dialysis.

Patient Areas

Dialysis

Treatment Area[1,9]

- The treatment area should be separate from administrative and waiting areas.
- The treatment area should be permitted to be an open area
- Open treatment areas should be designed to provide privacy for each patient.
- Renal dialysis, bed station, private—150 NSF (14.0 NSM).
- Renal dialysis, chair station, cubicle—80 NSF (7.5 NSM). Individual patient treatment areas of at least 80 sqft (7.44 sqm). With a clear dimension of at least 4 ft (1.22 m) between beds and/or dialysis lounge chairs.
- Exam/treatment room—120 NSF (11.2 NSM).

Support Areas for Patients[1,9]

- Toilet, Patient—50 NSF (4.7 NSM)
- Toilet, Patient, Private—50 NSF (4.7 NSM)
- Toilet, Patient, Isolation—50 NSF (4.7 NSM)
- Locker room, Patient—50 NSF (4.7 NSM).

General Support Areas and Facilities[1,9]

- Utility room, Soiled—80 NSF (7.5 NSM)
- Utility room, Clean—100 NSF (9.3 NSM)
- Storage, Clean supply—80 NSF (7.5 NSM)
- Storage, Sterile supply—80 NSF (7.5 NSM)
- Storage, Clean linen—40 NSF (3.8 NSM)
- Storage, Equipment—1 00 NSF (9.3 NSM)
- Medication preparation—110 NSF (10.3 NSM)
- Alcove, Crash cart—20 NSF (1.9 NSM)
- Dialysate Preparation Room—150 NSF (14.0 NSM)
- Water Treatment Room—200 NSF (18.6 NSM)
- Alcove, Wheelchair/Stretcher—50 NSF (37.2 NSM)
- Housekeeping Aids Closet—50 NSF (37.2 NSM).

Staff and Administrative Areas[1,9]

- Nurse station—110 NSF (10.3 NSM)
- Office, Physician—120 NSF (11.2 NSM)
- Office, PA/Resident/Intern—120 NSF (11.2 NSM)
- Room, ANS/Sister-in-charge—120 NSF (11.2 NSM)
- Cubicle, Education Coordinator—60 NSF (5.6 NSM)
- Cubicle, Dialysis Support Technician—30 NSF (2.8 NSM)
- Conference Room—300 NSF (29.9 NSM).

Facilities for Staff[9]

- Locker room, Staff—80 NSF (7.5 NSM)
- Toilet, Staff—50 NSF (4.7 NSM)
- Lounge, Staff—80 NSF (7.5 NSM).

Heating, Ventilation, and Air-conditioning

- All air supply and air-exhaust systems should be mechanically operated. All fans serving the exhaust system should be located at the discharge end of the system. The ventilation rates shown in Table 3 should be minimum rates and should not be considered as precluding the use of higher ventilation rates.
- Duct linings should not be used in HVAC systems

Table 3: General pressure relationships and ventilation of certain dialysis areas.

Area designation	*Pressure relationship to adjacent areas*	*Minimum of changes of outdoor air per hour supplied to room*	*Minimum total air changes per hour supplied to room*	*All air exhausted directly to outdoors*
Patient treatment area	P	2	6	Yes
Office(s)	E	Optional	2	Yes
Examination and treatment room	V	Optional	6	Optional
Waiting room	N	2	6	Optional
Medication room	P	Optional	6	Optional
Isolation room	N	2	2	Yes
Isolation room alcove or anteroom	N	2	10	Yes
Soiled workroom	N	Optional	10	Yes
Clean workroom	P	Optional	4	Optional
Equipment maintenance room	P	Optional	4	Optional
Toilet room	N	Optional	10	Yes
Equipment storage room	V	Optional	2	Optional
Environmental services closet	N	Optional		Yes

Continued

Continued

Area designation	Pressure relationship to adjacent areas	Minimum of changes of outdoor air per hour supplied to room	Minimum total air changes per hour supplied to room	All air exhausted directly to outdoors
Sterilizer equipment room	N	Optional	10	Yes
Laboratory	N	Optional	6	Yes
Soiled linen	N	Optional	10	Yes
Clean linen storage	V	2, Optional	2	Optional
Dialyzer reuse room	N	2	12	Yes
Central batch mixing room	N	2	12	Yes

(P: positive; N: negative; E: equal; V: varying)

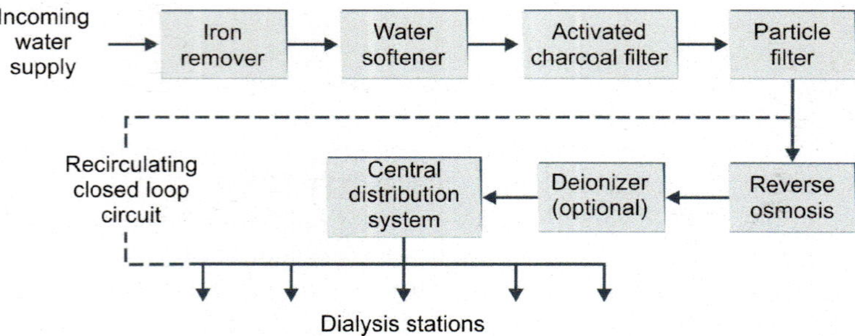

Fig. 11: Schematic diagram of a water treatment system.

- All central ventilation or air-conditioning systems should be equipped with filters having efficiencies no less than 80%.
- HVAC temperature and humidity should provide the following—temperature, 70–76°F; relative humidity 30% minimum –50% maximum.

Water Distribution and Storage

- Water distribution systems should be constructed of plastic pipes because metal pipes could contaminate the treated water with chemicals such as copper, lead, or zinc.
- The minimal number of elbows and T joints should be used and outlets should be at the highest point of the system to allow adequate contact of all parts of the system with germicide.
- As long as possible, storage tanks should not be used because they increase the amount of water and surface area available for bacterial contamination.

WATER TREATMENT PLANT AND DISTRIBUTION SYSTEM

Design Guideline (Figs. 11 to 13)

Water treatment systems that supply hemodialysis machines remove contaminants through various treatment stages, which for any given system, can include filtration, adsorption, deionization, and/or reverse osmosis. Each of these stages is limited in the amount of contaminant that it can remove. In some instances, a stage must be repeated one or more times to be effective; this can require added equipment.

The most frequently used components are represented by mechanical filters, oxidizing filters, cartridge filters, ultrafilters, carbon filters, ion exchanger and reverse osmosis units. To ensure removal of all possible contaminants (particulate matter, soluble and insoluble inorganic compounds, soluble organic substances, heavy metals, trace elements, bacteria and pyrogens) the system is composed of several serially oriented components usually divided into a pretreatment section and a final production unit.

Mechanical filters are used to remove large particles and turbidity from the incoming water, and therefore they protect the following components from clogging or being damaged by particulate matter (Fig. 11).[10]

Oxidizing filters remove excessive iron, manganese and sulfides by oxidizing and adsorbing these ions.

Cartridge filters are used to protect components from small particles and they usually work in the range from 50 to 3 microns.[10]

Ultrafiltration cartridges remove bacteria, pyrogens and other macromolecular compounds, by a combined mechanism of filtration and absorption. They are used to obtain ultrapure water or to avoid

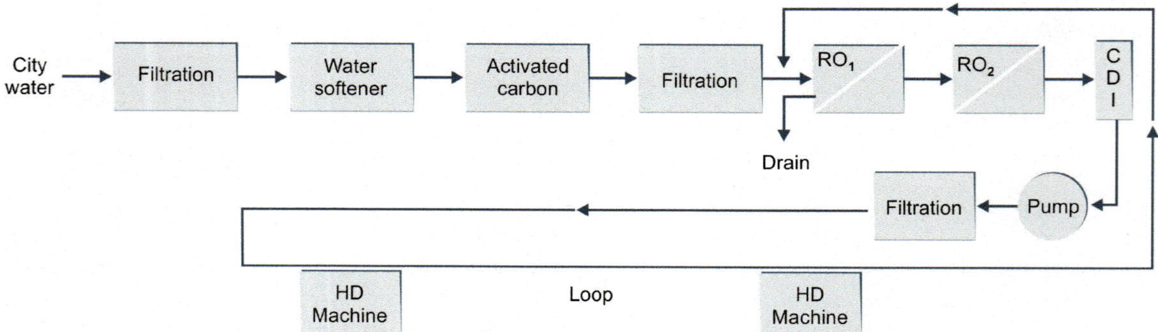

Fig. 12: Schematic diagram of a water treatment system. Ultrapure water treatment plant. (CDI: capacitive deionization; HD: hemodialysis)

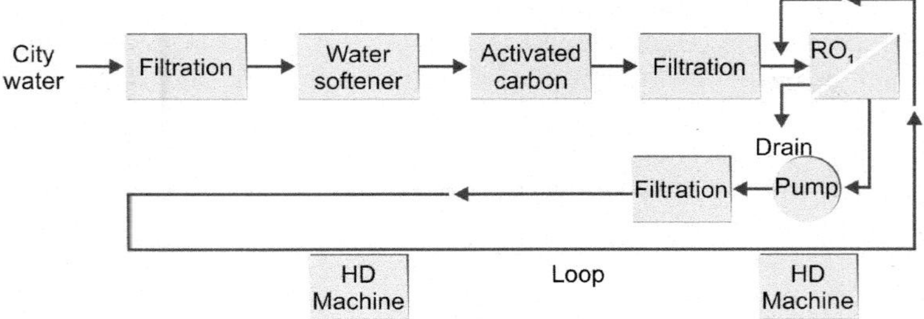

Fig. 13: Simplified schematic diagram of a water treatment system. Conventional water treatment plant.

back contamination from distribution loop to the final osmosis unit (Fig. 12). Ultrafilters reject contaminants in the range of 1000 Dalton to 0.1 µm particles, allowing most ions and small organics, such as glucose, to permeate the porous structure.[10]

Carbon filters absorb low-molecular-weight organic compounds such as chlorine, chloramines and some pyrogens from the water.[10]

The most common ion-exchangers used in dialysis are water softeners; they exchange calcium and magnesium present in the water with sodium salts, thus changing hard water to soft water with a proportional increase in sodium ions.[10]

Similarly ion-exchange deionizers use two types of synthetic resins—one to remove the positively charged ions (cations) and another to remove the negatively charged ions (anions). Resins have limited capacities and need to be regenerated upon exhaustion. A demineralization or deionization unit is typically used on water that has already been prefiltered and uses a two-stage process to remove virtually all ionic material remaining in water.[10]

Deionizers have usually two-bed or mixed-bed configuration in which the cationic and anionic resins are in a separate or single tank, respectively. Recently, an electrical current has been used to reduce the ionic content of water, using special semipermeable membranes based on the charges of the ions. This component is called electrodialysis, which improves the efficiency of the classic deionizers, avoiding the troubles of using chemicals for regeneration. Two flat-sheet membranes, to preferentially permeate cations and anions, respectively, are stacked alternatively with flow channels between them. Cathode and anode electrodes are placed on each side of the alternating stack of membranes to draw most ions through the membranes. This leaves much lower concentrations of the ions in water in the alternate channels. A recent development has improved the efficiency of electrodialysis by reducing scaling and fouling problems on membranes. This has been obtained by reversing the polarity of the electrodes periodically and is called electrodialysis reversal.[10]

Reverse osmosis removes virtually all organic compounds—90% to 99% of all ions, and 99.9% of viruses, bacteria and pyrogens. Reverse osmosis membranes represent the heart of any water treatment system. They may, sometimes, differ in the efficiency of rejection or resistance to disinfectants. The membranes are sensitive and can be easily damaged by excessive hardness, iron and chlorine in the feeding water; hence a correct pretreatment is essential for the membranes to function properly.[10]

Selecting a water purification system requires care. Institutions may find an analysis of the local water supply helpful in establishing a baseline for specific contaminants that must be removed. Facilities should contact their respective water departments to acquire quality data (i.e. ranges in contaminant levels) for their supply water. This information must be interpreted with caution, however, because municipal water may come from a variety of supplies with different levels of contaminants that are likely to vary over time. Additionally, facilities should periodically monitor the quality of their water before and after treatment through a comprehensive preventive maintenance program (including testing—performed in-house and/or by an outside laboratory—and correcting for conductivity, flow, water temperature, and chlorine levels).[10]

Manufacturers should supply, with their systems, specifications listing the maximum allowable concentration that can be efficiently removed by their water purification systems. If a facility's intake water supply might or does exceed these limits, one or more additional pretreatment devices should be considered when purchasing the dialysis system. The water filtration company's sales representative should be able to design a system based on the hospital's flow rates, intake water quality, and demand level requirements.[10]

Technical Design of the Water Treatment System

The key elements to be considered for choosing the most appropriate components to include in the water system are the feed water contamination levels and the maximum allowed or wished—for levels of contaminants in the final product water.[10]

One has also to take into account the amount of water required and the flow rate for each device. Based on removal ratio, that is the ratio for each known contaminant of feed water value to the standard level, it is possible to select the most appropriate component. Starting from the tap water-a pressure reducer is sometimes needed to enter water into the pretreatment section which includes a 25 µm cartridge filter, dual water softener with brine tanks, two carbon adsorption filters in series and a final 5 µm cartridge filter. The next two components are a double reverse osmosis in series, where rejected water from the second osmosis is not discharged but is sent back to the pretreatment section to spare it. The final component is a loop distribution system, where sampling points are included between the 0.2 µm-antibacterial microfilters to avoid back contamination of the loop or of the osmosis membrane. This is a general description of the commonly used water treatment plant. Different plants, however, can achieve, in special situations, better results. In general, a pretreatment with filters, softeners and activated carbons is always necessary. Placement of the activated carbon, as the last component, ensures a higher level of chlorine to disinfect softeners. However, the carbon resins will last less, and, therefore, it represents a solution with a higher maintenance cost. For the final treatment section, the combination of a single reverse osmosis with ultrafiltration or a deionizer unit has been reported. The first combination is especially active on bacterial contamination, while the second one on chemical contaminants. The combination of the two reverse osmosis units in series is preferable since in case of breakdown of any single osmosis component, the remaining unit can still serve to get reasonably good water quality while awaiting repair. The water treatment system should thus consist of pretreatment and RO modules feeding directly the dialysis machines. Storage tanks should be avoided. Pipe tubing material and plumbing should be designed to prevent bacterial contamination and to be easily disinfected. Water engineering consists of the optimal assembly of the different components of the water treatment in terms of size, position, and purity to guarantee the appropriate quality of the water product. A combination of water pretreatment (softener, activated carbon, down-sizing microfiltration), RO module, and a direct delivery pipe system (no storage tank, if possible) represents the minimal technical configuration intended to produce pure water and to prevent microbiological contamination.[3,10]

An alternative option to produce higher quality grade water consists of a system to 'polish' the water by passing through a second RO module and or electrochemical continuous deionizer in series. Such a technical configuration is used in the semiconductor industry and is able to produce ultrapure water with very stringent purity criteria. In this case, resistivity exceeds 1.5 MOhms and bacterial contamination is <0.1 CFU/mL. To prevent bacterial contamination and biofilm formation, the water distribution circuit should be particularly well-engineered. Suitable materials for pipe network are made of stainless steel, polyethylene tubing, acrylonitrile-butadiene-styrene plastic, polyvinylidene fluoride, polypropylene, or polyvinyl chloride of sanitary grade. High shear stress should be maintained by means of small internal diameter pipes and high flow rates. The greatest effort should be made to obtain an adequate plumbing of the water distribution loop, with a linear pipe configuration favoring continuous high-speed water circulation and preventing water stagnation by avoiding dead space and lateral arms.[3,10]

Design Requirements for a Water Distribution System in a Hemodialysis Center

- *Introduction*: Once it passes through the purification process, the water needs to be distributed to the dialysis equipment. There are certain requirements for distributing water to each individual station (dialysis machine, reprocessing equipment, bicarbonate-filling area, etc.), as well as many drawbacks with delivering this large a quantity of water.[11]
- Each station requires a specific water flow rate, along with a minimum and maximum pressure. If only the minimum pressure and flow rate were supplied, the result would be a very low flow velocity. There would even be areas within the supply system that were completely stagnant; this is especially true with a direct distribution system (no storage tank). Therefore, it is imperative to build in extra flow capacity above what is needed, creating a "scrubbing" velocity. Along with routine disinfection, this will aid in preventing bacterial adhesion that can lead to biofilm and its consequent problems. For this reason, there are minimum flow requirements.[11]
- *Loop-flow design:* Both with indirect (storage tank) and direct-feed systems, the water should flow in a loop. This means that the water travels in a continuous circle throughout the facility without any branching off. The unused, expensively purified water is then returned to either the RO or the storage tank and not discarded to drain. Furthermore, with a loop design, along with proper piping size, you can achieve higher flow rates through the system, which give higher flow velocities.[11]
- *Determining the loop flow velocity:* The flow rate is described in terms of cubic ft per minute. This then gets converted to the flow velocity in ft per second (FPS).[11]

For a direct feed system, a minimum flow velocity of 1.5 FPS is required, as measured at the "end" of the loop and during peak demand (all systems operating and drawing water).

For indirect feed systems, the minimum flow velocity would be 3 FPS, with an average range of 3–6 FPS.

If the flow velocity is too high, there may be excessive noise in the system, as well as excessive heat, not to mention the increased wear and tear and electrical costs of running the pumps at an excessive speed. Consider, however, that in ultrapure applications outside of dialysis, flow velocities of 8–10 FPS are not uncommon. When designing a system, it is important to remember that the flow rate within the piping system will vary. It will be very high at the beginning of the system and will decrease as the water moves through the pipe. The reason is that the various hemodialysis equipment demand certain amount of water from the loop as the water passes by, decreasing the volume as each piece of equipment collects its requirement.[11]

When designing a system and loop, it is imperative to take into account the flow requirements of each individual hemodialysis machine, piece of reuse equipment, bicarbonate-fill station, machine repair station, etc.[11]

Build-in space and options for future expansion of facility so that the new water system and loop are not obsolete in a few years and so that the capital investment is not lost.[11]

Construction Considerations

The way in which the water distribution system is installed is critical and requires attention to certain details that a local plumber might not understand. Typically, the material of choice in the US is polyvinyl chloride (PVC) schedule 80. However, there is some movement toward more pristine materials such as polyvinylidene fluoride (PVDF), polypropylene (PPE), etc. When using these types of specialty piping, it should be assured that the installer understands how to correctly weld the material. When using PVC, the pipe should be cut using an approved PVC pipe-cutting method (a PVC pipe cutter, for instance, looks like a knife and cuts the pipe square). The pipe should not be cut with a hacksaw, as this will leave a rough edge to which bacteria can adhere. Once the pipe is cut, a chamfering tool should be used that will round off the inner and outer diameter of the pipe. Chamfering the edges will reduce the burrs, thus allowing the glue to be more evenly distributed; it will also decrease the occurrence of stress points so that the pipe will be less likely to crack. All solvent welds should be primed prior to the gluing process. Primer comes both with and without a blue tint. If it has a blue tint, the solvent-weld can be inspected after it has been completed. Where possible, all connections should be solvent welded; however, the overuse of glue should be avoided, as the excess glue can hang down and provide place for bacteria to attach.

Threaded joints also should be avoided, as they will have spaces where there will be stagnation, thus increasing the possibility for bacterial growth. Ninety-degree turns in the loop should be accomplished through the use of two 45-degree angles. This will provide a more even flow through the turn and prevent the stagnation that occurs when a 90-degree turn is used. The connections to the stations should be kept as short as possible. In this way, when a station is not in use, the stagnant area will be kept to a minimum. The connection to the station should be maintained at as high a flow velocity as possible. Nonetheless, it will probably not be possible to achieve the minimum flow velocity of the distribution loop for this short segment.[11]

PHYSICAL ENVIRONMENT

Color

Everyone perceives color somewhat differently because of personal likes and dislikes of certain colors but, in general terms, light, warm colors increase light reflectivity and enhance the feeling of space, whereas dark, rich colors absorb light and make a space feel smaller and more intimate. Dark colors may be appropriate for a small intimate lounge or a home entertainment area but should not be used in a patient care environment. Yellows and light oranges should also be avoided, as they may make skin appear yellow and jaundiced, not a good idea for dialysis patients.[12]

It is better to use light shades of secondary or tertiary colors to add accents in order to help to maintain the perception of light and to make the space feel larger. Staff need a high light level, as reading fine print and working with small needles is a big part of their work. Even though white enhances light reflectivity and provides a sense of cleanliness, it is sterile and quickly becomes boring.[12]

Color is still one of the best ways to enhance a cheerful, homelike environment, which also makes patients feel better about the time they spend in the clinic and about the treatment they must undergo.[12]

Wall Coverings

Vinyl wall coverings are a very good way to introduce color, patterns, and texture to a wall surface. A dialysis facility has at least four major zones within it public, office staff, patient treatment, and maintenance/service areas. Each needs a different type of finish treatment. Areas that require constant industrial cleaning may need a seamless or heat-sealed wall covering. Ceramic tile and plastic laminate are also very durable wall coverings, with numerous design options that can create a very pleasant environment, at a cost.[12]

Flooring

Flooring is another area with almost limitless options in the types of floor systems available, depending on esthetic desire, durability needed, and budget limits. Vinyl composite tile (VCT) is one of the most economical and relatively durable surfaces. One drawback to VCT is that it is typically available in 120 × 120 tile, which has the disadvantage of creating numerous seams that can harbor bacteria and enable water to get in, which can ruin the floor.[12]

Linoleum is in vogue again, but as a 120 × 120 tile, it has advantages and disadvantages similar to VCT. A commonly used alternative to tile is sheet vinyl (SV), which can be installed in 10- or 12-foot-wide rolls with only one seam along the edge of each roll. The joints of a SV floor can be chemically seamed or heat welded to create an almost seamless installation. Like vinyl wall coverings, SV comes in an unlimited number of colors and patterns.[12] However self levelling epoxy flooring is well suited for function.

Engineered wood flooring and artificial wood flooring made from plastic laminated material are now used in certain clinic environments but because of the potential for water spills, a dialysis unit probably should not use these types of material.[12]

Dividing Walls

Dividing walls can also be used to introduce variety and color. By using a modular box theme, the dividing walls can be stepped to vary their heights in a manner that allows more light and visibility at one end of a cul-de-sac, with lower walls, and more privacy and sound at the other, with walls stepped up to the ceiling. Dividing walls can also have shelves that can have artwork and plants, creating a warmer, more homelike atmosphere that is so important in the healing process. The modular boxes can be of different colors and materials for visual variety, which can be a stimulus to help patients stay more alert and for staff to take pride in their workplace. The dividing walls can be used much like a modular furniture system to create storage cabinets that keep most medical supplies out of view while keeping them immediately accessible. It is important to make a treatment area as homelike as possible and to hide the clinical elements without hampering the medical service delivery process. Sensitive design can go a long way toward accomplishing both a homelike atmosphere and an efficient medical treatment area.[12]

The glass wall is used to separate an isolation station from the general treatment and work area, while still allowing for visual contact from staff.

MECHANICAL SYSTEMS

The following should be provided:

Plumbing[9]

- Plumbing for the unit should be designed to provide a minimum water pressure adequate to the needs of the equipment used with wastelines serving the dialysis equipment designed to prevent backflow and necessary check valves and shutoff valves appropriately located in the plumbing system.
- In so far as possible, drainage piping should not be installed within the ceiling or exposed. Where exposed, overhead drain piping in these areas is unavoidable, special provisions should be made to protect the space below from leakage, condensation, or dust particles.
- Floor drains should not be installed in operating rooms
- Backflow preventers (vacuum breakers) should be installed on hose bibbs, janitor's sinks, bedpan flushing attachments, clinical sinks, and all other attachments to which hose or tubing can be attached.
- If a centralized dialysate delivery system is utilized, each distribution line should be clearly labeled and color-coded to identify its contents.
- All dialysis system piping should be readily accessible for inspection and maintenance. Design consideration should be given to the disposal of liquid waste from the dialyzing process to prevent odor and backflow.
- Handwashing stations—in new construction and renovation where hemodialysis or hem perfusion are routinely performed, handwashing stations should have a separate water supply and drainage facility that does not interfere with hemodialysis piping.
- When the functional program includes hemodialysis, continuously circulated filtered cold water should be provided.
- Water treatment equipment room—the water treatment equipment should be located in an enclosed room.

Electrical Service

- There should be a minimum of two duplex receptacles on each side of a patient bed or lounge chair. Additional receptacles may be located where convenient for use.
- Receptacles should be located at least 36 inches and not more than 54 inches above the finished floor and be of "hospitalgrade" construction. At least one of these receptacles should be connected to the emergency power system. Electrical receptacles supplied from the emergency systems shall be distinctively colored or marked for identification. There should also be a receptacle at the head of each bed/chair location for the purpose of powering the bed/chair. There should be no less than one receptacle on each wall located at least 18 inch above the finished floor.
- Duplex receptacles for general use should be installed approximately 50-ft apart in all corridors and within 25-ft of corridor ends. All electrical receptacles within 36 inches of a plumbing fixture should be equipped with ground fault interrupting protection.
- Include in the prefabricated bedside patient unit (PBPU), a dedicated single receptacle for the dialysis machine. Power the receptacle from its own circuit fed from an emergency source (critical). Mount this receptacle approximately 1000 mm (40 inches) above the floor and distinctly identify it by an engraved wall plate on the PBPU. Plate should read "Dialysis Machine Only" in minimum 6 mm (¼-inch) letters.

- Services, switchboards, panel boards and transformers should be located in an area separate from plumbing and mechanical equipment and should be accessible to authorized persons only. Switchboards, panel boards and transformers should be convenient for use, readily accessible for maintenance, and located in dry, ventilated spaces free of corrosive or explosive fumes, gases, or any flammable material. Overload protective devices should operate properly in ambient room temperatures. Panel boards serving normal lighting and appliance circuits should be located on the same floor as the circuits they serve. Panel boards serving critical branch emergency circuits should be located on the same floor. Disconnects or electrical panels should be remotely located from any potentially hazardous equipment, including boilers, sterilizers, and generators being served to allow for the safe shutdown of the equipment.

Emergency Electrical Service (Fig. 14)

- *General*: To provide electricity during an interruption of the normal electric supply that could affect the nursing care, treatment, or safety of the occupants, an emergency source of electricity should be provided and connected to all circuits for lighting and power.[10,16]
- At least two primary electrical feeds served from separate substations or on-site back-up electrical source with 24 hours fuel supply to serve the entire facility demand should be considered.
- *Source:* The source of this emergency electrical service should be as follows:
  An emergency electrical generating set, including prime mover and generator, equipped with an automatic transfer switch (which will transfer within 10 s), should be located on the premises and shall be reserved exclusively for supplying the emergency electrical system. The emergency generator set should be of sufficient kilowatt capacity to supply all lighting and power load demands of the emergency system. The power factor rating of the generator should not be less than 80%.

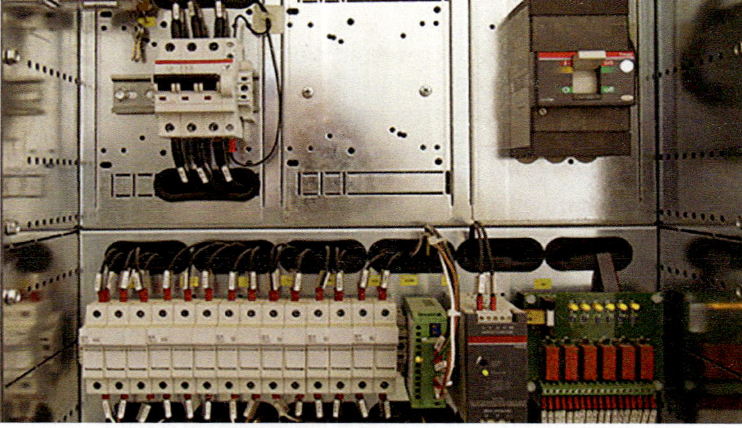

Fig. 14: Emergency electrical service (Electric panel).

- Battery-powered lighting should be provided for operating rooms, procedure rooms, dialysis rooms, intervention labs, etc. The battery should provide illumination for a period of 90 minutes after the loss of normal and emergency power.
- The reliance on emergency power in healthcare facilities continues to increase. Equipment and electrical systems on emergency power are escalating equally as fast. It is no longer unusual to find the patient care information system on emergency power. It is incumbent on the electrical system designer to anticipate the effect on the healthcare facility of scheduled and unscheduled downtime of the emergency power system. Install bypass-isolation switches for emergency power automatic transfer switches (ATS) so maintenance can be performed while they are de-energized on the throw-over mechanism without interrupting power to the essential load. Bypass isolation switches eliminate downtime for maintenance of the emergency power transfer switches as well as provide an alternate method of transfer in the event the emergency power transfer switches are damaged. Facilities should be designed to be self-sufficient for up to 72 hours following a regional disaster.

Emergency Electrical Connections

Emergency electrical services should be provided to circuits as follows:

- *Lighting*
  - All task lighting, exit ways, exit signs, exit directional signs, exit doorways, stairways, corridors, lobby, dialysis distribution systems and related equipment, and, if provided, the water treatment system.
  - Patient treatment rooms/cubicles, nursing station, medication preparation area, clean workroom, soiled workroom, equipment storage and waiting room.
  - Generator-set location and switch-gear location.
- *Equipment*
  - A minimum of one duplex receptacle on each side of patient bed/chair, or line isolation monitor panels connected to a dedicated circuit of a minimum of 20 amperes.
  - One duplex receptacle in the equipment maintenance room
  - Corridor receptacles in the patient treatment area
  - Essential refrigerators
  - Telephone equipment, nurses' call and intercom systems which depend upon electrical power supplied by facility.
  - Central batch delivery, water treatment, and related systems and equipment
  - Dialyzer reuse equipment
  - Ventilation equipment.

CONCLUSION

The contemporary designs having standardized, international dialysis protocols, including the unique water testing protocol, combined with a meticulously clean environment and other comforts like reclining chairs, Wi-Fi connectivity and personal LCD screens for a relaxed dialysis experience is a step towards making dialysis a stress-free patient-friendly procedure.[13] Proposed indicative diagram in Figures 15 and 16.

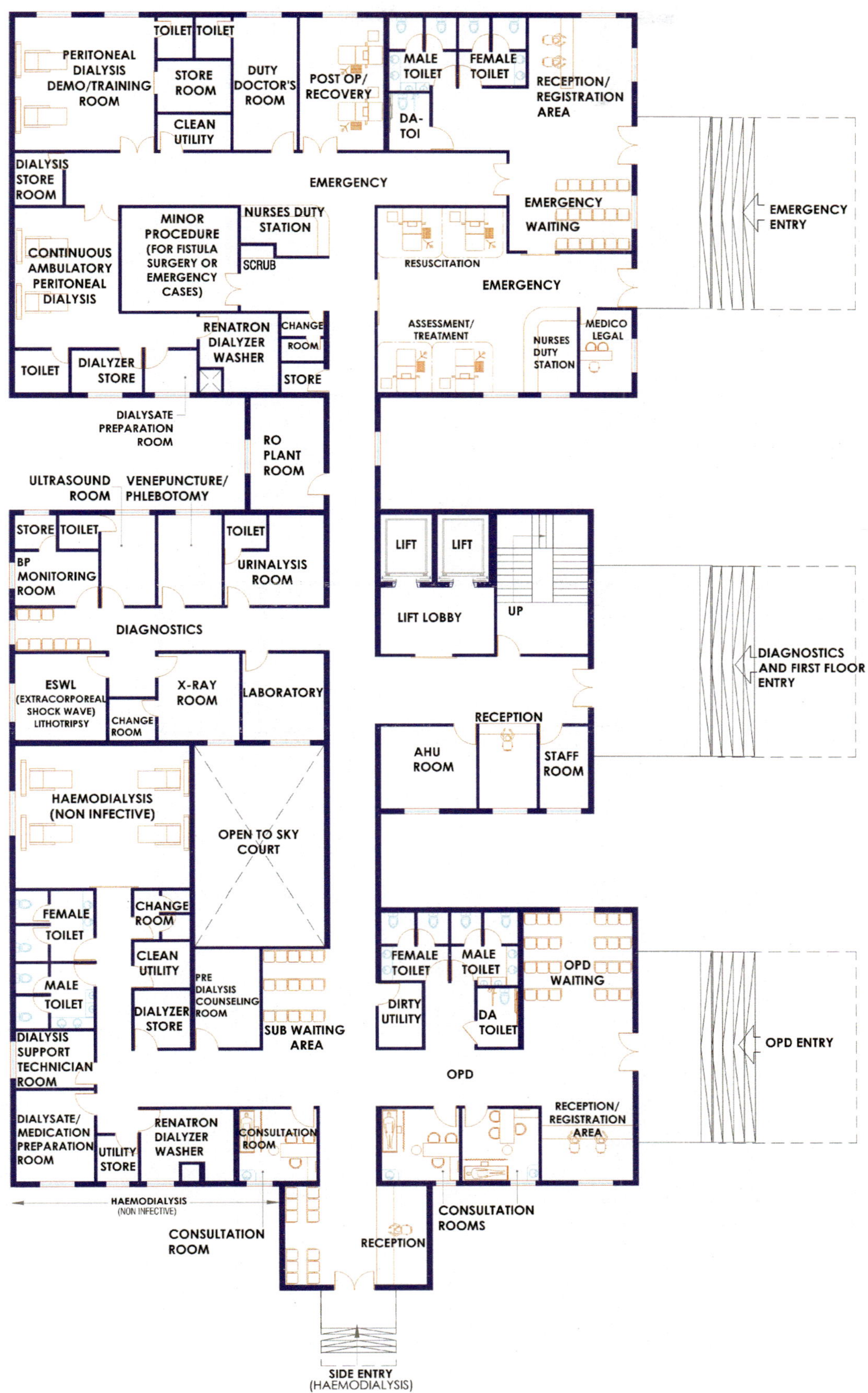

Fig. 15: Ground floor plan.

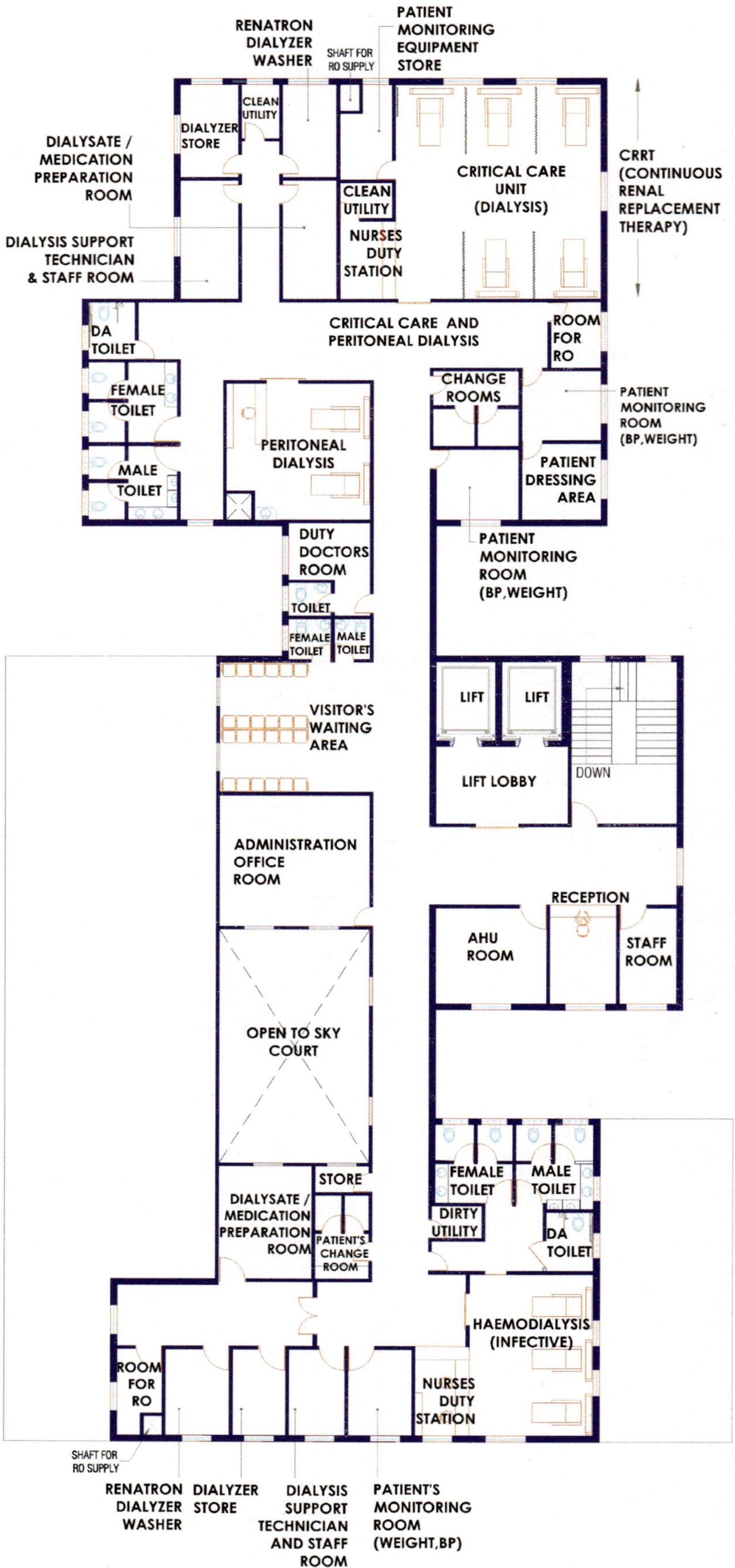

Fig. 16: First floor plan.

REFERENCES

1. www.cfm.va.gov
2. advancedrenaleducation.com
3. www.ndt-educational.org
4. https://www.ncbi.nlm.nih.gov/
6. www.wbdg.org
5. www.nmji.in
7. http://mercuryhealthcare.net/
8. Steven B. Bower. "Dialysis facility design—part I: Developing a strategic and financial plan", Dialysis & Transplantation, 08/2006.
9. dianousgroup.com
10. www.sjkdt.org
11. www.vdt.org
12. onlinelibrary.wiley.com
13. www.fortishealthcare.com

OTHER REFERENCES

- Graham T. The Bakerian lecture: Osmotic force. Philos Trans R SocLond 1854;144:117-28.
- Graham T. Liquid diffusion applied to analysis. Philos Trans R SocLond. 1861;151:183.
- Eggerth AH. The preparation and standardization of collodion membranes. J Bio Chem. 1921;48:203-21.
- Ferry J. Ultrafilter membranes and ultrafiltration. Chem Rev. 1936;18:3.
- Richardson BW. Practical studies in animal dialysis. Asclepiad 1889;6:331-2.
- Bigelow G. Collodion membranes. J Am Chem Soc. 1907; 29:1576-89.
- Abel J, Roundtree L, Turner B. On the removal of diffusible substances from the circulating blood of living animals by dialysis. J Pharmacol Exp Ther. 1914;5:275-316.
- Hess J, McGuigan W. The condition of the sugar in the blood.Pharmacology. 1914;6:45-55.
- Haas G. Versuche der BlutauswaschungamLebendenmitHilfe der Dialyse. KlinWochenschrift. 1925;4:13.
- Benedum J. Pioneer of dialysis, George Haas (1886-1971). Med Hist. 1979;14:196-217.
- Thalheimer W. Experimental exchange transfusion for reducing azotemia. Use of the artificial kidney for this purpose. Proc Soc Exp Biol Med. 1937;37:641-3.
- Quinton W, Dillard D, Scribner BH. Cannulation of blood vessels for prolonged hemodialysis. Trans ASAIO. 1960;6:104-7
- Lysaght MJ. Maintenance dialysis population dynamics: current trends and long-term implications. J Am Soc Nephrol. 2002;13:37-40.
- www.bmj.com
- Ansell D, Feest T (Eds). UK renal registry report 2004. Bristol: UK Renal Registry, 2004.
- lib.bioinfo.pl
- www.tulukootakuwait.org
- Guidelines for Dialysis Centre. Directorate General of Health Services, Govt. of India, 2017.
- www.sgacos.com
- www.michigan.gov
- www.drguide.mohp.gov.eg
- mdsr.ecri.org
- "IV.2 Technical design of the water treatment system", Nephrology Dialysis Transplantation, 07/01/2002.
- www.eneph.com
- www.readbag.com
- Steven B. Bower. "Dialysis facility design—Part IV: Color, sound, and materials", Dialysis & Transplantation, 11/200.
- www.fgiguidelines.org
- www.apicgd.org
- www.sots.ct.gov
- Mani MK. Experience with a program for prevention of chronic renal failure in India. Kidney Int. 2005;67:75-8. (Suppl) [PubMed].
- Agarwal SK, Dash SC, Irshad M, Raju S, Singh R, Pandey RM. Prevalence of chronic renal failure in adults in Delhi, India. Nephrol Dial Transplant. 2005;20: 1638-42.
- Modi GK, Jha V. The incidence of end-stage renal disease in India, a population based study. Kidney Int. 2006;70:2131-3. [PubMed

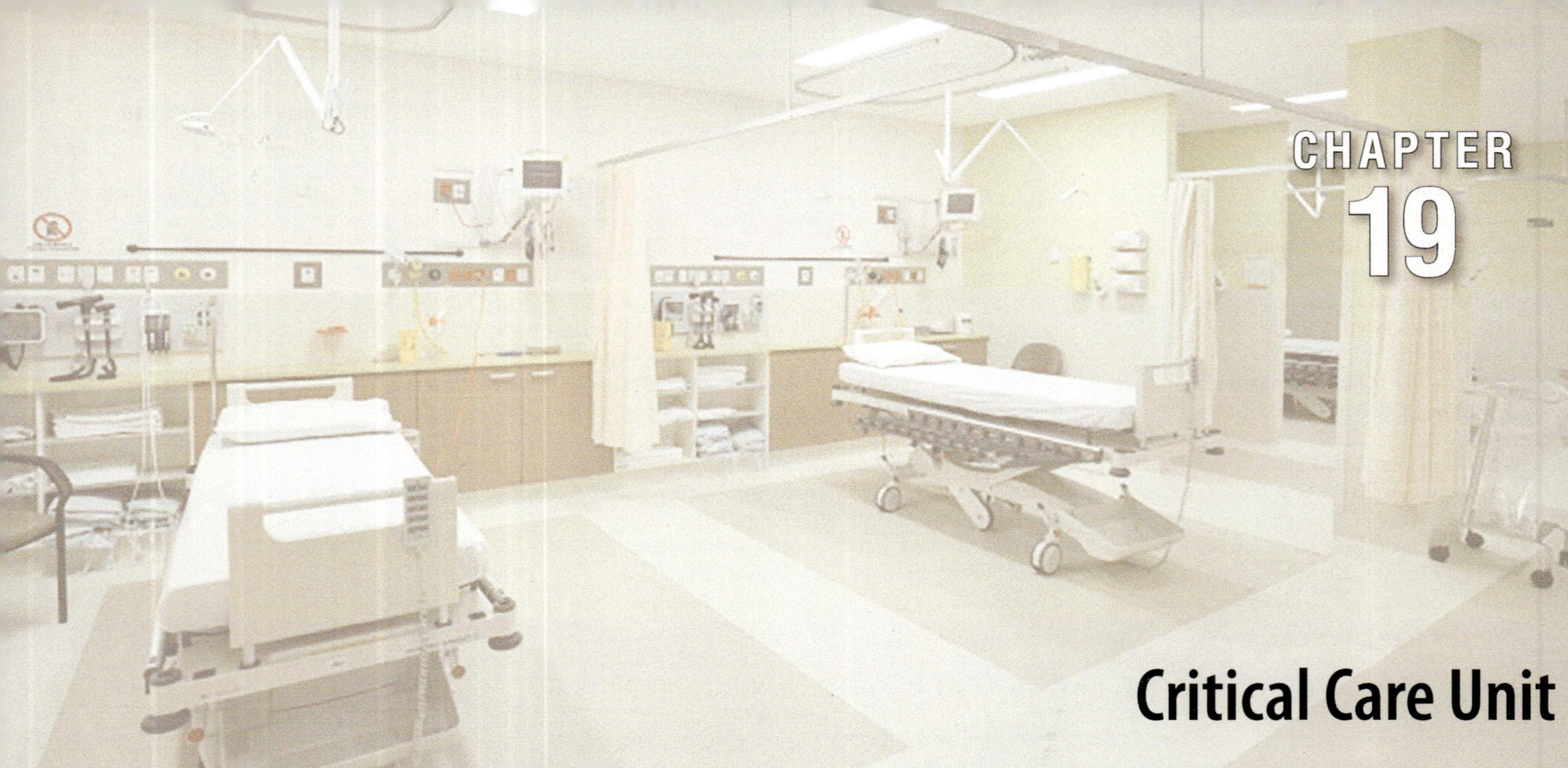

Critical Care Unit

Pankaj Arora, Shakti Kumar Gupta, Sunil Kant, R Chandrashekhar

INTRODUCTION

Critical care or intensive care, highest level of care in the continuum of progressive patient care, has assumed an important role in the delivery of hospital care, especially in the tertiary care settings. Life-expectancy has increased tremendously over the last few decades due to improved healthcare delivery. This has resulted in more and more people living longer and some of the countries have been labeled as "aging countries" due to negative growth rate of population and increasing geriatric population. Developed countries have by and large overcome the menace of communicable diseases but are faced with increasing burden of noncommunicable diseases like cancer and lifestyle diseases like diabetes mellitus, and hypertension, etc. At the same time, traffic accidents resulting in significant morbidity and mortality have attained alarming proportions.

The development and advancements in the techniques of healthcare delivery has meant that more and more lives can be saved but this entails an intensive level of care for the very sick. Critical care unit (CCU) in any hospital provides the opportunity and resources to provide such a level of care to the patients. CCU can be defined as a especially equipped hospital area designed for the treatment of patients with sudden life-threatening conditions. CCUs contain resuscitation and monitoring equipment and are staffed by personnel especially trained and skilled in recognizing and immediately responding to cardiac and other emergencies.[1,2]

FUNCTIONS

The very nature of the patients being cared for in any CCU implies that it has to be a part of a hospital providing the full spectrum of care or "progressive patient care". The level of services being provided will depend upon the nature of the hospital and the availability of resources both in terms of men and material. The Indian Society for Critical Care Medicine in its guidelines has proposed three levels of intensive care units ICUs, i.e. Level 1, Level 2, Level 3 based upon the type of hospital whether small, large or tertiary care, type of services being offered and the resources available.[3] Similar stratification of the ICUs has been suggested in the UK as well as Australia. The functions of any CCU will depend upon various factors. Some of them are listed below:

- Level and mandate of the hospital, e.g. rural hospital or a superspecialty hospital.
- Type of services being offered, e.g. general surgery or subspecialty like neurosurgery.
- Type of accident and emergency services being offered
- Expertise available or availability of trained manpower
- Availability of supportive facilities, e.g. blood bank, MRI and CT scan
- Networking with other hospitals usually higher level hospitals.

Based on the above factors, the functions of a particular critical care facility can be determined. For example, in a rural hospital setting where intensivist may not be available and other supportive facilities are also scarce, the CCU may be used to stabilize a sick patient before he is referred to a higher center. On the other hand, a tertiary care hospital, where complex procedures are being undertaken, many subspecialty ICUs may be functioning, e.g. NICU, neuro-ICU, etc. The protocols for a CCU in a hospital will also depend upon these factors. Underlying all the possible functions of a CCU is the effort to provide intensive care to the patients who cannot be managed in a routine ward so as to improve their chances of recovery from the disease they are suffering from.

KEY PLANNING AND DESIGNING PARAMETERS

The factors which will affect the planning of a CCU will again depend upon the functions of the facility as mentioned above. Besides, other key parameters are:

- Whether the facility is being created afresh as a part of a new hospital or is being renovated in the existing hospital.
- In case of renovation or a new facility, the space available for the proposed facility.
- The proposed operational model for the CCU
- The number of beds in the CCU
- Establishment of a high-dependency unit (HDU).

High-dependency unit is one step down from the ICU whereby the patients can be managed by the level of care less intense than an ICU but still cannot be managed in the general ward, i.e. an intermediate level of care between an ICU and a ward. This unit can also admit patients on its own depending upon the policy of the hospital as well as acting as a step-down facility. This will lower the pressure on the ICU as well as improving its throughput.

Operational Model[4]

Single/general critical care unit: This model is suitable for small- or medium-sized hospitals which do not have subspecialties or have a few subspecialties. All the patients requiring critical care are admitted in this unit irrespective of the specialty they belong to. The unit is headed by an intensivist and the admitting specialty provides the consultation but the primary responsibility for the care remains with the intensivist. This type of approach results in the optimum utilization of the beds and resources. The protocol for the admission can be decided by the hospital administration.

Hot floor: The CCU is composed of many ICUs belonging to different subspecialties, e.g. neurosurgery, cardiology, pediatric surgery, etc. and HDUs located on the same floor. Each subspecialty ICU may be headed by the respective department or by the intensivist depending upon the policy of the hospital but the Director of CCU should be an expert in critical care or an intensivist. It has been seen that the association of the critical care expert with an ICU has resulted in better outcomes as far as the patient care is concerned. The advantage of such an arrangement is the better utilization of the resources and manpower. The nursing staff can be rotated among different subspecialties resulting in capacity-building and depending upon the workload can be rationally deployed. The support services like ABG lab can be optimally utilized and duplication can be avoided.

The disadvantage is the nonavailability of the alternative place for accommodating these patients in case of internal disaster like fire. Another difficulty arises in the case of outbreak of an epidemic in the hot floor due to deficiency in infection control measures since all the patients are highly susceptible to hospital-acquired infection (HAI).

Segregated critical care unit: Different ICUs comprising the CCU are located in different parts of the hospital. This type of arrangement is more suitable for tertiary care hospital with organ-based units/centers separated by physical distances, where these are not a part of a single composite hospital.

Number of beds: Because of the realization of benefits of critical care beds, their numbers in any hospital have increased over the passage of time. It has been generally said that 5–10% of hospital beds should be critical care beds with numbers increasing up to 20% in case of some subspecialties like neurosurgery or cardiothoracic surgery. According to the Indian Public Health Standards (IPHS) for a 500-bedded hospital, 2–5% of the beds shall be critical care beds which will be equally divided between ICU and HDU.[5] The number of beds in CCU will depend upon variety of factors including existence of such facilities in the other hospitals in the community, availability of trained manpower, and policy of the hospital.

The formula given by Bridgman[6] can be used to calculate the number of beds:

No. of critical care beds =

$$\frac{\text{No. of patients admitted to intensive care in 1 year} \times \text{ALOS}}{\text{(where ALSO : Average length of stay) } 365 \times \text{desired occupancy rate}}$$

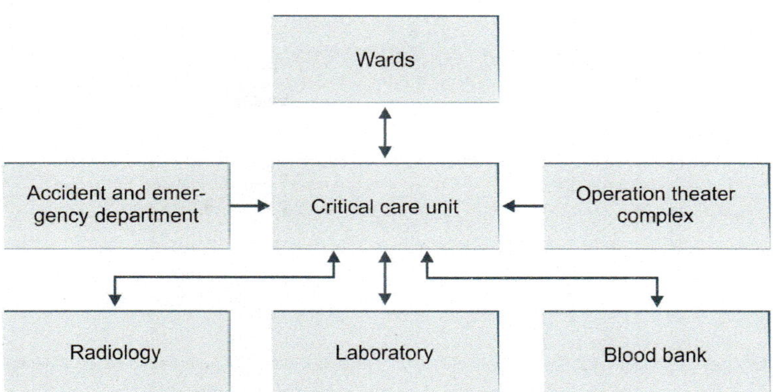

Fig. 1: Functional relationships of critical care unit.

Location: The CCU should be located in close physical and functional relationship with the areas from which it will receive patients. These are accident and emergency (A & E) departments and operation theater (OT) complex. Simultaneously, it should be ensured that the support services which will be most frequently used are in close proximity. These are radiology, laboratories and blood bank. With the advancements of technology like PACS, mobile CT scan, pneumatic tube system for transportation of samples and results, this requirement of proximity to the support services may be suitably modified depending upon the availability of the resources.

Functional Relationship

The access to the CCU must be controlled for better infection control. It should be attempted that the patient transportation routes are segregated from the transportation route of the general public. Since the patients will be predominantly received from the A & E department and OT complex, dedicated lifts can be earmarked for the transport of patients from these two areas. The same is shown in Figure. 1.

PLANNING CONSIDERATIONS

Patient Care Areas

The bed of the patient is the hub of all the activities in the critical care area, literally. Ideally, the bed should be located in direct line of vision from the nursing station. Simultaneously, the privacy of each individual should be maintained so that other patients and visitors may not be able to view the patient. This can be ensured by having curtains, screens, or partitions between the beds.

The pros and cons of each option have to be weighed before deciding upon the best according to the hospital management. The curtains and curtain rods/rails accumulate dust and can be a potential a source of infection. Hence, their cleanliness may be an area of concern. The screen may look clumsy resulting in poor state esthetics. The partitions may hamper the flexibility around the bed so that an alteration in the space around the bed cannot be made easily. This problem can be overcome by having moveable partitions and turned into an advantage by having lead incorporated in them. This helps in minimizing the inadvertent exposure to X-rays for the adjacent patients since a lot of these patients will require portable X-ray investigation.

Open Plan Area versus Single Rooms

A considerate decision has to be taken regarding the plan of the unit whether to have beds in an open area or to have single rooms. Both the approaches have advantages and disadvantages.

Single Room (Fig. 2)[7]

Advantage	Disadvantage
• Improved patient satisfaction • Better infection control • Increased privacy • Less sensory overload • Less anxiety	• Decreased visibility and access to patients • Difficult to manage • Decreased communication • Patient anxiety, boredom and depression

Open Plan Area (Fig. 3)[7]

Advantage	Disadvantage
• Increased visibility • Easier access to patients • Communication and teamwork increased • Management easier • Stimulation for patients • Sense of security and support for inexperienced staff	• Noisy • Busy environment • Decreased concentration • Sensory overload for patients and staff

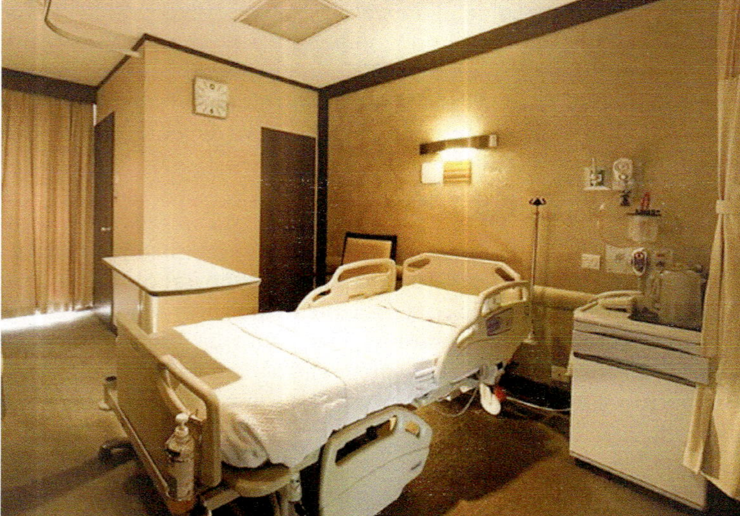

Fig. 2: Single room.

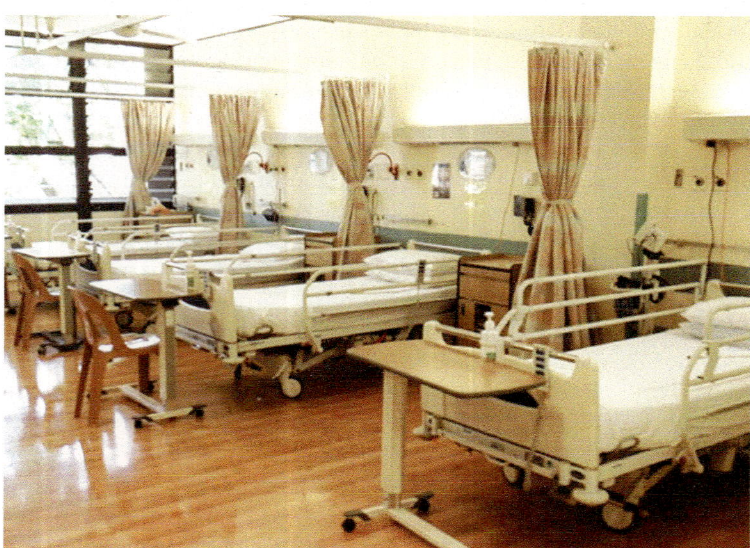

Fig. 3: Open plan area.

In case of a general CCU (mentioned above) an equal mix of open plan area and single room accommodation would be appropriate so that different variety of patients can be handled in the same unit with optimal utilization of resources. This has become essential since a number of patients may be suffering from infectious diseases rendering other susceptible patients more vulnerable.

If the hospital has a hot-floor concept it may be more appropriate to have a dedicated intensive care area consisting of only single room accommodation. Since all the patients requiring critical care are housed on the same floor, transferability between the units will not be an issue. All those patients requiring isolation care can then be housed in a single area decreasing the vulnerability of all other patients in the critical care unit.

A segregated CCU should be located in different parts of the hospital based on the subspecialties, the tradeoff between the open plan area and single room accommodation will be based on the subspecialty. Those handling more number of infectious cases need to have more single room accommodation and vice versa. The exact number can be arrived at based on the brainstorming, current trends and past experience.

Whatever may be the arrangement of the beds; different authors have suggested that a particular unit should not have less than six beds or more than fourteen beds. Any number less than six makes it uneconomical to run while a number greater than fourteen will be difficult to manage. Though 8–12 beds may be taken as accepted figure but larger units may be designed if the adequate resources in terms of men and material can be provided. Additionally, a staff station is required for every 12 beds.

Patient visibility: A lot of stress has been placed on the patient visibility and the arrangement of beds is done to facilitate direct visibility from the nursing station. This is however not always feasible with the single room accommodation and privacy issues. Video monitoring is a viable alternative to the direct visibility. A dedicated CCTV can be mounted at vantage point for each patient and the feed can be beamed to the monitor at the nursing station. All the patients can be simultaneously monitored from the nursing/staff station. The system can be linked with the telemedicine facility and the feed can be visualized at multiple portals simultaneously. This will render offsite expertise available in case of emergency or referral or for teaching purposes. This model of eICU is most useful in case of segregated CCU or a network of CCUs in a community whereby services of intensivist can be utilized without causing physical stress. It is stressed here that the technology is not intended to replace the direct patient monitoring but to supplement it. Further the pictures can be beamed to the waiting lounge for the attendants so that they can also be updated about the condition of the patient.

Patient monitoring: Since the patients are acutely ill, the care is equipment intensive. The patient will have ventilator, cardiac monitor, probably a dialysis machine, or any other equipment required for the monitoring of the patients. The equipment should be easily accessible to the healthcare workers without impeding the patient visibility. Traditional approach of having all the equipment on the head side of the patient may not be the most appropriate since it may obstruct the approach to the head end of the patient bed in case of emergency. Pendants may be used to mount the equipment as well as for the electrical and manifold outlets. If rails are used, then they must be sturdy enough to hold the weight of equipment. These approaches may offer more flexibility and reduce the cluttering of wires around the bed, hence *Media Bridge* helps in resolving these issues (Fig. 4).

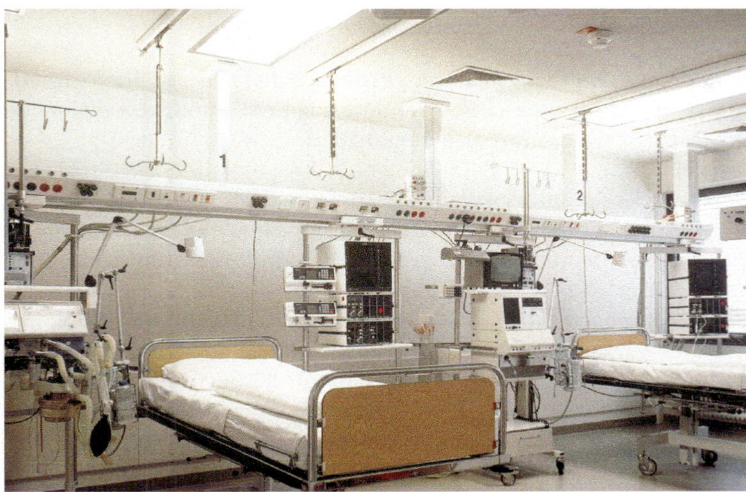

Fig. 4: Media bridge.

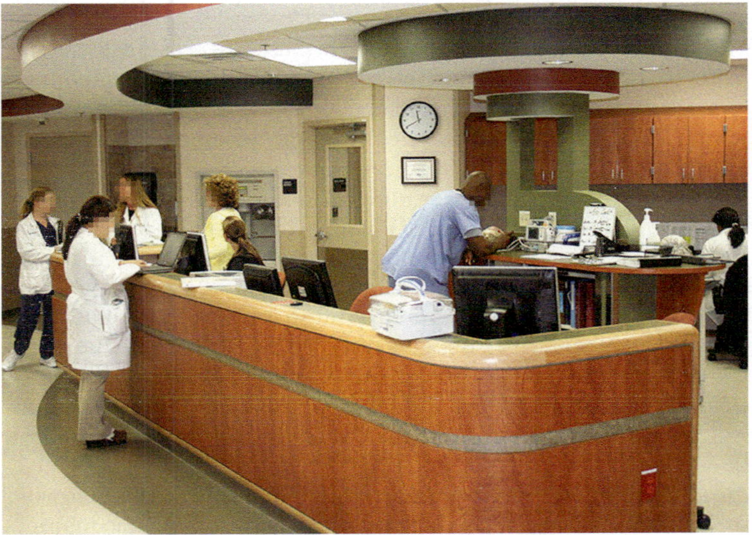

Fig. 5: Nursing station.

Space requirement: As mentioned above, the amount of gadgets placed around the patient bed implies that the space required per bed will be higher than in a general ward. Hence, CCUs must be spacious with 20–22 sqm area per bed and a clear corridor space of 2.5 m beyond the working area. Besides these a gowning lobby of 6 sqm should be provided. In case of single room accommodation the area required per bed is 22–24 sqm with isolation rooms requiring an additional anteroom of 2–2.5 sqm for hand washing and gowning. An unobstructed clear space of 750–900 mm should be left between the head end of the bed and the wall to allow for resuscitation in case of emergency. Similarly a clear space of 1–1.5 m should be left between the sides of the patient bed and any fixed structure.

Nursing station: Staff station or nursing station should be well equipped to facilitate the patient-care activities (Fig. 5). Adequate storage space should be provided for storing different items required for discharging the activities. These include space for resuscitation cart, drugs refrigerator and stationery. Working area should have monitor for viewing patients electronically as well as computer for entering data. X-ray-view box should be there at the station even if the PACS facility is available. Patient beds should be visible from the station as mentioned above.

Environmental Considerations

Noise: Various equipment in the CCU emit sound continuously in the form of beeps or alarms. Since the number of instruments can be very high, this may result in a very noisy environment. Additionally, the manpower working in the area may be another source of noise. Hence, it is necessary that the measures be taken to reduce or absorb the noise. The International Noise Council has recommended that noise levels in the hospital acute areas not exceed 45 dB(A) in the daytime, 40 dB(A) in the evening and 20 dB(A) in the night. Hence, floor coverings that absorb sound should be used keeping in mind the constraints of infection control and movement of equipment. Walls and ceilings should be constructed of materials with high sound absorption capabilities. Ceiling soffits and baffles help in reducing echoed sounds.[8,9]

Daylight: Daylight has a healing effect on the patients and helps in restoring the circadian rhythm. Windows or skylight should be provided so that the patients have view of the outside. Patient beds should be placed near the windows for this purpose. Furthermore, the use of daylight will help in decreasing the requirement for the artificial light during the daytime saving the energy considerably.

Clock/calendar: A clock and a readable calendar should be visible from every patient bed as it helps in maintaining proper orientation for the intubated patients.

Architectural Considerations

Floor: Floor should be nonslippery, joint-less (if possible) coved and easy-to-clean and sturdy so as to be capable of bearing the load of equipment. Vinyl flooring may be used keeping in mind the necessity to change it if it cracks from any part.

Walls: Similarly, walls should be easy to clean and suitably protected at places where they may get damaged due to trolleys or other equipment.

Engineering Considerations

Lighting: Adjustable lighting must be available so that the light intensity can be regulated according to the time of the day as well as requirement of the patient and the staff. Provision should be made for glare-free focused light for the patient bed in case some bed-side procedure is required to be done. This can be achieved by having a mobile light or wall-mounted light with long swivel arms so that only one fixture is sufficient for 3–4 beds.

Type of interior, task or activity	*E_m in lux*	*UGR_L*	*R_a*
General lighting	100	19	90
Simple examinations	300	19	90
Examination and treatment	500	19	90
Night watch	20	19	90

HVAC

Sl. No	*Parameter*	*Value*
1.	Temperature	22 ± 2°C
2.	Air changes	10–15 per h
3.	Filtration	Hepa filters–99% efficiency
4.	Relative humidity	45 ± 5%

(HVAC: heating, ventilation, and air conditioning)

Electrical fittings: A range of electrical outlets from 10 per bed to 15 per bed has been suggested for the ICU. Because of ever-increasing changes and advancements in technology, instrumentation is bound to increase in the future hence higher number (15) may be appropriate. Electric outlets/inlets should be common 5/15 amp pins, should have pins to accommodate all standard International Electric Pins/Sockets, so that all the equipments can be used. These include portable X-ray machines, warmers, computer terminal and such equipments as radio or television depending upon the policy of the hospital. Few of the outlets should be on UPS for uninterrupted supply and must be distinctly colored or marked for easy identification.

Medical Gas Pipe Systems

- *Oxygen*: 3–4 outlets per bed are required
- *Compressed air*: 2 outlets per bed are required
- *Vacuum*: 2 outlets per bed are required.

Other Considerations

Communication: Different communication systems should be used which can act as complementary to each other. These include telephone, PA system, visual alarms, etc. Duress alarm should be provided at each bed site so that a patient may be able to seek assistance in case of need. This alarm can be an audiovisual alarm which can be fitted at the nursing station. Similarly, an emergency alarm blowing off simultaneously at several places in the critical care complex, i.e. doctor's duty room, seminar room, and nursing station signifying code blue should be provided.

The healthcare staff should have access to internet, hence computer terminal may be provided at the nursing station along with accessories like printer, etc. to facilitate the work.

Information kiosk: An information kiosk will help the healthcare staff in finding out necessary information for the patient care from the reference material. The reference material may be in the form of e-books, online journals.

Ergonomics: Critical care unit is inherently stressful because of the nature of patients and services being provided. Hence, every effort should be made to reduce stress—both physical and mental. The ward should be designed ergonomically so as to minimize musculoskeletal stress. It is known that physical stress can be an important factor in staff turnover.

Infection control: The patients admitted to this facility are sick or immunecompromised or have undergone procedures, which render them susceptible to infections, hence infection control is of paramount importance. The infection control measures must be incorporated at the planning stage and carried through the designing phase to the formation of standard operating procedures (SOPs) for the facility.

Nonpatient Care Areas

Stores: For keeping the linen, drugs, housekeeping material, etc.

Duty rooms: For the doctors, nurses and other staff.

Visitor's lounge: Usually 1–2 seats per patient are sufficient. There should be a small cafe or a tea/coffee-vending machine. Public conveniences like drinking water must also be provided.

Dormitory: A dormitory may be built near the facility for the attendants who have to stay overnight. This will earn the hospital revenue, propel the image of the hospital and provide comfort to the attendants.

Disaster management: Since the patients admitted in the facility are very sick and usually immobile, an internal disaster like fire can cause a huge problem as far as evacuation of the patients is concerned. This aspect must be taken care while designing the facility so that in case of any such disaster, the loss of lives can be minimized. Proper air scavenging system should be in place and needs to be monitored periodical as use of O_2 to abundance in this area.

CONCLUSION

Critical care unit is designed to provide a highest level of care to the sickest patients admitted in the hospital. A lot of life-saving and complicated procedures have been developed and are being performed due to the advancements in the critical care medicine. A well-functioning CCU with acceptable mortality statistics cannot only help to save lives but also can be an immense image builder for the hospital.

Depending upon the level of the hospital, expertise available and policies governing the hospital, different levels of the CCU can be developed. They will vary in terms of equipment available and the types of patients who are admitted in these units.

Since the critical care is highly resource-intensive in terms of men and material, the provision of care is very costly. The facility has unique spatial requirements which are different from the general ward. All efforts must be made to optimally utilize the facility for economical throughput.

Design features also have to step into consideration of critical aspects, such as infection control, patient safety and disaster management.

REFERENCES

1. www.sccm.org
2. kpjkluang.com
3. www.isccm.org
4. Australasian health facility guidelines. Sydney: Centre for Health Assets Australasia (CHAA); 2009.
5. http://nrhm.gov.in./images/pdf/guidelines/iphs/iphs-revised-guidelines-2012/district-hospital.pdf
6. Miranda DR, Williama A. Loirat Management of intensive care: Guidelines for better use of resources. Springer; 1990.
7. www.baccnconference.org.uk
8. sccs-sa.org
9. Guidelines for intensive care unit design. Critical Care Medicine. 1995;23(3):582-8.

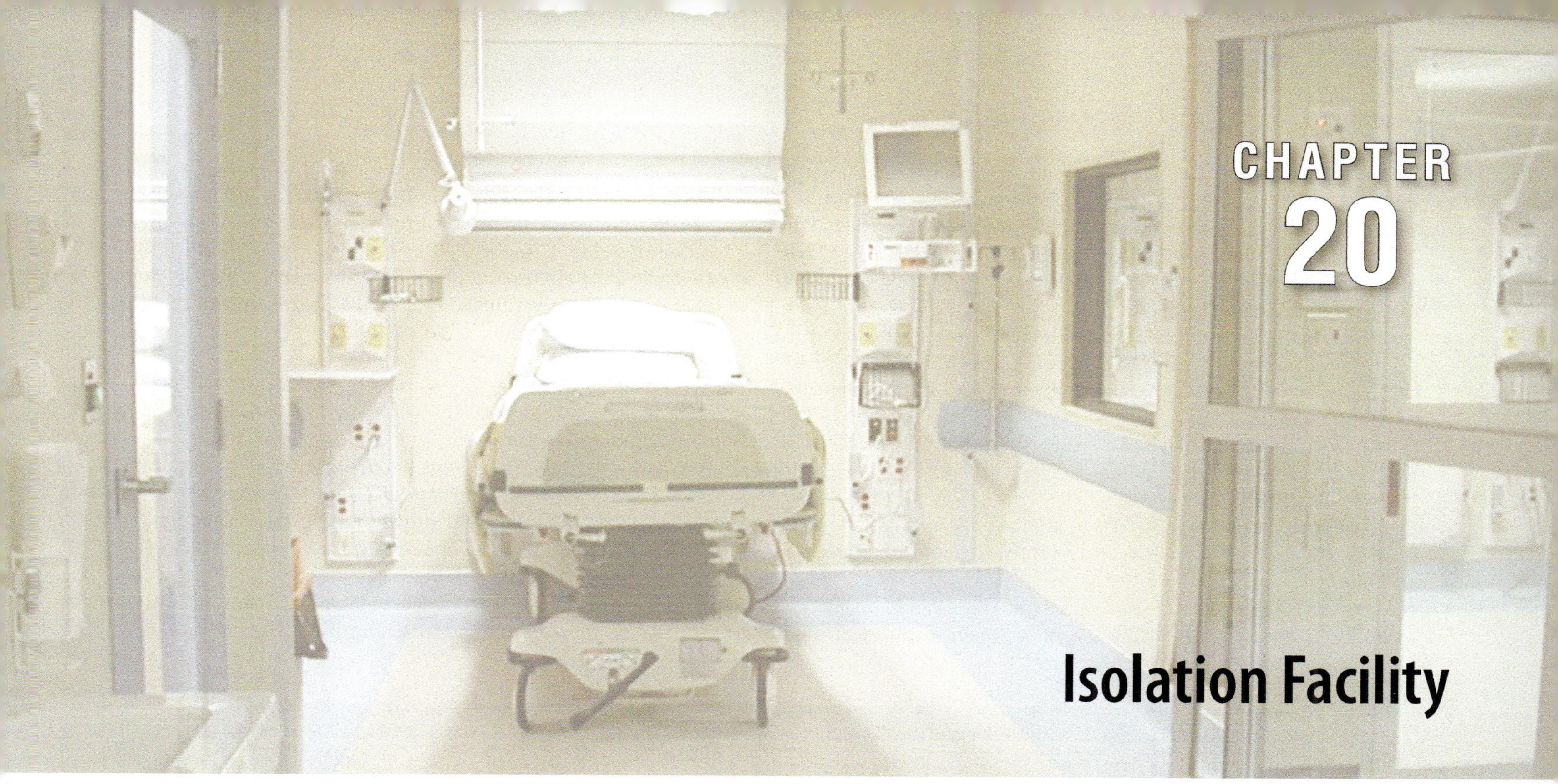

CHAPTER 20

Isolation Facility

Kumari Shweta, Shakti Kumar Gupta, Sunil Kant, R Chandrashekhar

INTRODUCTION

Infection control is emerging as a biggest challenge to health services around the world. All hospitals knowingly or unknowingly admit patients with communicable diseases. In recent years, the transmission of healthcare associated infections has become a serious threat for healthcare facilities. Technically, healthcare associated infections relate to those who are hospitalized, but healthcare professionals may themselves be at risk.[1]

Eliminating transmission can never be guaranteed but certainly the built environment can help to minimize and reduce the risks along with sound deployment of clinical. Occupational Safety and Health Administration (OSHA) states that, "The most effective way to prevent or lessen transmission of nosocomial infection (hospital acquired) is to isolate the airborne contaminant and to provide an environment that will promote reduced exposure to contaminant". The role of infection control in the design of hospitals is increasing everyday with emergence of communicable diseases like tuberculosis, immunocompromised conditions like HIV/AIDS and multidrug resistant organisms.[2,3]

FUNCTIONS[4]

The main functions of the facility are:
- To separate patients who are likely to be infectious to other persons.
- To provide an environment that will allow reduction of the concentration of airborne particles through various engineering methods.
- To prevent escape of airborne particles from such rooms into the corridor and other areas of the facility using directional airflow.
- To protect patients who are immunocompromised from potential harmful pathogens.

There are two types of isolation rooms—viz. airborne infection isolation (AII) rooms and protective environment (PE) rooms.
- *Airborne infection isolation* refers to the isolation of patients infected with organisms spread via airborne droplet nuclei <5 µm in diameter. These include patients suffering from measles, chickenpox and tuberculosis.
- *Protective environment* is a specialized area for patients who have undergone allogeneic hematopoietic stem cell transplant (HSCT).

PLANNING PREMISES OF ISOLATION ROOMS (FIG. 1[1,3,5-7]

General Planning Considerations

Location: The isolation rooms should be located at one end of medical and surgical wards/critical care units/pediatric care units/newborn intensive care units/emergency service areas/also other areas such as dialysis. Isolation wards for infectious cases to be kept out of routine

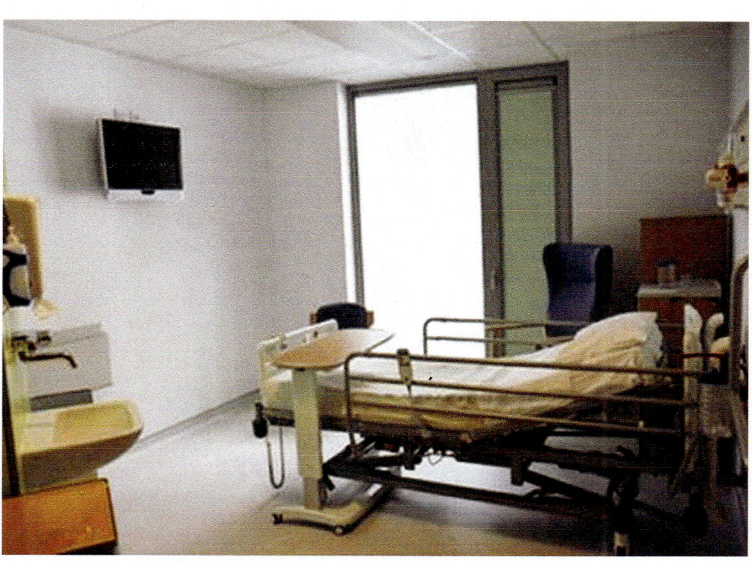

Fig. 1: Isolation room.

circulation. The location of the proposed isolation room such as those near elevator banks or doorways should be avoided.

- *Number of beds for isolation beds*: About 2.5% of the beds of a large hospital in a special unit would probably be adequate except during periods of unusually high demand.
- *Space*: An isolation room has to provide uncluttered space around the bed for equipment and the increased number of personnel involved in emergency care. A room area of about 22 sqm is adequate within an isolation unit.
- Adequate number of wash hand basins should be provided within the patient care areas and nursing stations with a view to facilitate hand washing practice.
- Separate arrangements for garbage and infectious waste removal from wards and departments in the form of separate staircases and lifts.
- One to two standard isolation rooms per ward unit should be planned throughout the hospital with wash hand basin in room, shower, toilet and wash hand basin in bathroom. Door with self-closing device and a central air-conditioning with desired air changes is recommended.
- Gasketing should be provided at the sides and top of the door, and at ceiling and wall penetrations such as those around medical and electrical outlets.

LAYOUT (FIG. 2)[2,7]

Bed management system:

- Bed centers should be at least 3.6 m apart
- Beds in a cohort should be kept to a minimum number possible as this will greatly assist in the prevention of cross-infection.
- Design, accessibility and space in patient areas all contribute to ease of cleaning and maintenance.
- Spacing must take account of access to equipment around the bed and access for staff to hand wash facilities.

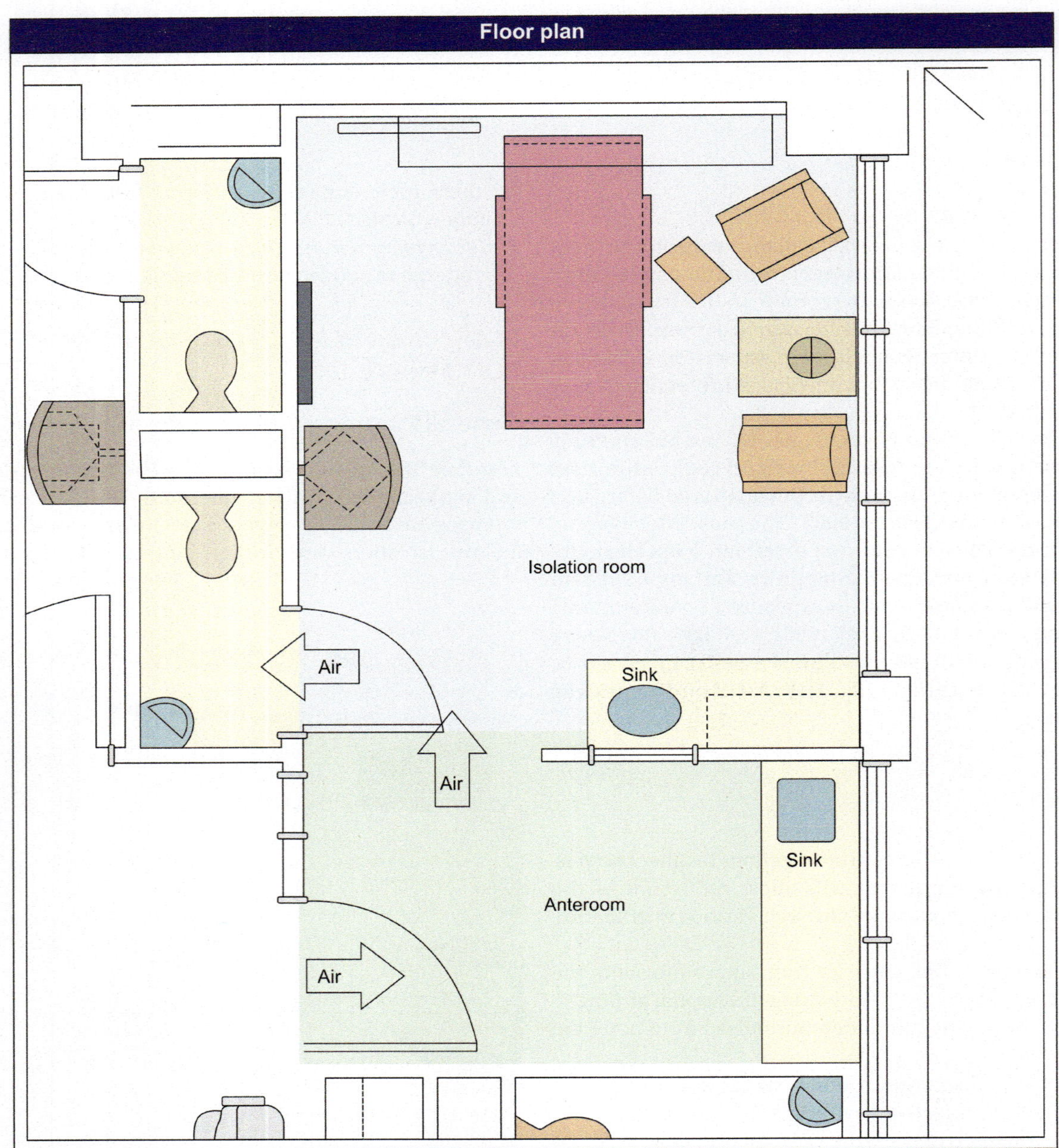

Fig. 2: Layout of an isolation room.

- Consideration can be given to permanent screens between bed spaces as an aid to prevent frequent traffic and thus, the potential for microorganism transfer.

Classification of Isolation Rooms (Table 1)[8]

Isolation Room: General Planning Considerations

The design, materials and construction of the interior surfaces of an isolation room are critical to the performance of the room in containing infections.

- Continuous impervious surfaces such as welded vinyl, epoxy coatings or similar durable surfaces.
- Welded vinyl floors coved up the walls, and wall finishes that are durable and easy to clean; for example, welded vinyl. Isolation rooms also need smooth finishes, free of fissures or open joints and crevices that retain or permit passage of dirt particles. The use of carpet is discouraged because it is difficult to clean.
- Minimization of horizontal surfaces.
- Guard rails to protect the walls from damage by beds and mobile equipment.
- Epoxy-coated or stainless steel joinery that is easier to clean than uncoated timber
- Windows designed to avoid pelmets and dust collection areas
- Washable curtains
- Wall-hung toilet pan and basin with non-hand operated taps
- *Window setting (Fig. 3)*: Isolated patients can distinguish day and night by looking through the window panes at the isolation room. This is particularly important to the elderly as it relieves symptoms of disorientation
- *Signs and labels*: All isolation room ductwork systems should be labeled with appropriate warning signs. Appropriate signage should be prominently placed outside the door of isolation rooms. The bedside and other charts should also be labeled once isolation has been ordered for a patient (Fig. 4)
- *Doors (Fig. 5)*: Sliding doors are not recommended but if space is an issue, sliding doors should only used as a last resort due to difficulties

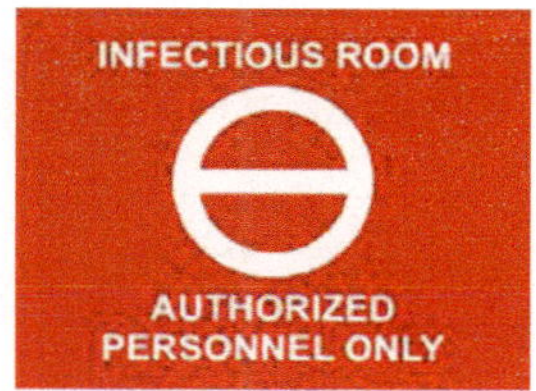

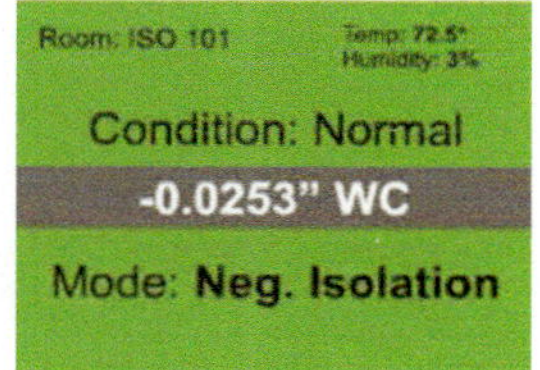

Fig. 4: Signage.

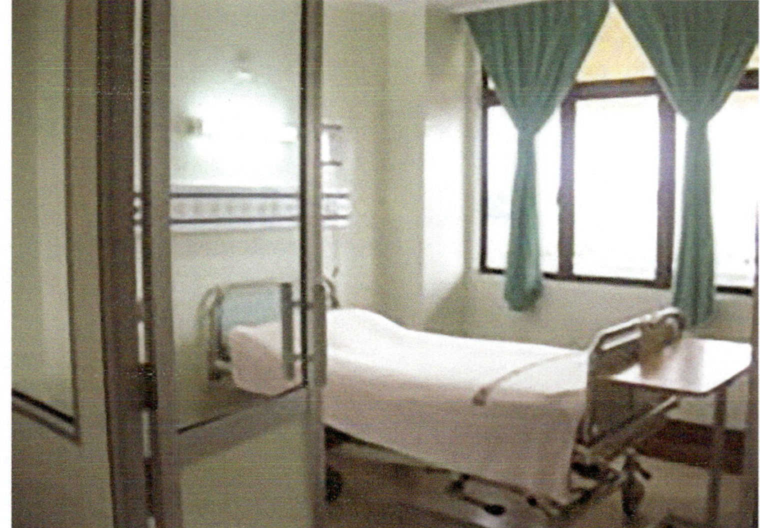

Fig. 3: Window setting.

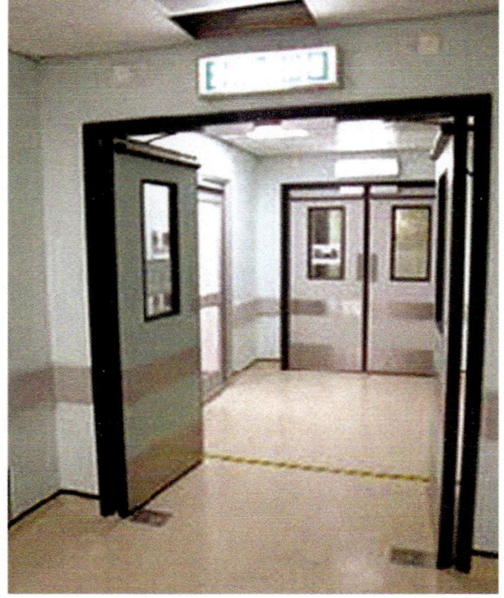

Fig. 5: Doors should open out of a negative pressure to positive pressure.

Table 1: Functional classification of isolation rooms.[1,8,9]

	Class S (Standard)	*Class N (Negative) (Fig. 7)*	*Class P (Positive) (Fig. 8)*	*Class A (Alternating)*
Key ventilation criteria	No air pressure difference between the room and the adjacent corridor	Lower air pressure in the room than in adjacent corridor	Greater air pressure in the room than in the adjacent corridor	Ventilation controlled to achieve either positive or negative pressure in the room
Transmission-based precautions	To prevent contact or droplet transmission	To prevent airborne transmission	To prevent transmission of pathogens from outside environment to immunosuppressed patients	Not recommended
Examples	Hepatitis A, meningococcal infection	Measles, chickenpox, tuberculosis	Prevention of infection in bone marrow or organ transplant recipients	Not recommended

with maintenance and maintaining a seal. The pressure differential should force swing doors into the seal, i.e. doors should open out of a negative pressure room or open into a Positive pressure room. An alternative arrangement can be to have both doors swing into the anteroom. If doors have an interlocks mechanism fitted (Fig. 6), an emergency breakout system must be provided.

- Communication system.
- A nurse call system with the capacity for direct communication between the nurse and patient should be available in each room.

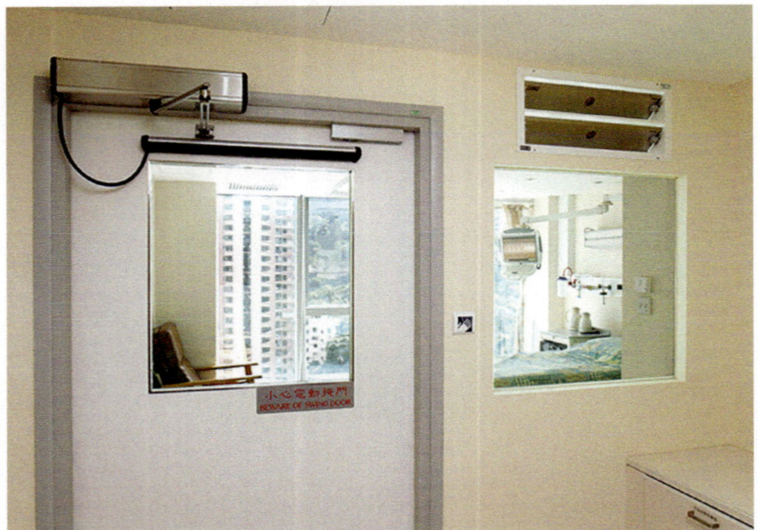

Fig. 6: An air tight door.

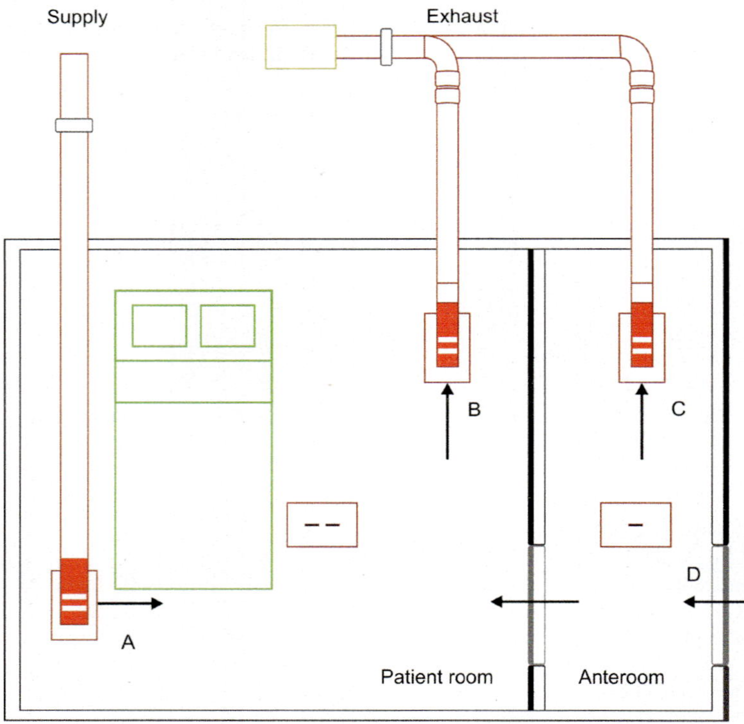

Fig. 7: Negative pressure isolation room.

CLASS N: NEGATIVE PRESSURE ISOLATION ROOMS[4,9]

Air in an open Class N room, for example, should flow from corridors into the isolation room to prevent the spread of airborne contaminants from the isolation room to other areas. The purpose of this design is to eliminate the spread of infectious contaminants and pathogens into the surrounding environment via the airborne route. Other patient treatment areas that can also be benefited from in-room negative pressure isolation with HEPA-CARE systems include:

- Bronchoscopy suites
- Endotracheal intubation and extubation
- Open suctioning of airways
- Invasive vascular procedures
- ER triage and treatment rooms
- Waiting areas
- Morgue/autopsy.

The schematic above shows HVAC air flow arrangement for class N rooms. An anteroom designed to provide an "air-lock" (no mix of air) between the infectious patient and the common space is placed adjacent to the patient room. The air would flow from the anteroom to the isolation room. Pressure control is maintained by modulating the main supply and exhaust dampers based on a signal from a pressure transducer located inside the isolation room.

Infection: Control and Ventilation Requirements for Rooms[4]

According to American Institute of Architects (AIA) guidelines, recommended elements include:

- Ensure that the airborne infectious isolation rooms are designed to maintain negative pressure.
- Maintain continuous negative air pressure no less than [2.5 Pa (0.01 inch water gauge)] in relation to the air pressure in the corridor. This is accomplished via a separate exhaust system sized to remove at least 15% more air than that of the supply system (Fig. 8).
- Monitor air pressure periodically, preferably daily, with audible manometers or smoke tubes at the door (for existing AII rooms), or with a permanently installed visual monitoring mechanism.

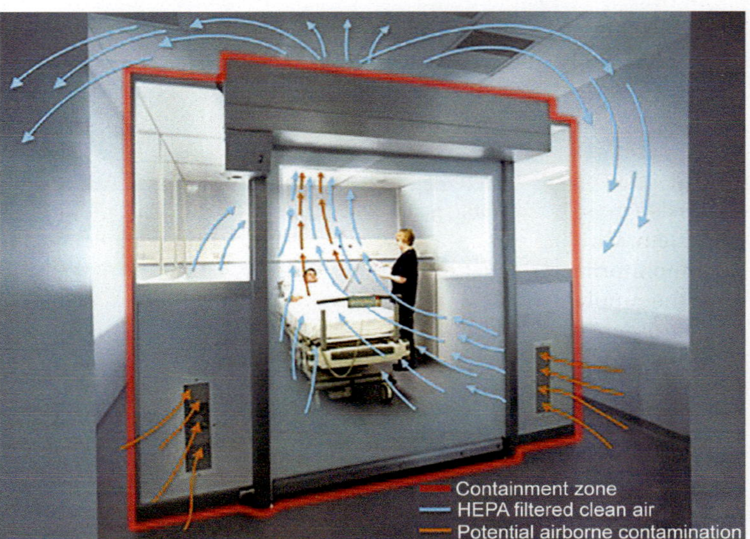

Fig. 8: Negative pressure room.

- Provide ventilation to ensure ≥12 ACH for renovated rooms and new rooms, and ≥6 ACH for existing AII rooms, when supply or exhaust air filters are at their maximum pressure drop.
- The recommended air filtration for the Class N, airborne infectious isolation rooms is MERV 14 rating air filters (90% dust spot test filters) on the supply side and high efficiency particulate air (HEPA) (99.97% @ 0.3 μm DOP) on the exhaust side.
- Recirculation of exhausted air is discouraged, from Class N rooms. The exhaust air should be directed to outside, away from air-intakes and populated areas. However, where recirculation may be deemed acceptable in some circumstances, HEPA filters (99.97% @ 0.3 μm DOP) capable of removing airborne contaminants on the supply side must be incorporated.
- The disposal of effluents should not create a hazard to persons outside or the staff maintaining these systems. Where supplemental engineering controls for air cleaning are indicated from a risk assessment of the 'AII' area, also install ultraviolet germicidal irradiation (UVGI) units in the exhaust air ducts of the HVAC system to supplement HEPA filtration.
- Consider UVGI fixtures on or near the ceiling to irradiate upper room air. Note that UVGI, may be used to augment HEPA filters, but cannot be used in place of HEPA filters, as their effectiveness on airstreams is limited.
- The supply air should be located such that clean air is first passed over the staff/other occupants and then to the patient. Air distribution should reduce the staff's exposure to potential airborne droplet nuclei from infectious patients, accounting for the positions of the staff and the patient, and the procedures undertaken in the isolation room.
- Insider patient room, the supply air should be from the ceiling diffuser located at the perimeter near to the entry and the exhaust air should be drawn at lower levels approximately 6 inches above the floor in the room.
- Exhaust air ducts should be independent of the building's common exhaust air system to reduce the risk of contamination from back draught.
- Locate the exhaust fan at a point in the duct system that will ensure the duct is under negative pressure throughout its run within the building.
- The makeup air intakes should be located so that no contaminated air from nearby exhaust stacks or any sources of air contaminants is drawn into the makeup air system.
- Ensure supply air ducts are independent of the building's common supply air system. If sharing of supply ducts with other isolation rooms is unavoidable, provide the ducts with terminal HEPA filters (or other fail safe back draught prevention system). Install a high efficiency bag filter as a prefilter to protect the HEPA filter.
- Design the supply air and exhaust systems to be of a constant volume system. Variable air volume (VAV) systems are not recommended.
- A monitoring system should be provided to signal any malfunction of the supply/exhaust air system. Consider differential low-pressure instrumentation in a prominent location outside the room along with a local audible alarm in case of supply/exhaust failure.
- Ensure that rooms are well-sealed for better maintenance of pressure gradients that will also eventually reduce load on the air handling plant. Ensure air tightness by:
  - Properly constructing windows, doors, and intake and exhaust ports
  - Maintain plasterboard ceilings that are smooth and free of fissures, open joints, and crevices
  - Sealing all penetrations on the walls above and below the ceiling
  - Monitoring for leakage and making any necessary repairs
- Install self-closing devices on all 'AII' room exit doors considering the direction of door swing in relation to room pressure.
- Provide a staff hand wash basin in the anteroom and include personal respiratory protection for persons entering these rooms and for staff who lack immunity to airborne viral diseases [e.g. measles or varicella zoster virus (VZV) infection].
- Do not use a room with a through-the-wall ventilation unit unless it can be demonstrated that all required 'AII' engineering controls are met.
- Maintain backup ventilation equipment (e.g. portable units for fans or filters) for emergency provision of ventilation requirements for AII rooms, and take immediate steps to restore the fixed ventilation system.
- Label the area as being a negative pressure isolation room.

Emergency Rooms and Reception Areas

The likelihood of airborne contaminants leaving these rooms is reduced by keeping these rooms under negative pressure, relative to surrounding areas. Air is exhausted from these rooms either directly to the outside or through HEPA filters.

CLASS P: POSITIVE PRESSURE ISOLATION ROOMS (FIG. 9)[4]

Class P—positive pressure isolation rooms are set at positive pressure relative to ambient pressure, meaning that air flow must be from the "cleaner" area towards the adjoining space (through doors or other openings). This is achieved by the HVAC system providing more air into the "cleaner" space than is mechanically removed from that same space.[4]

In the schematic diagram above an airlock or anteroom is provided adjacent to the patient room. For a positive pressure room, air would flow from the isolation room to the anteroom and then to the corridor. Pressure control is maintained by modulating the main supply and exhaust dampers based on a signal from a pressure transducer located inside the isolation room.

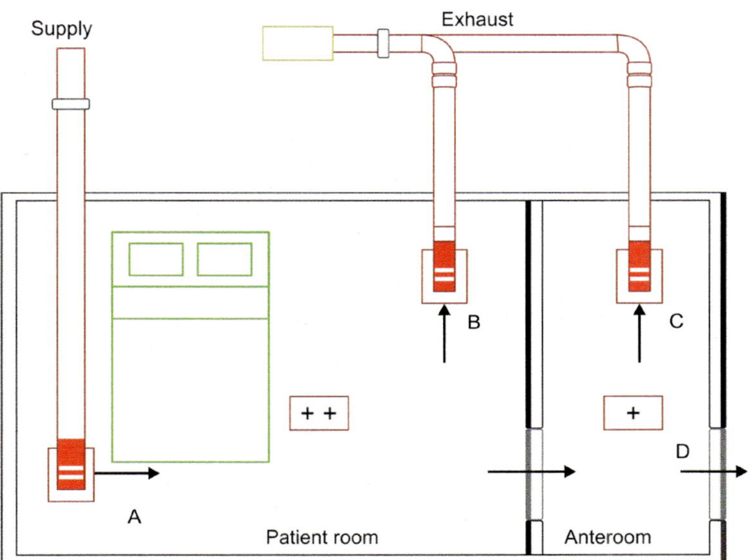

Fig. 9: Positive pressure isolation room.

Infection Control and Ventilation Requirements for PE Rooms

According to AIA guidelines, recommended elements include:

- Ensure that the PE room is designed to maintain positive pressure.
- Maintain positive room air pressure [≥2.5 Pa (0.01-inch water gauge)] in relation to the corridor. Ideally it should be >8 Pa (0.03 inch-water gauge).
- Ventilate the room to maintain ≥12 ACH or 145 liters per second per patient (whichever results in the greatest air quantity), when the supply air filter is at the maximum pressure drop.
- Class P rooms can be either 100% fresh air or can use recirculated air usually a 60/40 mix of outdoor air/recirculated air. As rule of thumb, air pressure should be maintained positive with respect to any adjoining rooms by supplying 10–15% excess airs.
- The recommended air filtration for the Class P, protective rooms is HEPA (99.97% @ 0.3 μm DOP) on the supply side and no filtration is needed on the exhaust side. The HEPA filter could be centrally located at the air handling unit or point-to-use HEPA filters may be used. A terminal HEPA filter at the point of use is recommended.
- UVGI systems are sometimes used in conjunction with HEPA filters (Fig. 10). When UVGI is used as a supplemental engineering control, install fixtures (1) on the wall near the ceiling or suspended from the ceiling as an upper air unit; (2) in the air-return duct of an 'AII' area; or (3) in designated enclosed areas or booths for sputum induction.
- The supply air should be located such that clean air is first flows across the patient bed and exits from the opposite side of the room. Air distribution should reduce the patient's exposure to potential airborne droplet nuclei from occupants.
- Positive pressure rooms may share common supply air systems.
- Differential pressure indication device should be installed to permit air pressure readings in the rooms and provide a local audible alarm in case of fan failure.
- Ensure that rooms are well-sealed for better maintenance of pressure gradients that will also eventually reduce load on the air handling plant. Ensure air tightness by properly constructing windows, doors, and intake and exhaust ports
  - Maintain plasterboard ceilings that are smooth and free of fissures, open joints, and crevices
  - Sealing all penetrations on the walls above and below the ceiling
  - Monitoring for leakage and making any necessary repairs.
- Maintain airflow patterns and monitor these on a daily basis by using permanently installed visual means of detecting airflow in new or renovated construction, or by using other visual methods (e.g. flutter strips or smoke tubes) in existing PE units. Plan for automatic documentation of the monitored results.
- Install self-closing devices on all room exit doors in PE rooms. All emergency exits (e.g. fire escapes, emergency doors) in PE wards should be kept closed (except during emergencies) and equipped with alarms.
- Do not use laminar air flow systems in newly constructed PE rooms.
- Do not use a room with a through-the-wall ventilation unit as PE room.
- Install an en suite bathroom along with a staff hand wash basin in the anteroom.
- Label as a positive pressure isolation room.

Special Challenges

A unique challenge occurs when a patient needs both the positive and negative room isolation.

Caution: Avoid designing systems to switch between positive and negative pressure.

ANTEROOMS (FIG. 11)[1,4]

If space and budget permit, an anteroom should be provided between the negative/positive pressure isolation room and the corridor. It is always recommended for both positive and negative isolation rooms for three main reasons:

- To provide a barrier against loss of pressurization, and against entry/exit of contaminated air into/out of the isolation room when the door to the airlock is opened.
- To provide a controlled environment in which protective garments can be donned without contamination before entry into the isolation room.
- To provide a controlled environment in which equipment and supplies can be transferred from the isolation room without contaminating the surrounding areas.

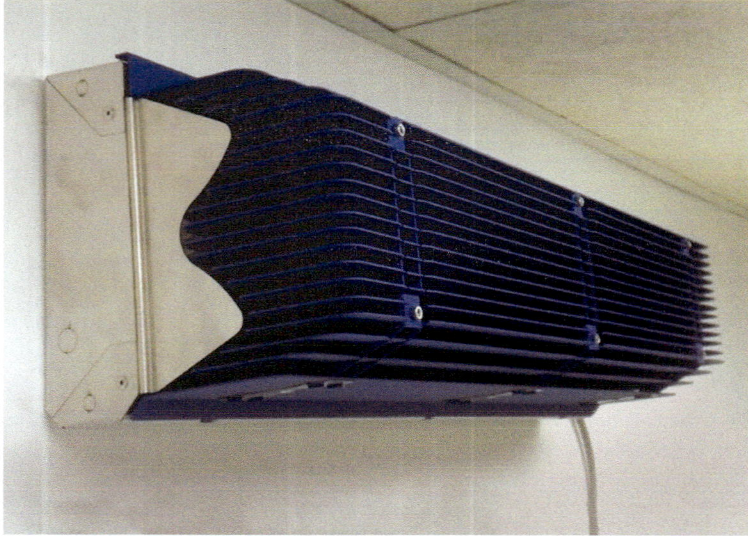

Fig. 10: Ultraviolet germicidal irration (UVGI) supplemental engineering.

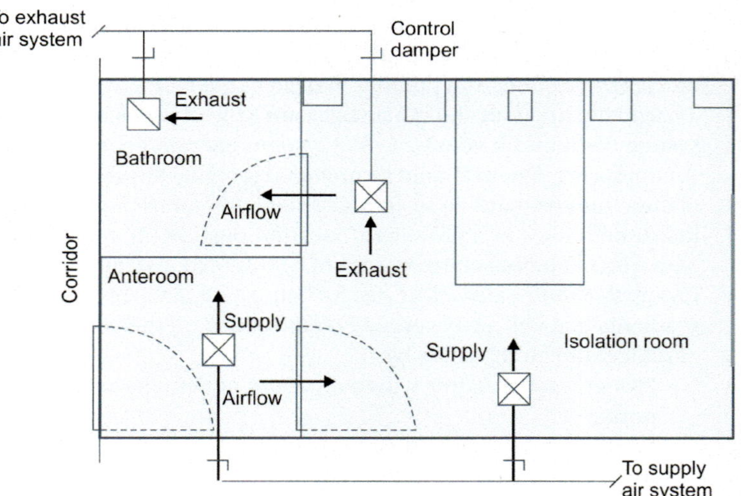

Fig. 11: Anterooms.

Other requirements of anteroom:

- Provision of a sink, cabinets, and work counter
- Provision of a view window in the door to the isolation room
- Alignment of door to corridor with door to isolation room
- Maximum of two isolation rooms per anteroom.

There are three possible airflow/control designs which differ in pressure relationship of anteroom to the isolation room and the corridor:

Design 1: Anteroom negative to both isolation room and corridor

Design 2: Anteroom positive to both isolation room and corridor

Design 3: Anteroom net neutral; negative to isolation room and positive to corridor.

In case of space constraints, Inflatable Emergency Anteroom Module are there, which inflates in minutes using the compressor. It can be mounted inside the doorframe to minimize corridor intrusion, or placed entirely in the corridor and sealed around the doorframe. Fits any 1200 mm to 500 mm wide, 2100 mm tall doorway. Large windows with roll-up covers at either end.

ISOLATION ROOM CHECKLIST (TABLE 2)[4,8,9]

Specific Design Considerations for Isolation Rooms

Ventilation Strategy (Fig. 12)

Environmental control in an isolation facility aims to control the airflow and so reduce the number of airborne infectious particles to a level

Table 2: Isolation room checklist.[8,10-13]

Features	*S standard*	*N negative*	*A alternating*	*P positive*
Non-hand operated hand-basin in room and anteroom	Yes	Yes	This isolation room type is not recommended	Yes
Ensuite bathroom (shower, toilet and hand wash-basin)	Yes	Yes		Yes
Pan sanitizer (near room)	Optional	Optional		Optional
Door on room with door closer	Yes	Yes		Yes
Anteroom		Yes		
Sealed room, door grille for controlled airflow		Yes		Yes
12 ACH/h or 145 liters per patient		Yes		Yes
100% outside air ventilation		Yes		Yes
Local differential pressure monitoring		Yes		Yes
Independent supply air		Yes		
HEPA filters on supply air				Yes
Low-level exhaust 150 mm above floor		Yes		Yes
Independent exhaust discharging vertically at 10 m/s according to AS 1668.2 Type A exhaust		Yes		
Exhaust duct under negative pressure within building with duplex fans		Yes		Optional
HEPA filters on exhaust for retrofit		Optional		

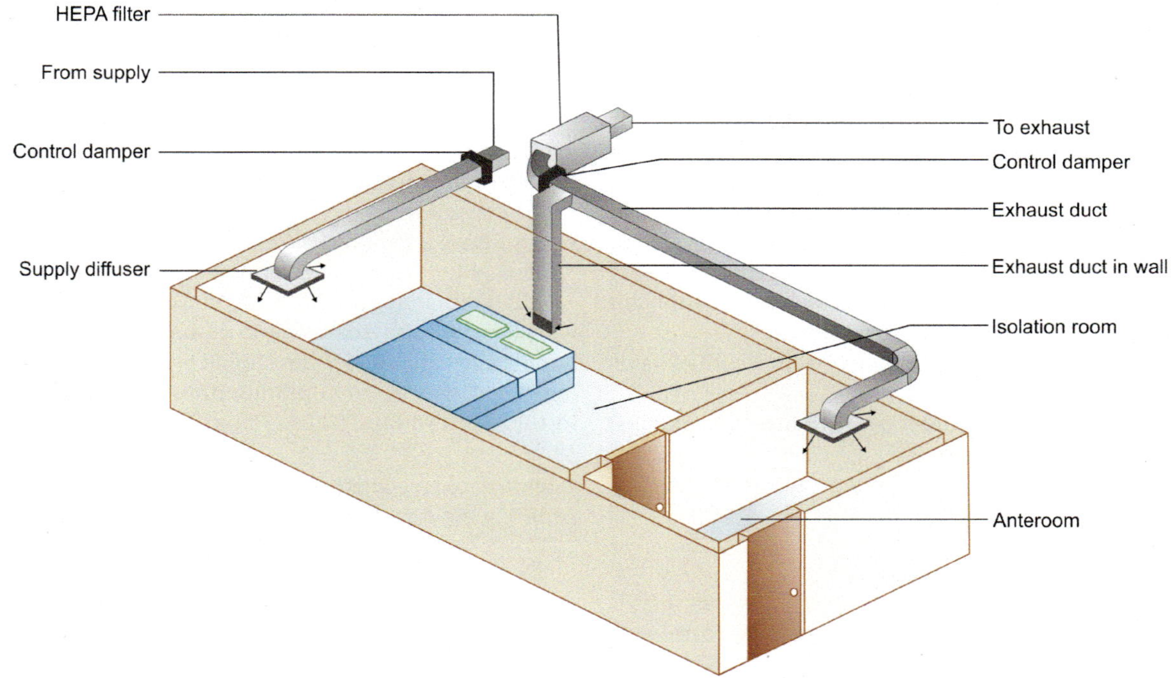

Fig. 12 : Ventilation strategy.

that ensures infection of another person within the healthcare facility is unlikely. This is achieved by:

- Controlling the quality and quantity of intake and exhaust air
- Diluting infectious particles in large volumes of air;
- Maintaining differential air pressures between adjacent areas
- Designing patterns of airflow for particular clinical purposes.

These design parameters are:

- Air change rates
- Pressure gradient appropriate with class of isolation
- Appropriate air distribution in the compartments being air-conditioned
- High quality air filtration including absolute filtration
- Precise temperature and humidity control ensuring maintenance of the intended microclimate.

AIR CHANGE RATES[4]

The ventilation rates for healthcare facilities is expresses as air changes air per hour (ACH), which is a measure of how quickly the air in an interior space is replaced by outside (or conditioned) air. For example, if the amount of air that enters and exits in one hour equals the total volume of the space, the space is said to undergo one air change per hour. Air flow rate is measured in appropriate units such as cubic ft per minute (CFM) and is given by

$$Q = \frac{(\text{ACH}) \times (\text{room volume})}{60\ \text{min/n}} = \text{cu ft/min}$$

In this equation,

Q is the volume flow rate of air being calculated, and ACH is the number of air changes per hour.

To determine the airflow required to adequately ventilate an area.

1. Calculate the room volume to be ventilated
   Width × Length × Height = ft^3 (cubic ft)
2. Calculate the air volume requirement by multiplying the room volume by the air change rate per hour = $ft^{3/h}$.

Studies carried out by AIA, indicate that just one air-change with fresh air can remove 63% of suspended particles from the room air. If a ventilation system can perform 10 ACH, it takes 14 minutes to remove 90% of airborne contaminants in a room and 28 minutes to remove 99%. Thus, increased number of fresh ACH is effective for cleaning airborne contaminants. However, the higher air change rate (>20 ACH) may cause turbulence and the cost for ventilation itself will be too high. Therefore, a recommended compromise of 12 ACH is proposed which should be achievable when the filters have reached their maximum pressure drop. Higher ACR also equates to higher energy use.

Healthcare facilities without specific ventilation standards should follow ANSI/ASHRAE Standard 62, *Ventilation for Acceptable Indoor Air Quality* or otherwise in the absence of any specified supply air change/hour following guidelines may be used:

- For the space to be maintained under negative pressure exhaust 10–15% more air than the supply.
- For the space to be maintained under positive pressure, exhaust 10–15% less air than the supply air.

AIR LEAKS[8,9]

Planned Leakage (Controlled Air Path)

Planned leakage provides a controlled air path from the corridor to anteroom, and from the anteroom to the patient room in an isolation suite. The planned air leakage into a properly sealed isolation suite normally occurs through or around the doors between these spaces.

Unplanned Envelope Leakage

Unplanned envelope leakage refers to airflow into an isolation suite or room that occurs because of insufficient tightness in joints and penetrations through the suite or room envelope. Common unplanned leakage points include electrical and plumbing outlets, and wall-ceiling and floor-wall joints.

ROOM PRESSURE CONTROL[4,9]

Building room pressurization is a critical factor to monitor in a hospital as it can greatly affect the controllability of the environment. Building room pressure gradient is achieved by controlling the quality and quantity of intake and exhaust air, maintaining differential air pressures between adjacent areas, and designing patterns of airflow for particular clinical purposes.

Pressure Gradients (Table 3 and Figs. 13 to 15)[8,9]

The minimum differential pressure between the isolation room and adjacent ambient pressure areas should be 30 Pa if the room has an anteroom, and 15 Pa if the room does not have an anteroom. The gradient between successive pressure areas should not be less than 15 Pa. It is recommended that the ensuite entrance is not located in the anteroom.

Air Filter Efficiencies[8]

Air filtration should comply with the requirements as documented in the Department of Human Services, Design Guidelines for Hospitals and Day Procedure Centers.

Class N[12]

- Optional terminal HEPA filter on exhaust only to prevent back draught.
- High-efficiency prefilters before HEPA filters.

Class P[12]

- Terminal HEPA filter on supply air. Integrated fan-assisted terminal HEPA units are not recommended due to potentially high noise levels. Use of a separate inline centrifugal fan in the ductwork should be considered.
- Optional terminal HEPA filter on exhaust only to prevent back draught.
- High-efficiency prefilters before HEPA filters.
- Supply air and exhaust duct design.

Supply and exhaust systems should be designed as fail safe and duplex fans used to prevent contamination of any area within the facility in the event of fan failure. Fans should be interlocked to provide

Table 3: Recommended isolation room pressures.

Room type	*Room*	*En suite*	*Anteroom*
Class N	–ve 30 Pa	–ve 30 Pa	–ve 15 Pa
Class P	+ve 30 Pa	+ve 30 Pa	+ve 15 Pa
Class P room with negative pressure anteroom	+ve 15 Pa	+ve 30 Pa	+ve 15 Pa

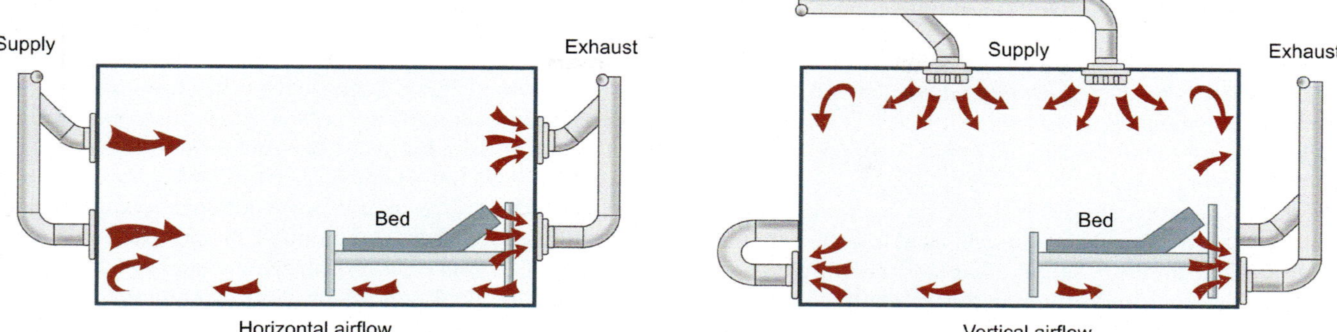

Fig. 13: Room air distribution in isolation rooms.

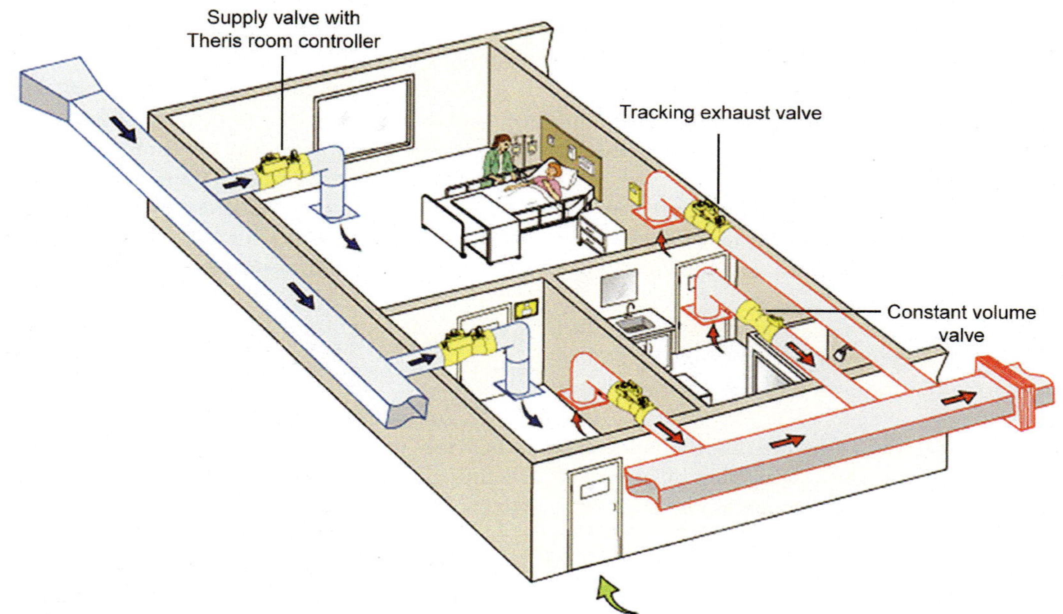

Fig. 14: Air distribution in isolation facility.

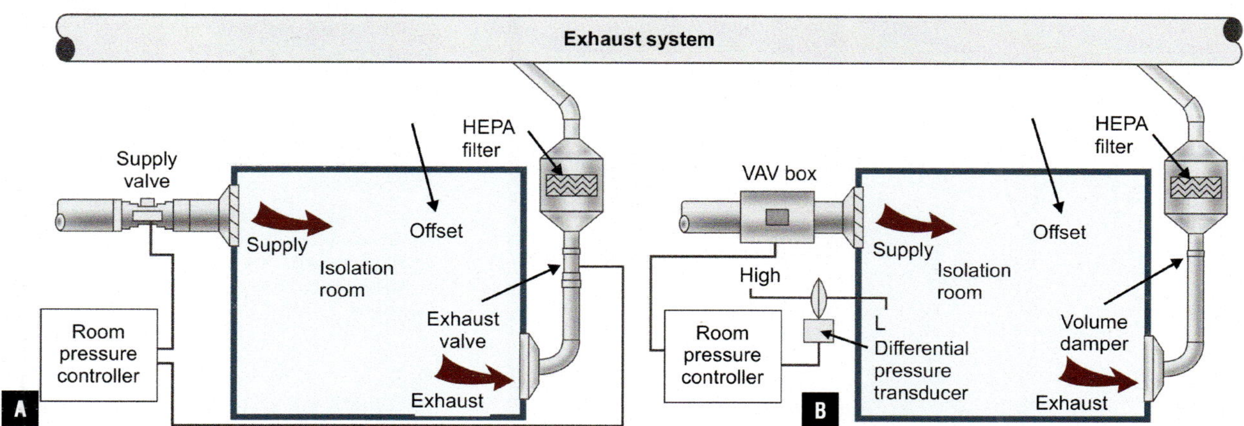

Fig 15: Isolation room differential pressure contol measurements: (A) Flow-tracking measurement and control; (B) Differential pressure management and control.
(VAV: variable air volume)

automatic shutdown in the event of failure; for example, the NPR supply fan should shutdown in the event of exhaust fan failure. The exhaust fan should be located at a point in the duct system that will ensure the entire duct is under negative pressure within the building.

- Pressure differential between rooms (door closed)
- Ventilation supply air volume (outside air) ventilation supply air to the patient room is filtered, conditioned outside air supplied directly to the patient room, and does not include outside air that has first been supplied to the corridor or anteroom before being transferred to the patient room.

- Ventilation exhaust-supply differential volume
  - Air distribution
  - Within the room, the air should follow similar principles:
    - ◊ In a Class N room, the air should pass over first the staff then the patient
    - ◊ In a Class P room, the air should pass over first the patient then the staff
    - ◊ Air distribution should reduce the staff's exposure to potential airborne droplet nuclei from infectious patients, accounting for the positions of the staff and the patient, and the procedures undertaken in the isolation room.
- Use of HEPA filters on ventilation exhaust and supply air-related considerations.

Several other important design considerations for isolation room are discussed below:

- *Thermal comfort*: Isolation rooms have relatively high air exchange rates in relation to other patient rooms. This implies high ventilation air supply and exhaust rates as well. Potentially uncomfortable air velocities (draughts) within the patient room can result, and therefore, special attention must be given to thermal comfort, particularly for the patient, as a design issue.
- *Control strategy*: There are two fundamental control strategies that reflect the basic ventilation strategy discussed above of achieving containment between the patient room and anteroom, and the anteroom room and corridor.
- One strategy is to maintain constant exhaust-supply flow differentials under changing conditions and accept that the pressure differentials between the patient room and anteroom and the anteroom and corridor will vary.
- Second strategy is to maintain constant pressure differentials under changing conditions by varying the exhaust-supply flow differentials. Alternatively, a combination of the two approaches can be used.

Supply and Exhaust Ductwork and Outlets Location[4,10,14]

The bottom of the exhaust grille should be located approximately 150 mm above the floor. Because the grille does not direct air, its face pattern is not as important as that of the diffuser. The vertical exhaust duct should be installed in the Airborne infection isolation room (*AIIR*) wall. An enlarged wall cavity will be required and should be coordinated with the architect. To reduce noise, dampers should be located at a point in the duct far from the outlet. The area in front of the exhaust grille should be kept clear of obstructions, such as furniture and supply carts. The individual air ducts providing supply and exhaust air for the AIIR suite should have control dampers to adjust the airflow quantity. These dampers are usually manually operated, but may be automatic. To ensure access, the handles for the dampers should not be above the AIIR ceiling. They should be either accessible from above the corridor ceiling, or remote, tamper-proof handles should be provided in the ceiling or wall of the AIIR.

Proper room pressurization can be checked using a smoke stick or smoldering match at doors held open approximately 10 mm to visually see which direction air is moving. Care must be taken when checking this to make sure that the door is not moving during the test since a door swinging can move more air than the design ventilation differential in the room. An alarm system (visual/audible) should be installed to warn of pressurization failure.

RENOVATING OR CONVERTING A ROOM (FIGS. 16 AND 17)[8,9]

When an isolation room is being incorporated into an existing facility, it is rarely possible to create the ideal room. Physical and financial factors often constrain the construction. It is critical to create a room that is fit for its purpose.

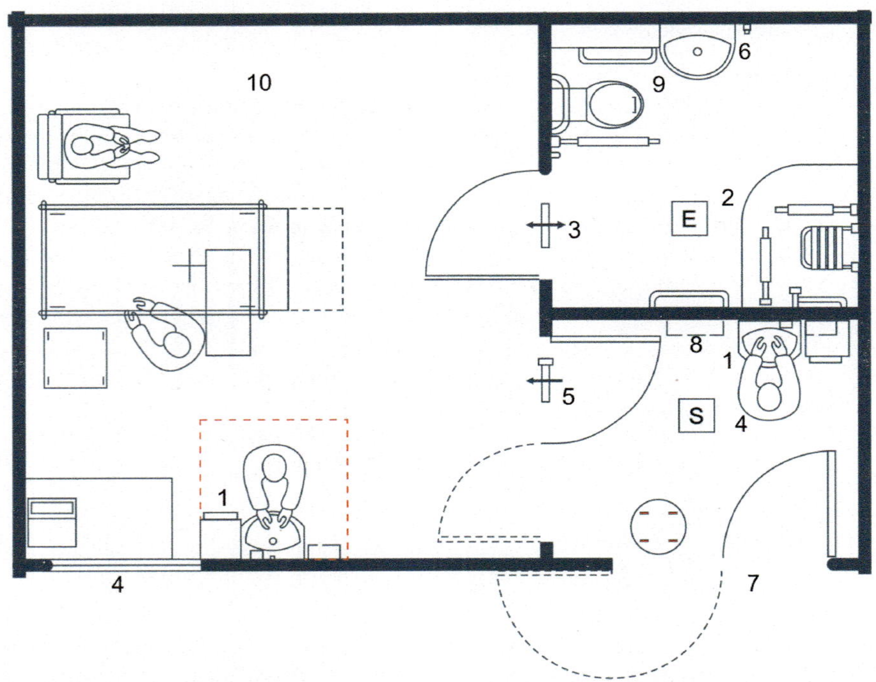

Minimum requirements:

1. Clinical hand wash basin with non-touch, fixed temperature mixer tap
2. Provide suitable extract fan
3. Install transfer grille to en suite door
4. Supply air
5. Pressure stabilizer
6. Observation window in corridor wall with integral privacy blinds to allow for staff observation and patient views out
7. Double door for personnel and bed access
8. Disposable apron dispenser
9. Ensuite WC to be non-touch flush and wash basin to have single tap with flow and temperature control
10. Ceiling to be sealed solid construction, external window to be sealed

Fig. 16: Newly built single isolation room with anteroom.

Minimum requirements to upgrade existing facilities:

1. Add clinical hand wash basin with non-touch, fixed temperature mixer tap
2. Provide suitable extract fan
3. Install transfer grille to en suite door
4. Observation window in corridor wall with integral privacy blinds to allow for staff observation and patient views out
5. En suite WC to be non-touch flush and wash basin to have single tap with flow and temperature control

Fig. 17: Upgrading three existing single rooms to provide two single anteroom in common.

When converting existing accommodation into Class N rooms, the easiest and least expensive option is to adapt existing single rooms with en suite facilities. The following requirements should be met in any conversion:

- Furnishing and fittings
  - Clinical hand wash basin with non-touch, fixed temperature mixer tap
  - Wall-mounted soap dispensers
  - Disinfectant hand rub dispensers
  - Disposable towel holders
  - Glove dispensers
  - Storage for clean personal protective equipment
  - Clean waste bins
- Observation window in corridor wall with integral privacy blinds
- Investigate the use of a pressure stabilizer above the bedroom door
- Compliant exhaust system
- Compliant air supply
- Sliding transfer grille in room door
- Sealed, monolithic ceiling with sealed access panels
- Windows to the exterior to be locked shut and sealed
- Provision of two-way intercommunication system between the patient's room and the nurses' station.

Fire Strategy (Fig. 18)[15]

- The isolation suite is intended to be built as a single fire compartment. The positive pressure in the lobby will detect smoke originating in the corridor from entering the room. Smoke from a fire in the room will be contained within the suite and extracted via the en suite extract. Hence, the ventilation system serving the isolation facility should be kept running in the event of a fire.
- Ductwork thickness should be such that ducts can be considered an extension of the isolation suite. Fire dampers, where the ducts penetrate walls and floors will not then be required.
- A motorized smoke/fire damper should be fitted at the discharge of the supply air handling unit (AHU). The damper should close in the event of an AHU or intake fire under the control of a smoke detector mounted in the AHU.

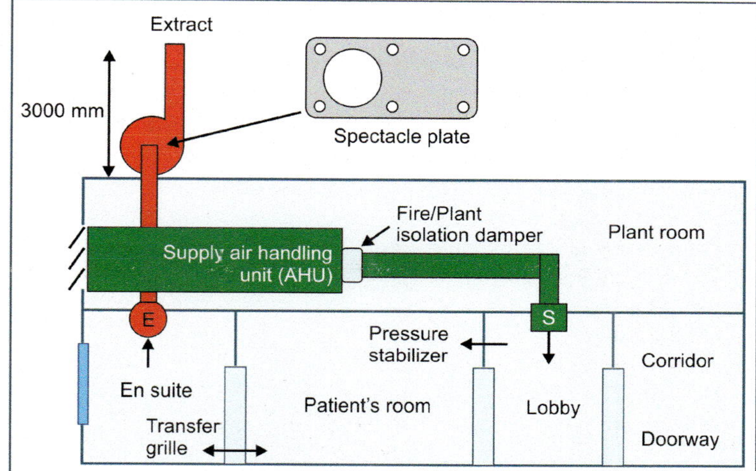

Fig. 18: Fire strategy.

CONCLUSION

The physical design of a hospital is an essential component of its infection control measures to minimize the risk of transmission of any infectious disease. Today, with a more progressive outlook, it is the fundamental requirement to adopt a holistic view of the design and management of hospitals.[23]

With the challenges of new and emerging infectious diseases as well as higher public expectations and awareness of healthcare-related issues, much consideration has to be given to these in the planning phase of building hospitals. For existing institutions and hospital buildings, renovation and upgrading plans must incorporate the necessary changes. Among the various methods for infection control two important environment factors are isolation and ventilation. Infected patients or those highly susceptible to infection need to be isolated in private rooms with proper ventilation systems in order to stop spread and reduce the possibility of developing a new infection.[15]

REFERENCES

1. www.hvacindia.org.in
2. www.dhsspsni.gov.uk
3. https://www.aer1.org/
4. www.cedengineering.com
5. www.indmedica.com
6. Putsep E. Modern Hospital: International planning practices. Lloyd- Luke Ltd., London; 1979.
7. CB DHC. Isolation Rooms (including Mechanically Ventilated Rooms): Best Practice Standards for Capital Planning: Northern Ireland; 2004.

8. health.vic.gov.au
9. www.abatement.com
10. Review of Hospital Isolation and Infection Control Related Precautions Report of the Joint Working Group of the Hospital Infection Society, 2002.
11. Recommendations for Isolation Precautions in Hospitals (Part II), CDC, Hospital Infection Control Practices Advisory Committee-HICPAC) http://www.cdc.gov/ncidod/hip/ISOLAT/isopart2.htm
12. Mosby's Medical Dictionary, 8th edition. Elsevier. 2009.
13. Julia S, Garner R, MN. Guidelines for Isolation Precautions in Hospitals. In: Committee tHICPA, editor.01/01/1996.
14. www.nationaltbcenter.edu
15. www.ncbi.nlm.nih.gov

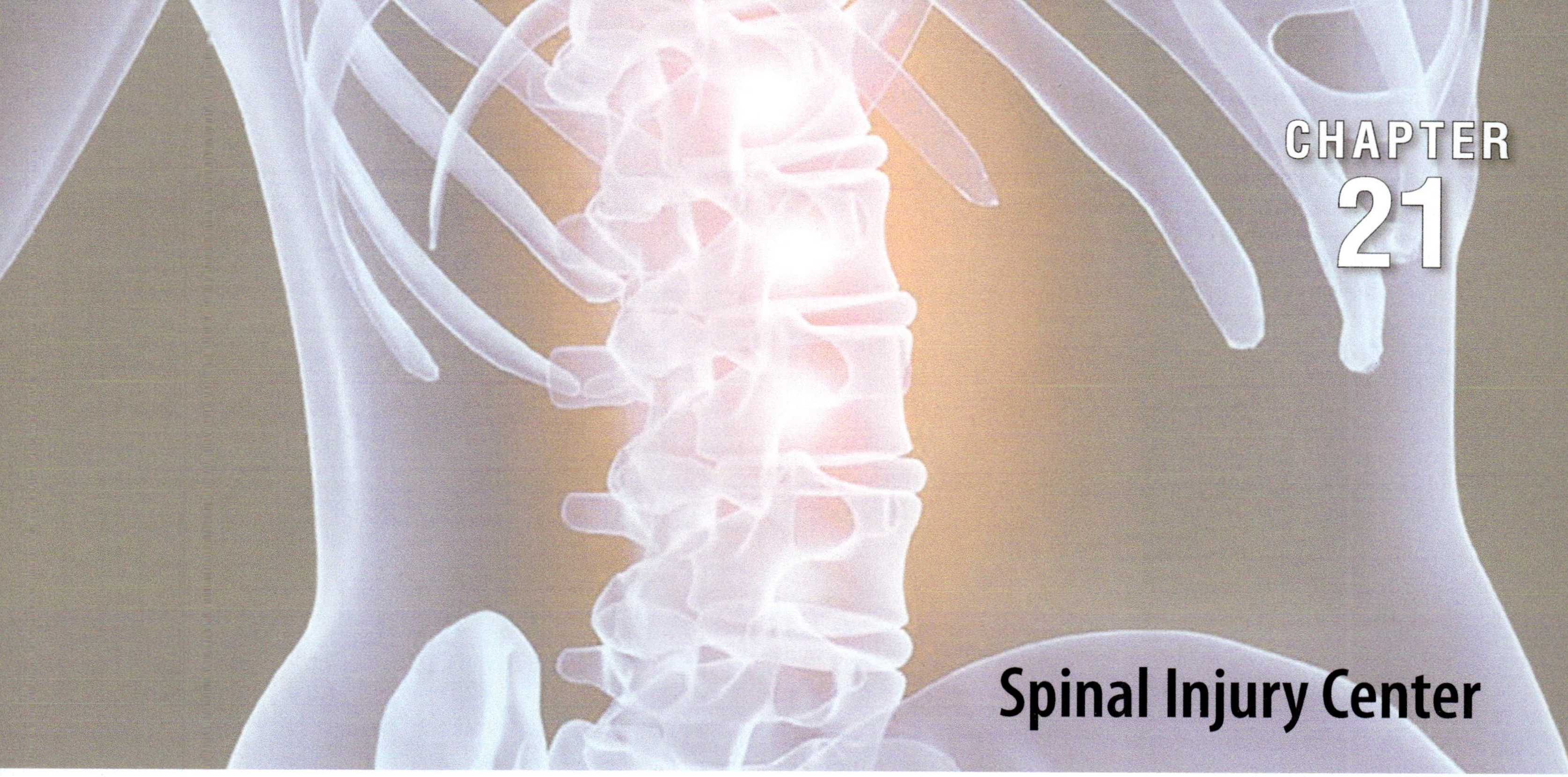

Spinal Injury Center

Sudhin Kurien, Shakti Kumar Gupta, Sunil Kant, R Chandrashekhar

INTRODUCTION

Spinal disorders are a wide and heterogeneous range of specific diseases and nonspecific musculoskeletal disorders involving the spinal column. Specific diseases of the spine include trauma, mechanical injury, spinal cord injury (SCI), inflammation, infection and tumor. Nonspecific musculoskeletal disorders of the spine include maladies affecting the muscles, nerves, inter-vertebral disks, joints, cartilage, tendons and ligaments of the neck and back. Complaints about pain involving the neck and back are the primary manifestation of most spinal disorders. The incidence of spinal disorders varies with age, most conditions being distributed throughout the life span.[1]

Spinal Cord Injury/Disorder Patient

A patient with a spinal cord injury or disorder (SCI/D) is one who has sustained a lesion or disease of the spinal cord or cauda equina resulting in either paraplegia or tetraplegia (quadriplegia).[2]

Spinal Cord Injury/Disorders Center[2-8]

A spinal cord injury/disorders center (SCI/DC) is a specialized medical facility designed to provide a full range of care for patients who have sustained a lesion of the spinal cord and/or cauda equina resulting in either paraplegia or tetraplegia.

The World Health Organization states that musculoskeletal conditions are the most common causes of severe pain and physical disability, affecting hundreds of millions of people across the world. The concept of the specialist spinal injury center (SIC) was first conceived in the 1930's and 1940's by Sir Ludwig Guttmann in the UK and by Donald Munro in the USA. In the UK, the National Spinal Injuries Centre (NSIC), based at Stoke Mandeville Hospital, became operational in 1944 as the first SCI center.

Spinal cord injury is a rare and complex impairment which will result in some degree of loss or reduction in voluntary muscle activity, sensory deprivation and disruption of autonomic function related to the level and severity of the cord damage.

Various studies in India have placed, "fall from height" followed by "road traffic accidents" as the major cause of SCIs. There are many facilities functional presently world over that cater exclusively to SCI.

Spinal centers need to be set up that provide the finest comprehensive and state-of-the-art care for patients with spine disorders, with the goal of restoring normal function and relieving spine-related pain.

PLANNING

The treatment for patients that sustain SCI/D fall into two major groups, viz:

- *Acute*: Acute care involves medical stabilization immediately after injury and is usually provided at the nearest trauma center, with later transfer to an SCI/D Center as soon as possible. After the patient is stabilized a period of rehabilitation of 4–8 months begins, with the goal of enabling the individual to return to independent living. Correct surgeries are undertaken at these centers after assessing the stage in which they report as well as the progress of the patient evolves over a period of time.[2,3]
- *Sustaining care*: Involves the care rendered when problems arise medical, surgical, rehabilitative and SCI/D homecare services subsequent to independent living.

Hence, the general planning for a SCI/DC should incorporate provisions for—Adequate space allocation, infection control, selection of private room versus wards, noise reduction, views of nature/day lighting and disabled accessibility and mobility. The fact that paraplegic/quadriplegic patients will use assistive devices viz wheelchairs or motorized vehicle should always be borne in mind.

Considering the above, the key elements required in a SCI/DC may be broadly classified into:

- The direct patient care units:
  - Short stay area
  - Outpatient department (OPD)

  - Inpatient department
  - Physical medicine and rehabilitation unit
  - Operation theater (OT).
- Diagnostic services
  - Radiology
  - Laboratory medicine
  - Blood transfusion services.
- Support services
  - Central sterile supply unit/theater sterile supply unit
  - Laundry
  - Manifold
  - Heating ventilation and air-conditioning (HVAC).

GENERAL PLANNING CONSIDERATIONS

Location and Access

A center of this nature should be located in a major city. The approach should be wide enough to accommodate two-way traffic. Further emergency access is required to be provided on to the grounds of the center for ambulances, fire and rescue and law enforcement vehicles. A space of 6 m around the building for fire tenders is mandated by the law.[4]

Covered Entry

Provisions for a covered entrance at the primary access point to the spinal center are required. Enough covered area to accommodate two vehicles, one behind the other are to be provided. The width of the roadway or motorable area under the covering also should be designed to accommodate an accessible van to park at the entrance while allowing a separate vehicle to pass by. Height of covered entrance is to be designed to allow clearance for large emergency vehicles. Ample space for seating and circulation should be planned in the spinal center.[3,7]

Parking Areas

Space should be marked for parking for diffreantly abled, parking for ambulances and parking for the staff. While the space allocation for parking for the staff and ambulances should be as per the regular norms, there should be a dedicated lot for patients with accessible parking spaces (2 spaces/bed) with safe and easy access to buildings. Site roadways to and from parking areas should be capable of accommodating two-way traffic. Proper signage and direction arrows may enhance clarity of destinations and paths.[2]

Signage

Signage in a spinal center should be designed to indicate, firstly whether the facility is accessible to the differently abled and secondly to provide information. The international symbol of accessibility should be used as an integral part of the facility (Fig. 1).

Further, there should be "site signage" for visitors, staff and service accommodations. The letters and numbers should be of adequate height, width and spacing and should contrast with their background. A person on a wheelchair is less than 1200 mm high. The signage exclusively for wheelchair users should be between 750 mm and 1200 mm. Self-illuminating signage is preferred in the areas exterior of the building.[11]

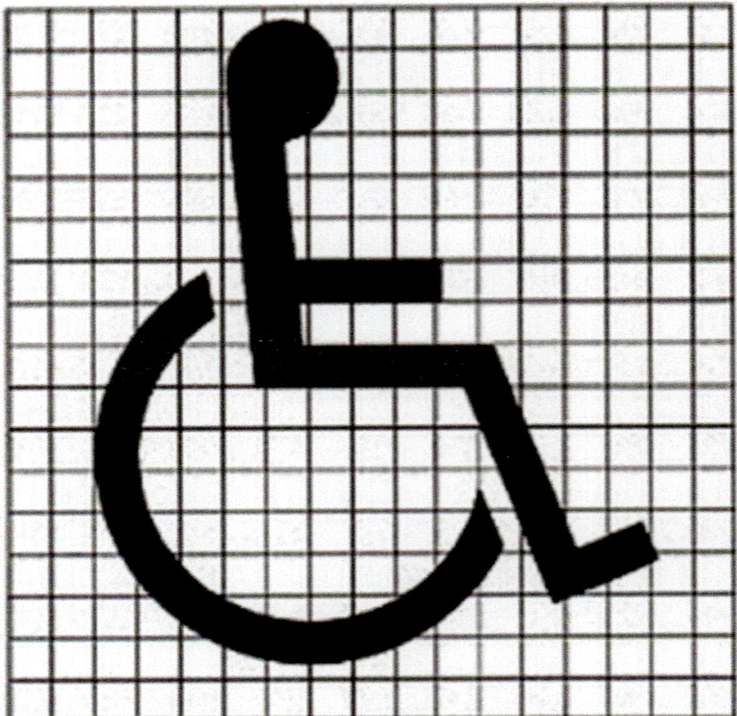

Fig. 1: Signage for differently abled.

Ramps[2,9,10]

Any part of an accessible route with a slope greater than 1:20 should be considered a ramp. The function of a ramp is to provide accessible building entrances across steep topography where a gradual incline is not possible.

Requirements

- *Slope*: The recommended slope of the ramp in the new construction should be 1:12
- *Width*: The minimum width of a curb ramp should be 1200 mm. The ideal ramp width of a regular ramp is 2100–2400 mm.
- Department of veterans affairs USA, recommends landings distanced as per the gradient. However, it is convenient to have a landing planned every 9 m. Landing length shall be a minimum of 1524 mm clear. If ramps change direction at landings, the minimum landing size shall be (1524 mm × 1524 mm).

Handrails installed on both sides and mounted at a height of 838 mm and extend 304 mm beyond beginning and end of ramp. About 101 mm high × 203 mm wide curbs on each side to prevent wheelchairs from scuffing walls or catching on railing posts. Such curbs also enable a person to stop a wheelchair that is out of control quickly by turning one wheel against the curb.[2] Smooth transitions between vehicular pathways and pedestrian walkways should be ensured by means of curb ramps.

Walkways

The walkways provide a continuous and accessible surface free of any steps or change in levels. The surface should be slip resistant and the surface slope be conducive for the patients movement. A minimum width sufficient for two individuals in wheelchairs to pass each other comfortably must be provided for 2.1 m.[3]

Lifts/Elevators

The elevator door should facilitate the movement of beds, trolleys and multiple wheelchairs. A set of double handrails is recommended. The dimensions that take into consideration the SCI patients are:

Length	:	2400 mm
Breadth	:	1850 mm
Door opening	:	1200 mm

Doorways and Passages

Doorways to rooms should be 1500 mm wide or wider to accommodate patient beds, electric wheelchairs and other personal mobility devices. A level space should extend on either side of the doorway for facilitating opening/closing by a wheel-chaired person (450 mm long × 1520 mm broad space). The entrances and exits of passages should be wide enough to move to heavy machinery, beds and trolleys in and out. The corridor width should be in the range of 2100–2400 mm considering the new age motorized wheelchairs that are bigger than standard wheelchairs. Automatic doors as an option at doorways should be actively considered wherever possible.[3]

Wall Protection (Fig. 2)

Measures to protect the wall should be employed to reduce damage caused by wheelchairs, stretchers, and carts. A crash rail located 200 mm above the floor is beneficial, as well as one located at chair rail height. This upper bumper guard may be combined with a handrail to provide additional assistance to patients traveling along corridors. In areas that experience only cart traffic, the upper rail may be eliminated. Solid sheet products installed between the upper and lower crash rails can protect this area from dents and marks caused by rolling equipment and wheelchairs.

Engineering Services

Water supply: The water requirement in the hospital is 500 L/bed/day for inpatients, excluding fire-fighting needs. There should be separate tank for water for fire-fighting. A 3 days reserve should be available at all times.

Heating ventilation and air-conditioning: The entire center should be provided with a central HVAC system. This is a necessity considering the climate of the subcontinent and the fact that spinal injury patients stand a risk of pressure sores and infection. This will be located in the basement.

Electric supply and power back-up: The requirement of electricity is 5 kW/bed/day for as for super specialty hospitals. This will be from 2–3 grids. The proper wiring and earthing should be done in accordance with the state electricity board. A suitable generator back-up should be provided.

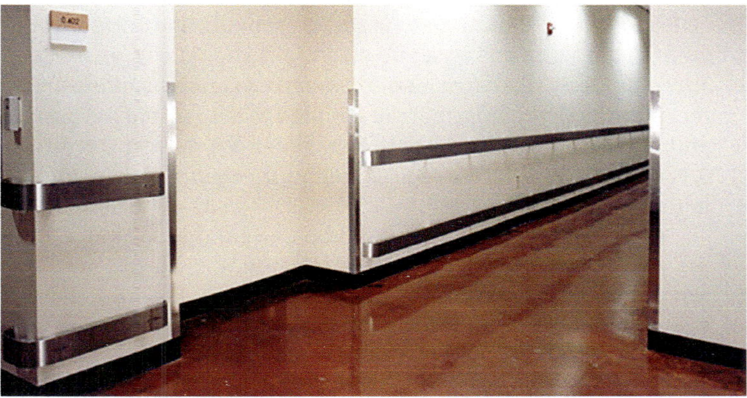

Fig. 2: Wall protection.

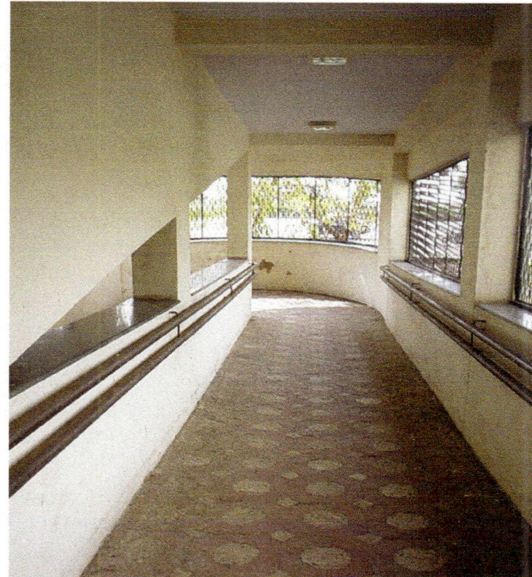

Fig. 3: Fire safety ramp.

Fire Safety (Fig. 3)

The building should be constructed incorporating the fire safety features as per National Building Code 2016. It is preferred to have the inpatient facility up to first floor with external ramp connectivity to the ground floor. This area requires attention considering the general bedridden state of the patients. An external ramp provision is required from the first floor ward area to augment the lift access.

General Design Considerations[10]

The spinal cord center should be designed and developed around the needs of the patient as an individual. Design should follow function. Each patient's perceptions, expectations, and needs should be considered to maximize the benefit especially from SCI service care. Individuals who have sustained SCIs face many challenges, including such medical issues as pressure wounds and infection, loss of bowel and bladder control, and requirement of ventilator-aided breathing. They may also experience low self-esteem, depression, poor body image, and tension in their personal relationships and work environments. The quality of life for people with a SCI can be dramatically improved with facility design that addresses their needs in the form of use of space and materials, technological and lighting considerations and so forth (Table 1).

Table 1: Design considerations.[2]

Description	*Key features*	*Dimensions*
Covered entry	Allow clearance for large emergency vehicles	
Ramp		
Slope	Any part of an accessible route with a slope greater than 1:20 shall be considered a ramp	1:12
Width		Ideal width 2100–2400 mm
Handrails	Both sides	Height of 838 mm and extend 304 mm beyond beginning and end of ramp
Walkways	A minimum width sufficient for two individuals in wheel-chairs to pass each	2.1 m

Cont'd...

Cont'd...

Description	*Key features*	*Dimensions*
Lifts/elevators	Should facilitate the movement of beds, trolleys and multiple wheelchairs	Length—2400 mm Breadth—1850 mm Door opening–1200 mm
Doorways and passages	A level space should extend on either side of the doorway	Doorways to rooms minimum 1500 mm wide
Corridor		2100–2400 mm
Wall protection	A crash rail located 200 mm above the floor is beneficial	
Water supply	A 3 days reserve should be available at all times	500 L/bed/day
Heating ventilation and air-conditioning	Necessity considering the climate of the subcontinent	5 kW/bed/day
Electric supply and power back up	Proper wiring and earthing should be done in accordance with the state electricity board	5 kW/bed/day for as for super specialty hospitals

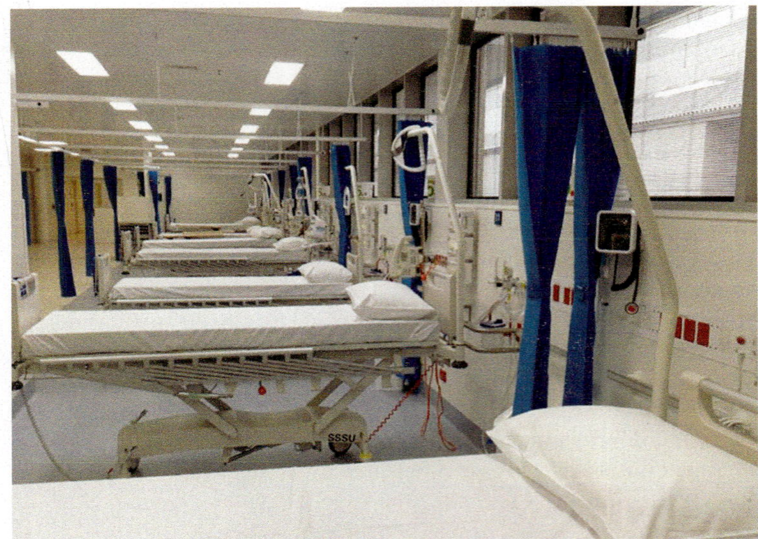

Fig. 4: Short stay area.

Materials Considerations

The development of a homelike environment should be the primary goal. In view of the long stays involved for SCI patients, all components should be hospital-grade and easy to maintain to ensure cleanliness and durability. Materials with antimicrobial properties (e.g. antimicrobial copper for touch surfaces like bed rails, stair rails, faucet handles, IV stands) are ideal because patients with SCIs are at higher risk for developing infections. The introduction of color, texture, light, sound, and smell are additional tools and bedrooms must be designed to provide privacy and dignity by shielding the patient from direct view into the room. Space requirements in the patient room for wheelchair battery charging must be considered, in addition to adequate storage space for personal possessions.

Design in Technology

New designs in technology that promotes additional independence for SCI patients, such as remote control devices to adjust artificial lighting levels, window treatments that admit or filter natural daylight, and individual thermostats to control room temperature. Sip-and-puff technology—a straw-like pneumatic switch that allows the use of one's breath to perform mouse clicks—has been developed to aid individuals with quadriplegia. The signals generated from sip-and-puff are also used in conjunction with wireless transmitters that interface with various devices to control the patient environment.

MAIN BLOCK

Ground Floor

Short Stay Area (Fig. 4)

The major proportion of the traumatic spinal disorder patients accessing the service of the hospital would have been referred to from other centers after initial stabilization. Lone spinal injury cases *per se* without other co-existing morbidities are less in number. Acutely presenting patients that may require to be initially evaluated while contemplated for further course of treatment. This warrants that an easily approachable and accessible area be present. This may be located in the ground floor adjacent to the OPD so that the facilities of imaging and investigation can be adequately utilized and the trained professionals are at hand.

This area is proposed to be used for staging (i.e. receiving an acute patient, stabilizing and managing) till he is admitted to the ICU. The short stay area should have minimum 6–8 beds. An area of 15 m per treatment area is required. The area should be able to fit standard mobile bed with able storage and usage space for essential equipment. The inter bed distance should be at least 2.4 m. Each treatment area is to be provided with curtain systems to provide privacy. Every bed shall have its own bed head panel with adequate power sockets, examination lights, wall mounted sphygmomanometer and hand wash dispenses. A hand washing bay as well as a bay for mobile equipment will be earmarked. Adequate stores space for consumables and nonconsumable stores need to be catered.

A fully equipped nursing station which is centralized is better suited. Separate rest/changing rooms for doctors and nurses with separate toilets are required.

Reception and waiting area: A reception consisting of helpdesk, admission counter, waiting area and waiting area with washroom facilities for the attendants of the patient needs to be located outside the short stay area in the central lobby.

Outpatient Department Complex (Fig. 5)

The OPD complex should also be on the ground floor and located adjacent to the short stay area and essentially should comprise of:

- *Reception area*: This area should consist of general waiting areas, reception, toilet rooms, that are planned to help orient the patient and accompanying persons to the center. An area at the rate of 0.1 m^2/bed will suffice in the spinal injury center. This should be in the central lobby.[2,3]
  - The reception counter should be designed to accommodate persons using wheelchairs and trolleys.
- *Waiting area*: The general waiting area should be spacious enough to accommodate people on wheelchairs also. It would be prudent to plan SCI patients on different days than for other spinal disorders. An area of approximately 60 m^2 is appropriate considering 0.8 m^2/bed.

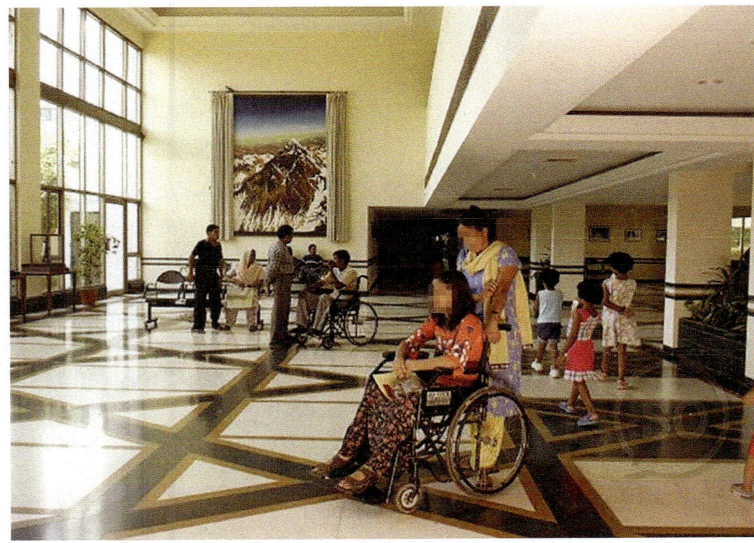

Fig. 5: Outpatient department.

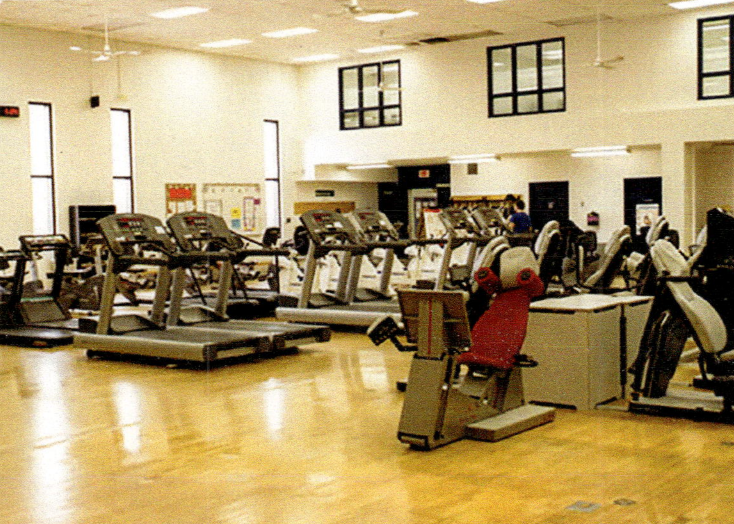

Fig. 6: Physical rehabilitation.

- *Consultation rooms:* About 5 consultation rooms are required with one each for orthopedics, neurosurgery and spine surgery and one for medicine and allied disciplines and one for surgery and allied disciplines. The minimum area required will be 12.5 m^2/room.
- *Toilet*: Disabled friendly toilets (5 m^2) for patients use and common toilets for accompanying persons should be provided. There should be separate staff toilets in the OPD complex.
- *Exam/treatment room*: Exam room for SCI/D patients must accommodate patients on a trolley, which requires a larger space than the normal exam/treatment room. These rooms (15 m^2 each) should also include provision for patient lifting hoist.[2,3]
- *Pharmacy*: There should be a pharmacy to cater to the requirements of the clientele in the OPD.
- *Sample collection room*: A sample collection room of size 7 m^2 in the OPD is recommended.

Radio Imaging Services

The three main radio imaging services required are X-ray, magnetic resonance imaging (MRI) and computerized tomography (CT) facilities. Since they need to be accessed by the short stay, OPD and inpatients the imaging services are better located on the ground floor next to the short stay area with adequate waiting area for patients. Provision of lifts close to the same will make the area accessible to the other floors also. For the three facilities of MRI, CT scan and X-ray an area of 200 m^2 is required. A common waiting area in the imaging area is prescribed. An area of 40 m^2 each is required for the MRI and CT machine room alone excluding the console rooms and waiting rooms. The urodynamics lab should also be located here so as to make use of the imaging facilities if required. The imaging facility can have option of being functional on an outsourcing model with the space being leased out to the players who will be allowed to staff and run their machines to make the enterprise cost effective.

Physical Medicine and Rehabilitation (Fig. 6)[2,3,11,12]

This department is the bedrock on which spinal disorder treatment rest upon. The emphasis in any modern spinal center is "back to activity" as soon as possible. Hence, one of the most crucial components to creating a spine center of excellence is building an inviting workout facility for patients to use through every step of the recovery process. Open gym environment encourages collaboration and teamwork between physiatrists, surgeons and spine manual therapists—rather than isolationism and treatment biases. The spine center of the future will in many ways resemble a health club environment that is an attractive place to get active and fit. An area of 100 m^2 is ideal.[11,12]

However, the space can vary a lot depending on the type and model of equipment an institution will establish. The main components involved are:

- *Physical/occupational therapy*: Physical therapy concentrates on gross neuromuscular and skeletal activity. Physical therapy components are treatment areas and a gymnasium configured to accommodate portable equipment. This may include mats, platforms, giant training, parallel bars and weights, as well as other resistive equipment and orthotic and prosthetic training services. Occupational therapy focuses on strengthening and optimizing a patient's independence while concentrating on finer physical movement. Both simulated and actual training age to be included. Additional activities may also include vocational training with special adaptive equipment such a computers and telephones. Physical therapy departments should be designed to that therapists can reach all four sides of patients on PT mats or other similar equipment.[2,3]
- *Kinesiotherapy*: A separate space for kinesiotherapy or it may be combined with PT/OT. Kinesiotherapy combines exercise and education to motivate and assist patients in maintaining physical skills. Previously called corrective therapy, kinesiology focuses on large motor exercises and activities (Fig. 7).[2,3]
- *Aquatic therapy*: A therapeutic/exercise pool as part of the initial therapy for acute SCI/D patients is recommended (Fig. 8). Therapy pools allow patients to move and exercise while suspended in water, thus reducing the impact of body weight during therapy. Self-contained aquatic therapy pools should allow adequate space for several patients with trained staff. The SCI patient requires 33°C water temperature, while the MS patient requires 28°–33°C water temperature. The pool equipment should be designed to accommodate quick water temperature change, where both patient types can use the same pool on a given day based on schedule. Careful consideration to the shape of the pool, water supply,

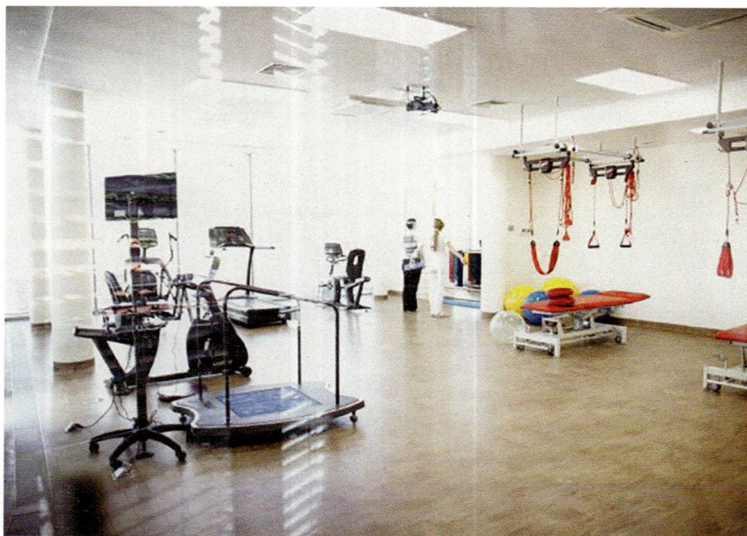

Fig. 7: Kinesiology therapy area.

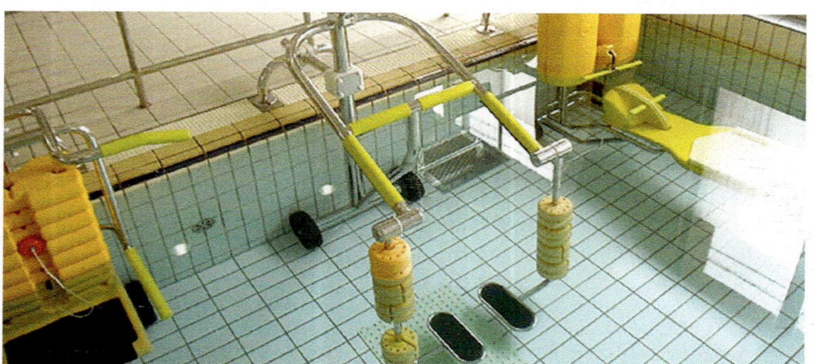

Fig. 8: Aquatic therapy.

drainage, chlorination plant, changing and heating of water, should be given. The hall housing the bath should approximately 18 m × 10.5 m × 5.5 m. The size of the pool itself should be approximately 12 m × 5.5 m and the depth should vary from 1 m to 1.5 m. The additional accommodation for the staff as well as storage space is also to be catered for. A pool size of 2000 m^2, is recommended.[2,3]

Activities of Daily Living (Fig. 9)

These are activities that individuals need to master in order to live independently. The activities include bathing, physical ambulation, grooming, dressing, eating and toileting. Activities of daily living (ADL) facilities provide a mock kitchen and bathroom arrangement. This space will be combined with PT/OT area on the ground floor.[2,3]

Home Environmental Learning

The concept of evidence-based design will be behind the creation of this area. The purpose of this suite of rooms is to teach and promote independence for the SCI/D patient who is transitioning from the center setting to the home environment.[3]

Lighting

Proper lighting (preferably shadow-free) is a necessity in a hospital especially in case of SCI/DC. All entry and exits as well as pick up and drop-offs should be adequately lighted. Critical areas for lighting

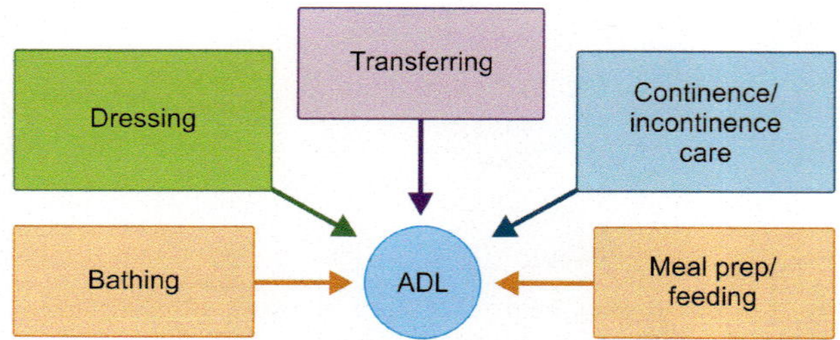

Fig. 9: Activities of daily living.

are ramps, steps and hazardous areas. The diagonal projection of light from one outlet should overlap the diagonal projection from the other. Lights should be arranged so that they form a straight line over the center of the ramp or path so that it can be a guide for a patient with visual perception only. The lights in the patient care areas should be recessed and should be glare-free.[3]

LEVEL-WISE DISTRIBUTION OF AREAS (FIGS. 10 AND 11)

There should be two blocks, the main block and the ward block. The ward block which will be of two floors from the floor should extend from the corresponding floors of the main block through passages. The main block will comprise of basement, ground floor, first and second floors. The ward block should have two floors with the general ward on the ground floor and rooms on the first floor. The blockwise as well as floorwise distribution should be as mentioned.

Basement

The basement of the main block should house the following establishments:

- Medical records
- Main stores—medical, surgical, stationary and IT stores
- Heating ventilation and air-conditioning
- Mortuary.

Ground Level

Main Block

- Reception
- Short stay area
- Outpatient department
- Radio imaging and urodynamics laboratory
- Physical medicine and rehabilitation unit.

Ward Block

- General ward area (ward block)
- Dietary services.

Level One

Main Block

- Intensive care unit
- Step-down ward [high dependency unit (HDU)]
- Laboratory and blood storage center.

Ward Block

- Private/semiprivate ward area (single and twin sharing).

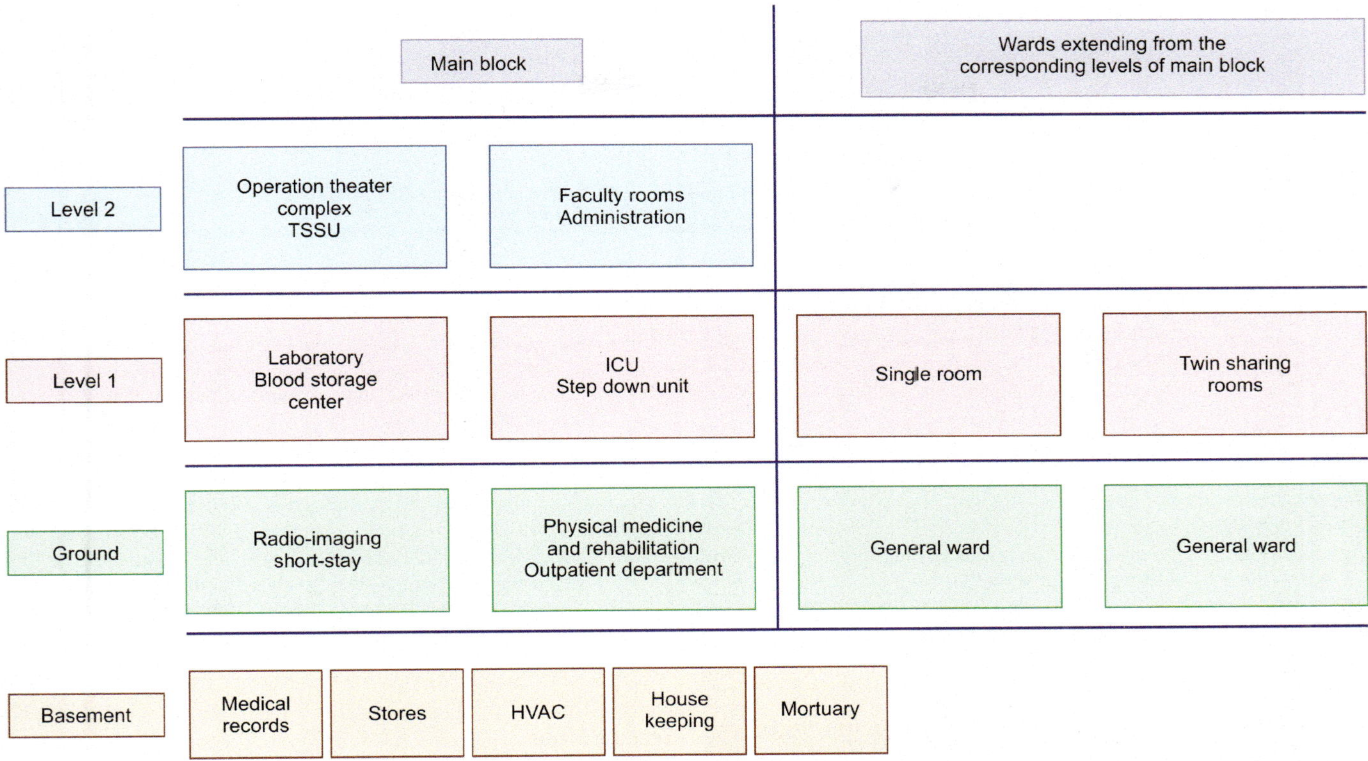

Fig. 10: Stack diagram of spinal injury center.

(TSSU: theater sterile supply unit; ICU: intensive care unit; HVAC: hearting ventilation and air-conditioning)

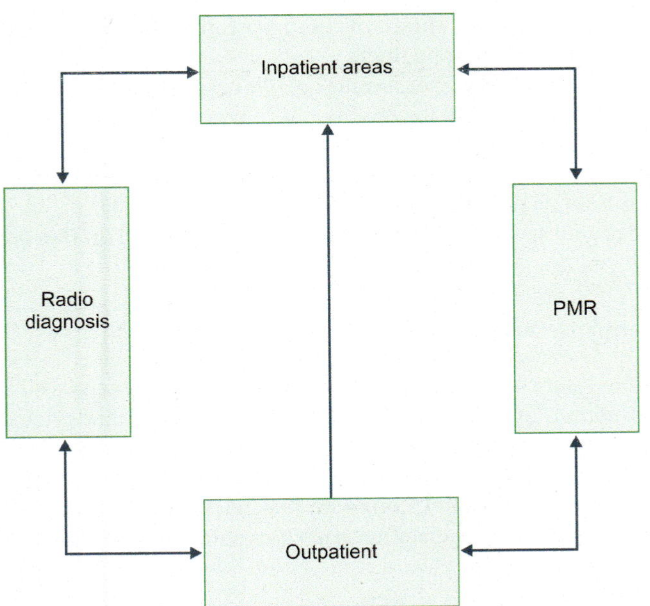

Fig. 11: Ground floor—functional relationship.

(PMR: physical medicine and rehabilitation)

Level Two

- Operation theater complex (with theater sterile surgical unit, pre- and postoperative areas and waiting area)
- Faculty rooms
- Administration
- Telemedicine.

The floors should be connected by two sets of lift banks at opposite ends as well as an internal ramp instead of stairs. The ward lock should also be connected by lifts. Further, the first floor of the ward side should be provided with an external ramp to the outside to facilitate mobility of the beds *per se* outside in case of disasters.

SCHEDULE OF ACCOMMODATION SCI (TABLE 2)

Main Block

First Floor

Intensive care unit and step-down unit (Fig. 12)

- A 10-bedded ICU would be sufficient for 80–100 bedded hospital.
- However, it would be ideal for the ICU to be supported by a step-down unit of 10 beds.
- Separate cubicles/bedrooms should have dimensions of 20 m^2/cubicle.
- *Environmental control*: The room should be adequately sound proofed. HVAC should ensure RH 50 ± 5% and maintain temperature in the range of 20–25°C. The number of air changes required is 8–10/h. The ICU shall be at a positive pressure.
- *Beds*: The beds should be mechanically or electrically operated beds capable of adjusting various therapeutic positions. Provisions for individual bedside patient monitors have to be made available.
- *Bed head unit (BHU)*: The BHU should have provisions for power socket (15 Amp), multisockets for medical devices, 2 oxygen outlets, 2 suction inlets, one compressed air outlets and nurses call system.
- *Patient lift hoist*: There should be provisions for patient movement in the form of a portable lift or permanent ceiling-based tracked patient lift hoist system.
- *Nursing station*: The pattern that may be adopted that gives optimum visual observation of patients with due consideration for nurse

Table 2: Spinal cord injury schedule of accommodation.

Ground floor		
Description	***Key features***	***Dimensions***
Short-stay area	Minimum 6–8 beds	An area of 15 m^2 per treatment area
OPD complex		
Reception area	Should provide a pleasant and welcoming environment	Area at the rate of 0.1 m^2/bed
Waiting area	Should be spacious enough to accommodate people on wheelchairs	Approximately 60 m^2 is appropriate considering 0.8 m^2/bed
Consultation rooms	About 5 consultation rooms are required with one each for orthopedics, neurosurgery and spine surgery and one for medicine and allied disciplines and one for surgery and allied disciplines	The minimum area required will be 12.5 m^2/room
Toilets	Disabled-friendly toilets	5 m^2 for patients use and common toilets for accompanying persons to be provided
Exam/treatment room	Must accommodate patients on a trolley	15 m^2 each should also include provision for patient lift hoist
Pharmacy	To cater to the requirements of the clientele in the OPD	10 m^2
Sample collection room	In the OPD itself to avoid unnecessary inconvenience	7 m^2
Radio imaging services	On the ground floor next to the short stay area with adequate waiting area for patients	For the three facilities of MRI, CT scan and X-ray an area of 200 m^2 is required. An area of 40 m^2 each is required for the MRI and CT machine room alone excluding the console rooms and waiting rooms
Physical medicine and rehabilitation	On the ground floor where they are easily accessible to both the OPD and inpatient services	An area of 100 m^2 is ideal

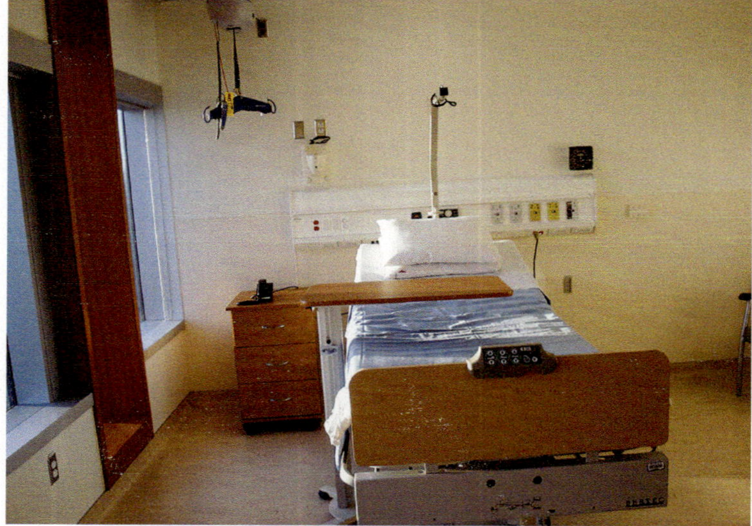

Fig. 12: Step down unit.

fatigue factor. Centralized monitoring will increase the efficiency of monitoring.

- *Duty rooms*: There should be duty rooms for doctors with toilet facilities. Staff changing rooms with separate toilets for male and female staff should be present.
- *Private/semiprivate rooms*: These rooms should be located as a block over the general ward block as described earlier.

Laboratory and Blood Storage Center

The laboratory and blood storage center should be co-located on the first floor. However, to reduce unnecessary traffic and allow accessibility, the collection rooms and donor room (with counseling room) are to be located on the ground floor near to the OPD and short stay area. The laboratory should be connected to all the collection points by pneumatic tube systems. There should be scope for expansion.

Second Floor

Operation Theater Complex

- The integrated OT complex is preferred on the second floor consisting of one be hybrid OT and one general OT.
- OTs should be modular in nature.
- There should be preoperative and postoperative patient holding areas also on the same floor.
- The area of hybrid OT should be 100 m^2 and that of the general OT should be 60 m^2 for enabling it to be used for orthopedic and neurosurgeons.
- An augmented theater sterile surgical unit should be located on this floor as part of the OT.
- Adequate space for expansion should be provided on this floor.

Third Floor

Administrative and Faculty Wing

The third floor should have all the administrative offices as well as the departments other than radiology, laboratory medicine and critical care which should be functionally located. The faculty rooms for orthopedics, neurosurgery, spine surgery, neurology, respiratory medicine and urology should be located along with seminar rooms. This wing should be provided with lift and staircase access to the ground floor separate from the OT access.

Ward Block

Inpatient Services (Wards and Private Rooms)[13]

It is prudent to locate the wards for quadriplegic/paraplegic on ground and first floors. The first floor should be connected to ground level by an additional external ramp to the outside for evacuation of these immobile patients in case of disasters.

The long-term care patients should comprise of predominantly the SCI patients who have some of residual weakness. The need to have the private/semiprivate wards separate from the general ward in the hospital should be considered. Each of the blocks to have a minimum of 5 cubicles of 4 patients each is advisable. An area of 12 m^2/bed is to be followed here. The general ward block may be provided with 4 toilet with litter bath facility (each of 15 m^2).

Similarly a private ward block comprising 10 single private rooms and 5 twin sharing semiprivate rooms with attached disabled-friendly litter bath/toilets are recommended to be located above the general ward block. The single rooms should be of 15 m^2 and twin rooms should be of 35 m^2.

Bed head unit (BHU): All the beds in the spinal center should have BHU with provisions for power socket (15 Amp), multi-sockets for medical devices, 2 oxygen outlets, 2 suction inlets, one compressed air outlets and duress call system. Having BHU will make available space also without the suction machines and other equipment interfering with the mobility of the patient.

Patient lifting hoist: There should be provisions for patient movement in the form of a portable lift or permanent ceiling-based tracked patient lifting hoist system (Fig. 13).

Toilets: Patient toilet/showers (private litter baths) are larger to allow staff and other caregivers to assist patient with toileting and showering, as needed (15 m^2). The ceiling lift hoist system if used in the patient bedroom is extended to the private litter bath to provide mobility for patient with staff assistance.[3]

A toilet cubicle for a wheelchair user should have clear internal dimensions of not less than 1500 mm × 1750 mm. It should be equipped with grab bars as under:

- One horizontal grab bar should be provided on the wall closest to the water closet, extending from the rear wall to the 450 mm to the front of the closet seat.
- One horizontal grab bar on the wall behind the closet and be at least 750 mm long.
- A vertical grab bar may also be provided on the side wall closest the water closet.

Wash basins in the toilets should be the accessible type for wheelchair bound patients. The top edge should be between 800 mm and 840 mm from the floor, knee space of 750 mm (wide) × 250 mm (deep) × 680 mm (high) and toe space of 750 mm (wide) × 250 mm (deep) × 230 mm high. The mirror in the bathrooms also should be accessible to the height of the wheelchair bound patient.

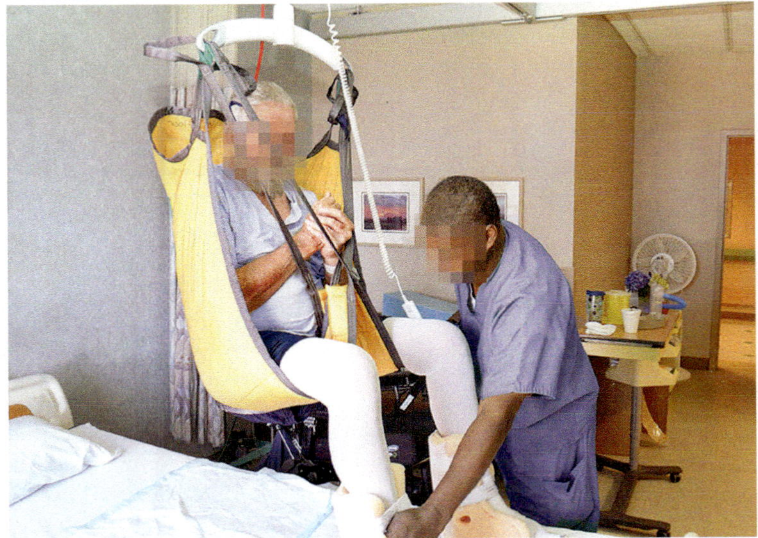

Fig. 13: Patient lifting hoist.

Basement

The following establishments should be located in the basement:

- Medical records
- Stores
- Mortuary
- Engineering services and HVAC

Line diagrams of ground and first-floor are shown in Figures 14 and 15.

SCALE OF ACCOMMODATION

Refer Table 3.

Table 3: Scale of accommodation.

Area	*Dimension (m^2)*
Short stay area	
Treatment area	15 (per bed)
Reception	7
OPD complex	
Reception	7
Waiting area	60
Consultation room	12.5
Treatment room	15
Toilet (disabled-friendly)	5
Toilet common	4
Pharmacy	10
Sample collection room	7
Radio diagnosis	200
PMR	300
Laboratory	80
Blood storage center	10
ICU treatment cubicle	20
HDU cubicle	20
Operation theater	
Hybrid	100
Integrated	60
Faculty offices	12
Administration	
CEO office	20
Office single person	12
Office workstation	6
Inpatient area	
Single room	15
Twin sharing room	35
Patient toilet/shower (ceiling lift hoist)	15
General ward/bed	12

CONCLUSION

Spinal injuries center are facilities receiving patients for stabilization or corrective surgeries of the spine. The development of the spinal surgeon apart from the orthopedic and neurosurgeon as well as the advance of the technology that has made minimally invasive spinal surgery (MISS) possible has given the concept of spinal center increasing credence. Such centers will be rendered more cost-effective by making use of the outsourcing model for various facilities like the radioimaging. Developing such centers in staggered fashion initially on a state level to start with will definitely provide the much needed succor to the patients as well as help in decongesting the tertiary centers which are hard-pressed for rendering this time-taking and dedicated skilled care.

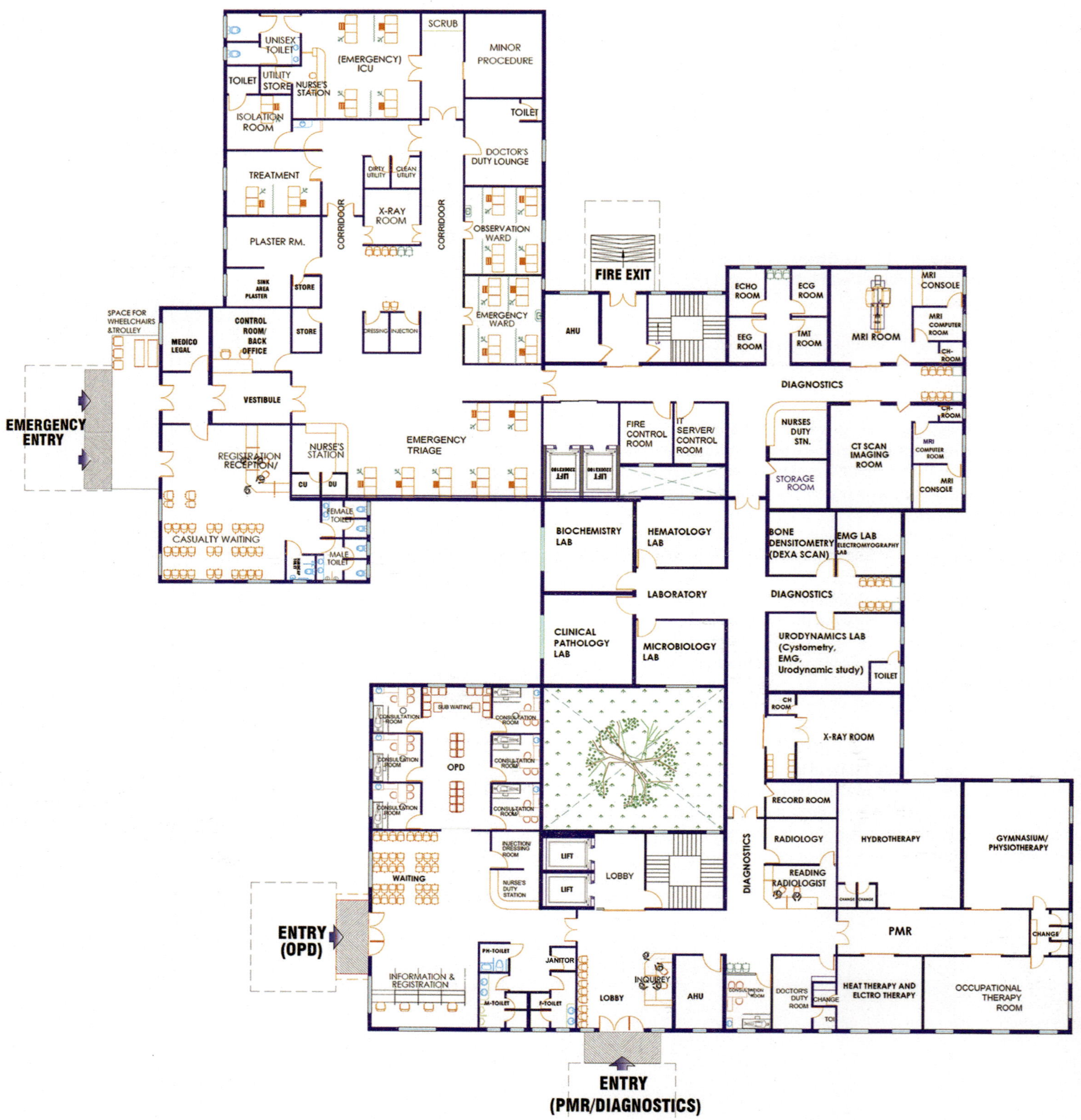

Fig. 14: Ground floor plan.

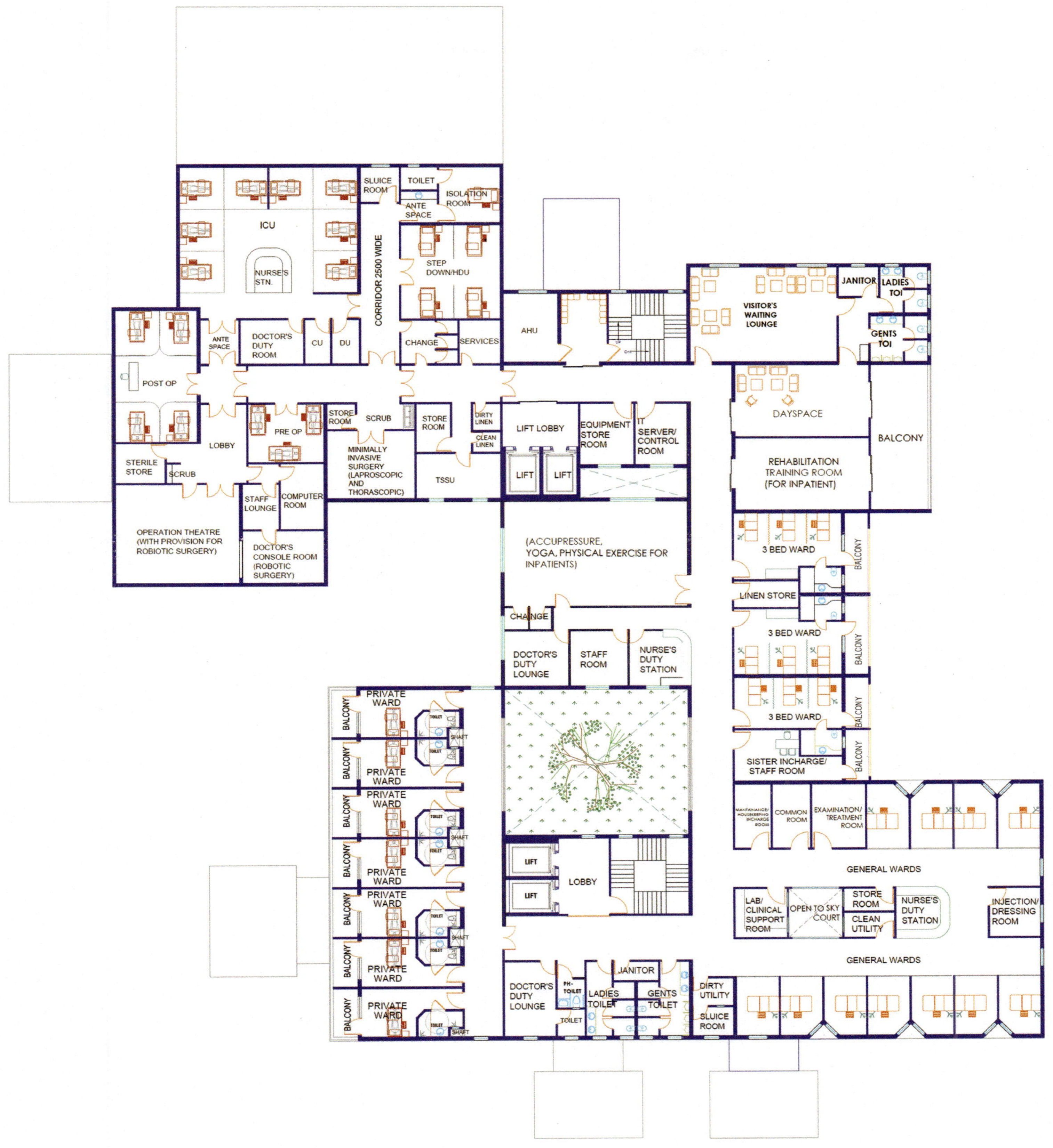

Fig. 15: First floor plan.

REFERENCES

1. www.emro.who.int
2. www.cfm.va.gov
3. www.spinal.co.uk
4. L Jones. "Spinal injuries units (SIUs) for acute traumatic spinal cord injury", Cochrane Database of Systematic Reviews Reviews, 2003.
5. worldspinecare.com
6. Chacko V, Joseph B, Mohanty SP, Jacob T. Management of spinal cord injury in a general hospital in rural India. Paraplegia. 1986;24(5):330-5.
7. Agarwal P, Upadhyay P, Raja K. A demographic profile of traumatic and non-traumatic spinal injury cases: a hospital-based study from India. Spinal Cord. 2006;45(9):597-602.
8. www.wbdg.org
9. www.va.gov
10. www.access-board.gov
11. www.prizmdevelopment.com
12. archive.samj.org.za
13. www.ideasbuilt.ca

OTHER REFERENCES

- Donovan WH, Clifton G, Carter RE. Developing a system of comprehensive care for the spinal cord injured patient in Houston, Texas, USA. Paraplegia. 1982;20(3):174-9.
- Nwadinigwe CU, Iloabuchi TC, Nwabude IA. Traumatic spinal cord injuries (SCI): A study of 104 cases. Niger J Med. 2004;13(2):161-5.

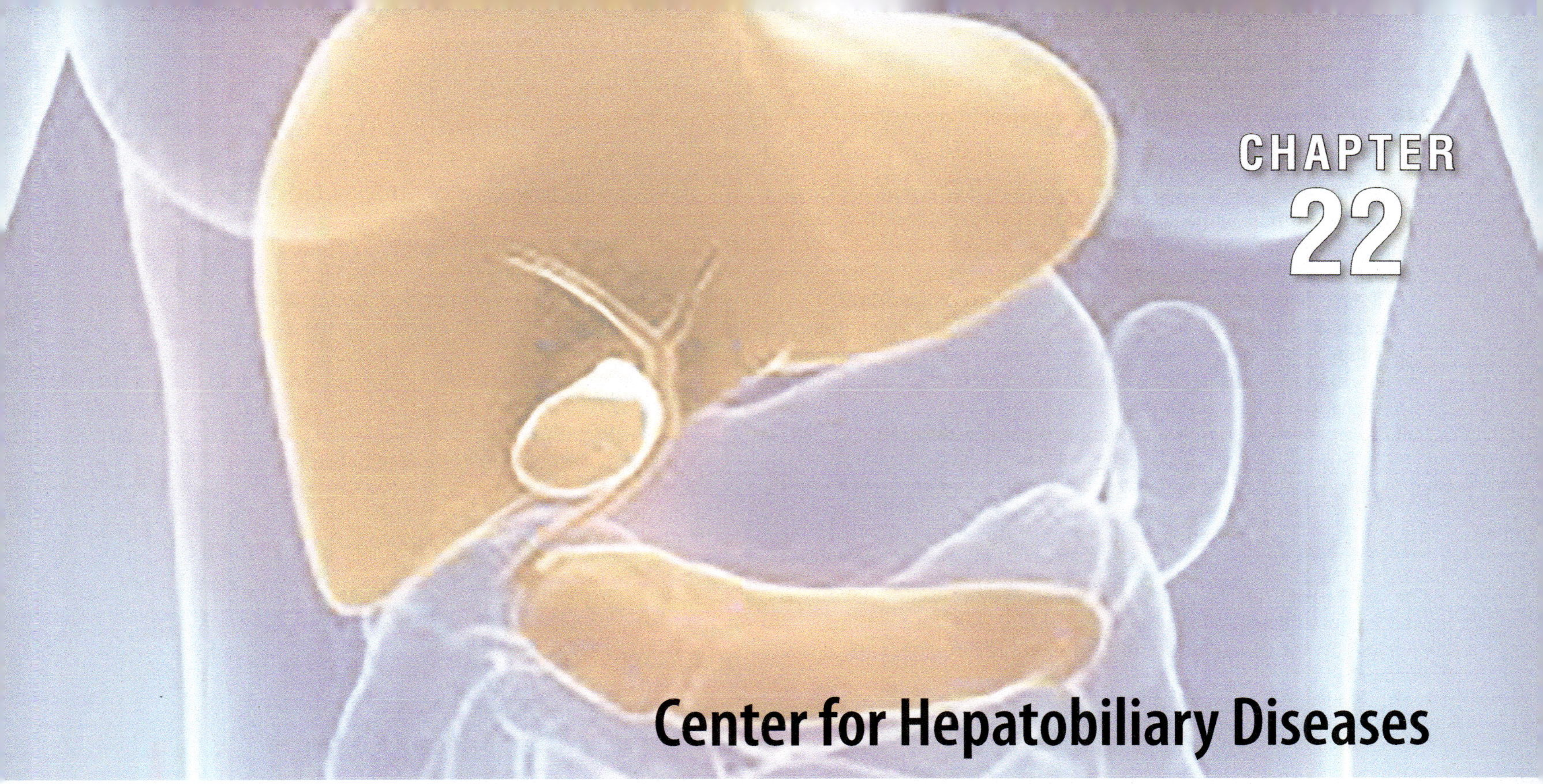

CHAPTER 22

Center for Hepatobiliary Diseases

Sunil Verma, Shakti Kumar Gupta, Sunil Kant, R Chandrashekhar

INTRODUCTION

In the recent past, gastroenterology (GE) and hepatology as a subspecialty have taken rapid strides with explosion of knowledge in the areas of pathogenesis, diagnosis and treatment, providing benefit to innumerable patients. Rapid advancement in this area is evidenced by:

- Establishment of postdoctoral courses in GE and gastrointestinal surgery (GIS) worldwide, including India.
- Each country has distinct professional societies in GE and many countries have additional professional societies in liver diseases.
- Therapeutic innovations in this area include liver transplantation, various endoscopic surgical treatments, therapy for liver cancer, hepatitis B, hepatitis C, improved surgical techniques and various image-guided therapeutic interventions.

Starzl performed the first human liver transplant in 1963. Since then, the evolution of immunosuppression and the development of new surgical approaches have led to the establishment of 100 transplant

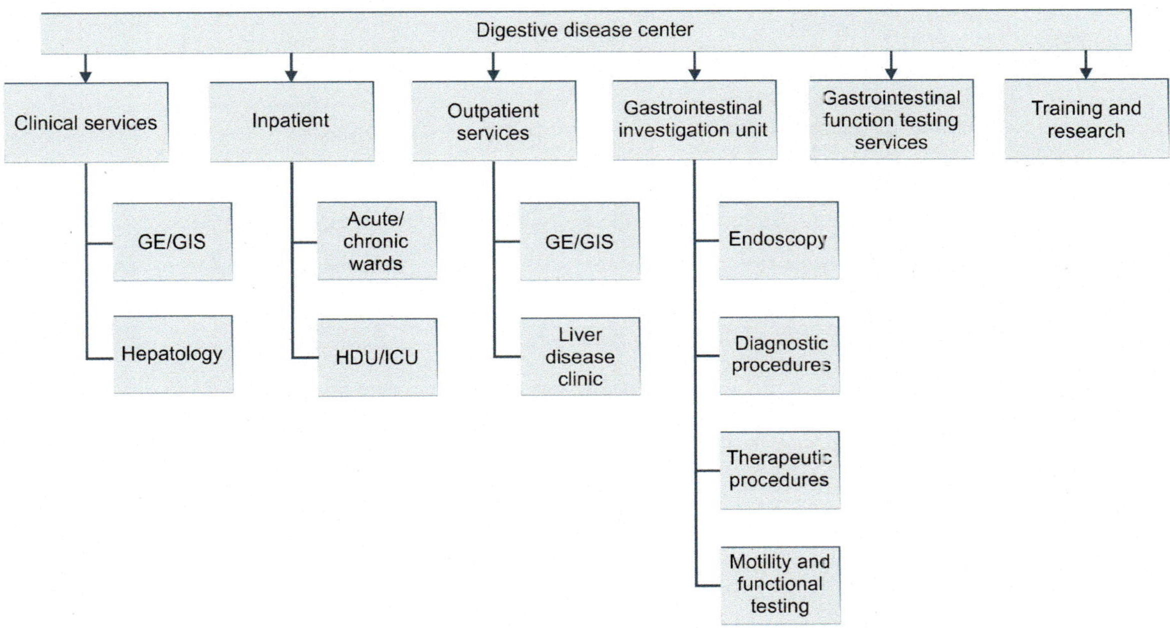

Fig. 1: Subunits of digestive disease center.
(GE: gastroenterology; GIS: gastrointestinal surgery; HDU: high-dependency unit; ICU: intensive care unit)

centers in the United States. Liver transplantation is a major surgical procedure whereby a diseased or failing liver is replaced by a healthy liver form a donor. This can be done in two ways.[1]

1. *Cadaveric (dead donor) liver transplantation (DDLT)*: This is where a liver is harvested from a cadaver (a deceased individual).
2. *Living donor liver transplantation (LDLT)*: This is also sometimes known as split-liver transplantation and is where a portion of a healthy liver is taken from a live donor and transplanted into the recipient.[1]

A comprehensive hepatobiliary center is a desirable entity (Fig. 1).

FUNCTIONS

Clinical Services

The department of GE, GIS and hepatology provides specialized assessment and care of patients with problems of the gastrointestinal tract and liver, in both acute/chronic inpatient, outpatient and daycare settings.[2]

Gastroenterology[2]

- Gastrointestinal bleeding disorders
- Inflammatory bowel disease (IBD: Crohn's disease and ulcerative colitis)
- Peptic ulcer and reflux disease
- Malabsorption syndrome
- Gastrointestinal motility and functional disorders
- Biliary and pancreatic diseases.

Hepatology[2]

- Chronic hepatitis
- Metabolic liver diseases (e.g. hemochromatosis)
- Cirrhosis
- Portal hypertension
- General hepatobiliary diseases (HBD)
- Fibroscan
- Liver biopsy.

PLANNING

Floor-wise Plan of Space in a Proposed Center for Digestive Diseases

Refer Figure 2 and Table 1.

Stack Diagram of a Liver Disease Center (Standalone Setup) (Fig. 2)

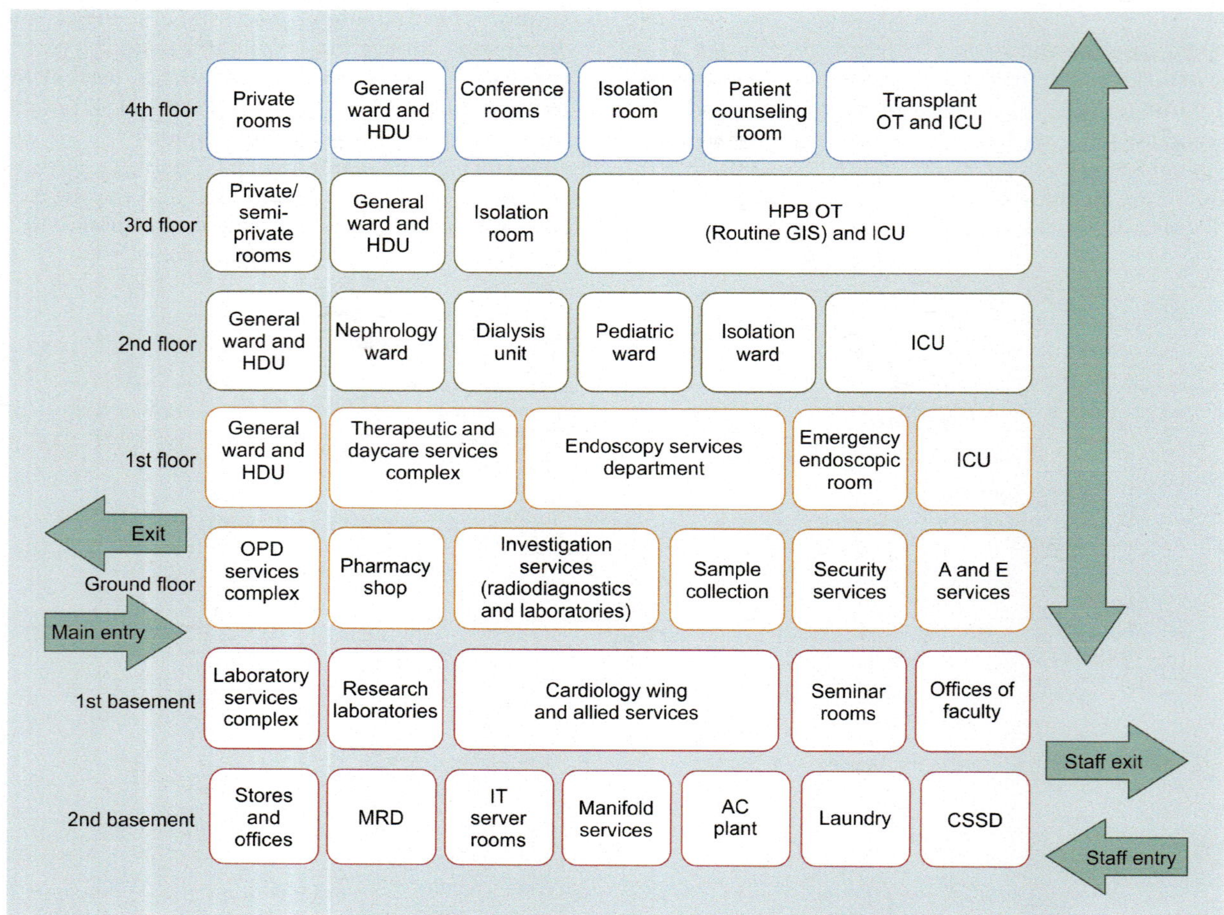

Fig. 2: Stack diagram of digestive disease center.

(HDU: high-dependency unit; OT: operation theater; ICU: intensive care unit; HPB: hepato-pancreato-biliary; GIS: gastrointestinal surgery; OPD: outpatient department; A and E: accidental and emergency; MRD: medical record department; IT: information technology; AC: air-conditioning; CSSD: Central sterile services department)

Table 1: Floor-wise plan of space for digestive diseases center.

Floor	Suggested facilities
Lower	• Stores and offices of various store officials
	• CSSD
	• IT department and server rooms
	• Security guard office
	• MRD
	• Laundry
	• AC plant
	• Manifold services
Upper basement	• Accommodation (offices)
	• Conference hall/seminar rooms
	• Various laboratories (microbiology, virology, pathology, histopathology, clinical pathology, biochemistry, immunology laboratory, tissue culture laboratory, hematology)
	• Research laboratories
	• Blood bank
	• Cardiology wing and ECHO
Ground floor	• Central reception and registration
	• OPD complex and consultations rooms
	• Accident and emergency services
	• Pharmacy shop
	• Radiodiagnostic services (general and specialized radiological services)
	• Security services rooms
	• OPD sample collection room
First floor	• Daycare services complex and its allied segments
	• Endoscopy services complex and allied services (for routine and booked cases)
	• Separately demarcated endoscopy room for emergency cases
	• General in patient ward
	• HDU
Second floor	• General in patient wards
	• Nephrology ward and dialysis unit
	• Pediatrics ward
	• ICU/HDU and isolation wards
Third floor	• Semiprivate rooms and allied facilities
	• Private rooms and allied facilities
	• HPB OT complex and allied facilities (to be used for the routine surgical procedures)
	• Surgical ICU and allied facilities
	• HDU and isolation wards
Fourth floor	• Private rooms and semiprivate rooms and allied facilities
	• General inpatient ward
	• OT complex dedicated for liver and organ transplantation
	• Transplant ICU complex
	• Patient counseling rooms
	• Conference/seminar room
	• Doctor duty rooms
	• Cafeteria

(CSSD: central sterile services is department; IT: information technology; MRD: medical record department; AC: air-conditioning; OPD: outpatient department; HDU: high-dependency unit; ICU: intensive case unit; OT: operation theater; ECHO: echocardiogram; HPB: hepato-pancreato-biliary)

DISTINCTIVE FUNCTIONAL AREAS OF A HEPATO-PANCREATICO-BILIARY DISEASE CENTER

Diagnostic and Therapeutic Endoscopic Services: Requirements for Endoscopic Devices (Figs. 3 and 4)

Endoscopy forms and integral and essential part of modern GE services. From largely being a diagnostic tool, endoscopy has advanced rapidly and steadily as an important and effective therapeutic procedure. Endoscopic assessment of almost the entire (GI) tract is now possible through upper (GI) endoscopy, colonoscopy and enteroscopy. Difficult to diagnose lesions are now being picked up with the help of newer endoscopes with advanced technology. Even some of the newer technology is being evaluated to complement visual image with microscopic tissue characterization to give an equivalent of histological diagnosis. Therapeutic endoscopy encompasses a large number of procedures for treating both acute and chronic disease that obviated the need for open surgical operations.

The functional requirement of an endoscopic suite is given in the Figure 5.

Therapeutic Procedure Facility

Modern GE and GI surgical center is expected to perform a variety of therapeutic procedures on a large number of patients. These procedures

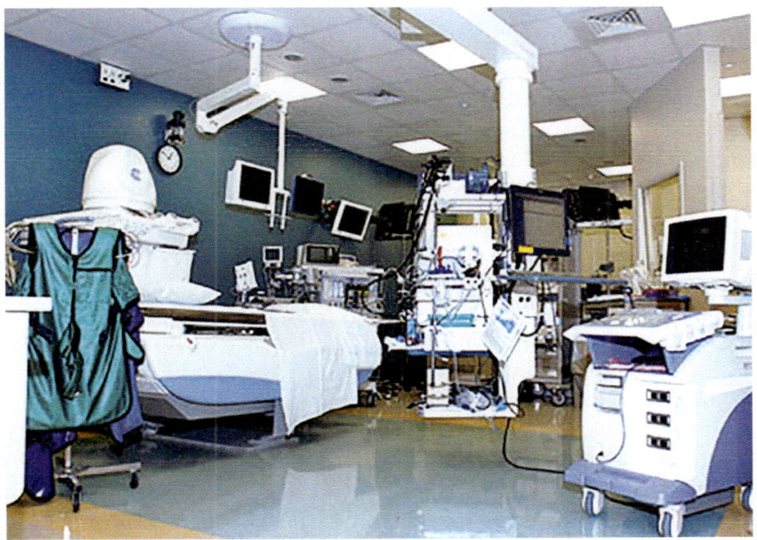

Fig. 3: Theraputic endoscopy services facility.

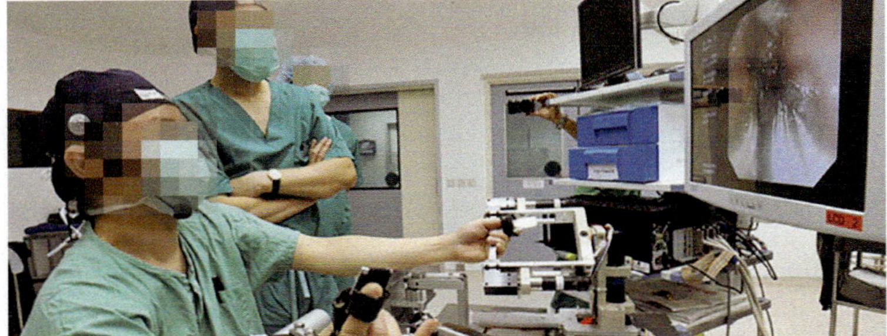

Fig. 4: Therapeutic endoscopy.

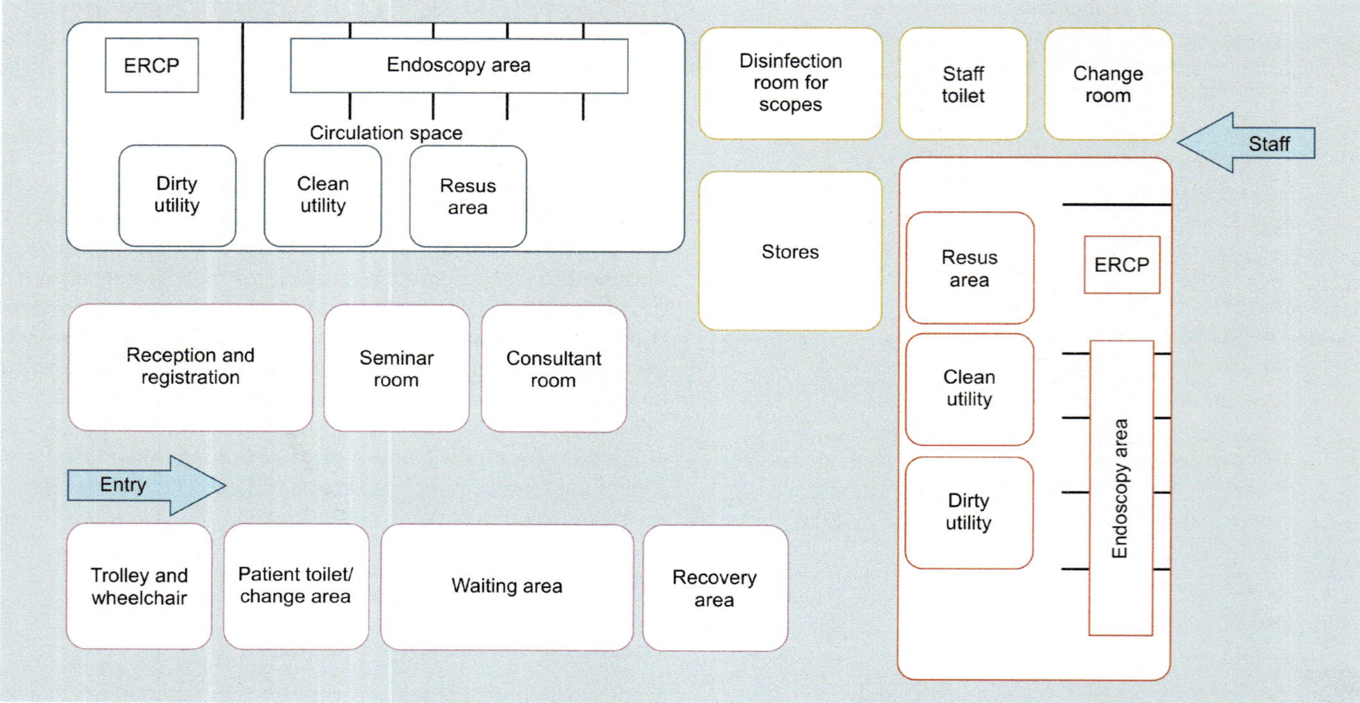

Fig. 5: Functional diagram of integrated endoscopic suite.
(ERCP: endoscopic retrograde cholangiopancreatography)

are aimed at both curative and palliative treatment of various GI and liver diseases. The nature of these procedures varies from ultrasound guided percutaneous procedures to treatment of cancers. The procedures and their utility are as follows:

- *Ultrasound-guided procedures*: These include liver and abdominal abscess drainage, percutaneous biliary drainage, FNAC and biopsy.
- *Radiofrequency ablation (RFA)*: This is a special type of treatment for liver cancers (Fig. 6).
- *Percutaneous alcohol injection (PAI)*: This is a treatment modality for liver cancers and liver hydatid cyst (Figs. 7A and B).
- *Gastrointestinal motility*: It is an important component in the diagnostic algorithm for various motility disorders of the GI tract.
- *H_2 breath analyser*: This is an important test for malabsorption.
- Liver biopsy.
- Large volume paracentesis for tense ascites in patients with cirrhosis of the liver.
- Special ultrasonography includes Doppler and color ultrasound in patients with portal hypertension.

New facilities: The newer therapeutic facilities include:

- *Hemodynamic monitoring and angioplasty*: This has become an essential part of the medical management of patients with portal hypertension. It paves the way for planning further treatment. Angioplasty is the standard treatment for patients with IVC and hepatic vein block that leads to Budd-Chiari syndrome (Fig. 8).
- *Leukapheresis*: This is a specialized treatment for patients with severe inflammatory bowel disease through a special apheresis machine.
- Extracorporeal shock wave lithotripsy (ESWL) has become standard treatment for breaking stones in patients with chronic pancreatitis. This coupled with therapeutic endotherapy gives results that are comparable to surgery (Fig. 9).

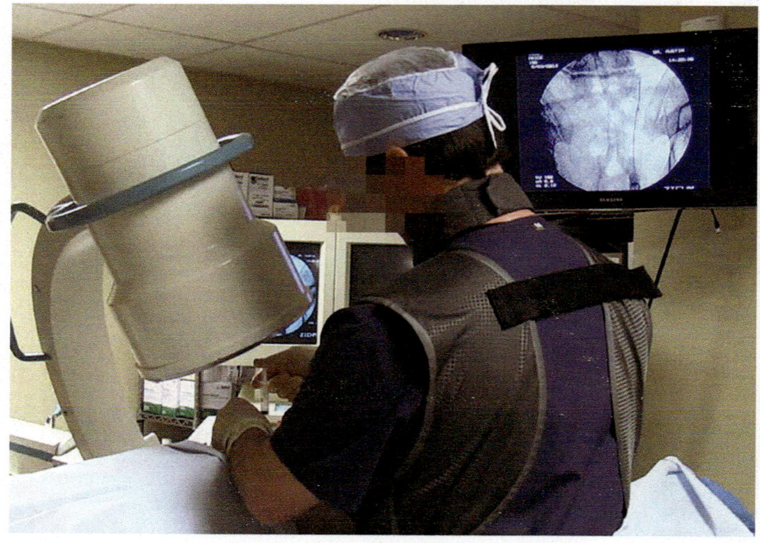

Fig. 6: Radiofrequency ablation.

A layout for the planning of therapeutic procedure facilities is depicted in Figure 10.

Intensive Care Unit (Figs. 11 and 12)

Patient area: There should be at least 15 sqm with 0.9 m of free space on head end and 1.2 m of free space at the foot end. Patients must be situated so that direct or indirect (e.g. video monitor) visualization by healthcare providers is possible at all times. The preferred design is to allow a direct line of vision between the patients and central nursing station.[3]

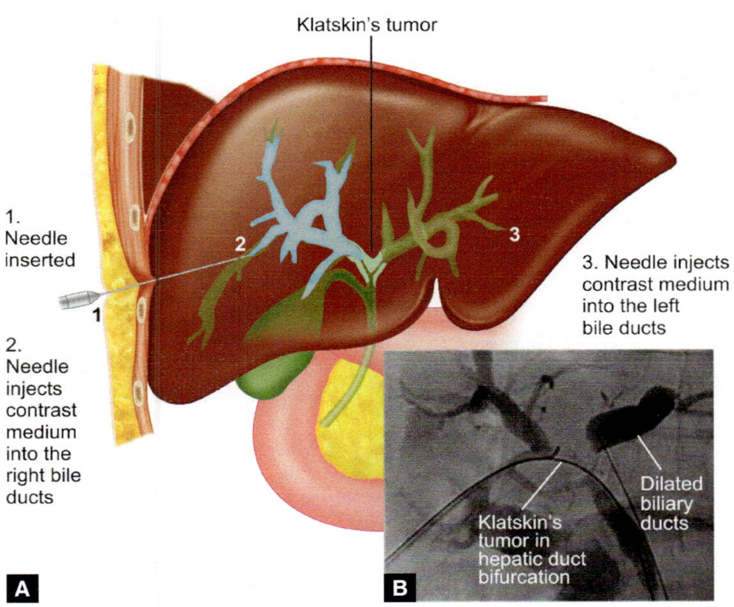

Figs. 7A and B: Percutaneous injection.

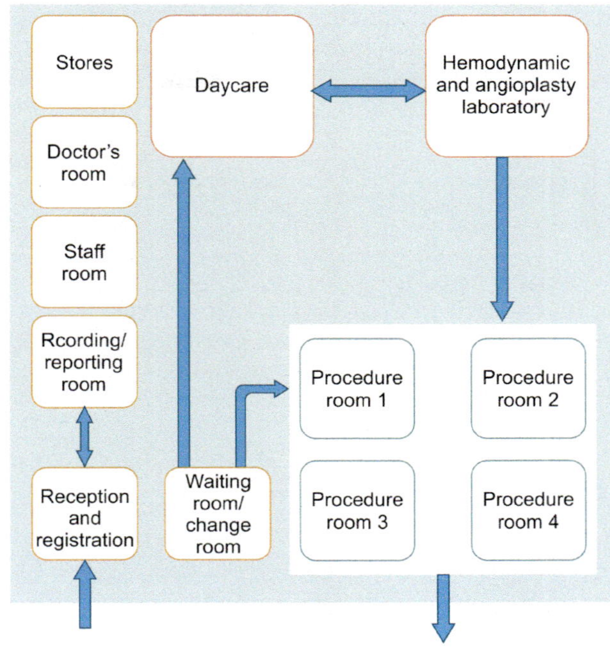

Fig. 10: Layout for the planning of therapeutic procedure facility.

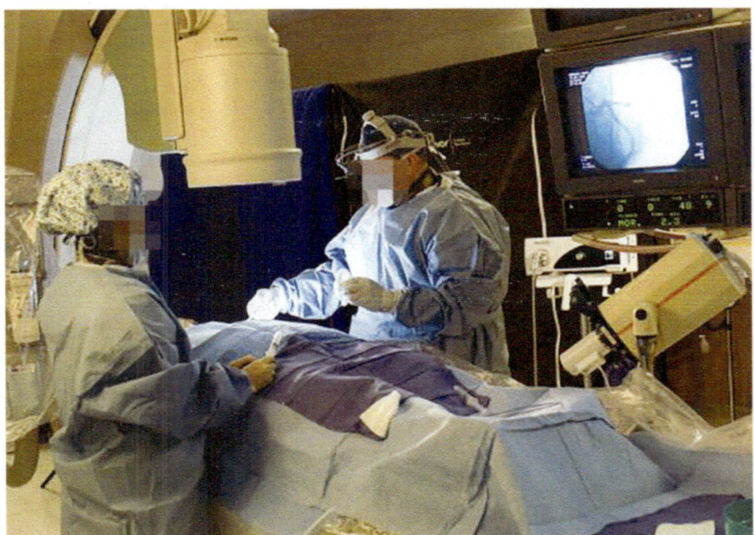

Fig. 8: Hemodynamic monitoring.

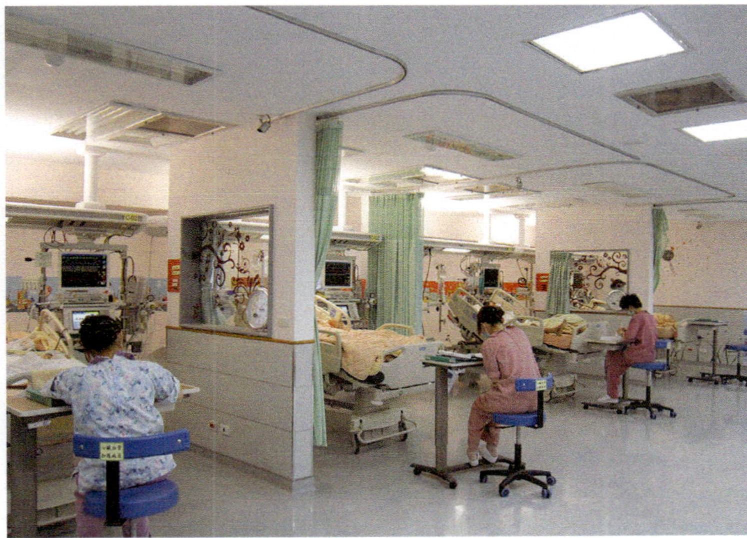

Fig. 11: Intensive care unit.

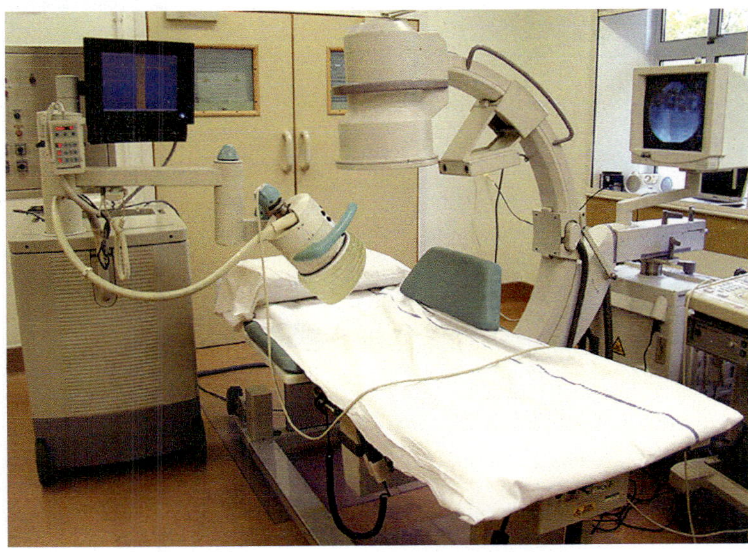

Fig. 9: Extracorporeal shock wave lithotripsy.

- *Individual patient module:*[3] Two isolation patient modules will be required for each module and a minimum width of 4.5 m excluding ancillary space (anteroom, toilet, storage).[4]
- The design should consider natural illumination and light. As many windows as possible should be provided to reinforce day/night orientation.
- The stress, while constructing the center, should be on the energy efficiency and conservation and all necessary aspects of green design should be incorporated at the very beginning of project.
- Space and surfaces for computer terminals and patient charting should be incorporated into the design of each patient module.
- Walls and ceilings should be constructed with high sound absorption capabilities to reduce the noise levels in ICU which are usually high.

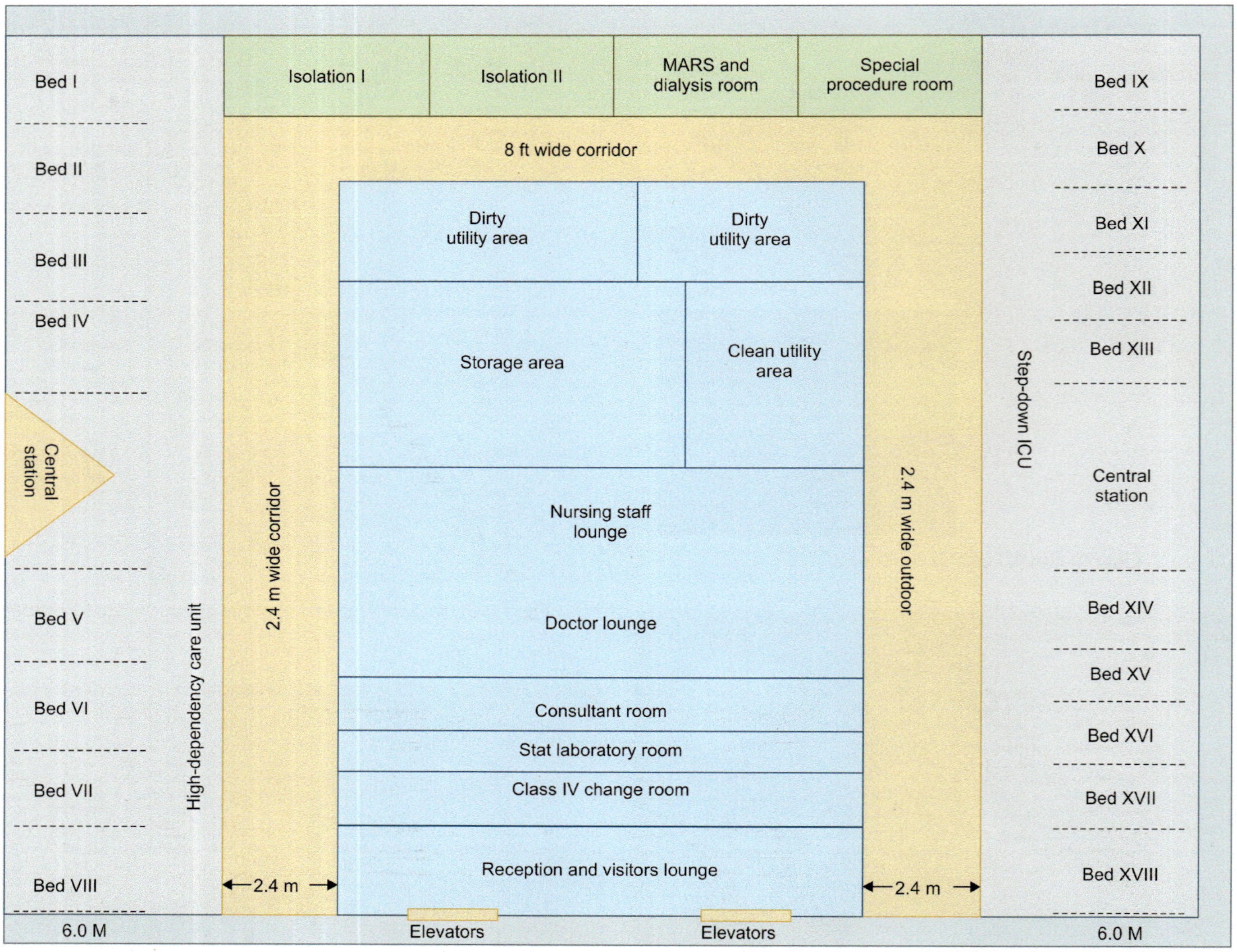

Bed I
Isolation I
Isolation II
MARS and dialysis room
Special procedure room
Bed IX
8 ft wide corridor
Bed II
Bed X
Dirty utility area
Dirty utility area
Bed XI
Bed III
Bed XII
Bed IV
Storage area
Clean utility area
Bed XIII
Step-down ICU
Central station
2.4 m wide corridor
Nursing staff lounge
2.4 m wide outdoor
Central station
Bed V
High-dependency care unit
Doctor lounge
Bed XIV
Bed XV
Bed VI
Consultant room
Bed XVI
Stat laboratory room
Bed VII
Class IV change room
Bed XVII
Bed VIII
2.4 m
Reception and visitors lounge
2.4 m
Bed XVIII
6.0 M
Elevators
Elevators
6.0 M

Fig. 12: Layout of an intensive care unit.

- There should be 3 cubicles of 6 beds each and 2 isolation rooms. These cubicles are required for the purpose of breaking the infection chain and providing ICU facilities in relative isolation.
- *Minimum number of simultaneously accessible outlets*: Oxygen 2; air outlets 2, suction outlets and electrical outlets 4 should be available for every bed.
- One wash basin for every 2 beds.
- Sliding glass doors in cubicles for isolation.

Central station: A central nursing station should provide a comfortable area of sufficient size to accommodate all necessary staff functions (Fig. 13). Zones must be provided for medication preparation and cabinets for storage of medication and supplies.[4]

- There should be facility for computerized charting. These systems provide for 'paperless' data management, order entry and nurse/physician charting. Bedside terminals facilitate patient management by permitting nurses and physicians to remain at bedside during the charting process.[4]
- *Voice intercommunication system*: A voice linkage system between the central nursing station, patient modules, physician-on call rooms, conference room and staff lounge.[4]

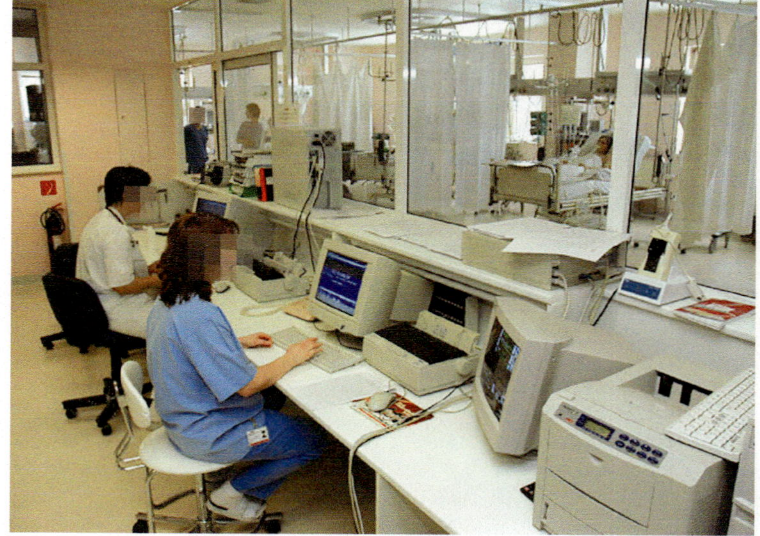

Fig. 13: Central station intensive care unit.

- *The work area*: Medication preparation area, file storage area, computer terminals, essential medicine storage area, emergency medicine storage area, X-ray viewing area.

Receptionist area: To control visitor access.

Special procedures room: Changing room and wash stations.

Clean and dirty utility room: The clean utility room should be used for storage of all clean and sterile supplies and linen. The dirty utility room must contain sinks.

Staff lounge/consultation lounge

Visitor's lounge/waiting room

Supply/service corridor
Environment control systems: Suitable and safe air quality must be maintained at all times. A minimum of 6 air changes per room per hour are required with 2 air changes per hour composed of outside air. Central air-conditioning system and recirculated air must pass through appropriate filters. Adequate isolation facilities (at least 1 cubicle for every 6 beds) should be available.[4]

Dialysis and MARS room: As patients admitted to ICU will require molecular adsorbent recycling system (MARS) *(liver dialysis)* and renal dialysis, a room dedicated to this purpose is required with facility for continuous RO system. A dedicated nephrology ward and associated Dialysis room is also envisaged (Fig. 14).

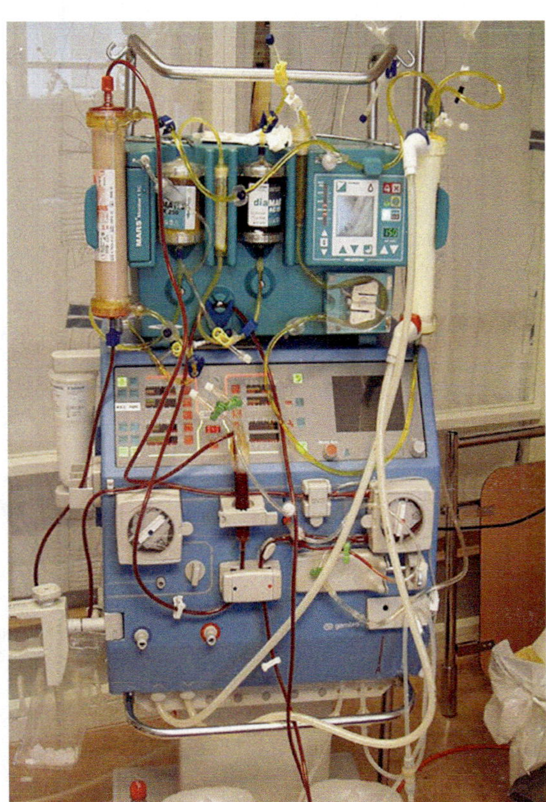

Fig. 14: Molecular adsorbent recycling system.

Stat laboratory facilities which will include arterial blood gas analysis machine. Figure 15 shows the interdepartmental relationship of an ICU and Table 2 shows the scales of accommodation.

Research Laboratories

These laboratories are in addition to the routine laboratories which are also stationed on the same floor. Two toilets and research officers' room should be placed at the beginning of the floor.

Daycare Area for Investigative and/or Therapeutic Procedures

Refer Table 3.

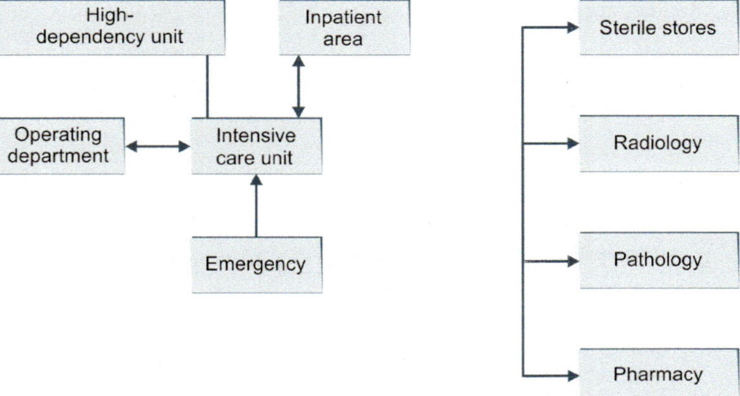

Fig. 15: Interdepartmental relationship of intensive care unit.

Table 2: Scales of accommodation in intensive care unit.

Room/space	*Area (in sqm)*
Bed bay	20
Isolation room	22
Mobile equipment bay	4
Janitor's closet	2
Clean utility	12
Dirty utility	10
Disposal room	8
Medication room	10–12
Staff station	14–20
Store room (for equipment)	15–20
Toilets	
• Patients	3
• Disabled patients	5
• Staff	2
Meeting room (where doctors will meet the relatives of patients)	12
Office (single occupancy)	9
Conference room	15–20
Circulation space	35%

Table 3: Scales of accommodation in daycare facility.

	Area (in sqm)
Operating area	1
• Bays for hand wash	4
• Bays for mobile equipment	2
• Trolley bay	2
• Change cubicle for patients	2
• Change cubicle for disabled	5
• Clean utility	12
• Dirty utility	10
• Operating room (minor)	36
• Operating room (major)	54
• Treatment room	9
Recovery area	
• Patient holding	9
• Recovery stage 1/2/3	9
• Staff station	14
• Store for equipment	9–20
• Stores for linen	2
• Cleaners' room	4
• Toilet with change facility	4
Staff and support area	
• Consultation room	12
• Waiting room	6–18
• Reception	10
• Toilet (staff)	2
Shared area	
• Change room—staff	8–10
• Disposal room	8
• Conference room	20

OPERATION THEATER(S)

General Consideration for an Organ Transplantation Operation Theater (Fig. 16)

The general features are as following:[5,6]

- A continuous flow of highly filtered 'bacteria-free' air is circulated under positive pressure into the operating field and air contaminants generated during surgery are removed from the site
- Seamless floor and walls
- Easy-to-clean steam cleaned, electrometric (ideal for high humidity areas)
- Vapor permeability (allows substrate moisture to escape) protects against growth of bacteria, mold and yeasts
- Moisture resistance, freeze/thaw resistance.

In an operating department for which the most integrated function is required, cleanliness must be kept and the safety of facilities, equipment and devices must be maintained any time. Furthermore, the working environment for medical staff such as doctors and nurses must be considered from the view point of human engineering. The operating theater satisfying those conditions consists of wall, ceiling and slanted panels, and is capable of incorporating not only electrical equipment, medical gas system and lighting gears but all the necessary functions and equipment at need.

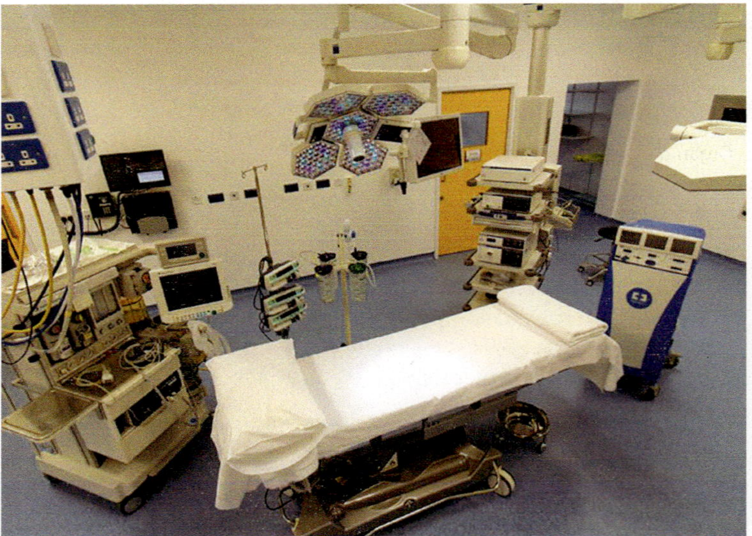

Fig. 16: Organ transplant operation theater.

In addition, the modular theater has a high availability of extension providing for the introduction of new facility in the future, establishing as well an operating environment with high work ability and enough function.

The most complex and challenging area of hospital construction is the operating department. The prefabricated operating theater integrated approach to the construction and coordination of operating theater. The prefabricated operating theater offer the advantage of speedy construction combined with design, future expansion and development in surgical technique whilst simultaneously providing a structure of the highest quality and standards. Modern equipment as follows must be incorporated.[7]

- Plenum unit (laminar air flow)
- Wall and ceiling
- Air and light
- Pendants
- Hermetically sealed door
- Operation theater control panel
- X-ray viewer
- Pressure relief damper
- Scrub sink
- Operation theater table
- Anti-static flooring
- Writing board
- View window
- Hatch box
- Equipment storage unit
- Pressure stabilizer.

Designing an operating theater outlines the intricacies of the hospital design process. An operating theater suite consists of the theater, the anesthetic room, scrub room and the dirty utility (or just utility) room. The size and room dimensions vary but as an indication, it should be about 7 m wide by 8 m long (56 sqm). Scales of accommodation are at Table 4.

The over-riding principles while designing an operating theater are:

- Flexibility of use of the space.
- Ease of cleaning the theater—including the floor, walls, surgeon's panel and any equipment such as pendants and theater lights.
- Ease of use of surgeon's panels, theater lights and pendants.

Table 4: Scales of accommodation in operation theater.

Room/space	Area (in sqm)
Reception	10
Anesthetic induction room	15
Organ translations operating room	52–56
Scrub up/gowning area	6
Support area	
• Anesthetic room	10–15
• Mobile equipment bay	4
• Janitor cupboard	2
• Stores (anesthetic/equipment/sterile/non-sterile)	20–40
Recovery area	
• Patient bay	9
• Linen bay	3
• Hand washing bay	1
• Clean utility bay	12
• Dirty utility bay	10
• Staff station	6–14
Administrative staff area	
• Change room	10–30
• Toilet staff	4
• Office (single occupancy)	9
• Staff lounge	10–30
Shared area	
• Meeting/conference room	20–30
• Waiting area	4
• Circulation space	35%

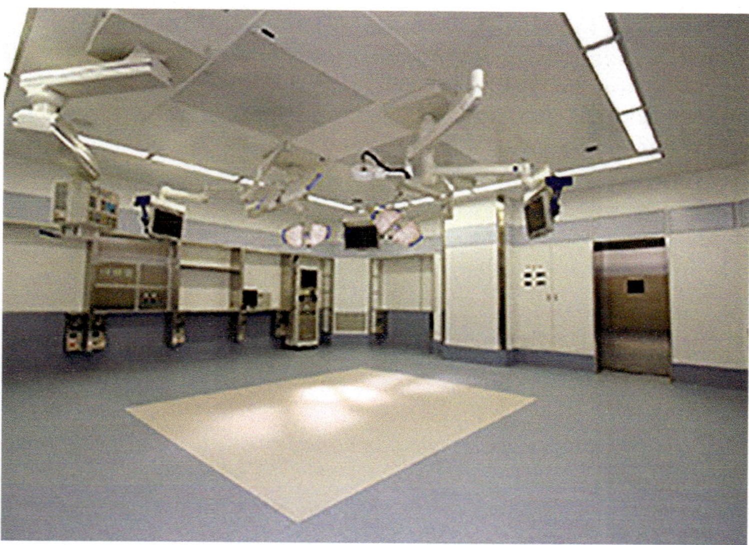

Fig. 17: Wall and ceiling in an operation theater.

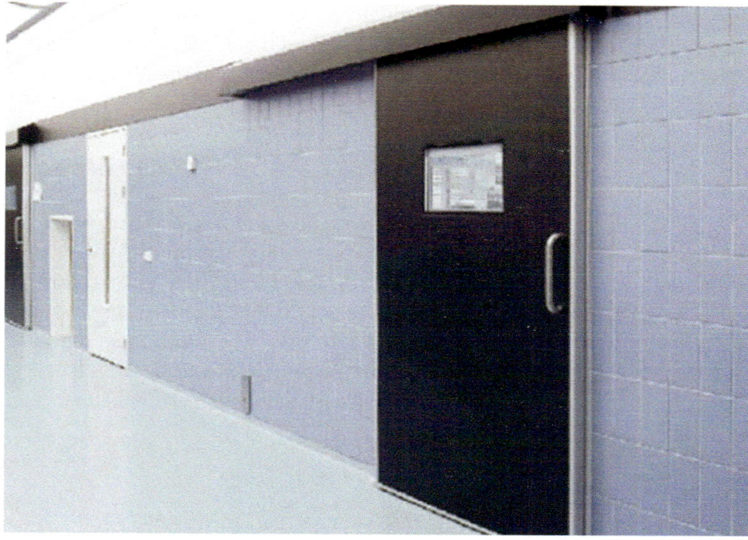

Fig. 18: Hermetically sealed door.

The equipment and instruments maybe either on mobile trolleys to allow 100% flexibility on use of the theater and ease of cleaning the theater or mounting a great majority of equipment on ceiling mounted theater pendants. The ceiling slab must be able to hold the weight of the theater lights, pendants and the equipment if mounted on the pendants.

Plenum Unit (Laminar Air Flow)

Bacteria cause infection within operating theater. Specialized ceilings are supplied with optional air-conditioning and control systems, either independent or as part of an existing mechanical services systems, and thus reduce the risk of postoperative infection. They provide optimum comfort through the use of conditioned, filtered clean air. The system is designed to allow the user to select from a variety of lighting and diffuser arrangements to suit the specific requirements of the operating team.

The ceilings consist of a plenum box supplied with conditioned air from the central system via "S" class high efficiency particulate air (HEPA) filters mounted on the inlet to the supply ceiling. All HEPA filters and housings should be certified in accordance with DIN: 1946 and DIN: 4799. All ceilings incorporate supports to secure them to the main structural frame of the modular operating theater, or structural slab.

Wall and Ceiling (Fig. 17)

The fabricated operation room should be designed as a free standing structure. All the four corners have return air duct outlets and grill for the same made of steel duly powder coated with the color choice to suit the hospital. Distance between the walls and panels should be around 100 mm. Antibacterial paint does not leach out so that its antimicrobial properties remain active throughout the life of the product. They tolerate harsh cleaning. Filling of all joints and cavities is done with metallic epoxy filler and sanded flush provides a jointless finish.[6]

Air and Light

The air/light diffusers consist of 2 layers of monofilament precision woven polyester of uniform porosity, with an open area of sufficient resistance to create laminar air flow from the diffuser face. Integral lighting provides an illumination level in excess of 1300 lux at the wound site and electronic steeples dimming down to 3% without flicker.[6]

Hermetically Sealed Doors

Hermetically sealed sliding doors (Fig. 18) are intended to maintain sterile environment and the correct air pressure in the room, which requires less valuable space than hinged doors. The door can be operated manually or automatically with microprocessor based electronic automation system. The door frame is made out of high quality anodized aluminum extrusion and the door panel is made out of compact laminated board that can withstand high abrasions. The controller will be capable of either being operated by elbow switches/ foot switches, radar switch (touchless sensor). All doors should be able to be operated manually easily in the event of power supply failure or the automation unit.[6]

View Window

The view window of specified size to be provide consisting of double insulated fixed glazing with not less than 5 mm thick toughened glass. Window frame to be powder coated aluminum of approved shade flush mounted with wall paneling.

Pressure Relief Damper

Pressure relief dampers are provided in each operating room to prevent cross-contamination of air from clean and dirty areas. Suitable sized air pressure relief damper are strategically placed. They enable differential room pressure to be maintained and ensure the same when doors are opened between clean and dirty area. Counterweight balancing system is provided to maintain positive pressure inside the operation room.[8]

Operation Theater Control Panel

All the controls for the modular operation theater are provided on a membrane type, microcontroller-based electronic control panel mounted in the theater wall. Control panel meet the electrical safety codes for high and low voltage systems. The control panel is user-friendly and case of operating and maintenance purpose. The fascia is made with superior quality UV resistance membrane with sterilization feature. The control panel (Fig. 19) may consist six tiles or nine tiles. These are:

- Time of day clock
- Elapsed time clock
- Temperature display/control
- Humidity display/control lighting control/dimming
- Medical gas alarm systems
- Hands-free telephone
- HEPA filter status indicator
- OT pressure indicator
- Music control.

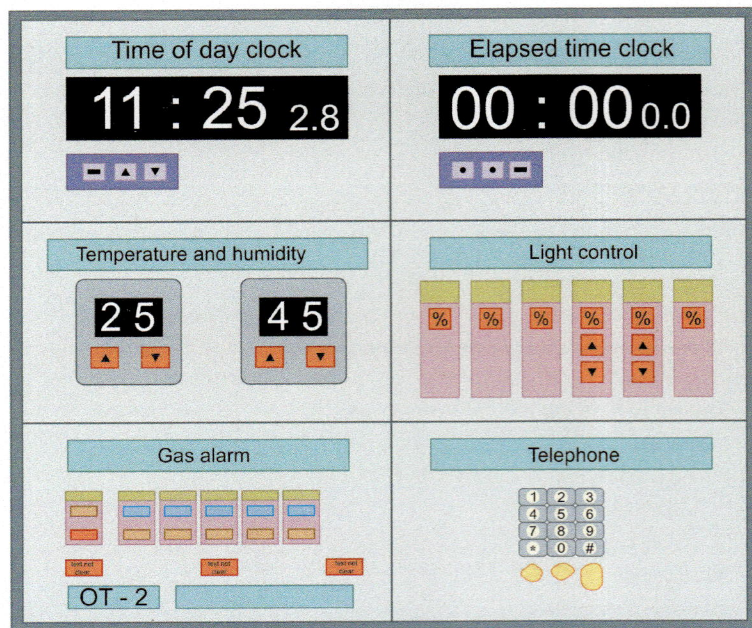

Fig. 19: Operation theater control panel.

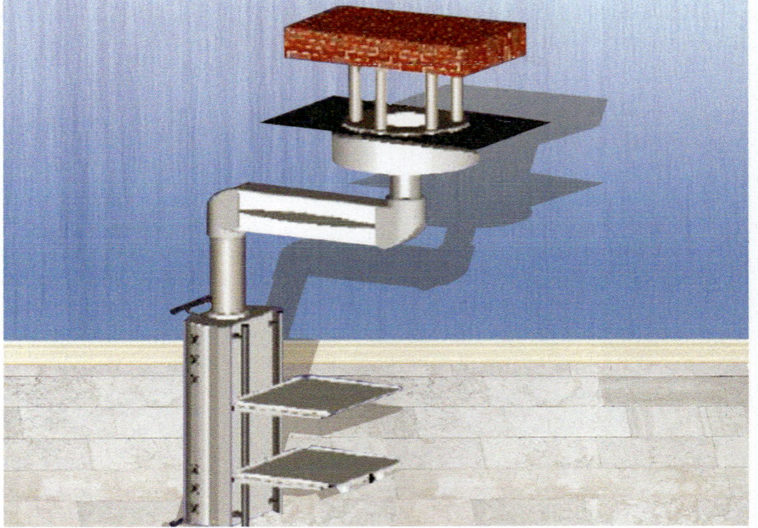

Fig. 20: Pendant.

Ceiling-mounted Equipment

Pendants (Fig. 20) can be rigid, retractable or fully articulated. Theaters require fully articulated pendants for maximum flexibility. A lot of coordination is required between medical gas, electrical and pendant trade contractors together with electrical, mechanical and structural engineers/consultants while installing pendants to ensure all structural steel support is in place, gas pipes are properly connected and power and data cables run at the correct programmed dates. In case of power failure during surgery. Various lifesaving equipment must be supplied uninterrupted power socket(s).

Theater lights[9] *(Fig. 21)*: Earlier there were gas discharge lights or halogen lights. Aspects to consider were bulb life, costs associated and theater down time while bulbs were changed. The new and more suitable technology for the OT lights is LED. Although it is about 30% more expensive compared to the existing technology yet it brings along with its numerous advantages. These are:

- Long life bulbs (over 20,000 hours)
- Ease of maintenance (couple of minutes to replace an LED)
- Cheap cost of replacement (fraction of older technology)
- Ability to vary light temperature hence helping to diagnose cancerous cells, etc.

Theater lights must be backed up by a battery backup in case of power failure during surgery. Suggested time can be 3 hours backup. It should be noted that general lighting and emergency escape lighting should also be on similar battery/UPS back-up time.

Camera, in a teaching and research facility, and microphone is also required for 1-way video (from operating theater to lecture theater and/or seminar rooms) and 2-way audio for surgeons and students to communicate. The camera can either be installed in the handle of

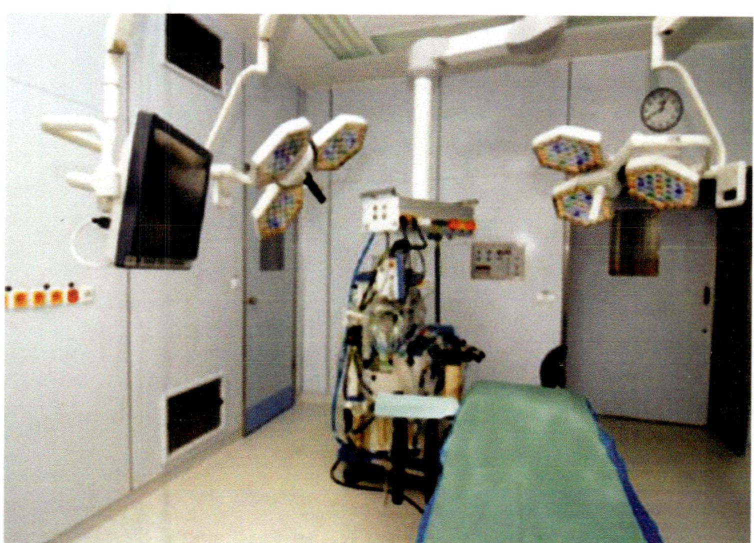

Fig. 21: Operation theater lights.

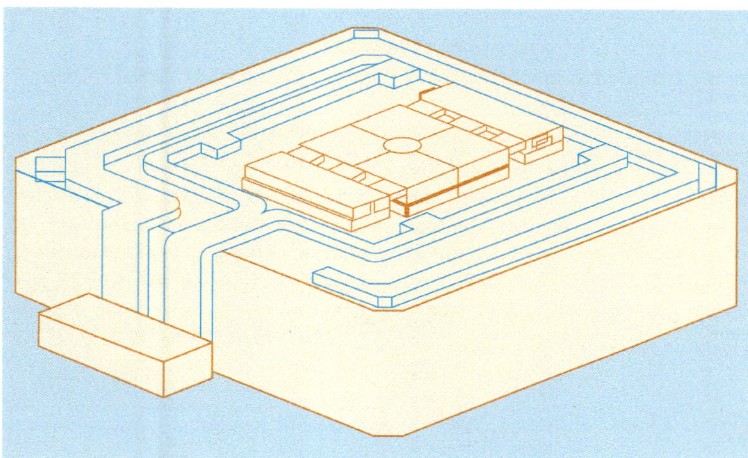

Fig. 22: Clean air canopy in organ transplant operation theater.

the main theater light of installed on a separate ceiling-mounted arm. In organ transplant theaters consider the largest ceiling-mounted item—the laminar flow or the ultra clean ventilation (UCV) Canopy (Fig. 22).

Floor-mounted Equipment[5]

Theater table generally are rechargeable and do not necessarily require power socket close by.

Trolleys are used for instruments and equipment such as video endoscopes and anesthetic equipment.

To achieve maximum infection control walls should have special plastic enamel paint to allow chemical cleaning if required in case of disinfection. The ceiling is generally constructed of plaster board or special metal to ensure it is air-tight and easily cleaned. Airflow regime is an important part of moving the air from clean areas towards dirty and out of the operating theater suite to ensure the theater is the cleanest environment for operating on the patients.[8]

Functional Classification of Isolation Room (Table 5)[10,11]

Table 5: Functional classification of isolation room.

	Class S (standard)	*Class N (negative)*	*Class P (positive)*	*Class A (alternating)*
Key ventilation criteria	No air pressure difference between the room and the adjacent corridor	Lower air pressure in the room than in adjacent corridor	Greater air pressure in the room than in the adjacent corridor	Ventilation controlled to achieve either positive or negative pressure in the room
Transmission based precautions	To prevent contact or droplet transmission	To prevent airborne transmission	To prevent transmission of pathogens from outside environment to immunosuppressed patients	Not recommended
Examples	Hepatitis A, meningococcal infection	Meales, chicken pox, tuberculosis	Prevention of infection in bone marrow or organ transplant recipients	-

Air Filtration

For infectious isolation rooms, where recirculation of room air is allowed, the return air should be HEPA filtered. For protective isolation, the supply air should also be HEPA filtered. HEPA filtration can be used as a method of air cleaning that supplements other recommended ventilation measures. HEPA filters should be used:

- When the HVAC system configuration dictates recirculation of air from the isolation room to other parts of the facility.
- When it is impossible for air from an infectious isolation room and/or local exhaust devices to be exhausted directly outdoors.
- When air is being recirculated into the same infectious isolation room.

Newer Trends in the Air Filtration for Effective Control of Infection in a HBD Center

Ultraviolet germicidal irradiation (UVGI) (Fig. 23) is a disinfection method that uses ultraviolet (UV) light at sufficiently short wavelength to kill microorganisms. It is used in a variety of applications, such as food, air and water purification. It utilizes short-wavelength ultraviolet

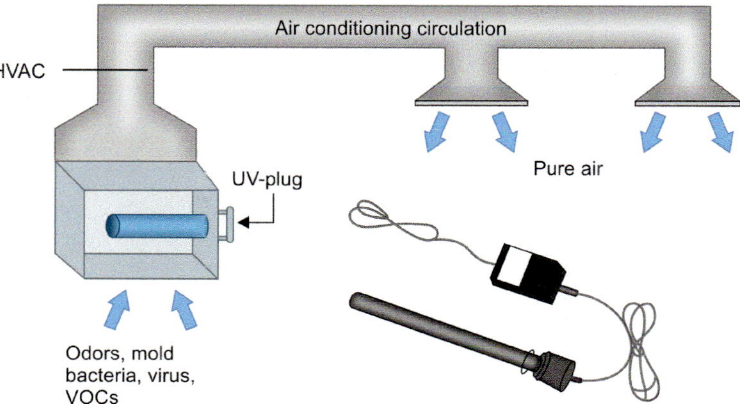

Fig. 23: Ultraviolet germicidal irradiation.

radiation (UV-C) that is harmful to microorganisms. It is effective in destroying the nucleic acids in these organisms so that their DNA is disrupted by the UV radiation, leaving them unable to perform vital cellular functions.[9,12]

HEPA–MD

High efficiency particulate arrestance-Microbial destruction (HEPA-MD) This technology is an innovative system originally developed for space technology. It causes inactivation and destruction of a large spectrum of microorganisms when exposed to the combined action of electrostatic fields and nonthermal plasma. It causes sequential rupturing of the protective membranes and inactivation of the microorganisms. Unmatched one-pass up to 99.999% efficacy on airborne germs (fungi, bacteria, virus and spores).

CONCLUSION

Rapid advancement in the knowledge and therapeutic modalities in different areas such as endoscopy, hepatology, luminal GE, pancreatic biliary diseases and nutritional therapy have made these areas into exclusive sub-branches under GE. Similarly, several sub-branches of GIS have come up recently these include pancreatic biliary surgery, colorectal surgery, liver transplantation, etc. For proper development of patient care, research and training facilities in these areas, it is important to develop a separate center for further development of these subspecialties in GE and GIS.

REFERENCES

1. emedicine.medscape.com
2. www.rah.sa.gov.au
3. www.authorstream.com
4. home.cmcvellore.ac.in
5. www.hospitaldesigntips.com
6. www.imscare.net
7. www.abhiskhospital.com
8. www.creativeoperationtheatre.com
9. www.mitchellewis.com
10. m.bhasinsons.com
11. bariatrictimes.com
12. https://www.rgf.com/rgf-biocontrols/

OTHER REFERENCES

- Harper PR, Shahani AK. Modelling for the planning and management of bed capacities in hospitals. J Opera Res Soc. 2002;53-1:11-8. Available at http://*www.palgravejournals.com/doifinder/10.1057/palgrave/jors/2601278*
- Ninomura P, Rousseau C. Design and construction of hospital and health care facilities. 2006;48. Available at (*www.ashrae.org*).
- Singh CR, Sharma UUV. Design and implementation aspects of operation theatre management module in HMIS; 2012.pp.181-90.
- Gupta SK, Kant S, Chandrashekhar, Sathpathy S. Modern trends in planning of hospitals: Principles and Practice. Jaypee Brothers Medical Publisher Pvt. Ltd; 2005.
- Putsep E. Modern Hospitals, International Planning practices; Critical Care units; Lloyd Lukes Ltd; London; 1979. pp. 354-405.
- BIS; Recommendations for Basic requirements of general hospital ital.ding, IS: 10905 (Part 2); 1984.
- Phillips DA, Sinclair RJ, Schuyler GD. Isolation Room Ventilation Design Case Studies; Available at *www.ashrae.org.*
- Geramizadeh B, Malek-Hosseini SA, Bahador A, Salahi H, Nikeghbalian S, Sharijan M, et al. Post-transplantation Lymphoproliferative Disorder after Liver Transplantation: Report of 5 Cases among more than 550 Liver Transplants in Iran; Available at *www.sid.ir* § Emerging trends in health care. A Journey from Bench to Bedside. Feb 2011. Available at *www.kpmg.com*

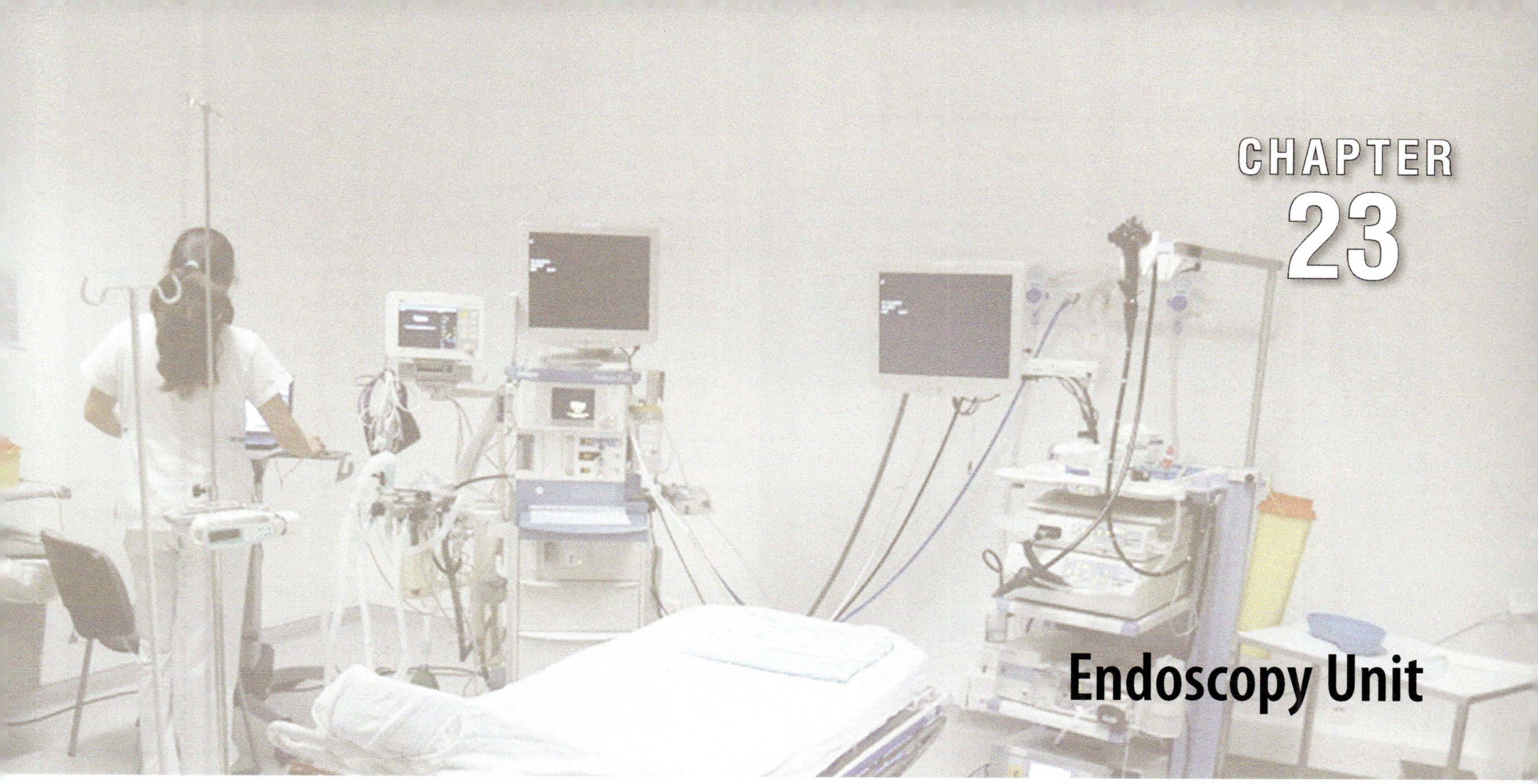

CHAPTER 23

Endoscopy Unit

RY Asangi, Pramod Garg, Aarti Vij, Shakti Kumar Gupta, Sunil Kant, R Chandrashekhar

INTRODUCTION

Endoscopy is a procedure of looking inside the body by inserting endoscope through natural orifice. It started as a diagnostic tool but now has a key role in day-care procedures. Endoscopic unit may be a part of the hospital or a stand-alone unit.

BENEFITS OF ENDOSCOPY

The important benefits of endoscopy are described in Table 1.

EVOLUTION OF ENDOSCOPE (FIGS. 1 TO 3)

The earliest mention of endoscopy and endoscope (attempt to look inside the rectum by use of rectal speculum) has been made by Hippocrates of Greece (460–375 BC). But the modern-day endoscopes began to take shape only after 1800 AD.

Advantages of a single standalone endoscopic facility rather than decentralized endoscopic facilities, are:

- Need for fewer supervisory staff.
- Greater ease in overcoming staff deployment in cases of absenteeism.
- Optimum equipment utilization and no need of duplication of equipment and trained manpower in various departments.

Table 1: Benefits of endoscopy.

To patients	*To staff*	*To hospital*
• Smaller incision • Improved cosmetics • Reduced possibility of infection • Reduced postoperative pain • Reduced blood loss • Return-home quicker	• Improved patient care • Procedures can be quicker • Better view	• Higher bed turnover • Patients go home quicker • Reduced cost (overall)

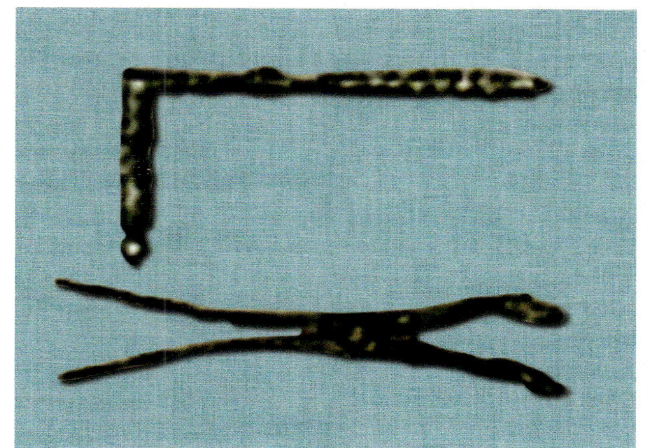

Fig. 1: Evolution of endoscope.

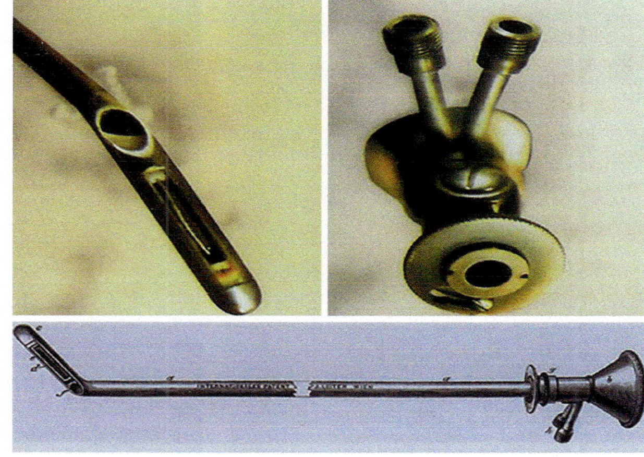

Fig. 2: Nitze cystoscope.

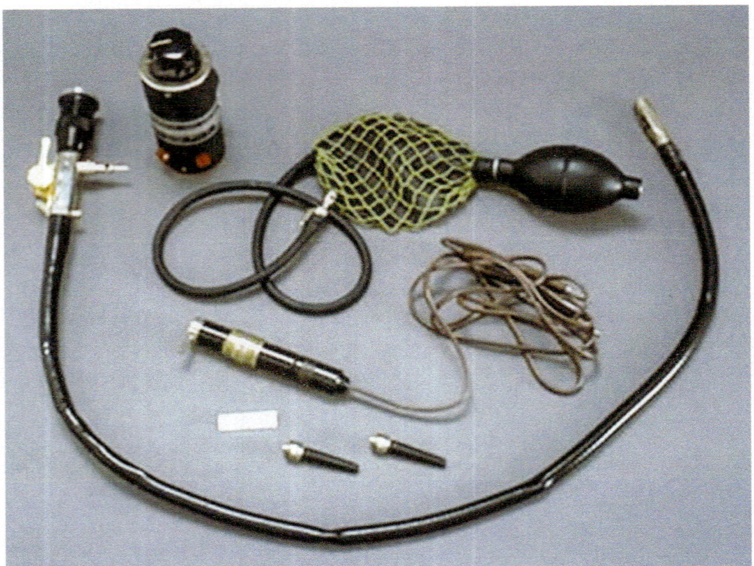

Fig. 3: Hirschowitz fiber gastroscope.

- Smaller capital and power costs.
- Greater flexibility in procedural planning.
- Overall economy.

There could be some disadvantages like:

- The facility cannot be near to all the departments hence there could be difficulties in shifting the patients to the facility in cases of emergency.
- The more is the number of users, more difficult is to schedule the procedures and hence to plan for the optimal utilization of the facility.

OBJECTIVES OF THE FACILITY[1]

- To provide all the departments with possibly specified and limited exceptions, adequate access to endoscopic treatment facilities to the patients.
- To decrease the average length of stay.
- To reduce the workload of OT.
- To pool the equipment resource of the hospital, so as to ensure their economical and effective utilization under adequate managerial and technical supervision.
- To provide for adequate training in the field of endoscopy to postgraduate and undergraduate students and to assist in medical education.
- To utilize the available manpower efficiently and effectively through training in precise endoscopic procedures.
- To provide facilities for in-service training of nursing and ancillary personnel in endoscopy.
- To ensure quality control of the services rendered by the department.

FUNCTION OF THE FACILITY

It will be catering to the comprehensive diagnostic and therapeutic endoscopic needs of the outpatient department (OPD) and inpatient department (IPD) patients.

KEY PLANNING AND DESIGNING PARAMETERS OF THE FACILITY

Location: If within the hospital, should be nearer to the radiology department so that there could be equipment sharing and should have an easy access from OPD. It should also have easy accessibility to emergency and intensive care unit (ICU) due to the frequent need to perform endoscopy in these areas.

Various rooms/spaces of the facility and space criteria: Space projections should include the likelihood for growth in volume and potential expansion of services over 5–8 years, allowing for construction of a facility that can either accommodate growth or expand into adjacent space.[2] The facility is equipment intensive (Figs. 4A and B).[2-4]

Reception/Waiting Area for the Patients

- Should accommodate normal chairs/wheelchairs/stretcher for the patients.
- About 4–5 chairs/procedure room and each chair will require 1.5 m^2 (area) while each wheelchair and stretcher will utilize 2.5 m^2 and 4 m^2 of area respectively.[3] This also should have space to accommodate 1–2 stretchers per procedure room depending on the inpatient load who are recumbent for whom the waiting time should be as less as possible. (These recumbent patients need not wait since they have been already examined and preparation has been done in the wards).
- Should have at least 10 m^2 which will accommodate 3 normal chairs, one wheelchair and one stretcher. Depending on the number of procedure rooms, expected recumbent patient load, the required area may be decided. Apart from minimum of 10 m^2, additional 5 m^2 (2 normal chairs and one wheelchair) will be required for each EGD/colonoscopy, ERCP, gastric (esophageal) motility procedure room; per each digital fluoroscopic, screening: proctoscopy/sigmoidoscopy examination room, and per each gastroenterology laboratory greater than two.[4]

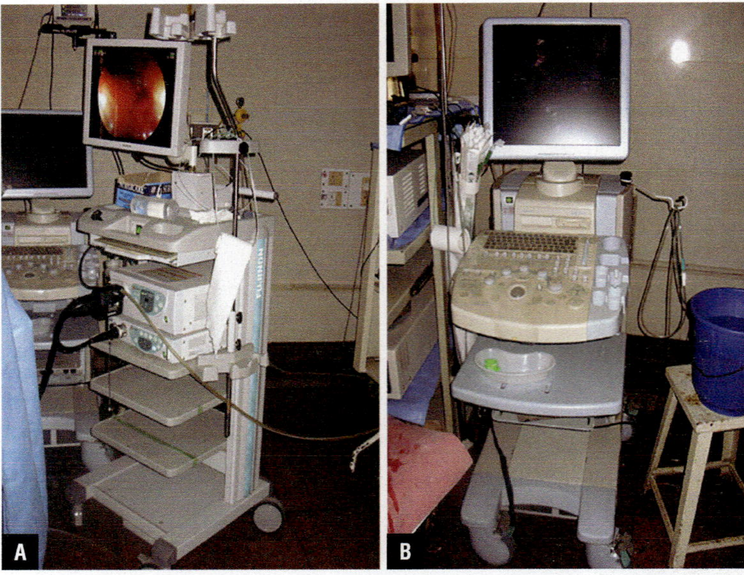

Figs. 4A and B: (A) Endoscopy trolley; (B) Endoscopic ultrasound.

- Waiting room should be connected to the patient entrance corridor and be under visual control of the receptionist.
- Should have public toilet facilities separate for males and females. The number of toilets should include additional one each toilet for the expected routine number of colonoscopy and sigmoidoscopy cases since the preparation (colon lavage) for these procedures is best done in the endoscopy unit itself so as to ensure proper preparation which requires about 3–4 hours.[4]

Appointment Desk and Record Room (Fig. 5)

- This room is necessary where the volume of procedures is high (e.g. tertiary care facilities). Here the scheduling of procedures is done depending on the policies for the efficient utilization of the procedure rooms. The concepts of procedure room unit and weighted value are to be applied here. The patient records are also maintained in this area.
- This should have at least 10 m^2 of area; and, for maintaining of records additional 1 m^2 area per each physician and per each four gastrointestinal assistants. Total requirement may be of 20 m^2 of area.

Examination/Interview Room

This is equal to routine examination room of any clinic where patients will be examined and given appointment for endoscopy.

Dressing Room/Changing Room/Preparation Area

- Patient changes his/her clothes to the hospital attire and waits for the procedure.
- About 1–2 intake beds/stretcher bays per procedure room,[2] each separated from the other by soft partition. It should have lockers for ambulatory patients to keep their clothing and valuables.
- There may be carts instead of beds. After changing to hospital attire, the patient lies over the cart which itself is wheeled into the procedure room and then to the recovery area. These carts should have lockers to keep the belongings of the patients. A monitor is set up in the preparation area for blood pressure and pulse oximetry and this monitor follows the patient into the procedure room. A monitor that attaches to the gurney is best so that only one person instead of two (one for the gurney and one for the monitor stand) can transport the patient into the procedure room and back again. This also makes the procedure safe which avoids shifting the patient to and from the procedure table.

Recovery Room (Fig. 6)

- Patient is monitored here till recovery (normally requires 30 min) and interviewed before giving the discharge.
- There should be 1.5–2 recovery beds per procedure room and each separated from the other by soft partition. Each recovery bed will require 12 m^2 (120 sq ft) of space.
- Each recovery bed should have adjacent access to monitoring capabilities, emergency call systems, pulse oximeter, oxygen and suction outlets and full electronic access to databases and the electronic medical record.
- The recovery area should be easily visible from the nursing station.
- There should be 1 toilet (5 m^2) for every 6 recovery beds.
- In larger facilities, it is often considered desirable to have a three-stage recovery area. The first stage involves intensive supervision, the second stage has changing facilities in more casual surroundings and in the third stage, the patient is fully mobile and can meet the relatives/visitors. Supervision of the patient is vital at each stage. This three-tier approach appears more suitable since complete recovery becomes a vital before the patient can leave the facility.[6]
- These areas also need to have piped oxygen, full monitoring facilities (including pulse oximetry), suction, resuscitation equipment and emergency drugs.

Procedure Room

Room size will vary based on:[7]

- Use of video equipment
- Electrosurgical laser treatment
- Fluoroscopy
- Multiple scope activity
- Multiple observers.

Basic endoscopy with video equipment will require about 40 m^2 sized procedure room[8] and should be preferably rectangular in shape with

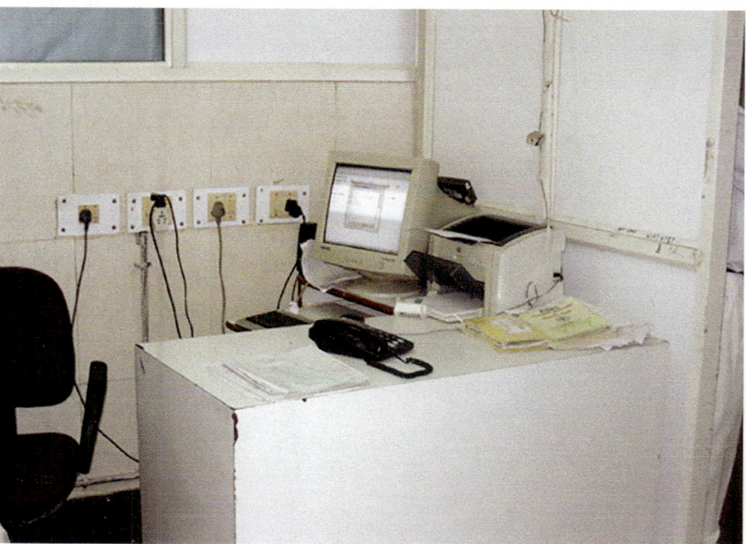

Fig. 5: Appointment desk.

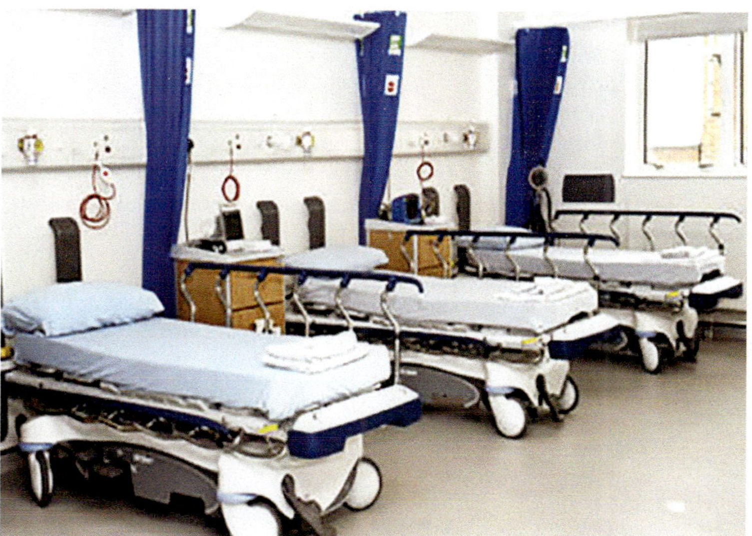

Fig. 6: Recovery room.

the procedure table at the center so that there is access to the procedure table from at least three or even from all four sides. The room size, where possible, can be still larger so as to accommodate flexibility and future developments. The ceiling height should be minimum 3 m. A room of this size will accommodate the endoscopy cart with video monitor will require about 12 m^2 of space, considerable storage for clean linen and supplies. Hampers for soiled linen and a resuscitation cart will require 2 m^2 of space. Procedure rooms should have a minimum of 20 sq of clear floor area and minimum clear width should be 3.6 m. Floor covering should be monolithic, joint free with an integral coved base. The door must be wide enough to accommodate gurney traffic.[5,8,9]

Rooms need central oxygen and suction, ideally ceiling type. There should be typically two monitors on the endo-cart—one for performing the procedure and the other for patient information.

A clinical scrub-up basin shall be provided outside the entrance to the endoscope room.

- *Fluoroscopic examination room*: Fluoroscopic procedures room should be larger than other procedure rooms so as to accommodate C-arm/digital subtraction angiography machine. The fluoroscopy room can also be used to perform the urological procedures if the facility is catering to the urology patients.
- The various other kinds of procedure rooms include:
  - Screening proctoscopy/sigmoidoscopy room—may require about 15 m^2 of area excluding that required for gurney storage.
  - Gastroenterological laboratory (and other routine hematological, biochemical and radiological investigation facilities based on the requirement). For performing gastric analysis and esophageal manometry tests, may require about 30 m^2 of space.[3]

Number of Procedure Rooms Required

Annual procedures per room–Operating days/year × hours of operation/day minutes per procedure/60 minutes.

Considering operating days - 300/year, 8 hours of operation/day and room efficiency factor 80%, (for ERCP, room efficiency factor of 75% will be taken since the resources are often shared with either radiology department or else there will be less back-up for these equipment) the total number of procedure rooms required will be calculated.

Minimum Annual Workload to Generate One Room

The prescribed minimum annual workload to generate one room is given in Table 2.

Store Room

Should have adequate space to store:[2]

- Linen
- *Biological samples containers*: Preparation, storage and transport
- Reprocessing fluids for endoscopes
- Disposables, i.e. personal protective ware, etc.
- Medications; controlled and noncontrolled substances
- Disposables used during the procedure.

Table 2: Minimum annual workload to generate one room.

Procedure	*Average procedural time*	*Utilization rate*	*Annual procedures per room*	*Minimum annual workload to generate a room (30%)*
Flexible sigmoidoscopy	30	80%[1]	3840	1152
EGD	30	80%	3840	1152
Colonoscopy	60	80%	1920	576
ERCP	90	75%	1200	360

Reprocessing/Cleaning-disinfection Room/Workroom for Cleaning Endoscopes (Fig. 7)

This room should have minimum size of 2.4 × 4.2 m, i.e. 10 m^2. Here the endoscopes and accessories are cleaned, disinfected, and dried. The guidewires are also cleaned with soap and water and then sterilized by ETO which will take 3-12 hours. It should have a larger dirty area and a smaller clean area.

The room should have the following:

- Deep, large sinks placed at 750 mm height (lower than the standard 850 mm height) for washing endoscope with foot pedal control for water and countertop (worktop) on either side. There can be separate sinks for washing different types of scopes:
  - ETO
  - Autoclave
  - Automatic reprocessors
  - Suction
  - Air-leak tester
  - Air compressor to provide air to blow the endoscopes.
- Drying cabinets with endoscope-hanging facility. These must be tall enough so that the endoscopes can be hung fully extended within the cabinet.
- There should be facility for filtration of water since the tap water is contaminated.
- The room should have a good temperature control.
- Adequate storage space for boxes of gloves, masks, disinfectant solution and disposable gowns, which provide a better barrier than linen.
- The glutaraldehyde ventilation if same is being utilized
- Staff room
- Office complex (Director office/Nurse Incharge or Chief Endoscopy Assistant room).
- *Janitor closets*: Janitor closet to be used primarily by the housekeeping staff, should include a service sink, shelving for a limited amount of housekeeping supplies, and floor space for housekeeping equipment, such as a vacuum cleaner and/or mop bucket. This may be either specific to the endoscopic facility or else shared between the departments.[4]

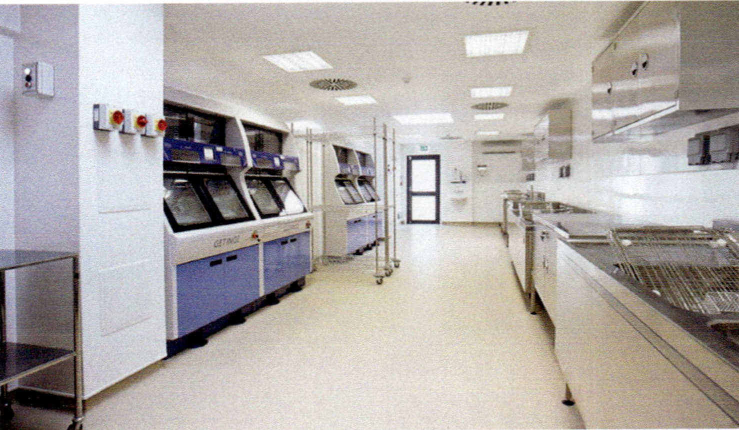

Fig. 7: Reprocessing/cleaning-disinfection room.

Circulation Requirements[4,10,11]

Patient flow within the procedure room is largely dictated by door and equipment location. Large units seeking to separate pre- and postprocedure patients employ separate doors at each end of the room for arrival of alert ambulatory patients and departure of wheeled sedated patients on gurneys. This requires additional space for dual hallways. Similarly, larger rooms for complex or fluoroscopic procedures should have an entry at each end for arrival and departure of staff or equipment during the procedures.

Unique Design Requirements

A suitable database which interfaces with the institutional EMR and several other systems should be used for maintaining the patient records. This should be designed individually or purchased from several vendors as per facility requirements.

Structural Requirements[4,11]

Electrical and plumbing and suction is standard for healthcare facilities. Vacuum capacity may need local boosters or auxiliary units to accommodate the number and spectrum of active rooms in a unit at any one time. Most facilities use standard 'medical' or 'clean' in-wall vacuum suction attached to disposable waste traps in the room. A useful alternative that may reduce supply expenses, room clutter, and nursing tasks, is use of a wet vacuum system which evacuates fluid waste directly into the sewage system. These systems eliminate the need for suction canisters and the infection control issues related to their emptying or disposal. Periodic flushing of lines (1–3 times per week) with a cleaning agent is recommended.

Mechanical System such as Heating, Ventilation and Air-conditioning (Table 3)[11]

- Operating room HVAC systems should be in continuous operation.
- Exhaust systems serving the endoscopy suite should be in continuous operation.
- Air changes may be reduced during nonoperational hours provided room pressurization is maintained.
- Return air systems should be ducted.

Glutaraldehyde Ventilation Strategies

Glutaraldehyde used for sterilization and high-level disinfection of endoscope, is an irritant that can be absorbed by inhalation, by ingestion, and through the skin. It has a strong odor. The Society of Gastroenterology Nurses and Associates, Chicago, have recommended the following strategies for safe and effective handling of glutaraldehyde solutions.

Table 3: Conditions for mechanical ventilation systems.

Inside design conditions	21–24°C dry-bulb temperature 30–50% humidity
Supply air changes/h	8 to 10
Return air	Not permitted
Exhaust air	100%
Room air balance	Negative (–), i.e. exhaust air or return air = (Supply air + 15%)

- About 10 air exchanges per hour
- A room large enough to ensure adequate dilution of vapors.
- Exhaust vents located at the source of glutaraldehyde vapors, i.e. automated reprocessor outlet or a plain tray.
- Additional exhaust vents at floor level (glutaraldehyde vapors are heavier than air and this pulls the vapors down away from the breathing zone).
- Fresh air supply at ceiling across (opposite) from exhaust vents.
- Consideration of outside air intakes, windows, or other openings to prevent re-entry of discharged vapor or exposure to other occupancies, i.e. this air must not be circulated.
- Employing scope cleaning procedures and taking air samples to monitor vapor levels at completion of construction.

Lighting

Procedure room lighting: Room lighting is preferably darkened during the procedure. Indirect perimeter lighting, which could be dimmed, combined with standard 2×4 fluorescents overhead or LED lights, when more light is required, would be ideal.

Special Equipment and their Space Requirements[3,4,11,12]

- *Endoscopy setup, endoscope, light source and image-management systems*: One colonoscope, gastroscope, and sigmoidoscope for every 350 procedures per year; one duodenoscope and EUS scope for each 150 procedures per year; one light source and processor per endoscopic procedure room; and one scope reprocessor for each 1000 procedures per year. Some specialty endoscopes such as pediatric and therapeutic instruments, may be needed to provide complete basic services. The procurement should be such that there should not be any delay in adopting latest technology.[11]
- *Fluoroscopy units, patient gurneys, and databases*: These all take space in the procedure rooms and the setup should be such that all wiring is concealed and not on the floor with impeding dangers of hazards.

Space for storage and drying should also be considered (Figs. 8 and 9).

Functional Layout

It is shown in Figure 10.

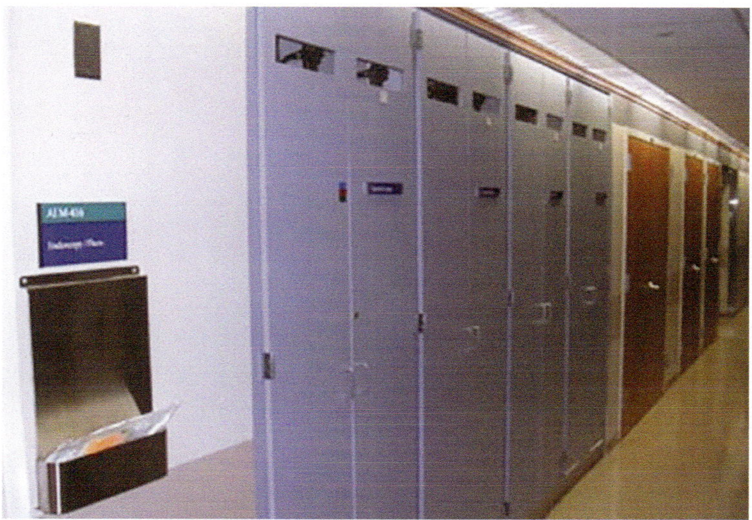

Fig. 8: Storage space.

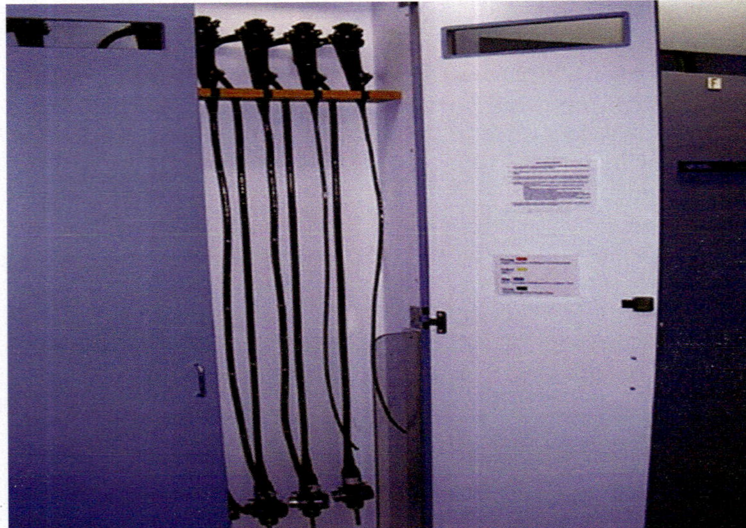

Fig. 9: Drying cabinet.

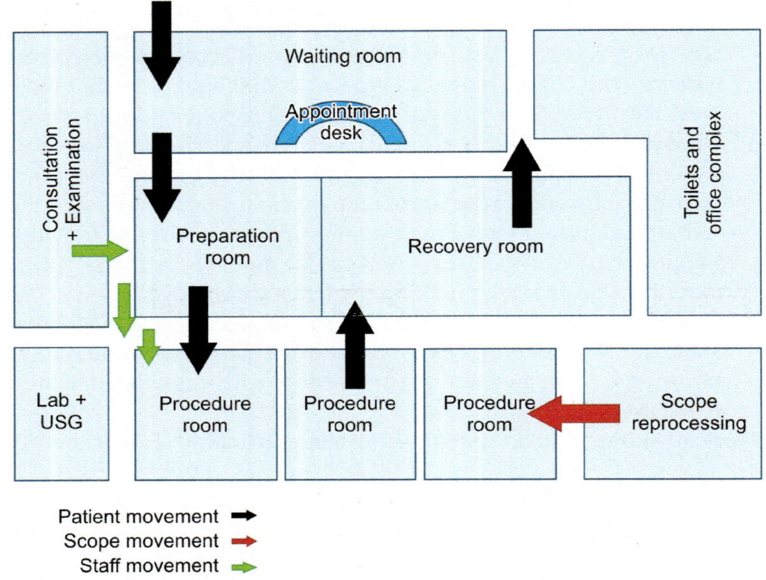

Fig. 10: Functional layout.

CONCLUSION

Endoscopy units may be part of a hospital, where emergency procedures may be performed on ill patients admitted to the hospital; however, most endoscopies are performed on ambulatory patients in the outpatient setting.

The growth in this field has been exponential and has replaced the many of the traditional diagnostic and treatment modalities. The decrease in length of stay and early recovery has resulted in economy to the patient as well as the hospital.

REFERENCES

1. www.rfhha.org
2. https://onlinelibrary.wiley.com/
3. VA Space planning criteria- March 2008, United States Department of Veterans Affairs.
4. www.wbdg.org
5. Guidelines for design and construction of Health care facilities American Institute of Architects.
6. DiMarino AJ, Benjamin SB. Gastrointestinal disease, Chapter 7. The Endoscopy Unit. SLACK Incorporated, 2002. ISBN 978-1-55642-511-0.
7. www.health.wa.gov.au
8. Design Guidelines for Hospitals and Day Procedure Centres by Health Projects International, Victoria, Australia.
9. Minimum Physical Plant Standards For Physician Owned – Single Specialty Ambulatory Endoscopy Treatment Centres, Department of Community Health, Georgia.
10. Brennan, Melissa A. "Appendix A - The Procedure Unit". Handbook of gastroenterologic procedures. Douglas A Drossman, Ian S. Grimm, Nicholas J Shaheen. (4th edn.). Lippincott Williams & Wilkins. 2005. p. 371. ISBN 978-0-7817-5008-0.
11. https://onlinelibrary.wiley.com/journal/14781239
12. HVAC design manual, United States Department of Veteran Affairs.

OTHER REFERENCES

- Anthony J DiMarino, Stanley B Benjamin. Gastrointestinal disease, chapter 7. The Endoscopy Unit. SLACK Incorporated, 2002. ISBN 978-1-55642-511-0.
- American Society for Gastrointestinal Endoscopy. ASGE guidelines for clinical application. Establishment of gastrointestinal endoscopy areas. American Society for Gastrointestinal Endoscopy. Gastrointest Endosc. 1999;50(6):910–2. PMID 10644189. doi:10.1016/s0016-5107(99)70193-8.

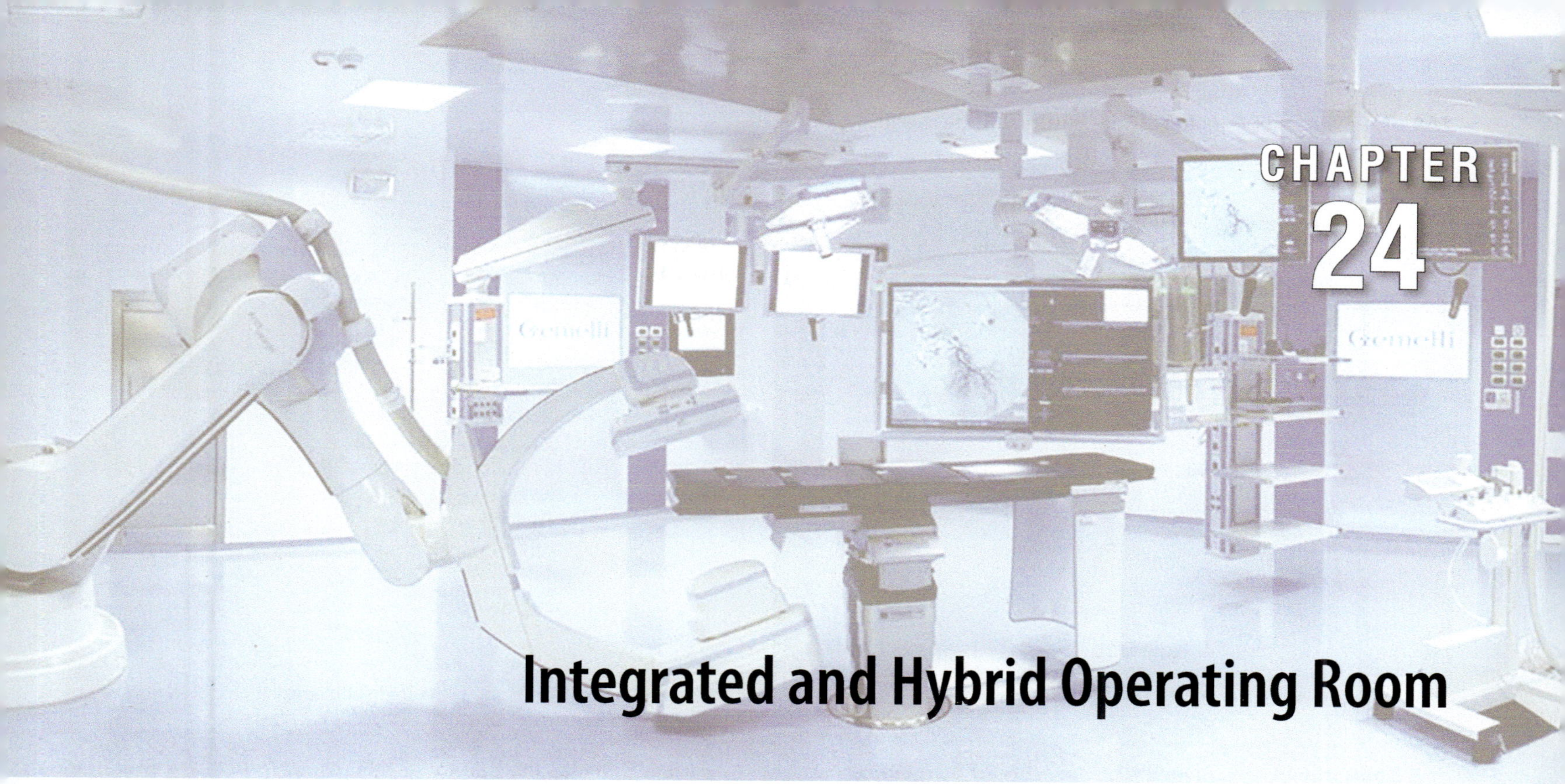

CHAPTER 24

Integrated and Hybrid Operating Room

Vijaydeep Siddharth, Shakti Kumar Gupta, Sunil Kant, R Chandrashekhar

INTRODUCTION

Operation Theater (OT) has been defined as that specialized facility of the hospital where lifesaving methods under strict aseptic conditions in a controlled environment by especially trained personnel to promote healing and cure with maximum safety, comfort and economy.[1]

The hybrid operating room (OR) can be defined as the combination of imaging system and operating table installed in an OT room, e.g. use of an angiography imaging system and operating table in an OT or use of an operating table in angiography room.[2] Conventionally, integration in OT, usually refers to systems integration, which means functionally connecting the OT environment, i.e. OT equipment, OT light, audio and video devices, hospital information system, OT environment, etc.

HYBRID OPERATING ROOM

The word 'hybrid' originally refers to the result of interbreeding between plants or animals of two different species, it has been more recently used to mean combination of two different methods to achieve higher performance as in case of hybrid cars. The hybrid OR can be defined as the combination of imaging system and operating table installed in an operating theater (OT) room, e.g. use of an angiography imaging system and operation table in an OT or use of an operating table in angiography room.[1]

The hybrid operating theater is a combined operating theater and interventional radiology suite. It can function as either a conventional operating theater, or as a radiology facility, but crucially allows intra- and postoperative on-table imaging and intervention, and overcomes many of the limitations of standard facilities (Figs. 1 and 2).[2]

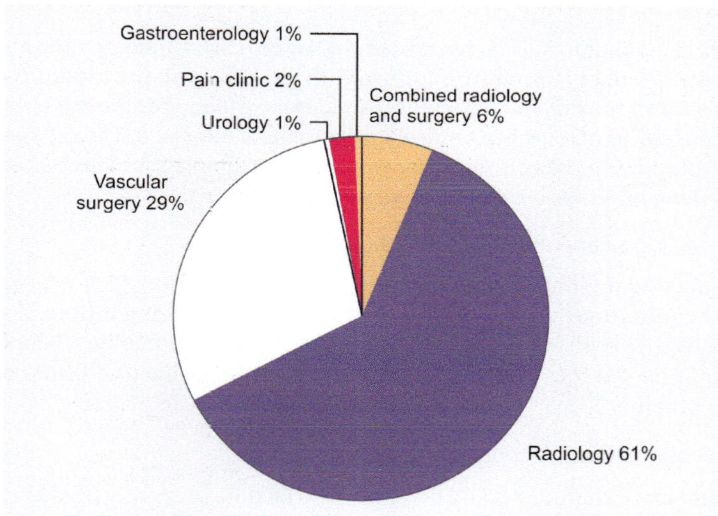

Fig. 1: A graph to demonstrate multispecialty usage of the hybrid operating theater.

Planning and Design Considerations

Planning Premises[3-5]

Compliance with Statutory and Other Requirements

The building should comply with all the statutory and other legal requirements of the country, e.g. building laws and regulations, Environment Protection Act, etc.

Infection Control

Infection control teams should be consulted from the outset and should remain integral planning team members throughout. In a

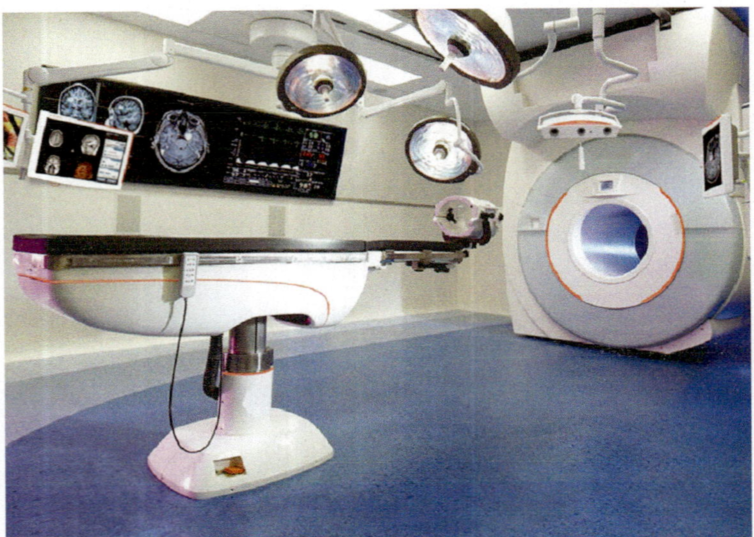

Fig. 2: Duke University Medical Center's hybrid operating room.

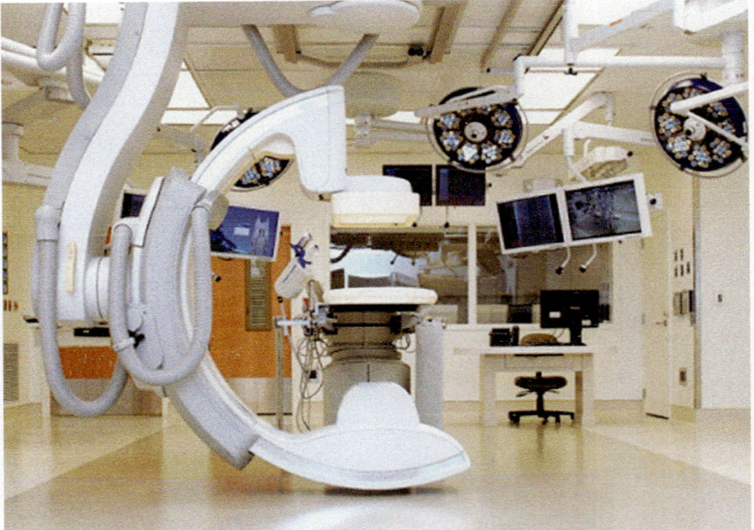

Fig. 3: The hybrid room—planning and designing challenges.

new-built project, this means that they should be members of the team that develop project report from its inception.[4,6] OR managers have special responsibilities to reduce the chances that patients will develop an infection during their stay.

Sterilization Practices

Sterilization practices, as recommended by the CDC, Atlanta, Infection Control Society should be followed to prevent any postoperative infection or any hospital-acquired infection. Strategy pertaining to the reprocessing of reusable surgical instruments is that local reprocessing should be the exception rather than the norm and that automated washing methods are preferred to manual cleaning.

Protecting a Patient's Privacy and Dignity

Protecting the dignity of a patient is a critical function. This is even more important when the patient is unconscious, being induced or recovering from an anesthetic. A number of measures can be taken to minimize the invasion of privacy, including the design and fitting of the building.[4]

Environmental Impact/Sustainable Design

Operating departments and other surgical facilities annually produce a large amount of waste. Much of this is categorized as biomedical waste and should be treated in an appropriate manner as a legal requirement.[4]

Design Considerations

Designers should aim to create an environment that is conducive to making patients feel at ease and giving them confidence, thus aiding the healing process.[4]

Child-friendly Environment

In view of the small number of children that require certain types of surgery, separate facilities for them will be hard to justify. However, provision should be made for children and young people to be segregated away from adult patients, and to have their parents or attendants with them, for example, in the anesthetic room and recovery unit.[4]

Artificial Lighting

The positioning of artificial lighting should be carefully considered. Ceiling-mounted lighting should not be installed directly overhead in patient areas in the operating department. If ceiling-mounted fittings are used, they should be two-directional so that they can be adjusted to prevent unwanted glare. The lighting should be dimmable without flicker. Artificial lighting should include clinical task lighting in anesthetic rooms and at each bed space in the recovery unit.[4]

Way Finding

Each operating theater, anesthetic room and recovery bed space should be clearly numbered to avoid any possible confusion.[4]

Planning and Designing Challenges (Fig. 3)[4,5]

The following are the challenges associated with designing of hybrid OR:

- Multiple stakeholders
- Space
- Multivendor coordination
- Lighting
- Monitors and video switching
- Parking X-ray system
- Other OR requirement
- X-ray dose
- Cost.

Location

The main inpatient operating theater department should be located centrally within an acute hospital. Ideally, all the operating theaters in the hospital should be in one location with one recovery unit. Figures 4 and 5 describe the physical and functional relationship of OR with different hospital services.[4]

Layout

Clustering of Accommodation[4,5]

The following accommodation should be an integral cluster with access through a single, and secure entrance:

- Communications base
- Operating theaters (with associated ancillary accommodation (Figs. 4 and 5)

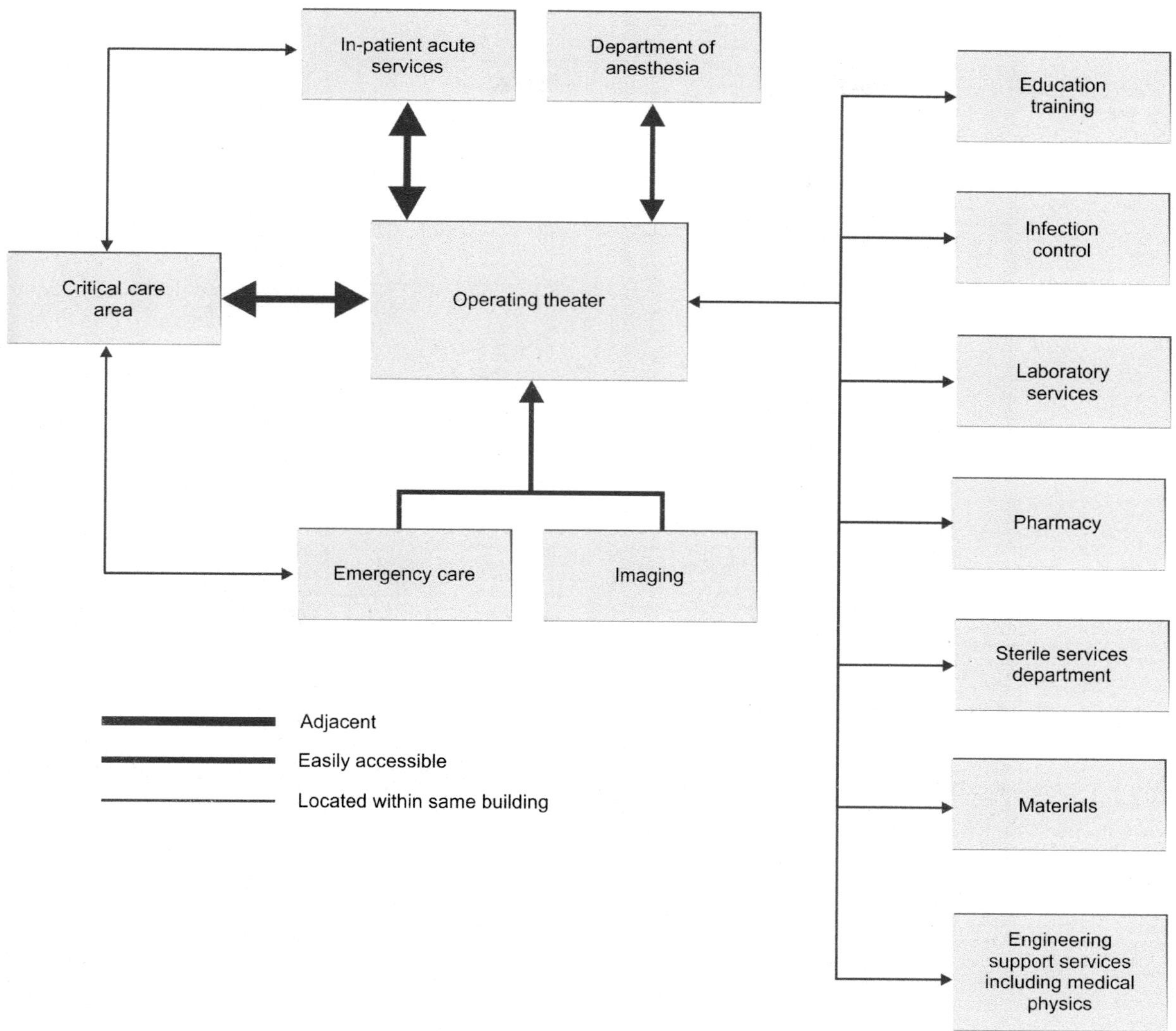

Fig. 4: Operating theaters—relationships with on-site services.

- Anesthetic rooms (equal to total number of operating theaters)
- Patient support facilities
- Recovery unit (with associated ancillary accommodation)
- Staff support facilities
- Storage areas (equipment, bulk store)
- Disposal areas (dirty utility, disposal hold, housekeeping room).

The following accommodation could be integral or collocated with access through the main entrance or with its own secure entrance adjacent to the operating department

- Education and training facilities
- Anesthetic department
- Administrative offices.

Main Entrance: Control of Access

Patients and staff, all will use the main entrance to the department. Supplies and disposals will also be carried through this entrance. Security measures are needed to prevent unauthorized access to the theater suite. It is recommended that visitor access to the suite be controlled by use of an entry-phone or intercom system with closed circuit television (CCTV), information technology (IT) enabled access control system (biometrics), linked to the communications base located in the entrance lobby. The security measures chosen should not inhibit emergency escape from the department in case of fire.[4,5]

The entrance should be wide enough for the transfer of patients on beds, supplies, equipment and waste. An electronic automatic double-door, with a minimum clear opening width of 1.5 m, will be suitable. Care should also be taken with the design of corridors in the department to ensure they are of sufficient width to allow the passage of two beds and accompanying equipment and staff simultaneously.[4,5]

The main entrance lobby should contain the communications base, the administrative office, the porters' base and a waiting room for visitors to the department (including members of a patient's family, if appropriate). The entrance area, including the communications base, should be warm, welcoming and well lit. The furnishings and fittings should be easy to clean, disinfect and maintain.[4,5]

Communications Base

The communications base should be located so that it commands a clear, unobstructed view of the main entrance, the waiting room, the entrance to the main theater corridor and the access route to the staff support areas. Entry to the operating theater suite should be controlled from this base.[4,5]

The operating department receptionist will be located here. All general information for the operating department, including fax and computer links, arrives at the base. The design of the reception desk should allow access for people with disabilities. The countertop

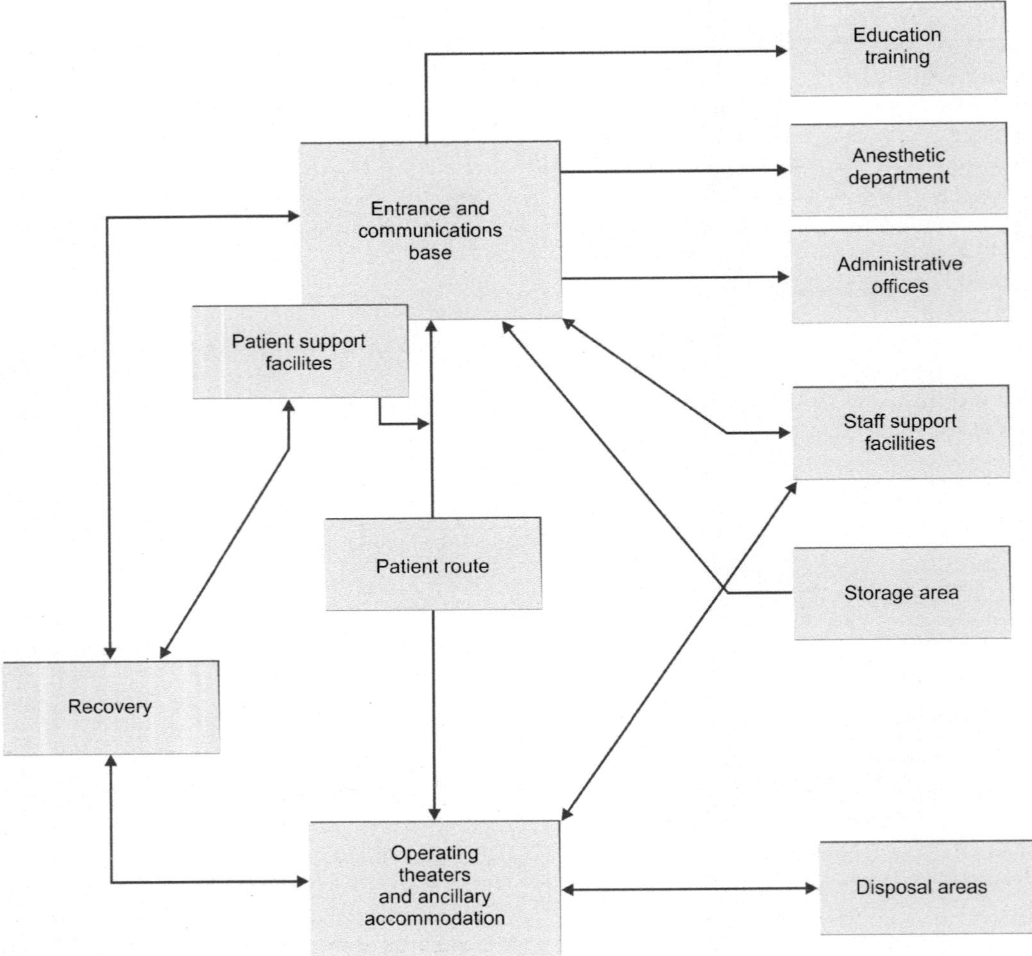

Fig. 5: Functional relationships.

should have two heights—one for wheelchair users and children, and the other for adults at standing height for occasional writing. The communications base should have access to an integral administrative office. A wall-mounted staff emergency call lamp should be located at the communications base to alert the reception staff of a problem within the department.[4,5]

Administration Office

This office should be large enough to accommodate two people along with computer and telecommunications equipment. A small safe where patients' valuables can be held when necessary, should be located in the office. A wall-mounted staff emergency call lamp should be located here.[4,5]

Dedicated Operating Department Porters' Base

Locating their base in the main reception area will give them easy access to the main hospital and to the operating theater corridors. A wall-mounted staff emergency call lamp should be located in the base.[4,5]

Waiting Room

A waiting room should be provided for patient's attendants. The room should be large enough to accommodate up to six people at one time. The décor should be selected carefully to reflect a calm and relaxing atmosphere. People may wish to wait here for long periods of time, so comfortable seating is essential. Daylight should be provided if possible; however, soft lighting is an acceptable alternative. Beverage-making facilities should be available at all times. A television should be provided. An en-suite wheelchair-accessible water closet (WC) is essential.[4,5]

Admissions Lounge

Patients arriving in the admission lounge will have had their preoperative assessment and examination previously, and should only require minimal physical assessment on the day of surgery. A small number of consulting/changing rooms with an examination couch will be required, with entry from the waiting area and a separate exit to the operating suite. All doors will require secure access and should be wheelchair accessible. The patients' clothing will be transferred to their inpatient accommodation via the recovery unit.[4,5]

Each consulting/changing room will require a clinical hand wash basin with non-touch taps, desk with computer facilities, and internal telephone. Shower and bathing facilities will not be required. Patients will walk, or be taken by wheelchair, to the anesthetic room/operating theater.[4,5]

Interview Room

A small room should be designated for this purpose. In common with the general waiting room, this room should portray an area of calm and comfort. A telephone should be provided. An en-suite wheelchair-accessible WC should be included.[4,5]

Anesthetic Room

The minimum space required in each anesthetic room is 15 m. One set of double doors should open from the corridor into the anesthetic room, with another set opening into the operating theater. Installing either sliding or automatic doors is a project option. Each set of doors should be wide enough to admit the patient and associated equipment, minimum clear opening width of 1.5 m, and close quietly. Obscured vision panels are required in both sets of doors. An electronic "in-use" sign should be located outside the main corridor entrance into each anesthetic room. Automatic doors should be capable of standing in the open position.[4,5]

A lockable controlled drugs cupboard is required in each room, as well as a lockable refrigerated drugs store. Storage units should not impinge on the working area required during the preparation and induction of the patient. An adjustable ceiling-mounted examination lamp is required for clinical procedures. All work surfaces should be lit. It should be possible to vary the level of general lighting. A radio-controlled clock with sweep seconds hand should be located on the wall above the patient's feet. A clinical handwash basin with no-touch taps should be provided. It should be sited at the end of the room opposite to the normal position of the patient's head.[4,5]

Every anesthetic room should be child-friendly. Patients of all ages report less anxiety, and are physiologically more stable, if they can listen to music preoperatively. A music system should be provided for this purpose. Anesthetic rooms can be sited at right-angles to the operating theaters. A wall-mounted push-button staff emergency call with reset and indicator lamp should be located in each anesthetic room, linked to the recovery unit and the staff rest area. A telephone capable of ring or silent/light indication should be appropriately located.[4,5]

Scrub and Gowning Room

One scrub and gowning room can be shared between two operating theaters, both of which should be directly accessible with sufficient space for a minimum of six people and space between to prevent contamination (minimum size–16 m^2).[4,5]

No-touch taps, scrub solution and nail brush dispensers are required. Sensor taps are now available that allow a sufficient run-on time for the scrub protocol to be completed. The recommended length of the tap is 250 mm with a sensing range of 200–250 mm, and the run-on time should be a minimum of 20 seconds. Wall-mounted paper towel holders should also be provided. The height of the scrub sink should be 1000 mm to the rim from floor level. The rim of the scrub sink should not have an internal lip as this is a control of infection concern, as contaminated water during the scrub procedure drains from the elbows back into the sink.[4,5]

Preparation Room (Fig. 6)

The preparation room should provide storage and suitable work surfaces for the laying-up of instrument trolleys. A room of area between 12 m^2 and 15 m^2 will be required to open packs and maintain a sterile field. There will be a minimum of two members of staff (scrub and circulating personnel) in this area. The work surfaces should be of sufficient height to store 870 mm high trolleys beneath in order to conserve space.[4,5]

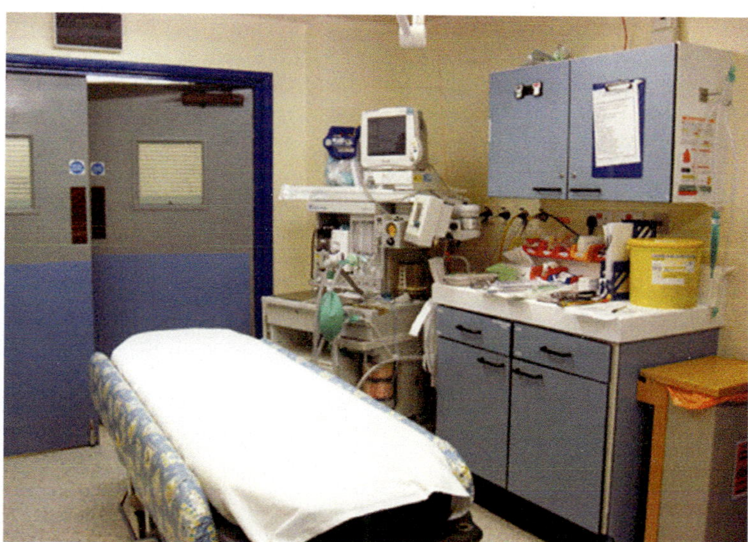

Fig. 6: Preparation room.

Music System

Many patients undergo surgery without the need for a general anesthetic and remain awake during the procedure. They may wish to listen to music. Some staff also find music beneficial in an operating theater. Integral music systems are the preferred option, as there are potential hazards from cross-infection and interference with the existing power supply from standalone systems.[4,5]

Doors within the Operating Suite

Doors through which beds or trolleys will pass should be wide enough to allow easy passage with attachments, including sterile drapes. It should be possible for them to stand in the open position. All doors should be fitted with vision panels capable of being obscured. If manual swing doors are used, care should be taken to prevent the possibility of repetitive strain injuries. A number of the doors to the operating suite will be lead-lined for X-ray purposes and can weigh more than 100 kg per leaf. The use of a cam action door closer is recommended. These units are adjustable, allowing minimum opening resistance.[4,5]

Ceilings

In operating theaters, a minimum clear height of 3 m between the finished floor level and ceiling is required to allow unrestricted adjustment of the operating luminaries and other ceiling-mounted equipment. The building structure should be capable of supporting the loads generated when the ceiling-mounted medical supply unit is installed. Powered medical supply units allow unrestricted access to the patient and enable staff of all heights to operate them easily.[4,5]

Lighting

Care should be taken when selecting the correct operating lamp, especially when the theater has ultraclean ventilation, to maintain minimal interference with downward airflow patterns.[4,5]

Swab-count Board

A dry-wipe wall-mounted marker board at least 800 mm × 600 mm is required. This board should be fixed permanently to the theater wall and be at a height and in a position that facilitates access and visibility during the procedures. Weighing scales should be located on a trolley positioned in close proximity to the marker board. Two "kick about" stainless steel bowl stands should also be available.[4,5]

Theater Warning Light

Each theater requires a light warning when laser surgery and X-rays are being undertaken. The lights should be located in the corridor above the theater doors. Windows should be fixed. This is essential to assure the clean environment, and assist the air-conditioning by maintaining positive/negative airflow.[4,5]

Theater Ventilation

Theater ventilation is a crucial issue at the initial design stage. The planning team should agree the principle for delivering a clean environment to each theater.[4,5]

Finishes and Fittings

If laser surgery is being undertaken in the operating theater, it is important that there are no reflective surfaces or bright door handles.[4,5]

Exit Bay

An exit bay may be shared between two theaters; single exit bay may be more efficient because it will be less likely to get blocked with storage equipment. The area should be sufficient for the parking of two beds with additional circulating space. Walls should be protected against heavy traffic in this area. Ideally, the controls for lighting, heating and medical gas isolation valves should be located in each dedicated exit bay. The bay may contain a local equipment store.[4,5]

Reporting Room

A small room is required for surgeons to record each completed operative procedure. The room should be located close to the operating theaters and can be shared by several people at one time. A desk with a computer terminal and external telephone is required.[4,5]

Imaging Equipment Bay

An open bay should be provided close to the operating theaters for the storage of imaging equipment and protective lead aprons. A suitable socket-outlet should be provided for charging the imaging equipment. The bay should be 5 m^2 to accommodate one mobile imaging machine and a single ultrasound unit. A larger storage area (8 m^2) is required if mobile image intensifiers are used. It is a statutory requirement that the regulations pertaining to the use of ionizing radiations are complied with.[4,5]

Emergency Trolley

One emergency trolley with defibrillator should be sited within easy access of all operating theaters. In addition, space will be required for a fiberoptic bronchoscope light source trolley for emergency use. Both pieces of equipment should be located within a recess of the theater main corridor. A second cardiac arrest trolley should be sited within the recovery unit.[4,5]

Theater Dirty Utility Room

It is common to provide an individual dirty utility with every theater. As a project option, a dirty utility can be provided for every two or four theaters. Size of dirty utility shared between four theaters, is 18 $m^2 \times 2$.[4,5]

The room should be large enough to enable cleaning of theater equipment, and disposal of the contents of bedpans, urine bottles, vomit bowls, washbowls, etc. A disposal unit consisting of sink and hopper with concealed cistern should be provided. Mechanical extract ventilation and hand washing facilities should be provided. The dirty utility may also be used for urine testing. This should be zoned separately within the room.[4,5]

Disposal Hold

Bagged refuse, clinical waste, soiled linen and materials for recycling are held here safely and securely while awaiting collection. This lockable room should be accessible from the hospital. Full "sharps" containers from the anesthetic rooms, operating theaters and recovery unit will also be stored in the disposal hold. Other distribution trolleys will be stored in the hold while awaiting collection by the CSSD. These trolleys can be extremely large (1.5 m × 0.75 m). When planning the size of the hold, the approximate number of trolleys to be stored following an operating session and frequency of collection should be taken into consideration.[4,5]

Storage Areas

- Bulk store
- Clinical equipment store
- Linen store
- Blood storage refrigerator
- Satellite pharmacy.

Recovery Unit

Staff will need 360° access to a patient; therefore, an island solution is required in each bed space. The main overhead lighting should be dimmable. A wall-mounted clock with a sweep seconds hand is required, visible from all bed spaces. Every bed space should be separated by lead-lined solid partitions with a lead-lined curtain at the foot end of each bed space. Four of the 16 recovery spaces should be single cubicles.[4,5]

Consideration should be given to the use of hoists in the recovery unit. For maximum flexibility, a hoist in every bed space is the ideal solution for new facilities or a major refurbishment. A clinical handwash basin with no-touch taps is required. Each bed space should be provided with:[4,5]

- About 12 socket-outlets, six to be located on either side of the bed, which may be from IPS circuits
- About 1 medical air outlet
- About 1 oxygen outlet
- About 2 vacuum outlets
- Adjustable examination luminaire
- Push-button staff emergency call linked to an emergency call repeat lamp in the communications base and each theater
- Flat-screen monitor with recording system for patient records.

The recovery room should be mechanically ventilated with low-level extraction, since exhaled anesthetic gases pollute the air. Patient scavenging masks are impractical.

The recovery unit requires a dedicated communications base. It should be closed in a partition of wired fireproof double-glazed glass, from which all bed spaces are visible to reduce noise levels. A minimum of three telephone lines plus data access, computer facilities also required. Some units have a large, raised central station, enclosed by partition walls.[4,5]

Recovery Unit Clean Utility Room

The clean utility provides storage for clean disposable items and equipment. It may also accommodate lockable controlled drugs cupboard; drugs refrigerator; and warm blanket storage facility. Shelf space is needed for items of equipment, such as infusion pumps, ventilator accessories, monitoring equipment and suction apparatus. Electrical socket outlets are required for charging equipment. One anesthetic machine and a cardiac arrest trolley with defibrillator should also be located here.[4,5]

Recovery Unit Dirty Utility Room

The equipment in this dirty utility room will be identical to that described in the theater dirty utility room with the exception that if disposable bedpans, vomit bowls, etc. are used, a macerator is required. If reusable bedpans, etc. are used, a steam-washer/sterilizer is necessary.[1-5]

Equipment Service Room

The space provided should be sufficient to park and maneuver equipment and to accommodate a work-bench with integral lockable cupboards, preferably in a self-contained room or space. A clinical hand wash basin should also be provided. The supply to socket-outlets should be provided via a dedicated residual current-protected circuit device, and emergency power isolation buttons should be installed at the work-bench and adjacent to the room entrance. Medical gas outlets supplying oxygen, medical air and vacuum should be provided.[4,5]

Housekeeping

Adequate space should be provided for the convenient local storage of cleaning equipment and materials. A lockable storeroom is required for the storage of cleaning supplies and domestic equipment. Extract ventilation will be required. Floor space is required for a minimum of two floor-scrubbing machines. Dry storage space is required for clean disposable cloths, new mop heads and additional unused bags. Facilities should be provided in this space for filling and emptying cleaning equipment via a bucket sink with hot and cold running water. A sluice hopper for the disposal of soiled mop water, a sink for washing soiled mop buckets and a drainer should be provided, along with a hand wash basin.[4,5]

Switch Room

Accessible directly from a circulation area but not generally on a route used by beds or trolleys, providing clear and safe access for the maintenance staff (accessible space may be part of the circulation area); sited away from water services; and lockable.[4,5]

Uninterruptible Power Supply Room

A room of at least 9 m^2 is required to house the back-up system for essential electrical supply to the operating theaters and recovery area. The room should be well-ventilated, and should be kept locked at all times, with access only for permitted staff. The room may also be used to house the data hub for the operating department. Monitoring of all the UPS status is advised. This may be connected to the communications base monitoring equipment where appropriate and/or the theater control panel.[4,5]

Integrated Operating Room: Specific Design Considerations[4-9]

A high-quality, magnified video, projected on a flat-screen monitor, gives the surgeon an optimal view of the surgical field. As minimally invasive surgery continues to grow and robotic surgery and telemedicine become more common, integrated operating room (I-ORs) will become an industry standard.

Design Features for Integrated Operating Room (Fig. 7)

In addition to housing a large amount of technology, I-ORs impact workflow. Factors that must be considered in the design of an I-OR, include:[9]

- Total room size
- Best placement of lights, cameras, monitors, and the AV equipment
- Ceiling structures
- Articulating display arms, and

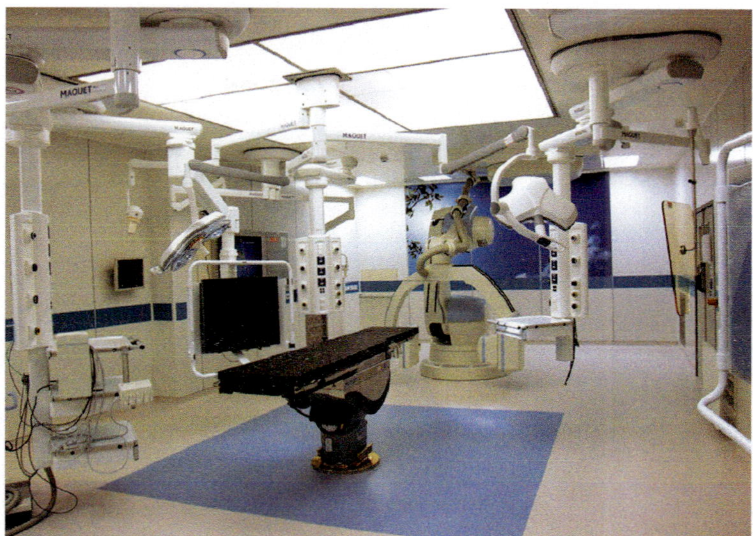

Fig. 7: Integrated operation theater.

- Equipment booms should be designed to allow for added capabilities in the future.

Additional space is required for the infrastructure and electronics to support the components outside the I-OR.

Room Size

In general, I-ORs are 15% larger than their nonintegrated counterparts. It is true that some equipment is smaller than ever before, but an in-room control or documentation center adds about 10 m^2 to an OR. With integrated technology, a general I-OR is about 60 m^2, a cardiovascular I-OR or one that includes robotics may approach 80 m^2 or more, and I-OR with in-room imaging equipment requires at least 100 m^2.[4-9]

Media Bridge

Media bridge provides OR team's an easy access to power supplies, manifold supplies, communication technologies and data transfers customized or moved as per the requirement for different surgical procedures (Figs. 8A to D).

Technology Room

The I-OR support hardware has invaded the telecommunications closet. This closet is now a 10′ × 15′ walk-in technology room that houses teleconferencing and A/V equipment, blade-server computers in racks, fiberoptic network electronics, and fiberoptic cables to the work area.

The I-OR's video-integration technology is often housed in a 3′ × 3′ × 6′ rack. In addition, there may be three or more additional computers to support picture archiving and communication system (PACS), hospital information data, electronic medical records, and/or care plan documentation.[9]

Hybrid Operation Room: Specific Design Considerations

Location[4,5]

The following things should be considered while deciding on the location of hybrid OR:[8]

- Relative ease of access to/from emergency department, radiology department, intensive care unit, inpatient beds, etc.
- Proximity to blood bank, labs, pharmacy, etc.

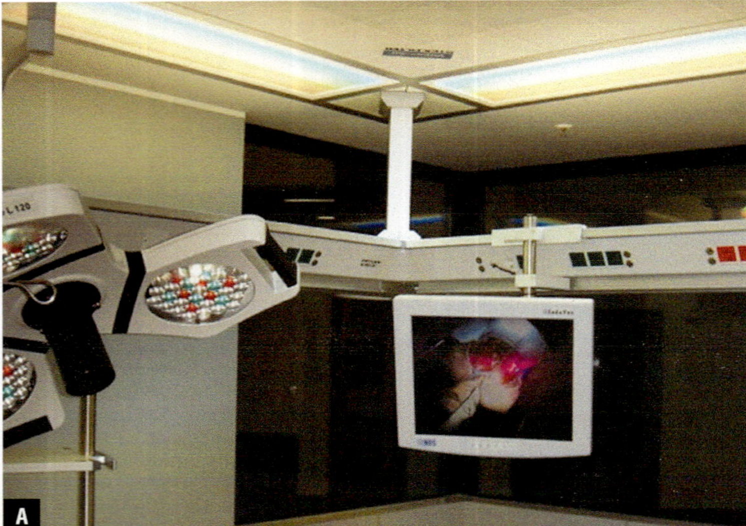
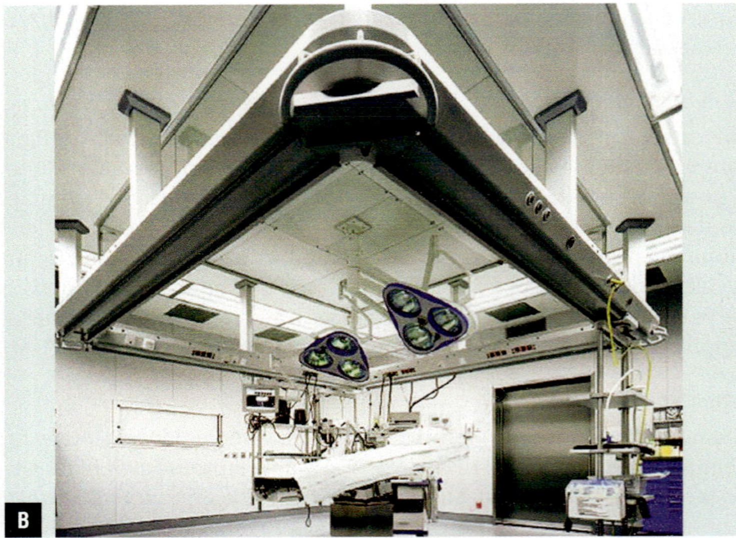
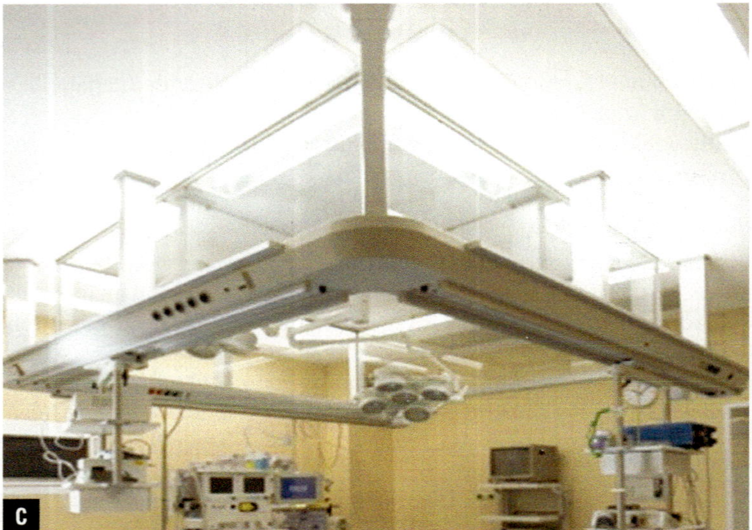
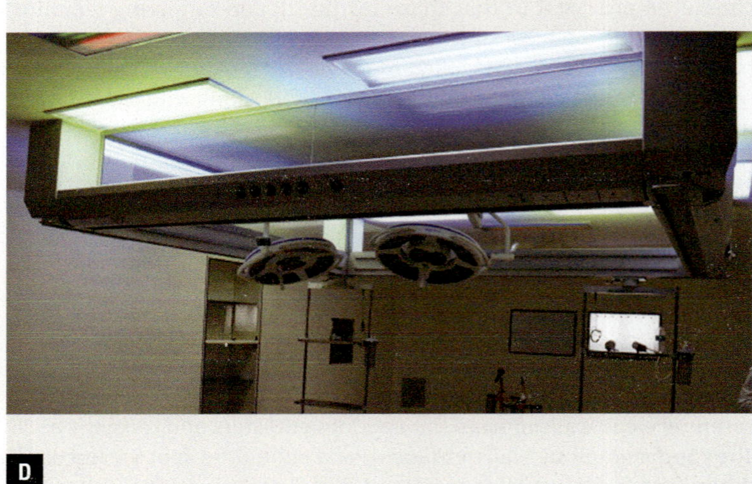

Figs. 8A to D: Media bridge of an integrated operating room.

- Materials support
  - Supply restock support
  - Standardized inventory
  - Mobile or stationery storage.
- Flow management
  - Ease of patient entry/exit
  - Away from heavy traffic areas for sterility reasons
  - Adequate electrical service to support new imaging equipment.

Size of the Hybrid Operating Room (Figs. 9 and 10)[8-11]

The OR should ideally be between 60 m^2 and 100 m^2 with a minimum clear area of 40–50 m^2. Efficient functioning hybrid ORs require between 100 m^2 and 120 m^2 for both the operating theater and control area.

Floor to ceiling height should be at minimum 3 m to accommodate floor- or ceiling-mounted C-arms capable of rotational angiography for volume-rendering 3D CT-like images achieved with advanced biplane imaging systems, usually hybrid operating theater has a procedure room of 80 m^2, equipment room of 10 m^2 and control room of 12 m^2.

Storage room: Space for storage for the special procedure-related equipment, such as stents, wires, balloons and stent grafts should be available. Size of storage room should be approximately 20–50 m^2.

Radiation Protection[9,12-14]

The equipment in interventional/hybrid surgeries can emit radiation. Positioning closer to the patient will lead to less scatter and radiation exposure for OR personnel, while improving image quality most standard ORs have lead-covering 0.5 mm, which is not sufficient for the radiation dose generated by a fixed unit. Lead-lined walls in the range of 2–3 mm for the fixed units may be needed. In addition, ceiling-mounted transparent shields are available for optimal scatter protection of the operator's upper body and face. Moreover, the newer portable C-arm units are less restricted as to the energy they can deliver, compared to fixed systems. This implies an increasing imaging quality, but the boost setting on these units delivers radiation doses with intense scattered radiation.

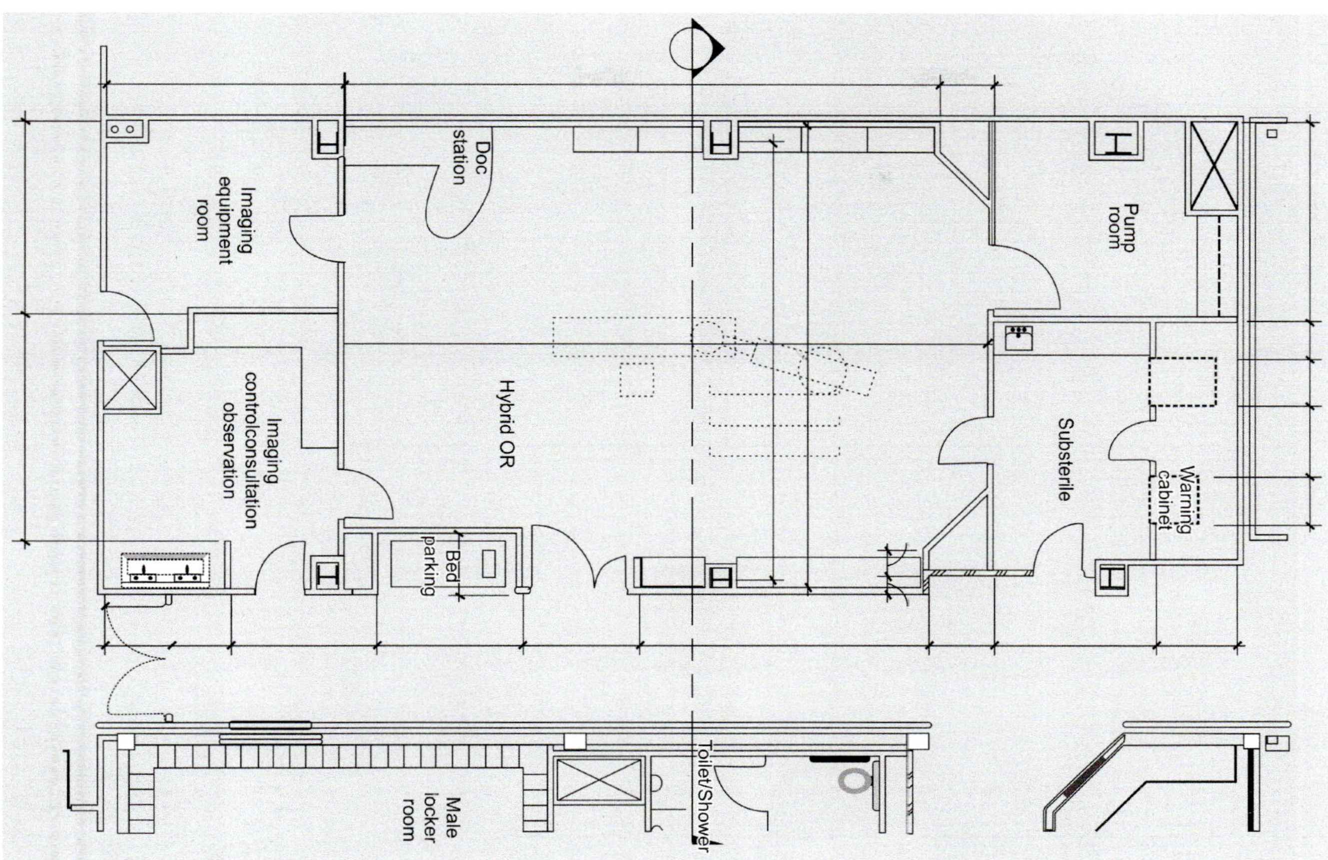

Fig. 9: Hybrid operating room layout.

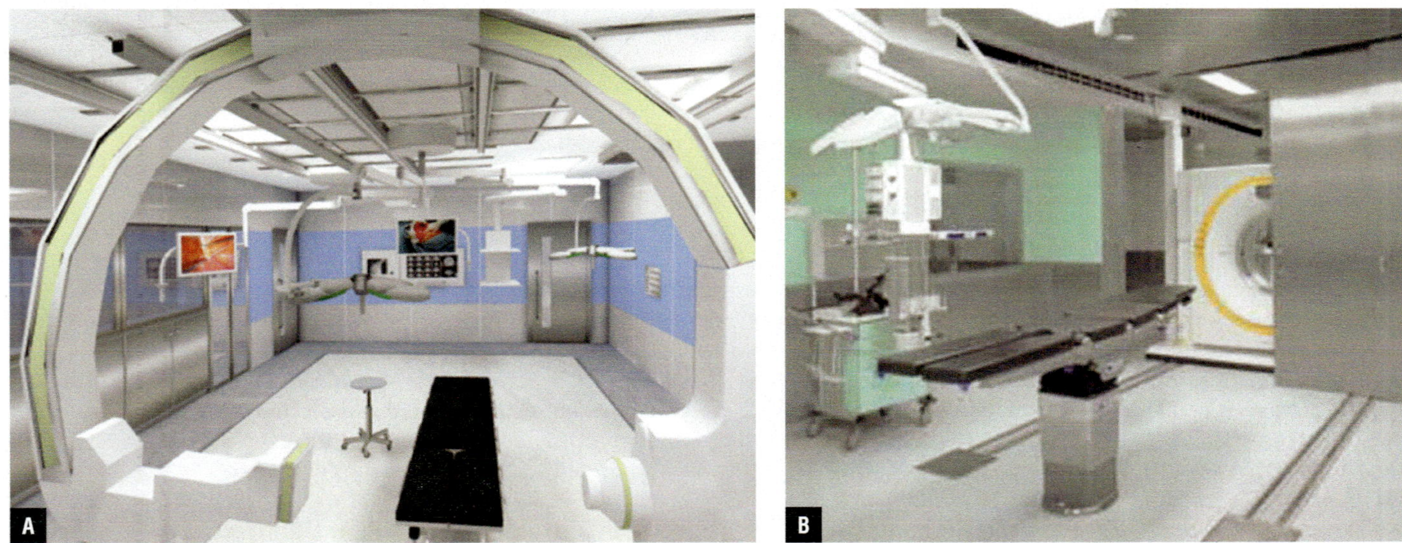

Figs. 10A and B: Fully magnetic resonance technology (MRT) compatible operating table.

BARN OPERATING ROOM (FIGS. 11 TO 13)

The Barn concept provides a single space for many operating stations. Each station within the larger space has its own air-handling system (laminar flow), duct work, lighting, controls, and shares preparation and cleaning facilities. This arrangement allows some team members, such as anesthetic and radiology staff to move between cases, supervise staff and be easily on-hand if problems arise. This concept may be considered as part of overall service planning and in the development of a facility model. It will need to address the number of work areas and the procedures to be undertaken.[7,15-17]

The theater walls, by Modular Multilevel Converter Modular Systems, are modular stainless-steel panels with built-in equipment that can be replaced when it becomes obsolete and membrane control panels are easy to clean.

Each operating table has a 3.2 m × 3.2 m glass-sided canopy (Fig. 12) which delivers clean air in a laminar flow, a streamlined current

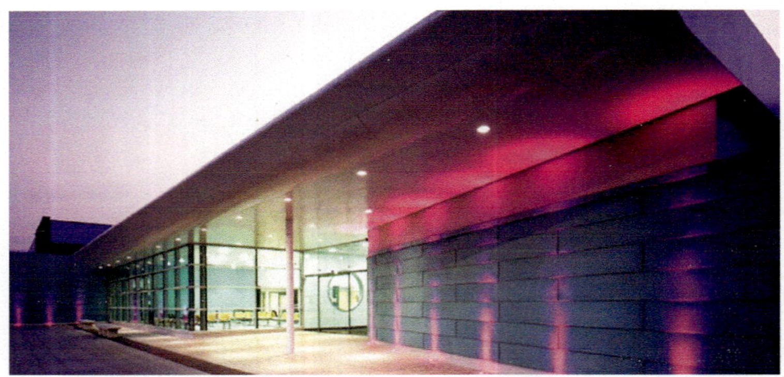

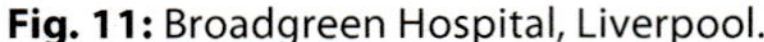

Fig. 11: Broadgreen Hospital, Liverpool.

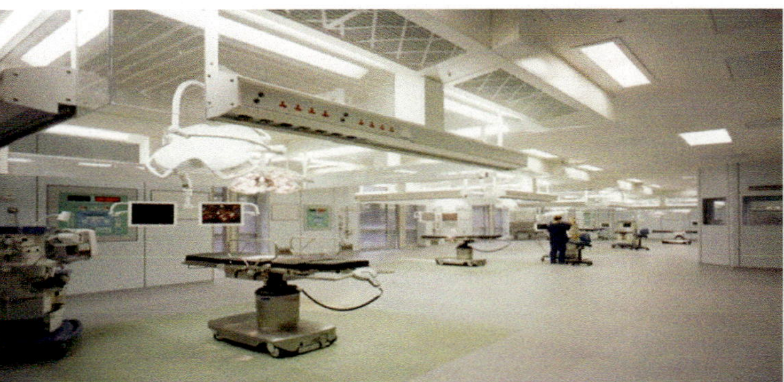

Fig. 12: Barn operating theaters, Broadgreen Hospital, Liverpool.

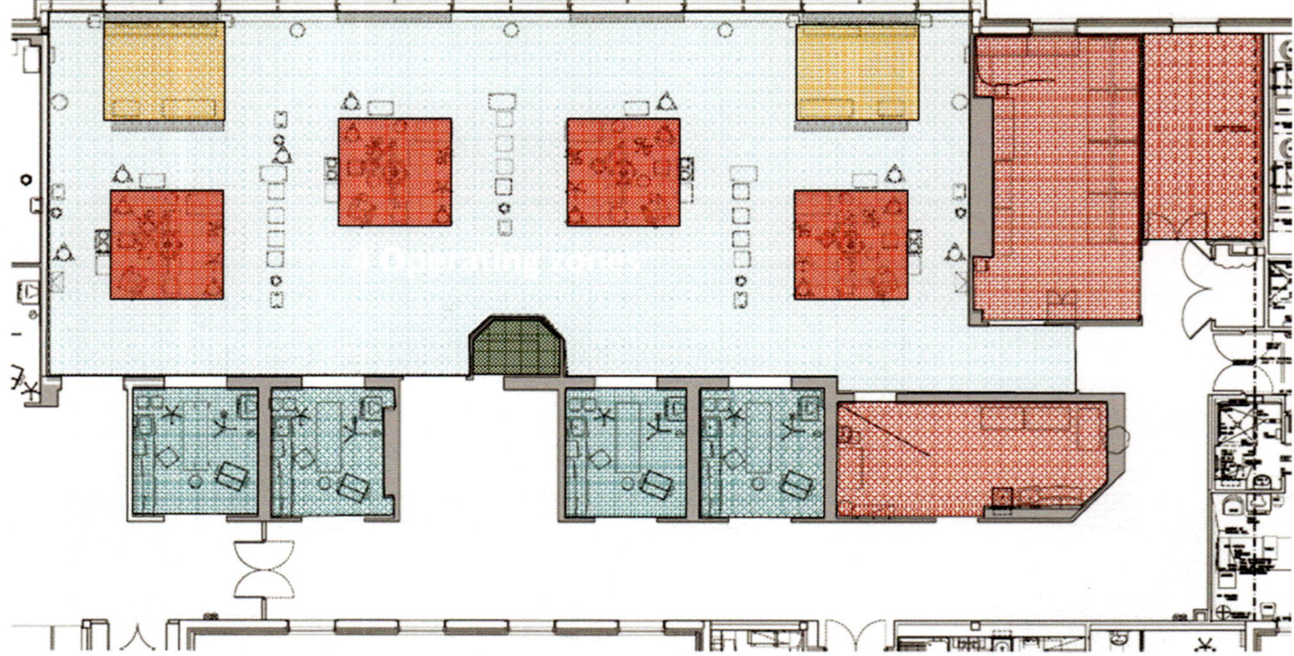

Fig. 13: Barn operating theater layout, Broadgreen Hospital, Liverpool.

with no turbulence producing a positive pressure around the table compared to the rest of the room. Extract grilles in the ceiling between the tables draw dirty air away to be recycled. The theater, in turn, has a higher pressure than adjoining rooms which is maintained by weighted dampers in grilles (Fig. 13) and doors that only open under a given pressure. All doors are sliding doors to minimize air disturbance.

Infections do not travel on their own volition but require a carrier particle of at least 0.5 microns diameter. HEPA filters, or high-performance paper-based filters, mounted in the canopy, remove all particles larger than 0.3 microns diameter. The extracted air is prefiltered to remove lint and any larger contaminants picked up in the theater before being recycled (Figs. 11 to 13).

SUPPORT FACILITIES: GENERAL AND SPECIFIC FUNCTIONAL AND DESIGN REQUIREMENTS[4,5,13]

Staff Accommodation

There are five main categories of staff facilities, all of which should be designated clearly as nonclinical areas:

- Rest facilities
- Changing rooms and associated facilities
- Office accommodation
- Facilities for education and training
- Storage.

Rest facilities and changing rooms should be located within the operating department. Ways of preventing access to staff areas other than by authorized staff, should be implemented.[4]

Rest Facilities

A rest room is required where staff can relax and take beverages and snacks. The room should have windows with a pleasant outlook, be comfortably furnished and have a telephone. The room should have direct access to the beverage bay and should be located close to the operating theaters. A dining table and chairs should be provided to enable staff to eat and drink in comfort. An appropriate number of male and female WCs should be located within the rest and recreation facilities as well as in the staff changing rooms. WCs, including provision for disabled people, should be located at strategic points throughout the department as well as in the staff changing rooms. Each WC will require a hand-wash basin with no- touch taps and a WC with a no-touch flush valve. Extract ventilation should be provided.[4]

Beverage Bay

Facilities are required for the safe handling of food, including the preparation of beverages and light snacks, for washing and storing crockery and cutlery, for storing a limited quantity of dry goods, and for the refrigerated storage of milk, etc. A hand wash basin should be provided. Drinking water should be supplied.[4]

Changing Rooms and Associated Facilities

Changing facilities should be located close to the operating theaters to minimize the movement of staff in their theater clothing. Provision should be made for separate male and female changing facilities. The sanitary and shower facilities should be provided in self-contained, full-height rooms to provide maximum privacy. Separate male and female staff WCs should be provided in association with other facilities for staff. A WC should also be provided that is accessible for disabled people.[4]

Office Accommodation

Some office accommodation will be required within the department. Where space is at a premium, it is suggested that a number of offices are located adjacent to, rather than within, the operating department. Planners should consider including, as an alternative to more offices, one small informal room that is comfortably furnished and can be used for interviewing staff and visitors, and one larger interview/meeting room that could be utilized by members of staff when required. Where possible, every office should have a window and natural ventilation, and should be equipped with a computer terminal with access to full IT services and internal and external telephones.[4]

Education and Training Facilities

Staff should be given every opportunity to use any quiet times to undertake prearranged or spontaneous personal or group learning. Facilities should include a seminar room and library along with access to a large multifunctional education and training room. Where appropriate, these facilities may be shared with the anesthetic department. All staff will need access to IT facilities.[4]

Additional Office Space/Audit Office

Anesthetic departments increasingly take on a teaching role and accommodate students and trainees. Additional office accommodation will be required for these and other staff who may not be permanent members of the team but may still spend substantial period of time in the department.[4]

On-call Facilities

Anesthetist on-call facilities are required within the department. Facilities should include a bed, en suite shower/WC, clothes storage, a hand wash basin, a desk and chair, and a computer with connection to IT services. This space should be linked into the staff communication system.[4]

OTHER DESIGN CONSIDERATIONS

Communications

Provision of effective communication system is essential for the efficient management of the operating department.

Telephones

In the waiting area, where public telephones are provided, at least one should be mounted at a height suitable for wheelchair users and the handset fitted with an inductive coupler to assist people using a hearing aid. Where telephones are provided for reception use, in theaters, anesthetic room and recovery, consideration should be given to hands-free systems.[4,5]

Patient-to-staff and Staff-to-staff Call Systems

Patient-to-staff call systems should be provided in all spaces where patients may be left alone temporarily, such as recovery, admissions lounge or patient WCs. Staff-to-staff call systems should be provided in all spaces where staff consult, examine and treat patients. It is preferable that these systems work on the principle of flashing lights rather than ringtones.[4,5]

Noise and Sound Attenuation

Sound transmission can be reduced by use of sound-reducing partitions and doors. The use of soft floor coverings and acoustic treatment to walls and ceilings will improve sound absorption in a space. Sound absorbers, for examples acoustic ceilings or walls, are able to absorb a varying percentages of the sound hitting the surface and improve speech intelligibility by reducing the spread of airborne sound in the room.[4,5]

Finishes

Finishes should be robust enough to withstand accidental impact, and additional protection should be provided at likely points of contact. Wall protection is recommended in all corridor and heavy traffic areas, plus storage rooms and bays. Cleaning regimes should be considered when materials are selected.[4,5]

Color

Colors of surfaces in spaces occupied by patients should not adversely affect the color rendering of light sources. It should be possible to clearly define and easily identify changes to a patient's skin tone and color. Décor should be light and attractive.[4,5]

Floors

Floors should be able to withstand harsh treatment, including: the rolling loads of heavy mobile equipment; frequent spillages with subsequent "mopping-up"; and regular hard cleaning.[4]

The floor finish should be properly anchored to the underlying surface, and carpets are not acceptable anywhere in the operating department. Vinyl, linoleum or rubber are examples of slip-resistant flooring and should have welded joints. The flooring should be at least 2 mm thick. In theaters with ultraclean ventilations, the floor area enclosed by the hood should be marked with lines or a contrasting colored area of flooring. In all theaters, floor markings can be used to indicate where specific equipment should be located for different procedures within the operating theater.[4,5]

Walls Paneling

Careful selection of materials as it can limit the costs and time needed to prepare the OT room for surgery. The following are the different paneling options available (Figs. 14 to 18):

- Stainless steel
- Glass
- High pressure laminates
- Mineral acrylic solid materials.

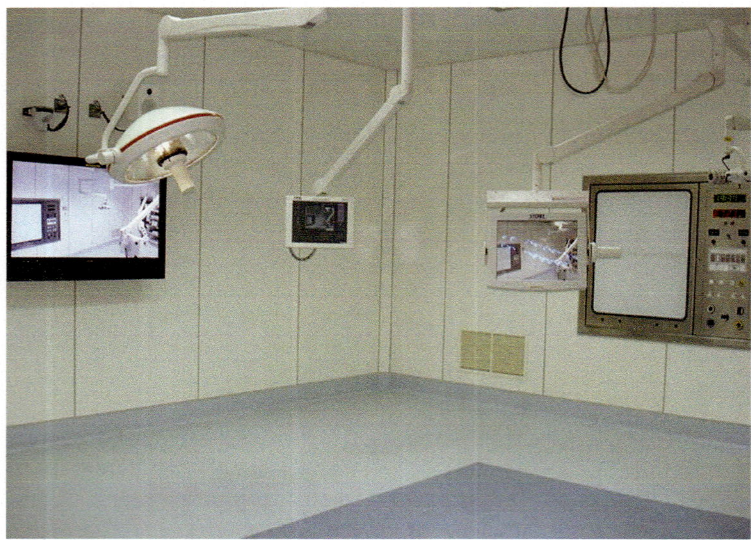

Fig. 14: Galvanized steel paneling.

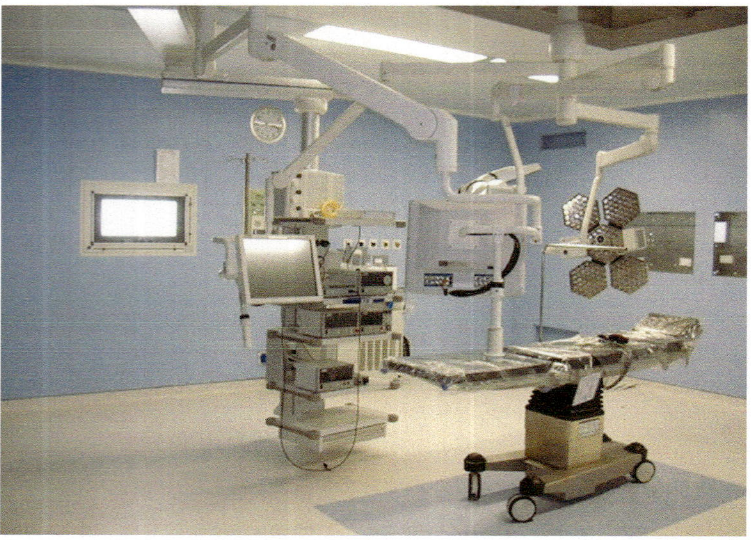

Fig. 15: Stainless steel paneling.

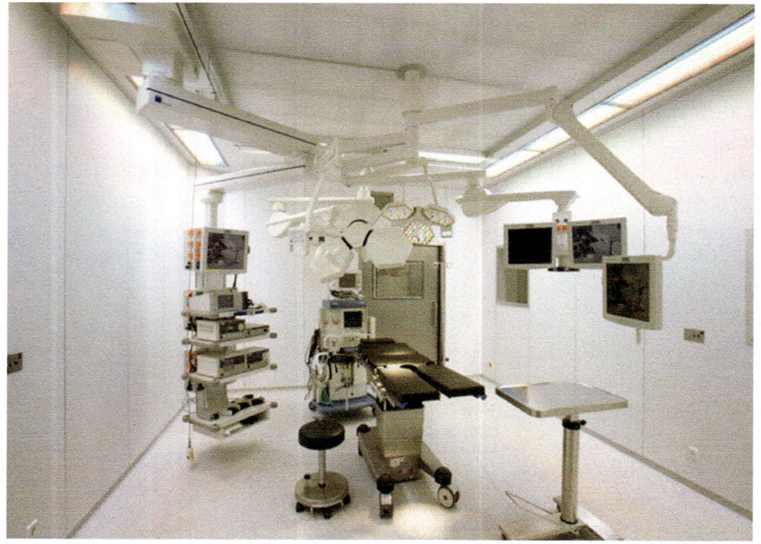

Fig. 16: High-pressure laminate.

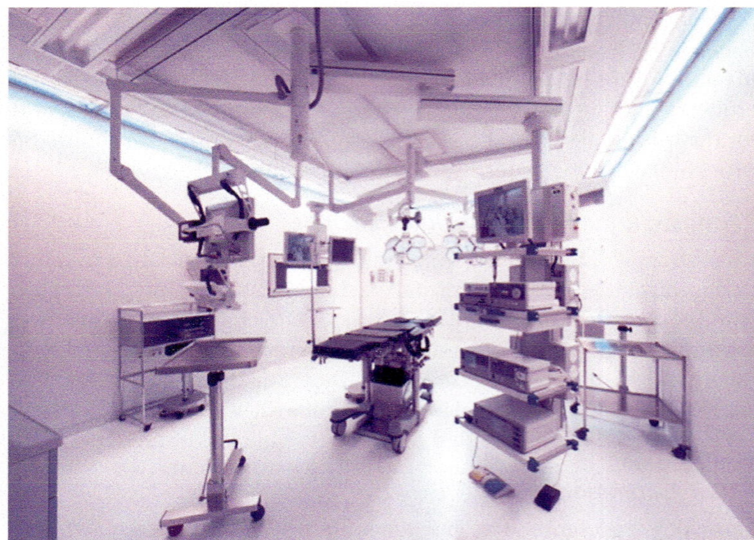

Fig. 17: Thermoplastic panel.

Stainless Steel

Stainless steel is a ferrous alloy containing at least 10.5% of chromium. The use of other alloy elements such as nickel, molybdenum, copper, titanium, as well as nonmetals, especially carbon or nitrogen, results in stronger structures and can improve such qualities as flexibility and durability. Stainless steel, due to its parameters, compares favorably with other materials in both technical and economical aspects. It also has additional high aesthetic value and is environmentally friendly.[18]

Glass

Glass has become very in-demand in hospitals due to its high safety and hygienic qualities as well as interesting design. Custom design graphics make the hospital environment more patients friendly.[18]

High Pressure Laminates

High pressure laminates (HPL) are also known as plastic laminates. HPL consists of several layers of paper impregnated with resin and pressed under heat and high pressure between embossing steel plates, to produce a homogeneous board. The core papers give it the resilience necessary for further processing. The decor paper soaked with melamine resin, one of the hardest resins, and the transparent overlay form an indestructible surface and facilitates that inexhaustible design versatility which at the same time is unique to this product.[18]

Solid Mineral Surface

Mineral-acrylic surfaces are hygienic due to their non-porous structure, so they resist bacteria, mold, and moisture from penetrating the surface. As a result, the solid surfaces are appreciated in medical facilities.[18]

Ceilings

The ceiling in the operating theater should also be able to withstand an occasional wash and have completely sealed finish to maintain microbiological standards. If access hatches are required, they should be of the sealable type. The choice of ceiling construction and finish should reflect the necessary compromise between sound control and the control of infection.[4]

Doors and Door Frames

Materials used for doors and frames should be able to withstand frequent impact from mobile equipment. All double-swing doors should incorporate clear glass vision panels; however, privacy, safety and other considerations may require that panels can be obscured. Automatic door openers can be provided to aid the movement of patients through the area.[4]

Windows

The following issues require consideration:
- Daylight and natural ventilation
- Insulation against noise
- User comfort
- Energy conservation
- Prevention of glare
- Provision of a visual link with the outside world.

Windows should be completely weather-tight, with the correct thermal performance so as not to affect microbiological standards and to prevent airflow pattern distortion and condensation. All windows should be at least double-glazed as a minimum, to provide thermal and sound insulation. Where required, blinds should be installed between the glass that can provide "black-out", which is essential for ultrasound examinations and other imaging procedures. It may be necessary to provide triple glazing to allow the blinds to be maintained. The windows should be easily accessible for cleaning, disinfection and maintenance.[4,5]

Clinical Hand Wash Basins

The basins should be placed in a prominent position to remind the staff of the importance of hand washing. All basins should have curved sides with no plugs, have no overflows, and be fitted with infrared no-touch taps, which should not be placed over the waste outlet. Mixer taps should be used, as very hot or very cold water discourages handwashing. There should be sufficient space around the basin to wall-mount alcohol gel, liquid soap, hand disinfectant and paper towels.[19]

Shelving and Storage

The tops of cupboards should be fitted to ceiling height or should have sloping tops to prevent the accumulation of dust. Monitors should be fitted at a height where they can be cleaned easily. Items should not be stored on the floor. Paper towel wall dispensers are required. Sharps boxes should be wall mounted.[19,20]

Work Surfaces and Bins

All work surfaces should be smooth and easily washable, coved to the wall, and preferably unjointed with integral sink. Joints should be sealed. The surface covering should be hard-wearing and should not damage easily. Edges should be rounded. Damaged work surfaces should be replaced rather than repaired. Foot-operated bins are essential.[4,5]

SCHEDULE OF ACCOMMODATION

The scheduling of accommodation for hospital areas is described in Table 1. The line diagram of hybrid operating unit is shown in Figure 18.

Table 1: Schedule of accommodation.

Area	*Space*
Reception	10 m^2
Operating room	40 m^2 (60 m^2 for integrated OT and 80–120 m^2 for hybrid OT)
Anesthetic room	15 m^2
Scrub and gowning room	10 m^2
Preparation room	15 m^2
Support areas	
Theater dirty utility room	10 m^2
Anesthesia store	15 m^2
Equipment store	20 m^2
Sterile store area	15 m^2
Nonsterile item store	15 m^2
Linen bay	3 m^2
Image equipment bay	8 m^2
Uninterrupted power supply room	9 m^2
Disposal room	10 m^2
Minimum clear ceiling height	3 m (4 m for hybrid OT)
Door width	1.6 m
Other areas	
Changing area	15 m^2
OT-incharge room	9 m^2
Staff lounge	30 m^2
Nursing incharge room	9 m^2
Circulation area	35%

(OT: operation theater)

CONCLUSION

Careful planning and professional expertise is a key factor for every hybrid room project. Before planning a hybrid OR, a clear vision for the utilization should be established. Today's ORs require concepts that address the requirements and needs of different surgical specialties and procedures. Workflow efficiency is a key success factor for the hospital and the surgical program. Minimal turnover times and optimal processes throughout the entire surgical workflow and the actual surgical procedure, are required. Therefore, a hybrid OR should ideally be integrated into an existing OR suite. All aspects and steps starting with patient transfer from the ward to anesthesia and OR preparation are important. Additional aspects for planning are material supply processes, i.e. of materials necessary for the procedure, and postoperative intensive care surveillance and treatment.[21-23]

Layout and design should be ergonomic- and workflow-driven. For the hybrid OR, with the addition of an angiography system to the room, it becomes even more important, because this often involves nonstandard installations, or nonstandard functionality, or nonstandard products. During the entire planning and implementation process, clear, frequent and comprehensive communication of all parties involved, is vital.[21]

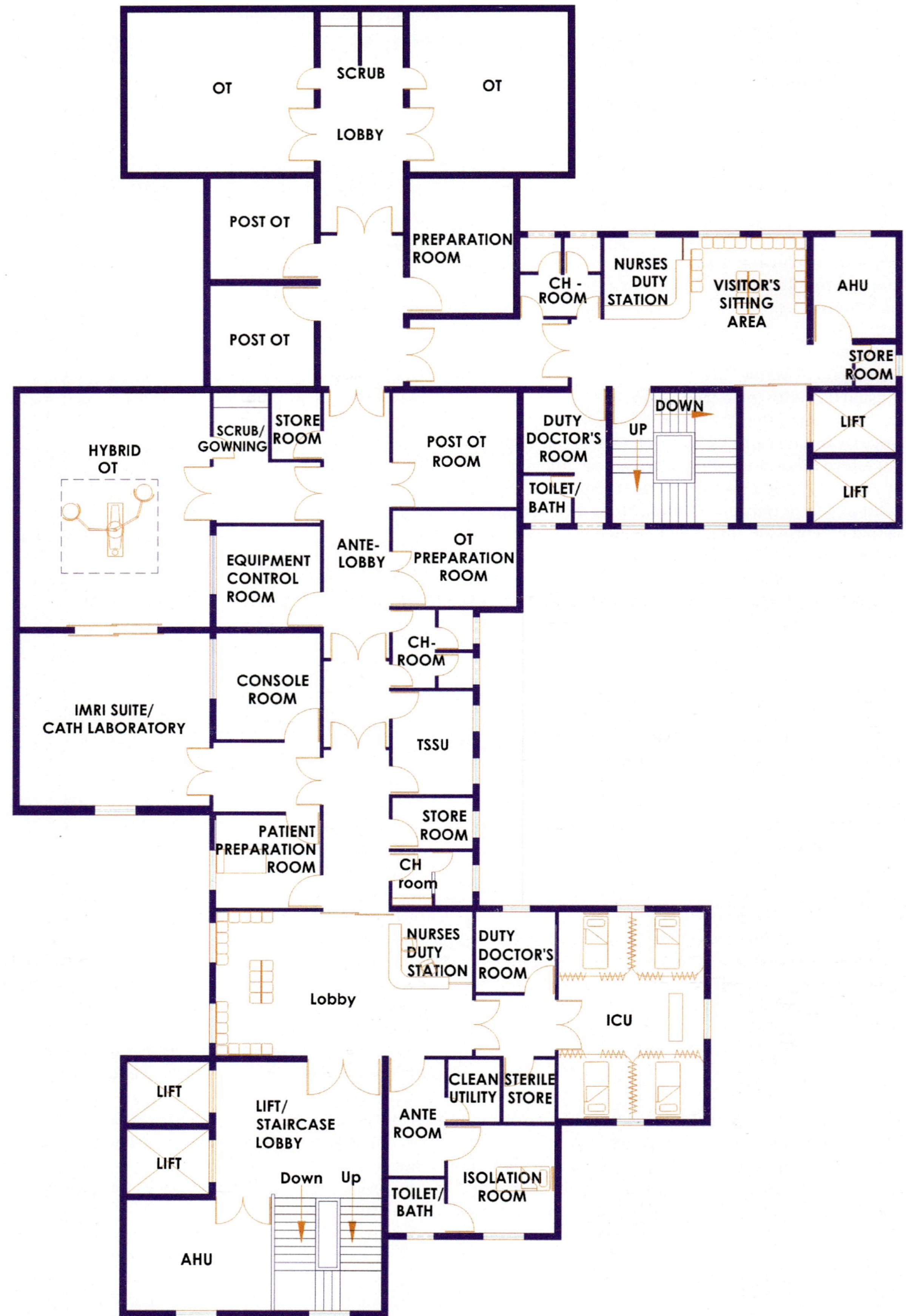

Fig. 18: Hybrid operating unit.

REFERENCES

1. Gupta S, Kant S, Chandrashekhar R. Operating unit—Planning essentials and design considerations. Journal of Academy of Hospital Administration [Internet]. 2005 [cited 2012 Oct 15]; Available from: *http://www.indmedica.com/journals.php/12?journalid=6&issueid=72&articleid=907&action=article*
2. Towers M. The modern conception of an operating theatre suite. South African Medical Journal [Internet]. 1967;41(8):181–6. Available from: *http://www.ncbi.nlm.nih.gov/pubmed/6024606*
3. Systems Integration—Operating Room [Internet]. VTS Medical Systems. [cited 2012 Oct 15]. p. 2. Available from: *http://www.vtsmedical.com/pdf/datasheets/SystemsIntORrevB.pdf*
4. www.wales.nhs.uk
5. www.wales.gov.uk
6. Kpodonu J, Raney A. The cardiovascular hybrid room—a key component for hybrid interventions and image-guided surgery in the emerging specialty of cardiovascular hybrid surgery. Interactive cardiovascular and thoracic surgery [Internet]. 2009 [cited 2012 Oct 15];9(4):688-92. Available from: *http://www.ncbi.nlm.nih.gov/pubmed/19622541*
7. Juett S, O'Connor P. The Integrated Operating Room [Internet]. Healthcare Design Magazine. 2006 [cited 2012 Oct 16]. Available from: *http://www.healthcaredesignmagazine.com/article/integrated-operating-room*
8. Naus H. Designing the Hybrid OR Considerations & Recommendations. Philips Healthcare. p. 1–10.
9. Kpodonu J. "Hybrid Cardiovascular Suite: The Operating Room of the Future", Journal of Cardiac Surgery, 2010.
10. Kpodonu J. Hybrid cardiovascular suite: the operating room of the future. Journal of Cardiac Surgery [Internet]. 2010 Nov [cited 2012 Oct 15];25(6):704-9. Available from: *http://www.ncbi.nlm.nih.gov/pubmed/20796084*
11. Belkin M. The Design and Implementation of Hybrid Operating Rooms [Internet]. [cited 2011 Dec 29]. p. 3. Available from: *www.veithsymposium.org/pdf/vei/2761.pdf*
12. Sikkink CJJM, Reijnen MMPJ, Zeebregts CJ. The creation of the optimal dedicated endovascular suite. European Journal of Vascular and Endovascular Surgery: the official journal of the European Society for Vascular Surgery [Internet]. 2008 [cited 2012 Oct 15];35(2):198-204. Available from: *http://www.ncbi.nlm.nih.gov/pubmed/17964193*
13. Estates N. HBN 26 Facilities for surgical procedures : Volume 1. Leeds; 2004. p. 92.
14. Mansour M. The new operating room environment. The Surgical Clinics of North America [Internet]. 1999; 79(3): 477-87. Available from: *http://www.ncbi.nlm.nih.gov/pubmed/10410682*
15. Australasian Health Facility Guidelines—Health facility briefing and planning [Internet]. [cited 2012 Nov 14]. Available from: *https://aushfg-prod-com-au.s3.amazonaws.com/HPU_B.0340_6_IPU_0.pdf*
16. Bizley, Graham. "Barn operating theatre, Broadgreen Hospital, Liverpool.(IN DETAIL)", Building Design, April 22, 2005 Issue Publications.
17. healthfacilityguidelines.com.au
18. http://paramedica-bg.com/
19. johnsonmedical.com
20. https://www.intechopen.com/
21. *http://cdn.intechopen.com/pdfs/30184/InTech-The_hybrid_operating_room.pdf*
22. Van Pelt J. Hybrid ORs: what's behind the increasing demand? OR Manager 2011 May; 27(5): 7-10. Available at: http://www.ncbi.nim.nih.gov/pubmed/21678825
23. Siddharth V, Kant S, Chandrashekhar R, Gupta SK. Integration in operation theatre: Need of the hour. Int J Res Foundation Hosp Healthc admin 2015;3(2): 123-128.

OTHER REFERENCES

- Babb JR, Lynam P, Ayliffe GA. Risk of airborne transmission in an operating theatre containing four ultraclean air units. The Journal of Hospital Infection [Internet]. 1995 [cited *2012, Nov 14];31(3):159-68. Available from: http://www.ncbi.nlm.nih.gov/pubmed/*8586784
- Barn operating theatre, Broadgreen Hospital, Liverpool [Internet]. 2005 [cited 2012, Nov 14]. Available from*: http://www.bdonline.co.uk/buildings/technic*al/in-detail-43-barn-operating-theatre-broadgreen-hospital-liverpool/3050105.article
- Broadgreen Hospital, Liverpool Best Practice Data Sheet [Internet]. [cited 2012, Nov 14]. Available fro*m: http://www.ihprojects.co.uk/best-practice/E1633_IHP B*est Practice sheets_Broadgreen.pdf
- Cardiovascular imaging. Cardiovascular Journal of Africa [Internet]. 2009 [cited 2012, Oct 17];20(4):258-9. Available from: http://www.cvja.co.za*/onlinejournal/vol20/vol20_issue_4/index.html?pageNumber=48*
- *Field ML, Sammut J, Kuduva*lli M, Oo A, Rashid A. Hybrid theatres: nicety or necessity? Journal of the Royal Society of Medicine [Internet]. 2009 [cited 2012, Oct 15];102(3):92-7. Available from: http://www.pubmedcentral.ni*h.gov/articlerender.fcgi?artid=2746850&tool=pmcentrez&rendertype=abstract*
- *Fillinger MF, Weaver JB.* Imaging equipment and techniques for optimal intraoperative imaging during endovascular interventions. Seminars in vascular surgery *[Internet]. 1999 [cited 2012, Oct 17];12(4):315-2*6. Available from: http://www.ncbi.nlm.nih.gov/pubmed/10651460
- Fornell D. Planning for a Hybrid Suite *[Internet]. 2010 [cited 2011 Dec 17]. Available from: h*ttp://www.healthcare.philips.com
- Hankel A. OR of the future [Internet]. www.surgicalproductsm*ag.com. 2011 [cited 2012, Oct 16].* pp. 9-10. Available from: https://www.ecri.org/Documents/Reprints/OR_of_Future (Surgical_Products)_JanFeb_2011.pdf
- Healthcare *design insights [Internet]. Surgical Innovation and A/E/C* Impacts. 2010 [cited 2012, Oct 17]. p. 3. Available from: http://www.mahlum.com/pdf/MahlumHDISpring2010Issue02.pdf
- Jolesz F. *Future perspectives for intraoperative MRI. Neurosurgery Clinics of North America [*Internet]. 2005 [cited 2012, Oct 6];16(1):201-13. Available from: http://www.ncbi.nlm.nih.gov/pubmed/15561539
- Matsumae M, Fukuyama H, Osada T, Baba T, Mizokami Y, Atsumi H, et al. Fully functional MR-compatible flexible operat*ing table resolves the neurosurgeon's dilemma* over use of intraoperative MRI. The Tokai Journal of Experimental and Clinical Medicine [Internet]. 2008;33(1):57-60. Avail*able from: http://www.ncbi.nlm.nih.gov/pubmed/21318967*
- *Myiari T. Reducing invasive*ness by employing therapeutic approaches combining catheterization and surgery [Internet]. Toshiba Medical Systems. [cited 2012 Oct 16]. Available from: https://www.yumpu.com/en/document/read/39825255/a-new-era-with-hybrid-operating-systems-toshiba-medical-
- *Operating Theatres. Elliott [Internet]. [cited 2012, Nov 14]. Available from: http://www.*elliottuk.com/operating-theatres
- Perry J, Katz A. Planning a hybrid operating room [Internet]. Health Facilities Management. [cited 2012 Oct 16]. Available from: http://www.hfmmagazine.com/hfmmagazine/html/WebExclusives/WebExclusives_TwoInOne.html
- Portou MJ, Browne TF, Prionidis I. Th*e vascular hybrid operating theatre: The Broo*mfield Hospital experience [Internet]. RAD Magazine; 2011 [cited 2012 Oct 16]. pp. 29-31. Available from: http://www.radmagazine.co.uk/ScientificPDFs/October 2011—The vascular operating theatre - Dr M J Portou.pdf
- Pre*venting infections during construction [Inter*net]. OR manager. [cited 2012 Oct 16]. Available from: http://www.ormanager.com/issues-articles/#.UH2YKaCQTV9

- Samson RH. Setting up an imaging center, adding *computed tomographic, magnetic resonance, and* an angiography suite to vascular labs. Journal of Vascular Surgery [Internet]. 2009 [cited 2012, Oct 17];49(4):1073-6. Available from: https://www.ncbi.nlm.nih.gov/pubmed/19056758Stanbridge DD, Fried GM. Current Developments in Operating Room De*sign [Internet]. Operating Room; 2007. p. 8-9.* Available from: http://www.touchbriefings.com/pdf/2742/fried.pdf
- Uhl E, Zausinger S, Morhard D, Heigl T, *Scheder B, Rachinger W, et al. Intraoperative computed tomography with integrated navi*gation system in a multidisciplinary operating suite. Neurosurgery [Internet]. 2009 [cited 2012, Oct 6];64(5 Su*ppl 2):231-9; discussion 239-40. Available from: http://www.ncbi.nlm.nih.gov/pubmed/19404103*
- *Van Pelt J. Hybrid ORs: what's beh*ind the increasing demand? OR manager [Internet]. 2011;27(5):7-10. Available fr*om: http://www.ncbi.nlm.nih.gov/pubmed/216788*25
- Yrjänä SK, Katisko JP, Ojala RO, Tervonen O, Schiffbauer H, Koivukangas J. Versatile intraoperative MRI in neurosurgery and radiology. Acta Neurochirurgica [Internet]. 2002;144(3):271-8; discussion 278. Available from: h*ttp://www.ncbi.nlm.nih.gov/pubmed/11956940*

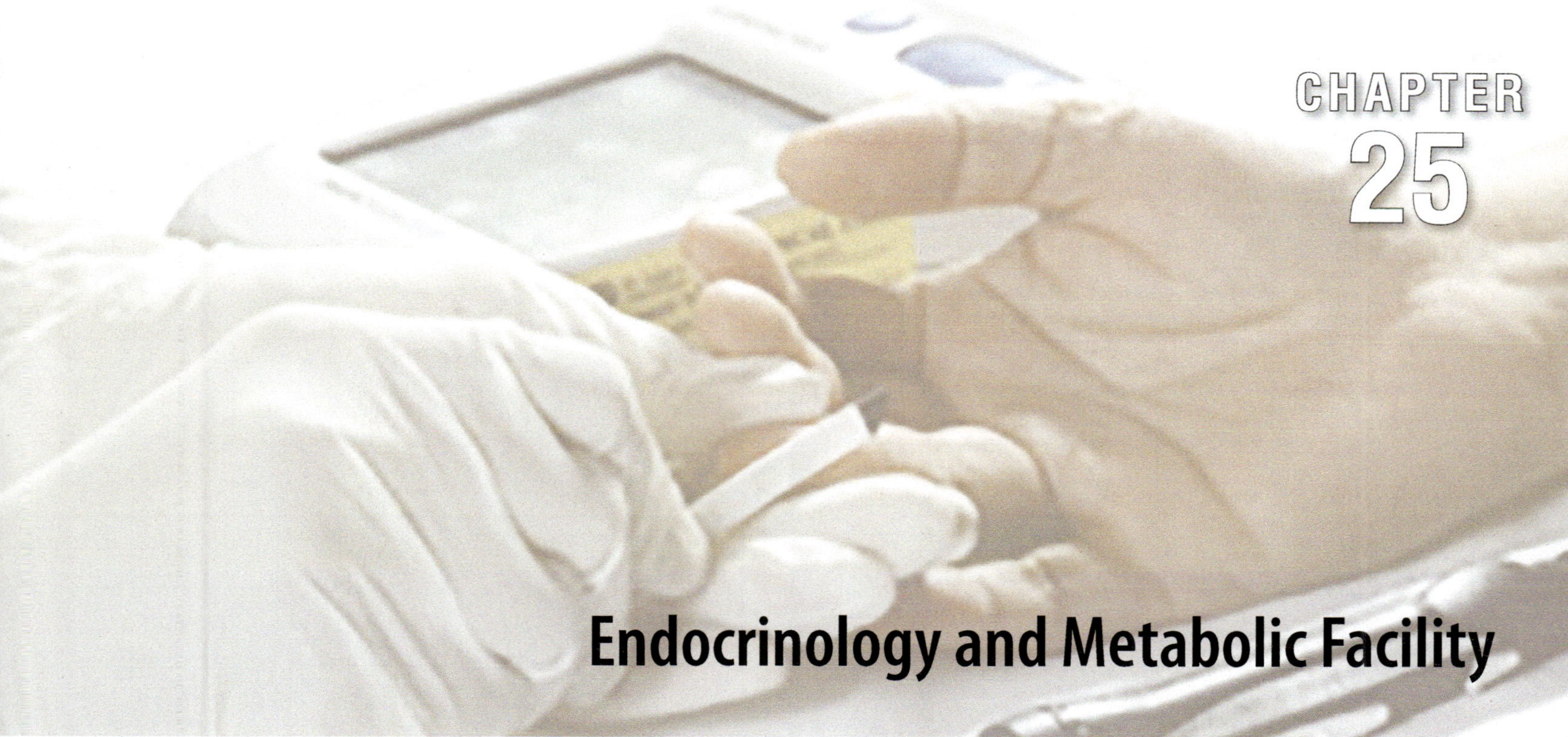

Endocrinology and Metabolic Facility

Shilipi Verma, Shakti Kumar Gupta, Sunil Kant, R Chandrashekhar

INTRODUCTION

Endocrine and metabolic diseases are among the most common contemporary human afflictions. The prevalence and incidence of certain disorders, such as diabetes and obesity, have been well defined in large population-based studies. There has, however, been no comprehensive survey and compilation of data regarding the epidemiology of endocrine and metabolic disorders to serve as a unified source of information about these conditions.[1,2]

The term endocrine was coined by Dr Starling. It is used to describe hormones secreted internally compared to those secreted externally or into the lumen. The word hormone is derived from Greek word, *Hormao* which means to set in motion or having property of stimulating. This is based on the ability of hormones to elicit a cascade of physiologic responses by acting on target tissues.[1,2]

HISTORY OF ENDOCRINOLOGY

The current understanding of endocrinology as we know now has evolved over last 150 years. However, ancient Indian text Sushruta Samhita dating back 5000 BC has a detailed description of diabetes including its various types and its symptoms. Ancient Chinese texts have also elaborated on endocrine disorders like goiter and its therapy using seaweed which we know now is rich in iodine.[1,2]

There have been references to hormones and its disorders in medical literature during the middle ages. Andreas Versalius the anatomist in 1543 had drawn drawings of major glands and ducts in his famous book De Humani Corporis Fabrica (The Structure of the Human Body). In 1849, Berthold, recorded physiologic effects of castration. Claude Bernard, in 1855 noted two secretions from liver, the external secretions like bile and internal secretions like glucose. In 1888 William Ord gave the classical description of myxedema (mucinous edema) related to hypothyroidism.[1,2]

The beginning of 20th century heralded endocrinotherapy. Clinical manifestations of Graves disease, acromegaly, Addisons disease was described. The landmark event was the discovery and isolation of insulin by the famous duo of Banting and Best in 1922. The singular event enabled doctors to treat endocrine cases in a scientific manner.[1,2]

The other landmark was the invention of radioimmunoassay (RIA) for estimation of hormone levels. This allowed the clinical to accurately diagnose the disorders and monitor the therapy. The last few decades has seen the advent of recombinant DNA technology in the field of endocrinotherapy. Recent work in endocrinology focuses on the molecular mechanisms responsible for triggering the effects of hormones. Future therapies will target hormone receptors and postreceptor effects to treat various endocrine disorders.[1,2]

FUNCTIONS

The function of 'Endocrine and Metabolic Diseases Facility' is to provide comprehensive care for metabolic and endocrine disorders. To achieve this purpose the facility must deliver the entire range of interventions[3] viz.—promotion of health, prevention of disease by specific protections, early diagnosis and treatment in active phases of disease, limitation of disability that could result from the disease and rehabilitation required to enable the patients to return to family, society and vocation.

PLANNING AND DESIGN CONSIDERATIONS

The foremost aspect of facility planning and design that needs to be considered is whether the facility would be standalone or will be an integrated part of a multispecialty care institution. An integrated facility has distinct advantages (Box 1). The stack diagram is shown in Figures 1A and B and the functional relationship diagram in Figure 2.

The practice of endocrinology involves following aspects:

Box 1: Integrated facility.

- Only cases requiring specialized endocrinology management are managed all others get filtered at medicine department
- Endocrine cases pose complex problems of management in clinical terms. Multidisciplinary approach is the most desirable way care of the endocrinology patients
- A standalone unit will need to cater for all the support services that would otherwise be available in an integrated facility

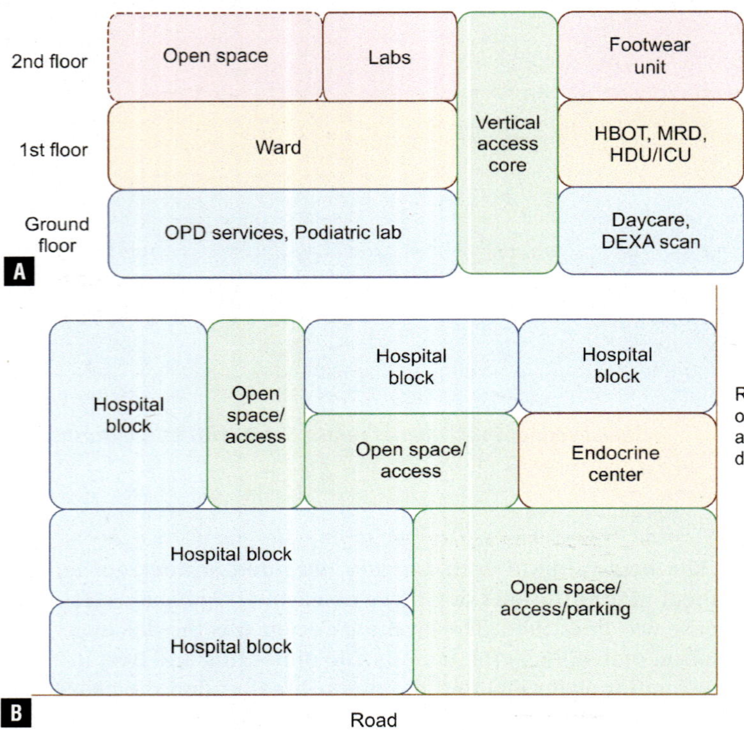

Figs. 1A and B: Stack diagram.
(HBOT: hyperbaric oxygen therapy; MRD: medical record department)

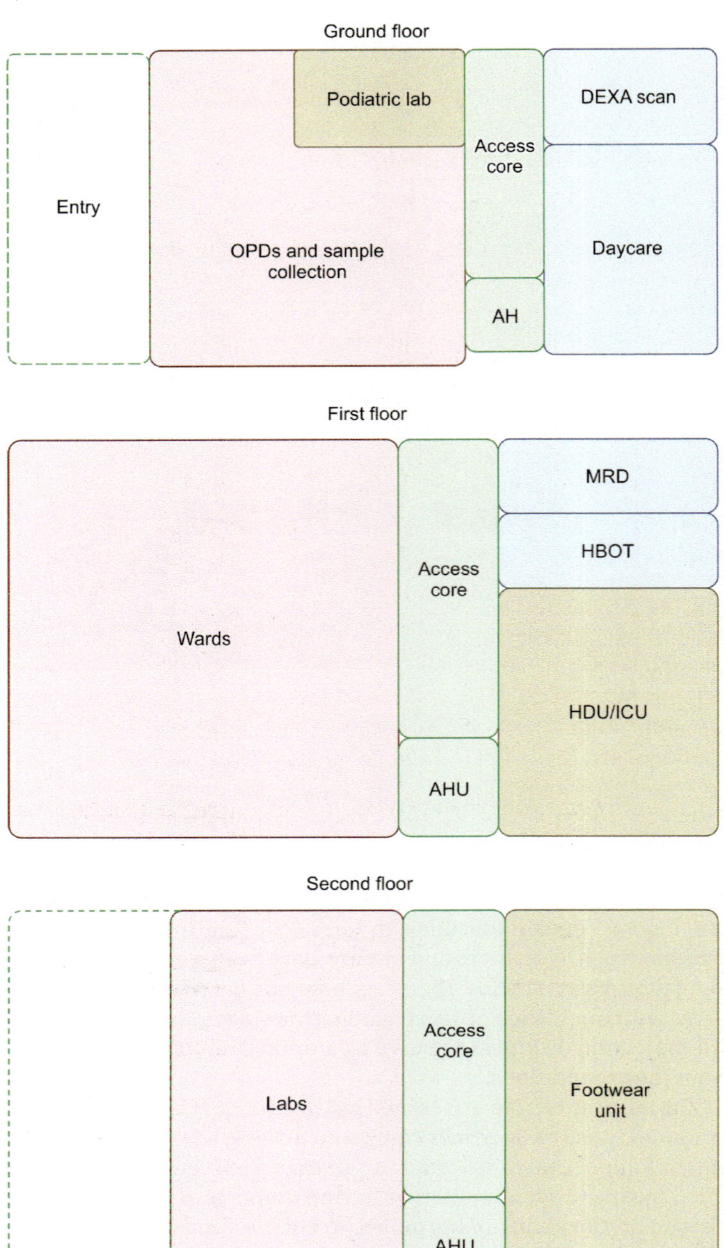

Fig. 2: Functional relationship diagrams.

- *Clinical endocrinology*: This covers the clinical diagnosis of endocrine disorders. The endocrine diseases can be grouped into those which occur due to excess or deficiency or resistance to the action of hormones. Most endocrine disorders are chronic in nature and require life long therapy.
- *Endocrine laboratory*: Endocrine services in any center need to be supported by a well established endocrine laboratory. The various types of endocrine laboratories are:
  - *Radioimmunoassay-based labs*: These laboratories use RIA kits and are regulated by guidelines laid down by Atomic Energy Regulatory Board.
  - *Chemiluminescence immunoassay (CLIA)*: The CLIA kits are designed to detect glow based chemiluminescent reactions.
  - *Enzyme-linked immunoassays (ELISA)*: These are old technologies and the results are not very accurate.

The diagnosis of endocrine disorders involves use of excitation/stimulation or inhibition/suppression testing of hormones. In addition there is requirement of other diagnostic services. These include:

- *Dual-energy X-ray absorptiometry (DXA) scan*: The DXA scan previously known by the acronym DEXA is an important and integral element for an endocrine center. It is used for estimation of bone density. Measurement of bone density is useful to diagnose and monitor therapy for disorders like osteoporosis. This equipment would be integral to the endocrine center.
- *Imaging services*: The following services are required for diagnostic support. These are normally available in a tertiary care hospital and do not form part of the endocrine center.
  - *Ultrasound*: Required usually for imaging of thyroid gland.
  - *CT/MRI scan*: Required for imaging for various endocrine glands.
- *Nuclear medicine center*: Nuclear medicine plays an important role in management of endocrine disorders. It is required both for imaging of thyroid, parathyroid, adrenal glands and for treatment of disorders like Graves disease.
- *Surgical support*: Hormone deficiency disorders are treated by appropriate hormone replacement. Disorders of hormone excess are managed by suppressive therapy. However, certain disorders like acromegaly, Cushing's syndrome, and toxic goiter require surgical intervention. Therefore surgeons trained in endocrine surgery form an important part of the endocrine team.

COMPONENTS OF THE FACILITY

This includes:
- Outpatient department
- Inpatient including daycare facilities
- HDUs and ICUs
- Hyperbaric oxygen therapy unit
- Specialized facilities—RIA lab, DEXA scan, Podiatric laboratory
- Footwear manufacturing unit.

The description here is limited to the extent that pertains to the specific requirement for endocrinology and metabolic disease facility.

Specialized Facilities for Outpatients Department

Diabetic eye clinic: This is required to be separately provided as the requirement is to permanently position equipment eye slit lamp biomicroscope, indirect ophthalmoscope, auto refractometer, keratometer and a scan bimetry.[3]

Weight management clinic utilizes the services of endocrinologist, diabetologist, nutritionist, physiotherapist, physician assistant and pharmacist for providing integrated weight management care to patients. Since obesity is one of the major risk factors for diabetes, this clinic advices solution for weight management. This is a type of functional arrangement and no separate space is provided for this.

Nutritionist/dietician room: For counseling of patients regarding dietary intake in diseases like diabetes, thyroid dysfunction, lipid dysfunction, etc.[3]

Patient Counselors and Clinical Psychologist

The various types of counseling required are:
- IDDM counseling
- Lifestyle modification counseling
- Obesity counseling
- Adherence counseling.

Transition clinic: Transition clinics are OPDs which aimed at ensuring a smooth transition of the patient between the pediatric and adult services. It also caters for those patients who will need long term endocrinology follow-up treatment.

Pulse electromagnetic fields [PEMF (Fig. 3)] facility is to be provided in the treatment rooms in the OPD area. PEMF promotes tissue healing and provide relief from pain and inflammation, especially long standing uncomplicated diabetic ulcers, vascular ulcers, post surgical non-healing/delayed incision wounds and neuropathy.[3]

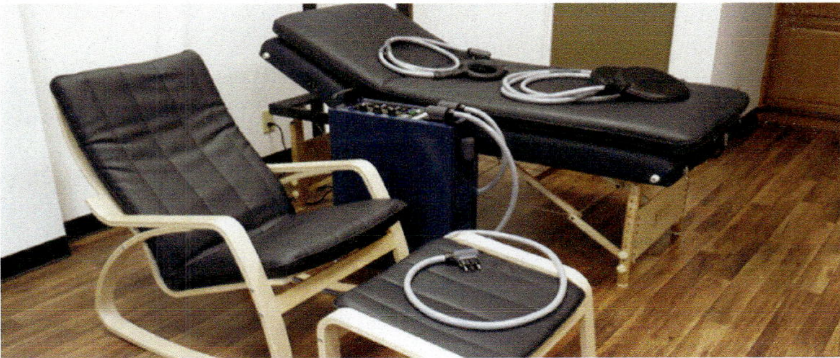

Fig. 3: PEMF facility.

Podiatric Unit

Diabetes affects feet and causes loss of sensation on the feet due to peripheral neuropathy. Patients are vulnerable to injury on the feet. This unit provides specialized podiatric services including advice of the types of footwear to be used. Separated footwear unit helps design special footwear for patients with high risk foot.[3]

HYPERBARIC OXYGEN THERAPY UNIT

Introduction

Hyperbaric oxygen therapy (HBOT) is breathing 100% oxygen under increased pressure. HBOT is a drug that treats disease processes and not a specific disease. The primary action of HBOT is at the DNA/chromosome level. HBOT is an effective treatment for acute and chronic damaged tissue. The underlying causes can be trauma, infection, autoimmune, ischemia, hypoxia or toxins. Among endocrine diseases delayed wound healing, stumps infections, diabetic retinopathy and diabetic ulcers are treated by HBOT.[4]

Chambers

There are two types of chambers (Figs. 4A and B)—for single patient. Monoplace (Class B) or for multiple patients—Multiple (Class A) chamber. In addition there are common space and safety requirements as given below.[4]

Planning Parameters

Location: Since HBOT requires continuous monitoring for 8–10 hours therefore unit should be planned within inpatients department so that resources can be shared.

Floor space: Minimum floor space for monoplace chamber would be 16 m^2 with length of the room not less than 5.60 m.[4] The functional relationship diagram is shown in Figure 5.

Emergency Exit Requirements[5]

- Must allow rapid or emergency removal of patients and staff.
- In the case of multiple chambers emergency removal of a patient or personnel from one chamber/compartment should not restrict in any way the rapid and simultaneous removal of patients of personnel from all other chambers or compartments.
- A minimum of two exits to be provided. In only one single entry, it must open directly to a primary evacuation corridor.
- Exit doorways to be 1.30 m wide.

Minimum Clearance Around the Chambers

Class 'A'[5]

- Chamber entry for gurney/stretcher access: 3.00 m. Entries for wheeled gurneys should have access ramps those are flush with the chamber entry doorway

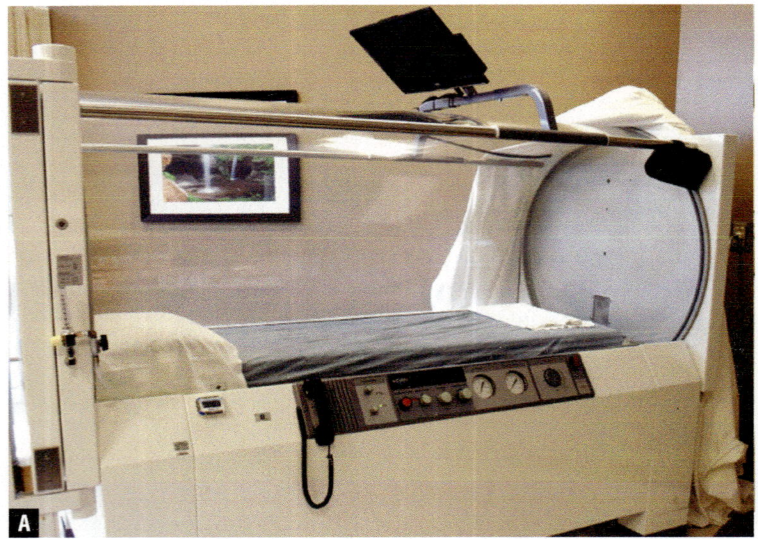

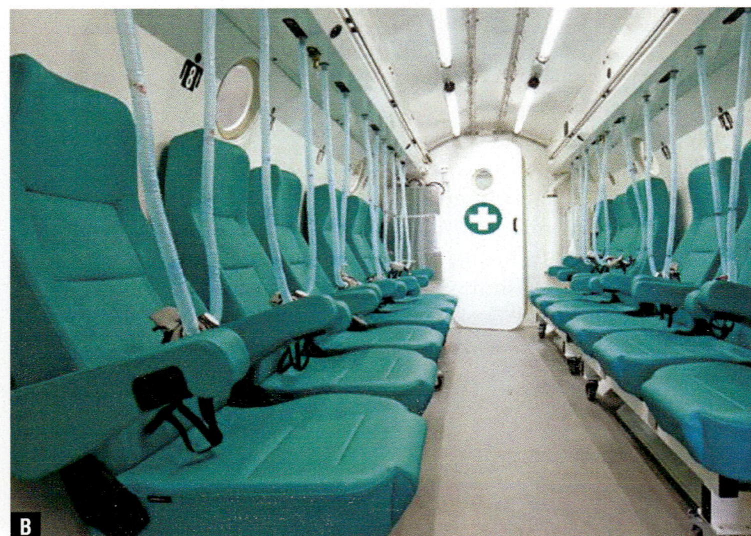

Figs. 4A and B: Class 'A' and Class 'B' HBOT chambers.

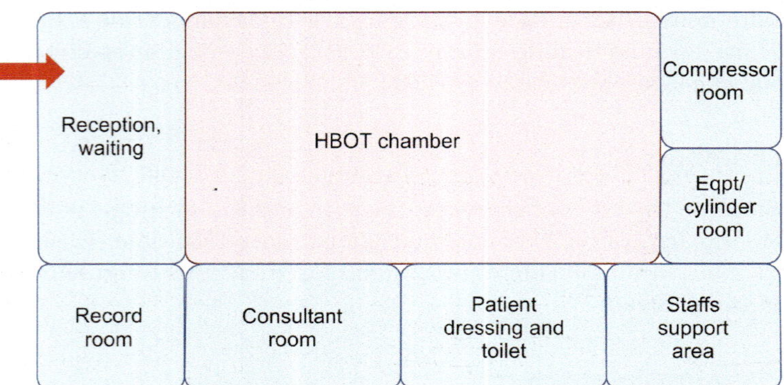

Fig. 5: Functional relationship diagram—HBOT.

- Chambers having fixed internal stretcher frames and transfer gurneys should allow immediate removal of the patient upon chamber depressurization.
- Chamber main lock entries or compartments utilizing circular entry hatchways: 1.21 m.
- A minimum of 1.21 m of clearance all the way around the chamber, except as specified for entry areas.
- If chamber control console is adjacent to the chamber, a minimum passageway of 1.21 m to be provided between the control console and any obstruction.

Class 'B'[5]

- Chamber and side wall—0.45 m. (*Exception*: If any chamber controls, ventilation valves, or other operator-adjustable devices are located on or under the chamber adjacent to the side wall, minimum clearance should be 0.90 m)
- Between control side of two chambers, 1.20 m
- Between back side of two chambers, 0.60 m
- Minimum passage of 0.36 m should be provided at the foot end of each chamber. An oxygen shut-off valve should be provided for each chamber and should be unobstructed by the chamber and located as to be immediately accessible to the chamber operator.
- A minimum space of 2.60 m should be available at the head end of the chamber to allow for the safe insertion and removal of the patient from the chamber.
- Any electrical service outlets located within 3.00 m of the Class B chamber entrance should be site on less than 0.91 m above floor level.

Support Area

The following support areas should be provided for the hyperbaric facility. If the hyperbaric facility is integrated within a hospital, the support areas may be shared.[5]

- Reception/control desk
- Patient waiting/holding area. The area should be under staff control and should have seating capacity in accordance with the workload. When the hyperbaric chambers are used for outpatients and inpatients at the same time, separate waiting areas should be provided with screening for visual privacy between the two classes of patients. A holding area should accommodate inpatient on stretchers or beds. Stretcher patients should be out of the direct line of normal traffic. The patient waiting/holding area may be omitted for two or less individual Class B units.[5]
- Consultation/treatment rooms
- Patient record storage area.
- *Compressor room:* This area should be large enough to house the chamber compressors, accumulator tanks, fire suppression system. The reserve breathing gases could also be housed here if it is in close proximity to the chamber room.[5]
- Soiled holding area with waste receptacles and soiled linen receptacles.
- Equipment and supply storage.
- *Gas cylinder room*: This room should be large enough to accommodate the storage of enough cylinders and manifolds for the reserve breathing gases required for chamber operations. The minimum room size should be able to house eight cylinders and two gas manifolds, consisting of at least two cylinders on each manifold. It must meet the requirements of Gas Cylinder Rules 1984.[5]
- Housekeeping room—can be shared with another department.
- Support areas for staff—Toilets with hand-washing fixtures.
- Patient dressing rooms with facilities for securing valuables. It should accommodate wheelchair patients.
- Patient toilet rooms with hand-washing fixtures with hands-free controls. It should also accommodate wheelchair patients.[5]

ENDOCRINE LABORATORY

The laboratory services integrated with this facility will only provide specific endocrine centric diagnostics. All other services are to sources from main laboratory of the hospital with which the facility is integrated.

Biochemistry Lab

- This is to be planned as standard biochemistry lab with automatic and semi-automatic analyzers.
- The number, type and sophistications of the equipment will depend upon the patient profile of the facility, expertise available for handling the equipment and availability of services support for the equipment.

Radioimmunoassay Lab

The RIA lab carrier out hormonal assay for management of endocrine patients. RIA work involves the handling and use of very small quantities of radioisotopes, usually not exceeding 3.7 mBq of Iodine-125 and Tritium (3H). Atomic Energy (Radiation Protection), Rules (2004) promulgated under the Atomic Energy Act, 1962 requires that the user should obtain authorization from Atomic Energy Regulatory Board (AERB) for handling radioisotopes.[6]

Planning Requirements[3,7,8]

Location

Lab to be away from main traffic of patients and visitors.

Areas

For RIA lab the area/floor space is to be as per AERB Guidelines.[3]

Safety

Provisions for safety including eye flushing devices, emergency shower and fire extinguishers are to be made. The safety provisions are required to be in line with the safety program in the hospital as well as AERB safety guidelines.

Work Stations

Work counters with space for equipment under the counters and overhead cabinets is to be provided. Work stations to be equipped with services like electricity, has and vacuum as needed. Counter sinks with hand washing, glass lined iron traps and pipes for drainage to be provided.

Lighting

Stores and reception—200 lux, Offices—300 lux and work stations—500 lux. Natural lighting may be advantageously used.

Doors

Minimum 1.20 m in width. In rooms where large sized equipment will be installed the door must of appropriate size.

Benches

Countertop heights vary depending whether the work will be carried out standing or sitting. For standing—900 mm, sitting —750 mm. Depth of the wall tables should be 700 mm. Length of the bench ranges from 1.6 m to 1.8 m. Each laboratory bench should have a sink with swan-neck fittings having cold-hot water supply. Bench tops to acid/alkali resistant.

Ergonomics

This is a frequently neglected area in any design consideration. In the laboratory, the relationship between works and their tools of the trade is very close. A productive laboratory is the one designed to enhance the harmony of this relationship by means of good illumination, well-designed benches and work space, noise control, proper tools and an overall pleasant environment. These factors serve to reduce stress experienced by the workers, contributing to an overall productive and safe environment.[8]

Ventilation

Mechanical ventilation with 10-15 air changes in areas where fumes are expected and 8-10 changes in other areas.

Equipment

- Geiger counter—for monitoring spillage on work surfaces and in the centrifuge after each assay.
- Gamma counter—Gamma multidetector RIA system counter is used for measurement of activity in RIA and IRMA assays performed in this laboratory. It can measure counts in 12 tubes at a time. All assay protocols are programmed into the computer, which can then automatically calculate the analyte concentration based on the counts measured.
- Centrifuge—For heterogeneous assays (to separate bound from free isotope). This low speed centrifuge can be temperature-adjusted (range 0-30°C), and is capable of reaching a maximum speed of 6000 rmp (±9800 G).
- Refrigerators (2-8°C)/Freezer (-20°C)—For storage of kits. Reconstituted internal quality control specimens are stored in the freezer.
- Air extractor unit (Fume hood)—To maintain high-speed laminar airflow. Fume hood is one of the necessary facilities for laboratory. It will discharge poisonous, harmful, flavors air caused in experiment.
- Other instruments—Vortex Mixers (Used for mixing of reagents/sample during assay procedure), Shaker incubator (For shaking IRMA tubes during incubation), Pipettes (used for transferring specific amounts of reagent or sample into tubes), timer/stopwatch, venturi aspirator (used to aspirate supernatant in heterogeneous assays) and thermometers.

The layout of RIA is shown in Figure 6.

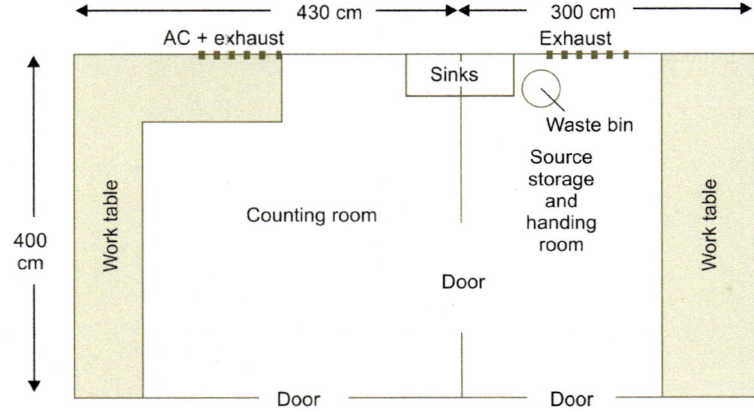

Fig. 6: Layout of RIA lab (As per AERB guidelines).

Chemiluminescence Immunoassay Lab

Chemiluminescence is the generation of electromagnetic radiation as light by the released of energy from a chemical reaction. CLIA using microplate luminometers provides a sensitive, high throughput, and economical way to quantitatively measure antigen in cell lysates plasma, urine, saliva, tissue and culture media samples.

The CLIA kits are designed to detect glow based chemiluminescent reactions. The kits provide broader dynamic assay range, superior low-end sensitivity, and a faster protocol than the conventional colorimetric methods. CLIA is one of the detection method used in clinical chemistry laboratory.

DUAL-ENERGY X-RAY ABSORPTIOMETRY (FIG. 7)

It is quick, painless and preferred technique to measure bone mineral density (BMD). Two X-ray beams with different energy levels are aimed at the patient's bones. When soft tissue absorption is subtracted out, the BMD can be determined from the absorption of each beam by bone. Dual-energy X-ray absorptiometry is the most widely used and most thoroughly studied bone density measurement technology.

Planning and Design Considerations

- Location—DEXA scan should ideally be located on ground floor and conveniently accessible to inpatient, outpatient and HDU.
- Adequate sub-waiting area and having washrooms in close proximity
- Cater for efficient record keeping
- Safety features as DEXA scan room is part of the complex. The design and construction of room must cater to the guidelines of AERB such as thickness of the wall, lead lining and measurement of exposure to the staff, etc.
- Wide entrance and wide doors for the moment of trolleys and equipment.

PODIATRIC LABORATORY

This lab performs biothesiometry and doppler tests. Biothesiometry test checks the nerve sensation in the hands and the feet. Doppler test assesses the blood flow in arteries and veins and checks the blood pressure in both the limbs. Foot clinic also provides information about special footwear requirements. Footwear manufacturing unit may be provided along with the facility (Fig. 8).[4]

Location

Planned at the ground floor as a number of diabetic patients are expected to frequent this lab. Floor space required for this lab is 35 m^2 (Biothesiometry facility including Doppler (7 m^2), monofilament test (7 m^2), nerve conduction studies (7 m^2), electronic baro-pedometer (7 m^2), podoscope/luminoscope (7 m^2).

Lighting

Stores and Reception - 200 lux, Offices - 300 lux and work stations - 500 lux. Natural lighting may be advantageously used.

Walls and Floors

To be made of material that can be cleaned easily, acid/alkali resistant, joint-free (or with minimal joints).

Doors

No door should be less than 1.20 m in width.

Instrumentation

Doppler

Doppler test assesses the blood flow in arteries and veins and checks the blood pressure in both the limbs. These noninvasive vascular tests can be used for—diagnosis and quantification of peripheral vascular disease, predicting wound healing of a diabetic foot ulcer, follow-up and control of treatment.[4,9]

Biothesiometry Test (Foot Vibration Test) (Fig. 9)

This study is done to determine vibration perception which is a good indicator of diabetic neuropathy.

Monofilament Test (Fig. 10)

About 10 g monofilament is used for this test. Inability to perceive the 10 g monofilament at the toes or dorsum of the foot predicts future occurrence of a diabetic foot ulcer.[4,9]

Nerve Conduction Studies

Slowing of nerve conduction velocity is one of the earliest neuropathic abnormalities in diabetes mellitus. This test quantifies nerve conduction and help to localize the lesions.[4,9]

Electronic Baro-pedometer (Fig. 11)

For preparing therapeutic insoles for footwear. *Podoscope/Luminoscope*—for qualitative analysis for therapeutic insoles for footwear.[4,9]

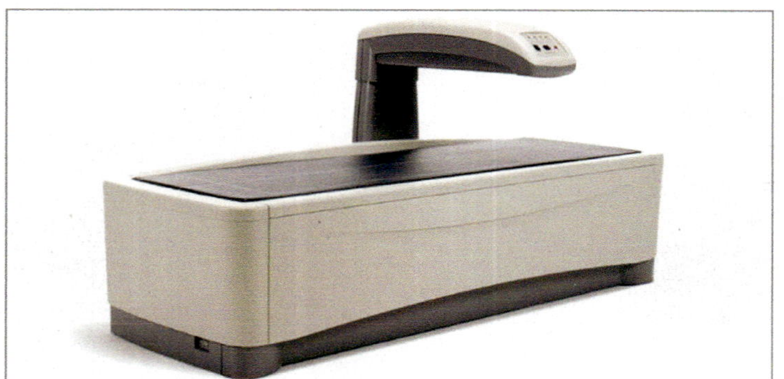

Fig. 7: DEXA scan.

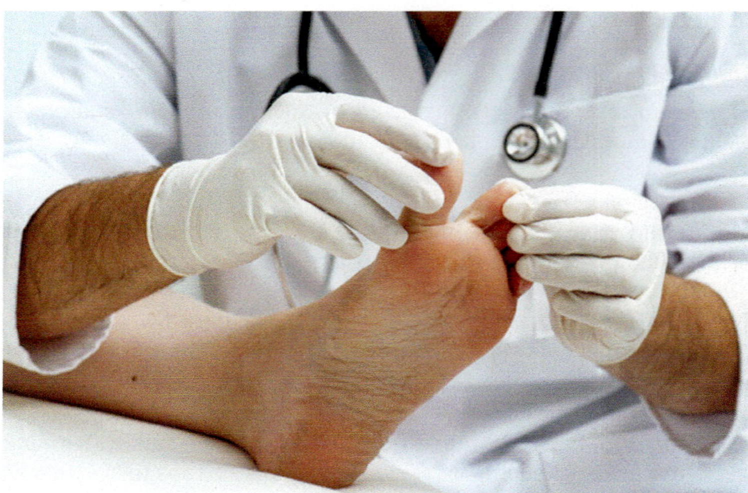

Fig. 8: Podiatric care area.

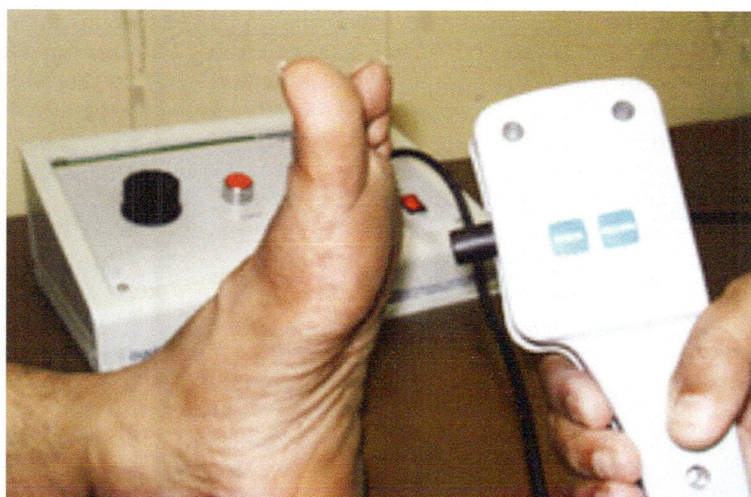

Fig. 9: Biothesiometry.

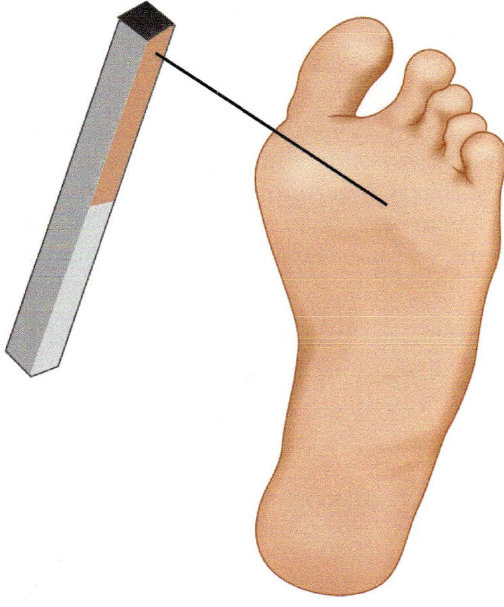

Fig. 10: Monofilament test.

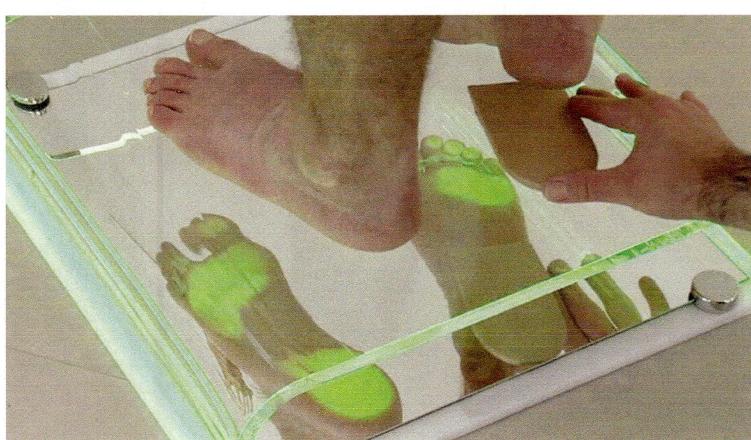

Fig. 11: Baro-pedometer.

FOOTWEAR MANUFACTURING UNIT

The high incidence of foot problems and lower limb amputations associated with diabetes means the issue of foot care has become important in diabetes treatment. More often foot care entails use of specialized footwear to protect feet. As such the need for specialized footwear is met by foot manufacturing unit.

SPECIAL CONSIDERATIONS

Infection Control

General Considerations

- Infection control in the facility is critical requirement for favorable outcomes in any healthcare facility. Therefore, the infection control principles must be applied and monitored scrupulously.
- Infection control should aim at prevention of spread of infection by any means within the facility.
- Apart from various design and planning considerations, the most effective and efficient means of preventing infection is hand washing.
- Sluice rooms should be provided in such a manner that there is separate entry and exit. These rooms should not be dependent on the AHU (air handling unit) covering a patient care area.
- All surface that come in contact with hands and have the potential to harbor pathogens should be made of copper alloys as this has been proven to have anti-microbial properties.[10,11] Some of these are door handles, hand rails, bed rails, faucets, etc.

Hand Washing (Fig. 12)

- Hand-basins for hand washing should be available within each treatment area and should be accessible without traversing any other clinical area.
- They should be available at a ratio of one for every four beds and at the ratio of one to one for every procedure/consulting room.
- Several types of hand wash units could be deployed:
  - Surgical scrub station—For areas requiring hand washing for sterile procedures, dressing rooms, ICU, etc.
  - General staff hand wash units—For staff and visitors/attendants to use. These are to be provided in all clinical areas. These can be wall mounted units.

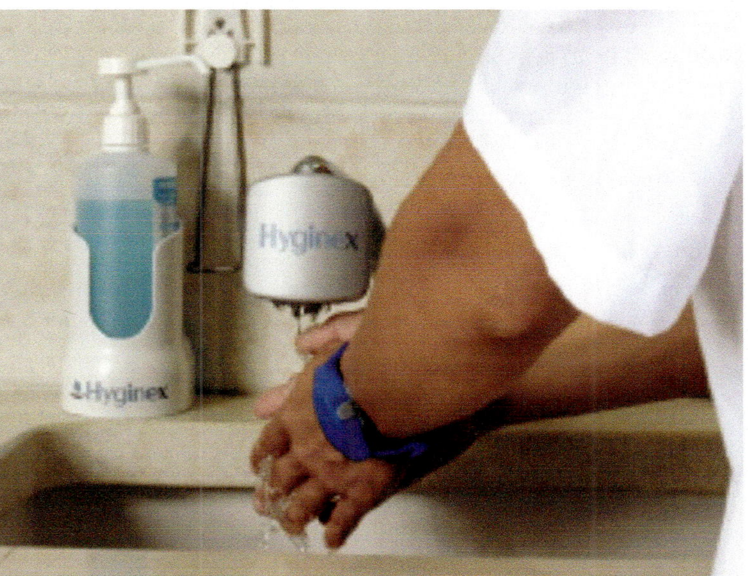

Fig. 12: Antiseptic dispensers.

- Number of hand wash units required are—for ICU/HDUs —One per enclosed room, one per bed, OPD—One per consultant and for other areas—under no circumstances a person requiring to use a hand wash unit should be more than 10-12 m away from a wash unit.
- In place of hand wash units, antiseptic lotion dispensers can be provided for each bed to avoid the plumbing and water disposal connection which can also be a source of infection in case of poor maintenance.

Space Standards and Dimensions

Corridors

All corridors should be at least 2.7 m high and 2.4 m wide. Where doors have been provided in the corridors, it must be borne in mind that the effective usable width reduces by at least 25 cm. Where storage bays have been provided to store trolleys/wheel chairs, etc, these should be outside the corridor width, i.e. should be recessed. Corridor dimensions[12] and usage are shown in Table 1.

Ceiling Heights

All areas—2.7 m height; in recesses/storage bays—up to 2.25 m.

All exposed ceilings and ceiling structures in areas occupied by patients or staff, and in food preparation or food storage areas, should be finished so as to be readily cleanable with equipment routinely used in daily housekeeping activities.[12]

In areas where dust fall would present a potential problem such as clinical areas, supply and storage areas and sterile stock storage, there should be a finished ceiling that covers all conduits, piping, ductwork and open construction systems. Light fittings shall also be recessed, flush fitted and sealed to prevent dust ingress.[12]

Floors

Flooring should be impervious, smooth, nonstainable and should allow easy movement. It should be without carpets or any other similar covering that would allow accumulation of dust and dirt. Floors are to be anti-slip in all the areas. In wards and ICU vitrified tiles or marble can be used. Joints in the floor can be thermo-sealed. Epoxy can be used as material for making joint-less, antistatic floor.

Wall and Skirting

Walls in clinical areas should be water resistant, scrubbable, smooth joint free and with coving of 3 inches diameter. The color should be nonreflecting type and of soothing shade. Skirtings should have same finish as floors, be integral with floors, be tightly sealed against the wall and constructed without any voids or cracks.

Ceramic wall tiles are considered the best for areas where liquids splashes a wall surface, potentially overcoming a damp or hygiene problem. Alternatives to ceramic wall tiles include PVC wall cladding systems, resin wall coatings and screed mortars, epoxy based finished with antibacterial paints.

Plumbing

Plumbing too should be as per specifications.[13]

Ergonomics and Human Engineering Aspects

No patients care area will be designed in a manner that would pose avoidable risk to the patient and staff. At all places principles of ergonomics should be kept in mind. For keeping the facility disabled friendly and barrier free it is important to consider this issue at the time of planning. For this, ramps and rails, etc. should be provided. Adequate number of lifts should be provided. The height of each step on a staircase should be such that enables easy climbing and descend. Staircases width—1500 mm; Tread—300 mm; riser—150 mm.

Security

The building plan should facilitate secured housing of the patients, staff and equipment. It must cater the requirements of access control and should have provisions for preventing thefts and other such incidents. Intruder/duress alarms should be provided in suitable places. In critical areas online camera based monitoring can be considered. Adequate guard post should be built-in in the plan.

Communication System

There should be an effective communication system.

Building Codes/Regulations

Building codes and regulations to be complied with are local and National Building Code—2016 and norms for fire safety.

Air-conditioning

Air-treatment plants are required to fulfill two unrelated set of requirements: first that of guaranteeing certain ideal microclimatic conditions (temperature, humidity, dilution of smells, etc.) while keeping noise to a minimum, and second that of reaching and maintaining required levels of asepsis in the air.

Table 1: Corridor specifications.

Category	*Usage*	*Dimension*	*Specification*	*Remark*
Corridor	Patient on trolley/bed/regular use	Width	2400 mm	Width between hand grab rails
Corridor	Only staff, on trolley	Width	1000 mm	–
Wall low protection	Wheel chairs	Height of protection	150–350 mm	Kick boards required
Wall mid protection	Trolleys	Height of protection	900 mm	Trolley protection
Wall corners protection	Trolleys	Height of protection	150–900 mm	Trolley protection
Hand rails	For patients	Height	900 mm	32 mm thick
Eqpt bays	For eqpt	Recessed bays	On one side	–
Wall phones	–	–	–	In long corridors

Lighting

Adequate lighting is an essential requirement and glare free lighting should be provided as follows:

General illumination—100 lux, nursing station—300 lux, Examination area—500 lux.

The LED lighting fixtures should be used as these are not only environment friendly, these also last longer and consume least electricity for equivalent brightness.

Parking

Adequate parking space need to be provided for the additional patient flow that the facility will attract. This could either be enhancement of the parking facilities in the existing hospital for creation of sub-parking area near the facility. Norms applicable are:

Space per car—2.5 m × 5.0 m;[20] Scale for parking—1 per 5 beds.[14]

Safety Considerations

Fire Safety

For fire safety norms the requirements of NBC part 4 must be adhered to.

Barrier Free Design

For barrier free design, the "Guidelines and Space Standards for Barrier Free Built Environment for Disabled and Elderly Persons - 1998" published by Central Public Works Department, Ministry of Urban Affairs and Employment, Government of India are applicable and need to be implemented. In addition each aspect of the facility planning, design and construction must consider the requirements of safety for patients, staff and visitors.

Energy Efficiency Rating

Green Rating for Integrated Habitat Assessment (GRIHA)/Indian Green Building Council (IGBC) is the National Rating System of India. With GRIHA/IGBC guidelines, the buildings are designed around nature, not against it. A green building depletes as little of the natural resources during its construction and operation.

The Scales of accomodation, DEXA scan, HVAC and lighting requirement are tabulated in Tables 2 to 5 respectively.

The floor plans are depicted in Figures 13 to 15.

CONCLUSION

In todays' healthcare scenario the endocrine system holds a very important place in view of the rapidly increasing number of endocrine related cases such as diabetes and obesity. India has significant number of these diseases. It is thus essential that comprehensive and scientifically planned endocrine centers are made available in the healthcare delivery systems.

Table 2: Space data sheets.

Outpatient department	m^2
Common areas – (Figures in parenthesis show area in m^2)—reception (7), Trolley/wheelchair bay (7), officer in-charge room (12), treatment room (15), injection room (10), ECG/EMG (10), sluice room (7), playroom (10)	78
Consultation room—health educator/counselors room/Medico-social guide/worker (15), thyroid clinic (12), vocational counseling unit (12), nutrition intervention/counseling clinic (12), diabetes clinic including transition clinic for adolescent (12), podiatric clinic (12), opthalmology room (12)	75
Waiting area including sub-waiting area	45
Consultation rooms—other specialized clinics—pediatric endocrine clinic, metabolic diseases clinic, reproductive endocrinology clinic, adrenal clinic, lipid clinic (2 room × 12 m^2; to be used by time sharing)	24
IPD—wards, HDU, daycare	
Inpatient wards—One 30 bed ward (@ m^2 per bed)	240
High dependency unit (HDU)—One 06 beds unit (@ 14 m^2 per bed). This should be an integrated part of ward complex and share ancillary services with ward	84
Inpatient rehabilitation care needs would be fulfilled by the physical medicine and rehabilitation medicine department of the hospital with which this facility is integrated. In case of standalone facility, this unit will need to be provided	
Daycare facility—A daycare facility of 10 beds is to be provided for carrying out short-admissions (up to 6–8 hours) for monitoring patients	80
Hyperbaric oxygen therapy (HBOT)	16
Support services area	
Lab common area—(Figures in parenthesis show area in m^2)—reception (15), specimen collection (10), specimen reception and sorting (12), stores (10), cleanup/sterilization (12), staff change room (6), toilets (staff—4 and patients—14, waiting (15), Office (10)	
Diagnostic facilities for biochemistry only (Office—12, Lab—30)	42
Radioimmunoassay, hormone assay lab (RAI Lab)	30
Bone density (DEXA scan)	15
Foot lab—Biothesiometry facility including Doppler (7), monofilament test (7), EMD (7), electronic podometer, electronic baro-pedometer (7), podoscope/luminoscope (7)	35
Medical record	16
Footwear manufacturing unit for special footwear (only if considered essential and space can be provided)	25

Table 3: DEXA scan data sheet.

System weight	*353 kg (Approx); varies depending upon the model*
Power	100-127 V/200-240 V; must meet IEEE 519-1992 standards
Temperature/humidity	18–27°C (65–81°F) 45 ± 5
Heat output	150 BTU per hour when idle; 1500 BTU per hour when actively scanning; The host PC (PC with 17 inch monitor) will output approximately 400 BTU per hour when powered on
Radiation	Only AERB type approved equipment to be use. Opearator must be minimum 1 m away from scanning table
AERB licensing requirements	Layout for installation of X-ray unit, valid NOC/Type approval, RSO approval, list of protective accessories, list of qualified/trained personnel with TLD badge numbers, QA report

Table 4: HVAC system data sheet.

Area	*Air pressure*	*Air changes per hour*	*Relative humidity (%)*	*Temperature (°C)*
Outpatient	Normal pressure	8–10	45 ± 5	24 ± 2 - 27 ± 2
Ward/daycare	Positive	6–8	45 ± 5	22 ± 2 - 29 ± 2
Pantry (ward)	Negative	10	45 ± 5	25 ± 2 - 29 ± 2
Disposal room (ward)	Negative	10	45 ± 5	25 ± 2 - 29 ± 2
HBOT	Positive	6–8	45 ± 5	22 ± 2 - 25 ± 2
Lab services	Negative except in biochemistry	6–8	45 ± 5	22 ± 2 - 27 ± 2

Table 5: Lighting data sheet.

Area	*Light intensity*
OPD patient area	300 lux
OPD corridor and waiting area	200 lux
Ward nursing station	300 lux
Ward corridor	200 lux
Ward support area	200 lux
Daycare	300 lux
Administrative areas	200–300 lux
Lab and DEXA scan	500–300 lux
HDU clinical observation	500 lux
HDU patient care area	300 lux
HDU corridor	200 lux
BOT	500 lux

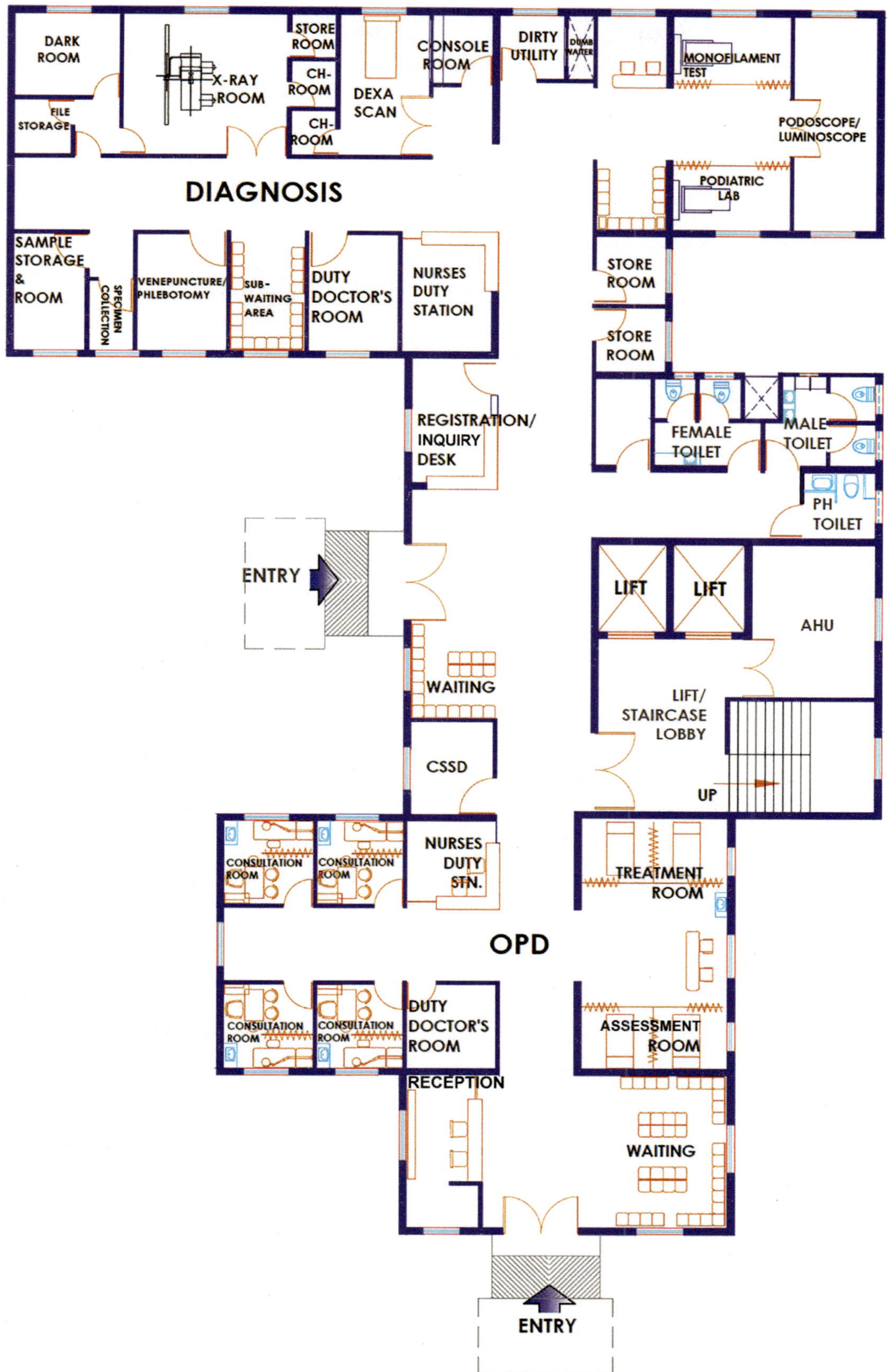

Fig. 13: Ground floor plan.

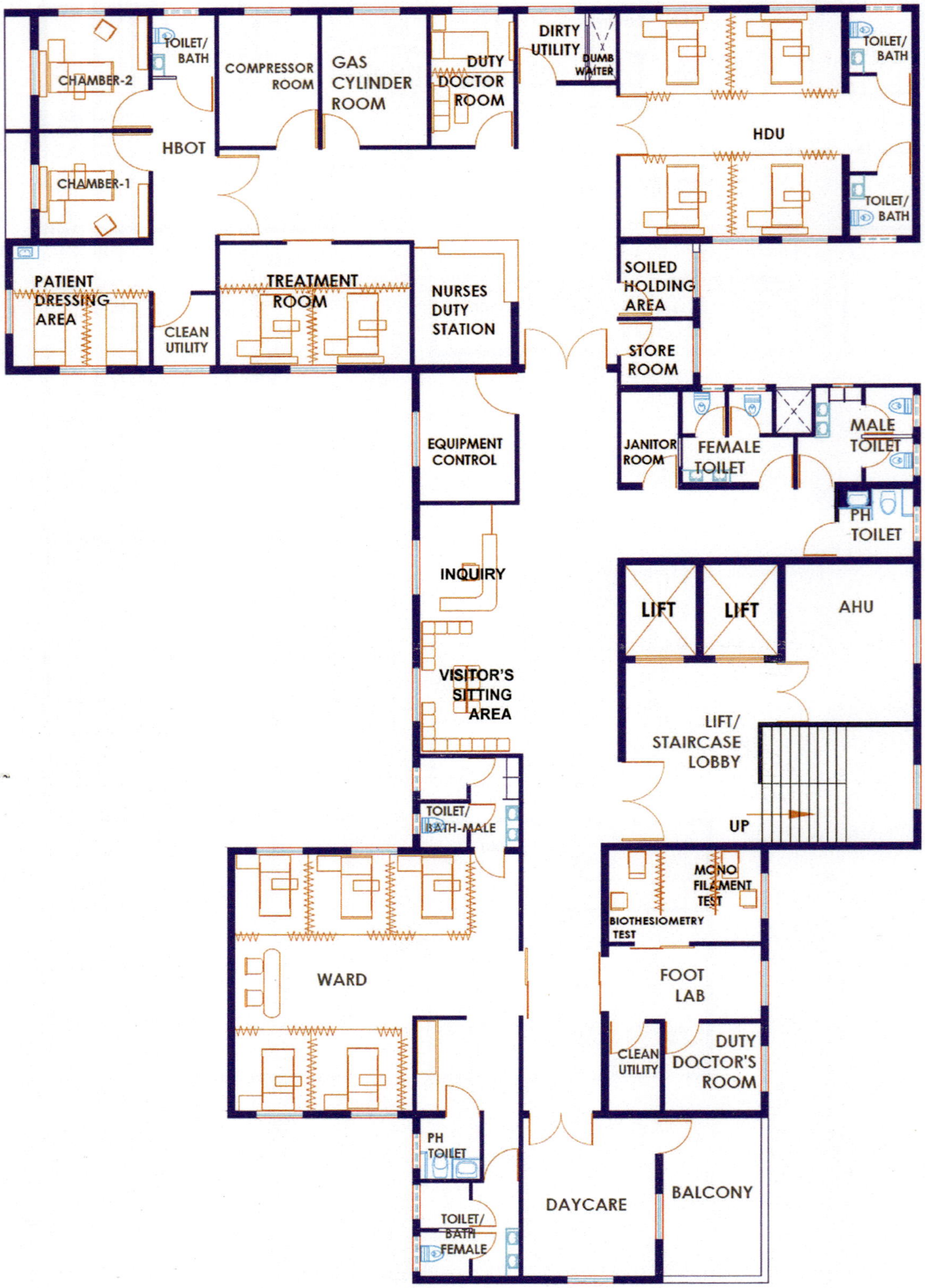

Fig. 14: First floor plan.

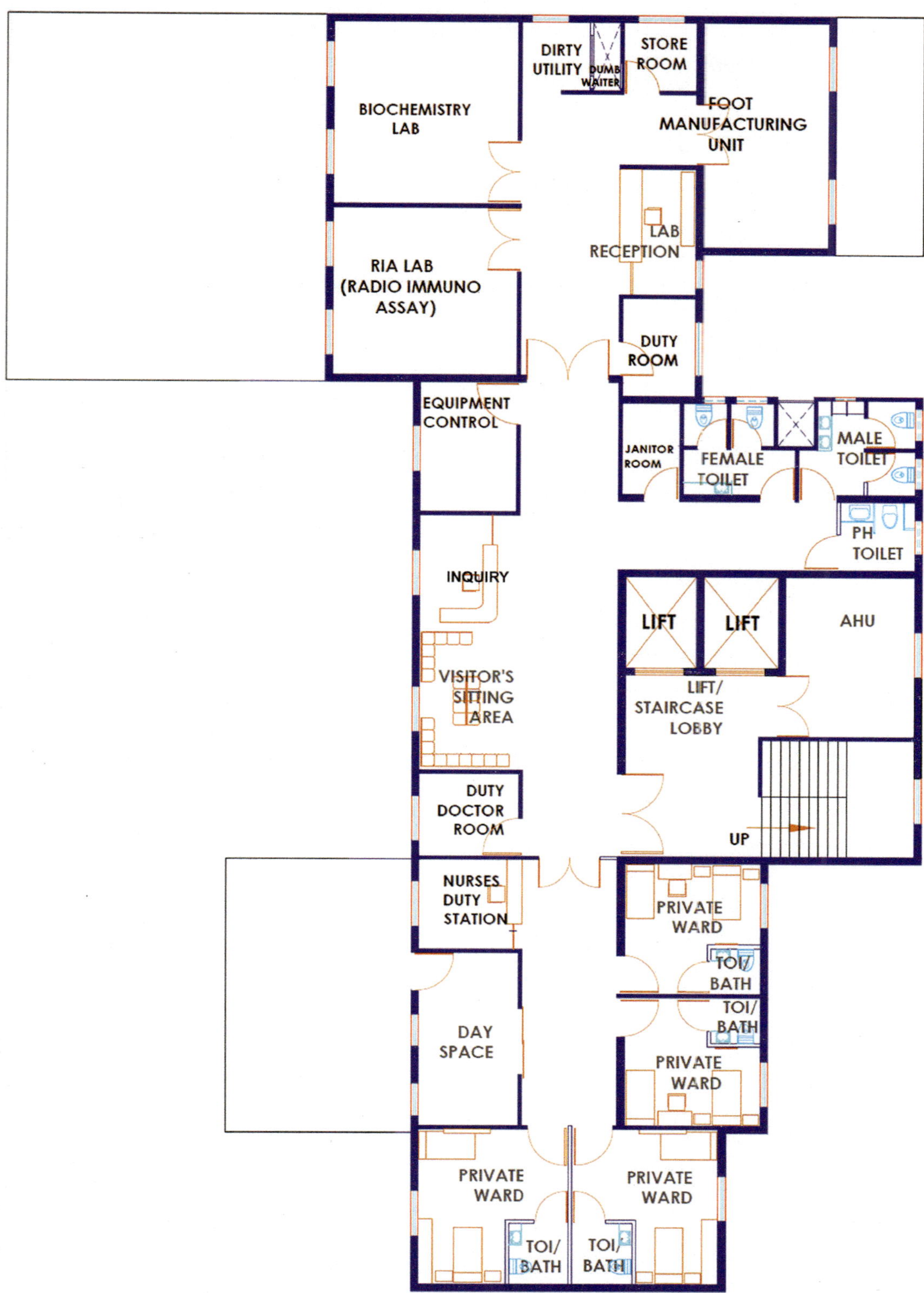

Fig. 15: Second floor plan.

REFERENCES

1. Golden SH, Robinson KA, Saldanha I, et al. Prevalence and Incidence of Endocrine and Metabolic Disorders in the United States: A Comprehensive Review. J Clin Endocrinol Metab, 2009;94(6):1853-878.
2. jcem.endojournals.org
3. www.mvdiabetes.com
4. Guidelines for Design and Construction of Health Care Facilities. The Facility Guidelines Institute, Dallas Texas. 2006;pp.96-76.
5. www.fgiguidelines.org
6. www.aerb.gov.in
7. Guidelines to setup RIA Lab, AERB, India
8. Wood, Wayne. "Laboratory Safety", Handbook of Modern Hospital Safety Second Edition, 2009
9. www.mvdiabeticfoot.com
10. Noyce JO, Michels H, Keevil CW. Potential use of copper surfces to reduce survival of epidemic Methicilin-resistant Staphylococcus aureus in the healthcare environment. J. Infec. 2006;63(3):289-97.
11. Maraisa F, Mehtar S, Chalkleya L. Antimicorbial efficacy of copper touch surface in reducing environmental bioburden in a South African community healthcare facility. J Hosp Infec. 2010;74(1):80-20.
12. International Plumbing Code 2009 [Accessed from www.iccsafe.org on 24 Jul 2012].
13. Central Public Works Department Specifications 2009, Volume 2.
14. Manual on norms and standards for environment clearance of large construction projects, Ministry of Environment & Forests, Govt of India [Accessed from http://envfor.nic.in/divisions/iass/Construction_Manual.pdf on 22 Jul 2012]

CHAPTER 26

Respiratory Medicine Facility

Surajeet Kr Barua, Shakti Kumar Gupta, Sunil Kant, R Chandrashekhar

INTRODUCTION

A standalone Respiratory Medicine center offers emergency management of patients with respiratory problems requiring intubation, mechanical ventilation (IMV) as well as noninvasive ventilation (NIV); inpatient care and outpatient reviews and investigations for patients with a range of problems associated with their lungs.

Clinical Procedures Involved in Respiratory Medicine

- Laboratory investigation of blood (blood tests). Sometimes arterial blood gas measurements are also required.[1]
- Spirometry (the determination of lung volumes in time by breathing into a dedicated machine; response to bronchodilators and diffusion of carbon monoxide).[1]
- Bronchoscopy with bronchoalveolar lavage (BAL), endobronchial and transbronchial biopsy and epithelial brushing.[1]
- Chest X-rays
- Computed tomography (CT) scanning (Magnetic resonance imaging (MRI) scanning is rarely used).
- Scintigraphy and other methods of nuclear medicine
- Positron emission tomography (especially in lung cancer)
- Polysomnography (PSG) (sleep studies) commonly used for the diagnosis of sleep apnea.

FUNCTION

The importance of this field of medicine has received new attention on an urgent basis with the fast pace of industrialization and urbanization, which has led to environmental and atmospheric pollution, thereby causing a myriad of respiratory diseases.[2]

Special Feature of a Respiratory Medicine Unit—The Noninvasive Intermediate Respiratory Intensive Care Unit (Fig. 1)

An intermediate Respiratory Intensive Care Unit (RICU) or noninvasive respiratory care unit is an area for monitoring and treating patients with acute or exacerbated respiratory failure caused by a disease that is primarily respiratory. The essential aim is adequate and appropriate cardiorespiratory monitoring and/or treatment of insufficiency by NIV. A RICU (Fig. 2) also provides continuous monitoring of patients after thoracic surgery or of those undergoing invasive IMV through tracheostomy and treats critical patients whose weaning from IMV is difficult. NIV or noninvasive monitoring techniques should be the main therapeutic approaches of such a unit.[2]

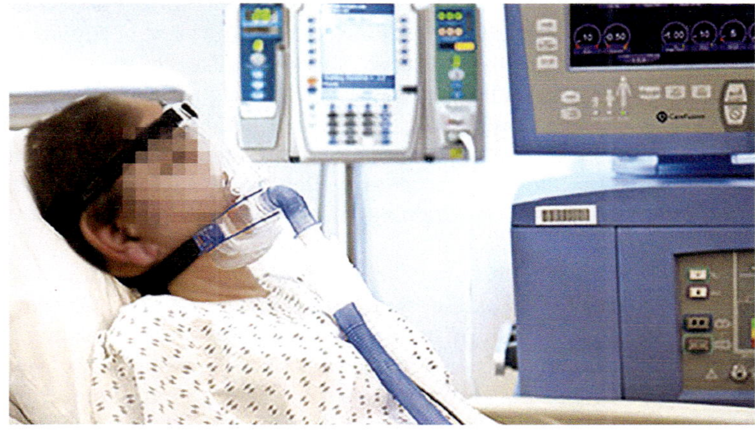

Fig. 1: Noninvasive intermediate respiratory intensive care unit.

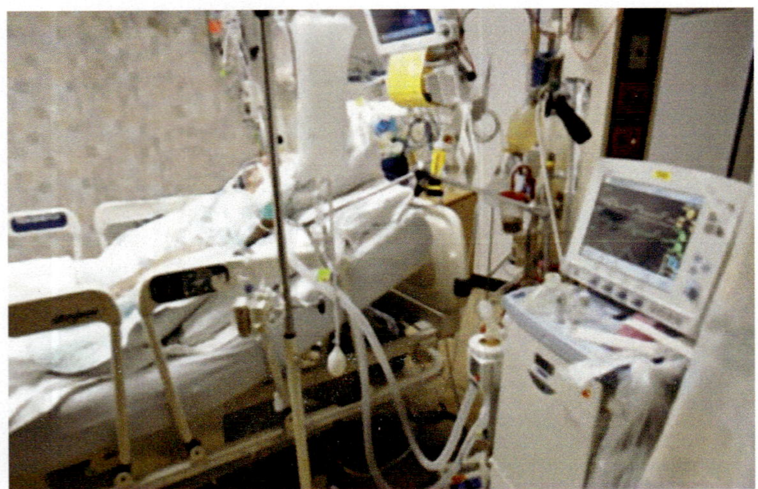

Fig. 2: Respiratory intensive care unit.

A RICU is designed to care for respiratory patients whose illness is at a level of severity that is intermediate between that which requires intensive care unit (ICU) facilities and that which can be managed on a conventional ward. Therefore, the function of a RICU is essentially for monitoring severely ill respiratory patients noninvasively and providing better weaning from IMV.[2]

KEY PLANNING AND DESIGN CONSIDERATIONS

Intermediate Respiratory Intensive Care Unit Location and Infrastructure

Currently, there are no guidelines or standards describing the best placement, configuration or makeup of RICUs. Since admitted patients have respiratory diseases and the main treatment is NIV, the responsible physicians should be pneumologists and the support staff should come from a pneumology department.[2]

Various locations have been proposed for hospital RICUs:

- *Independent location*: This model has the advantage of greater operating independence and adequate support for numerous patients, given that mixed cases will be better managed. The unit should have good access to the respiratory medicine department and/or the ICU. The main disadvantage of this model is loss of efficiency if the RICU is small or if large units have low occupancy. For RICUs following this model, staff and space use is less integrated and, hence, less flexible, possibly leading to higher costs.[2]
- *Parallel model*: Locating an intermediate RICU adjacent to an ICU offers greater privacy for the RICU patient and allows for greater flexibility, both in terms of team availability and rotation of staff between the two units. The main disadvantage is low occupancy for large RICUs.[2]
- *Integrated model*: A RICU that forms a part of the ICU or a pneumology ward, within a more or less specifically dedicated space, offers the advantage of continuity of patient care within the same department or unit and facilitates transfers when a patient's condition improves or worsens. This arrangement also offers integration of medical, nursing, physical therapy, auxiliary and administrative personnel. A disadvantage is that workloads are highly variable in terms of complexity, calling for adjustments in nursing assignments. Other constraints that can arise are high costs for equipment per bed and for staff training. A variation of this last model would be a RICU that is adjacent to and functionally integrated with a sleep laboratory. Such spaces have resources with which to monitor breathing that are not normally used during the day. Since intermediate RICUs specialize in NIV, these spaces can be used as a day hospital for initiating home ventilation in certain chronically-ill patients and for monitoring chronically ventilated patients to diagnose and solve problems that arise during home respiratory therapy. Some monitoring resources available in sleep laboratories can also be used for patients admitted to RICUs. This model facilitates the integration of NIV for acute conditions and for home respirator titration. Although integrating an intermediate RICU into a pneumology ward is the usual pattern, such placement will depend on a hospital's characteristics.[2]

LAYOUT

General Considerations

Safety and Risk Reduction[3]

- *Plan to control cross infection*:
  - *Hand washing and controlled access*: To enhance infection control, hand washing station is to be ensured and circulation paths organized so that entrances to invasive procedure rooms are from a non-public, controlled access corridor.[3]
  - *Avoid clean/dirty circulation conflicts*: System to avoid circulation conflicts between patients and service traffic and between soiled and clean areas.
- *Adequate visualization of patients*: Where prep and recovery are required for invasive procedures, well-planned locations of nurse work areas will support this objective since caregivers will be closer to patients during pre- and post-procedure. For bronchoscopy and pulmonary test and exam areas, nurse positions are to be planned to observe patient waiting and travel to exam and test areas.[3]
- *Specific materials and finishes that enhance infection control to be used*: Use materials, finishes and casework that resist microbe growth and are easily cleaned. Specify antimicrobial materials and finishes to the greatest extent possible. Minimize seams in floor and wall finishes and at floors to walls. To limit dust accumulation, avoid horizontal surfaces which are not work surfaces. Provide storage for all unpackaged items in enclosed casework.[3]
- *Fully integrated electronic medical records*: Implementation of electronic medical records with established protocols for their use. Electronic tools reduce risk and raise efficiency. This promotes quick access to comprehensive records, including imaging and test results, and consistency of patient documentation across all services. Benefits include the ability to locate nurses closer to patients and enhance opportunities for more time with patients. Space efficiency benefits include a decreased need for records storage, both at departmental service locations and at central storage spaces.

Efficiency and Flexibility

Standardization of key room plans, so that items like equipment and sharp containers are always in the same location in procedure rooms, can reduce errors and speed services as staff provides care in different rooms. Where size permits, planning of procedure areas, adjacent to each other with appropriate links, will provide an opportunity to share resources among two or more services. Shared resources can include prep and recovery, waiting, linen storage, housekeeping, general storage, waste storage and staff support areas.[3]

Planning Accommodates Program Growth

Planning for larger scale long-term growth for key program components should be identified early in the design process. Space needed to accommodate projected growth can be addressed by first identifying the ideal direction for planned growth to occur. For procedure platforms where there is often a service access corridor parallel to a patient access corridor on opposite sides of the procedure rooms, the growth direction would be in the direction of the long axis (i.e. the direction of the service and patient access corridors). At the end, furthest from patient access to the procedures platform, locate "soft" or nonclinical program space, such as offices or storage, since they can most easily be relocated to permit conversion of the space to accommodate clinical growth needs (Fig. 3).[3]

Response to Human Needs

Patient dignity and self-determination must be accommodated while considering operational efficiencies. Besides this, patients' vulnerability to stress from noise, lack of privacy, poor lighting, and other causes, and the subsequent harmful effects they can have on the healing process to be taken care of.[3]

Functional Considerations

Pulmonary medicine service incorporates a range of examinations, investigations and procedures, all of which require specific planning consideration.[3]

Functional Organization

This service is usually organized into eight functional areas:[3]

- Reception area
- Pulmonary medicine/respiratory care patient area which includes:
  - Pulmonary function testing (PFT) with related rooms
  - Bronchoscopy, an invasive procedure examining upper airway function
  - Sleep study area which examines breathing and other biophysiological issues related to sleeping.
- Bronchoscopy patient area
- Sleep study patient area
- *Support area*: Pulmonary medicine/respiratory care
- Prep and recovery area
- Staff and administrative area
- Education area.

Functional Relationships

- *Reception area*[3]
  - Reception area accommodates the initial processing and admission of all scheduled and unscheduled outpatients. These areas include registration functions, waiting, and opportunities for patient education. The reception control area should be strategically located to give the receptionist clear observation of waiting areas to facilitate control of outpatient traffic entering the suite and secure the department from unauthorized access. On the day of the procedure, ambulatory patients will register at the reception area. Functional considerations include location of workstation monitor screens to protect patient information, access to lockable files, and accessibility-compliant workstations. Outpatient processing areas should be separate from inpatient circulation and holding areas when both outpatients and inpatients use the same exam rooms.
  - The consultation room should be located adjacent to the waiting room.
  - When possible, access to natural daylight, views of nature, and other positive distractions should be provided to improve the human experience in these spaces.
  - For smaller size services, sharing functions associated with reception and waiting with other similar and adjacent services should be considered on a per facility basis.
- *Pulmonary medicine/respiratory medicine patient care area*[3]
  - The primary function in this area is to test respiratory function.
- *Test rooms include:*[3]
  - Testing laboratory pulmonary function
  - Testing laboratory extended pulmonary function
  - Physiology laboratory pulmonary exercise, which includes a treadmill for exercise testing.
  - In or adjacent to this area, a walking area should be provided for a 6-minute walking test, which includes marked distance measurements.

  Patients can move directly from the waiting room to the test room and return for post-test consultation or discharge. The consultation room should be located between waiting and the exam and test rooms.
- *Bronchoscopy patient area*: The primary function in this area is to provide bronchoscopy procedures, an invasive procedure which includes the need for mild sedation. The room includes special equipment accommodated on articulated ceiling-mounted booms to keep the floor area around the procedure table as clear as possible of equipment and cables for unimpeded provider access. The room is organized with a centrally-located patient stretcher under a dual articulated arm ceiling-mounted boom system, specifically designed to support medical equipment. One arm includes an equipment carrier for endoscopic imaging equipment with provisions for medical gases, data, video, and print capabilities for use with fiberoptic (direct vision) endoscopes and power outlets. This system takes optical images from a single endoscope and directly records them or converts them to digital signals for recording. The other arm supports a flat screen monitor for video and data displays.[3]

  Several clean scopes can be stored in a cabinet in the room in addition to the storage area listed in support area below. An electrosurgical unit is accommodated in each room for sterile therapeutic interventions using argon plasma coagulation.[3]

  The room is best organized with a patient access side providing direct access from/to prep and recovery, and a service access side, with a door to a service corridor accessing the equipment cleaning room.[3]
- *Sleep study patient area (Fig. 4)*: This area, often called a sleep laboratory, includes monitoring over unusually long test times. It should be located in a quiet zone away from other clinic and hospital activity. Patients who require sleep laboratory testing generally

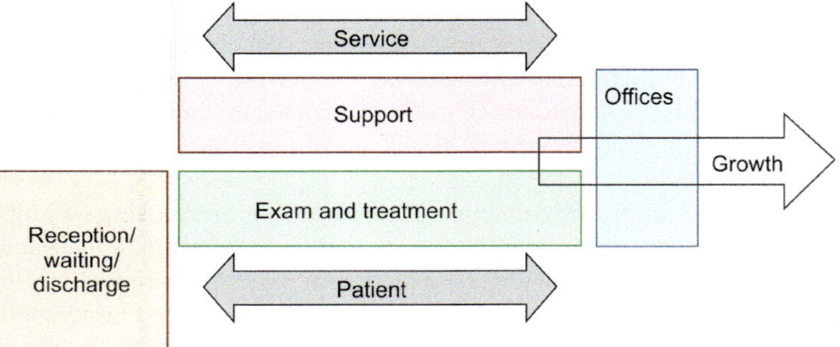

Fig. 3: Functional planning spaces.

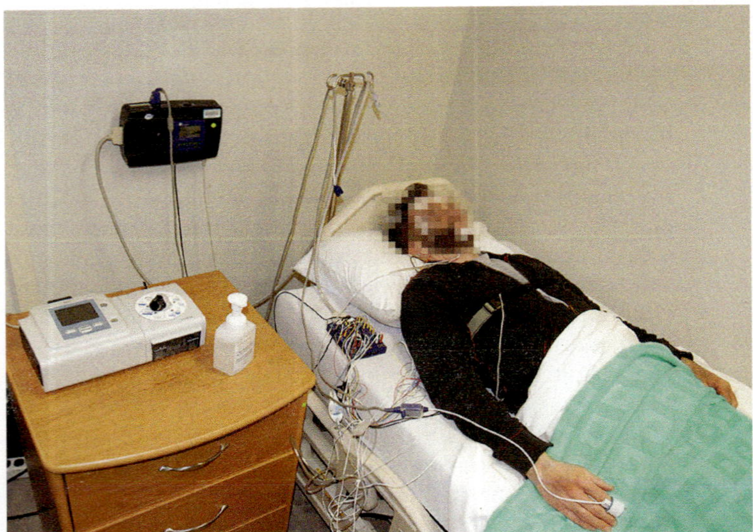

Fig. 4: Sleep laboratory area.

access the test area after normal clinic hours and go directly from waiting to the sleep study prep room.[3]

Sleep study patients are prepped in the prep room with the application of electrodes before entering the sleep study room. The sleep study room is organized like a normal bedroom with a bed, side table, wardrobe and chair. A private patient toilet is directly accessed from the room.[3]

The suite of tests used in sleep studies is called PSG (Fig. 5).

It is a comprehensive recording of the biophysiological changes that occur during sleep. While usually performed at night, when most people sleep, some labs can accommodate people with circadian rhythm sleep disorders and do the test at other times of the day.

The PSG monitors many body functions during sleep including (Fig. 6):[3]

- Brain, using electroencephalography (EEG)
- Eye movements, using electrooculography (EOG)
- Muscle activity or skeletal muscle activation, using electromyography (EMG)
- Heart rhythm, using echocardiography (ECG).

A polysomnogram will typically record a minimum of twelve channels requiring a minimum of 22 wire attachments to the patient. These channels vary in every laboratory and may be adapted to meet the doctor's requests.[3]

Wires for each channel of recorded data lead from the patient and converge into a central box, which, in turn, is connected to a computer system for recording, storing and displaying the data. During sleep, the computer monitor can display multiple channels continuously. In addition, there is a small infrared video camera in the room, so a technician can observe the patient on a monitor from the sleep study monitoring room.[3]

The sleep study monitoring room accommodates the providers and technicians running the tests. The room includes the PSG printer, the monitor for patient viewing and a computer. The room and its equipment can be used to monitor up to four multiple sleep study room tests simultaneously. Other spaces include a nourishment room for patients and staff, a clean linen storage room, and a housekeeping aides closet.[3]

- *Support Area*:
  - *General*: Support functions include rooms for gas cylinder storage and ventilator storage. Gas cylinder storage must be provided with two rooms—one for full and one for empty cylinders.[3]

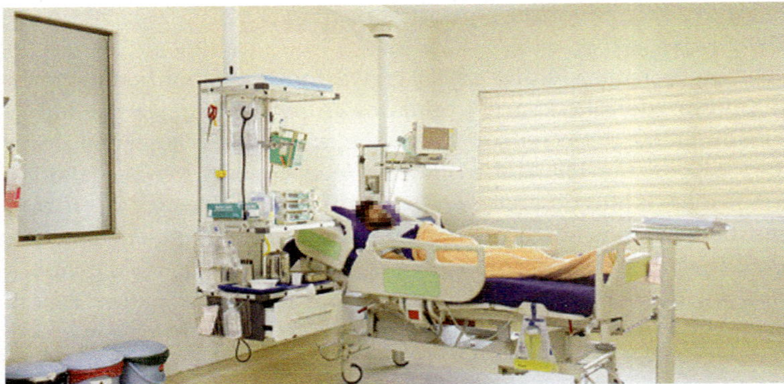

Fig. 5: Polysomnography.

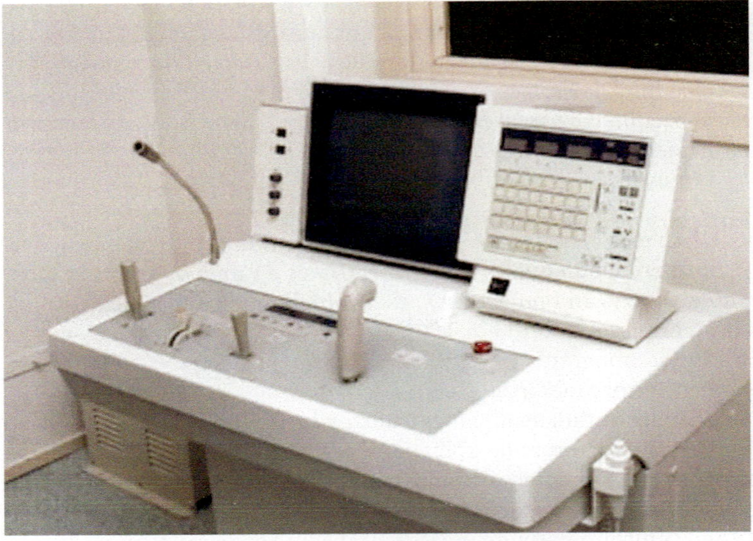

Fig. 6: Polysomnography monitors body functions.

- *Bronchoscopy patient area*: Equipment cleaning room where scopes are cleaned and packaged for transport to the sterile processing department (SPD) for reprocessing.[3]
  - Respiratory therapy room where instruments and components for pulmonary tests are stored, tracked, tested and adjusted.
  - Storage room for argon plasma coagulation equipment
  - Storage room for C-arm equipment
  - Storage room for other equipment
  - Housekeeping aides closet
  - Soiled and clean utility rooms.
- *Sleep study patient area*: Soiled and clean utility rooms should be provided.
- *Prep and recovery area*: Prep and recovery is the bridge for patients between public areas and the controlled environment that supports the bronchoscopy invasive procedures area. It is comprised of patient rooms or cubicles, depending on facility needs and monitored from a nurse station. Rooms are different from cubicles because they include sliding glass doors which permit visibility with acoustic privacy.[3]

A nurse station provides positions for nurse monitoring of prep and recovery positions as well as work and charting areas. This space should be located to provide visualization of patient positions in prep and recovery and permit nurses to monitor patients who may be agitated both pre- and post-procedure, and may become unstable postprocedure. Nurses also monitor patient movement to and from procedure rooms.

In prep and recovery areas with many patient positions, to reduce nurse travel and enhance nurse visibility of patients, nurse stations may be decentralized as long as the total program net sq ft for the function is not exceeded.[3]

Ergonomically designed work areas should be provided for all staff to reduce staff fatigue and support peak performance.

Inpatients will generally require preprocedure preparation in prep and recovery and are generally monitored in recovery before being returned to their room. Inpatients' status may be at a higher acuity level than outpatients and may require closer observation. For both reasons, rooms or cubicles in prep and recovery, which are slated for inpatients, pre- and post-procedure should be identified and allocated in close proximity to nurse positions.[3]

Prep and recovery includes support spaces within its area. These include medication and nourishment spaces, clean and soiled utility rooms, equipment storage room, and a housekeeping aides closet[3]

- *Staff and administrative areas*: Enclosed office spaces and technician cubicles shall be provided per number and sq ft authorized for the facility.

Key offices include those for:[3]

- Director of respiratory therapy
- Physician offices
- Nurse manager
- Chief technician
- Conference room.

Cubicles may be provided for:[3]

- Home care coordinator
- Polysomnographer
- Respiratory therapist
- Administration staff.

In planning for future flexibility of spaces, it is beneficial to plan for a modular (i.e. same size/same proportion) approach for offices to allow the spaces to be reallocated without significant reconfiguration. Access to and control of natural light should be considered in designing these spaces for staff satisfaction and stress reduction.[3]

Administrative areas include reading, interpretation, and consultation areas that are accessible to physicians and nursing staff and located near the procedure area.

The staff lounge and staff locker room are important as respite areas which reduce stress and enable staff to maintain a high level of quality service when clinics are active. The staff lounge should be conveniently located to staff work areas but separate from patient areas. Provision of a separate locker room from the staff lounge is desirable for staff privacy and noise reduction. Staff toilets should be located with immediate adjacency to the staff lounge but should not open into it. These staff support functions should be considered for sharing with other adjacent services as appropriate.[3]

- *Education area*: Spaces for education are required when a residency program is authorized. They include a conference/classroom, and office and cubicles for interns.

  Line diagram are shown in Figures 7 and 8.

Other Functional Considerations

General considerations: The planning approach should locate high volume short duration services closer to patient waiting areas. This will decrease patient travel time and distance and reduce staff travel time and distances permitting more staff time with patients. Procedures with low volume or longer duration time may be further inside patient areas.[3]

Technical Considerations

- *Architectural*:
  - *Interior design*: Key functional and design considerations include:[3]
    - ◊ Durability and cleanliness
    - ◊ A timeless quality for materials and colors
    - ◊ Creation of a distinctive, clear lead for the planning and selecting of furnishings and art.

  Elements which create nonfunctional horizontal surfaces, like decorative moldings, which become dirt catchers, or wall coverings that cannot be washed down, should be avoided.
  - *Way-finding*: It should become an integral part of the overall design. Examples of design strategies to achieve way-finding goals include:
    - ◊ Use of graphic signages
    - ◊ Use of specific color, pattern, or artwork cues for different components in a unit or service.
    - ◊ Use of artwork can signal a department entrance
    - ◊ Treat corridor ends and junctures as way-finding opportunities.[3]

  Where possible, corridor ends can be the sources of daylight or special graphic or color panels can be used to cue destination information from a distance.[3]
  - *Partitions*: Partitions should generally be gypsum wallboard. Provide sound attenuation and noise transmission control.[3]
  - *Corner guards*: Incorporate corner guards in corridors and other areas where the potential for wall damage from wheeled patient and cart traffic is anticipated.[3]
  - *Floors*: Floor finish for most spaces, including exam rooms, corridors and supply and storage spaces, should be a resilient tile with a high rubber base. Floors in all bronchoscopy procedure rooms should be welded seam resilient flooring with integral cove base manufactured specifically for invasive healthcare settings. For all clean and soiled utility rooms, decontamination, and clean storage rooms, floor finish should be welded seam resilient flooring (WSF) with integral cove base. Floors in toilet rooms should be porcelain tile with a porcelain tile base.[3]
  - *Ceilings*: In most spaces, including toilet rooms, lay-in acoustic ceiling tile should be used. Where required for sanitation or moisture resistance, such as in all bronchoscopy procedure rooms, clean and soiled utility rooms, decontamination, and clean scope storage rooms, acoustical ceiling tile should have a washable sprayed plastic finish
  - *Interior doors*: Doors should be 40 mm thick, solid core, flush wood doors or hollow metal doors in hollow metal frames. Hollow metal doors should be used where high impact is a concern and where fire rated doors are required. Door width of 1200 mm is recommended for all wheeled traffic and for bariatric wheelchair access to all patient spaces. Doors in the decontamination and clean scope storage rooms should be fully clad in solid vinyl guard sheets to allow for daily cleaning with chemical disinfectants.[3]
  - *Millwork*: Key locations, such as nurse stations and departmental reception points, will be well served with the use of custom millwork to respond to individual facility designs and configurations. Millwork should be used as an architectural encasement for standard modular components, such as files and

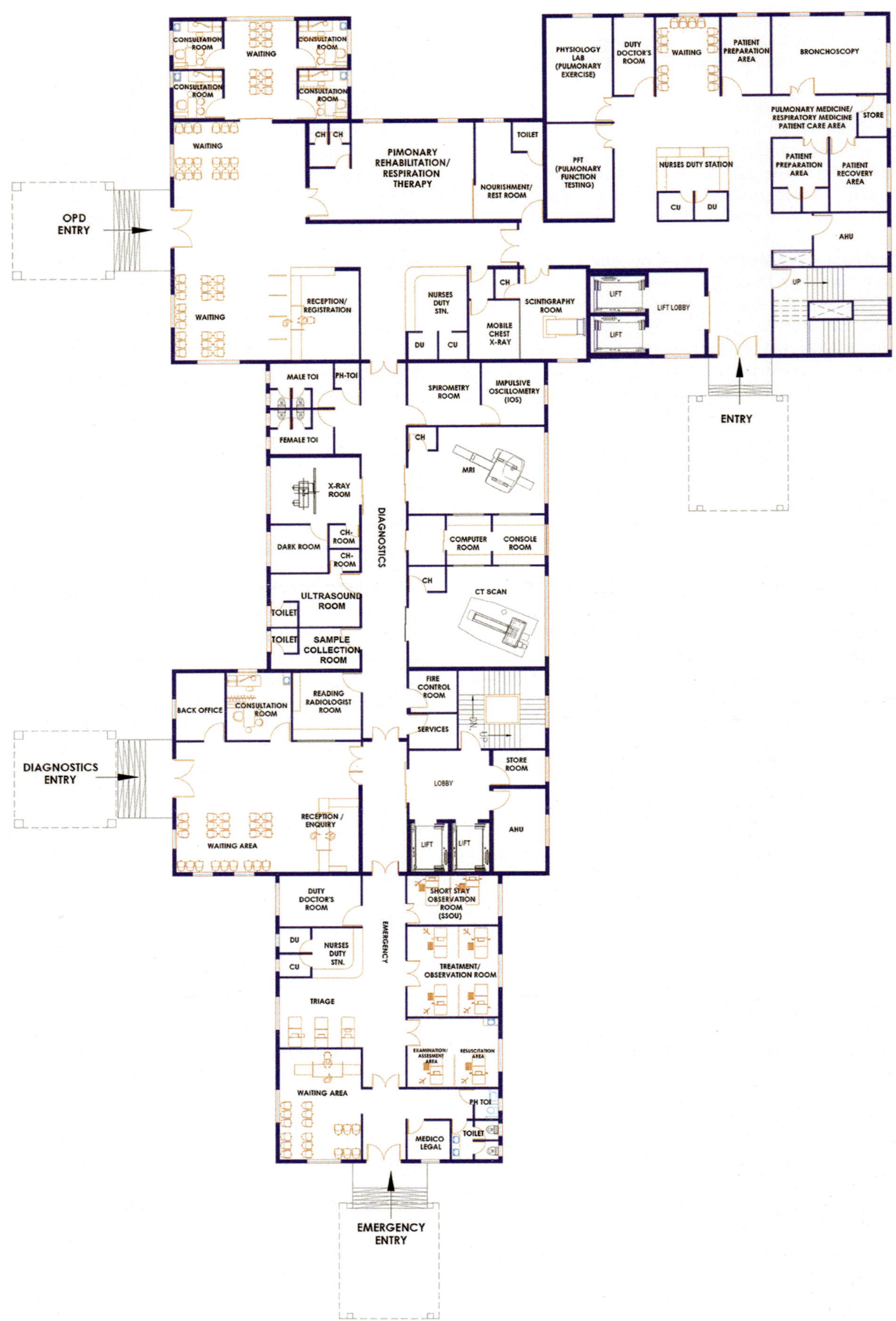

Fig. 7: Ground floor plan.

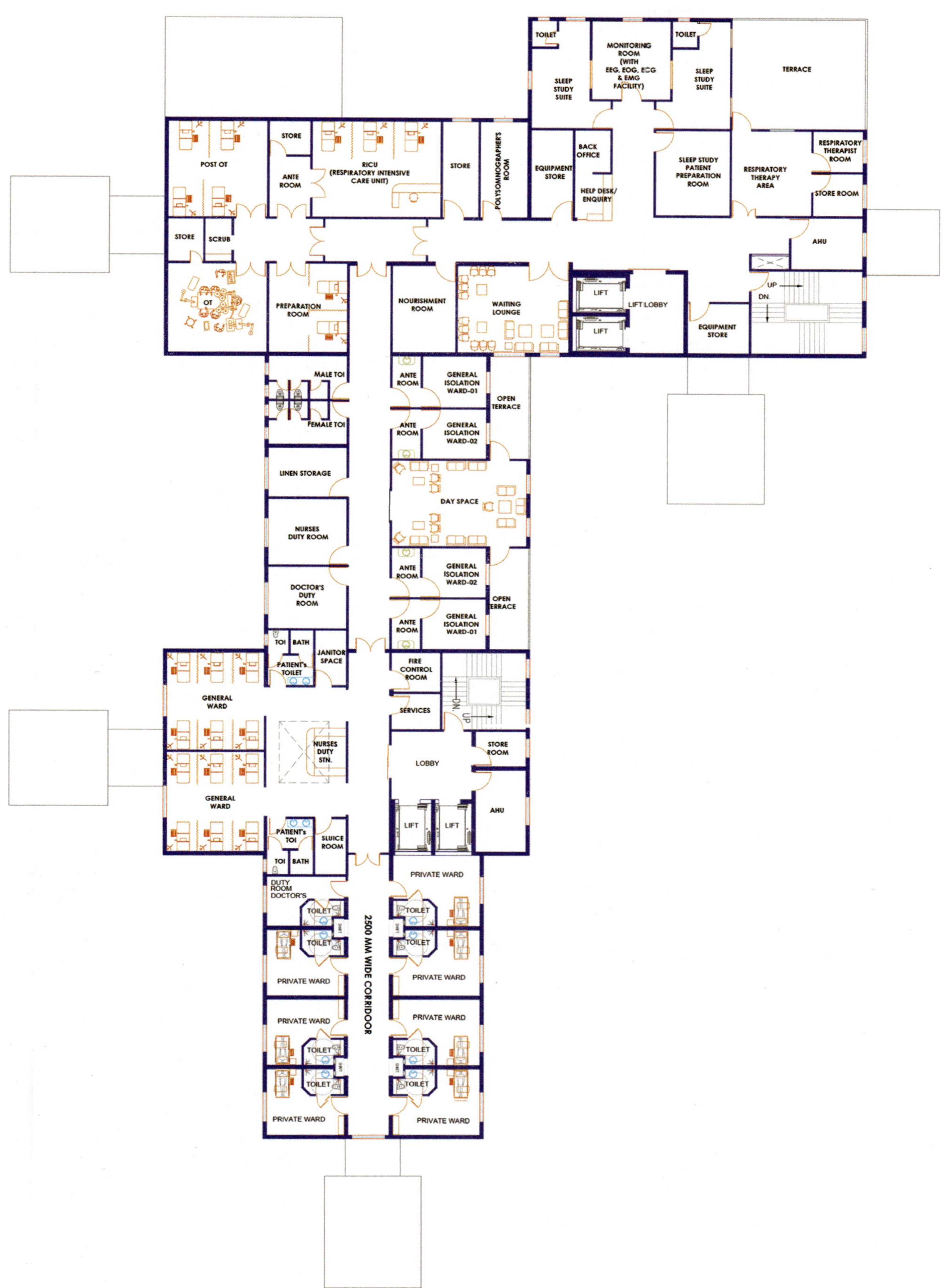

Fig. 8: First floor plan.

storage cabinets, which are listed in the equipment list for each relevant space. Millwork would provide both the transaction surface at stand up height as well as the work counter at normal desk height for a receptionist or nursing staff. Transaction counters should be made of solid mineral surface materials which resist chipping and staining. Work surfaces at desk height may be constructed of solid mineral surface materials or plastic laminate with flush let-in vinyl edges. Consider including task lighting built under the transaction counter. Coordinate locations of computers, printers, keyboards and power and data ports as required by facility needs.[3]

- *Structural:*[3]
  - *Reinforced concrete design*: Bronchoscopy rooms include ceiling-mounted booms which require structural framing above the ceiling to support them.
  - National Building Code
  - Bureau of Indian Standards for buildings
  - Seismic design requirements.
- *Equipment:*[3] Casework systems should be planned to avoid corner installations and filler panels.
- Information management systems
- *Heating, ventilation and air-conditioning:*[3]
  - *General*: Air-conditioning systems should be provided to heat, cool and ventilate the pulmonary medicine service as required.
  - *Air quality and distribution*: In general, clean areas should be maintained at positive air balance and soiled areas should be maintained at negative air balance with respect to adjoining areas. Bronchoscopy procedure rooms require negative air pressure to reduce the risk from airborne infectious agents. Specific pressure requirements are noted on the room data sheet for each guide plate room.

    Corridors should not be used to supply or exhaust/return air from adjacent rooms, except that they may be used to ventilate housekeeping aides closets (HACs) and small electrical or telephone closets opening directly onto them.

    Care should be taken to minimize the short-circuiting of air between supply and return or exhaust openings in rooms, with careful placement of supply registers and return grills inside rooms such as bronchoscopy procedure and pulmonary test rooms.
  - *Exhaust system:*[3] Controlling odor with proper exhaust is critical within the pulmonary medicine service. The HVAC design should provide for exhaust air from spaces to control the transfer of odors and provide proper room pressurization and proper air changes per hour. A dedicated exhaust system is required for spaces housing TB patients. The dedicated exhaust shall not be mixed with any other exhaust and should be discharged outdoors as per specifications.
  - *Mycobacterium tuberculosis (TB)*: Centers for disease control (CDC) requirements for the design of public areas within buildings which accommodate *Mycobacterium tuberculosis* patients must be addressed by architectural and mechanical disciplines.
- *Plumbing:*[3]
  - *General*: Plumbing systems should be provided for the pulmonary medicine service as required to satisfy.
  - *Water systems*: Domestic cold and hot water should be piped to all plumbing fixtures and equipment requiring these utilities. A hot water return system should be provided to ensure the design temperature is met at the fixture furthest from the source.
  - *Waste water systems:*[3] Plumbing fixtures and drains should be drained by gravity through sanitary waste stacks, including required vent stacks. Fixtures located below gravity drain line shall be pumped as required by a duplex ejector system. Any special acidic waste should be drained through corrosion-resistant, flame-retardant piping into either a local or centralized acid dilution tank.
  - *Medical gas systems:*[3] Specific quantities and locations should be determined on project basis.
- *Electrical:*
  - *General*
  - *Lighting*: Lighting is typically provided utilizing recessed fluorescent luminaires with acrylic prismatic lenses. Recessed fluorescent fixtures with parabolic louvers may be used at the nurse station, reception and offices to control glare on monitor screens. Consider providing under-cabinet or under-shelf fluorescent lights above counter work surfaces for task lighting. Lamps should not be of high output, and should have a minimum color rendering index (CRI) of 70 and a color temperature of 3500° Kelvin (K).

    Lighting in PFT laboratories should be controlled by ceiling mounted dual technology (ultrasonic/infrared) occupancy sensors. Lighting in pulmonary exercise physiology and bronchoscopy procedure rooms should be controlled by wall mounted dimmers located at the entrance to each room.

    Lighting load densities should be verified for the actual design, as they may vary depending on the room configuration, fixture types, lamps, and ballasts used.

    Supply power to selected light fixtures in physiology laboratory, pulmonary exercise and bronchoscopy procedure rooms from the critical branch of the emergency power system to allow for continued operation during a power failure. Emergency generators have to be provided.
- *Power:*[3]
  - *General*: Special receptacles are to be provided for select pieces of equipment. Emergency power outlets are also to be installed to allow for continuous operation during a power failure outage. Provide dedicated duplex receptacles energized from the emergency power system in areas where crash carts are stored.
  - *Special purpose*: Dedicated duplex or special receptacles are provided for select pieces of equipment in procedure room and bronchoscopy. Dedicated power outlets and outlets for emergency circuiting are mounted at service boom.
    Workstations with personal computers (PCs) are typically provided with quadruplex receptacles for the PC, monitor and printer. Junction boxes are to be provided for equipment requiring a hardwired connection.
  - *Telephone*: Telephone outlets are typically provided at each workstation or in each room.
  - *Information Technology (IT)*: Computer data (telecom) outlets are typically provided at each workstation or in each room.
  - *Nurse call and code one system*: The nurse call and code one systems should be PC-based, and consist of patient call stations, staff stations, duty stations, dome lights and head-end equipment located in signal closet. The actual system configuration is dependent on the overall layout of the department and should be coordinated with the functional design.
  - *Television*: Television outlets are provided at the select areas as determined by function or local facility policy.

- *Public address system*: The public address system is usually part of the telephone system. Speakers are generally located in corridors and public spaces as per the overall design layout and functional requirements. The pulmonary medicine service may/may not have an independent PA system depending with the policies of the institution. Determine whether pulmonary medicine will be included as part of the hospital-wide or clinic-wide PA system or have an independent system.

- *Fire and life safety systems*:[3]
  - *Fire protection/sprinkler systems*: Fire protection/sprinkler systems should be designed as per the fire safety norms of the state and as required to meet the needs of the pulmonary medicine service and individual rooms. Fire/smoke alarm systems should be designed as required to meet the needs of the pulmonary medicine service and individual rooms.
- *Waste management*:[3] Space requirements for waste holding areas will vary with the selection of waste collection and recycling methods and systems, and need to be analyzed to determine the method to be considered for new facilities or coordinated with existing facilities.
  - *General and biomedical waste*: Biomedical waste is generated in most patient care spaces as well as instrument clean up areas where it is segregated, collected and transported to the soiled utility rooms. There, it is held in separate containers pending transport to the medical waste handling facility or disposal by contract.
  - *Recyclable waste*: Methods for sorting, collecting, transporting and disposing of recyclable products must be specifically analyzed for each facility and location. The optional use of disposable and reusable products is an important consideration in recycling and waste disposal alternatives.
  - *Reusable medical equipment (RME)*: Reusable utensils and instruments which are used in patient care areas are handled in different ways within the pulmonary medicine service. For pulmonary function test rooms, they are precleaned on the unit in a decontamination Room for bronchoscopy procedures, they are pre-cleaned on the unit in an equipment cleaning room. For all other areas, they are precleaned in a soiled utility room. Utensils and instruments which require sterilization prior to reuse are packaged for transport from their precleaning areas. Specific protocols for utensil and instrument reprocessing shall be confirmed with each individual facility.
  - *Soiled linen*: Soiled reusable linens will be generated in examination rooms, procedure rooms, sleep study rooms, and patient and staff gowning areas. Soiled linens are collected in carts or hampers (depending on volume) and are held in soiled linen rooms or in linen carts in soiled utility rooms pending transport to the laundry facility. Disposable linens are included with recyclable waste or biomedical waste as appropriate.

CONCLUSION

Respiratory related ailments are on the rise. It is essential that specialized facilities related to management of these are constructed. These will enable appropriate processes to be implemented and consequently result in optimum outcomes.

REFERENCES

1. www.medicalexpert.com
2. Intermediate Respiratory Intensive Care Working Group of the Spanish Society of Pulmonology and Thoracic Surgery (SEPAR). "Intermediate Respiratory Intensive Care Units: Definitions and Characteristics", Archivos de Bronconeumologia (Internet), 200509.
3. www.cfm.va.gov

OTHER REFERENCES

- http://www.archbronconeumol.org/en/unidades-cuidados-respiratorios-intermedios-definicion/articulo/13079312/
- http://www.cfm.va.gov/til/dGuide/dgPulmonary.pdf
- www.wbdg.org

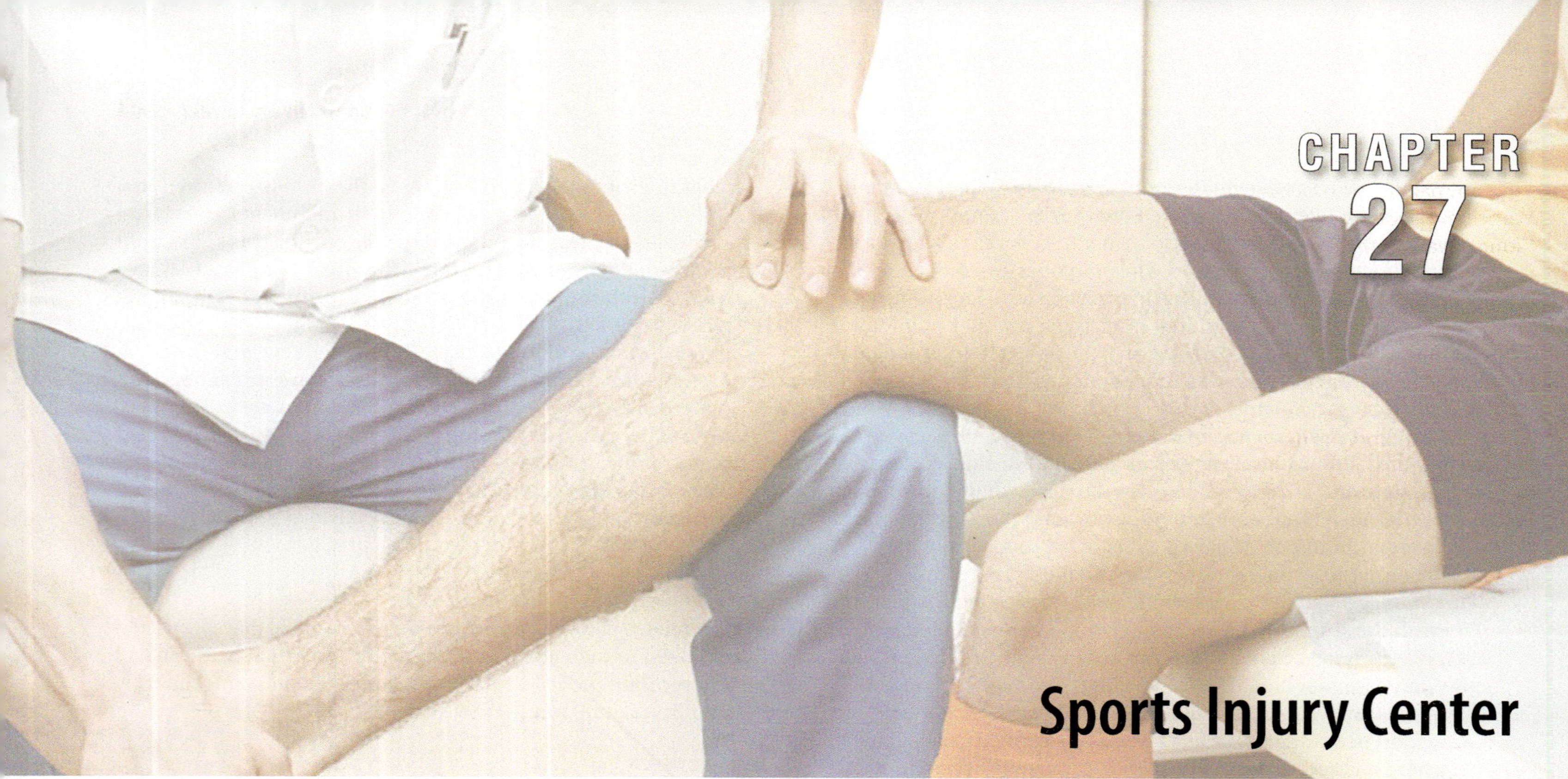

Sports Injury Center

Anki Reddy Jangamreddy, Shakti Kumar Gupta, Sunil Kant, R Chandrashekhar

INTRODUCTION

The injuries which result from acute trauma or repetitive stress associated with athletic activities are defined as sports injuries. Sports injuries can affect bones or soft tissues (ligaments, muscles, and tendons). Many types of injuries that affect athletes may also occur in workers in certain occupations; for example, many people in the building trades develop tennis elbow or golfer's elbow. The principles of sports medicine can be applied in the treatment of most common musculoskeletal injuries.[1,2]

Sports medicine endeavors to achieve following goals:
- Maintenance of health and physiological function
- Improvement of performance
- Prevention of injuries through training and education
- Treatment and rehabilitation from injuries.

A sports injury center is, thus, needed for providing comprehensive surgical, rehabilitative and diagnostic services under one roof for specialized treatment of sports and related joint disorders. The benefits would not be limited only to the sports persons but would also be extended to general patients sustaining similar and related joint injuries. The sports injury center is a permanent asset and besides catering to the needs of the sports person, will continue to provide its specialized services to the general patients sustaining similar injuries and disorders as well.[3,4]

FUNCTIONS OF SPORTS INJURY CENTER

The goal of a sports injury center is to improve bodily function and quality of life through provision of the best possible physical therapy assessment and treatment. It is done by thorough assessment to achieve accurate diagnosis prior to initiating treatment. Then the treatment decisions are chosen to select the most appropriate treatment for a particular problem. The sports injury center covers all types of sports injuries of all varieties including fresh and recurring injuries:
- Manual physiotherapy
- Rehabilitation exercise routines.

The main functions of a sports injury center can be summarized as management of the following:[5-7]
- Soft tissue injuries
- Muscles, tendons and ligaments
- Disorders of the back and neck
- Back and neck pain, sciatica, disk prolapse, osteoarthritis
- Rehabilitation postsurgery
- Cartilage or ligament repair, discectomy
- Whiplash injuries
- Muscular tension and headaches
- Work-related repetitive strain and overuse injuries
- Postural dysfunction
- Fitness and training programs
- Shoe assessments and advice
- Electrotherapy and core stability programs.

GENERAL PLANNING CONSIDERATIONS[8-10]

User Mix

A sports medicine center's users are at any given time associated with one particular function of the center, be it physical therapy, fitness training, testing or medical treatment. Thus, the same facility must accommodate a variety of needs simultaneously.

Convenient Access

A center that is conveniently located, visible from the street, and easily accessible from the parking area will both enhance its marketing plan objective and meet users' expectations for convenience. A physical therapy patient, who faces an intensive 6- or 8-week course of treatment, may be discouraged by difficult access or parking that involves too long a walk to the building entrance.

Flexibility and Future Expansion

The need to create flexible healthcare environments has never been greater. Flexibility can be increased by using:[8]

- 'Open plan' construction system
- Demountable partition systems
- Standard sized rooms for consulting, treatment, counseling, etc.
- Locations which can grow laterally
- Just in time (JIT) stock systems can be employed to alleviate floor pressures.[8]

Synergy with Local Climate and Vernacular Architecture

Although, India is a tropical country, the extremes of weather make this a very important factor. Due to harsh and long summers and humid monsoons, most hospitals have to be air-conditioned to provide proper comfort.

Visual Impact of Hospital

Primarily, the architectural inputs to the design will affect the visual impact of the hospital. It is important for the architect to amalgamate both the science and art components of architecture, so as to meet the functional requirements in an esthetic manner.

Natural Light

Sunlight enhances color and shape, and helps to make a room bright and cheerful. Wherever possible, spaces to be occupied by patients, visitors or staff should have natural daylight with an outside view. Bay windows that allow seating in comfort may be suitable. Consideration should be given, however, to the need for privacy.[8]

Natural Ventilation

Natural ventilation is preferred unless there are internal spaces or clinical reasons that call for mechanical ventilation or comfort-cooling systems.

Art in Health Building

Works of art can make a significant contribution to the environment. Specialist advice should be sought regarding the effect of different types of art on the emotional state.[7]

GENERAL DESIGN CONSIDERATIONS[10,11]

Location

Location near a medical complex or hospital is very common for a source of patient referrals.

Way Finding

People receive, see and look for information that helps them find their way. Four types of information help people to complete their journey—Previsit, enroute, onsite and location information.

Car Parking

Car parking spaces should be preferably covered and provided immediately adjacent to the unit and as near to the entrance of the emergency unit of sports injury facility as possible. It is recommended that there should be at least one dedicated car parking space for every 25 inpatient beds.

Helipad

There are three principle options for siting a hospital helipad—At ground level, roof-top and a low level structure or a raised mound. While planning a helipad facility, following points should be kept in mind:

- Surrounding area free of obstruction
- Licensing
- Hospital noise level
- Safety of general public
- Night flying.

INTERNAL LAYOUT

Need for Visibility

A pool and spa, if provided, could be either indoors or outdoors, depending on the locale's climate. The pool and spa generally command a high visual profile from an image-building standpoint and they should be adjacent to the fitness area and locker/shower facilities.

The aerobics area can be separated completely, needing no direct visibility from staff other than the instructor conducting the session. The aerobics floor should be well- cushioned. There are specific products designed for this purpose, but success can also be achieved with a very dense, thick foam rubber pad under an 88 oz/yd^2 face weight cut pile carpet. The pile need not be high, but must be dense.

Lockers and showers will be used mostly by fitness and pool patrons, but should be convenient to other areas as well. These should be directly accessible from the lobby area to avoid unnecessary traffic through other activity areas.

Noise

Several functions cause considerable noise and should be separated by distance or mass (walls) without unduly restricting visual access where needed. Hydrotherapy generates some noise. This area may be separated by partially glazed partitions to reduce noise transmission to the adjacent physical therapy area. Jacuzzi pump noises can be reduced by surrounding pumps with an isolation closet.

The aerobics area should be fully separated by well-insulated partitions that run above the finished ceiling, since exercisers usually enjoy feeling the beat of the music.

Esthetics

The esthetic character of a sports medicine facility depends on the marketing philosophy, target population, locale and budget.

Wet Areas

All wet areas, including locker and dressing rooms adjacent to showers, toilet rooms, spa and hydrotherapy, should be supplied with floor drains.

Shower and steam rooms should have threshold water stops or dams of half inch maximum height (which must be beveled, maximum slope not to exceed 45°) on the wet side or the entry, with a floor slope that directs water away from the entry.

Linen Storage

Copious amounts of linen are used in the daily routine of a sports medicine facility. Clean and soiled towels must be accommodated in locker rooms, as well as the hydrotherapy area. The physical therapy area uses linen sheets on the tables, pillowcases and towels. All of this linen must be delivered, stored before and after use, and later picked up by the linen service. Thus, adequate storage space for linen must be provided along with additional ventilation to prevent soiled and damp linen from becoming a nuisance.

Interior Finishes

The floor surface in wet areas should be slip-resistant and consistent in texture. The user should not be challenged with changing from one material to another, because he or she will not be concentrating on the difference. This change could provide a hazardous surprise.

Vinyl wall covering is ideal in a sports medicine facility because it offers great variety in texture as well as ease of cleaning. If paint is used, it must be semi-gloss or eggshell enamel, fully washable. Painted wall graphics can be especially appealing in this type of facility.

Lighting

Treatment areas within the facility normally require broadly distributed lighting of 300 to 500 lux. Under ideal conditions, the physical therapy area would have indirect or ambient lighting. Fixtures might be suspended from the ceiling, with the light shining on and bouncing off the ceiling, creating an overall high level of diffused illumination without casting glare in the eyes of patients lying on physical therapy tables. In the hydrotherapy area, fitness gym and aerobics room, on the other hand, the standard 2 × 4 ft fluorescent troffer with a parabolic low-brightness lens would be appropriate. The reception area, lobby or corridors might benefit from accent lighting focusing on wall graphics, special artwork or educational exhibits.

SPECIFIC DESIGN CONSIDERATIONS

Accident and Emergency

Entrances

There should be two separate entrances to an accident and emergency (A&E) department, the "main entrance" for those arriving by their own means and the "ambulance entrance" for patients arriving by ambulance on a stretcher.[9,12]

Both the entrances should have canopies. The ambulance canopy should be high enough to clear lights and aerials. The area should be well lit. The entrance should be bright and easily identifiable from entrance roads, with good signage. Both the entrance should have a suitable draught lobby, with two sets of automatic sliding doors that ensure the heat is retained within the building.[9,12]

A wheelchair bay should be provided adjacent to the main patient entrance lobby for immediate use. There should be a designated trolley/wheelchair storage area located close to the ambulance entrance lobby.[9,12]

There should be a telecommunications link from the lobby to the central porters' base. Ambulance crews should have access to changing and hand wash facilities.[9,12]

Reception Area

The main function of the reception area is to meet and greet patients and direct the majority of them to an assessment room or, if necessary, the waiting area. It should be possible to transfer a patient immediately to a resuscitation room, or to a treatment room.

The risk of violent behavior in the form of physical or verbal abuse is very high in A&E departments, with reception and waiting areas being particularly vulnerable. It is not normal practice for security officers or police to be a permanent presence in the A&E department, as this may serve only to worry patients and visitors unnecessarily. CCTV should be installed in strategic places linked to monitors situated in the central security office.

The reception area should be located in an open space directly inside the entrance. The position of the reception area should allow staff to see all patients and escorts entering the department and have vision to the main waiting and children's waiting/play areas.

Space should be provided behind the reception desk for photocopying, faxing, printing equipment and the disposal of confidential waste paper, etc.

Security of the reception area should include the use of personal alarm transmitters. Office chairs with castors should be used for ease of movement.

Waiting Facilities

A waiting area may be required to accommodate some patients during very busy periods and for family and friends, who accompany the patient to the hospital.

The design of the waiting area and all subwaiting areas should include:

- Circulation space for wheelchair and pushchairs users
- Space around seating for parking pushchairs and wheelchairs without impeding circulation areas.
- Public and/or free phones
- Information boards
- Drinking water dispensers
- Optimal use of natural lighting
- Appropriate heating and ventilation
- Secure environment.

The preassessment waiting area should be close to water closets (WCs), a wheelchair-accessible WC, nappy change and baby feeding area. Each subwaiting area should have access to WCs.

A telephone with a phone taxi service should be provided. Ideally, this would be located within the vestibule between the entrance lobby and reception. Provision should also be made for a vending bay and display systems for healthcare information.

Assessment Rooms

The assessment rooms should be located next to the reception area. Each of these rooms should have a set of lockable doors on each of the front and rear walls (linked to a personal attack alarm) and should accommodate:

- An emergency care trolley
- A clinical hand wash basin
- A ceiling-mounted adjustable examination/minor operating luminaires
- Provision for manual blood-pressure monitoring
- A wall-mounted auroscope and ophthalmoscope
- A lockable cupboard for the storage of drugs, needles and syringes

- A mirror and coat hooks
- A computer workstation for recording clinical information and viewing digital images, with an adjustable-height office chair.
- If digital imaging is not part of whole-hospital policy, an X-ray viewing screen will be required.
- A dressings trolley
- Two small upright chairs
- Personal alarm transmitters for the security of staff
- A staff call system for use of patients
- A clinical emergency call for use by staff
- Bin holders for waste disposal (clinical including sharps, used sterile supplies and general waste).

It is essential that sharp bins are wall- or trolley-mounted in any area where children may be present.

Treatment Room (Fig. 1)

The required number of treatment rooms should be determined locally. A proportion of these treatment rooms will be multifunctional and equipped and furnished identically to enable clinical staff to consult, examine and treat the majority of patients. One should be equipped to deal primarily with patients who have head and neck injuries.

Head and Neck Treatment Room

The equipment required in this room is identical to that listed above, with the exception of the trolley. An ENT patient chair, which can also be used for patients with dental problems, and an adjustable anatomic stool will be required. An ophthalmic slit lamp mounted on a desk may also be required.

Resuscitation Room (Fig. 2)

Each resuscitation bay should be contained by retractable lead/PVC-protective curtains or lead-lined screens. This will allow several patients to be assessed, treated and resuscitated simultaneously in visual privacy. Space is required in each resuscitation bay for a minimum of five staff to work at speed and under stress. Accurate temperature control is very important for many resuscitation patients. The trolley should be capable of being rotated through 360°. Fixtures and fittings required for each resuscitation bay include:

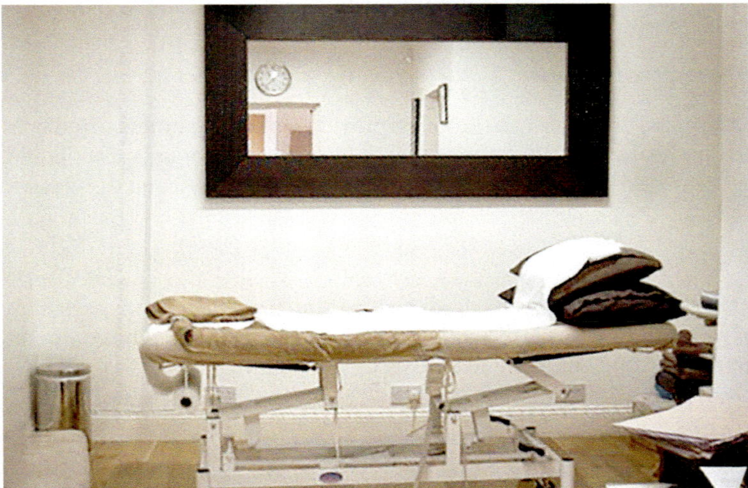

Fig. 1: Treatment room.

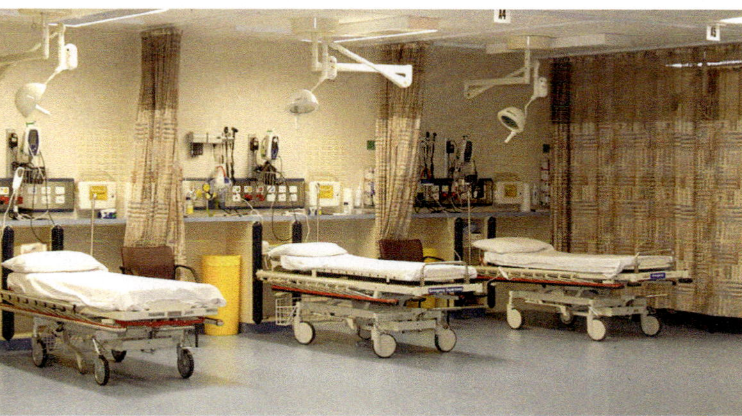

Fig. 2: Resuscitation room.

- Ceiling-mounted examination lamps
- Ceiling-mounted piped oxygen, nitrous oxide, medical vacuum and medical air (4-bar) outlets
- An adequate number of electrical socket-outlets, on the ceiling-mounted medical supply unit, to minimize obstacles and danger from tangled and trailing leads. A minimum of 12 twin sockets in each resuscitation bay is required. These must be connected to the essential supply. A "grab" board at the head of the trolley, with "shadows" of small items of equipment, instruments and medical and surgical sundries stored there.
- A workstation for preparation, and for monitors and a computer and keyboard
- An imaging viewer
- A hands-free telephone, either wall-mounted or attached to the medical supply unit
- Bin holders for waste disposal (clinical—including sharps—used sterile supplies and general waste)
- Boards to record progress, drugs, etc.
- Screens for posting algorithms
- Space for ventilator/anesthetic equipment
- Space and shelving for immediate supplies, such as fluids, oxygen masks, etc.

Furniture, fittings and other equipment that can be shared in a resuscitation room include:

- Ceiling-mounted and mobile imaging equipment
- Drugs (including the controlled drugs) cupboards
- Shelving and racking for medical and surgical sundries, including sterile packs
- Refrigerator
- Clinical hand wash facilities
- Storage and recharge of drug pumps
- X-ray gown storage
- Linen storage and disposal
- Bier's cuffs for intravenous (IV) anesthesia
- Portable monitors and ventilators to transport patients following resuscitation.

Clinical Decision Unit/Observation Unit

It should be an appropriate environment where patients' needs are met and essential care can be provided, for example, privacy and dignity, access to refreshments and meals (if appropriate), toilet and washing facilities, as well as being suitably equipped to support the observation and monitoring of the patient's condition. Medical gases (normally oxygen, air and suction) should be provided.

Interview Room for Distressed or Disturbed Patients

It should contain easy chairs and an occasional table, arranged as informally as possible. Personal alarm transmitters should be installed. A telephone should be provided with direct access to an outside line. This space may also function as a small group room. Ensuite WC facilities made of stainless steel should be included.

The facilities should be located in a quiet place, away from the general distractions of the department, with an external view.

Rooms should be decorated in calming colors, with comfortable seating. Care should be taken in choosing furniture and fittings that present the least risk of causing deliberate or accidental injury to the patient and the supervising staff. The need for rapid and thorough cleaning of these rooms is essential. Interior designers with expertise in furnishing such facilities are invaluable and should be consulted at the initial planning stage.

If a special room is provided for patients who are susceptible to self-harm, a mattress on the floor may be the only furniture. None of the fittings in the room should be able to be used as a weapon. Walls should have a nonabrasive finish decorated to achieve a calming environment. Ceiling tiles should not be installed. A stainless steel ensuite toilet and handwash basin should be installed. The room should have two exits which are lockable from the outside and can provide easy escape for staff from inside. Consideration should be given to noise reduction, alternative means of entry and egress. Concealed heating and recessed lighting of a nonfluorescent type should be provided. The room should be located to provide good observation by staff.

Sitting Rooms for Family and Friends

Two sitting rooms with a nonclinical atmosphere should be provided. These should be sensitively decorated, bright, well-lit and homely, where people accompanying seriously ill and injured patients or the recently bereaved may sit and talk, make telephone calls, prepare and consume beverages, and wash their hands and faces.

Each sitting room should be:

- Located adjacent to the visiting/viewing room and near the resuscitation room but not within earshot of any sounds which may be disturbing.
- Accessible from the resuscitation room without having to pass through public areas of the department.
- Accessible by, and with space to accommodate, a person in a wheelchair.
- Close to a WC (ensuite an option)
- Provided with tea- and coffee-making facilities
- Well signposted.

Near-patient Testing Area

A near-patient testing area is required for blood gas, electrolyte and glucose analysis and other tests carried out within the unit. The main requirements are for a sink, laboratory benching and adequate bench space on which equipment will be placed, electrical socket-outlet provision, a blood gas machine, a specimen fridge, and sufficient space for staff to perform tests and use computer equipment. Separate clinical hand washing facilities are also required.

Digital Imaging Suite

At least two general imaging rooms will be required within easy access of the A&E department, with an associated sub-waiting area. Local circumstances will determine the exact number required. At least one of the general imaging rooms should be equipped with an orthopantomogram. Every room should be able to accommodate both trolley patients and mobile patients. This will avoid unnecessary delays.

Dirty Utility Room

At least one dirty utility/sluice room should be provided where the analysis of specimens can be completed. It should be easily accessible from all areas used for treatment. A storage fridge should be provided for urine samples.

Water closets should be located adjacent to the dirty utility/sluice room for patients, who are requested to supply a specimen of urine or feces. A hatch should be provided to enable specimens to be passed from the WC to the dirty utility/sluice room. Hatches should be designed to ensure patients' privacy at all times.

Unused (clean) disposable bedpans, urine bottles and vomit bowls should not be kept in the dirty utility/sluice room because of the risk of cross-infection from dirty equipment. Such equipment should be stored in an appropriate storage room or within a closed cupboard in each treatment room.

Equipment Service Room

The space provision should be sufficient to park and maneuver equipment and accommodate a workbench with integral lockable cupboards, preferably in a self-contained room or space. There should be sufficient socket-outlets protected by residual current devices. A hand wash basin should also be provided. It is recommended that manufacturers' user manuals be kept in this room.

Medical gas outlets supplying oxygen, medical compressed air and vacuum should be provided. The provision of nitrous oxide together with gas scavenging facilities is a local decision.

Storage and Supplies Rooms

One storage room will be required for the holding of sterile equipment and supplies, and refrigerated storage. Double-sided cupboards that can be stocked and emptied from the corridor and accessed from within every assessment and treatment room are recommended.

Storage of Drugs

Controlled drugs storage should be provided for the treatment of patients attending the A&E department. In addition, secure storage space should be provided for take-home drugs when the main pharmacy is closed.

Plaster Room

The room should have the double-sided couch access with the inclusion of a plaster sink and associated ventilation for plaster dust. The computer must be suitable for use in a dusty environment.[13]

Clinical Hand Wash Basin

The basin should be fitted with nontouch taps. The recommended fixing height of a lever tap on a clinical hand wash basin is 1095 mm.

Where a lever tap is used, the fixing height of the dispensers should be chosen to reduce any possible conflicts in use.[13]

Plaster Sink

The space requirement for a plaster sink is 1200 mm long and 600 mm deep. However, plaster sinks range in length from 1000 mm to 1600 mm. The underside of the sink and area beneath it should be designed for ease of cleaning and to avoid dirt traps.[13]

Clinical Workstation

The clinical workstation is intended for accessing and updating patient records within a clinical environment. It should only be used for short periods of time.[13]

Functional Relationship Diagram of Emergency Care Unit

There are depicted in Figure 3.

OUTPATIENT DEPARTMENT

Location

Ideally, outpatients should be located at the fringe of the sports injury center and be on the ground floor. It should be immediately adjacent to the emergency and minor OT. The outpatient areas should have covered links with other hospital departments, particularly radiology, ward, laboratory services and physical therapy. Access to the adjacent areas that lead off the outpatient areas should be fitted with disabled access facilities.[11,12]

Reception/Waiting Area

Reception Office

Secretarial and other administrative staff is based in this office. Duties of administrative staff may include management of the patient appointment system, management of the patient transport systems, general correspondence, and liaison with other parts of the healthcare system, preparation of reports and analysis of statistics.

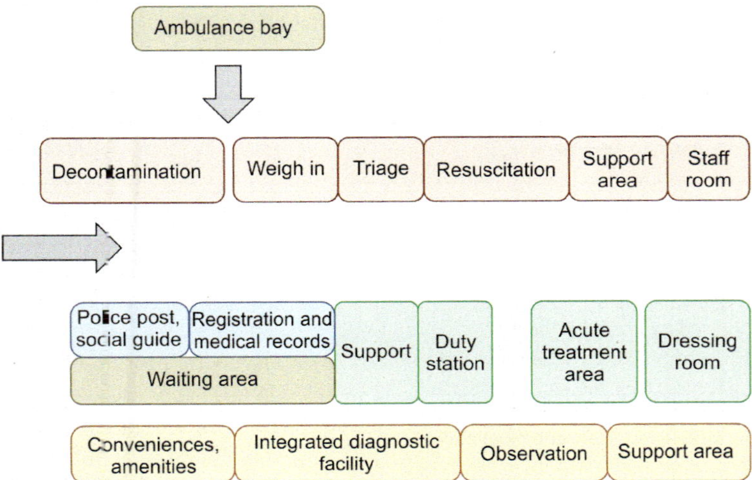

Fig. 3: Functional relationship diagram of emergency care unit.

Waiting/Refreshment Area

A waiting area should offer a comfortable and relaxing environment with domestic-type finishes and furnishings. The layout should be informal. There should be space for patients in wheelchairs to continue sitting in their wheelchairs while waiting, and for people using walking aids. There should also be a children's play area.

The waiting area is an important social space. The provision of notice boards and posters can help to lend a sense of identity to the facility. A supply of general reading material should be available.

There should be a next-patient call system to alert the waiting patients. This could take the form of both an audible and a visual display system.

A vending machine for hot and cold drinks is an option. A public telephone with an acoustic hood should be provided in accordance with hospital policy. A free phone for taxis should also be considered.

Outpatient Waiting Area

WC for Patients and Escorts

Separate male and female WCs with hand wash basins should be provided close to the waiting area for use by all patients and escorts/carers. There should also be a separate accessible toilet.

Examination/Treatment Room

Treatment Room

One or more treatment rooms will be needed for examining, assessing and treating patients. Patients may arrive in a wheelchair, on a stretcher trolley or in a bed. There should be enough room for one patient and three other people. Data points should be provided for picture archiving and communication systems (PACS). A worktop is required where sterile packs, lotions and drugs for immediate use are stored and prepared for use, and where dressing/instrument trolleys can be prepared for use and/or held. An emergency call point and clinical hand wash facilities are also required.

Combined Consulting/Examination Room(s)

Sports injury center houses various disciplines. Each discipline will need space to hold its own clinics (although not necessarily separate space).

Venepuncture/Phlebotomy

This area will be used for the taking and testing of blood specimens.

Interview/Counseling Room

A room should be provided where patients and relatives can be interviewed in a relaxed environment that ensures that their privacy and dignity are maintained. Acoustic privacy is important. Semi-easy chairs and a desk space for one person should be provided.[11]

Office Accommodation

Nurse Manager's Office

This office is the administrative base for the outpatient area. It should be sufficiently private for confidential discussions among staff. The office should accommodate a workstation with computer and keyboard, seating for up to three other people, and storage for books and files.

Nurses' Office

A separate administration office may be needed will depend on the size of the outpatient area. It may be possible for its functions to be carried out in the manager's office and/or the reception desk/area.

Support/Utility Services

Staff Restroom

Provision of restroom facilities in the outpatient area, where staff can relax and take beverages and snacks, can be shared with other departments within the sports injury center. However, local considerations, including the length of clinics, may mean that such facilities should be included. Pantry facilities for staff may be needed if staff cannot easily use other hospital facilities for consuming or preparing food and beverages. Equipment should include a stainless steel sink and drainer, an electric water boiler, a microwave oven, a worktop with cupboards, and a hand wash basin.

Staff Change/Locker Room

Separate male and female staff change/locker rooms should be provided where staff can change into a uniform and store outdoor clothing and other personal items. Personal full-length lockers for the secure storage of dry outer and middle garments, footwear and small personal belongings are required. Hanging rails, with security, for the storage of wet outer garments and lockers for large personal belongings should be provided.

Staff Sanitary Facilities

Gender-specific sanitary facilities, including WCs with hand wash basins and a WC accessible to the disabled, should be located adjacent to the staff change/locker room.

Patients' Sanitary Facilities

Separate male and female sanitary facilities, including WCs with hand wash basins, should be provided.

General Storage Area

A backup store specifically for sterile supplies, such as bulk dressing packs, syringes and needles, will be required to supplement supplies held in the clean utility room and working supplies held in individual spaces within the department.

Clean Utility

A clean utility room is required for storing and preparing drugs, medicines and lotions, and for holding a working supply of clean and sterile supplies. A controlled drugs cupboard—attached to a load-bearing wall and alarmed–may be located here. A refrigerator will be required to store specific drugs. The clean utility should be adjacent to the treatment room. Clinical hand wash facilities are required. The floor should have an impervious finish.

Dirty Utility

A dirty utility room should be provided, where items of equipment may be cleaned and for the disposal of liquid and solid waste. If a disposal room is not provided, the dirty utility should be large enough to temporarily hold materials for disposal and those items that need to be reprocessed. The room should be fitted with a sluice sink, a sink-unit with drainer, a hand wash basin, a work surface, cupboards and shelves. Bedpan disposal facilities are required. Space should be available to park trolleys and for temporarily holding bags of soiled linen, etc. Pedal-operated sack-stands are also required. The floor should have an impervious finish. A secure collection area for clinical waste and nonclinical waste should be provided. There should also be separate external access for clinical waste bins.

Disposal Room

The disposal room is the temporary storage point for all items of supplies and equipment which have to be removed for cleaning, reprocessing or disposal, for example, linen, waste disposal and sharps. The room should allow for cleaning of any spillage from the clinical waste bags. The floor should have an impervious finish.

Cleaners' Room

This could be shared with those available in other functional areas of the sports injury center. Space and facilities must be sufficient for parking and maneuvering cleaning machines and a cleaners' trolley, cleansing of cleaning equipment, and disposal of fluids and used cleaning materials. Hand washing facilities are also required. Shelving and vertical storage should not encroach on the working space or restrict access to the cleaners' sink.

Electrical Distribution Cupboard

An electrical distribution cupboard, with lockable doors, housing the main isolators and distribution fuse switchgear should be:

- Accessible directly from a circulation area (access space may be part of the circulation area)
- Sited away from water services
- Lockable.

Functional Relationship of Outpatient Department

This is depicted in Figure 4.

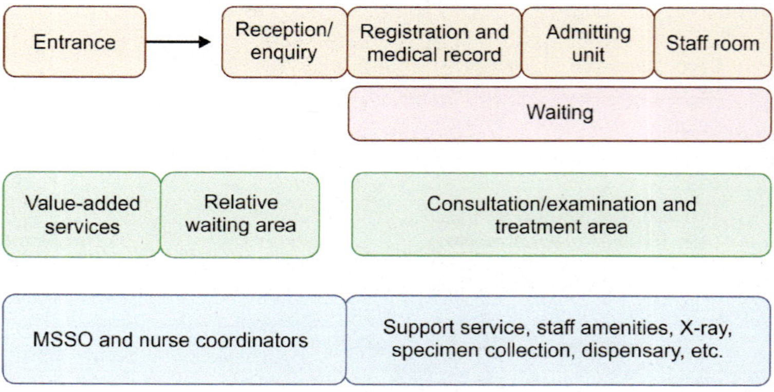

Fig. 4: Outpatient department function relationship. (MSSO: medical staff service office)

SPORTS INJURY WARD[8-12]

Location

The inpatient ward should be located on the floor which has covered, bed-accessible links with other hospital departments, particularly radiology, laboratory services, OT and physiotherapy unit.[11,12]

Functional Areas

Inpatient Accommodation

Consideration should be given to the following:[11,12]

- A high-dependency area should be provided in the ward
- An area of the ward is provided for simple diagnostic investigations and procedures that may be done on a daycare basis or which require an overnight admission, suitable waiting and recovery areas should be considered.
- Where possible, consideration should also be given to the provision of single bay.

Bed Spaces

There should be enough space in each bay or room for appropriate weighing equipment to be brought to the bedside or into the bay. There should also be enough space to use a hoist, as there will be a greater number of wheelchair users in the sports injury center.

Bed Provision

The total number of beds in the ward will need to be arrived at through local consultations, with assessment of current and projected demand.

Bed Head Services

Every bed head should have a nurse call button which can be reached by patients, and an emergency call button for staff. A communication and entertainment system with individual TV, radio, video and stereo headphone systems, and a telephone handset, that allows patients to both make and receive calls, should be provided. Televisions may be mounted on walls.

Isolation Room(s)

The exact provision of isolation room for patients with infection is likely to vary considerably. Where an isolation room is provided in the ward, a negative air pressure facility may be needed. The room should be accessible from the main ward and have a window through which patient and staff can view one another. The door to the isolation room should be kept close as much as possible so that the required direction of air movement is minimally disturbed. An emergency call button is needed in each isolation room. An ensuite shower and WC should be provided within the isolation room.[11,12]

Staff Base

The staff base/bases should be located so that staff sitting at the base can observe the patients in the bed bays/rooms under their care. Staff bases should not, however, be a source of disturbance to patients. The likely numbers of nursing staff, the choice and location of monitoring and computing equipment, storage policies and requirements for notes (with due regard to patient confidentiality), forms and other stationery must be considered.[11,12]

Waiting Area

A waiting area should offer a comfortable and relaxing environment, with domestic-type finishes and furnishings. Different types of seating are required, and should include those suitable for older people. There should be space for patients in wheelchairs and for people using walking aids. Refreshment facilities offering hot and cold drinks should be provided. A public telephone with an acoustic hood should be provided in accordance with hospital policy.[11,12]

Day Room

A small day room for patients should be provided. Patients may sit and rest here after meals, watch television and listen to the radio. A bookcase with various reading materials should be provided, and an occasional table. The day room should be accessible, with a variety of seating heights to help ambulant disabled people.[11,12]

Minor Operation Room(s)

Facilities for recording patient data, and enclosed storage and disposal of dressings and other disposables should be provided. A theater-standard examination light should be provided. A clinical hand wash basin is required. A surgical scrub sink should be installed. This should be large enough to accommodate at least two people scrubbing up simultaneously. An emergency call system should be installed. The minor operations room should be located adjacent to the bed areas and clean utility room.[11,12]

Treatment Room

A worktop is required where sterile packs, lotions and drugs for immediate use are stored and prepared for use, and where dressing/instrument trolleys can be prepared for use and/or held. An emergency call point and clinical hand wash facilities are also required.[11,12]

Clinical-quality color-rendering light sources should be provided, and walls, ceilings and floors should be of suitable color and reflectance. The room should be sound-attenuated. Natural light is preferred but not essential.[11,12]

The treatment room should have easy access to both the clean utility and the dirty utility, and have enough space available for the disposal of clinical and nonclinical waste bins.[11,12]

Multidisciplinary Interview Room

This office space may be shared on a sessional basis by dieticians, physical therapists, social workers, pharmacists and other members of the sports injury center.

It should be equipped with a desk, chairs, a computer terminal, and storage for medical forms and information leaflets, etc., although it will not need a full range of office equipment.[11,12]

Offices/Other Accommodations

Multidisciplinary Office

This office space may be shared by physical therapists, dietitians, social workers, pharmacists, nursing and other members of the team for administration purposes. It should be equipped as an office, with workstations with computers and keyboards, printers, photocopier, fax, seating for the number of people likely to use it at any one time, and storage for books and files.[11,12]

Ward Sister's Office

This is the administration base for the ward sister. It should be sufficiently private for confidential discussions among staff. The office should have a workstation with computer and keyboard, printer, photocopier, fax, seating for up to three other people, and storage for books and files. There should be space for a secure, controlled drugs cabinet to be installed on a load-bearing wall. This office should be near the staff base.[11,12]

Doctor's Office

A doctor's office should be provided in which medical staff can hold confidential discussions, make telephone calls and write up medical notes. It should be near the staff base.[11,12]

Support/Utility Services

Resuscitation Trolley Bay

A resuscitation trolley bay, with space for parking a resuscitation trolley (with defibrillator), a mobile suction unit and a cylinder of oxygen on a trolley should be located with easy access to all spaces used by patients.[11,12]

Clean Utility

Same as outpatient department.

Dirty Utility

Same as outpatient department.

Disposal Room

Same as outpatient department.

Staff Rest Room

Same as outpatient department.

Staff Pantry

Pantry facilities are needed for the safe handling of food including the preparation of beverages and light snacks, for washing and storing crockery and cutlery, for storing a limited quantity of dry goods, and for the refrigerated storage of milk, etc. Equipment should include a stainless-steel sink and drainer, an electric water boiler, a microwave oven, a worktop with cupboards and a hand wash basin.[11,12]

Equipment Store

The store will require lockable and alarmed double doors to the exterior for receiving delivered goods. Additional storage space is required for the storage of equipment (chairs, drip-stands, etc.) and of disposables.[11,12]

Fluid Store

A store room for bulk liquid deliveries should be considered. This room is optional accommodation.

Cleaners' Room

Same as outpatient department.

General Storage Area

Same as outpatient department.

Electrical Distribution Cupboard

Same as outpatient department.

FUNCTIONAL RELATIONSHIP OF INPATIENT AREA

This is depicted in Figure 5.

PHYSIOTHERAPY UNIT[7,8,10]

The gym floor must have sufficient open space to be used as a gait lane to visualize patients' ambulation and also to provide room for patients to exercise with elastic ankle bands or straps or other devices. A quieter, or less active, part of the gym should have one or more small rectangular tables for a hand therapist who sits across from the patient. A nearby work area will provide space to fabricate braces to immobilize the hand. This requires storage for the Velcro straps and other splint materials as well as a small device to heat the material, so it can be molded.[14,15]

Physical Therapy Modalities

There are eleven basic modalities of physical therapy:
- Hydrotherapy
- Heat or cold
- Massage
- Exercise
- Ultrasound
- Traction
- Electrical stimulation
- Transcutaneous electrical nerve stimulation (TENS)
- Iontophoresis
- Continuous passive motion
- Mobilization.

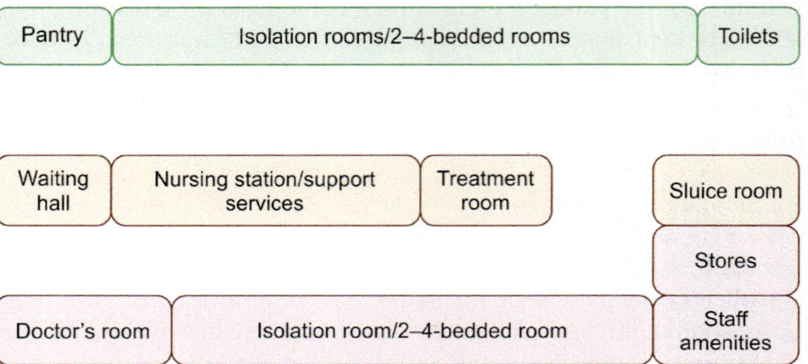

Fig. 5: Inpatient area functional relationship diagram.

Hydrotherapy (Fig. 6)

Hydrotherapy involves immersion of a limb or, at times, even the entire body, in water. The tank may be a portable whirlpool or a full-body hubbard tank. The latter is more apt to be found in a hospital physical medicine department. Mobile whirlpool tanks may be filled and drained with a hose. The patients sits in a high chair and swings a leg over into the whirlpool. The full-body whirlpool in requires permanent water and waste connections. Since large amounts of hot water release a lot of steam, the walls of rooms with large tanks should have at least a 5-foot-high ceramic tile wainscot with commercial vinyl wall covering above. The preferable flooring material is ceramic tile or else commercial-quality sheet vinyl.

Occasionally, physical therapy suites have built-in whirlpools, but most will have a couple of small portable tanks suitable for an arm or a leg. Floor sinks must be provided for portable tanks, which have to be drained and filled for each patient. A hose connection to a nearby tap may suffice for filling the tank. Whirlpool rooms or enclosures are usually 6 × 8 ft in size and may be closed off on the open side by a cubicle drape. Depending on the location of walls and circulation between hydrotherapy tanks, larger space may be needed.[14,15]

There are several ways of designing the hydrotherapy area:

- A large hydrotherapy room can be designed to accommodate several portable whirlpools, plus the Hydrocollator units (steam packs), the cold pack unit, and the ice machine
- Individual privacy cubicles can be created, each having a sloped ceramic tile floor with drain and plumbed for hot and cold water to fill the mobile whirlpool tank
- Fiberglass or stainless steel mobile whirlpool tanks may be enclosed to appear built-in. They may be placed in either a large open room or individual privacy cubicles.

If whirlpool tanks are placed in privacy cubicles, the walls of these enclosures should have a 3- to 4-foot-high wainscot of ceramic tile and the wall above the tile must have a waterproof enamel finish or commercial vinyl wall covering.

Heat or Cold

Heat is produced by a variety of methods, ranging from a simple electric heating pad to hot steam packs to soaking the affected part of the body in hot water or placing it in hot paraffin. The unit must be filled with water by a hose from a nearby faucet. It plugs into a standard 120V AC grounded outlet. The steam packs must be wrapped in several layers of terry cloth towels/terry cloth covers.[14,15]

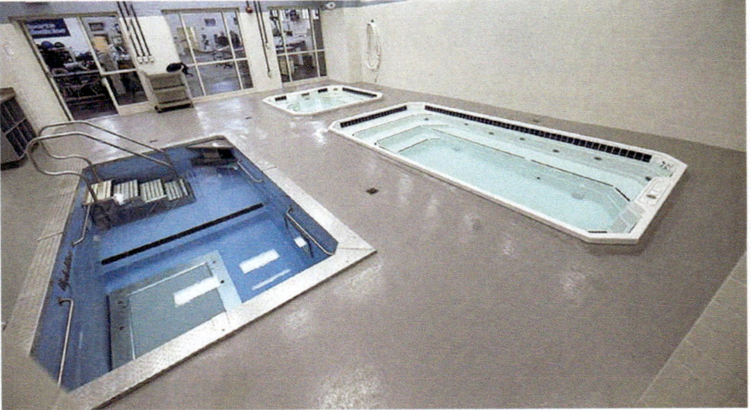

Fig. 6: Hydrotherapy.

Suitable storage must be provided for clean linen, a large hamper for soiled lines, and a drying rack in a ventilated louver-door closet for drying wet towels unit the linen services picks them up.

Cold is normally produced by cold pack or ice, which are applied to the affected part of the body. These units have the same electrical requirements as the steam pack units. Both the cold pack and the steam pack units may be positioned immediately adjacent to built-in cabinetry in order to provide a large countertop area for wrapping steam packs. The average height of these units is 33 inches.

The steam pack and cold pack units, along with an ice machine may be located in the hydrotherapy room with the portable whirlpools, or it may be located in a separate equipment room. This equipment room might also contain a storage area for small pieces of portable equipment when not in use, such as muscle stimulators and the ultrasound card.[14,15]

Massage

Massage is the oldest form of physical therapy. It is generally performed in private cubicles, which may be constructed of standard gypsum board partitions on three sides with a ceiling-mounted drape on the fourth side, or treatment cubicles may be contained in one large room, each one separated from the others, only by ceiling-mounted cubicle drapes. In either case, the treatment modules need to be approximately 8 ft wide by 9 ft long. A physical therapy treatment table is 27–30 inch wide and 78 inch long. It would be placed in the center of the room with space for the therapist to access either side of the patient. The room may also have a chair, wall mirror, hooks for patient's clothing, and a shelf for creams and ointments that may be used during the massage. Various types of portable equipment, such as a muscle stimulator or ultrasound unit, may be wheeled into the cubicles as needed.[14,15]

It should be noted that some physical therapists prefer that at least 50% of the treatment tables be arranged in an open area and that the therapists charting and workstations be similarly open, with an unobstructed view of the gym floor. A 42-inch-high-partition with a 34-inch-high work counter on the other side meets this goal.[14,15]

Exercise

A good deal of physical therapy involves the use of gym equipment. A large exercise room should be provided for exercise equipment, some of which is wall mounted and some of which stand on the floor. Although windows and a nice view make exercising very pleasant, considerable wall space will be required for positioning wall-mounted equipment such as stall bars, weights, and pulleys.[14,15]

The rooms may also have flat bars, exercise bicycles, barbells, an ambulation star-case, pulleys, and a shoulder wheel, as well as other gym equipment and mat tables. Note that physical therapy facilities sometimes have very sophisticated electronically integrated exercise equipment that can be calibrated to measure slight changes in a patient's progress. This equipment is designed to increased strength, flexibility and range of motion and records resistance and other measures of muscle function, often printing out a chart or graph for the patient's medical record.[14,15]

Wall-mounted equipment must be located before construction begins, since the walls will require plywood reinforcement to support the additional weight. The room should have a 9-foot ceiling height and large mirrors, which must be positioned so that people can see themselves using the equipment. Stylized wall graphics of people exercising add vitality to the room.

Consider the use of indirect lighting in the gym and exercise areas. It is especially appropriate when people are lying on their backs looking up at the ceiling. The glare from standard fluorescent fixtures is unpleasant.[14,15]

Ultrasound

Ultrasound involves an acoustic high-frequency vibration that is used to produce deep heat in muscle tissues. The ultrasound unit is small and can be wheeled on a mobile cart to a room as needed. It requires no special accommodation.[14,15]

Traction

Traction can be applied to various parts of the body. The procedure removes pressure from the muscles, ligaments, and tendons of the area being treated to allow the return of proper nerve flow and blood flow through the area, as well as to promote normal joint mobility patterns. The electronic control unit is affixed to the end of the table.[14,15]

Electrical Stimulation

Electrical impulses in milliamperages are delivered into the muscle to elicit external control of the muscle. Ranges of control extend from slight muscle tension to complete and extended muscle contraction. Electrical stimulation may be used to fatigue a muscle for treating spasm, for muscle re-education, to strengthen muscles, to stimulate debilitated muscles, and for pair management.[14,15]

Transcutaneous Electrical Nerve Stimulation

Transcutaneous electrical nerve stimulation (TENS) is the procedure of applying controlled, low-voltage electrical impulses to the nervous system by passing electrical current through the skin via electrodes placed on the skin. TENS therapy has been shown to interrupt or break the pain cycle, which facilitates control of spasms, inflammation, and pain.[14,15]

Iontophoresis (Fig. 7)

Iontophoresis is the process of driving medication topically through the skin by means of an ion transfer device. This is a small unit that may be stored in a cabinet.[14,15]

Continuous Passive Motion (Fig. 8)

Continuous passive motion (CPW) is a technique for rehabilitating a joint or muscle group that has become inhibited, weak, tight, or otherwise injured. These devices would typically not be used in an outpatient physical therapy setting but would, rather, be used post-surgically to keep the limb in motion after a total knee replacement.[14,15]

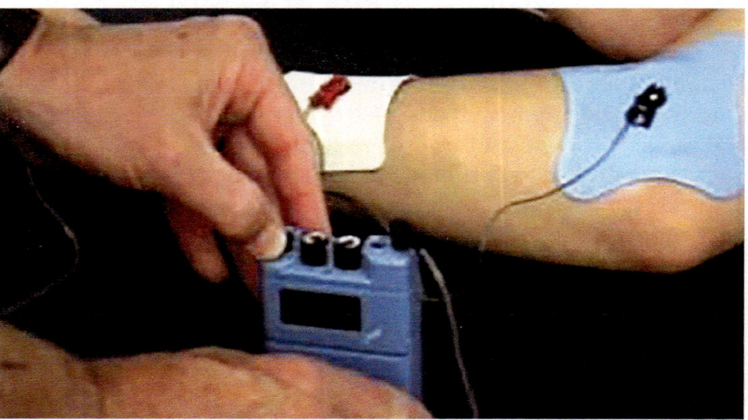

Fig. 7: Iontophoresis.

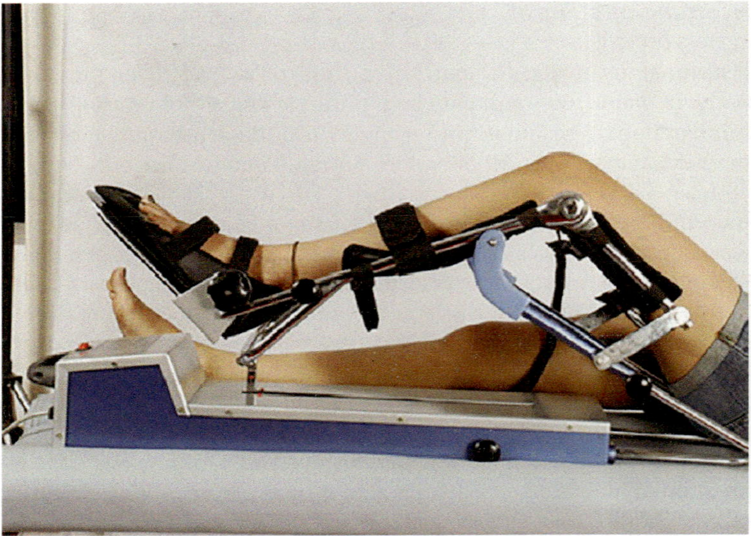

Fig. 8: Continuous passive motion.

Mobilization

Mobilization is a chiropractic-type manipulative therapy that mobilizes vertebral segments and other joints of the body to realign them to proper positioning and to restore normal joint motion. These procedures are sometimes called adjustment. A special segmented, adjustable table is used for these treatments.[14,15]

Offices/Other Accommodations

Physical Therapist's office

An office should be provided in which medical staff can hold confidential discussions, make telephone calls and write up medical notes. It should be near the staff base.[11]

Support/Utility Services

Resuscitation Trolley Bay

A resuscitation trolley bay, with space for parking a resuscitation trolley (with defibrillator), a mobile suction unit and a cylinder of oxygen on a trolley, should be located with easy access to all spaces used by patients.

Disposal Room

This disposal room is the temporary storage point for all items of supplies and equipment which have to be removed for cleaning, reprocessing or disposal, for example, linen and waste disposal. The room should allow for cleaning of any spillage from the clinical waste bags. The floor should have an impervious finish.

Patient Change/Locker Room

Separate male and female change/locker rooms should be provided where patients can change into a uniform and store outdoor clothing and other personal items.

Personal full-length lockers for the secure storage of dry outer and middle garments, footwear and small personal belongings are required. Hanging rails, with security, for the storage of wet outer garments and lockers for large personal belongings should be provided. The number of lockers provided should be arrived at following consultation with staff, bearing in mind any likely future expansion of the unit, and included in the design brief.

Separate male and female showers should be provided en-suite. The patient change/locker room door should be lockable.

Patient's Sanitary Facilities

Gender-specific sanitary facilities, including WCs with wash-hand basins and a WC accessible to the disabled, should be located adjacent to the change/locker room.

Equipment Store

Equipment store should be large. The store will required lockable and alarmed double doors to the exterior for receiving delivered goods.

Cleaners' Room

Space and facilities must be sufficient for parking and maneuvering cleaning machines and a cleaners' trolley cleansing of cleaning equipment, and disposal of fluids and used cleaning materials. Hand-washing facilities are also required. Shelving and vertical should not encroach on the working space or restrict access to the cleaners' sink.

Depending on the adjacency of the renal ward or hospital cleaning facilities, this would be essential complementary accommodation.

SPORTS INJURY CENTER OPERATION THEATER

The operating unit provides a controlled climatic environment for the operative and postoperative care of patients. The number of operating rooms and recovery beds and the sizes of the service areas shall be based on the expected surgical workload. In brief, the size, location and configuration of the surgical suite and support service departments shall reflect the projected volume of patients.[16,17] The total number of operating rooms for the center must be minimum:

- Arthroscopy OT-1
- Hip/Knee surgery/transplant-2
- Neurosurgery OT-1

At least two operating suites for 20 beds must be dedicated if it is a part of multispecialty/tertiary care hospital.

Location: The operating unit shall be located and arranged to prevent nonrelated traffic through the suite. As per the planning of this center, the operating room is preferably located on the last/top floor of the center.

Operating suite: Preference of modular theater for procedure area which consists of prefabricated units for operating suites complete with integrated mechanical and electrical service including air-conditioning should be utilized. In addition, the operating room must integrate with the telemedicine department of the center.

- It must be prefabricated jointless operation theater with all structural steel sections of grade 43 to BS 4360 or equivalent Indian standard.
- The floor should be of the type that does not promote bacteriological growth and the finish should be 2 mm static conductive PVC tiles, laid on a semiconductive adhesive base. The floor finish should be smooth, nonslip impervious material, seamless, welded and washable and terminate at the room perimeter passing over a concealed cover former and continuing up the wall for 100 mm. The doors of the OT must be 2100 mm in height and 1500 mm in width for patient entry and 2100 mm in height and 1000 mm in width for staff's entry. All the doors should be hermetically sealed to maintain sterility and correct air pressure. The edges should get sealed in closed position. All doors should be able to be operated manually in the event of power failure.[11,16]
- The ceiling must be impervious, soundproof and seamless and its height must be 3.0 m. The ceiling should provide optimum air distribution over the patient area, integrated with shadowless lighting. The ceiling should be constructed with a plenum box supplied with central air-conditioning system via 'S' class 8 Nos. HEPA filters mounted on the exit from the supply ducting. It should include integral lighting and composite air/light diffuser. The laminar flow ceiling should have illumination across its total area.
- The lighting should be evenly distributed throughout the room. General illumination is furnished by ceiling lights. To minimize eye fatigue, the ratio of intensity of general room lighting to that at the surgical suite should not exceed 1:5, preferably 1:3. It should be sufficient to provide an illumination level of 1500 lux (with 40 illumination lights) at the wound site and should be dimmable down to 3% of full lighting, without flicker. It is a combination of one major and one satellite light-head with intensity of about 110,000 for major and 100,000 for satellite light-head with individual intensity control arrangements for each light-heads. The color temperature is 3300 K and color rendering index is 95 Ra. Shadow reduction is to be achieved by prismatic optical system.[18]
- *Panels*: All controls within the theater should be located on a membrane control panel mounted in the theater wall. It must consist of time elapsed clock, standard clock, temperature and humidity indicators, temperature and humidity set points adjust, plenum lighting controls, medical gas alarms.
- *Medical gases*: Main storage of medical gases must be outside the facility and reticulated internally to gas outlets. Provisions shall be made for additional separate storage of reserve gas cylinders necessary to complete at least one day's procedures.
- *Others*: Writing board, equipment storage unit, pressure stabilizer and surgical scrub system.

Reception Area

To receive patients to the unit, with general overseeing of day-to-day operations, control of entry and exit from the unit and completion of general administrative tasks.

Holding Area

This area must be located away from the operation theater complex and, preferably, it can be located in the ward floor area. The area should be 7.5 m^2 and should have a clearance of 1.22 m which can hold a trolley/bed for the patient.

Patient Transfer Area

There must be an earmarked route for patient from the holding area and the operating theater and this can also be used for transfer of patients from different area of the hospital to operating room. It will be convenient to have a separate route/corridor for the transfer of patients from all areas of the hospital to operating theater. This will not only reduce the infection, but will also make easy segregation of unnecessary traffic movements towards OT.

Storage

Adequate equipment store room/s for equipment and supplies used in the operating unit should be provided. Equipment stores should be provided at the minimum rate of 10 m^2 per operating room. Store rooms are best designed in an elongated rectangular shape to allow easy access to all items. Storage bays should be provided for equipment such as portable X-ray machine, stretchers, warming devices and auxiliary lamps. Storage bays shall be provided at the minimum rate of 5 m^2 per operating room and minimum dimension of 0.8 m (1 m preferred). These areas should be out of corridors and traffic. This can be satisfied by recessing the bay and the corridor width. Adequate storage facility must be provided in the theater in the form of adjustable open shelving systems.

Equipment Room

An area for testing operating equipment also requires consideration in the planning stage of onsite facility needs. Part of the operating unit general store may be used for this function, or a dedicated room for this purpose may be necessary. Sometimes, it is referred to as the biomedical engineering room.

Recovery Area

The area should be 7.5 m^2 and should have a clearance of 1.22 m to accommodate a trolley/bed. Administrative and staff area includes change rooms, staff rooms, offices and administrative space for clinical staff.

Change Rooms

Appropriate change rooms should be provided for male and female personnel (nurse, doctors and technicians) working within the operating unit. The change rooms should contain adequate lockers, showers, toilets, hand wash basins and space for donning surgical attire and booting. The change room entrance door shall be provided with locks or electronic access devices to prevent the entry of unauthorized persons into the operating unit.[16,19]

Coffee Room/Lounge

It should be provided within the unit for staff to relax and prepare beverages. Inclusion of a window to the outside is desirable.[16] Staff room may be made separately for various categories of staff-like doctors, nurses, paramedical staff, etc. The air-conditioning of this area must be segregated by proper compartmentalization and connected to exhaust system.

Sterilizing Facilities

A workspace and hand washing facility should be included in this area. The facilities for processing and sterilizing reusable instruments may be located in another area of hospital unit such as Central Sterile Supply Department (CSSD).

Infection Control

A room must be provided for an infection control nurse with a table and chair along with the required stationery and also for taking samples for testing. A clinical hand wash basin should be provided within the room. The room must be 9 m^2 in size.

Preparation/Lay-up Room

This is the room in the operating unit where clean or sterile materials are held and arranged prior to use during the operation.

Toilets

Toilets should be provided at the minimum ratio of one per operating room but no fewer than two. Showers should be provided at the minimum ratio of one per two operating rooms but no fewer than two. The above toilets and showers are to be divided equally between male and female change rooms. It must be located in the nonsterile zone of the theater.

Security and Fire

The fire detection system should comprise of smoke detectors and heat detectors located at strategic locations in the OT and connected to a fire alarm panel at a convenient location.

Clean Utility Room

Clean utility shall be a minimum of 12 m^2 or 14 m^2 when access is required from two sides of the room. The clean utility is to have direct access from the unit corridor, with close proximity to the staff station and ready access to patient areas. Doors to the clean utility should be lockable.

Dirty Utility Room

It may be combined with a disposal room for space efficiency. It should be a minimum of 10 m^2 or 12 m^2 when access is required from two sides of the room. If combined with disposal room, the combined room shall be of 14 m^2. The dirty utility is positioned centrally to allow for ready access of operating suite and have easy access to hand washing facilities. The dirty utility must have direct access to the unit corridor and close proximity to the clean utility.

Equipment and Special Fluids

The operation theater must be fully equipped with basic equipment, such as anesthetic machines, pneumatic drills, diathermy, central line Hickman catheters, arterial blood gas machine with lactate test, thrombo elastic graph, intraoperative USG machine, Doppler, cardiac monitor, patient warming devices, refrigerator, deepfreezes and special perfusion/preservative fluids. These equipment must be provided with a room of 20 m^2 with good lighting and storage shelves can be retrieved easily as whenever required.

Operating Table

The OT table must be an electrohydraulic, operated on high storage capacity batteries and also must work on 220/240V AC single-phase power supply; it must be disinfectant resistant, radiolucent table top, with no crevices for ingress of liquids so as to enable proper infection control. It must comply with ISO 9001 and CE certificate.

MEDICAL IMAGING SERVICE[10,11]

Location

Radiology services should ideally be located on the ground floor and conveniently accessible to inpatient, outpatient and accident and emergency department.

Digital X-ray Room

Optimum size of X-ray room of 5.5 × 6 × 3 m is recommended. A control booth with adequate radiation exposure protection should be located in the room. It is recommended that 2–4 well-lit and ventilated cubicles for each X-ray machine should be provided. For each X-ray room, two toilets should be provided.

Ultrasound Room

Sonography is utilized to demonstrate soft tissue structures and to study physiological movements. The room should be minimum of 12 m^2. It should be located with access to patient toilet facilities from within the room. Facility for patient reception, registration and subwaiting should be provided based on workload.

MRI Room

Functional Areas

MRI computer room: It is required to accommodate the computer equipment. Recommend space is 35 m^2. It should be located adjacent to MRI scanning and console room.

MRI console room: It is required to accommodate the computer and other controls of the equipment. There should be a window to provide full view of the MRI room. A minimum space of 10 m^2 is recommended.

MRI room: This provides the area and equipment for MRI scanning procedures. It should be located with direct access to console room. Magnetic and radiofrequency shielding are required.

Other Areas

These include the patient bay offices, anesthesia induction hand washing bay and washroom.

CT Scan Room (Fig. 9)

Functional Areas

CT imaging room: This room should be located adjacent to CT control room. There should be clinical scrub facilities adjacent to the room. Area requirement is 38–42 m^2.

CT console room: It accommodates the computer and other controls for the equipment. A viewing window permitting full view of the patient should be provided. The room should be located with direct access to the CT imaging room and ready access to film processing areas. Area requirement is 6–8 m^2.

CT computer room: It provides area for the computer and generator modules associated with the CT scanning equipment and should be located adjacent to the CT scanning and console room. Area required is about 6 m^2.

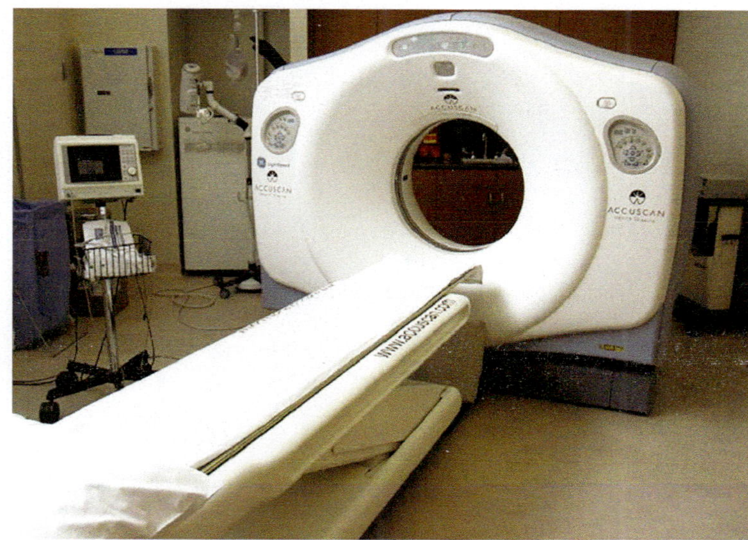

Fig. 9: CT scan room.

Scrub up/gowning area: An area of about 6–8 m^2 is required.

Patient holding area: A patient bay of approximately 9 m^2 is required for holding/recovery. Two bays per scanning room are recommended.

Patient toilet and change facilities: An approximate area of 4 m^2 is required. Along with this area, a staff toilet and change facility should also be provided.

Circulation area of 35% should be provided.

DUAL-ENERGY X-RAY ABSORPTIOMETRY (DEXA) SCAN (FIG. 10)

- The size of the examination room should be large enough to allow an adequate clearance for the operator's workstation and be an enclosed area with door(s) at the entrance(s). An appropriate X-radiation warning sign (such as those used for X-ray rooms) should be displayed at entrances accessible to patient/public.
- Standard drywall construction (two layers, each of 5/8 inch or 16 mm) is sufficient to provide radiation shielding for persons in adjacent areas, to within 1 m Sv/year, for a workload of up to 7,500 scans per year.[15,19,21]
- The operator's workstation is best positioned towards the patient's feet (and away from the head direction), keeping a clearance of not less than 1 m from the edge of the scanning table. If this cannot be achieved, the workstation has to be located with a minimum clearance of 2 m from the edge of the table.[19,20]
- A full-time worker in a new dual-energy X-ray absorptiometry (DEXA) facility should wear a quarterly personnel dosimeter for an initial period of one year to assess the annual occupational dose. This arrangement also applies to the existing facilities after a change of equipment or room layout, or when there is a significant increase in workload.[19,20]
- The operator's personal dosimeter should be worn at the upper body (i.e. chest) on the side facing the X-ray source. If worn on the opposite side, attenuation of the radiation received by the wearer's body will lead to under assessment of the operator's dose.

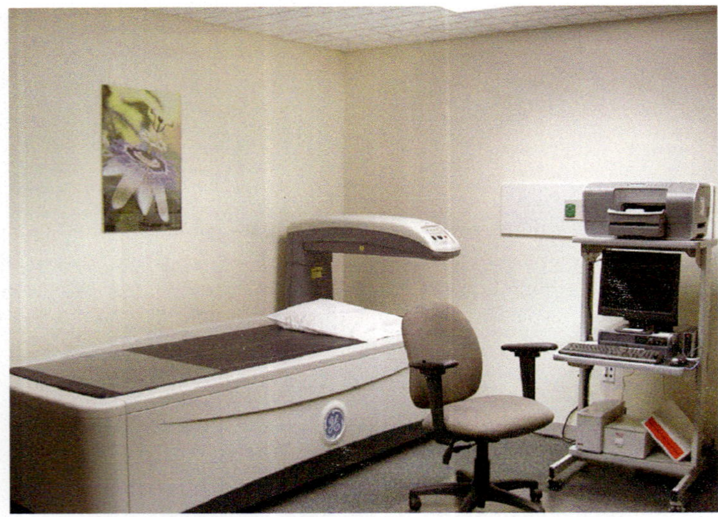

Fig. 10: Dexa scan.

LABORATORY SERVICES

The laboratory provides facilities and equipment for the examination of blood and fluids involving receipt of donors' and patients' specimens, testing and issue of reports.

Routine Laboratory

- Biochemistry
- Hematology
- Microbiology.

Each workstation must be provided with below and overhead cabinets. The workstation should be equipped with vacuum, gas, electrical services, sinks and water. A revolving adjustable stool/chair must be provided alongwith each workstation. Adequate storage facilities for reagents, standard supplies, stained specimen microscopic slides and separate for chemicals and flammable liquids. The floor must be made of moisture-resistant tiles, such as quarry or vitreous. The junctions of walls must be rounded and washable. The room must be provided with proper air-conditioning system, so that the windows can be closed, but it is important to ensure that the air circulation from the laboratory is not connected in any way with that of the reminder of the hospital.[15]

FUNCTIONAL RELATIONSHIP OF LABORATORY

This is depicted in Figure 11.

WORK HARDENING AND INDUSTRIAL MEDICINE[15]

The factory or workroom training module would be designed and equipped for tanks inherent in industries representative of the hospital's service area. Module task simulators may include a stud wall simulator, which is an open stud wall with predrilled holes at a variety of angles and heights permitting plumbing and electrical wiring simulations. A bending/range-of-motion exercises. A shelf system is designed to evaluate the ability to lift or reach, required for certain industrial tanks. Weighted containers in assorted sizes and shapes are also provided.[14]

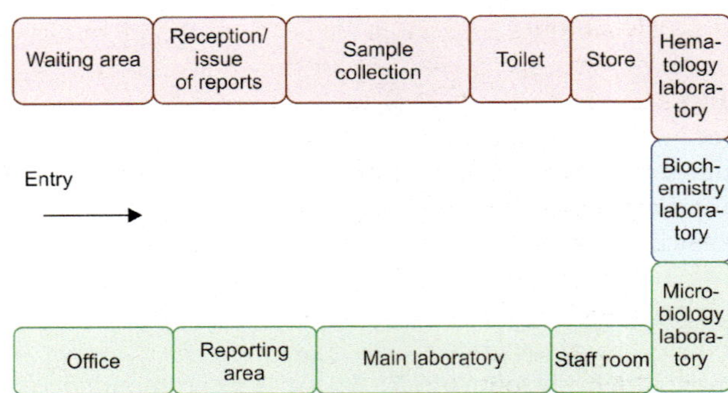

Fig. 11: Laboratory functional relationship diagram.

Special Issues

Structural support for freestanding equipment as well as hydrotherapy tanks (if large) must be evaluated with respect to floor load. Occasionally, specialized rehab equipment has such concentrated loads that the floor must be reinforced. Evaluating the final fixed positions of each piece of equipment, their individual and combined weights, against the structural system of the building looking at locations of beams, stairs, and sheer walls, is not only practical but also essential.[14]

All electrical outlets must be grounded, and codes usually require ground-fault interrupters on whirlpool tanks.

ENGINEERING SERVICES FOR SPORTS INJURY CENTER[5,9]

Specific Engineering Services for Hydrotherapy Pools

Heating

The chemically aggressive high humidity levels that are a persistent and inherent feature of the hydrotherapy pool hall, is an indicator that radiators or low-pressure hot-water radiant panel heaters should be avoided.[8]

Ventilation of Hydrotherapy Suite

The hydrotherapy pool hall should have a supply and extract ventilation system dedicated to this accommodation. The diffusion of high air temperature from the pool hall into the ancillary changing and recovery accommodation should be achieved by creating a positive air movement from the ancillary accommodation into the pool hall.[8]

Controls for Hydrotherapy Suite Ventilation System

The supply and extract ventilation fans to the hydrotherapy pool hall should be interlocked so that the supply fan will not operate unless an airflow is established within the extract system.[8]

The supply and extract ventilation for the hydrotherapy suite should be time-clock controlled to relate to the normal hours of the operations of the suite. A local override switch may be provided to permit staff to reactivate the plant on an extended day basis as required.[8]

Outside the normal hours of operation of the hydrotherapy suite, when the pool cover will be in place, the rate of evaporation from the pool surface will be greatly diminished but not completely eliminated. In order to prevent excessive condensation on the building fabric, especially glazing, the pool hall ventilation system should be provided with both a night setback temperature control and a high humidity control. Settings within a temperature range of 21–25°C and a relative humidity range of 60–75% are likely to be suitable.[8]

In order to assist the users with the day-to-day monitoring of the pool temperature and environmental conditions, consideration should be given to providing a remote indication panel, located in the pool hall, giving visual display of the pool water temperature and the pool hall air temperature and relative humidity.[8]

Plant Rooms

It is normally preferable for the pool water plant room to be at ground or semi-basement level. The shape and relative height of the pool hall may permit the ventilation plant to be installed within a roof level plant or enclosure adjacent to the pool hall, and such an arrangement could minimize the length of the ductwork routes to and from the pool hall and associated changing areas.[8]

Hydrotherapy Pool Water Circulation System

The pool water circulation system should ensure an even distribution of water through the pool and minimize any "dead" zones.[7]

Hydrotherapy Pool Water Treatment Plant (Fig. 12)

Continuous disinfection of the hydrotherapy pool water is essential to control water quality within the acceptable limits.

A pool water test kit should be provided which is suitable for manually sampling and testing the pool water for residual-free chlorine, pH level, alkalinity and hardness.[8]

Patient Hoist for Hydrotherapy Pool

A power-operated patient hoist, traversing over the pool, will be required. The hoist should give smooth lifting, lowering and automatic braking action and have upper and lower limit safety stops. An independent emergency stop control should be provided.[8]

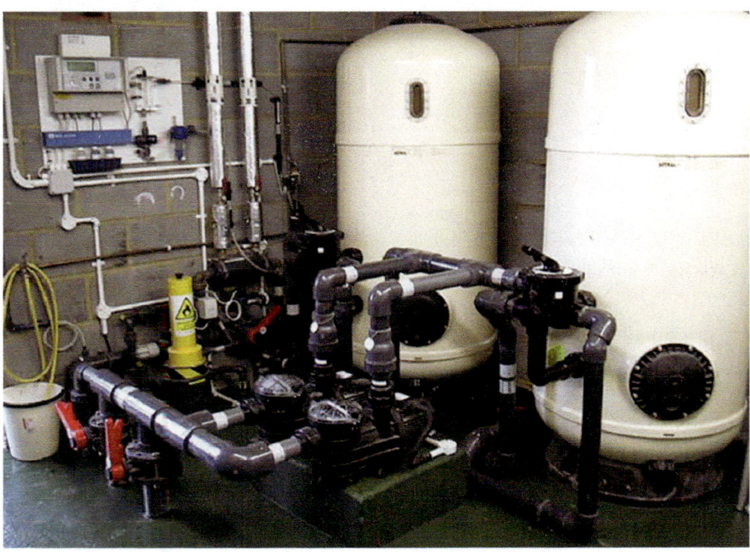

Fig. 12: Hydrotherapy pool water treatment plant.

Electrical Services

In practice the electrical switchroom for the hydrotherapy suite should be adjacent to the hydrotherapy pool plantrooms.[8]

Electrical Installations

Within the hydrotherapy pool area and associated water treatment plant room, any exposed services should be of PVC or similar finish to avoid corrosion by humid and chemically aggressive atmospheric conditions. Mineral-insulated PVC sheathed cables may be used providing cable glands are fully shrouded.[8]

Lighting

In the hydrotherapy pool area, the general lighting luminaires should be splash-proof and made from a noncorrosive material. With a high ceiling level in the pool hall, wall-mounted luminaires are one option, but care should be taken to avoid problems with glare.[8]

Internal Drainage Design Parameters

Depending on local circumstances, special consideration may have to be given to the size of the drainage connection from the hydrotherapy pool to deal with the flow rates associated with filter back-washing and pool emptying.[8]

HVAC OF SPORTS INJURY CENTER[15]

This is depicted in Table 1.

LIGHTING OF SPORTS INJURY CENTER[15]

This is depicted in Table 2.

Table 1: HVAC of sports injury center.

Area	*Air pressure*	*Air changes per hour*	*Relative humidity (%)*	*Temperature*
Outpatient	Normal	8–10	Normal filters	24 ± 2
Inpatient ward	Positive	6–8	45 ± 5	22 ± 2
Treatment room (ward)	Positive	6–8	45 ± 5	22 ± 2
Pantry (ward)	Negative	10	45 ± 5	22 ± 2
Corridor	Negative	6	45 ± 5	22 ± 2
Disposal room (ward)	Negative	10	45 ± 5	22 ± 2
Operating suite	Positive	20	45 ± 5	22 ± 2
OT preparation room	Positive	15	45 ± 5	22 ± 2
Recovery room	Positive	6–8	45 ± 5	22 ± 2
Corridor (OT)	Negative	6	45 ± 5	22 ± 2
Disposal room (OT)	Negative	10	45 ± 5	22 ± 2
TSSU	Negative	10	45 ± 5	22 ± 2
Radiology and lab services	Negative except in biochemistry and HLA lab	6–8	45 ± 5	22 ± 2

(HVAC: heating, ventilation and air-conditioning; HLA: human leukocyte antigen; OT: operation theater; TSSU: theater sterile supply unit)

AREA REQUIREMENT IN A SPORTS INJURY CENTER

Table 3 shows requirement of area in a sports injury center.

- *0.65/person*: Unit area per person occupying the space at one time[22,23]
- *5.02/staff*: Work area per staff that includes space for one desk and one chair, space for occasional visitor, and space for aisle[22,23]
- *1.40/person*: Unit area per person occupying the space at one time
- *7.43/bed*: Clear floor area per bed that includes space for one bed, space for occasional visitor, and space for passage of equipment
- *1.08/stretcher*: Clear floor area per stretcher that includes space for one stretcher.

The floor plans are given in Figures 13 to 16.

Table 2: Lighting of sports injury center.

Outpatient ward: • Patient area • Corridor and waiting area	 300–500 lux 200 lux
Inpatient ward: • Nursing station • Corridor • Support area	 500 lux 200–300 lux 200–300 lux
Operation theater: General illumination	 1500 lux
Emergency: • Clinical observation • Patient care area • Corridor	 500 lux 300 lux 200 lux
Laboratory and radioimaging services	500 lux
Blood storage and issue unit	200 lux

Table 3: Requirement of area in a sport injury center.

Space	*Area in m^2*
Administrative service	
Lobby	
Waiting area	0.65/person
Information and reception area	5.02/staff
Toilet	1.67
Admin office	5.02/staff
Medical records	5.02/staff
Office of the chief of hospital	5.02/staff
Laundry and linen area	5.02/staff
Maintenance and housekeeping area	5.02/staff
Parking area for transport vehicle	9.29
Supply room	5.02/staff
Waste holding room	4.65
Clinical service	
Emergency room	
Waiting area	0.65/person
Toilet	1.67
Nurse station	5.02/staff
Examination and treatment area with lavatory/sink	7.43/bed
Observation area	7.43/bed
Equipment and supply storage area	4.65
Wheeled stretcher area	1.08/stretcher

Contd...

Contd...

Outpatient department	
Waiting area	0.65/person
Toilet	1.67
Admitting and records area	5.02/staff
Examination and treatment area with lavatory/sink	7.43/bed
Consultation area	5.02/staff
Surgical service	
Major operating room	33.45
Sub-sterilizing area	4.65
Sterile instrument, supply and storage area	4.65
Scrub-up area	4.65
Clean-up area	4.65
Dressing room	2.32
Toilet	1.67
Nurse station	5.02/staff
Wheeled stretcher area	1.08/stretcher
Janitor's closet	3.90
Nursing unit	
Semi-private room with toilet	7.43/bed
Patient room	7.43/bed
Toilet	1.67
Isolation room with toilet	9.29
Nurse station	5.02/staff
Treatment and medication area with lavatory/sink	7.43/bed
Office of the chief nurse	5.02/staff
Ancillary service	
Primary clinical laboratory	
Clinical work area with lavatory/sink	10.00
Pathologist area	5.02/staff
Toilet	1.67
Radiology	
X-ray room with control booth, dressing area and toilet	14.00
Dark room	4.65
Film file and storage area	4.65
Radiologist area	5.02/staff

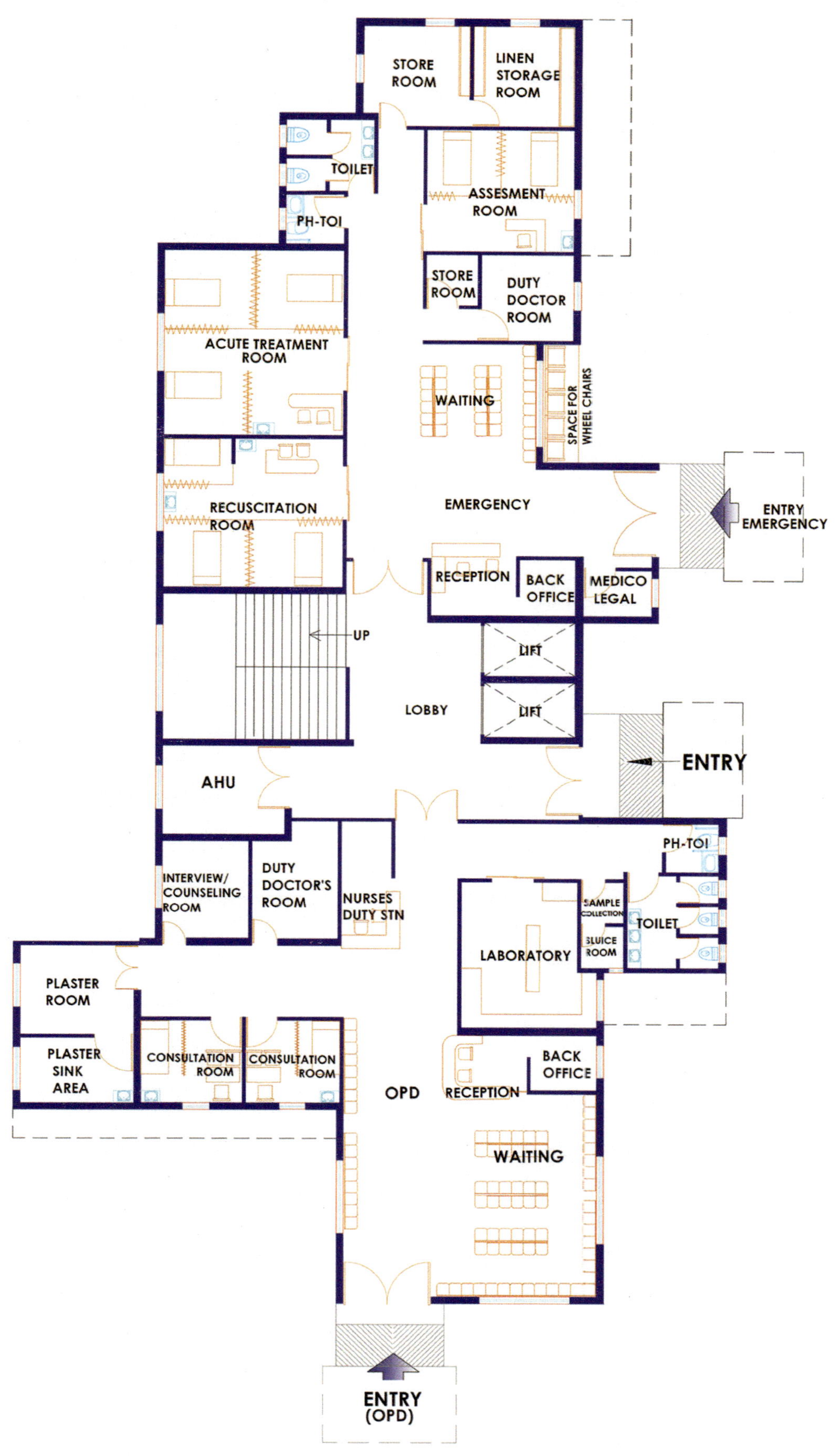

Fig. 13: Ground floor plan.

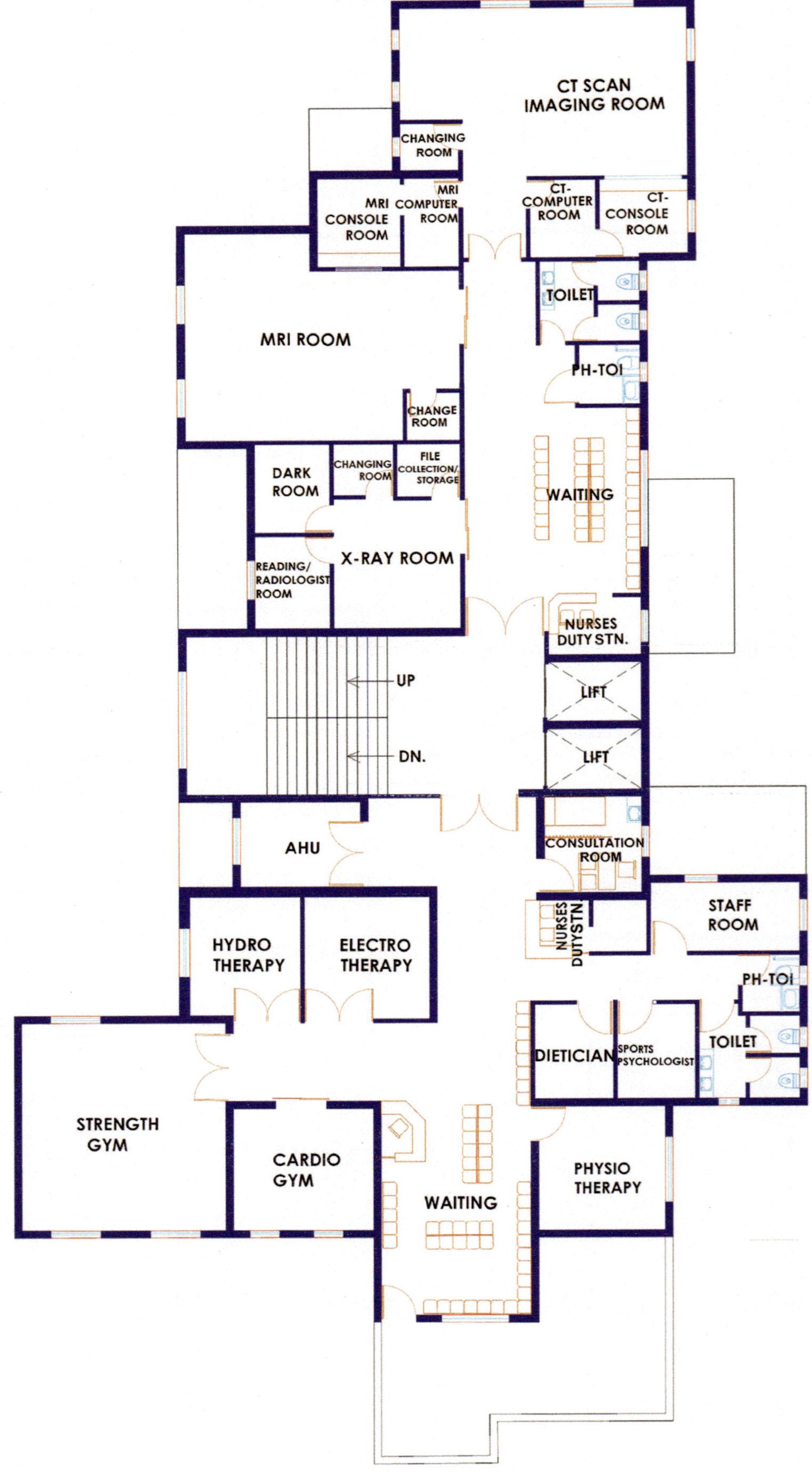

Fig. 14: First floor plan.

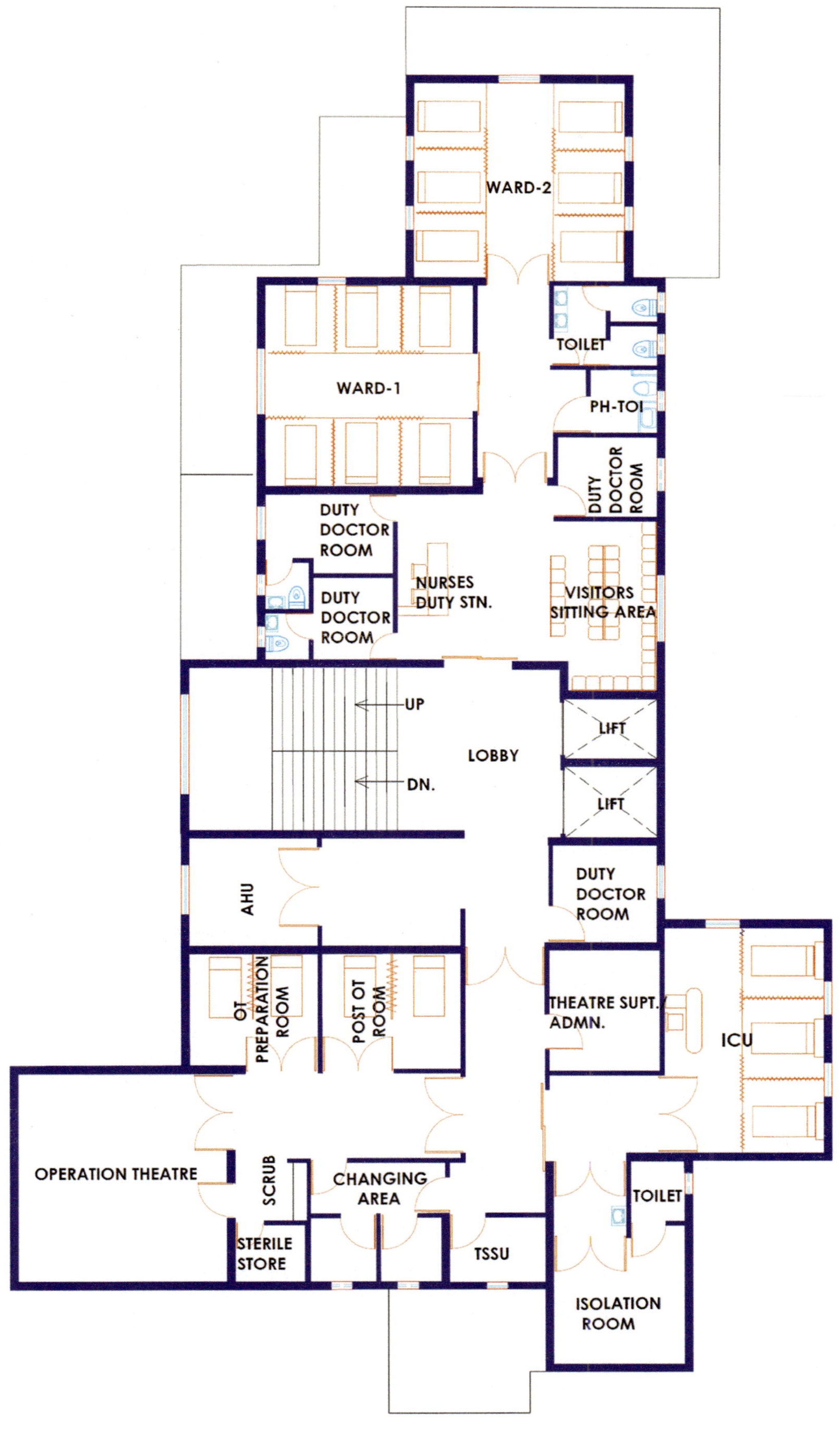

Fig. 15: Second floor plan.
(TSSU: theater sterile supply unit; AHU: air handling unit)

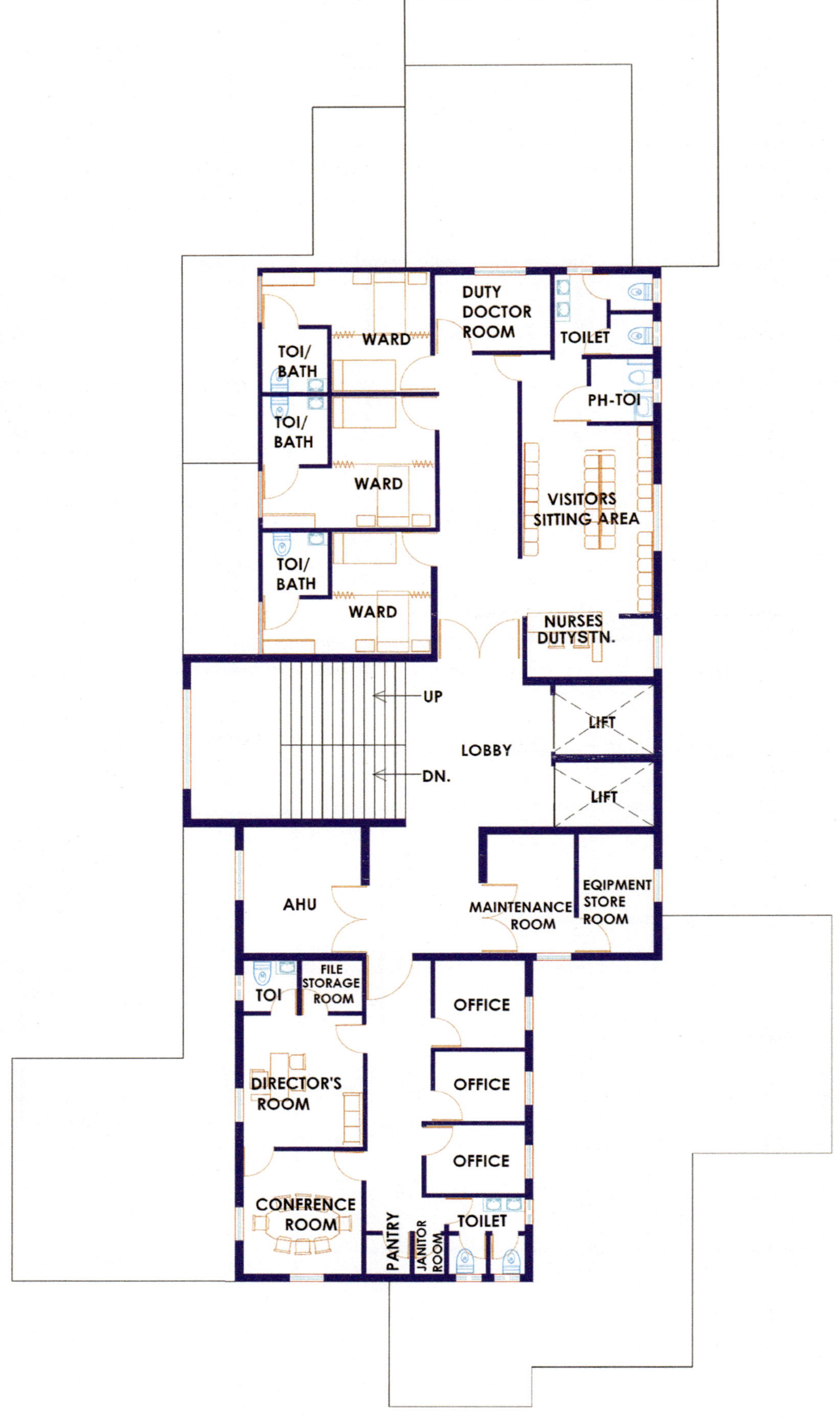

Fig. 16: Third floor plan.

REFERENCES

1. www.boneclinic.com.sg
2. saanichphysio.com
3. vmmc-sjh.nic.in
4. www.nitehawksfoundation.in
5. http://megrantphysio.goldenpages.ie/ms/ms/grant-dr-marie-elaine-sports-injuries-dublin-d4/ms-90037175-p3
6. http://www.sic.org.za
7. sic.org.za
8. www.wales.nhs.uk
9. www.cciffinquiry.org
10. www.wped.com
11. www.gov.uk
12. http://www.spaceforhealth.nhs.uk/articles/general-service-considerations
13. www.birmhealth.co.uk
14. Jain M. Medical and dental space planning: A comprehensive guide to design, equipment and clinical procedures/third edition, 2002. ISBN 0-471-38574-3.
15. Gupta SK, Kant S. Modern Trends in Planning and Designing of Hospital Principles and Practice, 2007. ISBN 81-8061-912-5. Jaypee Brothers Medical Publishers (P) Ltd.
16. www.healthdesign.com.au
17. www.statehealthsocietybihar.org
18. mohfw.nic.in
19. Beers MH, Berkow R, (Eds). "Common Sports Injuries." Section 5, Chapter 62 in the Merck Manual of Diagnosis and Therapy. Whitehouse Station, NJ: Merck Research Laboratories, 2004.
20. http://www.bccdc.ca/NR/rdonlyres
21. www.bccdc.ca
22. http://www.doh.gov.ph/system/files/planning_and_design_0.pdf.
23. www.chd11.doh.gov.ph.

OTHER REFERENCES

- "A Guide to Safety for Young Athletes". American Academy of Orthopaedic Surgeons, February 2002. Available online at <www.orthoinfo.aaos.org/brochure/thr_report.cfm?Thread_ID=34&topcategory=Sports%20%2F%20Exerse> (accessed 5th, January 2013).
- http://www.rightdiagnosis.com/s/sports_injuries/stats-country.htm.
- http://www.pearsonschoolsandfecolleges.co.uk/FE AndVocational/SportsStudies/FoundationDegree/Standaloneproducts/FoundationsinSportsTherapy/Samples/FOUND_SPORT_THERAPY_UNIT_2.pdf (accessed 5th January, 2013).
- "Paramedical Suites", Medical and Dental Space Planning, 2015.

CHAPTER 28

Facility for Nanomedicine and Nanotechnology

Uma Shankar Garg, Shakti Kumar Gupta, Sunil Kant, R Chandrashekhar

INTRODUCTION

Nanomedicine is the medical application of nanotechnology. The approaches to nanomedicine range from the medical use of nanomaterials, to nanoelectronic biosensors, and even possible future applications of molecular nanotechnology. A uniform international definition of nanomedicine does not currently exist. European Science Foundation (ESF 2004) took an extensive examination of the field of nanomedicine. The particular definition for nanomedicine that the Medical Standing Committee of the ESF compiled is "the science and technology of diagnosing, treating, and preventing disease and traumatic injury, of relieving pain, and of preserving and improving human health, using molecular tools and molecular knowledge of the human body" (ESF 2004). They defined five main disciplines of nanomedicine:[1-3]

- Analytical tools
- Nanoimaging
- Nanomaterials and nanodevices
- Novel therapeutics and drug delivery systems
- Clinical, regulatory, and toxicological issues.

FUNCTIONS

Nanotechnology is a field of applied science and technology involving control of matter on a scale smaller than 1 μm, normally between 1 nm and 100 nm, as well as the fabrication of devices on this same length scale. It is a highly multidisciplinary field involving many disciplines, including colloidal science, chemistry, applied physics, materials science, and even mechanical and electrical engineering. Two main approaches are used in nanotechnology—one is a "bottom-up" approach where materials and devices are built from molecular components which assemble themselves chemically using principles of molecular recognition; the other being a "top-down" approach where nano-objects are constructed from larger entities without atomic-level control. The impetus for nanotechnology has stemmed from a renewed interest in colloidal science, coupled with a new generation of analytical tools such as the atomic force microscope (AFM), and the scanning tunneling microscope (STM). Combined with refined processes such as electron beam lithography and molecular beam epitaxy, these instruments allow the deliberate manipulation of nanostructures, and in turn led to the observation of novel phenomena.[4]

PLANNING AND DESIGN CONSIDERATIONS[1-4]

Nanoscale research is a vast and complicated field of study that can engage a wide range of disciplines from both basic and applied science. Inherent in the nature of emerging areas of research, of program, and of a specific location are requirements that make each project unique—there is no standard design solution. In reality, many types of nanoscale research require specialized laboratories designed to meet an array of special criteria.

Sustainable Design Principles in Construction Sector

The design methods of sustainable construction identify, support and recommend evolution of practices and technologies that deal with all the sustainability aspects of the sector. The fundamental object of sustainable design is a bigger compatibility between the artificial and the natural environments without compromising the functional requirements of the buildings and their respective costs. The methods are to be developed to comprehensively account for all parameters of environmental, functional, economic and social impacts. Building construction affects each of the four topics of sustainable development, viz. ecological, economic, social and cultural development. Progress toward the sustainable construction requires novel technologies and policies; not only for the new buildings but also for the refurbishing processes. The subjective rating and valuation inside the current environmental assessment procedures complicates development of unanimous methods. Extension of evaluation to other sustainability aspects require indicators that are even more dependent on the context. As the evaluation of sustainability remains characterized by local and value-driven factors, the future building design methods need a generic basis with flexibility in implementation. The fundamental goal of sustainable development is to preserve the ecological systems that globally are the basis for human life and biodiversity of the nature. Environmentally, sustainable construction ensures more economical use of finite raw materials and reduces and prevents the accumulation of pollutants and waste. Methodologies to manage construction projects from design to use are nowadays of greater importance than ever due to increasing complexity of buildings and building processes, rapid changes of user needs and market environment, goals of sustainable development and demands for faster delivery schedules. The designers from architects to structural, mechanical and electrical engineers have to be educated and equipped to meet the challenges. Performance based building is an approach to building-related processes, products and services with a focus on the required outcomes.[5]

Environmental Life Cycle Analysis

The life cycle analysis (LCA) is internationally recognized as a usable approach to evaluate the environmental impacts of products or processes. An assessment of environmental impacts of a process or a product is an analysis that is made by identification of what has been taken from the environment and what has been brought back, by recognition of the potential harms due to these actions and by rating the significance of the impacts (Fig. 1).[5]

The complete cycle of sustainable construction activities comprise the ways in which built structures and facilities are procured and erected, used and operated, maintained and repaired, modernized and rehabilitated, and finally dismantled and demolished or reused and recycled.[5]

Some of the essential requirements which form a basis for consideration are thermal insulation, airborne and impact sound insulation, flexibility of natural illumination, structural stability and air permeability.[5]

Economic and Social Parameters

Economic and social indicators are combined in sustainability evaluation. Social indicators are accessibility, security, sense of well-being, movability and access to green areas, social services, health and comfort, cultural heritage, etc.[5]

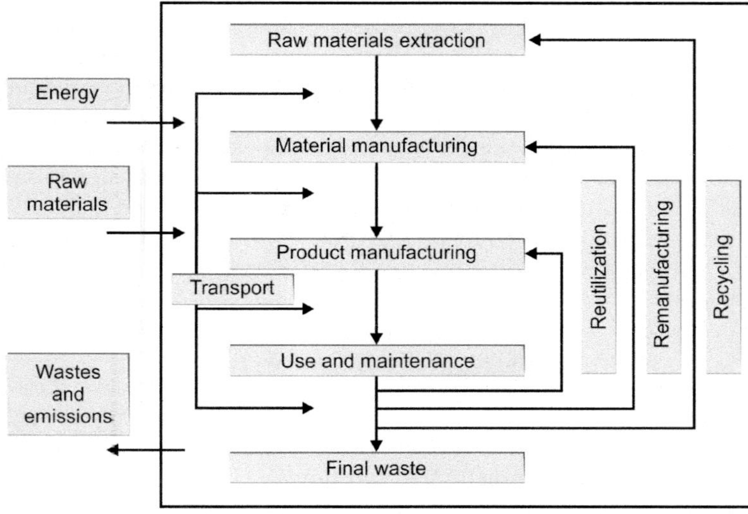

Fig. 1: Environmental life cycle analysis.

It requires a different breed of laboratories and clean rooms. As nanoscale research evolves and so, must the architecture and building technologies. Nanomedicine research facilities are divided into four parts:[5,6]

- A clean area, which can be either a major or minor portion of the structure
- The animal laboratory
- The utility systems necessary to support the clean area
- The rest of the building—everything from conventional labs and offices to conference spaces and public amenities.

Establishing Technical Requirements for a Project

Establishing technical requirements is the important first-step to designing a building that will not become prematurely obsolete. Nanoscale research is a vast and complicated field of study that can engage a wide range of disciplines from both basic and applied science. Inherent in the nature of emerging areas of research, of program, and of a specific location are requirements that make each project unique—there is no standard design solution. In reality, many types of nanoscale research require specialized laboratories designed to meet an array of special criteria. The complex mix of technical requirements for nanoscale research are aimed at creating an interior environment that is extremely controlled, to a degree far exceeding other research facilities, both for the science itself and for proper operation of equipment. Conducting atomic level measurements and characterization, as well as nanofabrication and other functions typically found in nanoscale research often require critical environments that demand tighter control of the fluctuation of environmental characteristics within the laboratory. These technical considerations might involve controlling temperature and humidity levels, isolating vibration and acoustic noise, reducing the quantity and size of airborne particulates, and shielding from electrical, electromagnetic, and radiofrequency interferences. Electron microscopes are most sensitive to many of the above 'noise' sources. Additionally, temperature fluctuation along the length of a laser beam could cause distortion and, therefore, lose focus and accuracy in measurements. The beam could also be misaligned by vibrations while electromagnetic interference causes the wavelength to change, introducing errors in measurements. The need for large air handling equipment used to control temperature and humidity in one area will affect the stringent vibration and noise limits required in other areas. The campus master plan may include a network of interconnected buildings designed as separate 'modules.' Each building module is dedicated to a particular measurement science, which in turn requires a high level of control over the various environmental criteria.

Temperature and Humidity Control

Achieving a certain temperature and keeping it constant can be difficult because work conducted in the lab can change the ambient temperature enough to interfere with the experiment. Temperature can be closely controlled and maintained by designing systems that circulate the volume of air inside the room with a high number of air changes per hour. In typical laboratories, temperature fluctuations are controlled to ± 1°C. Closer temperature control is sometimes needed and the tolerance can range from 0.5°C down to a range of ± 0.01°C in highly critical spaces. Similarly, humidity control, depending on the research requirements, may vary between ± 5% down to 1% of relative humidity (RH). The baseline average room air temperature for all laboratories is controlled to within ± 0.25°C. Some precision temperature control laboratories may be housed in underground wings requiring temperature control to within ± 0.1 or ± 0.01°C and humidity control to 1% of RH for laboratories designed to house highly specialized experiments such as the Molecular Measuring Machine. Arrays of high-precision thermistors and humidity sensors are used to control the temperature. These are individually calibrated to ensure a tolerance of less than ± 0.003°C. This extreme accuracy is necessary for input into the precision direct digital control systems.

Vibration Isolation

When measuring or capturing an image at the atomic scale, the slightest vibration can invalidate results; even extremely small motions can distort images created by an electron microscope. First, the level of vibration that can be tolerated must be determined. It is equally important to test the potential site at the outset to gauge ambient vibration levels, both during the day and at night. Once the threshold is set and the site's vibration level is identified, then building design options can be considered. The more stringent the requirement, the more expensive the structure will be. The building can be sighted at an adequate distance from the street to minimize the vibration caused by traffic or it can be located outside the perimeter of the main campus in order to provide more distance between the building and outside noise environment. Further, isolation of the building from potential noise generated from surrounding buildings and greater distance between the facility and vehicular traffic will reduce the vibrations. If quiet and ultraquiet laboratories are required within the same facility, the facility design can be in multiple wings. The most vibration sensitive laboratories are located the furthest from the wing where the research would generate the most noise. Vibration can be further reduced by building some of the facility's wings underground, minimizing the effects of predominant surface vibrations. With the sensitive area about 40 ft below the surface, the floor vibrations can be reduced by more than 50%. For ultraquiet spaces, rooms can be built on specially designed isolation slabs that are supported on a series of isolators, reducing the transmission of vibrations from the building to the slab where the experiment is mounted. The isolation slab is made of a concrete mass weighing about 10 to 30 tons and it is set on air spring isolators. The isolation slab is suspended about a quarter of an inch above the base, ensuring that people working in the lab and walking across the floor will not cause the instrument to vibrate.

Airborne Contamination

At the nanometer scale, some spaces may require the control of airborne particulates (dust particles), others may require the control of molecular contamination (biological matter). These two forms of contamination are distinct and each require different engineering and architectural solutions. These solutions may include segregation of spaces, in addition to air management systems that will provide positive or negative pressurization in the space where research or fabrication is conducted. Dust particles have a negative impact on the devices.

Electrical, Electromagnetic, and Radio Frequency Interference

Many of the instruments used by nanoscale researchers are highly sensitive to electrical and electromagnetic interference. Everything from a small fluctuation in the electrical power supply to electromagnetic interference (EMI) or radio frequency interference (RFI) can degrade research. At the outset of design, it is important to understand the specific requirements of the anticipated research in order to determine if EMI or RFI could be problematic. Sometimes, the source of interference

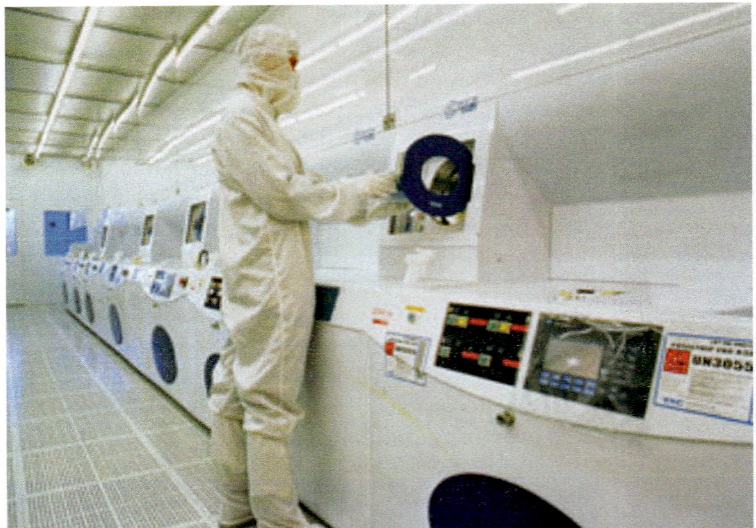

Fig. 2: Microelectronic lab.

comes from forces outside the building and steps to limit it are required. An outside interference issue during early planning phases should be resolved straightaway. The site should be specifically tested on this issue and the radio frequency (RF) interference (Fig. 2) should be handled with local attenuation. From an interior perspective, working to limit interference must take cognizance of how different types of labs can be arranged. Labs that are particularly sensitive to electromagnetic interference (Fig. 2) should not be located near elevators or lab equipment that will produce strong electromagnetic fields. Certain systems necessary for maintaining the building must be taken into account. Transformers, rotating equipment, and pumps are examples of equipment required to keep basic building systems operational, but can also wreak havoc with laboratories. These essential building systems should be located where they are as benign as possible; and if necessary, local shielding can help create an environment appropriate for nanoscale research. Generally, when designing the interior of a nanoscale research facility, components known to cause interference should be segregated from research areas as much as possible.

Nanotechnology Labs (Fig. 3)

Correctly sizing utilities is critical for nanotechnology labs. The size of utility systems is tied to the size of the building itself. In nanotech research, however, the process tools in the clean rooms drive the utility consumption; the tools, in turn, are determined by the research to be conducted in the lab and the mix of equipment needed to do it. The types of research or the discipline mix will drive the utility usage, based on how much each of the dependent disciplines are to be integrated. These labs are equipped with many utility-hungry tools, including horizontal furnaces; physical vapor deposition (PVD) and chemical vapor deposition (CVD) tools; and molecular-beam epitaxy (MBE). The number and mix of those tools is based largely on the size of the substrate.[6,7]

Categorization of Nanotech Facilities (Fig. 4)

Nanotech facilities are categorized by three sizes of substrates:[6,7]

- Large: 300 mm (12-inch) substrates
- Medium: 200 mm (8-inch) substrates
- Small: 150 mm (6-inch) substrates.

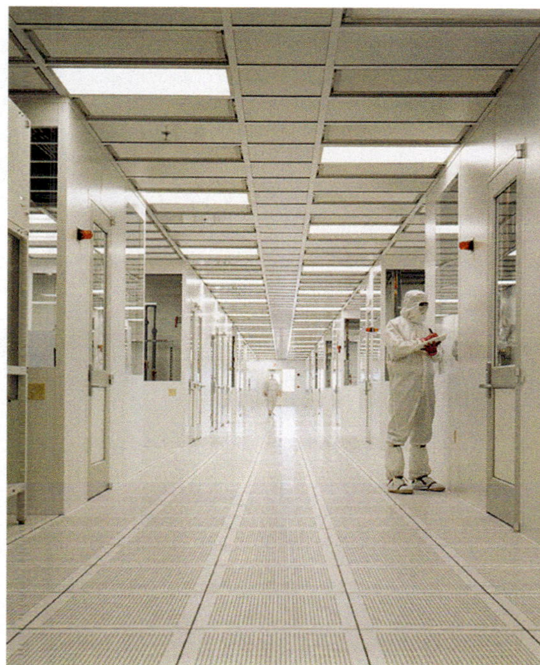

Fig. 3: Nanotechnology labs.

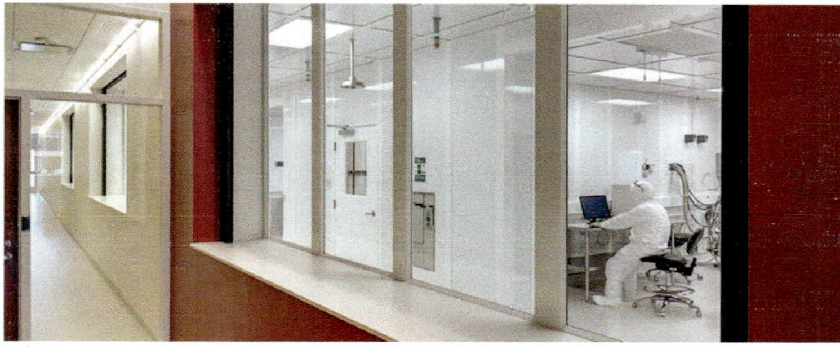

Fig. 4: Nanotech facilities.

Large Facility

The best-in-class layout for a 300 mm substrate nanotech research facility is a ballroom configuration, with the researchers working in one open cleanroom. A full floor below them, often called a subfloor, contains the support equipment, such as pumps, chillers, cryocompressors, etc. and the facility systems. The mechanical heating, ventilating, and air-conditioning (HVAC) units are typically located on the interstitial level or the penthouse above the cleanroom. Sizes for a 300 mm nanotech facility range from as small as 1,500 m^2 to as large as 3,500 m^2.[6]

Medium Facility

A medium-sized cleanroom facility is designed in the same fashion as a large facility with a configuration difference which may be a bay/chase or even a hybrid, which is a combination of ballroom and bay/chase concept. In the hybrid configuration, the cleanroom is organized to accommodate equipment that is extremely sensitive to environmental concerns, such as electromagnetic interference, vibration, and acoustics (EVA), typically located far away from the elevators, electrical switch gears, and other components in the cleanroom that generate EVA.[6]

Small Facility

Cleanrooms built for 150 mm substrates are commonly laid out like a series of wide-toothed combs. The 'dirty' sides of the room—the support chases—are the teeth of the comb, and the clean areas are the spaces between the teeth. There are several variations on this theme—labs with a center clean aisle; a clean aisle on one exterior wall and a chase aisle on the other; and chases and clean spaces that are either symmetrical or irregularly sized and spaced. The clean spaces are located where they fit in the process. The smaller cleanroom facility is heavily populated with utility-hungry tools that require higher use of power consumption as opposed to a disproportionate number of metrology and support tools in the larger facility, which requires less energy.[6]

Cleanrooms

The term cleanroom is used to describe a wide range of accommodation varying from areas with simple air-conditioning to the most sophisticated forms as can be found in wafer-fabrication plants. It is an environment, typically used in manufacturing or scientific research, that has a low level of environmental pollutants such as dust, airborne microbes, aerosol particles and chemical vapors. More accurately, a cleanroom has a controlled level of contamination that is specified by the number of particles per cubic meter at a specified particle size. Cleanrooms are areas within properties where higher than normal environmental standards are maintained. A cleanroom may, therefore, be defined as an area with environmental control of particulate contamination, temperature and humidity constructed in such a way as to minimize the introduction, generation and retention of particles inside the room. In terms of structure and internal finish, cleanrooms can vary significantly depending on purpose and design. The air entering a cleanroom from outside is filtered to exclude dust, and the air inside is constantly recirculated through high efficiency particulate arrestance filter (HEPA) and/or ultralow particulate air (ULPA) filters to remove internally generated contaminants. A clean-room may have laminar flow which is the preferred method of air changing and can be either horizontal or vertical. Air enters the room through a batch of HEPA filters that comprise the whole of one wall or ceiling and exits by corresponding ducts opposite. For effective laminar flow to take place, there should be minimal interruption by pillars, protruding light fittings, inset windows, furniture, etc. The most sophisticated cleanrooms have vertical laminar flow and is superior as lateral contamination is minimized, air being admitted through ceiling filters and extracted through perforated floor tiles. A conventional flow cleanroom has air entering the room through a bank of filters positioned such that ducting, after final filtration is minimal and leaves the room through outlets remote from the inlets. The air-conditioning method does not comply with laminar flow theory. A clean room has an air shower, an enclosed area at the entrance with air jets which remove loose particulate matter from personnel prior to entering the room. Clean work station, laminar flow benches or cabinets are working enclosures that have their own filtered air or gas supply. These areas have environmental standards much higher than the cleanrooms in which they are located.[7]

Cleanroom Performance

Cleanrooms are classified by the cleanliness of their air. This is done according to ISO 14644-1 which is an international standard adopted by the European Union in 1999 and the USA in 2001, revised and updated in 2015 (Table 1). However, the most easily understood classification of cleanrooms remains the British Standard (BS) 5295 (1989) equivalent of the USA Federal Standard 209(E), where the classification is determined by measuring the number of particles >0.5 microns in one cubic foot of room air (Table 2). The metric units used in the Federal Standard 209(E) have never become established. BS5295 (1989) nomenclature, therefore, continues to be the most widely used. Cleanrooms are thus, described

Table 1: ISO 14644-1:2015–Cleanrooms and associated controlled environments–Part 1: Classification of air cleanliness by particle concentration[8,9]

Class	Maximum particles[a]/m³						FED STD 209(E) equivalent
	≥0.1 μm	≥0.2 μm	≥0.3 μm	≥0.5 μm	≥1 μm	≥5 μm	
ISO 1	10[b]	[d]	[d]	[d]	[d]	[e]	–
ISO 2	100	24[b]	10[b]	[d]	[d]	[e]	–
ISO 3	1,000	237	102	35[b]	[d]	[e]	Class 1
ISO 4	10,000	2,370	1,020	352	83[b]	[e]	Class 10
ISO 5	100,000	23,700	10,200	3,520	832	[d,e,f]	Class 100
ISO 6	1,000,000	237,000	102,000	35,200	8,320	293	Class 1,000
ISO 7	[c]		[c]	352,000	83,200	2,930	Class 10,000
ISO 8	[c]		[c]	3,520,000	832,000	29,300	Class 100,000
ISO 9	[c]		[c]	35,200,000	8,320,000	293,000	Room air

[a]All concentrations in the table are cumulative, e.g. for ISO Class 5, the 10,200 particles shown at 0.3 μm include all particles equal to and greater than this size.
[b]These concentrations will lead to large air sample volumes for classification. Sequential sampling procedure may be applied.
[c]Concentration limits are not applicable in this region of the table due to very high particle concentration.
[d]Sampling and statistical limitations for particles in low concentrations make classification inappropriate.
[e]Sample collection limitations for both particles in low concentrations and sizes greater than 1 μm make classification at this particle size inappropriate, due to potential particle losses in the sampling system.
[f]In order to specify this particle size in association with ISO Class 5, the macroparticle descriptor M may be adapted and used in conjunction with at least one other particle size.

Table 2: BS 5295 (British Standard)-0:1989–Environmental cleanliness in enclosed spaces. General introduction, terms and definitions for clean rooms and clean air devices[10]

Class	Maximum particles/m³				
	≥0.5 μm	≥1 μm	≥5 μm	≥10 μm	≥25 μm
Class 1	3,000		0	0	0
Class 2	300,000		2,000	30	
Class 3		1,000,000	20,000	4,000	300
Class 4			200,000	40,000	4,000

Source: https://www.iso.org/standard/53394.html

as Class 1, Class 10, etc.—a Class 10 clean room for example having not more than 10 particles exceeding 0.5 microns in one cubic foot of air. It is not thought possible to operate a cleanroom better than Class 100 with human presence and any that do almost certainly require robot technology. Cleanroom specifications are continually advancing plants.

Animal Research Facility

Animal research and animal research facilities are critical to the biomedical research enterprises. Animal species are used in every stage of the research and development effort—from discovery, to development and safety testing, to clinical trials, and to manufacture—because their biological systems, genetic structures, and immunological responses, in various ways, closely mirror ours as a species. The animal research facility, also known as the *vivarium*, is a especially designed building type, which accommodates exquisitely controlled environments for the care and maintenance of experimental animals. Animal research facilities are distinct from research laboratories. The facilities are complex, and expensive to build and to operate, but they are vital to the support of a proper, safe, and humane research effort. Vivariums may be embedded within a lab building, or in a separate structure connected to a lab building, or may be independent free-standing structures.[7]

Components of a Vivarium

Animal Housing Rooms

They are designed to accommodate caging, bedding change stations, and sinks. Animal housing rooms (AHRs) can be organized as individual rooms accessed from a corridor system or multiple rooms could be organized into self-contained suites.[8,14]

Procedure Rooms

Proximate to AHRs and frequently interchangeable with them; they are a primary setting for research activity within the unit. The method of allowing researcher access under controlled conditions is a critical issue.[11]

Barrier Elements

Airlocks, lockers, pass-through autoclaves provide the primary barrier and access control that separates the controlled animal care environment from external influences.[11]

Cage Wash

They are the hubs for all cleaning, sanitizing, and husbandry activities. These areas are dominated by equipment-generated heat and moisture. The major equipment items include pass-through rack washers, tunnel washers, pass-through autoclaves, bedding dispensers and dump stations, and bottle washing and filling stations.

Cage Storage

It is a necessary function, but a space consumer, which should not be overlooked.[11]

General Storage

A necessary space and function for feed, bedding, and equipment has to be incorporated into the operational flow and space allocation.[11]

Quarantine

Isolated AHRs for suspect and incoming animals that could be a source of infection.[11]

Dedicated Receiving Dock

A dock specific to animal functions is generally required. An elevator dedicated to animal usage should be located near the dock.[11]

Necropsy/Perfusion

Critical support function used for postmortem procedures on sacrificed animals. It is a 'dirty' function that should not be proximate to 'clean' areas.[11]

Containment Facilities

These are the facilities for working with potentially infectious biological agents. They operate under negative pressure to prevent the escape of air to the general environment. Wastes and effluents are separately contained and decontaminated. Sophisticated control and monitoring systems and equipment are employed to achieve closely controlled and regulated air pressurizations and flows.[11]

Barrier Facilities

Facilities for working with immunocompromised species. These operate under positive pressure to keep contaminants out. As in containment facilities, control and monitoring systems and equipment are utilized in barrier facilities to maintain the required pressures and flows.[11]

Veterinary Care

Lab and care functions, e.g. surgery, clinical chemistry, and histology.

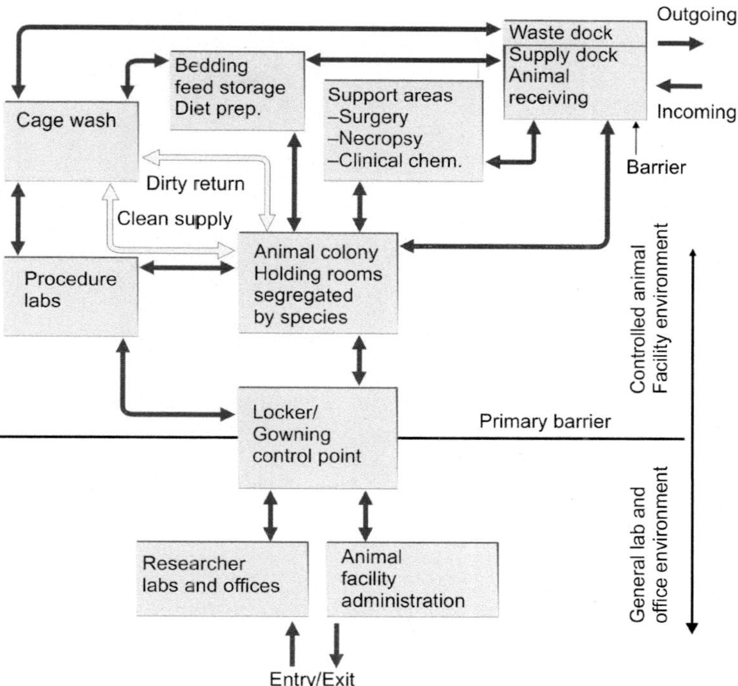

Fig. 5: Animal facility diagrammatic model showing basic flows and spatial relationships.[7]

Veterinary Office Space

Some provision for in-unit office spaces for veterinary care staff should be made.[8]

Staff Support Areas

Break area, cafeterias, workstation, lockers, and rest-room facilities. All are intended to support veterinary and research staff during their in-unit tours of duty.[11]

Mechanical/Electrical Equipment Spaces

Mechanical equipment rooms, electrical and telecom closets, rooms for terminal trim devices such as dampers, coils, humidifiers and controls, distribution shafts, and mechanical penthouses. A desirable goal is to locate the spaces and devices in a manner that allows the separation of maintenance functions from animal care functions.[11]

Corridors

These should be wide enough to accommodate animal rack, cart, and material traffic flow, not just egress requirements. They should have a clear width of 2.1 m to 2.5 m. Corridors should have impervious finishes so, that they are easy to clean and maintain. Protective components such as bumper and corner guards are frequently employed to protect walls and doors from heavy, abusive traffic. The general organization of a vivarium is illustrated in Figure 5.[11]

Important Attributes

Internal circulation systems need some form of control over clean versus dirty (or supply vs. return) traffic. Cage wash is divided between a clean, that is an incoming or supply side, and a dirty, that is an outgoing or return side. Presumed or inherent, dirty functions such as necropsy and quarantine should be located near the dock. The animal receiving areas should be subdivided to distinguished between incoming animals and receiving, and outgoing waste. HVAC is the dominant system. It is the maintainer of environmental control via regulation of airflow, air cleanliness via filtration, temperature, humidity, odor transmission, and contaminant control. Air changes per hour, a key benchmark of system capability, can vary from a minimum of 10 to greater than 20, which equates to 1.5 cfm/sf to more than 3 cfm/sf. Air quality, caging type and caging density are the primary determinants of airflow rate. Since HVAC is the life-sustaining system, consideration should be given to methods of providing redundancy and backup to maintain continual operation. Building automation systems (BAS) via direct digital controls (DDC), control and monitor the interaction of all elements of the HVAC system. BAS makes the HVAC system responsive and adaptive. Plumbing systems are pervasive, but are varied, discrete, and independent. The most important elements are animal watering and major water users such as cage and rack washers. Watering system vendors maintain reliable empirical databases on watering needs by species. For major equipment, load capacity is calculated system by system. Electrical systems are ubiquitous. The most critical issues are reliable power and redundancy and backup for critical systems and equipment via standby generators, weather-protected outlets in wet locations, and the increasing use of computers in procedure and holding rooms. Other critical electrical systems include—lighting cycle control, security, and monitoring of water usage.[11]

Lab Planning Concepts in a Nanotechnology Research Center (Fig. 6)

The laboratory module is the key unit in any lab facility. When designed correctly, a lab module will fully coordinate all the architectural and engineering systems. A well-designed modular plan should provide the following benefits:

- *Flexibility*: The lab module, should "encourage change" within the building. Research is changing all the time, and buildings must allow for reasonable change. It means the ability to expand easily,

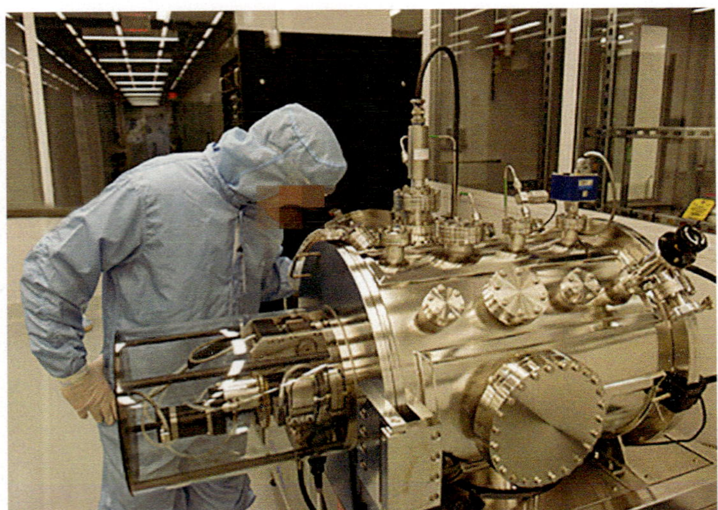

Fig. 6: Nanophysics lab.

to readily accommodate reconfigurations and other changes, and to permit a variety of uses.[11]

- *Two-directional lab module*: Design a lab module that works in both directions allows the casework to be organized in either direction.[11]
- *Three-dimensional lab module*: A three-dimensional lab module planning concept combines the basic lab module or a two-directional lab module with any lab corridor arrangement for each floor of a building.
- All vertical risers must be fully coordinated (vertical risers include fire stairs, elevators, restrooms, and shafts for utilities). Labs designed with overhead connects and disconnects allow for flexibility and *fast hookup of equipment*. The mechanical, electrical, and plumbing systems must be coordinated in the ceiling to work with the multiple corridor arrangements.[11]
- *Expansion*: The use of lab planning modules allows the building to adapt easily to needed expansions or contractions without sacrificing facility functionality.[11]
- The relationship of the labs, offices, and corridors is critical for the impact on the image and operations of the building.
- Natural light may not be desirable for special instruments and equipment, such as nuclear magnetic resonance *(NMR) apparatus*, electron microscopes, and lasers and vivarium facilities.[11]
- Zoning of the building between *lab and nonlab* spaces is essential.
- *Open labs versus closed labs*: An open lab concept encourages multiple teams to focus on separate research projects. The architectural and engineering systems are designed to affordably accommodate multiple floor plans that can easily be changed according to the research teams' needs. Closed labs are still needed for specific kinds of research or for certain equipment. NMR equipment, electron microscopes, tissue culture labs, darkrooms, and glass washing are examples of equipment and activities that must be housed in separate, dedicated spaces. The glass walls may be used which allow people to see each other, while also having their individual spaces.[11]
- *Flexible engineering systems*: Flexible engineering services—supply and exhaust air, water, electricity, voice/data, vacuum systems—are extremely important to most labs. They must have easy connects/disconnects at the walls and ceiling to allow for fast, affordable hookups of equipment. Engineering systems are designed to service initial demands and at least an additional 25% for anticipated future programs. All pipes, valves, and clean-outs are clearly labeled to identify the contents, pressure, and temperature.[11]
- *Separation of hot zones*: This is the space where equipment emit hot air (ovens) or fume hoods, etc. and large amount of toxic air is exhausted. This area does not need to be air conditioned and it reduces considerable load from HVAC system. A proper exhaust layout supported by forced draft fresh air ventilation is sufficient. This area is a dead space, which is visited only for the purpose of monitoring.
- *Equipment zones*: These are must in the initial design. Equipment zones are usually fitted out when the research team moves into the lab—that is, when the team knows exactly what will be needed to do the work.[11]
- *Mobile casework labs*: The labs are designed to accept the needed equipment easily. They allow a large volume of space for storage mobile carts make excellent equipment storage units. They allow computer hardware to be stacked and then moved to equipment stations as needed. Data ports are also located adjacent to electrical outlets along the casework. Mobile base cabinets are constructed with a number of drawer and door configurations and are equipped with an antitipping counterweight.[11]
- *Using the full volume of the lab space*: Many labs today are equipment intensive and require as much bench space as possible. Using the full volume of the lab space to stack equipment and supplies can be very helpful and cost-effective.[11]
- *Overhead service carriers*: An overhead service carrier is hung from the underside of the structural floor system. The utility services are run above the ceiling, where they are connected to the overhead service carrier. The utility services that are run above the ceiling should have quick connect and disconnect features for easy hookups to the overhead service carriers.[11]

Distribution Concepts (Systems)

- *Interstitial space*: An interstitial space is a separate floor located above each lab floor. All services and utilities are located here, where they drop down to service the lab below. This system has a high initial cost but it allows the building to accommodate change very easily without interrupting the labs.[11]
- *Service corridor*: Lab spaces adjoin a centrally located corridor where all utility services are located. Maintenance personnel are afforded constant access to main ducts, shutoff valves, and electric panel boxes without having to enter the lab. This service corridor can be doubled up as an equipment/utility corridor where common lab equipment like autoclaves, freezer rooms, etc. can be located.[11]
- *Electrical systems*: Three types of power are generally used for nanoresearch projects:
  - Normal power circuits are connected to the utility supply only in noncritical areas and general service areas, without any backup system.
  - Emergency power is created with generators that will backup equipment such as refrigerators, freezers, fume hoods, biological safety cabinets, emergency lighting, exhaust fans, animal facilities, and environmental rooms. Examples of safe and efficient emergency power equipment include distributed energy resources (DERs), microturbines, and fuel cells.
  - An uninterruptible power supply (UPS) is used in all critical areas for all kinds of facilities such as for data recording, certain computers, microprocessor-controlled equipment, clean room maintenance areas and possibly the vivarium area. The UPS can be either a central unit or a portable system, such as DERs, microturbines, fuel cells, and building integrated photovoltaics (BIPV).[11]

- *Dry and wet labs*: Research facilities typically include both dry and wet labs.[11]

Dry laboratory are usually computer intensive, with significant requirements for electrical and data wiring. Their casework is mobile; they have adjustable shelving and plastic laminate counters. Typical features of dry laboratory are:

- *Space attributes dry*: Laboratory space types are designed to accommodate project-specific work patterns and scientific equipment. As such, they tend to include design features that provide reliable working conditions in a somewhat mobile environment.[11]
- *Temperature and humidity*: As some equipment and experiments are temperature and humidity-sensitive, constant conditions are required in dry laboratory spaces to ensure that equipment can perform properly and that experiments produce accurate results. Laboratories are usually supplied with variable volume terminal reheat system with prefilters and after-filters for 90% efficiency. In general. laboratory spaces have positive pressure relative to other spaces with no return air from the laboratory to the other spaces.
- *Dust control*: Just as experiments and equipment may be sensitive to changes in temperature and humidity, so might they be to dust and other foreign particulates.
- *Laboratory occupancy*: Occupancy group classification for dry laboratory is B2, Sprinkler protected construction, as per IBC, with a GSA Acoustical Class C1 for enclosed spaces and Class C2 for open spaces.
- *Durable/flexible/mobile casework*: As working conditions will often change due to new projects and equipment, dry laboratories are usually fitted with mobile casework to allow for flexibility in the floor plan. This casework is generally a premanufactured laboratory metal casework system with cantilever support off of central service chase system. Counters are typically a plastic laminate with integral splash. The chase system has metal channel support with a horizontal distribution of wiring.
- *Reliable, easy to access, wiring system*: Due to the flexible nature of the dry laboratory, the distribution of critical wiring (power, voice data, and HVAC) should be clearly laid out, and easy to access and redirect. Thus, a raised floor system is the recommended system of distribution of critical services for this space type.
- *Fire and life safety*: All laboratory spaces typically will contain a hand-held chemical emergency fire extinguisher in an emergency equipment cabinet. There is generally one fire alarm pull station by each egress point and an audible and visible (strobe) alarm in each occupiable space (not including closets, storage rooms, or coat racks).

Wet laboratory have sinks, piped gases, and usually, fume hoods. Wet labs require chemical-resistant countertops and 100% outside air and are outfitted with some fixed casework. Typical features of a wet laboratory are:

- *Space attributes*: Wet laboratory space types are unique in that they must accommodate simultaneous and separate ventilation and utility connections at individual lab modules to ensure both the reliability and accuracy of results as well as occupant safety throughout the space.[11]
- *Surfaces*: Resilient surfaces are an integral part of the wet laboratory space type design. Use epoxy paint for lab walls and monolithic, seamless, chemical-resistant vinyl flooring with integral coved-based and mylar finish.
- *Separate laboratory modules*: A wet laboratory space is typically divided into separate laboratory modules that contain individually controlled connections to HVAC, utilities and safety devices. Modules are defined spatially by floor-to-ceiling structural slab with under-floor plenum divider.
- *Constant and reliable HVAC*: As some equipment and experiments are temperature- and humidity-sensitive, constant conditions are required in wet laboratory spaces to ensure that equipment can perform properly and that experiments produce accurate results. Laboratories are usually supplied with variable volume, terminal reheat system with prefilters and after-filters for 90% efficiency. In general, laboratory spaces have positive pressure relative to other spaces with no return air from the laboratory to the other spaces.
- *Dust control*: Just as experiments and equipment may be sensitive to changes in temperature and humidity, so might they be to dust and other foreign particulates.
- *Gas/utility services*: Utility connections in wet laboratory space types can include vacuum, pneumatic supply, natural gas, O_2 and CO_2, and distilled water. The fittings and connections for each module are connected to the building distribution system for six nominal piping systems.
- *Fume hoods*: Design wet laboratory space types to accommodate one 6 ft – 0 inch chemical fume hood for each laboratory module, and provide direct 100% exhaust. It is also typical of this space type to include an acid and corrosives vented storage cabinet located under the fume hood, as well storage for emergency equipment.
- *Laboratory occupancy*: Occupancy group classification for wet laboratory is B2, sprinkler protected construction, as per IBC, with a GSA acoustical Class C1 for enclosed spaces and Class C2 for open spaces.
- *Fire and life safety*: All laboratory spaces should contain a hand-held chemical emergency fire extinguisher in an emergency equipment cabinet. There is generally one fire alarm pull station by each egress point and an audible and visible (strobe) alarm in each occupiable space (not including closets, storage rooms, or coat racks). Also include toxic gas monitors in each lab module and a gas storage area with audio and visual (strobe) alarms both inside and outside the lab. Eyewash and deluge shower should be located at each module quad.

Design for the computer virtual labs: Areas in which virtual reality is playing a key role are:

- Virtual manufacturing
- Three-dimensional calibration for virtual environments
- Assembly path planning using virtual reality techniques
- Virtual assembly design environment
- Knowledge-based systems virtual environments for ergonomic design
- Telerobotics.

Planning and Designing of Office Spaces in a Laboratory

Office spaces a flexible environment that integrates technology, comfort and safety, and energy efficiency to provide a productive, cost effective, and esthetically pleasing working environment. It refers to a variety of spaces including: meeting spaces integrated into the office environment, reception, office support spaces such as work rooms, storage rooms, file rooms, mail rooms, copier areas, service units/coffee bar, and coat storage integrated into the office environment, and telephone and communications equipment rooms located in tenant suites containing tenant equipment.[11]

Characteristics of Office Space[11]

- Millwork other than service unit/coffee bar and coat storage.
- Meeting spaces and conference rooms that include special lighting systems, acoustical treatment, moveable partitions, mill work, or A/V systems.
- Secure storage, strong rooms, vaults, and hardened partitions located within the office suite.
- Large filing, library, or storage areas with concentrated floor loads.
- Enclosed spaces requiring acoustical separation higher than 40 STC, partitions to structure with acoustical insulation, and duct work sound baffling.
- Specialized window treatments (blackout shades, plantation shutters, motorized fabric draperies, etc.)—interior windows, glass block partitions, and glazed doors
- Humidity, pathogenic, or hypoallergenic air treatment systems.
- Upgrade or changes to standard items such as plaster or vaulted ceilings, specialty lighting, or upgraded ceiling tiles.
- Private toilets, elevators, or staircases.
- Office space plans can be arranged in several scenarios, including—100% closed office.

CONCLUSION

Mankind is still fighting against many complex illnesses like cancer, multiple sclerosis, cardiovascular diseases, Alzheimer's and Parkinson's diseases, diabetes as well as some inflammatory or infectious diseases (i.e. HIV). Nanotechnology raises hopes and expectations for millions of patients that suffer from those diseases. It is expected that doctors will be able to destroy the very first cancer cells and so stop the disease from growing. It is a field of applied science and technology involving control of matter on a scale smaller than 1 μm, normally between 1 nm and 100 nm, as well as the fabrication of devices on this same length scale. It is a highly multidisciplinary field cutting across many disciplines, including colloidal science, chemistry, applied physics, materials science, and even mechanical and electrical engineering. Both the technical criteria and human criteria that culminate in the design of nanotech laboratories and facilities can present astounding complexities to the architects and engineers involved in creating the design. Even the best planning effort cannot predict perfectly how spaces will be used, or anticipate technological advancements that may dramatically affect space requirements. Over time, spaces will be assigned to different researchers and programs, so architects and engineers should do what they can to build flexibility into any design. The fundamental object of sustainable design is a bigger compatibility between the artificial and the natural environments without compromising the functional requirements of the buildings and their respective costs and a challenge for the future. Given the limited amount of information about health risks that may be associated with nonmaterial, designing nano research centers with design guided measures to minimize worker exposures is prudent.[2-4,6,13,14]

Building a research center affects each four topics of sustainable development that are ecological, economic, social and cultural development. Progress toward the sustainable construction requires novel technologies and policies; not only for the new buildings but also for the refurbishing processes. As the evaluation of sustainability remains characterized by local and value-driven factors, the future building design methods need a generic basis with flexibility in implementation. The fundamental goal of sustainable development is to preserve the ecological systems that globally are the basis for human life and biodiversity of the nature. Environmentally, sustainable construction ensures more economical use of finite raw materials and reduces, and above all, prevents the accumulation of pollutants and waste. The Life Cycle Analysis (LCA) is internationally recognized as a usable approach to evaluate the environmental impacts of products or processes. An assessment of environmental impacts of a process or a product is an analysis that is made by identification of what has been taken from the environment and what has been brought back, by recognition of the potential harms due to these actions and by rating the significance of the impacts.[4,5]

REFERENCES

1. www.pubmedcentral.nih.gov
2. en.wikipedia.org
3. www.ncbi.nlm.nih.gov
4. in.answers.yahoo.com
5. repositorium.sdum.uminho.pt
6. www.tradelineinc.com
7. labquipasia.com
8. https://en.wikipedia.org/wiki/cleanroom cite-note-11
9. www.isranalytica.org.il
10. https://www.iso.org/standard/53394.html
11. www.wbdg.org

OTHER REFERENCES

- Bragança L, Heli K, Ricardo M. Sustainable design in construction sector. Balkema AA; 2005 [Online]. [cited 2011 Jan 02]; Available from: URL:http://hdl.handle.net/1822/5072
- Center for responsible Nano Technology. What is Nanotechnology. [Online]. [cited 2011 Jan 02]; Available from: URL: http://www.crnano.org/whatis.htm
- Center for Responsible Nanotechnology. What is Nanotechnology? [Online]. [cited 2011 Jan 02]; Available from: URL:http://www.crnano.org/whatis.htm
- Centers for Disease Control and Prevention, National Institute for Occupational Safety and Health. Managing the Health and Safety Concerns Associated with Engineered Nanomaterials. [Online]. [cited 2011 Jan 02]; Available from: URL:http://www.cdc.gov/niosh/docs/2009-125/pdfs/2009-125.pdf
- Cleanroom. [Online]. [cited 2011 Jan 02]; Available from: URL:http://en.wikipedia.org/wiki/Cleanroom
- Nano medicine center. History of Nano technology.[Online]. [cited 2011 Jan 02]; Available from: URL:http://www.nanomedicinecenter.com/article/history-of-nanotechnology/
- Nanomedicine. [Online]. [cited 2011 Jan 02]; Available from: URL:http://en.wikipedia.org/wiki/Nanomedicine
- New world encyclopedia. Nanotechnology. [Online]. 2008 [cited 2011 Jan 02]; Available from: URL: http://www.newworldencyclopedia.org/entry/Nanotechnology
- Phoenix C, Treder M. Applying the Precautionary Principle to Nanotechnology. Center for Responsible Nanotechnology [Online]. 2003 Jan [cited 2011 Jan 02]; Available from: URL:http://www.crnano.org/precautionary.htm
- Robert A, Freitas Jr. Nanotechnology, Nanomedicine and nanosurgery [editorial]. IJSU 2005;3/4:243-246. Available from: URL: http://www.nanomedicine.com/Papers/IntlJSurg Dec05.pdf
- Sohoni A. Basic architectural design considerations for a laboratory. Express Pharma [Online]. 2010 Feb 16-28 [cited 2011 Jan 02]; Available from: URL:http://www.expresspharmaonline.com/20100228/pharmaally02.shtml

- Soueid A. Nanotechnology Research Requires a Different Breed of laboratories and Clearrooms. Controlled Environments 2009 Dec 01; [Online]. [cited 2011 Jan 02]; Available from: URL:http://www.cemag.us
- Stahl NZ. Nanotech Planning Integrates Architecture and Engineering–Infrastructure Costs Are Often Underestimated. Tradeline 2003 Apr 23; [Online]. [cited 2011 Jan 02]; Available from: URL:http://www.tradelineinc.com/reports/98B4D97D-2B3B-B525-83282ABCB518461D
- Stark S, Petitto J, Darr S. Animal Research Facility. WBDG 2010; [Online]. [cited 2011 Jan 02]; Available from: URL:http://www.wbdg.org/design/animal_research.php
- Valuation of subjects containing Clean Rooms-Practice Note 5. SAA Industrial Committee-Revaluation 2005; [Online]. [cited 2011 Jan 02]; Available from: URL: http://www.saa.gov.uk/resources/148164/clean_rooms_pn_no5.pdf
- Webster Thomas J. Nanomedicine: what's in a definition? IJNM. 2006;2006(1/2): 115-6.
- Wesel L. Correctly Sizing Utilities is Critical for nanotechnology Labs – Bigger is Not Necessarily Better. Tradeline 2008 Nov 05; [Online]. [cited 2011 Jan 02]; 8A1875DD781CA265.

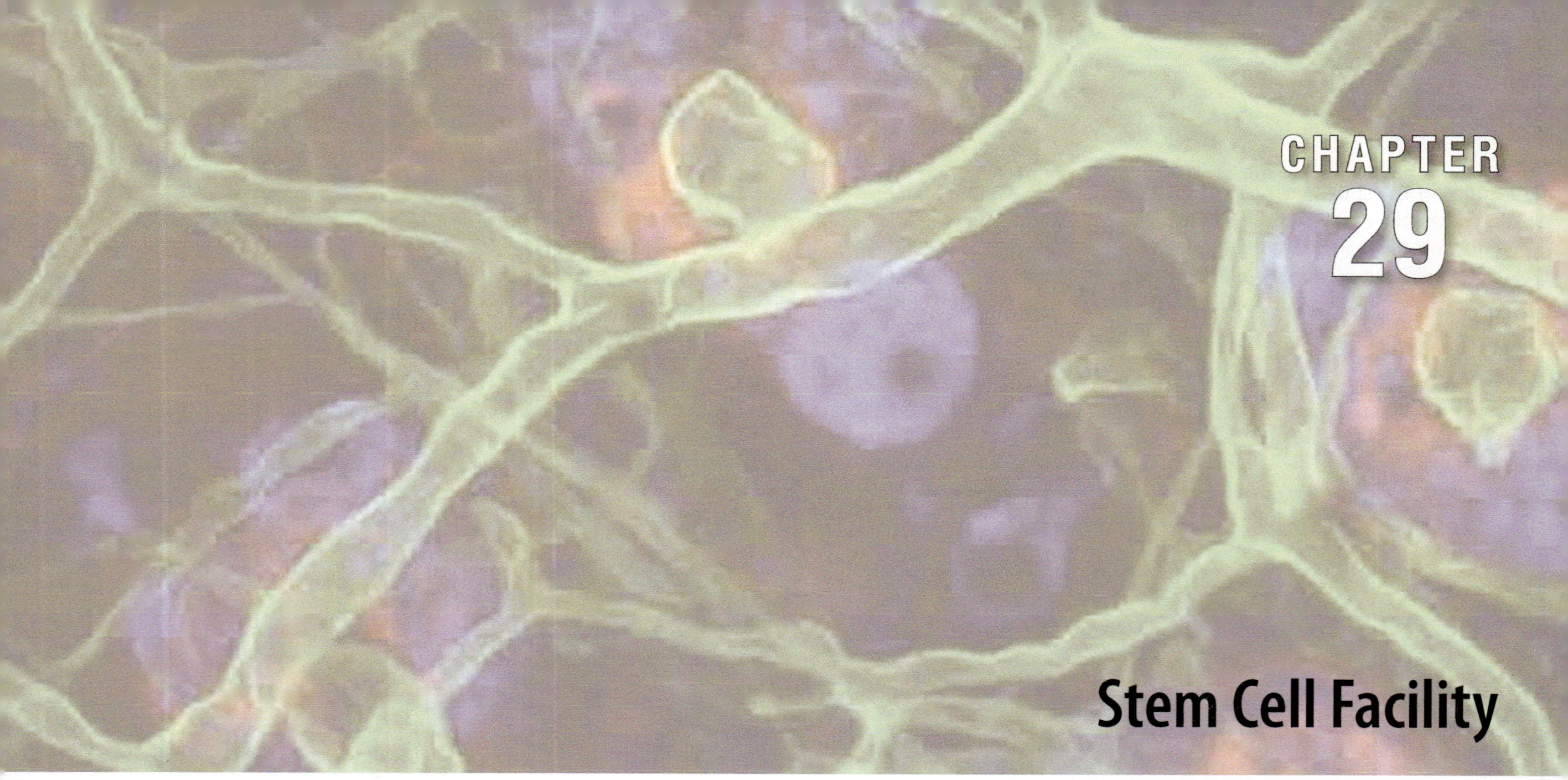

CHAPTER 29

Stem Cell Facility

Sapna Ramani, Sujata Mohanty, Shakti Kumar Gupta, Sunil Kant, R Chandrashekhar

INTRODUCTION[1]

Stem cells are undifferentiated biological cells with the ability to divide for indefinite periods in culture and to give rise to specialized cells. Stem cells have the remarkable potential to develop into many different cell types in the body during early life and growth. In addition, in many tissues they serve as a sort of internal repair system, dividing essentially without limit to replenish other cells as long as the person or animal is still alive. When a stem cell divides, each new cell has the potential either to remain a stem cell or become another type of cell with a more specialized function, such as a muscle cell, a red blood cell, or a brain cell.[1]

Stem cells are distinguished from other cell types by two important characteristics. First, they are unspecialized cells capable of renewing themselves through cell division, sometimes after long periods of inactivity. Second, under certain physiologic or experimental conditions, they can be induced to become tissue- or organ-specific cells with special functions. In some organs, such as the gut and bone marrow, stem cells regularly divide to repair and replace worn out or damaged tissues. In other organs, however, such as the pancreas and the heart, stem cells only divide under special conditions.[1]

CLASSIFICATION OF STEM CELLS

Until recently, scientists primarily worked with two kinds of stem cells from animals and humans—embryonic stem cells (ESCs) and nonembryonic "somatic" or "adult" stem cells.

Embryonic stem cells (Fig. 1) are derived from pre-implantation embryos. ESCs derived from the inner cell mass (ICM) are pluripotent, having ability to differentiate into derivatives of all three germ layers, viz. ectoderm, mesoderm and endoderm, but not placenta.[2]

Some specialized adult cells can be "reprogrammed" genetically to assume a stem cell-like state. This new type of stem cell, called induced pluripotent stem cells (iPSCs), as the name suggests are pluripotent in nature, quite similar to the ESCs but may not be exactly the same. They are capable of indefinite expansion and differentiation into ectodermal, mesodermal and endodermal cells. The iPS cells can be generated from somatic cells by a variety of genetic and epigenetic methods.[2,3]

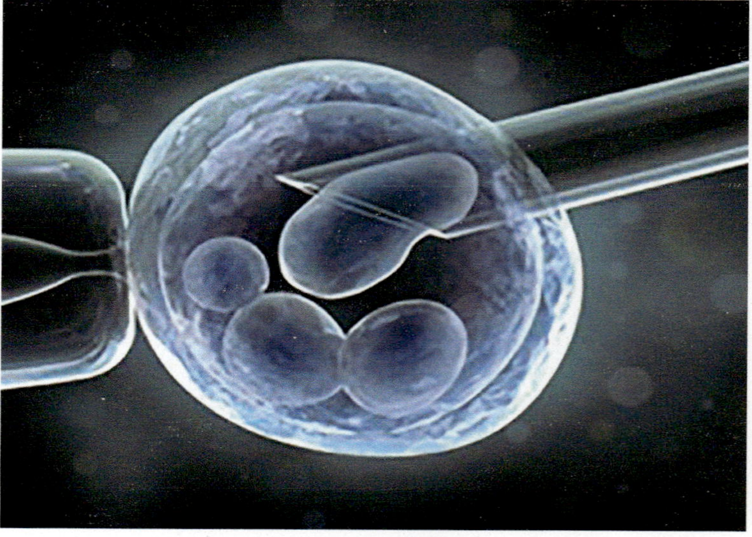

Fig. 1: Embryonic stem cells.

THE POTENTIAL USES OF STEM CELLS

Stem cell therapy is an emerging field with potential to alter the way we treat or prevent a disease or a condition. This is further providing new avenues in clinical research and drug discoveries.

There are many ways in which human stem cells can be used in research and the clinic.

A primary goal is to identify how undifferentiated stem cells become the differentiated cells that form the tissues and organs. Scientists know that turning genes on and off is central to this process.

Some of the most serious medical conditions, such as cancer and birth defects, are due to abnormal cell division and differentiation. A more complete understanding of the genetic and molecular controls of these processes may yield information about how such diseases arise and suggest new strategies for therapy. Predictably controlling cell proliferation and differentiation requires additional basic research on the molecular and genetic signals that regulate cell division and specialization.[4-6]

Human stem cells could also be used to test new drugs. For example, new medications could be tested for safety on differentiated cells generated from human pluripotent cell lines. The availability of pluripotent stem cells would allow drug testing in a wider range of cell types.[4-6]

Perhaps the most important potential application of human stem cells is the generation of cells and tissues that could be used for cell-based therapies. Today, donated organs and tissues are often used to replace ailing or destroyed tissue, but the need for transplantable tissues and organs far outweighs the available supply. Stem cells, directed to differentiate into specific cell types, offer the possibility of a renewable source of replacement cells and tissues to treat diseases including Alzheimer's diseases, spinal cord injury, stroke, burns, heart disease, diabetes, osteoarthritis, and rheumatoid arthritis.[4-6]

However, much work remains to be done in the laboratory and the clinic to understand how to use these cells for cell-based therapies to treat certain diseases, which is also referred to as regenerative or reparative medicine.

STEM CELL FACILITY

Stem cell research has come up in a big way in the past couple of years. The relevance of the research is well reflected by the enthusiasm of global scientific community. Stem cells have proved and are also being predicted to be the futuristic option for cell therapy because of its enormous therapeutic potential. However, the research in the subject is still in the juvenile stage and many efforts are still needed to fully understand the reason behind the stem cell magic.

The research of stem cell is multidisciplinary, i.e. it involves animal tissue culture, molecular biology, pharmacology, biophysics to name just a few. Apart from multidisciplines it has related components of research also. Animal studies and application of the findings to the humans is a crucial part of the whole research. To accomplish all the aspects of stem cell biology; all the components as discussed, should be under one roof to carry out quality research in this area.

An ideal stem cell facility should be composed of:

- Laboratory area for basic research
- Animal house including operating theater
- Area for patient care services which would include patient recruitment and registration corner, bone marrow aspiration room, operation theater (OT), and postoperation follow-up wards.

FUNCTION OF THE FACILITY

The stem cell facility is a multidisciplinary center for the scientists and clinicians to come together and explore the subject. Scientifically, it is involved in various studies related to the stem cells. Briefly, isolation, characterization, sorting and cryopreservation of stem cells from various sources are carried out in the laboratory along with cytogenetics and molecular studies are also done to study the properties of these cells at gene level.

Animal studies are the subsequent step for the application of the findings of the research before starting off with the human trials. Both scientists and clinicians would be responsible for the human trials, i.e. stem cell transplantation program and post-transplantation follow-ups.

The stem cell facility to function appropriately; the facility should be governed by certain regulations. The type of predicted work will be the deciding factor as to which category of regulation it will be adhered to; as architectural planning of the facility would much depend on the regulations. The designing of the facility is crucial to the good manufacturing process (GMP)/good laboratory practice (GLP) accreditation process. The two categories of regulations that are to be considered in this case are current good laboratory practices (cGLP) and current good manufacturing practices (cGMP). GLP deals with the organization, process and conditions under which laboratory studies are planned, performed, monitored, recorded and reported. GLP regulates all nonclinical safety studies that support or are intended to support applications for research. GMP facility is an ultra—clean, controlled environment where potent biological, cellular or other pharmaceutical products for administration in humans can be manufactured safely and reliably. For general research, not involving any manipulation or manufacturing of cells for therapeutic purpose can adhere to GLP regulations but in case of genetic manipulations in the stem cells or manufacturing of cells for therapeutic purpose GMP is mandatory.[7]

Planning and Designing of a Stem Cell Facility

The process of establishing a human pluripotent stem cell (hPSC) (Fig. 2) laboratory can be divided into two equally important parts:[1,8,9]

- One is establishing a hPSC laboratory involves the physical plant and includes design, equipment and personnel.
- The other part is completely administrative and includes developing protocols, seeking approval, and establishing reporting processes and documentation.

Proper planning of laboratory operations and proper design of the physical layout of the stem cell laboratory so that it meets the scope of planned operations is a major undertaking, but the time spent upfront will pay long-term returns in operational efficiency and effectiveness. A well-planned, organized, and properly equipped laboratory supports research activities by increasing efficiency and reducing lost time and wasted resources.[1,8,9]

Establishing a well-functioning laboratory for the culture of hPSCs provides the foundation for successful culture and experimentation. While the culture of hPSCs is carried out in a laboratory that is not much different than one used to culture other types of human cells, due to the special status of these cells, there is a higher degree of oversight, review, and reporting. It is found that a nearly equal amount of time and effort is required to establish initial protocols and seek approval for culturing and obtaining human pluripotent cell lines as is required to design and equip the laboratory (Fig. 3).[1,8,9]

This diagram indicates the interrelated nature of the four key elements in a stem cell laboratory.

Whether retrofitting an existing laboratory or designing a new laboratory from shell space, the basic issues are the same. One must consider the equipment, number of people, and type of activities to be performed in order to achieve the best design (within budget constraints). Using a modular design, both in terms of laboratory benches and equipment, allows the laboratory to be expanded as needed by adding additional tissue culture modules and personnel to manage the work load.[1,8,9]

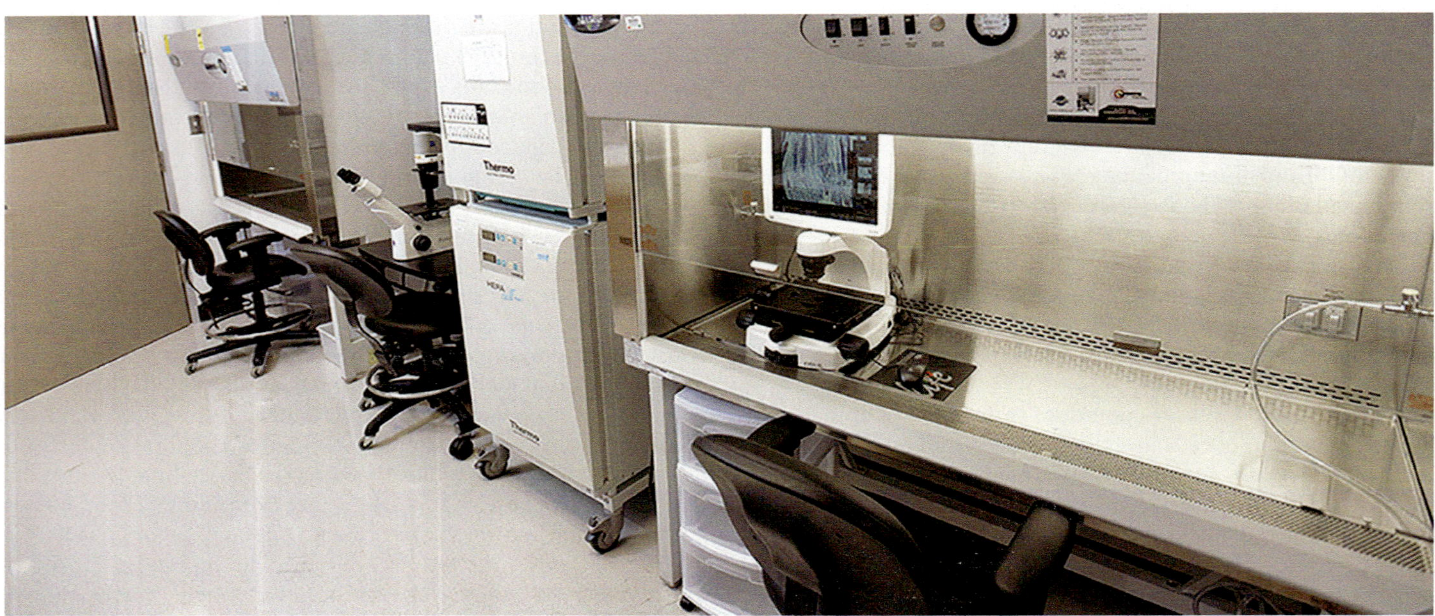
Fig. 2: Human pluripotent stem cell laboratory.

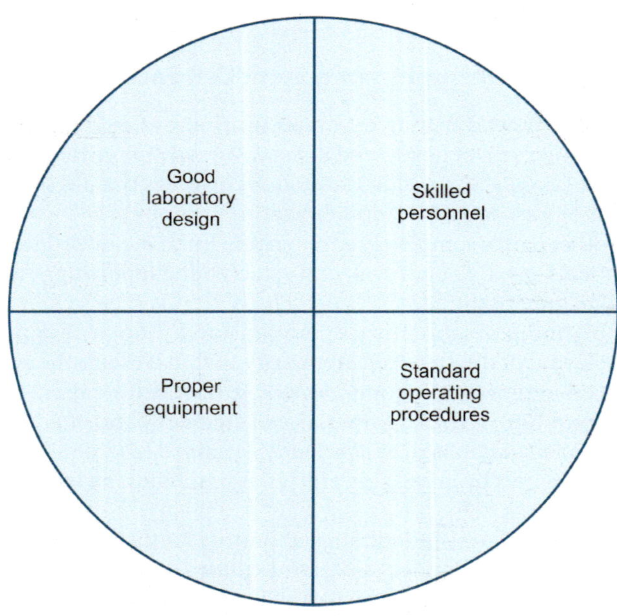

Fig. 3: Stem cell facility.

Laboratory Design and Layout

When building out new laboratory space, the design team usually includes an architect, a contractor, a builder, an electrician, a mechanical engineer, a plumber, and a laboratory director or manager. The design team for retrofitting existing laboratory space is usually smaller and less formal, but is still comprised a number of people with specialized skills including the builder, electrician, mechanical engineer, plumber, and the laboratory manager or director. Since the costs for building-out average laboratory space is 3–5 times that of office space, the budget is a key consideration and should be established as part of the preplanning.[1,8]

The dynamic nature of biomedical research and the cost of laboratory construction have resulted in the prevalent use of modular design that allows reconfiguration of the laboratory as needed while keeping construction costs to a minimum.[1,8]

Key Considerations for Planning and Design[1]

- Budget
  - How much money to spend and over what time?
  - Return on investment (what is expected to be gained through this investment). A resources land planning.
- Space
  - What type? Is it new construction, build-out of shell space, rehabilitation of existing laboratory or office?
  - How much space is available?
  - Phased construction, how do the phases relate to each other? Should the plan include drawings for eventual build-out of all of the space?
- Type and scope of work to be performed
  - Biosafety level of laboratory
  - Major equipment
  - Number of people.
- Major functional areas
  - Tissue culture laboratory
  - Quarantine laboratory (optional, but desired)
  - Molecular biology/quality control laboratory
  - Microscopy laboratory.
- Personnel
  - How many people?
  - In which functional area will they work?
  - How many offices?
  - How many desk spaces, shared or dedicated?
  - Break room.
- Freezer rooms
  - How many and what types of freezers?
  - Backup generator
  - Alarm system
  - A separate cryogenic freezer room with limited access.
- Storage areas in and adjacent to the laboratory
  - Cabinets
  - Shelves with 1-inch lip to prevent objects from falling
  - Closets.
- Information technology
  - IT closet.

INFRASTRUCTURAL CONSIDERATIONS

Space Requirements

Establishment of such a facility will require proper planning before establishment The selection of the location is foremost, as according to the allocated space, the layout of the laboratory has to be planned. The estimated space required would depend upon the predicted future workload and manpower. And also, the architecture planning committee should ensure that there is always a provision for upgradation of the facility. The architecture of the facility would much depend on the type of work being carried out.

The available space will be including all the components, i.e. research laboratories, animal house, and patient care service.

Research Laboratories

Ideally the whole laboratory area ought to be divided into three zone of nonsterile, presterile and sterile. The research laboratory area should be divided proportionally for different activities. The largest area should be allocated for culturing operations. The second largest space should be dedicated to wash up, sterilization and preculture preparations and third for storage purpose. The interiors of the rooms should be such that proper cleanliness is maintained. Wooden furniture are not recommended; as they accumulate dust and vast heat. The structural coating/finishing materials used for workbench should be of dust free grade and preferably of white or grayish shade for proper visualization of media etc. The furniture should be epoxy coated or made of solid mineral surface. It is always recommended that the flooring should be coved and its level of flooring should be slightly tilted towards the washing area to avoid sudden flooding of water under certain circumstances.

Patient Care Services

The service is for the stem cell transplantation patients of various disorders. This will be consisting of a bone marrow aspiration room, an OT and postoperation wards. The area would be separated still easy accessible from the laboratory area.

Animal House Facility

Animal house is a very important component of stem cell research as all the *in vivo* studies involving the stem cells are carried out on animals. The location of the facility should be within the premises not very far off from the main stem cell facility. The place should be well maintained in terms of cleanliness and environmental monitoring (EM). It should have a minor OT facility where high sterility is recommended. Moreover, there should be dedicated staff for the facility and the entry should be highly restricted.

Layout Plan (Fig. 4)

FACILITIES: BUILDINGS AND EQUIPMENT

Buildings

General Principles

Stem cell facilities should be of suitable size, construction and location to meet the requirements of the study and to minimize disturbances

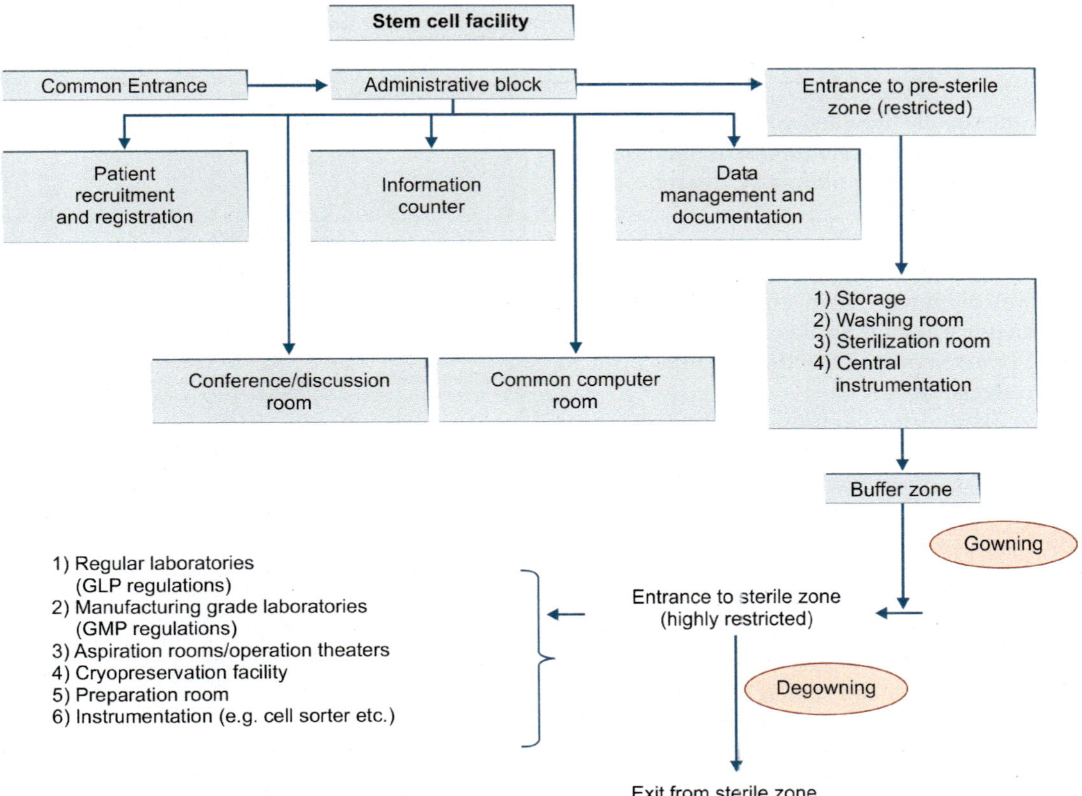

Fig. 4: The layout of stem cell facility.

(A common entrance to the facility should be leading to the administrative block. This block composes of patient recruitment and registration corner, an information counter and document management unit. The conference rooms and central computer access facility is located in this block. Next to the administrative block is the entrance to presterile zone, which further leads to the highly restricted sterile zone through the buffer area, where the personnel entering should undergo the process of complete gowning. The area of degowning preceds the exit from the sterile zone. In the premises are also central air-conditioner/power backup system, waste disposal management unit and central animal house facility).

that could interfere with the study. They should be designed to provide an adequate degree of separation of the diverse elements of the study. The purpose of these requirements is to ensure that the study is not compromised because of inadequate facilities. It is important to remember that fulfilling the requirements of the study does not necessarily mean providing the "state of the art" constructions, but carefully considering whether the objectives of the study can be achieved using the facilities available.[10]

Separation ensures that disturbances are minimized and that different activities do not interfere with one another or adversely affect the study. This can be achieved by:[10]

- *Physical separation*, e.g. walls, doors, filters or separate cabinets or isolators. In new buildings, or those recently renovated, separation will be part of the design.
- *Organizational separation*, e.g. carrying out different activities in the same area but at different times, allowing for cleaning and preparation between operations, maintaining separation of staff, or by establishing defined work areas within a laboratory.
- *Pharmacy and dose mixing areas*: Concerned with test material control and mixing with vehicles (although the same considerations would apply to other areas such as analytical or histopathology laboratories).
- Animal facilities.

Facility Premises

- Stem cell processing and storage facility should be situated and should have such measures as to avoid risk of contamination from external environment including open sewage, drain, public lavatory or any factory which produces disagreeable or obnoxious odor or fumes, excessive soot, smoke, chemical or biological emissions.[2,8]
- The facility should be secure to prevent the entrance of unauthorized persons.
- The facility should be adequately provided with working space to allow orderly and logical placement of equipment, material and movement of personnel so as to maintain safe operations and prevent contamination.
- The facility shall be developed to provide, safe, clean and hygienic environment.[6]
- The facility should be well illuminated and ventilated. It shall have 24 hour provision of potable water for drinking and hand hygiene. It should also have 24 hours supply of electricity, either through direct supply or from other sources.[6]
- The facility should be divided into defined areas of adequate size to prevent improper labeling, mix ups, contamination, cross contamination of cellular therapy products.[6]
- Provided with defined environmental conditions for temperature, humidity, ventilation, and air filtration. Classifications shall be defined and, if appropriate, monitored.[6]

Minimum Infrastructure Requirement

Facility areas: Separate dedicated and designated areas specifically designed for the purpose and the workload should be provided.[6]

- *Reception*: Reception area with space for transient storage of units and physical examination shall have adequate facilities for registration, data entry and generation of bar-coded labels.[2,8]
- *Cell processing areas (Fig. 5)*: The room should be clean and have an air handling system to provide a class 10,000 environment. Entry to this area should be through air lock. The room will house class 100 biological safety cabinets for umbilical cord blood processing. The temperature of the clean room should be maintained 20°–25°C and with a positive differential pressure of 10–15 pascal and relative humidity of 50–60%.[6]
- *Hematology and serology laboratory*: The laboratory should be equipped and utilized for the purpose of independently testing of cell therapy products for ABO grouping and Rh typing, total nucleated cell count, progenitor cell count and viability test. The room shall be air-conditioned.[6]
- *Transfusion transmissible disease screening laboratory*: The laboratory should be equipped and utilized for screening test on maternal blood for infectious diseases viz. human immunodeficiency virus I and II; Hepatitis B and C virus, syphilis, malaria, Cytomegalovirus and human T cell leukemia virus type 1 and 2. The room should be air-conditioned.[6]
- *Cryostorage room (Fig. 6)*: The cryogenic storage room should have provision for temperature monitoring of storage vessels, liquid nitrogen level in storage vessels and oxygen meter. The service space between each liquid nitrogen storage vessel, supply cylinders and

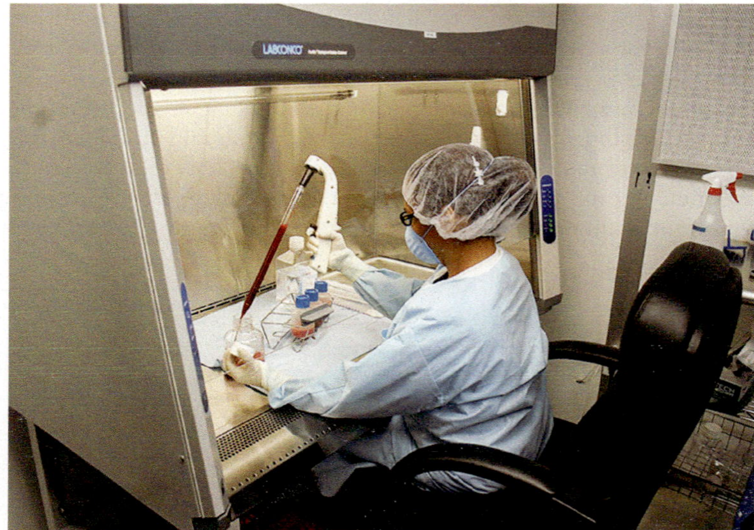

Fig. 5: Cell processing areas.

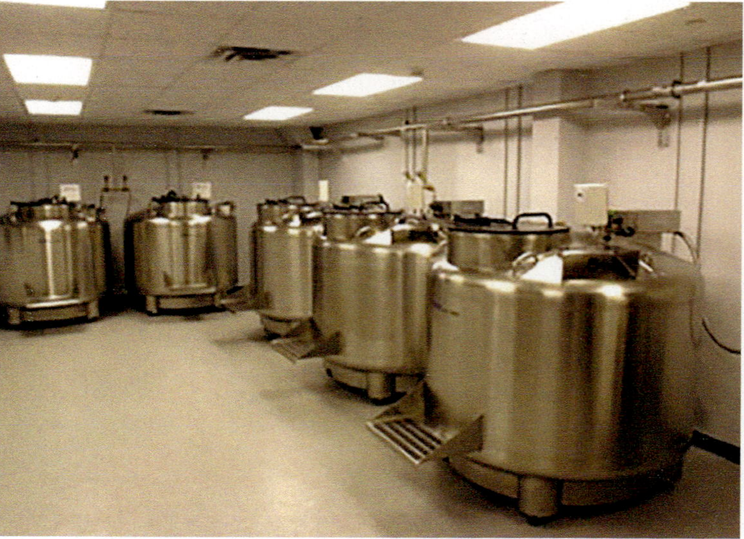

Fig. 6: Cryostorage room.

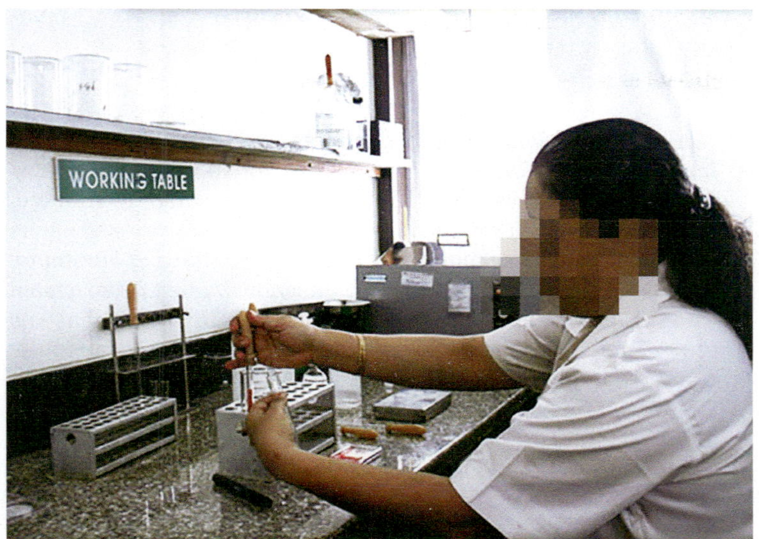

Fig. 7: Human leukocyte antigen typing laboratory.

connecting hose should be minimum 1.00 m^2. Separate storage space for other accessories required should be provided. The room should be air-conditioned.[3]

- *Sterilization-cum-washing*: Appropriate facility should be provided within the premises for proper washing and sterilization. This facility would be optional for laboratories using entirely disposable items.[3]
- *Human leukocyte antigen typing laboratory (Fig. 7)*: The cell processing unit should have arrangements for human leukocyte antigen (HLA) typing and genetic disease testing. In house testing can be done by providing a well demarcated laboratory from the processing area for evaluating of possible genetic disease and HLA typing. This facility would be optional for laboratories that are outsourcing these services for testing.[3]
- *General storage area*: It should be provided to store all the consumables, under conditions deemed optimum for storage by manufacturers.
- *Record room*: There should be designated record room permitted only to authorize persons. The room will have adequate protective facilities as the documents and records are to be preserved for long period.

Furniture

- Furniture and fixtures should be available in accordance with the activities and workload of the facility. They shall be functional and properly maintained.[6]
- Furniture should be placed in aseptic areas which are smooth, washable and made of stainless steel or any other appropriate no-shedding material other than wood.[6]

Equipment

The stem cell processing and storage facility is equipped for cell processing, isolation, testing, and cryopreservation. The facility shall ensure the availability of the accessories, spare-parts and backup/maintenance/service support for all equipment. This section lists the minimal equipment required for basic culture and characterization of hPSCs. A given program may require specialized culture equipment, such as incubators that allow culture in low oxygen tension, or characterization and analysis equipment.[6]

Tissue Culture Laboratory

- *Class II biosafety cabinet*: The type of biosafety cabinet (BSC) that one installs depends on the type of work being conducted in the laboratory. The Class II BSC is typically utilized in the hPSC laboratory. Class II BSCs are partial barrier systems that rely on the directional movement of air to provide containment. They provide protection to both the worker and the material that is being manipulated in the cabinet when properly maintained. They provide the microbe-free work environment that is necessary for cell culture. Class II BSCs are available in four different types—types A1 and A2 are recirculate the HEPA-filtered air back into the room. Types B1 and B2 are hard-ducted into a (preferably dedicated) exhaust system that carries the high-efficiency particulate air (HEPA)-filtered air to the outside. Class II A2 is the most common type of BSC installed in cell culture laboratories. Since the safe operation of the BSC relies on the HEPA filter, they are usually tested and certified on an annual basis or before any work commences following the relocation or movement of the BSC. Generally, Class II BSCs can be used to work with *nonvolatile* and *nonhazardous* chemicals or gases; however, only type A2-exhausted or types B1 and B2 can be used for preparing small amounts of volatile chemicals and minute quantities of hazardous chemicals, since they exhaust to the outside.[1,8]
- *CO_2 incubator*: It comes with a variety of options. Incubators can come as two-gas (CO_2:air) or three-gas models (CO_2:O_2:N_2), the two-gas being the most common and least expensive. Chamber temperature is maintained by a water jacket or an air jacket. It is important that the shelving and the hardware securing it be easy to remove and clean. Although copper shelving and interior walls can inhibit the growth of organisms, it is expensive and, unless all hardware components are of copper construction, thorough cleaning is still routinely needed. Routine cleaning with a disinfectant and ethanol rinse will help to reduce sources of contamination. The chamber, however, should be allowed to equilibrate overnight after a thorough cleaning prior to returning the cultures as the volatile components of the cleaning agents may kill the cells in culture. Use a portable RTD thermometer for accurate temperature determination and a Fyrite unit for CO_2 calibration.[1,8]
- Pipettors
- Vacuum flask/aspiration device
- Water bath (37°C)
- Low-speed centrifuge (clinical grade, for spinning cells).

Microscopy

- Phase-contrast microscope
- Dissecting microscope.

Storage

- *Cabinets and shelves for the storage of tissue culture supplies*: Storage cabinets for tissue culture supplies are usually overlooked when designing the laboratory; however, sufficient storage allows for smooth and safe laboratory operations. Sufficient space should be made available that accommodates large bulky boxes so that supplies can be properly stored off the floor and off the equipment, allowing for easy cleaning and accessibility.[1,8]
- Refrigerator (4°C)
- Freezer (–20°C, nondefrosting)
- Low-temperature freezer (–70 to –85°C)
- Cryogenic freezer (storage below –140°C, usually liquid nitrogen).

Molecular Biology Laboratory/Quality Control Laboratory[1,8]

- Reverse transcription polymerase chain reaction (RT-PCR)
- Flow cytometer (might be in a core facility)
- Fluorescence microscope (might be located in a microscopy core)
- Confocal microscope (might be located in a microscopy core).

Quarantine Laboratory[1,8]

- Class II biosafety cabinet
- CO_2 incubator
- Phase-contrast microscope
- Water bath (37°C)
- Low-speed centrifuge (clinical grade, for spinning cells)
- Pipettors
- Aspiration/vacuum flask
- Sink.

Additional Access to Common Equipment or Core Facilities[1,8]

- Microscopy
- Flow cytometry
- Microarray gene expression
- Genomics
- Proteomics
- Virus production[4]
- Vivarium.

KEY DESIGN CONSIDERATIONS (FIG. 8)

Facility Design

- The facility should be divided into two main work areas. The testing laboratory and processing laboratory which are clean rooms designed for GMP workflow. The clean rooms should be interlocked, with three interlock ante-rooms or change rooms. Once staff enters the clean room, they must exit either through the exit anteroom. Workflow through the anteroom is bidirectional, whereas movement through the waste-out room is unidirectional. Unidirectional flow of personnel, raw materials product, and waste product. Flow is restricted to the clean areas of the laboratory.[6]
- The processing facility should be divided into defined areas of adequate size to prevent improper labeling, mix-ups, contamination, or cross-contamination of cellular therapy products.[6]
- There should be a process to control storage areas to prevent mix-ups, contamination and cross-contamination of all products during quarantine and prior to release or distribution.[6]
- The processing facility should provide adequate lighting, ventilation, access to sink and air quality where applicable to prevent the introduction, transmission, or spread of communicable disease.[6]
- Pressure differentials of 0.05 inch w.c. between adjacent rooms with up to 60 air changes/hour.
- Rigorous control of room temperature, pressure and relative humidity.

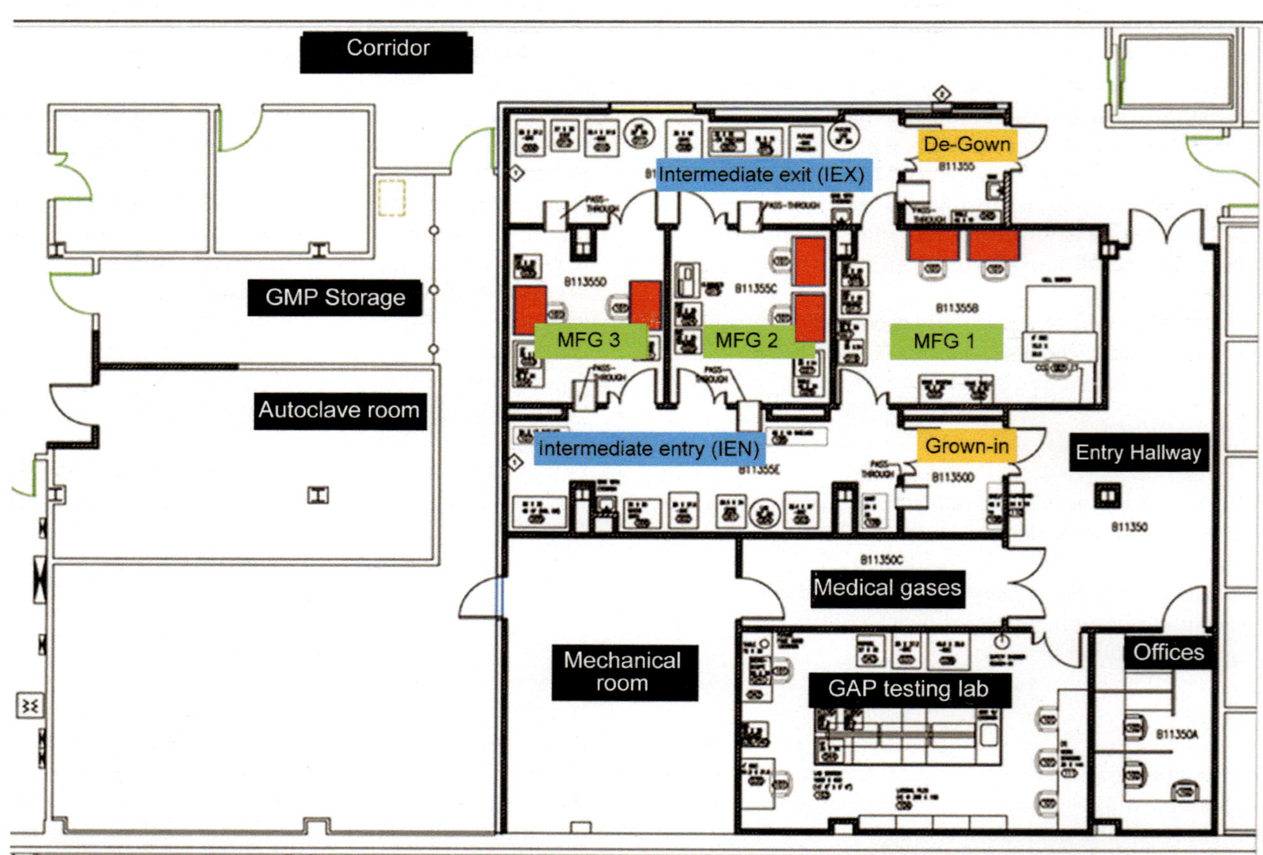

Fig. 8: Functional layout of stem cell facility.
Source: https:\\www.urmc.rochester.eduupstate-stem-cell-facilityour-facility.aspx

- Engineered for easy and effective cleaning, utilizing stainless steel surfaces, gel-coated polymer walls and ceilings, epoxy coated floors, minimal seams and ledges; and movable equipment and work surfaces.
- There should be documentation of facility cleaning and sanitation, EM for microorganisms, and inspection of environmental control systems to ensure adequate conditions for proper operations (Fig. 8).[6]
- Described and listed below are very high-level considerations that are meant to stimulate thinking by the laboratory manager and director as they begin working with their design or construction team to establish a new laboratory for the culture of human PSCs.[6]

Mechanical/Plumbing/Engineering[8]

- *Backup generators*: Dedicated or shared, alarms and controlled access.
- *CO_2 and LN_2 delivery*: Piped to the laboratory from "tank farm" or cylinders delivered to the laboratory and cryobank.
- Vacuum systems.

HVAC

The numbers and types of BSCs will play a major role in the build-out of a tissue culture laboratory[5] and can add greatly to the cost of the build-out. Air handlers must be sized to accommodate the numbers and types of BSCs, as well as any other heat-producing equipment such as incubators and freezers. Efficient and comfortable conditioning of the air in the laboratory is one of the more challenging issues of the design and operation of the laboratory. It can be very uncomfortable working in laboratories, where the heat cannot be controlled due to the installation of HVAC system that is not of sufficient capacity to handle the heat produced by the BSCs and incubators. Air flow and its direction (negative, positive, or neutral) is a key consideration when designing the laboratory and is critical to the safe operation of the cell culture laboratory. Maintain indoor air quality is the essence of designing.[1,8]

Electrical Capacity and Routing

Accurately predicting the number of BSCs, freezers, and other major equipment and determining how much electricity they draw and heat they produce is critical to calculating the correct electrical capacity to maintain and safe working environment. The power requirements for all equipments as well as the location of power outlets, light switches, the determination of emergency power requirements, proximity of outlets to water faucets (GFC), and the coordination of the placement of outlets with the modular furniture designer is part of the detailed design. There need to be sufficient and dedicated circuits to handle all current equipments as well as future expansion. Incubators and freezers must be on backup generator circuits and alarm systems.[1,8]

Environmental Monitoring[8,9]

As maintenance of asepsis is the most crucial requirement of such a facility; a proper EM program will be responsible for the management of environment in the stem cell facility. The aspects of an EM testing program will include sampling for non-viable air (particulates), viable air (microbial), surface (microbial), personnel (microbial).

Air handling systems: It is for sterile areas should be different from those for other areas. The filter configuration in the air handling system should be suitably designed to achieve the grade of air as given in the Table 1.[6]

The environmental microbiological monitoring of clean areas should be in accordance to the recommended limits (Table 2).[6]

Table 1: Maximum permitted number of non-viable particles/m^3 equal to or above.

		At rest		*At operation*	
Grade	Class	Size 0.5 μm	Size 5 μm	Size 0.5 μm	Size 5 μm
A	100	3,500	0	3,500	1
B	100	3,500	0	3,50,000	2,000
C	10,000	3,50,000	2,000	35,00,000	20,000
D	100,000	35,00,000	20,000	Not defined	Not defined

Table 2: Maximum limits for microbiological monitoring of clean areas during operation.

Grade	*Class*	*Air sample cfu/m^3*	*Settle plates (diameter 90 mm) cfu/ 2 hours*	*Contact plates (diameter 55 mm) cfu/plate*	*Glove points 5 fingers (cfu/glove)*
A	100	<1	<1	<1	<1
B	100	10	5	5	5
C	10,000	100	50	25	–
D	100,000	500	100	50	–

These are average, individual settle plates may be exposed for not less than 2 hours in grade B, C and D areas, and for not less than 30 minutes in grade A areas.

Ventilation and Lighting

The ventilation should be ideal, i.e. negative pressure should prevail in the culturing and preculture preparation area relative to the other working areas. The rooms should be supplied with filtered air. The lab airflow has to be on 24 hours a day, and so has to be the monitoring system. Proper ventilation is recommended in the liquid N_2 storage room as filling, dispensing or manipulation of stored samples in liquid N_2 makes liquid N_2 evaporate and lower the O_2 tension drastically which is risky for researchers working out there.

The whole area should be well lit. Incandescent lights are more preferred over fluorescent ones; as they have difficulty in lighting up in hot area and also interfere with the shelf life of stored media etc.

Interior Finishes[8]

- Antibacterial vinyl flooring—with thermosealing joint
- Nonporous ceilings
- Washable, impermeable paint and coatings
- Impermeable bench-tops and furniture.

Tissue Culture Area

The tissue culture area is comprised of a minimal set of equipment, referred to here as the "tissue culture module" (Table 3). It consists of one biosafety cabinet, one CO_2 incubator, one phase-contrast microscope, and a low-speed centrifuge, vacuum source, a water bath, two-2 L flasks, Pipet-Aid, micropipettors, and either a cabinet or cart next to the BSC for easy access to tissue culture supplies. If one keeps with the modular design concept, one can increase output by increasing the number of tissue culture modules in the laboratory design. In the hPSC laboratory, one tissue culture module can accommodate 1–2 technicians. Access to cryogenic storage, centrifuges, microscopes, refrigerators, and freezers is a must for a functional cell culture laboratory; however, these

Table 3: Tissue culture module.[11]

Item	Remarks
Biosafety cabinet	What class and type? Most commonly: Class II type A2
Incubator	Water or air jacketed One gas (CO_2 and air) Two gases (CO_2, N_2, and air) Three gasses (CO_2, N_2, and O_2)
Microscope	Phase–contrast Photo port
Water bath	37°C constant
Low-speed centrifuge	Refrigeration not required
Vacuum source	Portable Supplied by the building
2-L Erlenmeyer flasks, in series, with in-line filter	Collect aspirate and protect vacuum system
Pipet-Aid	Automatic pipettor, cordless, rechargeable
Micropipettors	2, 20, 200, and 1,000 µL

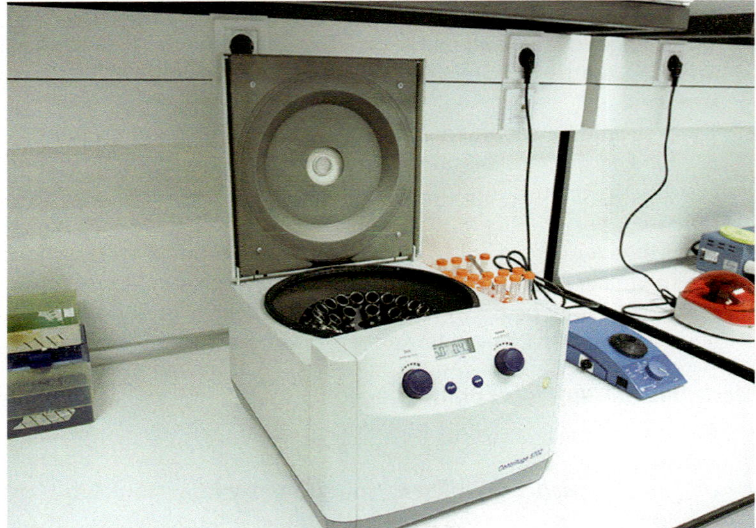

Fig. 9: Quarantine laboratory.

frequently can be shared between multiple modules or laboratories depending on the goals of the overall laboratory program. If setting up a PSC laboratory contained within an existing cell culture laboratory, at least one tissue culture module is required. This will greatly improve productivity and reduce the chances of cross-contamination.[1,8]

Molecular Biology Laboratory/Quality Control Laboratory

The molecular biology/quality control laboratory is comprised of the equipment and SOPs required to perform a predetermined list of characterization assays that allows one to systematically assess the quality of the cells in culture in the laboratory. Cultures are tested for the expression of specific markers, cytogenetic structure (karyotype or SKY), and the ability to differentiate.[1,8]

Quarantine Laboratory (Fig. 9)

The introduction of new cell lines into the laboratory is the major source by which cultures may become contaminated. Therefore, it is important that control systems are in place to minimize the potential for contamination. The quarantine control system may be a separate laboratory or cells can be quarantined through the use of a specific operating procedure where the incoming line is cultured at the end of the day by dedicated staff and grown in a dedicated incubator until it has been shown to be free of contaminates.[1,8]

Storage

The proper import and storage of materials and reagents, including cell stocks, is key to the long-term success of the laboratory. When setting up a new laboratory, one has the opportunity to establish systems for logging incoming supplies and documenting their testing and use. Many of the reagents used in the PSC laboratory are derived from animal sources and therefore are subject to lot-to-lot variability that may necessitate in-house testing to determine which lot is suitable for use for specific applications in the laboratory. In addition, tracking materials for expiration dates and keeping the laboratory properly stocked is a critical function that can be facilitated through the use of databases and bar-coded inventory systems. The banking and retrieval of large numbers of small vials of frozen materials such as cell stocks and reagents can be a challenging and is greatly facilitated by developing an efficient easy-to-use tracking system.[1,8]

Waste Disposal

Laboratory waste, including but not limited to, specimen cultures from medical and pathological laboratories, cultures and stocks of infectious agents from research and industrial laboratories, wastes from the production of biological agents, and culture dishes and devices used to transfer, inoculate and mix cultures or material which may contain infectious agents and may pose a substantial threat to health. All non-sterilized cultures should be presumed to be biohazardous.[12]

Data Management/Documentation[3]

Documentation is a part of GMP regulations. The documentation would include patient therapy data, equipment data etc. Written records should be maintained of all inspection, maintenance, testing, calibrating and/or standardizing operations. These records, containing the date of operation, should describe whether the maintenance operations followed written SOPs. Written records should be kept of non-routine repairs performed on equipment as a result of failure and malfunction. Such records should document the nature of the defect, how and when the defect was discovered, and any remedial action taken in response to the defect. Written records may be in logbooks especially designed for that purpose. The logbook should accompany the instrument when it is moved. Remedial action should include a review of effects on data generated before the defect was discovered. Proper protocol to be follow for digital data management.[7,8]

Quality Control

The laboratory should be designed, equipped, staffed, and operated in a manner that allows for the production of reliable and reproducible experimental results. While the research laboratory must operate with enough flexibility to allow discovery to take place, establishing standard operating procedures and a quality control system can provide the foundation on which new discoveries can take place (Fig. 10).[1,8]

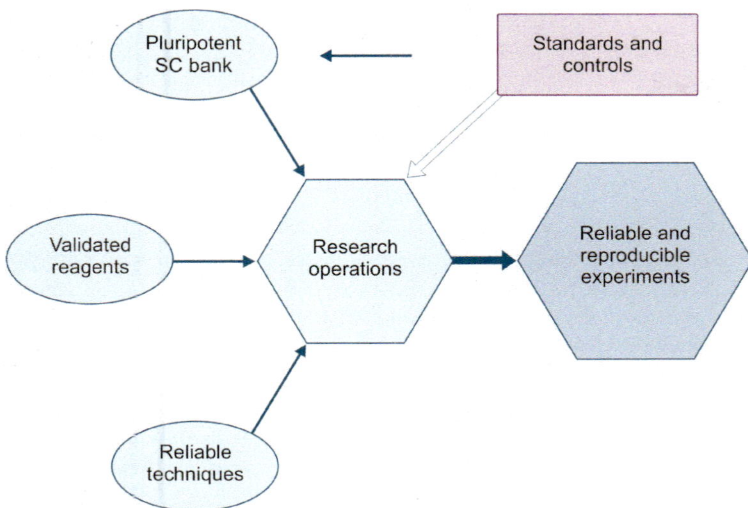

Fig. 10: Quality control in the stem cell laboratory.

Stem Cell Processing and Storage Facility

Stem cell processing and storage include all cells derived from the below sources:[2,6]

- Umbilical cord blood
- Bone marrow and mobilized peripheral blood
- Others including adipose tissue, etc.

The major objective for cellular therapy product/stem cell processing, storage and distribution is to promote quality medical and laboratory practice in hematopoietic progenitor cell transplantation and other therapies using cellular products. These standards apply to all processing, storage, and distribution activities performed in the processing facility on cellular therapy products obtained from living donors. These standards apply to hematopoietic stem cell progenitor cells, defined as self renewing and/or multipotent stem cells capable of maturation into any of the hematopoietic lineages, lineage-restricted pluri-potent progenitor stem cells, and committed progenitor stem cells, regardless of tissue source (bone marrow, umbilical cord blood, peripheral blood, or other tissue source). These standards include therapeutic cells, defined as nucleated cells from any tissue source (marrow, peripheral blood, umbilical cord, and placental blood) collected for therapeutic use other than as hematopoietic progenitor cells. Also, these standards apply to all phases of processing, storage and release of these cells that have been derived from marrow or peripheral blood, including various manipulations such as removal or enrichment of various cell populations, expansion of hematopoietic cell populations, and cryopreservation.[2,6]

Stem cell processing and storage facility means a place or organization or unit or institution or other arrangements made by such organization, unit or institution for processing and storage of stem cells derived from umbilical cord blood, bone marrow, mobilized peripheral blood etc. Stem cell processing and storage facility may be a standalone facility or be a part of the hospital services.

Scope of this Facility[3,6,13]

The scope of stem cell processing and storage facility includes collection, processing, testing, cryopreservation and distribution of stem cells derived from clinical umbilical cord blood, bone marrow, mobilized peripheral blood, and others for hematopoietic and nonhematopoietic transplantation. The stem cell processing facility shall establish and maintain policies and procedures, addressing critical aspects of operations and management. These documents shall include all elements required and shall address at a minimum.

- Donor and recipient confidentiality
- Transportation and shipping, including methods and conditions within the processing facility and to and from external facilities.
- Stem cell processing and process control
- Labeling and prevention of mix-ups and cross-contamination of samples
- Red cell compatibility testing and processing of ABO-incompatible products to include a description of the indication for and processing methods to be used for red cell and plasma depletion.
- Cryopreservation and thawing
- Release and exceptional release
- Cell therapy product disposal
- Reagent and supply management
- Equipment operation, maintenance, and monitoring, to include corrective actions in the event of failure.
- Facility management and environmental control to include a description of EM plan.
- Infection control, biosafety, and chemical and radiological safety
- Decontamination and disposal of medical and biohazard waste to include processing facility-specific requirements where these differ from institutional requirements.
- The quality management plan shall include, or summarize and reference, policies and procedures for documentation and review of cellular therapy product efficacy, and/or outcome analysis, as appropriate, including at least.
- For HPC products to be used for hematopoietic reconstitution, a process for documentation and review of time to engraftment following cellular therapy product administration.
- For other cellular therapy products, the criteria for product efficacy and/or the clinical outcome shall be determined and should be reviewed at regular time intervals.

The Stem Cell Market Scenario

It could be segmented as follows:[4,13]

- *Stem cell products*: Adult stem cell, human embryonic stem cell, and other stem cell types
- *Stem cell services*: Stem cell banking, stem cell acquisition and testing, drug discovery and target identification, isolation/characterization services, and molecular biology
- *Stem cell technologies*: Stem cell acquisition, stem cell production, cryopreservation, and expansion and subculture
- *Stem cell applications*: Regenerative medicine—neurological disorders, orthopedics, cancer, hematological disorders, myocardial infarction and cardiovascular diseases, injuries, diabetes, liver disorder, incontinence, and drug development.

At present, adult stem cell therapy dominates this segment, with almost 60% of total market share, due to its comparative uncontroversial nature. Further, in India most private players are primarily focusing in the area of stem cell banking, with a few notable exceptions.

CONCLUSION

Stem cell industry is a high-growth but nascent one, which has the ability to transform the field of diagnostics and therapeutics. With proactive governmental support and policies, private and public investments and public advocacy, this industry is poised to grow by leaps and bounds.[4,13]

REFERENCES

1. www.ncbi.nlm.nih.gov
2. www.focusonacure.org
3. docplayer.net
4. biofaba.org
5. www.cell-innovations.com.au
6. www.scripps.edu
7. apps.who.int
8. www.labcompliance.com
9. www.txstemcell.org
10. studylib.net
11. senior-hargreaves.co.uk
12. factwebsite.org
13. www.mohfw.nic.in

OTHER REFERENCES

- Establishment C, Standards A, Blood P, Çellsumbilical S, Cells C. (n.d.). Standard No. CEA/STL-036 Clinical Establishment Act Standard for Stem Cell Laboratory (Peripheral Blood Stem Cells and Umbilical Cord Cells) Standard No. CEA/STL-036, 1-18.
- Viswanathan S, Rao M, Keating A, et al. Overcoming challenges to initiating cell therapy clinical trials in rapidly developing countries: India as a model. standards, policies, protocols and regulations for cell-based therapies. stem cells translational medicine. Received January 31,2013; accepted for publication April 17, 2013; first published online in SCTM Express July 8, 2013.p 607-13.
- Griffiths T, Peto A, Thorogood J, et al. (n.d.). Conceptual design of a cutting edge stem cell research facility conceptual design of a cutting edge stem cell research facility. Cited from [internet]: Available from *http://www.engineering.leeds.ac.uk/e-engineering/documents/Griffiths_et_al_for_publication.pdf*
- Golan-mashiach M. The secret of stem cells, transcriptional profiling of human stem cells. 2003.
- Sekiya EJ, Forte A, Kühn TIBDB, et al. Establishing a stem cell culture laboratory for clinical trials. RevistaBrasileira de Hematologia E Hemoterapia. 2012;34(3):236-41. doi:10.5581/1516-8484.20120057
- Wesselschmidt RL, Schwartz PH. Human pluripotent stem cells. 2011;767(6),3-13. doi:10.1007/978-1-61779-201-4
- Placzek MR, Chung IM, Macedo HM, et al. Stem cell bioprocessing: fundamentals and principles. Biological Systems Engineering Laboratory, Centre for Process Systems Engineering, Department of Chemical Engineering, Imperial College London, South Kensington Campus, London SW7 2AZ, UK; Journal of the royal Society. J R Soc Interface. 2009;6:209-32.
- National guidelines for stem cell research. Indian Council of Medical Research. Department of Health Research and Department of Biotechnology. December; 2013.
- Stem Cells—An emerging Bio-Sector. Life Sciences Knowledge Banking Team, Yes Bank; 2012.
- "Human Pluripotent Stem Cells", Springer Nature, 2011.

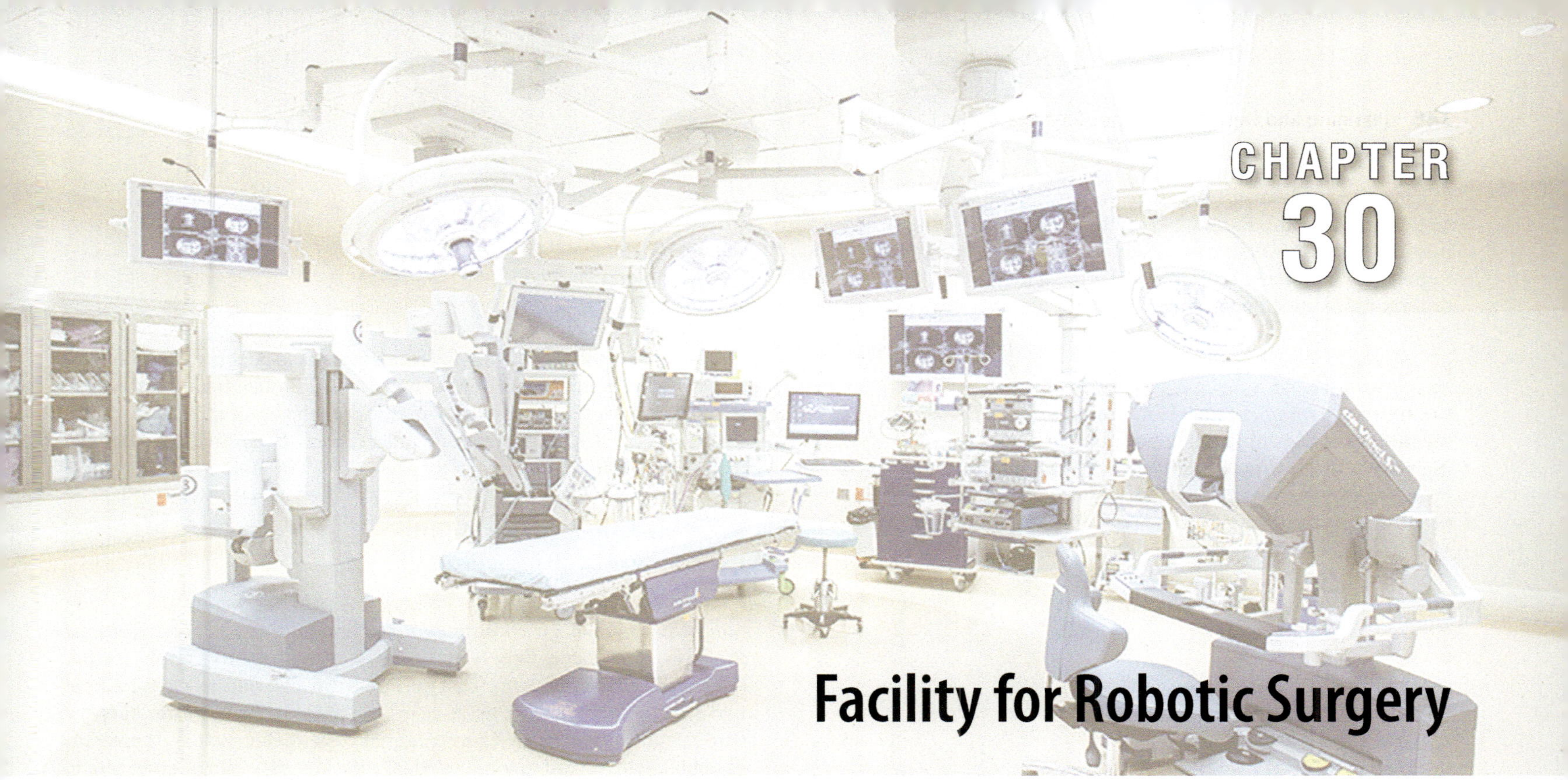

CHAPTER 30

Facility for Robotic Surgery

Mukunda Chandra Sahoo, NP Gupta, IB Singh, Shakti Kumar Gupta, Sunil Kant, R Chandrashekhar

INTRODUCTION

Advancements in communication, information technology, digital imaging, and robotics have aided the development of new surgical techniques, allowing surgeons to perform procedures with better outcomes, such as enhanced patient safety, less pain, shorter recovery periods, and reduced system-wide costs. Robotic surgery began as a technology-driven innovation but is now becoming a genuine method of improving healthcare effectiveness worldwide. Robotic assisted surgery brings new technologies into the operating room (OR). Details of the operation room design should facilitate optimal workflow for new surgical techniques, maintain a sterile environment, and provide flexibility to accommodate new technology over longer periods of time.[1-3]

Robotic surgery is often heralded as the new revolution and it is one of the most talked about subjects in surgery today. From their inception, surgical robots have been envisioned to extend the capabilities of human surgeons beyond the limits of conventional laparoscopy. Laparoscopic surgery is a type of intervention that may be considered a "transitional technology" bridging the gap between conventional surgery and more advanced forms of surgery.[4-6]

From laparoscopic surgery has evolved the revolutionary technology of robotic surgery, a computer-aided and image-guided intervention in which the surgeon has limited contact with either the patient's tissues or the surgical instruments. Instead, the surgeon works at a computer station, operating a set of finger controls while viewing an interactive three-dimensional (3D) representation of the intervention. The surgeon's finger movements are translated into actual instrument manipulation by a multi-armed robotic system that moves over the patient in the OR.[5]

The first surgical robot was approved for use in humans in 1994 (AESOP, Computer Motion, Goleta, California).[1] In 1997, the three-armed da Vinci robot (Intuitive Surgical, Sunnyvale, California) was approved for human surgery with additional capabilities allowing expansion of laparoscopic surgery.[7]

The da Vinci surgical system consists of three components (Figs. 1A to C):[6]

- The InSite™ Vision System
- Surgical cart
- Surgeon console.

The InSite™ Vision System provides the surgeon with a true minimally invasive 3D view of the surgical field including depth of field, magnification and high resolution. With its 3D view, the da Vinci System aids the surgeon in more easily identifying vital anatomy such as the delicate nerves and blood vessels surrounding specific anatomy.[5]

The surgical cart includes the EndoWrist™ instruments and four robotic arms whereby the laparoscope and three EndoWrist instruments are inserted. The EndoWrist instruments are designed to mimic the movement of the human hands, wrists and fingers. The extensive range of motion allows precision that is not available in standard minimally invasive procedures.[5]

The Surgeon Console is set away from the actual operating table and contains the master controls that the surgeon uses to operate. The handles translate the surgeon's natural hand and wrist movements into corresponding, precise and scaled movements.[5]

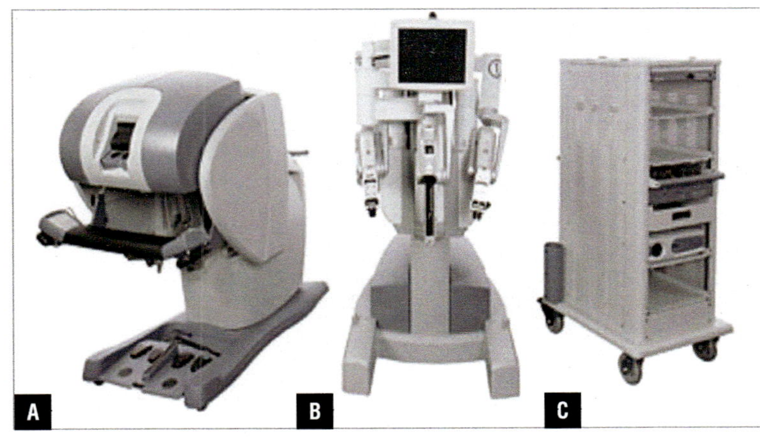

Figs. 1A to C: Da Vinci Surgical System: (A) A Surgeon Console; (B) A Surgical Cart; (C) The InSite™ Vision System.

The EndoWrist instruments are only able to move when commanded by the surgeon. The EndoWrist instruments provide the surgeon with the dexterity not available using conventional laparoscopic instruments to perform a delicate and precise surgical dissection, reconstruction or removal of specific tissue.[5]

PLANNING CONSIDERATIONS

Establishing a robotics facility requires more than transferring a surgical technique to one's hospital or acquiring a new piece of equipment. At the outset, the institution and surgeons should determine whether a robotic facility is feasible and identify champions of the endeavor. A multidisciplinary group is ideal and should include surgeons, nurses, and administrators. These groups should assess all components of a robotics program:[7,8]

- Surgical procedures to be performed
- Training
- Personnel
- Equipment
- Facilities
- Operational issues
- Research
- Finance.

It should begin before the purchase of a robot. The infrastructure needed to establish a robotics program is substantial, and may explain the suboptimal use of robotics at some institutions.[7,8]

Due diligence requires an assessment of current OR facilities, use, and manpower. At academic centers, training strategies for residents and fellows and research applications must be considered. A time line should be established that includes OR modification, equipment acquisition, hiring of personnel, and staff training.[7,8]

The OR room, the preoperative holding area and postoperative recovery room(s) in addition to other supportive facilities makeup the robotic facility.

FUNCTION OF THE FACILITY: STARTING A ROBOTICS FACILITY

For patients and surgeons, new medical technology generates various degrees of enthusiasm and will attract proponents even before demonstration of improved outcomes.[7,8]

The number of procedures that can be performed by robotic surgery is growing.

Procedures Performed with Robotic Surgery

Cardiac Procedures[7,8]

- Internal mammary artery take down
- Mitral valve repair
- Epicardial lead placement
- Beating heart totally endoscopic coronary artery bypass (TECAB) (single vessel)
- Arrested heart TECAB (single and multiple vessel)
- Esophagectomy
- Thymectomy.

General Surgery Procedures[7,8]

- Nissen fundoplication
- Gastric bypass
- Heller myotomy
- Colon resection
- Gastroplasty (gastric banding).

Urology Procedures[7,8]

- Prostatectomy
- Pyeloplasty
- Nephrectomy
- Cystectomy.

Another institutional benefit is the potential to become a training site or offer telementoring consistent with institutional educational objectives. The potential for research, including telesurgery, multimodality imaging, and design of new procedures, may be sufficient reason to establish a robotic facility.[7,8]

Key Planning and Designing Parameters of the Facility

Location

The best location for robotic suit is one which permits convenient and uncomplicated flow of patients, staff and clean supply traffic. Surgery receives inpatients from the floors through nonpublic corridors, elevators and ramps. In most cases, they are returned after surgery through the same route. Convenient access to elevators is, therefore, essential. With regard to services, ideal adjacencies would be emergency, radiology, clinical laboratories, intensive care units (ICUs), central sterile and supply department.

The separation of the robotic surgical suit from the rest of the hospital is important while planning the OR. It should be so located that there will be no traffic through it and no interference from the activities of other departments. The surgical suit may occupy a whole floor in a larger hospital—in others it should be placed at the end of a wing-its own *cul-de-sac* location.

Operating Room for Robotic Surgery (Fig. 2)

Objectives of Planning

A great deal of intelligent planning is necessary. The main objectives of planning should be:[9,10]

- Promote high standard of asepsis
- Ensure maximum standard of safety
- Optimize utilization of operation theater (OT) and staff time
- Optimize working conditions

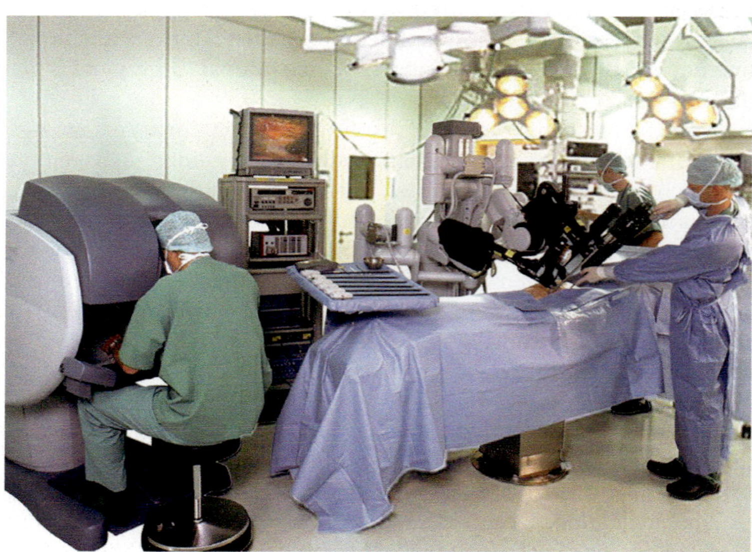

Fig. 2: Robotic surgery.

- Patient and staff comfort in terms of thermal, acoustic and lighting requirements
- Allow flexibility
- Facilitate coordinated services
- Minimizes maintenance
- Ensure functional separation of spaces
- Provide soothing environment
- Regulate flow of traffic.

PRINCIPLES FOR DESIGNING

The essential principles that should be followed in planning the physical layout of OR suite are exclusion of contamination from outside the suite with proper traffic patterns within the suite and separation of clean areas from contaminated areas within the suite.[9,10]

Operation Room Planning[7]

The operation room planning should include time and room availability, room size, room layout, availability of proper receptacles and circuits, imaging (either monitors or 3D room projection), and access to supplies. At least 52.2 m^2 is required to accommodate the staff, robot, anesthesia chart, table and 3D projection system (Fig. 2).[2] A dedicated room is optimal to avoid moving the robotic system and risking damage to the mechanical components or wiring. A dual digital projection system on a silver-coated screen to allow 3D viewing by the first assistant facilitates surgery and allows scrub nurses to follow the surgery and anticipate needs. New ORs with 3D projection systems are being designed to aid laparoscopic surgery. Meanwhile, assistants use two-dimensional flat-screen video monitors. There is a preference for the older cathode ray tube monitors, until flat-screen resolution and brightness are commensurate in quality.[3,7]

Cost effectiveness of robotic surgery is enhanced with reduced operative time and faster turnover. Thus, any modifications of procedure or technology that lower operative time are essential. Details as small as monitoring the percentage of gas remaining in the carbon dioxide tank allow anticipation of a change, warming of equipment to prevent fogging of the lens, and minimizing retrieval or changing robotic instruments. There should have an insufflator system with two tanks of gas that allows switching to a second tank when the first one gets low and then refilling the empty tank to be ready when the second tank empties. There should have enough instruments to perform two cases, which allow back-to-back procedures without having to wait for equipment to be cleaned. It is essential to maintain a supply of backup instruments that have been sterilized and are ready to use. Turnover times can be reduced by having a dedicated team that is rewarded for success. In addition, video monitoring of the OR by a surgeon so that inactivity between cases is observed may help minimize lost time.[3,7]

DESIGN PARAMETERS

Admission Area

The size of the admission area will vary according to the planned patient volume. There should be a spacious waiting room with comfortable seating, divided into sections by small partitions, pot plants, etc. to provide some privacy. The interior décor should be carefully designed to minimize anxiety, with special consideration for children in those centers providing pediatric services.[2,6]

The admission desk must be adequate to accommodate all the essential modern electronic office equipment with a connected staff room for the storage of office equipment, patient records, staff amenities, etc. The large majority of centers would require two or three admission staff.[2,6]

The nurse manager's office is adjacent to the admissions office and both of these open into a wide (1.5 m) passage way which connects the admission area to the discharge area. This facilitates the movement of staff and patient's relatives from the waiting room to the discharge lounge.

Operation room should be planned so as to ensure:[4,9]

- Avoidance of unrelated hospital traffic flow in the area.
- Convenient functional relationship and communication with surgical ward, ICU, central sterile services department, blood bank, medical imaging and laboratory services.
- Avoidance of outdoor source of noise.
- Provision for future expansion/alterations.
- If planning for modular theater, the walls should be galvanized iron, stainless steel panels, joints filled with epoxy and grinded. The final prepared surface is treated with antibacterial paint or use of solid mineral surface for wall paints.
- Doors should be of sliding type of minimum 1.2 m width in areas where patient movement is anticipated like OT, pre- and postoperative rooms. The sliding doors are preferred to the double action leaf type since they are more user friendly, saves space and prevents air turbulences. Ideally doors should be electrically operated hermetically sealed sliding doors to ensure sterilization and correct air pressure. The main advantages of a hermetically sealed sliding door are—that disinfection is quicker and safer, contamination risks are undercontrol, acoustic and noise control is easier and in case of failure of air handling unit temperature and humidity levels are brought within range more quickly.[1,9]
- Corridors should not be less than 2.85 m in width to facilitate movement of trolleys and stretchers.[1]
- Walls and ceiling should be esthetically pleasing nonporous, fire resistant, water and stain proof, seamless, nonreflective and easy to clean. They should not cause build up of a static electrical charge. They should be joint less or have joints capable of being sealed.[1,9]
- Floors should be smooth, nonslip, impervious material conductive enough to dissipate static electricity but not conductive enough to endanger personnel from shock. The flooring should either be inset mosaic with least possible joints and copper strips to carry away any static electricity produced or of joint less conductive tiles. Conductive copper mesh and self-leveling epoxy flooring may be done.[1,9]
- Ceiling should be painted with washable paint and corners of the rooms should be rounded off to prevent collection of dirt and dust.[1,9]
- Taps in the scrub room should be knee/elbow operated or preferably electronically controlled taps activated by infrared sensor. Power backup with provision of stand-by generating sets.[1,9]
- In ORs anesthetic room(s) recovery room, holding area, color of walls and ceilings should be such that they do not alter the observer's perception of skin color this will facilitate patient monitoring and management.[1,9]
- Operation theater should have facilities for high speed autoclaves/sterilizers for immediate/emergency requirements of sterilizing equipment. Essential pharmaceutical storage including refrigeration facilities should be available.
- There should be a waiting room with toilet facilities for patient attendants.
- Pass-through cabinets that circulate clean air through them while maintaining positive air room pressure allow transfer of supplies

from outside the OR to inside it. They help ensure the rotation of supplies in storage or can be used only for passing supplies as needed from a clean center core. There should be X-ray film illuminators preferably recessed into the wall[1,9]
- There should be emergency communication system that can be activated without the use of hands.[1]

Preoperative Patient Holding Area[6]

This should be able to facilitate stretcher as well as ambulatory patients not requiring stretchers. Each stretcher station should be of 80 sq ft (7.43 m^2) and should have a clearance of 4 ft (1.22 m) on the sides of the stretcher and foot of the stretcher.[1,9]

Postanesthetic Care Units

These should contain a medication station, hand washing station, nurse station, storage space for stretchers, supplies and equipment. Additionally 80 sq ft (7.43 m^2) for each patient bed clearance of 5 ft (1.5 m) between bed and 4 ft should be (1.22 m) between patient bed sides and adjacent walls.[1,9]

Service Area

These should include control station located to permit patient observation of all units into the suite:[1,9]
- A substerile area between two or more operating areas for flash sterilizer, sterile supply storage area and hand washing station
- Scrub facilities near the entrance of each OR
- Dirty utility for collection and disposal of solid material
- Clean supply room
- Operation room
- Medical gas storage facilities
- Anesthesia workroom for cleaning, testing and storing anesthesia equipment.

Staff Amenities[6]

Separate areas should be provided for male and female personnel containing lockers showers, toilets, lavatories and space for donning surgical attire should allow one way traffic, i.e. personnel entering from outside the surgical suite to change and move inside.[1,9]

Medical Gases[6]

The main storage of medical gases should be outside the facility and there should be provision for additional separate storage of reserve gas cylinders for a minimum of one day requirement.[1,9]

Anesthetic Work Room

It should provide space for anesthetic trolleys and equipment and should be located with direct access to circulation corridors and ready access to the OR. It is to provide cleaning, testing and storing of anesthesia equipment. It should contain work benches, sink(s) and racks for cylinder. It should have sufficient power outlets and medical gas panels for testing of equipment.[1,9]

Blood Store

There should be provision for refrigerated blood storage. The storage refrigerator may be in a dedicated or shared space.[1,9]

Set-up Room

It is the clean workroom where clean/sterile materials are held and arranged prior to use in the OR. Its functions include storage of instruments and materials, holding of sterile supplies and packs, preparation of dressing and instrument trolley, storage of drugs and where theater sterile supply unit service is not available flash sterilization of dropped or specialized instruments. It should be so located that it has direct access to ORs and central supply/theater sterile supply unit. Positive pressure to be maintained relative to adjoining rooms.[1,9]

Laboratory

An area for preparation and examination of frozen section may be provided. Depending on the operational policy this may be part of the main laboratory.[1,9]

Storage

For equipment and supplies utilized in the operating unit adequate store rooms should be provided. The design should allow ease of access to the storage areas for delivery of consumables. Controlled access from an external corridor is recommended. Store rooms are best designed in an elongated rectangular shape to allow easy access to all items. Part of the room may be utilized as an area for testing operating equipment. For this purpose, a separate room called as biomedical engineering room may also be planned. Storage bays preferably recessed into the corridor walls should be provided for equipment such as stretchers and portable X-ray.[1,9]

ZONING

Zones are area of varying degrees of cleanliness in which the bacteriological count progressively diminishes from the outer to the inner zones (operating area) and is maintained by a differential decreasing positive pressure ventilation gradient from the inner zone to the outer zone. They are of following types:[1,9]

Protective Zone

Areas included in this zone are:[1,9]
- Reception
- Waiting area
- Trolley bay
- Changing room.

Clean Zone

Areas included in this zone are:[1,9]
- Preoperative room
- Recovery room
- Staff room
- Store.

Sterile Zone

Areas included in this zone are:[1,9]
- Operating suite
- Scrub room
- Anesthesia induction room
- Set-up room.

Disposal Zone

Areas included in this zone are:[1,9]
- Dirty utility
- Disposal corridor.

The recommended schedule of accommodation is shown in Table 1.

Table 1: Recommended schedule of accommodation.[1,9]

Room/Space	Area (m^2)	Remarks
Reception	10	Many may be required depending on size of hospital
Anesthetic induction room	15	-do-
Operating room (major)	50–60	-do-
Scrub up/gowning	6	May be colocated between operating rooms
Support areas		
Anesthetic room	10–15	Many may be required depending on size of hospital
Mobile equipment bay	4	Many may be required depending on size of hospital
Bay Linen	3	-do-
Cleaners room	4	-do-
Clean-up room	10	-do-
Disposal room	8	-do-
Flash sterilizing	5–6	-do-
Laboratory/Frozen section	4–12	-do-(Optional)
Set-up room	20	-do-
Store anesthetic	20	-do-
Store equipment	20–40	Depending on size of hospital
Store sterile	20–80	
Store nonsterile	20–30	
Blood store	4	
Recovery area		
Bay patient	9	Many may be required depending on size of hospital
Bay Linen	3	Generally 2 bays for patient per operating room
Bay resuscitation trolley	2	
Bay hand washing	1	-do-
Clean utility	12	
Dirty utility	10	
Staff station	6–14	Depending on size of hospital
Administrative staff and shared areas		
Change room	10–30	Many may be required depending on type and size of hospital
Office single person	9	-do-
Store	10	-do-
Toilet staff	2	-do-
Shower staff	2	-do-
Staff lounge	10–30	Depending on size of hospital and staffing establishment
Shared areas meeting room	20–30	
Store general	9	
Waiting	4	
Circulation areas of 35% should be catered		

Ventilation[6]

Central air-conditioning should ensure temperature range of 18–24°C with 45 ± 5 humidity levels. A minimum of 20 air changes/h should be ensured. It is preferred to have 100% fresh air. Theater to maintain positive pressure and controlling of pressure is adhered to by providing pressure release dampers at the time of opening and closing of the door. The minimum bacteriological requirements are that the air should not contain detectable *Clostridium* spores of coagulase positive *Staphylococcus*. Aerobic cultures on nonselective medium should indicate not more than 35 bacteria-carrying particles in 1 m^3 of ventilating air. During surgical operations, the concentration of bacterially contaminated airborne particles in the operating theater averaged over any 5 minutes period should not exceed 180/ m^3 (5/ft^3), and special types of surgical operation, e.g. robotic and transplantation procedures, higher standards of air cleanliness must be ensured.[1,9]

Lighting

General illumination is furnished by ceiling lights. Lighting should be evenly distributed throughout the room around 300 lux. The anesthesiologist must have sufficient light, to adequately evaluate the patient's skin color. Electrical wiring should be in concealed conduit lighting both natural and artificial should be of appropriate illumination.[1,9]

Isolated power systems help prevent sparks from igniting flammables anesthetics and also help to protect patients and personnel from shock. Ground fault circuit interrupters (GFCIs) may be utilized which are designed to shut off the electric power within a few milliseconds of the occurrence of a ground fault, thereby preventing serious electric shock.[1,9]

To minimize eye fatigue, the ratio of intensity of general room lighting to that at the surgical site should not exceed 1:5, preferably 1:3. This contrast should be maintained in corridors and scrub areas, as well as in the room itself, so that the surgeon becomes accustomed to the light before entering the sterile field. Color and hue of the lights also should be consistent. The overhead operating light must make an intense light, within a range of 27,000–127,000 lux, into the incision without glare on the surface. The light may be equipped with an intensity control.[1,9]

- Provide a diameter light pattern and focus appropriate for size of the incision. Fixture should provide focused depth by refracting light to illuminate both the body cavity and the general operating field.
- Be shadowless. Multiple light sources and/or reflectors decrease shadows
- Produce the blue-white color of daylight
- Be freely adjustable to any position or angle by either a vertical or horizontal range of motion
- Should enable easy cleaning
- Should be aerodynamically designed to facilitate airflow
- Produce a minimum of heat. Halogen bulbs generate less heat than other types. LED bulbs are other alternative.

Auditory Effects

Sound level in OT should be limited to 25–35 dB. The reverberation time in OR should be reduced to below one second.[1,9]

Fire Safety

Both ionization and optical fire detectors should be provided in the OTs as against heat detectors, since equipment-oriented OTs are likely to create more smoke than heat in the eventuality of fire. Hydrants and fire extinguishers should be provided. Fire exist route should be clearly identified, earmarked and well illuminated.[1,9]

Water Supply

Besides normal supply of available water at the rate of 400 L/bed/day separate reserve emergency over head tank should be provided for OT. Modular industrialized systems are increasing with number of hospitals coming up. The advantage of these modular theaters is that they are predesigned and engineered with guaranteed performance and shorter duration of time.[1,9]

Modular Systems

Modular systems are available which consist of prefabricated units for operating suites complete with integrated mechanical and electrical services including air-conditioning are available and should be utilized.[1,9]

Various personnel have to be provided with lounges, lockers and toilet facilities. There should be a coffee room. Operation rooms have no fixed lunch hours. Quite often, personnel need to have their lunch or snacks in between operations. Arrangements must be made for their supply. A conference for meeting and in-service training program is necessary. All these areas should be removed from the strictly surgical areas and persons entering and leaving them in street clothes should not wander or penetrate into sterile areas without changing clothes and footwear.

The central sterilization and supply department, which is located elsewhere in the hospital, is responsible for preparing and autoclaving all surgical instruments, linen packs, gloves, syringes and needles. However, it is the responsibility of the surgical department to store it.

Postanesthesia Recovery Room

The surgical or postanesthesia recovery room located near the ORs, permit medical care and observation by anesthesiologist, surgeon and surgical resident in the first hours following operation through the use of special recovery room facilities. The size of this section will vary depending on the number of ORs. The rule of thumb is from one-and-half to two beds per OR.

Operating Room Requirements

- 30′ × 20′ minimum room size
- Optimally, a dedicated room for the robot
  - Decrease set-up time
  - Decrease risk of robot damage.

Equipment/Supplies

There are various questions regarding equipment and supplies. What supplies will be required? Where will they be obtained and how much will they cost? Whose budget will pay for them? How many will be kept in inventory? How many will be sterile and ready at a given time? Where will they be stored and who will be responsible for managing inventory and reordering? Some items may have to be approved by the clinical engineering department, and existing contracts with vendors may preclude purchasing from a competitor.[3,7]

The items needed to support a robotic facility, beyond those already available in the OR, for laparoscopic cases include hardware obtained from the robot vendor—reusable robotic accessories (e.g. sterile adapters, scopes, light guide cables, trocars), limited-life reusable robot arms that can be used for 8–20 cases depending on the instrument (e.g. needle drivers, forceps, scissors, cautery tools), and disposable robotic supplies (e.g. drapes, cannula seals).[3,7]

Other supplies include an insufflator. Necessary equipment includes a suction irrigator, a scope warmer, a surgeon's chair tall enough to see into the surgeon's console and made of a material suitable for the OR, and video equipment.[3,7]

The schedule of accommodation for an operating unit is given in Table 1.

Establishing the Robotic Team[7]

Robotic surgery is labor-intensive in terms of OR personnel. At least two surgeons, a scrub nurse, and an anesthesiologist are required. Usually a second assistant is necessary but sometimes can be replaced by a fourth-arm option formerly available on the da Vinci robot. The bedside surgeon must be a fully trained laparoscopic surgeon or surgical technician. Unlike open or other endoscopic surgeries, many robotic surgeries, especially radical prostatectomy, are nearly impossible without an accomplished first assistant. The academic medical center needs to decide whether the first assistant is a resident, fellow, faculty member, or surgical technician. This personnel and training decision is complex and has departmental morale and financial implications. Moreover, one scrub nurse may be insufficient to handle imaging, trips to the supply room, or communication with the company if a malfunction occurs. Thus, a robot company representative is often present. If many new patients are attracted to the institution, additional secretarial and office staff may be necessary. As per some institutes robotic team, excluding residents, includes 16 people.[3,7]

A dedicated team of surgeons and nurses is crucial to the successful implementation of robotics. Constantly changing assistants, nurses, and anesthesiologists delays starting times, turnover, and operative time. Optimal rotation time for trainees previously exposed to laparoscopic surgery on robotics should be determined, but at least 6 months is necessary. Defining goals, obtaining sufficient training, holding team events such as dinners, and encouraging joint continuing medical education programs will ease the stress when cases go overtime or problems arise. Continual communication among the team with newsletters and follow-up of patients is helpful to maintain esprit de corps.[3,7]

The adoption of robotic surgery by other surgeons helps ensure success of the program, although it limits urologic use. Originally developed for cardiovascular surgery, robotics has been used by general surgeons, microsurgeons, head and neck surgeons, and gynecologists.[3,7]

Integrated Operating Theater

Integrated operating theaters are now being developed (Fig. 3), in which all OR equipment, i.e. endoscopic camera equipment, robotics, operating tables, room lighting, surgical lights, digital documentation, data storage and teleconferencing technology can all be centrally controlled, either outside or within the sterile area as desired (Figs. 4 to 7).[8]

Integrated operating theater design allows for equipment (e.g. ceiling mounted suspension systems) to provide increased efficiencies and ergonomics in the OR. Endoscopic video systems are now interlinked with environmental room control where everything can be controlled via touch screen or voice activation in the sterile field or nurses work

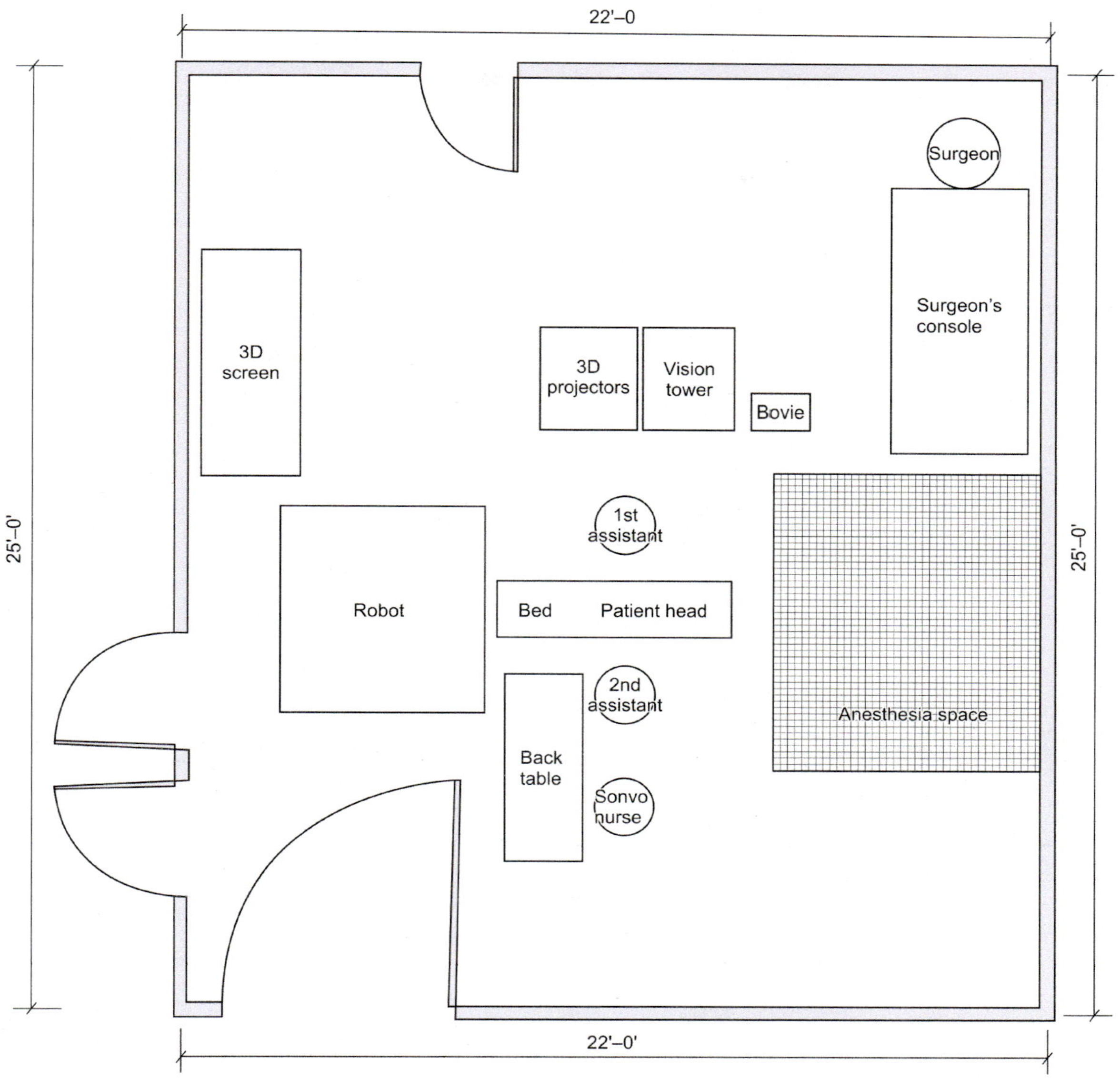

22'–0
25'–0'
Surgeon
Surgeon's console
3D screen
3D projectors
Vision tower
Bovie
1st assistant
Robot
Bed
Patient head
2nd assistant
Anesthesia space
Back table
Sonvo nurse
22'–0'

Fig. 3: Robotic operation room set-up.

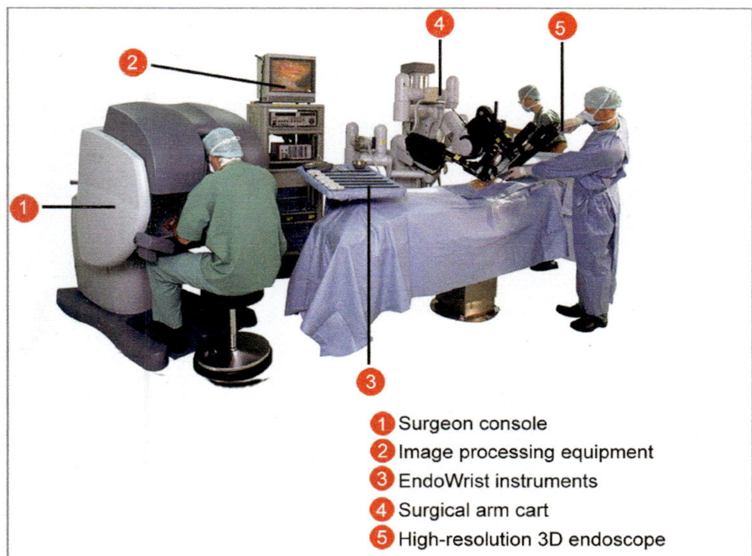

Fig. 4: Da Vinci robotic system.[5]

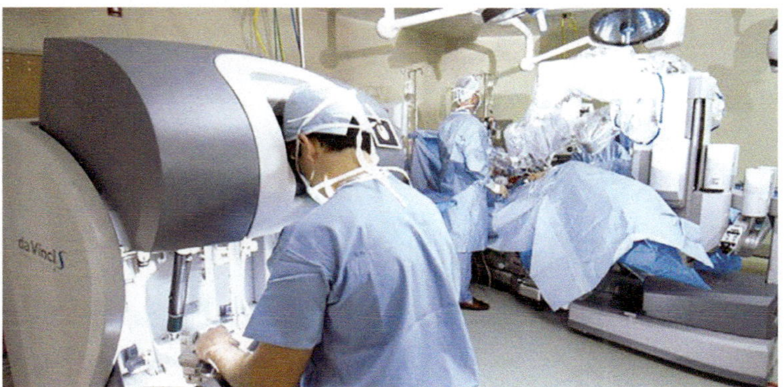

Fig. 5: Robotic urologic surgery at—In the da Vinci system, the surgeon sits at a viewfinder (left) and remotely manipulates probes and instruments on actuator arms over the operating table.

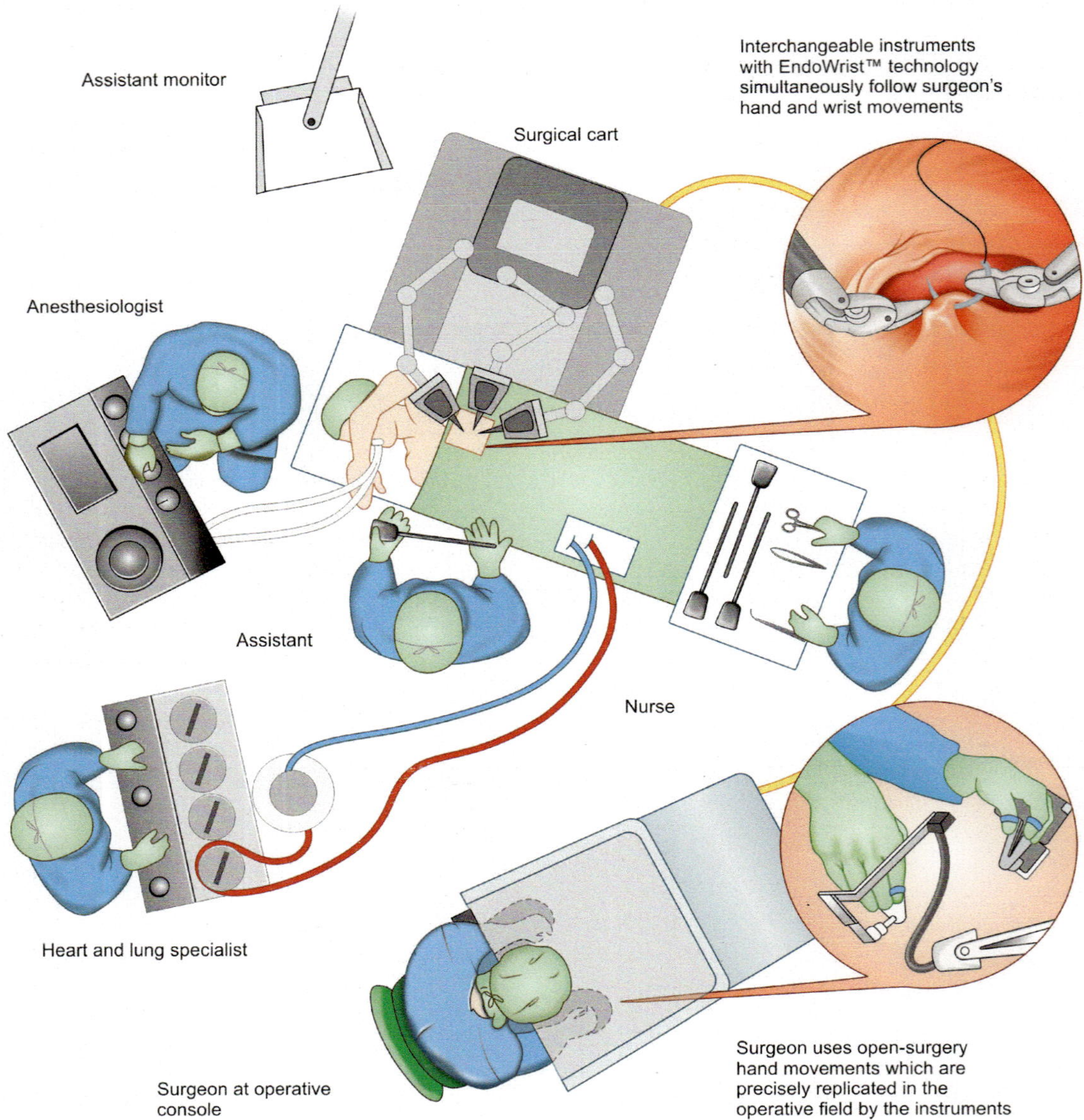

Fig. 6: Diagram illustrates how the da Vinci system is set-up in the operating room.[5,6]

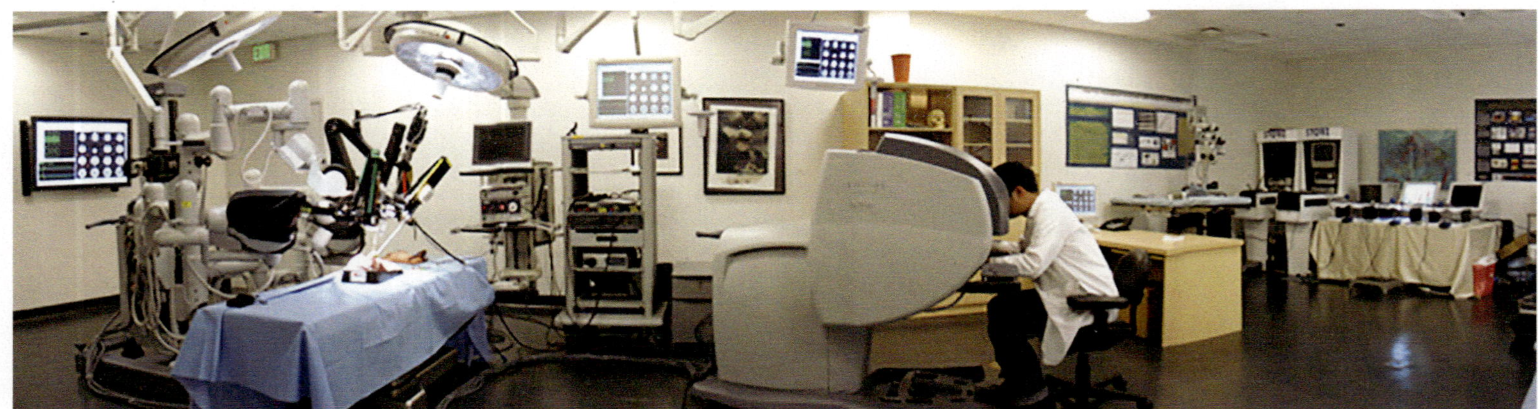

Fig. 7: Robotic operation theater set-up.

station at the touch of a button. Surgeons can now be in control of the camera, light source, insufflation, room lighting, room temperature and video conferencing. Communication from the sterile field to the entire world is at surgeons finger tips.[8]

CONCLUSION

The implementation of a robotics facility should include defining specific measurable objectives for case loads to be attained over the baseline volumes. The metrics to evaluate the success of the facility would be surgical volume compared with baseline. Outcome measures specific to the procedure such as continence, potency, blood loss, analgesic requirements, tumor margins, and prostate-specific antigen levels following prostatectomy at various intervals must be assessed. Additional quality assessment is based on—customer satisfaction, performance over time on internally designed quality performance measures, and overall quality-of-life instruments.[7-11]

The design of a robotic facility offer a challenge to the planning team to optimize efficiency by creating conducive environmental conditions, realistic functional traffic flow and flexibility of future expansion.

REFERENCES

1. www.incmedica.com
2. www.ncbi.nlm.nih.gov
3. www.aia.org
4. Corder CJ.'Preparation of the Operating Room, Back Table, and Surgical Team. Robotic Urologic Surgery; 2011.
5. gwhospital.com
6. www.aams.org.au
7. Steers W, LeBeau S, Cardella JB. Fulmer establishing a robotics program. Urologic Clinics of North America. 2004;31(4):773-80.
8. www.medicvision.com.au
9. www.jaoa.org
10. mohfw.nic.in
11. www.pubmedcentral.nih.gov

OTHER REFERENCES

- Kim H, Schulam P. The PAKY, HERMES, AESOP, ZEUS, and da Vinci robotic systems. Urologic Clinics of North America. 2004;31(4):659-9.
- Science.howstuffworks.com.
- Intuitive Surgical, Inc. - da Vinci® Surgical System Intuitive Surgical designs and builds the da Vinci Surgical System, the breakthrough platform for robotically assisted minimally nvasive surgery www.intuitivesurgical.com.
- Gupta SK, Kant S, Chandrashekhar R. Operating unit—planning essentials and design considerations. Journal of Academy of Hospital Administration;2005.
- Gupta SK, Kanta S, Cahandrashekhar R, Satpathy S. Modern trends in planning and designing of hospitals: Prin Prac; Jaypee Brothers Medical Publishers; New Delhi; 2007.
- Urologic Clinics of North America: Robotic Urologic Surgery. 2004;31:4.

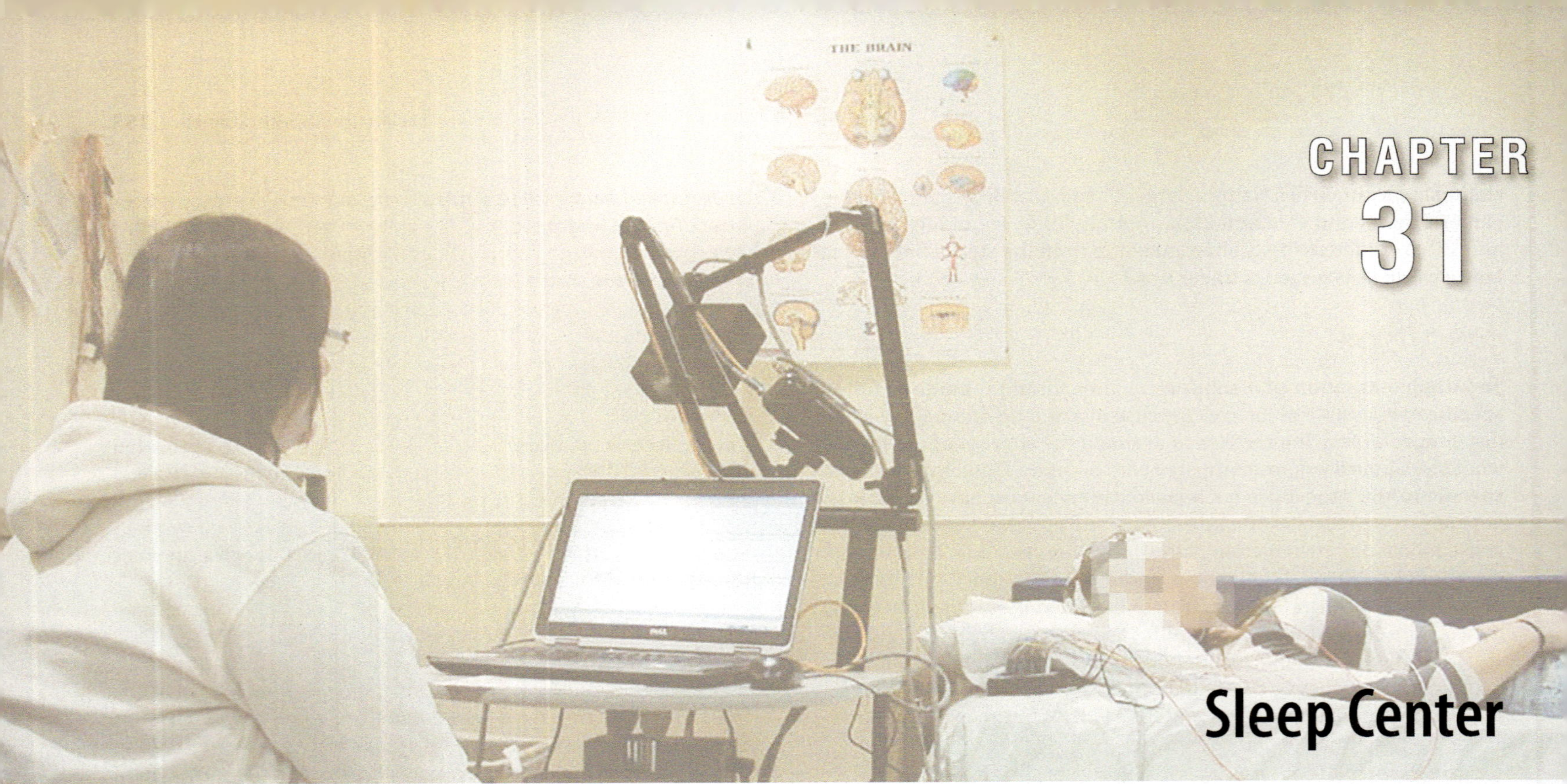

CHAPTER 31

Sleep Center

Saroj Kumar Patnaik, Shakti Kumar Gupta, Sunil Kant, R Chandrashekhar

INTRODUCTION

Sleep disorders have become common phenomena in today's world. The advent in technology in modern medicine has brought to surface a number of sleep disorders which earlier were accepted as normal. Sleep is more crucial than rest and it is a state of unresponsiveness brought about by nervous activities, which ensures that the whole body, including nervous system, recuperates.[1,2] Improvement in modes of travel has shrunk the world but has increased the number of patients who have sleep-related ailments. In the present environment, jet lag increases with age and number of time zones traveled through and is also affected by the direction in which you travel.[3]

The various sleep-related disorders are increasing at an alarming proportion. Bixler, Kales and Healey in a study conducted in the US found that the prevalence of sleep disorder is more than 50%.[4] Thus, it is imperative that planning and designing of a sleep center be done very carefully.

Sleep medicine is a medical specialty or subspecialty devoted to the diagnosis and therapy of sleep disturbances and disorders. From the middle of the 20th century, research has provided increasing knowledge and answered is many questions about sleep-wake functioning.[1,5] The rapidly evolving field has become a recognized medical subspecialty in some countries. The first sleep clinics in the United States were established in the 1970s by interested doctors and technicians; the study, diagnosis and treatment of obstructive sleep apnea (OSA) were their first tasks. As late as 1999, virtually any American doctor, with no specific training in sleep medicine, could open a sleep laboratory.[1,6,7]

HISTORY

The evolution of sleep medicine is pretty interesting. The practice of sleep medicine evolved in many centers in the 1970s. Although sleep clinics were established in the US and in some other countries in Europe in 1970, most of these were confined to diagnosis and management of OSA.[1,8] The use of patients complaining of insomnia in hypnotic efficacy studies brought a group of researchers in Stanford closely into relation with many insomnia patients, and demolished the notion that the majority of such patients were psychiatric subjects. One early question was, "How reliable are the descriptions of their sleep by these patients?" The classic all-night sleep recording could yield a great deal of information. The diagnosis of OSA in patients who had profound excessive daytime sleepiness nearly always was completely unambiguous. During 1972, the search for sleep abnormalities in patients who had sleep-related complaints continued; the intent was to conceptualize the pathophysiologic process as an entity and as the cause of the presenting symptom. With this approach, several phenomena seen during sleep rapidly were linked to the fundamental sleep-related presenting complaints. Toward the end of 1972, the basic concepts and procedures of sleep disorders medicine were established.[1,9]

TYPES OF SLEEP DISORDERS[1,10]

Breathing-related sleep disorders are syndromes in which the patient's sleep is interrupted by problems with his or her breathing. There are different types of breathing-related sleep disorders:

- *Obstructive sleep apnea syndrome*: This is the most common form of breathing-related sleep disorder that has been reported to occur in 2–4% of middle aged adults, it is marked by episodes of blockage in the upper airway during sleep. It is found primarily in obese people. Patients with this disorder typically alternate between periods of *snoring* or *gasping* (when their airway is partly open) and periods of silence (when their airway is blocked). Very loud snoring is a clue to this disorder.
- *Central sleep apnea syndrome*: This disorder is primarily found in elderly patients with heart or neurological conditions that affect their ability to breathe properly. It is not associated with airway blockage and may be related to brain disease (Fig. 1).
- *Central alveolar hypoventilation syndrome*: This disorder is found most often in extremely obese people. The patient's airway is not blocked, but his or her blood oxygen level is too low.

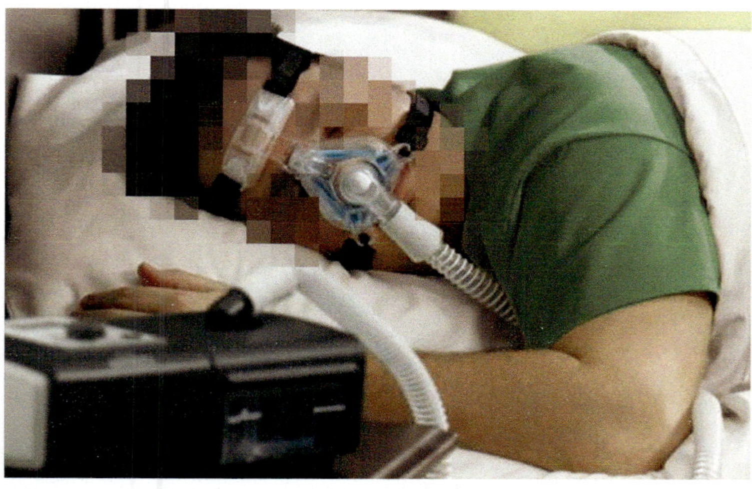

Fig. 1: Central sleep apnea syndrome patient.

- *Mixed-type sleep apnea syndrome*: This disorder combines symptoms of both obstructive and central sleep apnea.
- *Insomnia*: Inability to fall or stay asleep.
- *Daytime sleepiness*.
- *Restless legs syndrome*: Feel tingling or "crawling" sensations deep within your legs.
- *Narcolepsy*: Narcolepsy is a neurological disorder that affects the control of sleep and wakefulness. People with narcolepsy experience excessive daytime sleepiness and intermittent, uncontrollable episodes of falling asleep during the daytime. These sudden sleep attacks may occur during any type of activity at any time of the day.

SLEEP ASSESSMENT[1,11]

- The *Epworth sleepiness scale* (ESS), (Fig. 2) designed to give an indication of sleepiness and correlated with sleep apnea,[10] or other questionnaires designed to measure excessive daytime sleepiness, are diagnostic tools that can be used repeatedly to measure results of treatment.
- A *sleep diary*, also called sleep log or sleep journal, kept by a patient at home for at least two weeks, while subjective, may help to determine the extent and nature of sleep disturbance and the level of alertness in the normal environment. A parallel journal kept by a parent or bed partner, if any, can also be helpful. Sleep logs also can be used for self-monitoring and in connection with behavioral and other treatment.

PLANNING AND DESIGNING OF SLEEP CENTER[1]

Sleep centers are specialized centers where an individual is provided home-like environment and surroundings and his sleep cycle is monitored. Active therapeutic and diagnostic interventions are also done here. Mechanical ventilators, administering aerosols, monitoring the sleep pattern, recording of any abnormality, maintenance of equipment etc. are also undertaken here.

FACILITIES AND SPACE REQUIREMENT[1,12-16]

- *Reception*: A well-designated reception should be there in all sleep centers. Receptions should be planned to ensure privacy while conversing with the patient. They can be suitably planned in the entrance lobby of sleep center. Reception will require an area of 8–10 m^2 for smooth functioning. Sufficient number of drawers and shelves should be provided.
- *Patient rooms*: The most important part is the patient rooms, they are usually next to one another as they are quiet locations. Ideally, they are similar to the patient's rooms. Bed should be larger than standard. Night table, with small lamp for personal belongings should be available. An approximate area of 15 m^2/bed should be planned. *Patient testing rooms must not have any impediment. The rooms must be of sufficient size to accumulate emergency personnel access with a minimum of 24 inches available clear space on the three sides of bed.* A two-way communication system between the patient bedroom and center personnel should be maintained. A mechanism for visual monitoring and recording of patients during testing should be there. Polygraphic equipment capable of recording and storing a minimum of 12 channels of data should be there. Equipment for the delivery of continuous positive airway pressure (CPAP) (Fig. 3) and bilevel positive airway pressure, including remote control of pressure.

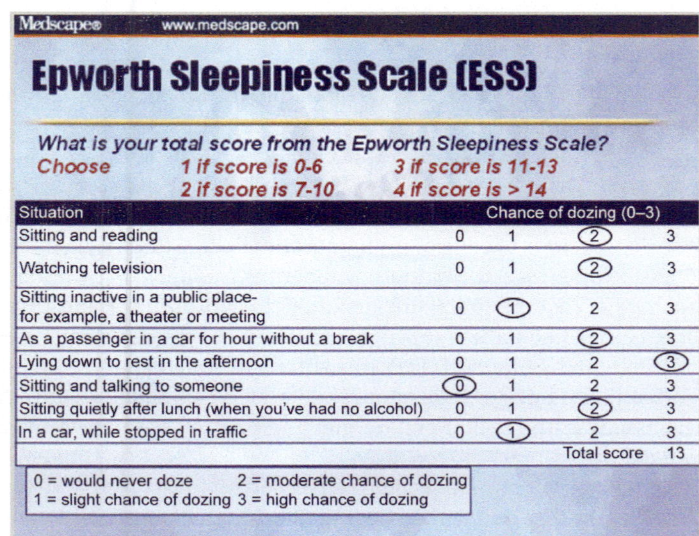

Medscape www.medscape.com

Epworth Sleepiness Scale (ESS)

What is your total score from the Epworth Sleepiness Scale?

Choose 1 if score is 0-6; 2 if score is 7-10; 3 if score is 11-13; 4 if score is > 14

Situation	Chance of dozing (0–3)			
Sitting and reading	0	1	(2)	3
Watching television	0	1	(2)	3
Sitting inactive in a public place-for example, a theater or meeting	0	(1)	2	3
As a passenger in a car for hour without a break	0	1	(2)	3
Lying down to rest in the afternoon	0	1	2	(3)
Sitting and talking to someone	(0)	1	2	3
Sitting quietly after lunch (when you've had no alcohol)	0	1	(2)	3
In a car, while stopped in traffic	0	(1)	2	3
			Total score	13

0 = would never doze; 1 = slight chance of dozing; 2 = moderate chance of dozing; 3 = high chance of dozing

Fig. 2: Epworth sleepiness scale.

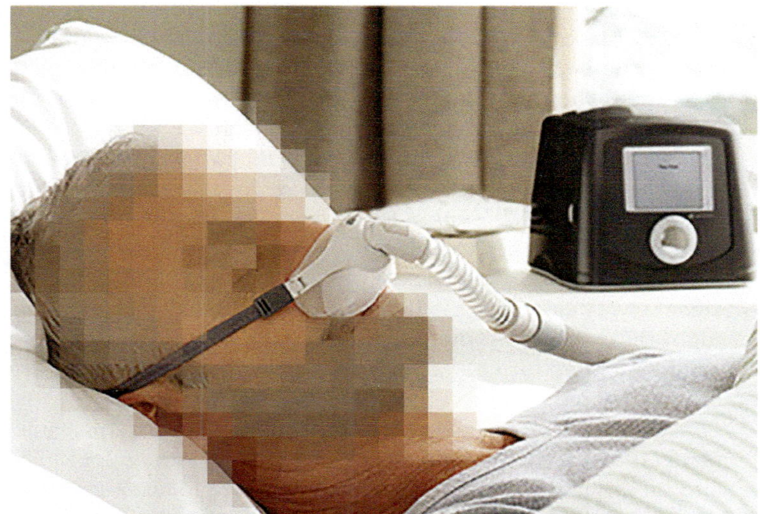

Fig. 3: Equipment for the delivery of continuous positive airway pressure.

Std 8-Accreditation of sleep disorder center of AASM (American Academy of Sleep Medicine).

- *Room acoustics*: Patients' room have special acoustic design wherein decibel level can be around 15–20 decibels. The most difficult aspect of space planning by clinicians for sound control is isolating operational noise sources. Operational noise is created by people and by machines brought into the building after it is constructed. Operational noise that can be isolated from business areas (desks, phones, printers), bulk storage, and pass-by foot traffic to other beds or common destinations (sinks, storage, entrances and exits). The best means of protecting from operational noise is a private cubicle. Light sleep, non-rapid eye movement (NREM) stage, show the greatest vulnerability to acoustic disruption. It is less protected than either dream sleep, rapid eye movement (REM) (Figs. 4A and B). However, some openings, for example-between two single-bed patient rooms, communication between quiet spaces that are used often but by few people have some non-disruption. Such communicating rooms without a door can meet permissible noise criteria if other aspects of the design offer sufficient protection. Automatic sliding doors are expensive and generate a good deal of noise in operation.
  If equipment such as a refrigerator are to be put in the sleep lab, it should be placed far from the bed in a housing that absorbs the condenser noise or be built specifically to produce little noise and vibration.[13,14]
- *HVAC*: Sleep centers should be centrally air-conditioned with total circulated air quantity should not be less than 12 air changes/h. Regulatory mechanism should exist with temperature monitoring panel in each room. Ambient temperature of 23–25° should be maintained at all times.
- *Lighting standards*: The surrounding should be pleasant and conducive to rest and relaxation. The light can be totally blocked out. Intensity of light should be controllable. Natural light is important to keep the patient in sync with the environment but adequate blinding facilities should be provided. Reading lights should be provided to each patient and intensity of 150–200 lux is recommended. Avoid white neon lights, and make sure the room can be made light-free.
- *Walls*: It should be painted with light colors and should be decorated to get it close enough to the feel of being at home. Corners of the wall should be protected against physical impact by stretchers.
- *Doors*: It should have minimum 90–120 cm clear opening to allow easy passage to patients and a level space of 152 cm wide should extend about 45 cm on each side of doorway for facilitating opening closing by a wheel-chaired person.
  The facility must afford rapid access to the patient by emergency personnel. Std 19-Accreditation of sleep disorder center of AASM (American Academy of Sleep Medicine).

- *Prep area*: The other important room is where the computers are placed, patients are usually prepared in this room, so that a signal check can be carried out. Technical staff also spends the night there in case something happens. A room of area 12 m^2 can be planned for Prep area. Prep area will be an integral part of sleep center.
- *Control room (Fig. 5)*: It is the area where technologists will reside for data collection. It should be very close to sleep rooms for safety and timely care. It should have adequate area to accommodate equipment and other computer peripherals. An area of 8 m^2 will be adequate for this control room. This area can be seamlessly merged with a glass partition to separate it from sleep suites and offer the patients, privacy.

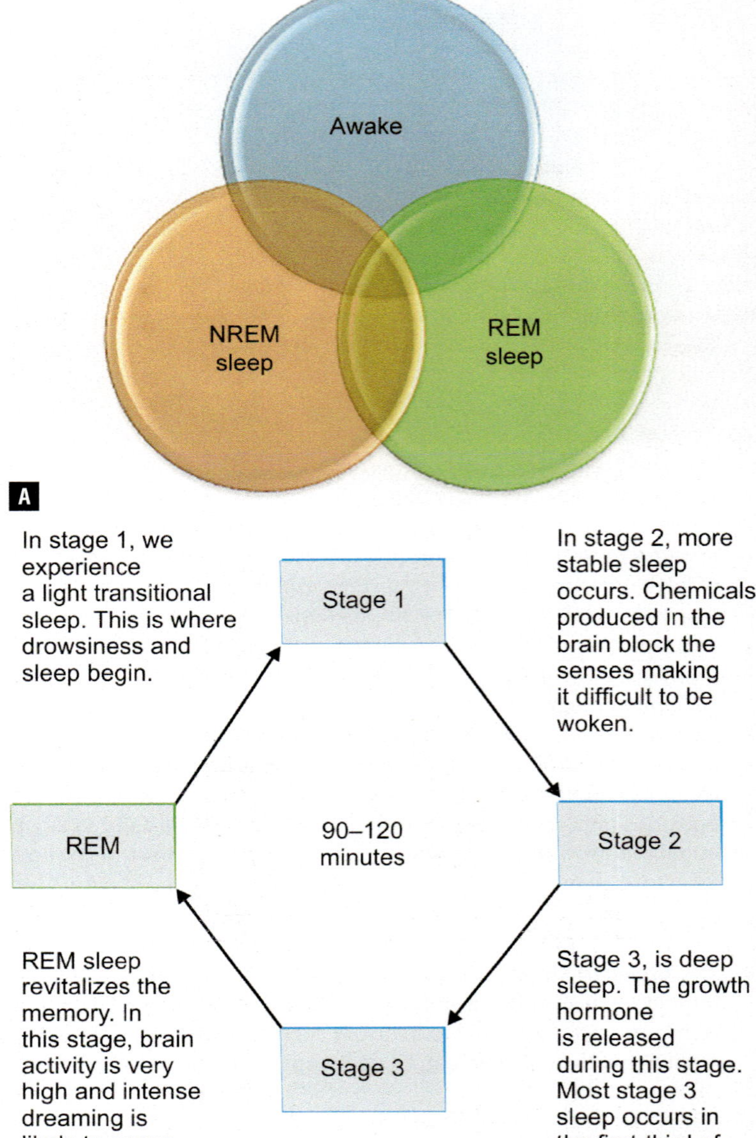

Figs. 4A and B: (A) Rapid eye movement; (B) Sleep cycle.

Std D-10[17]

- The demensions of control room must not be less than 40 sq ft total or 20 sq ft per testing bedroom, whichever is longer.
- *Storage area*: Adequate storage areas for equipment and other accessories like patient luggage and wheelchair, etc. Storage area of 15 m^2 can be planned. This area should preferably be on the exit end and can have a door opening to outside from where day-to-day needs of the center can be met and privacy of the patients is not disturbed.
- *Doctors' office*: It should be planned closed off from the rest, so that scoring can be done without being disturbed. Patients also come in to hear the diagnosis. This room can be planned in an area of 12 m^2. There should be adequate privacy.

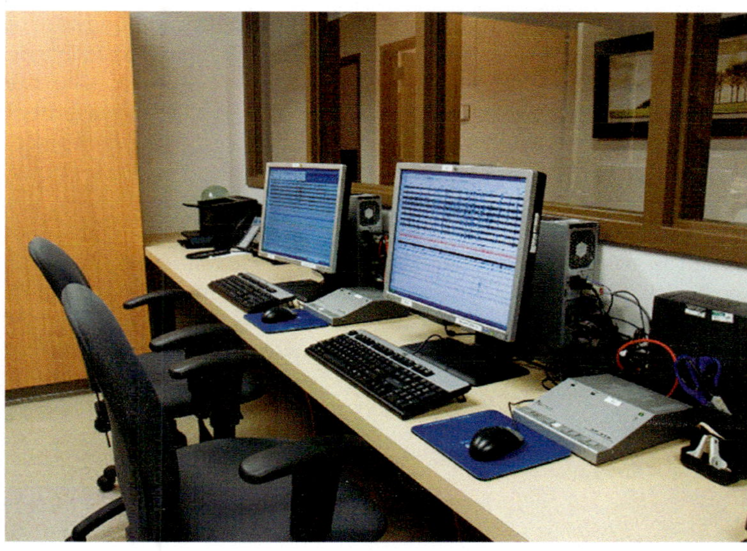

Fig. 5: Control room.

- *Toilets*: It can be planned as per the local needs of populace. An area of 10 m^2 should be earmarked. Toilets should have provision for wheelchaired patients also.

Std D-8[17]

- The facility must have clean bathroom with a minimum ratio of one bathroom for every testing room there, these bathroom must contain toilet and sink.
- *Waiting room*: There should be designated waiting area for patients' relatives. This area can be planned in an area of 20 m^2. This place can have magazine stands, TV, information kiosks, etc.

The line drawings are shown in Figures 6 and 7.

THE CHALLENGE FOR THE FUTURE[1,9]

The greatest challenge for the future is the cost-effective expansion of sleep medicine, so that its benefits will be available readily throughout the society. It will be very important to plan for customized sleep

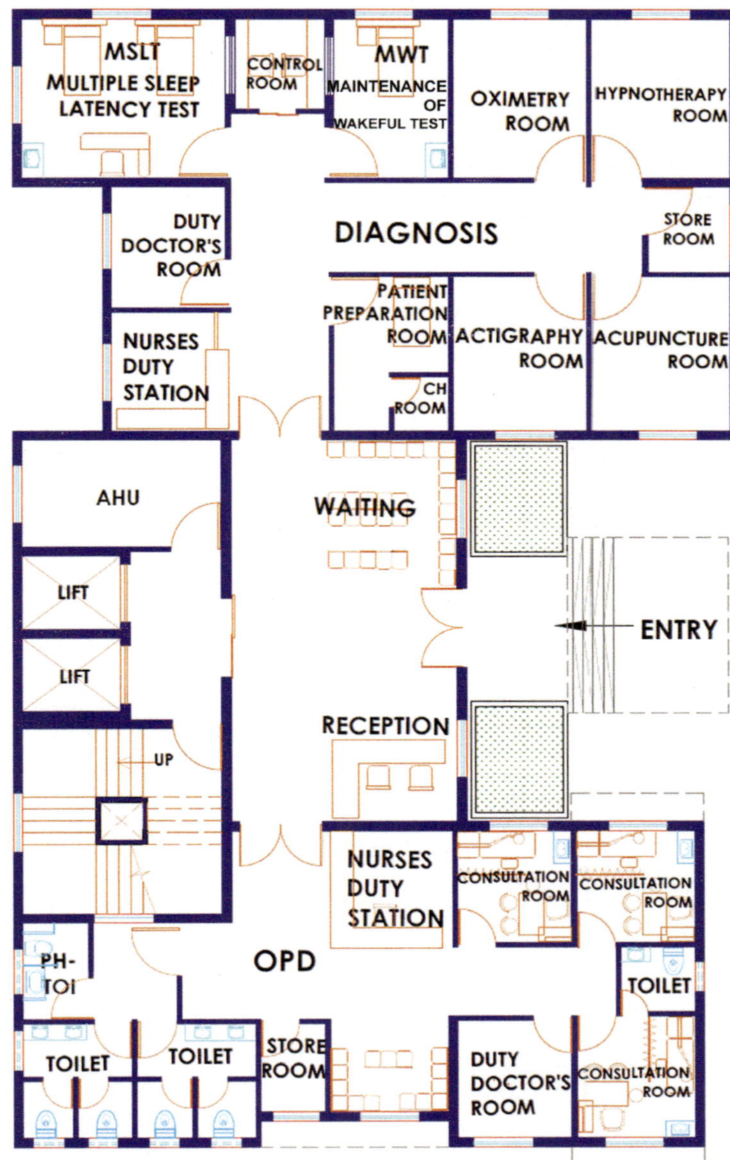

Fig. 6: Ground floor plan.

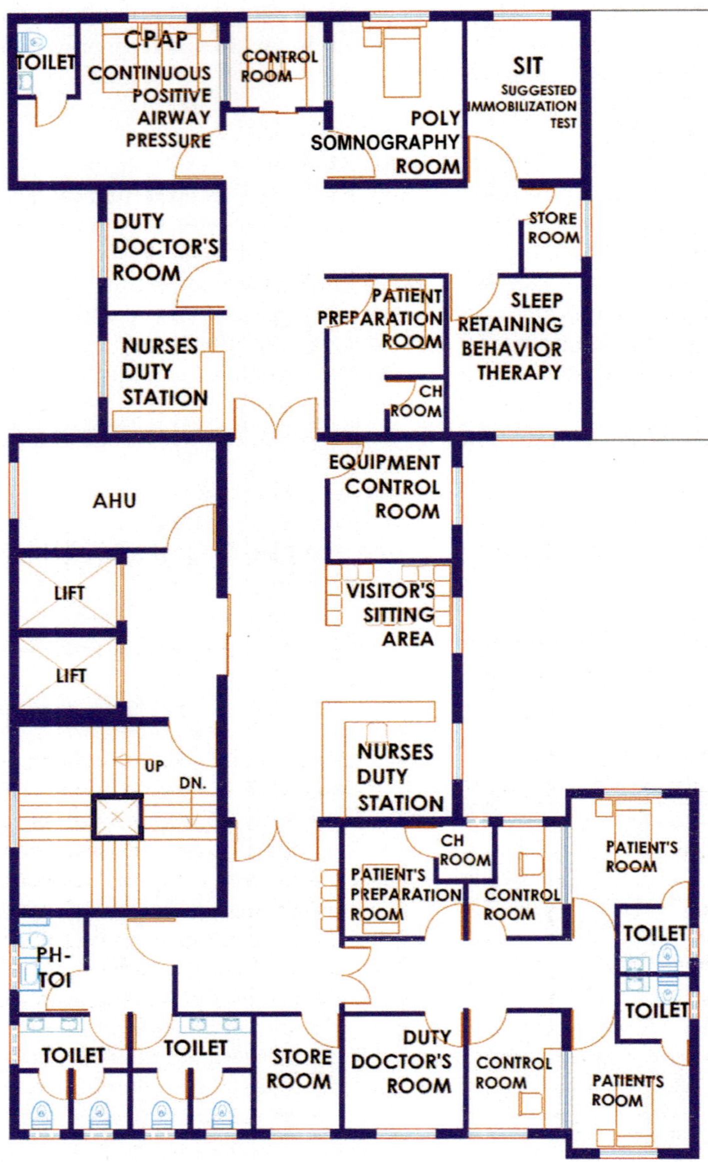

Fig. 7: First floor plan.

centers across the world as per the regional requirement. A major problem is the current failure of sleep research and sleep medicine to penetrate the mainstream educational system effectively at any level. As a consequence, the majority of human beings remain unaware of important facts of sleep and wakefulness, the fundamentals of biologic rhythms, and knowledge about sleep disorders, in particular the symptoms that suggest a serious pathologic process. The management of sleep deprivation and its serious consequences in the workplace, particularly in those industries that maintain sustained operations, is only beginning to be addressed comprehensively. Finally, the education and training of health professionals to be sleep specialists has far to go to reach adequate numbers. It has made a concern for the health of human beings a 24-hour enterprise and has energized a new effort to reveal the secrets of the healthy and unhealthy sleeping brain.

REFERENCES

1. www.cfm.va.gov
2. Ervin Putsep. Modern Hospital: International Planning Practices. London : Lloyd-Luke. 1979-80; 80p.
3. University of Glasgow Sleep Center: sleep matters, summer. 2009;2(1).
4. EO Bixler, A Kales, CR Soldatos, JD Kales and S Healey. Prevalence of sleep disorders in the Los Angeles metropolitan area. Am J Psychiatry. 1979 Oct;136(10):1257-62p
5. Roger B; Sejnowski T, Siegel J, et al. (February 2007). "Waking Up To Sleep" (Several conference videos). The Science Network. http://thesciencenetwork.org/programs/waking-up-to-sleep. Retrieved. 2008-01-25.
6. Collop NA. Conundrums in sleep medicine. Chest. March 1999; 115(3): 607–8p doi:10.1378/chest.115.3.607.
7. medlibrary.org
8. Bajaj JS. Annals of National Academy of Medical Sciences; Sleep Medicine Perspective, Potential and Prospect: 49(3)&(4). p. 75.
9. W Dement. History of Sleep Physiology and Medicine. Principles and Practice of Sleep Medicine. 2005
10. Vijayan VK. Annals of National Academy of Medical Sciences; Sleep-disordered breathing: OSA, CSA, Pathophysiology and Diagnosis. (49)(3-4); p. 92.
11. Johns MW. "A new method for measuring daytime sleepiness: the Epworth sleepiness scale". Sleep. 1991;14(6):540-5.
12. www.aasmnet.org
13. Accreditation of sleep disorder center of AASM (American Academy of Sleep Medicine) accessed on 27 Dec 18 at https://aasn.org
14. Putsep E. Modern hospitals International Planning 1970, p. 249.
15. Evidence-based design meets evidence-based medicine: The Sound Sleep Study, Wei Wang, Harvard Medical School, Division of Sleep Medicine. Jo M. Solet, Behavioral Medicine, Harvard Medical School, Division of Sleep Medicine Cambridge Health Alliance. pp. 17.
16. Planning and designing guideline, child care center. Ontario 2006.pp. 39-40.
17. www.sjkdt.org

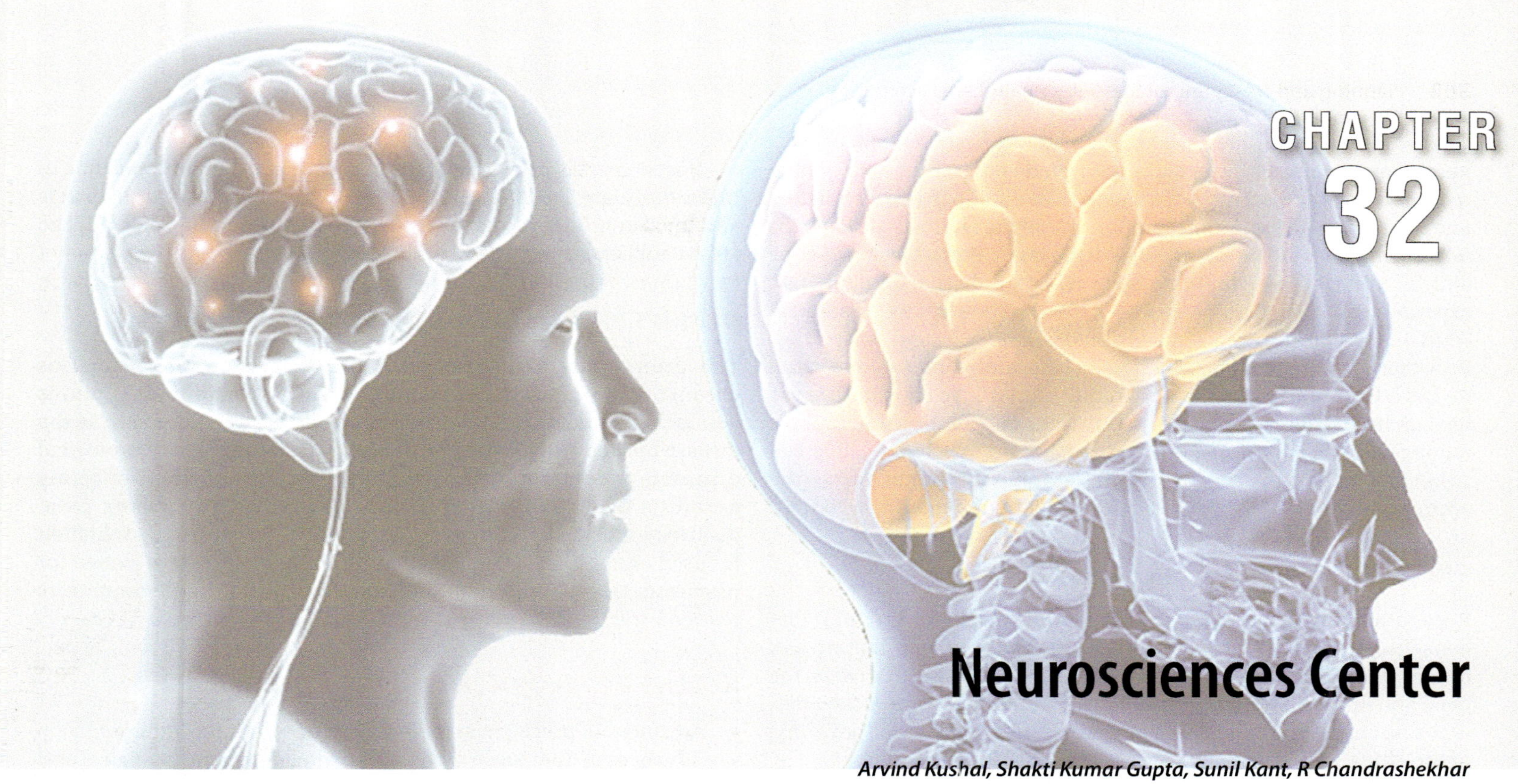

Neurosciences Center

Arvind Kushal, Shakti Kumar Gupta, Sunil Kant, R Chandrashekhar

INTRODUCTION[1-3]

From the 12th century Anatomical Amphitheater in Europe to the World War II style one/two surgical suite operation theaters to today's areas of prime action in modern hospitals, operation theaters have come a long way.

Rapid evolution in the technical support systems required for contemporary and advanced levels of neurological surgery, over the last quarter century, have completely changed the nature of the specialty. The advent of multiple refined imaging modes that define the concerned anatomical substrate of complex physiological monitoring methods, and of reliance upon microscopic and stereotactic techniques for precise operative control have created dramatic changes in neurooperative events and outcome.[1]

The ideal neurosurgical operating suite should provide the capability for optimal performance of the entire spectrum of neurosurgical procedures. The individual and integrated use of all technological adjuvants should be provided for, especially imaging modes, microscopic and stereotactic instrumentation. The entire setting should be self-contained and independent of external support services for critical intraoperative requirements. The design should provide an optimally functional environment for all surgical personnel, including anesthesiologists, surgeons, nurses, and staff. A hallmark of the entire system should be its ability to support fluid, refined, and precise operation with integration of team members and the technological adjuvants.[1]

The neuroscience center is a superspecialty center, which is dedicated to the effective diagnosis and comprehensive treatment of disease of the brain, spinal cord, muscle and nerves. The center is manned by a highly qualified team of neurologist, neurosurgeons, and neuropsychologist and is supported by neuroradiologist, dietician and a neurointensive care team. They work collaboratively with a skilled, multidisciplinary team of nurses, rehabilitation specialists and support staff who, are specialized in neurologic care. Neurologists diagnose diseases of the nervous system and brain.[2]

Patients may complain of headaches, epileptic seizures, damage suffered as a result of a stroke, or perhaps a cerebral palsy condition that has resulted in facial distortion, a distended jaw or a drooping mouth. Neurologists manage progressively degenerative diseases such as Parkinson's disease, Alzheimer's disease and multiple sclerosis, which involve considerable "trial and error" manipulation of drugs.[2]

The grossly inadequate number of neurologists and lack of infrastructure has deprived a large proportion of the patients of neurology care. Hospitals are traditionally designed for the average adult or child of normal physical and mental capabilities. However, persons with locomotion, sensory disabilities visit the neurosciences and it is inescapable to have appropriate facilities designed for them. It has been brought into focus that neurological disorders need to be recognized as a public health problem and advocacy be promoted to draw the attention of health planners and administrators in view of the magnitude of the problem of 30 million or more people with neurological disorders in the country.[3]

NEED FOR A CENTER

The concepts of brain functions have been continuously reshaped by the discovery of the new substances which are concentrated in neural pathways. The current upsurge of interest in the nervous system occurred only recently with the development of highly refined experimental and analytical techniques that enabled studies at levels of intensity and with a precision not possible previously. The contribution of one discipline was hardly known to the workers in other disciplines. Therefore, a need was felt to bring workers engaged in different disciplines— neuroanatomy, neurophysiology, biochemistry, biophysics, toxicology, psychology, psychiatry, pharmacology, etc. on a common platform, where they can share their knowledge and methodology and plan future strategy for effective collaborative research.[4]

In addition to above, considering vast and specialized field, latest advancement, research and special need for patients with neurological diseases, a separate dedicated center is an inescapable requirement. Neurosciences ICU needs to be equipped with ventilators and neurological monitoring equipment and the neurosurgical operation theater needs to be equipped with the latest operating microscope and OT tables along with other operative paraphernalia manned by experienced nursing staff and well-trained neurology/neurosurgical residents under the direct supervision of the neurosciences faculties. Provisions for all ancillary emergency laboratory, microbiology and neuroradiology investigations are required by above team to save the life and limb. There is a need for a very close cooperation and rapport amongst all the supportive departments for neurosciences. This will result in a quick and accurate diagnosis within the center and all the appropriate treatment accorded to the patient under a single roof.[5]

PRESENT SCENARIO[6]

Recognition of the magnitude of the burden, disability and mortality consequent to neurological disorders has led to global initiative of declaring them as a "global epidemic", the gross mismatch between the need and the available trained manpower and infrastructural facilities, is posing challenges to health planners and policymakers for providing neurological care to the community.[3-6]

Global Burden

Report published by the World Health Organization "Neurological disorders, public health challenges" states that about one billion people worldwide suffer from neurological disorders and that 6.8 million people die annually from these disorders.[7] The spectrum of neurological disorders include epilepsy, stroke, headache, Alzheimer's disease and other dementias, Parkinson's disease, multiple sclerosis, brain injuries, neuro infection, etc.[3,7-9]

An increase in mortality due to neurological disorders is anticipated.[7] Thus, neurological disorders can be considered as a global epidemic calling for a global campaign to promote advocacy, improve awareness, education and prevention and to enhance neurology care.[3,7-9]

Projections of the United Nations

Based on the projections of the United Nations that by 2025, there will be 1.2 billion elderly people in the world and 71% will be living in the developing countries, it is expected that neurological disorders in the elderly will show a significant rise, particularly in the developing world. Anticipated figures are as shown in Table 1.

Table 1: Prevalence of neurological disorders in the world.[7]

Year population disorder	*Per 1,000*
Epilepsy	6.38
Alzheimer and other dementias	5.56
Parkinson's disease	0.91
Multiple sclerosis	0.41
Migraine	52.15
Cerebrovascular disease	9.70
Neuroinfections	1.68
Nutritional and neuropathies	36.04
Neurological injuries	30.66
Total	143.50

Based on the prevalence studies, it may be estimated that in India there are 20–30 million people with neurological disorders and the common disorders include epilepsy (6–8 million), headache (10–12 million), strokes (1–2 million).[3,8]

Unique Characteristics of Neurological Disorders

The unique characteristics of neurological disorders such as chronicity, progressive degeneration, limited therapeutic options and lack of specific treatment for many diseases, contribute to the disease burden and morbidity. Disability consequent to neurological disorders is common and disabilities are categorized as affecting mobility, disturbance of cognition and behavior, causing pain, disturbance of consciousness and function.[10] Apart from rehabilitation focused on motor, sensory and cognitive deficits, there is a need for psychosocial rehabilitation and effective utilization of community resources.[3,10-12]

RECENT DEVELOPMENTS

- Advances in precision surgery with state-of-art brain suite.[3]
- Advances in diagnostic modalities of imaging, immunological and molecular tests.[3]
- Introduction of new therapeutic strategies, such as thrombolytic, immunoglobulin and interferon.[3]
- Use of new drugs for treatment of epilepsy, Parkinson's disease has enabled early diagnosis and more effective treatment leading to improved outcome of the disease.
- The future of neurosurgery will include increased usage of telesurgery, artificial intelligence and virtual reality.
- Neurorobotics and robots with ambidextrous abilities, more degrees of freedom, kinesthetic feedback and a more user-friendly interface.[13]
- Integration of artificial intelligence and nanotechnology will soon create surgical procedures that cannot be done without it, revolutionizing neurosurgical practices.[13]
- Emerging role of *ayurveda*, *yoga* and naturopathy in treatment of brain cognitive and neurological disorders.

Tertiary Center

The first institute of neurosciences came in India in Madras in 1959 followed by other institutes at Vellore and Mumbai. Facilities for neurology care are available in about 60 medical colleges, which may be considered as regional centers. All these figures pertain to the government sector only and since affordability is a major concern, the emphasis is on this sector. Increasing number of hospitals in the private sector are offering excellent care but at a prohibitive cost.[3]

Organization and Delivery of Neurology Services

The current scenario in the country is far from satisfactory with a gross mismatch of the burden of neurological disorders and the availability of trained neurologists, other essential health professionals and infrastructural facilities. The ratio of one neurologist for population varies widely among developed countries from one to two neurologists per 20,000–100,000; in developing countries the ratio is much higher at one neurologist for 3–5 million people; and in many regions of the world, there are no neurologists.[10] In the US, there is one neurologist per 26,200 and in Africa it is one per 5,009,908. In India these is one neurologist for 1,250,000.[3]

PLANNING AND DESIGN CONSIDERATIONS

Specific Design Consideration for Neurosciences Center

Building should consist of three floors with facilities distributed at various floor levels. All support services for center should be by main hospital of apex tertiary care center.

Basement Area

Basement should have parking for visitors and staff.

Ground Floor

Reception, lifts, OPD, pharmacy, waiting, radiology services, such as EEG, CT scan, MRI, sleep lab, pain management center, rehabilitation services, laboratory sample collection area, medical social worker, security office.

First Floor

The administrative office, laboratory, blood bank, private and general wards, and neuropsychiatric ward may be placed on the first floor.

Second Floor

Operating rooms, brain suites, ICU (both—critical care unit and postoperative intensive care unit), postoperative wards may be placed on the upper floor.

Design Guidelines

It is envisaged that neurosciences center would be holistic in nature, economical to build, respond to the local environment and create an environment which is user friendly. It should be cost- and energy-efficient building. This building should be 'Green' and environment friendly. Extensive use of natural light, provision of solar heating (having subsidy element) conservation of water and waste management systems, are being reflected in the design along with modular pattern of development, ability to expand to meet future needs.[13-18]

Physical Considerations in Design

Use of mobility aides such as walkers, canes and wheelchairs must also be considered when designing environments for persons with neurodisability. Patients may have movement disorders like ataxia, tremors, dystonia, dyskinesia and chorea, motor disorders such as spasticity and rigidity, hypo-tonicity or problems such as vertigo, lightheadedness and balance can also result.[19] Aforementioned deficits can significantly interfere with a person's ability to access their environments.[19-21]

Cognitive Considerations in Design

Brain injury may cause changes in cognition in multiple spheres of function, including memory, attention, and executive skills, such as organization, prioritization, and judgment and planning.[22] The design of the environment for such individuals needs to provide extra cognitive cues. Signage needs to be utilized as much as possible.

Visual and Visuoperceptual Considerations in Design

Visual and visuoperceptual impairments may lead to functional difficulties due to challenges in visual acuity, visual perception (such as depth perception, visual discrimination, visual closure, object constancy, visual matching), and balance.[23] For those with visual acuity and discrimination impairments, signs should be in large print and lettering should differ in color from the sign's background and lighting should be of the nonglare variety but allow for adequate illumination for both safety and function. The light should come from natural sources as much as possible, avoiding fluorescent lighting.[24]

Sensory Considerations in Design

Another challenging problem that can be associated is sensory neglect.[25] Persons with neurological disorder may completely ignore or may simply have decreased attention to sensory stimuli in one or both hemifields.[25] Therefore, environmental modifications are required to increase safety and function.

Acoustic Considerations in Design

Hearing problems may also accompany brain injury, and individuals with such may be under- or over- sensitive to sounds. Therefore, acoustics must be taken into consideration. Dry wall partition for noise reduction should be considered.[26]

Behavioral Considerations in Design

Behavioral problems are frequent after brain injury, often displayed as amplified behaviors such as irritability, aggression or a reduction in normal behavior, increased social reclusiveness, among the most common.[27] Breakable items should be out of reach of individuals with aggression and furniture should be heavy enough so that it cannot be picked up and thrown.

Mood affects one's ability to interact with one's environment on multiple levels. Brain injury has also been associated with neuropsychiatric disorders, such as depression.[28] One way to improve an individual's mood is to maximize natural light in the living environment through large windows, skylights and/or tube lights or alternatively with full spectrum lighting.

Designer should also consider the influence of color on behavior including mood. In general, in Western cultures, the use of blue is associated with calmness; however, too dark a blue hue may have the result of conveying "coldness". Light green has also been shown to have a calmative effect.

Universal Design Considerations in Neurosciences Center

Neurology patients are individuals struggling with the debilitating symptoms and changes in ability or functionality as a result of the condition with which they are afflicted. The principles of universal design will enable individuals to complete more tasks. While not competing with the benefits of rehabilitation design, universal designs focus on solutions that benefit multiple members of the social sphere. Universal Design is unobtrusive, even invisible.[29]

Washroom Accessories

- In each public washroom, provide at least one wheelchair/walker accessible modesty vestibule with enough space for a caregiver and room for mobility devices to be turned around.[30-32]
- Ensure flushing mechanism is easy to reach, easy to operate and that toilet paper is positioned within easy reach for people with limited mobility and dexterity (i.e. not behind the toilet).[30-32]
- Washroom doors that open outward and are at least 810 mm (2 ft 8 in) wide to allow space for a wheelchair/walker to pass through enables caregivers to enter washrooms and assist disabled or frail older adults. Provide space for full wheelchair turning radius 1500 mm by 1500 mm (5 ft × 5 ft) diameter.[31-33]

- Mount urinals 450 mm (18 in) above the floor or mount urinals without a step to reduce the risk of falls by older adults. Urinals should be at a lower height, conducive for use by pediatric patients. Use of adjustable urinals and wash basins are advised.
- Alarm switches/nurse call in all toilets is also recommended as neurology patients may not be physically capable of shouting for help in case of any requirement.
- Provide an appropriate chair for caregivers and so patients using walkers can sit when using wash basins.[34]
- For wheelchair access, wash basins 800 mm (32 in) high, and no higher than 860 mm (34 in). Provide a clear space under basins that is 680 mm (27 in) high and 200 mm (8 in) deep.[35,36]
- In at least some patient washrooms, install assist tubs and/or wheelchair/walker accessible showers with non-slip finish on standing/sitting surfaces. The bath and shower controls should be accessible from a wheelchair and operable with one hand.[36,37]
- Install towel dispensers and other accessories no higher than 1200 mm (48 in) from the floor to be accessible from a wheelchair.

Grab Bars

- To facilitate patients to shift from the crutches/wheelchair to the toilet seat, there should be grab bars at water closet.
- These should be slip-resistant with round ends and have a circular section of 30–45 mm in diameter.
- To promote independent voiding by older adults, place grab bars near urinals and adjacent to the toilet—on both sides.[38]
- All grab bars must be capable of withstanding a force of 2 kN and they should have a minimum clear space of 40 mm from the wall and be installed at a height of 800–900 mm.

Electrical Controls and Switches

- The operable part of electrical controls and outlets such as vending machines, electrical switches and intercom buttons should be located between 600 mm and 1200 mm from the floor.
- Switches should be operable by one hand.

Entrances

- Raised entrance poses problems for individuals needing the assistance of crutches, wheelchairs, and other mobility-assistive devices. Patients in wheelchairs require ramps with double handrails.
- There should be a landing planned after every 9 m long uninterrupted ramps and greater slopes are safety hazards and should be avoided.
- The gradient of a ramp should not be steeper than 1:12. The minimum clear width of a ramp should be 1200 mm. One inch in height for every foot traversed. So, if a ramp is supposed to traverse 10 ft, then the ramp should be 10 inches high off the ground at the higher end.

Parking

- Ensure bright, nonglare overhead lighting for security[31,32]
- Close to each entrance, provide wheelchair-accessible parking stalls designated with the International Symbol of Access. Accessible spaces should be 3900 mm (12 ft 9 in) wide on a level ground surface for safer transfers from vehicle to wheelchair and vice versa.[30,36]
- Equip some parking spaces with locking pincers to block wheelchairs and keep them in place when transferring the patients.[32,36]

Equipment-assistive Devices/Telephones

- Near each building entrance, in common areas, in special function areas, and in patient rooms, provide a variety of assistive mobility devices (i.e. wheelchairs, walkers, and canes).[36]
- At each information counter and reception area, provide hearing amplifiers, pressure reduction furniture and lumbar support cushions.[35,36,39]
- Locate public telephones close to each entrance. At least one telephone should be accessible from a wheelchair— with coin slot, dial and handset less than 1370 mm (54 in) from the floor, a handset cord at least 1000 mm (33 in) long, and partitions between phones at least 800 mm (32 in) apart.[30,31]
- Install a wandering system to monitor confused mobile older adults.[33,37]
- Use of patient transfer system to shift patients who are fully dependent due to neurological disability.

Furniture

- Arrange furniture to promote barrier-free access.[35,39]
- Provide sturdy framed, 4-legged furniture. Seat cushions and pads should provide a slight forward angle to support older adults as they raise themselves to a standing position. Avoid furniture with back tilting options and avoid furniture on castors as older adults with mobility problems will use furniture to steady themselves.[30,37,38,40,41]
- Provide stable tables with rounded corners that are accessible from a wheelchair.[35,37]
- To meet the diverse needs of older adults, provide diverse types of comfortable furniture (i.e. some chairs without arms to facilitate transfer to/from a wheelchair) in warm colors which contrast with the floor and walls.[30,31,38]

Elevators

- Locate elevators close to wheelchair/walker-accessible entrances and place them in visible areas that are directly accessible from main entrances and important circulation paths on each floor.[35,37,40]
- Outside each elevator, provide a waiting area that is 1600 mm by 1600 mm (64 in × 64 in) to enable easy wheelchair or walker maneuverability. Also, door openings should be at least 810 mm (32 in) wide, with an automatic reopen safety feature.[31]
- For all-purpose elevators, cabins should be at least 1300 mm by 1300 mm (4 ft 4 in × 4 ft 6 in).[31]
- To accommodate wheelchairs, cabins should be at least 1370 mm by 1725 mm (4 ft 6 in × 5 ft 9 in).[31]
- To accommodate stretchers cabin, should be at least 1300 mm × 2030 mm (4 ft 4 in × 6 ft 10 in).[31]

Way Finding and Signage[30-32,35-39,41-43]

- Include simple, explanatory graphics on signs using universal symbols wherever possible (i.e. the International Symbol of Access).
- Reception/information counters should be no higher than 840 mm (34 in) to allow access from wheelchairs or walkers.
- Place maps, including "you are here" maps, and large font informational handouts at reception areas.
- Use color coding to facilitate way finding and to indicate safe routes by using a standard color and texture throughout hospital grounds.

- Provide minimal information on all signs, ensure signage is uncluttered, logically structured, and use of consistent language on all signs. Aim should be to keep words and phrases within a sixth-grade reading level and avoid the use of technical and/or medical language; avoid jargon.[37]
- Use high-contrast color combinations on signs—preferably light letters on a dark (i.e. black, brown or red), matte finish background.
- For patients with vision deficiencies, the font size should be at least 16 mm (5/8 in) high on small signs and at least 40 mm (1-1/2 in) high on larger signs. Helvetica is the recommended font. Tactile letters should be raised 1 mm (1/20 in). Use a combination of capital and lower case lettering.
- Use very large signs visible to people with visual deficiencies and hang signs between wheelchair and standing heights—910-1320 mm (3-4 ft 5 in) high or as low as 50 mm (2 in) above handrails.

Flooring and Walls

- Ensure walls and floors are in a matte finish which reduce glare (consider using nonglare paint to achieve a glare index ≤20).[30]
- Keep the walls behind handrails smooth to prevent abrasion injuries to knuckles as patient navigates the hospital. Apply a nonabrasive finish to walls.[30]

Hallways, Doors and Windows

- At entrances, install automatic sensor doors; consider sliding doors equipped with an adjustable opening/closing delay system programmed to keep doors open for a longer duration than required by the code as patients with mobility impairments require additional time to clear the doorway.[30,31,44]
- Install doors equipped with lever-style handles that do not require twisting and can be opened with one hand. Doors require maximum 8 lbs pull force or 14 lbs push force; with closing mechanism to allow at least 4–6 seconds for patients with mobility problems to clear the doorway before it closes.[30,33,34]
- In all hallways, provide between 1470 mm and 1830 mm (4 ft 11 in–6 ft 1 in) handrails to allow 2 wheelchairs to pass.[36]
- Make hallway corners at least 1200 mm (4 ft) wide so older patients can turn a wheelchair/walker comfortably.[30]
- In patient rooms, install patient-controlled drapes, blinds, or an energy-efficient transparent sunscreen system to shade windows while letting in natural light. Controls should be easy to operate by people with limited dexterity and within reach from a wheelchair.[30]

Handrails

- When handrails are terminated or interrupted, consider a tactile signal (i.e. a notch cut into the rail) 100 mm from the endpoint or have the rail curve and connect back to the wall.[33,35,37]
- Install handrails 850 mm (3 ft) from the ground. Handrails should be between 40 mm and 45 mm in diameter with a non-slip texture.[37]
- Install handrails on both sides of stairways and hallways and on at least one side of ramps.[37]
- On ramps and stairways, extend handrails 300 mm (12 in) beyond the end of the ramp and consider installing a safety rail along with the handrail at 200 mm (8 in) above ground.[30,33,37]
- In elevators, provide handrails on both sides of the cabin at a height between 800 mm and 1000 mm (32–40 in).[31,38]
- Handrails should be in a color that contrasts with the floor and the wall to help older adults with visual impairments to locate the handrails; consider Braille on end of handrail.[30]

Walkways, Ramps and Stairways

- Avoid abrupt changes in ground levels keeping any surface relief (i.e. curbs) to under 25 mm high (1 in) with rounded edges.[31,37,39]
- Walkway and ramp surfaces should be firm and slip-resistant (i.e. rough concrete or treated cement).
- Keep grids or grates on the ground to less than 20 mm (4/5 in) wide for older adults using walkers, wheelchairs or canes, as mobility aides may become stuck in the grid.[35,37,39]
- Design walkways and ramps to be at least 1625 mm (5 ft 4 in) wide, providing space between handrails that allow two wheelchairs to pass or a walker; and with landings at a minimum of 1625 mm (5 ft 4 in) at the bottom and top of a ramp. Consider corners that are at least 1220 mm (4 ft) wide, to allow for a comfortable turning of a wheelchair/walker.[35,37]
- Avoid long or winding stairways, keeping to a maximum of 10 risers per flight. Provide rest areas landings every 10 risers (steps) on long flights of stairs and try breaking up long walkways or ramps with rest areas every 9000 mm (30 ft).[34,37,39]

Lighting

- Provide a minimum of 300 lux from overhead lighting
- Combine direct (i.e. ceiling-mounted fluorescents) with indirect lighting (i.e. high pressure, floor-standing up-lights or diffuse reflector and covered lamp shining down). Using multiple light sources reduces glare while increasing lighting beyond normal levels.[32,37]
- On way-finding cues and signage, provide direct, focused, nonglare lighting.[30,39]
- Just outside washrooms, place night-lights 300 mm (12 in) from the floor and install illuminated light switches in washrooms.[31,46]

Acoustics

- *Install*: Solid-core doors with sound stripping to reduce noise transfer; silent or quiet type switches; quiet heating and ventilation systems; and double-glazed windows which help reduce outside noises from penetrating the hospital environment.[33,37,38]
- Consider providing hearing amplifiers in all patient areas (i.e. Pocket Talker).[35,37,39]
- Single occupant patient rooms are preferable to multi-occupant rooms—less noise and fewer disruptions, which can exacerbate confusion and delirium in older adults.[32,37]

Colors

- Avoid bold patterns, especially on floors and walls, as the visual over-stimulation can exacerbate confusion.[35,37,43]
- Differentiate walls from floors by using different, contrasting colors for each surface.[37]
- Handrails should be in a color that contrasts with the floor and the wall to help the patients with visual impairment to locate the handrails.[37,39]

GENERAL PLANNING AND DESIGN CONSIDERATIONS[18,42,45-54]

- To configure the all-important norms, the service delivery of the entire center should be divided into three sections, viz., outpatient department (OPD) (where the patient is mobile while the doctors, paramedics and the equipment are fixed); wards (where the patient is fixed while the rest of the attendant facilities including physicians are mobile); operation theater and laboratory (where the equipment is fixed while the patients, paramedics and surgeons are mobile).

- Location of various departments has a very important role to play. All the departments are the 'activities' of the hospital and it is most important to rightly identify the 'activity' and 'activity sequence' in working out a functional program of spaces. In the words of Emerson Goble, "Separate all the departments yet keep them close to each other; separate types of traffic yet save steps to everybody. That is all there is to hospital planning."
- Keep patient as the focus of planning and designing.
- Patient flow—separate traffic flow for in- and outpatients as also separate access for physician and public.
- Material and services flow—it is also important to separate transport of clean and soiled material.
- Utilize energy saving/optimizing techniques such as solar energy, biogas units for lighting, heat reclaim from boiler exhaust and incineration.
- Use of eco-friendly materials (Green Building Concepts).
- Waste management to be planned for or to be outsourced.
- Inputs from equipment vendors, especially in specialty areas such as MRI, CT scan, and operation theaters will be essential to finalize the working plan of the neurosciences center. Public-private partnership (PPP) models for these services should be ventured.
- Essential to segregate the traffic, i.e. inpatients, outpatients, visitors, staff goods and waste.
- The development of heating, ventilation and air-conditioning (HVAC) and high-level artificial illumination has a significant effect. Pressurization zoning with HVAC for infection control is essential.
- Environment plays a dominant role in the healing process of a patient and selection of esthetically pleasing building material, which is also sustainable, and patient friendly, goes a long way in complementing patient healing.
- Value-added services—additional services may be added to add value to the neurosciences center like information kiosks, cafeteria—staff and visitors, flower shop, vending machine—tea, coffee, juice, communication facilities —STD, ISD, fax, and cyber cafe—internet, ATM facility, prayer room/facilities, etc.[18]
- Provide barrier-free environment that helps patient mobility and wellness by providing lounges, worship places, gardens, and kitchen activity rooms.[18]
- Use of copper as touch surface because copper has antibacterial nature.

Specialty organogram is shown in Figure 1.

OUTPATIENT DEPARTMENT

- The location should be such that an OPD shares diagnostic services, such as medical imaging, laboratory, pharmacy, blood bank with other departments of a hospital.
- Dignity and privacy of patients must be maintained.
- Design should cater for future expansion and must incorporate flexibility of space planning.
- Educational resource areas for patients education should be integrated in the lobby and waiting areas.
- Design of individual functional areas should not allow extraneous traffic to penetrate any work area. Design should be such that the flow of patients and visitors is unilateral.
- Waiting areas and public spaces should be large enough to accommodate patients and accompanying friends and family without causing congestion. Sub-waiting areas should be provided

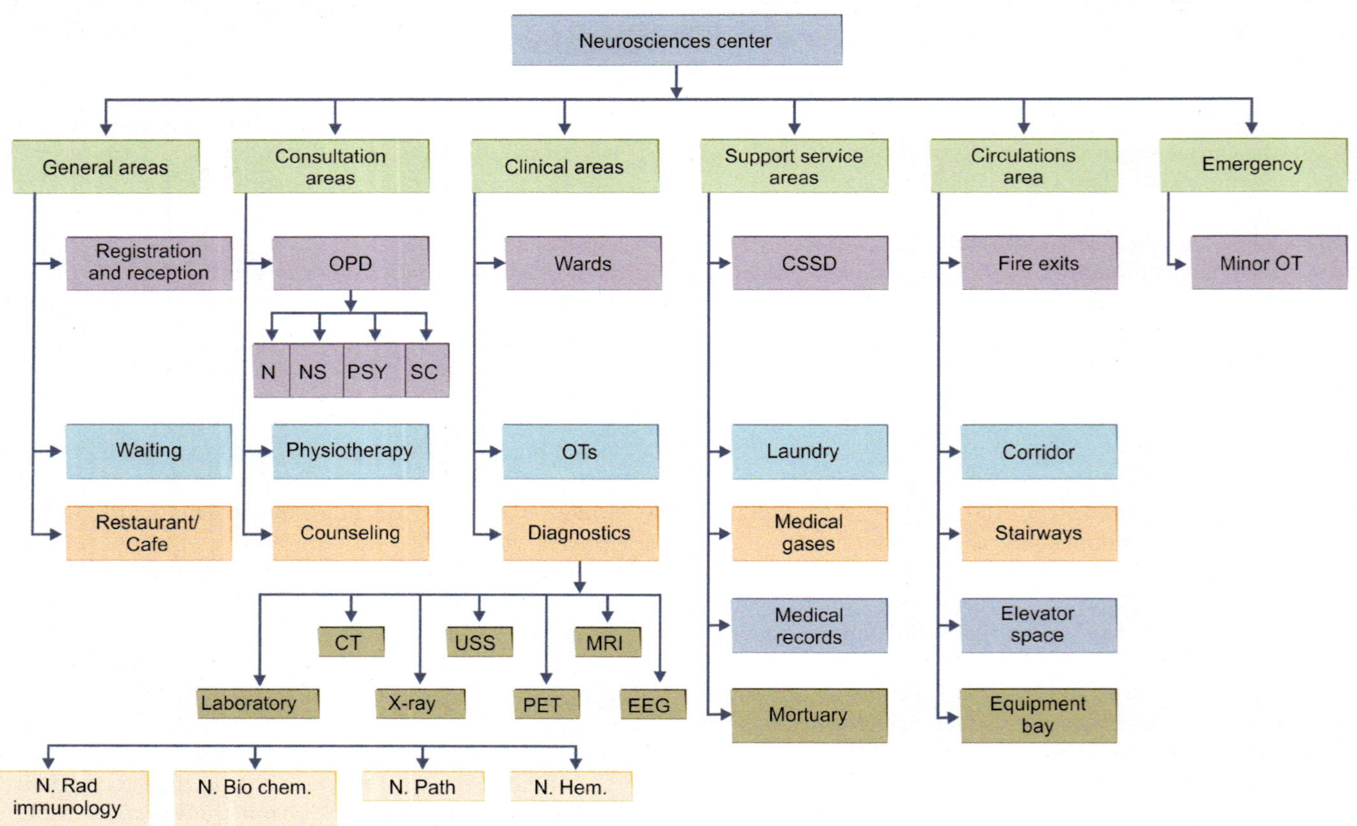

Fig. 1: Neurosciences center.

(N: neurologist; NS: neuro surgeon; PSY: psychologist; SC: specialist consultant) adjacent to various clinics. Space recommended is 0.8 m^2 per patient for one-third of the average daily number of the patients attending OPD in one session.

- Call center for appointments will reduce congestions in OPD and help in optimum utilization of space and proper management of time.

Physical facilities in OPD must include public areas, clinical areas, consultation rooms, special examination rooms, administrative area, circulation area, ancillary and auxiliary facilities.

Enquiry Desk or Reception Station

- The height of counter should be adapted to the needs of wheelchair patients.
- To ensure privacy of discussion between patient and reception staff, the reception should have counters.

Waiting Area

- Waiting area should be planned to accommodate more than the number of people expected during peak hours.
- Sub-waiting area may be shared between the various consultation rooms.
- Toilets should be close to the waiting area. Male and female toilets should be separate.

Neurologist Consultation Room (Fig. 2)

This is a low-volume specialty, with the taking of a preliminary history and an interview in the physician's consultation room or exam room requiring 20–45 minutes for new patients. Occasionally, there may be a small exam room opening off the consultation room. Two exam rooms per physician are generally adequate. A patient education room with TV and VCR and CRT with internet access is useful for patients and their families to learn about neurodegenerative diseases. Planning for patients in wheelchairs is mandatory. The waiting room and exam rooms must easily accommodate wheelchairs so a corridor width of 5 ft is optimal.[2]

After the patient interview, a series of tests may be performed. The most common test is the electroencephalogram (charting of brain waves), commonly known as EEG. This can be performed in a room as small as 8–10 ft if the technician does not remain in the room with the patient, but sits in an adjoining control room.[2]

A sink should be provided in the EEG room for hand washing. EEG requires the application of conductive paste at the temples before the leads are attached. The paste is messy and the patient must have access to a sink or a bathroom to wipe it out of his or her hair afterwards. Provide a vanity counter in the bathroom with a paper towel dispenser, a soap dispenser, and a place to hang a coat or handbag. The EEG procedure takes about 40 minutes to perform.[2]

Another commonly performed test is evoked potential, which tests the different pathways to the brain (auditory, visual, and somatosensory). Both EEG (Fig. 3) and evoked potential testing (Fig. 4) are done by a technician, and both units may be located in the same room. Provide large window so that the patient can be observed at all times. In the test room, locked storage is needed for drugs used to sedate the patients. Lighting in the test room should be able to be dimmed.[2]

Location for the EEG room is near the front of the suite so that these patients do not have to pass the consultation room or exam rooms in order to reach the test room.

Another office procedure is, electromyography, (EMG) which shows if a muscle is deteriorating, can be rehabilitated. It measures the strength

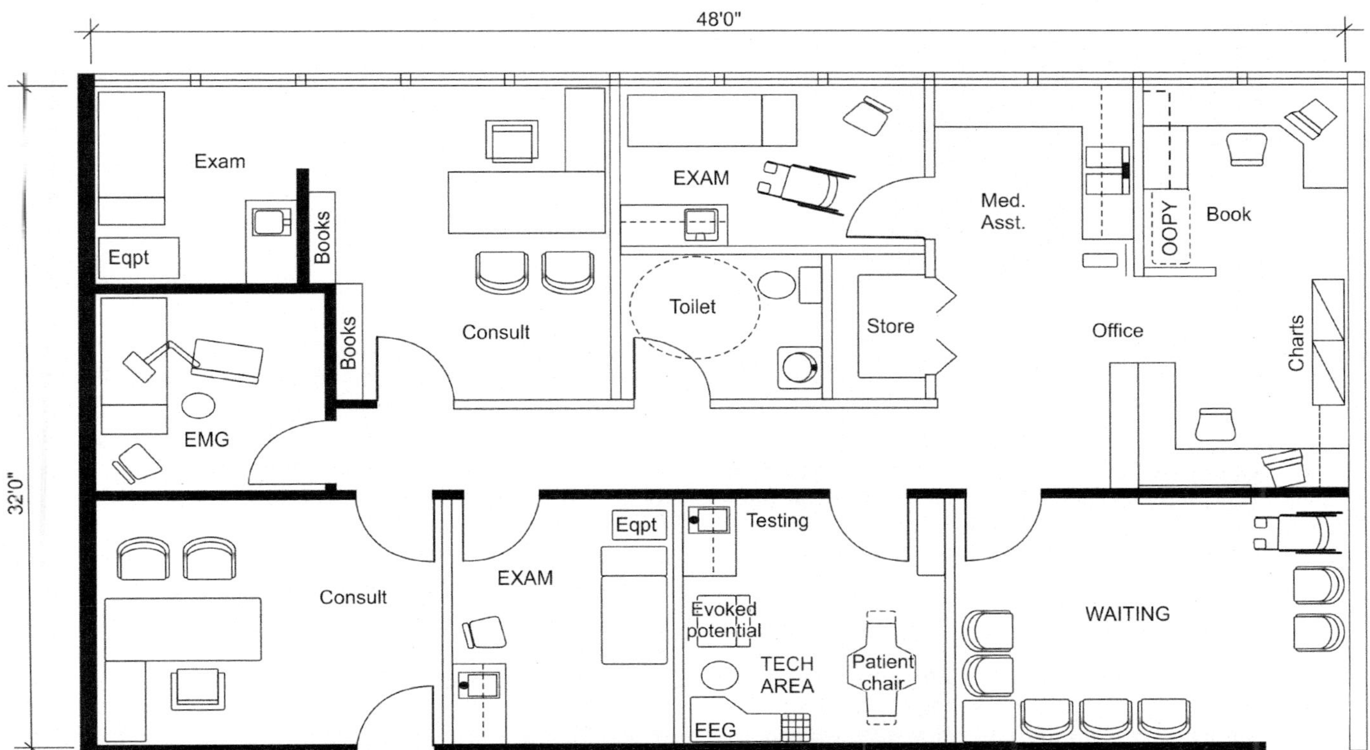

Fig. 2: Neurologist consultation room.
(EMG: electromyogram; EEG: electroencephalogram)

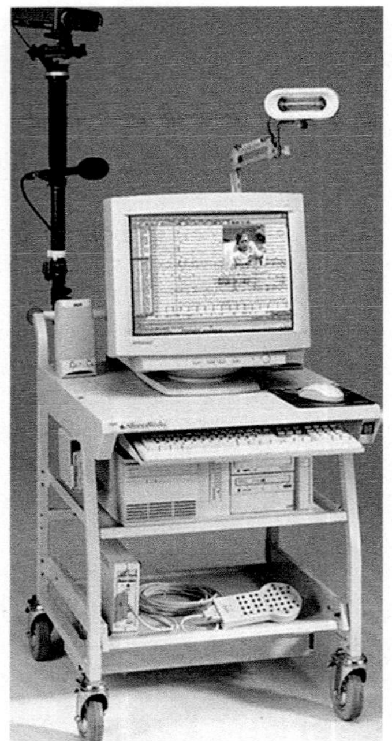

Fig. 3: EEG machine.

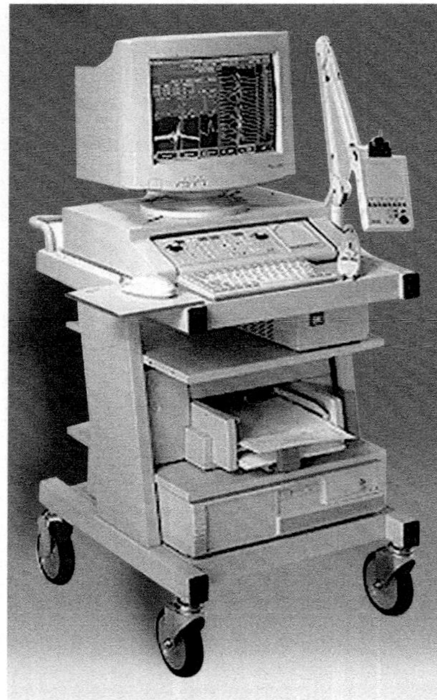

Fig. 4: Evoked potential machine.

of a muscle and indicates if the nerve has been affected. This test is performed by the physician, in a dedicated room, with a table placed against the wall. The procedure takes about half an hour, and the reason for putting it in a dedicated room is that it saves time in moving the equipment around and in setting up each patient. The room needs of only to be 10 × 10 ft. The equipment should be a mobile cart so that the physician can move it around the patient.[2]

Examination rooms will have a physical therapy-type table, a small sink cabinet, and a wall-mounted diagnostic instrument panel with ophthalmoscope, blood pressure cuff and otoscope. In addition, these rooms may have an eye chart and perhaps an X-ray view box. The patient's evaluation of his or her weight helps the physician gauge a patient's touch with reality. Maximum soundproofing is essential in the test rooms.[2]

All colors and patterns should be selected for their restful quality, anything bold is to be avoided. One must be particularly aware of patterns that have a figure-ground reversal or that have a visual rhythm. Such patterns may cause seizures in people with certain types of neurological disorders.[2]

Neurosurgery (Fig. 5)

A neurosurgeon's office does not include diagnostic testing equipment. All of the tests would be performed in the neurologist's office, and the neurosurgeon would mainly see patients for preoperative and postoperative consultations. Therefore, a small number of examination rooms are necessary, in addition to a business office, a book-keeping area, and a consultation room for each physician. The interior design of the waiting room should be soothing with careful attention to avoidance of geometric patterns or elements that may cause a figure-ground reversal or may "vibrate" or cause dizziness or possibly seizures in sensitive individuals.[2]

Pain Management Center (Figs. 6 and 7)

They involve a multidisciplinary approach to the treatment of pain. Frequently, one will find neurologists, nutritionists, deep-tissue massage therapists, psychologists, and biofeedback technicians working together in a holistic manner to change the patient's behavior or symptoms. There should be a recovery area because patients can get up after the procedure and fall. How patients feel after the procedure is very important and they might be interviewed in a consultation room or exam room after recovery.[2]

People who suffer from chronic pain need a relaxing and comforting environment in which to receive medical treatment. Lighting is especially important. Temperature control is very important, especially in a biofeedback room, physical therapy room, or massage room. With respect to the mechanical system, it is important to zone this suite very carefully and locate thermostatic controls in appropriate rooms. Interior design of a pain management suite may run the gamut from clean and clinical, for suites that are more procedure oriented, to "New Age"—serene spaces with soft lighting, soothing music or nature sounds, perhaps a fountain, nonclinical style of furniture—reflecting balance mind, body, and spirit.[2]

Psychiatry (Figs. 8 and 9)

Consultation room should be a minimum of 12 × 14 ft and preferably 14 × 16 ft. Illumination should be rheostatically controlled so that it can be dimmed. Patients are often nervous before therapy, thus the waiting room ought to have a relaxing color palette and feel comfortable, yet afford individuals some degree of privacy. Sound control is very important in this suite. All walls of consultation rooms and the group therapy rooms should have sound-attenuating construction.[2]

The ambience of this suite is of utmost importance. Colors and design should be tranquil and serve as a background rather than be stimulating enough to be distracting. Sharp contrasts in color or pattern should be avoided in favor of mellowness.[2]

Rehabilitation Department (Fig. 10)

The goals of a neurological rehabilitation program include helping the individual to return to the highest level of function and independence, and improving the overall quality of life for that individual physically, emotionally, and socially. Physical medicine and rehabilitation services should be located near the main entrance to the facility in order to

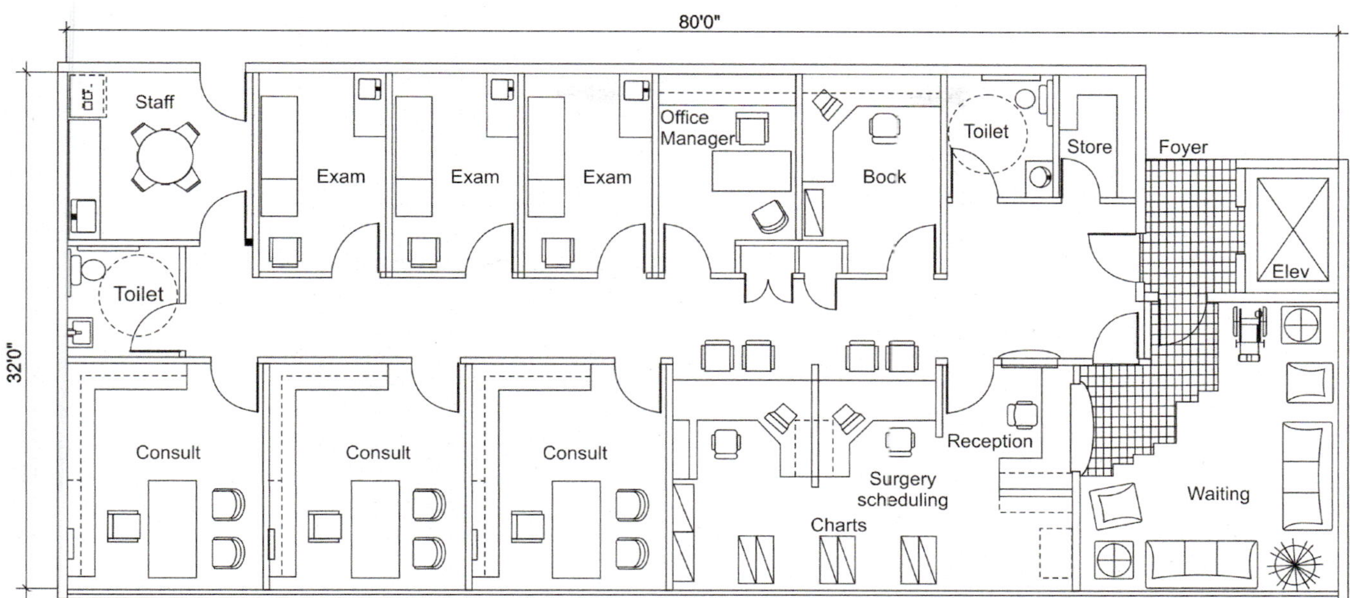

Fig. 5: Neurosurgery consultation room.

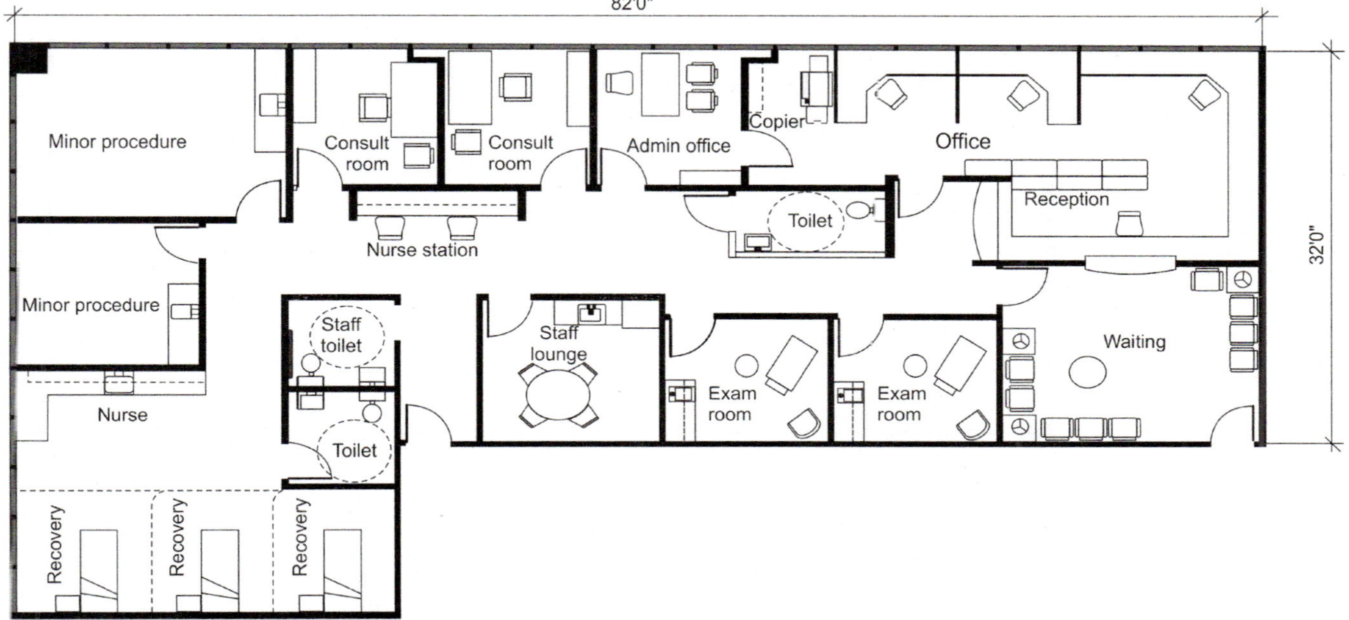

Fig. 6: Pain management center.

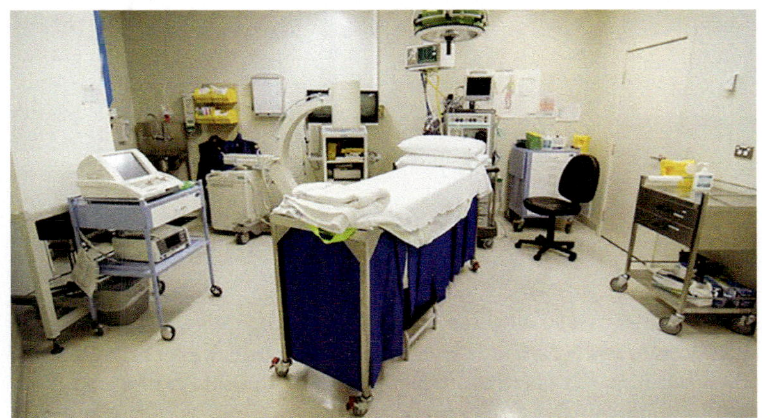

Fig. 7: Pain management center.

decrease the travel distance for patients with mobility limitations. A strong relationship between physical medicine and rehabilitation service, the SCI patient care unit, and prosthetics and sensory aids service should be maintained and these services should be located within close proximity to each other.[55,56]

Sleep Lab

A sleep lab or sleep clinic is a facility which has been designed for the purpose of studying sleep disorders; because the study of such disorders requires getting people to go to sleep, a sleep lab is designed to be a comfortable place to sleep in addition to being a scientific facility. Provision of beds and basic amenities are must to make sleep more natural and comfortable. Bathrooms/shower facilities should be there so that people can go directly from the lab to work in the morning or they may use shared bathroom facilities.[57]

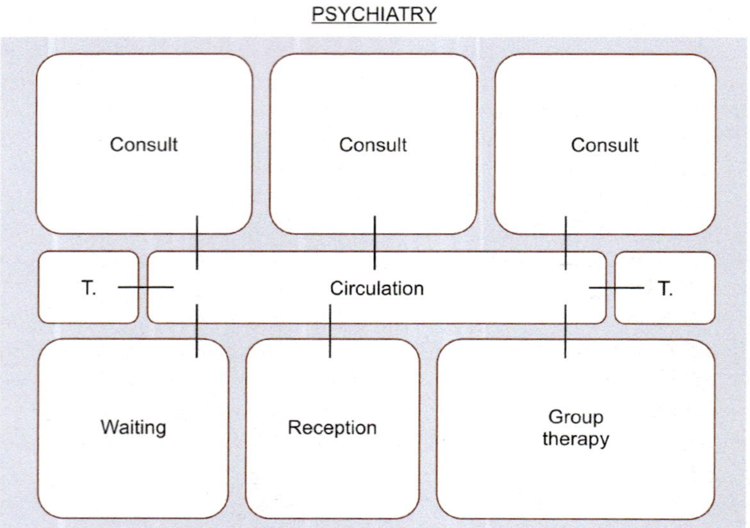

Fig. 8: Psychiatry suite—diagrammatic representation.

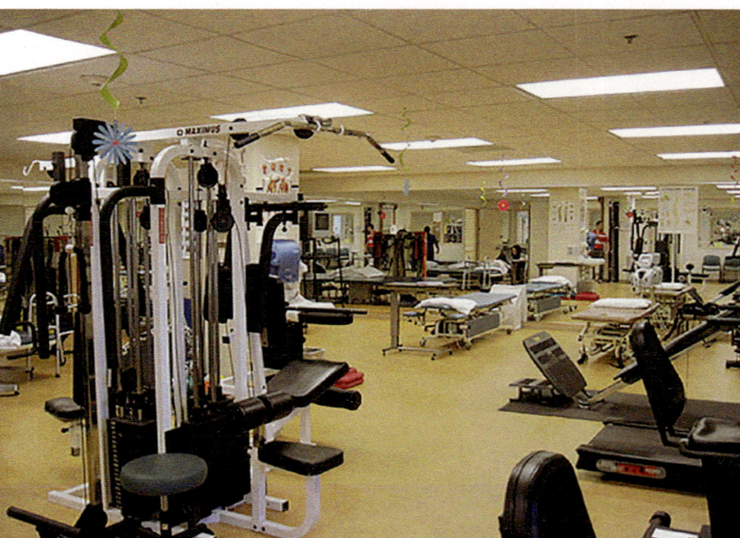

Fig. 10: Rehabilitation department.

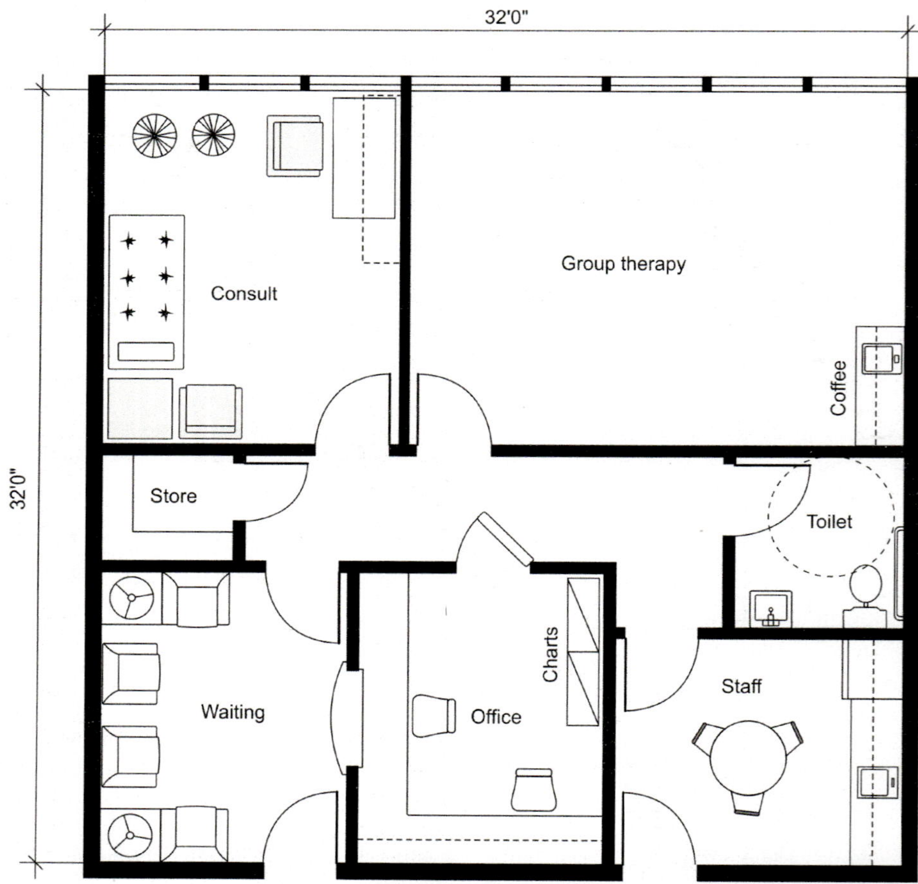

Fig. 9: Psychiatry suite—layout.

INPATIENT SERVICES

Design should follow the function and ensure privacy and safety for the patients. Efficient nursing care should be provided with minimum nursing fatigue factor. A view of the outside including those of elements of nature should be planned and designed for. Lighting illumination of 150–200 lux is recommended. Water requirement of 450–500 L/bed/day and electricity requirement of 2 kW/bed/day (5 kW/bed/day for superspecialty hospital) should be planned. This should ideally be from 2–3 grids.

Radioimaging

Ultrasound

Since ultrasound does not use radiation, there is no need for lead shielding. The room should not be smaller than 10–12 ft in size. The equipment is portable, approximately 27 inch, 34 inch deep, 54 inch high. The room is darkened for the procedure, and an ideal type of lighting would be indirect perimeter lighting that can be dimmed. An ultrasound room must have a toilet immediately adjacent to accommodate voiding studies of the bladder. A cabinet with sink should be provided in the ultrasound room.[58]

Nuclear Imaging (Fig. 11)

A nuclear imaging room does not require lead shielding, as the gamma camera emits no radiation; it picks up the small amount of radioactivity released by the organ being imaged. The patient prep room should be close to the hot lab where the radioactive material is prepared so that the technician never has to walk through patient circulation corridors carrying radioactive material. A sub-waiting area near the nuclear imaging procedure rooms is practical, as is a dedicated toilet since human waste discharged from patients who have ingested radioactive materials could splash on the floor or toilet seat; because the type (and amount) of radioisotopes used in diagnostic studies (as opposed to treatment) is minimal and decays quickly, the toilet waste can generally be discharged into the sewer system without being diverted to a holding tank; however, local codes should be consulted.[58]

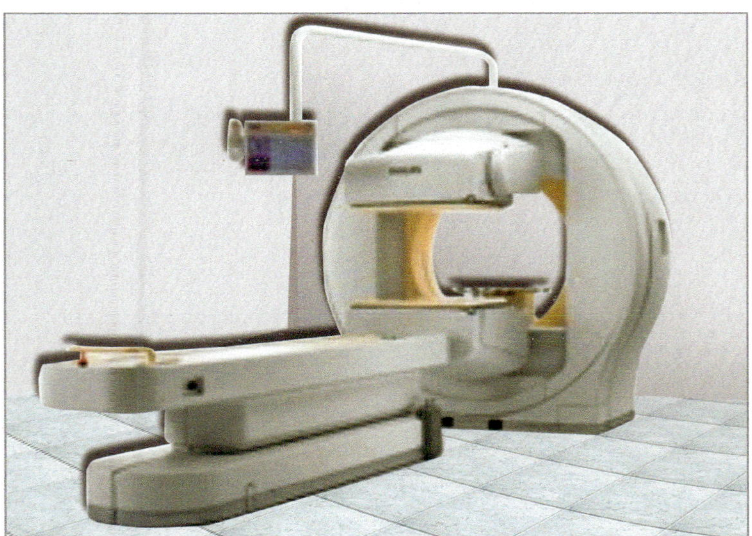

Fig. 11: Nuclear imaging.

Computed Tomography (Fig. 12)

Although there are slight differences between different models of CT scanners, generally a procedure room 18 ft long by 14 ft wide and an adjoining room for the operator's console 8–14 ft will suffice. There should be clinical scrub facilities adjacent to the room. The room needs a built-in cabinet and sink and storage for clean linen, contrast media, and IV materials.[58,59]

Ceiling of the room, it should normally be 9 ft 6 inch high. Door should be at least 48 inches wide, with a heavy-duty closer. The walls and door will have to be lead-shielded according to recommendations of a radiation physicist.[58]

The CT console room accommodates the computer and other controls for the equipment. It must have a lead-shielded window facing the procedure room so that the patient is always in view. Provision like scrub-up/gowning area, patient-holding areas, patient toilet and change facilities must be planned.[58]

Magnetic Resonance Imaging (Figs. 13 and 14)

Magnetic resonance imaging (MRI) uses computers and magnetic fields to provide noninvasive images of human anatomy. It does not involve radiation but, rather, uses powerful superconducting magnets to generate magnetic fields 8,000 times stronger than that of the earth. MRI computer room accommodates the computer equipment. Recommended space is 35 m^2. The room should be located adjacent to the MRI scanning and console room. MRI console room is required to accommodate the computer and other controls of the equipment. There should be a window to provide full view of the MRI room. A minimum space of 10 m^2 is recommended. It should be located with direct access to the MRI scanning room (Fig. 14).[58,59]

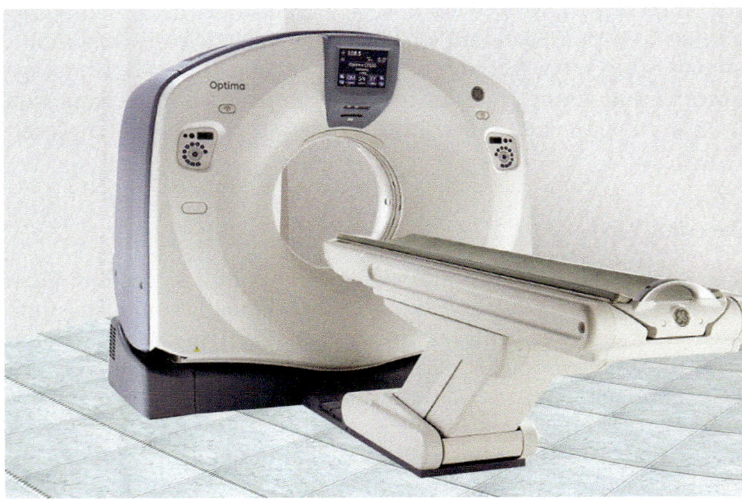

Fig. 12: Computed tomography.

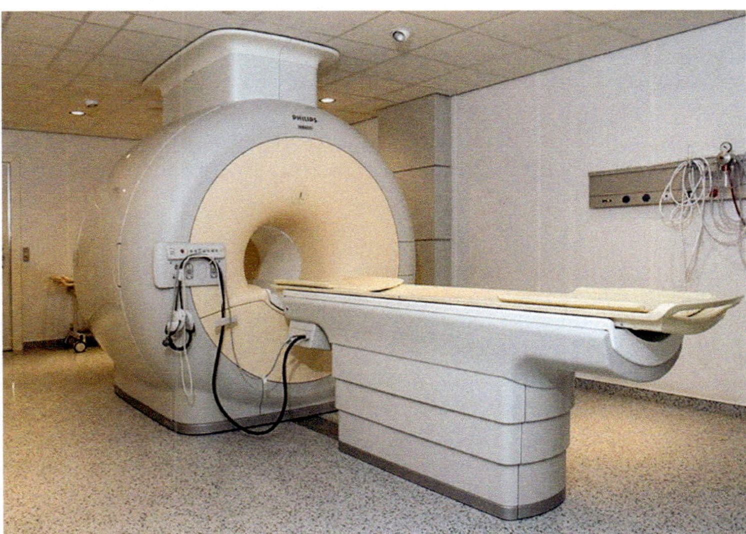

Fig. 13: Magnetic resonance imaging.

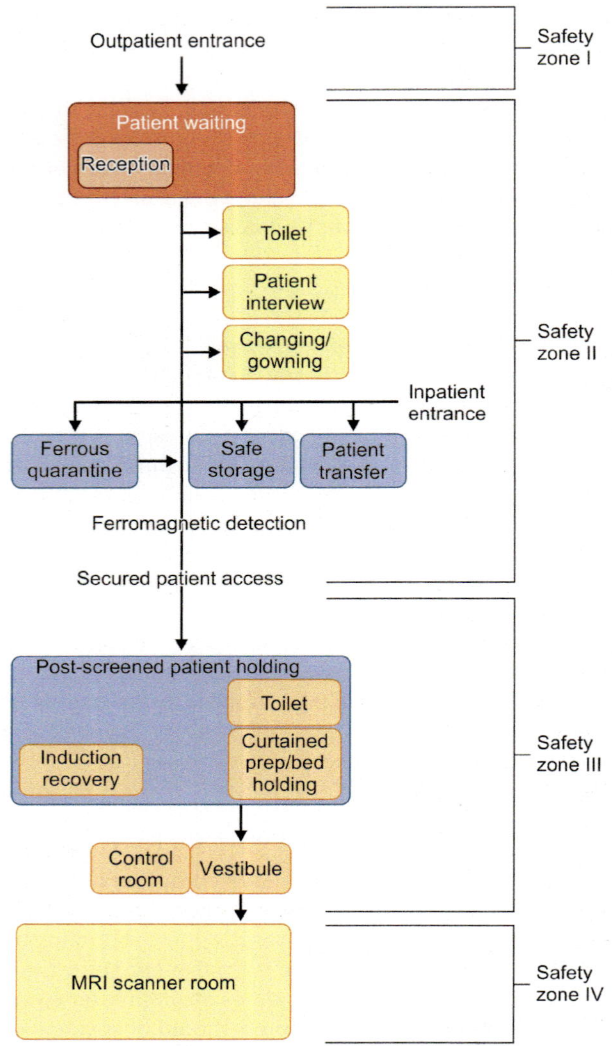

Fig. 14: MRI functional diagram.
(MRI: magnetic resonance imaging)

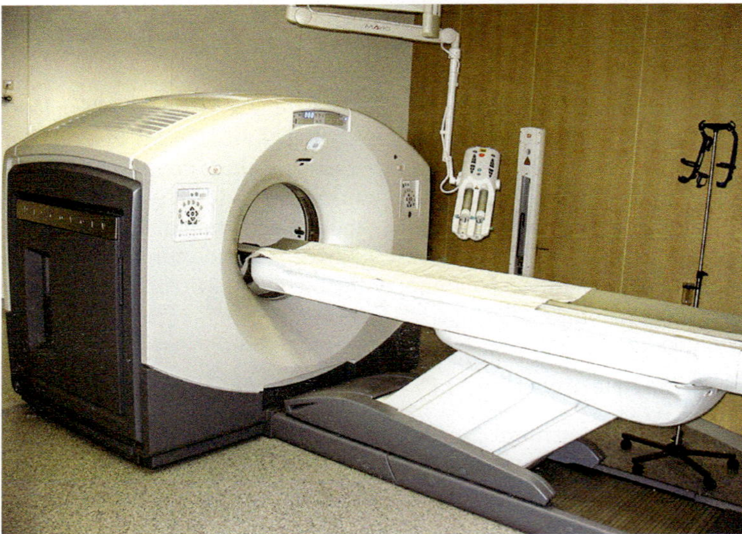

Fig. 15: Positron emission tomography.

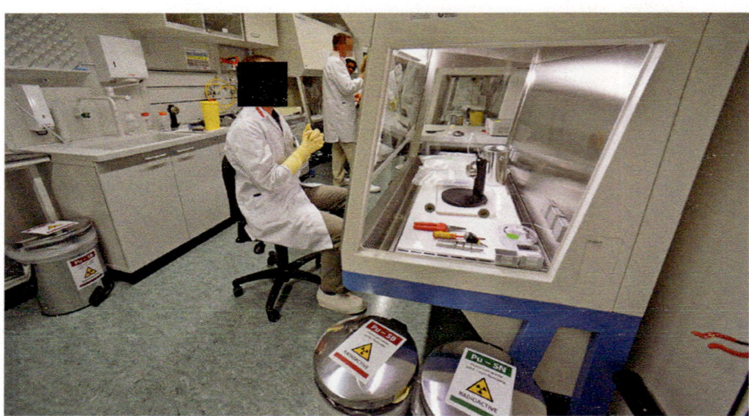

Fig. 16: Hot lab.

Consideration must be given to the transport of a magnet during installation. Corridor and door sizes, as well as floor strength, must be adequate to handle a 13,000-pound superconducting magnet or 29,000-pound open magnet. This piece of equipment cannot be broken down into smaller components. One might wonder how it arrives at the room. It is often brought through the roof or the side of the building. Use of latest theme-based MRI should be explored in which with help of technology, graphics of beech or sky with stars, etc. are created, with this the patient do not feel apprehensive during the procedure.[58]

Positron Emission Tomography (Fig. 15)

The positron emission tomography (PET) unit may be a part of the medical imaging unit or as a separate unit for PET imaging procedures using radiopharmaceutical agents. The unit should be located with close access to nuclear medicine unit, emergency unit, intensive care unit and operating unit. It would require a ground level location due to the weight of the equipment and for ease of installation and replacement. It should be noted that PET scan rooms do require lead shielding and that PET involves higher levels of radioactivity than with the standard nuclear gamma camera. A size of approximately 40 m^2 is recommended.[58]

Hot Lab (Fig. 16)

This is a room, perhaps no larger than 6 × 8 ft, where radiopharmaceuticals are prepared. This is best located in a part of the suite where there is no high traffic. The room would have 34-inch-high countertops with a single-compartment sink, and may have a lead-lined under counter refrigerator, with some open shelves and hinged-door storage under the countertop. Note that the countertop must be steel reinforced in order to support the interlocking lead bricks that will be placed on it.[58]

Gamma Knife (Fig. 17)

The *Gamma Knife* is a noninvasive neurosurgical/radiosurgical procedure that uses calculated doses of radiation to target and treat diseased brain tissue while leaving surrounding tissue intact. Gamma knife set-up must consist of the following compartments—central registration desk, patient waiting area, neurosurgeon's office, nurse's room, change rooms, procedure room and console room. The material used in construction of the walls of facility has cement with density 2.35 g/cubic ft to prevent scattered radiation beams from going out. The radiology functional diagram is shown in Figure 18.

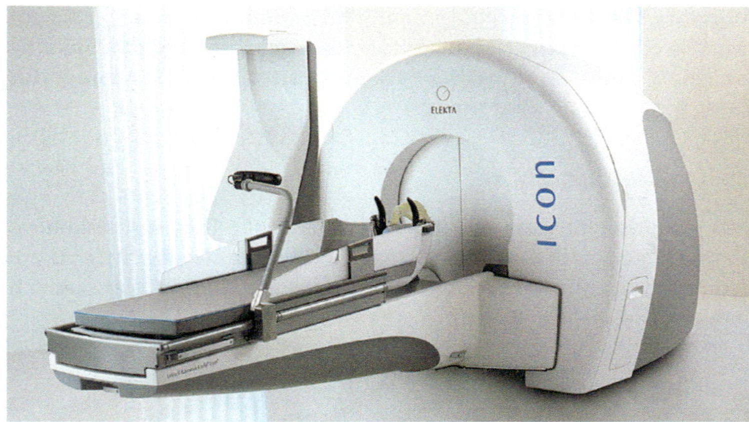

Fig. 17: Gamma knife.

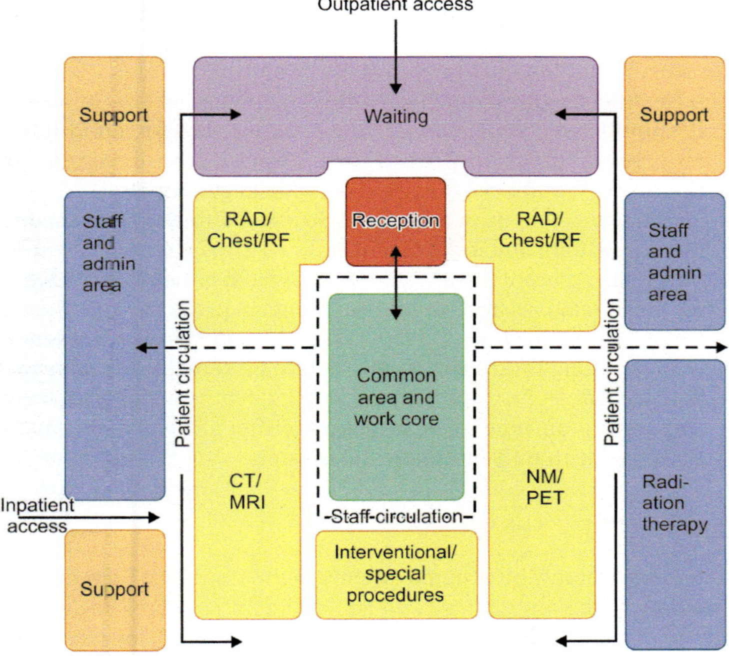

Fig. 18: Radiology functional diagram.

INTENSIVE CARE UNIT

Location: It is preferable to have the ICU in close proximity to the operation theaters, accident and emergency department and medical imaging departments.

Number of ICU Beds

It is recommended that at least 5% of total hospital beds may be designated ICU beds. However, in neurosurgical centers, about 10–15% beds may be ICU beds.

Size of Units

Depending on the requirement, an ICU of 6–12 beds is recommended. A unit of less than 6 beds is economically not viable; where the requirement is more than 12 beds, multiple units may be planned. The ICU may be planned as a large single room having multiple beds or individual single bed accommodation.

Bed Space

Requirement is 2–3 times more than general bed; 20 m^2 floor area for single-bed accommodation which is exclusive of service areas and 30 m^2 for multiple-bed accommodation is recommended.

Lighting

It is recommended to have a 300 lux light illumination for patient areas with anti-glare arrangement, 100 lux for corridor, 150 lux for staff area and floor lights for monitoring drainage seal and suction equipment. Appropriate and adequate lighting should be provided which is suitable for clinical observation. Provision of natural light should be made to the maximum. The color of the walls and ceiling should not affect perception of skin color by the staff.

Environmental Control

Rooms in the ICU should be sound-proof and air-conditioned with facilities of environmental control for each room. Air-conditioning should ensure 50 ± 5% humidity, and 20–25°C temperature. Ceilings, flooring and walls should be constructed of materials with high sound-absorption capabilities, the recommended noise level should be in the range of 35–40 dB. The following are recommended for ventilation in ICU:

- There should be 8–10 air changes per hour and positive air pressure maintained.
- Special provision of exhaust to eliminate any odor in ICU as and when required.

Doors

To facilitate easy passage of equipment, stretcher beds, etc. doors having width of 1.25 m are recommended.

Beds

Mechanically or electrically operated beds should be provided in the ICU. These should be capable of being readily adjustable to therapeutic positions and should have X-ray-transparent bedstead bottoms. The base of the beds should be firm to enable effective cardiac compression during resuscitative procedures as and when required. There should be detachable rails at the head end of the bed to facilitate tracheal intubation, if required.

Bed Head Panel (Fig. 19)

This should have a minimum of two oxygen outlets, two inlets for suction, one compressed air outlet per bed, nurse call button and wall-mounted blood pressure equipment.

Electrical Requirements

It is recommended that minimum six multi-sockets and one power socket (15 amps) for mobile X-ray unit should be provided per bed. These can be a part of bed head panel, or flush moulded in the wall. There should be backup source of power from an emergency generator in the event of a power failure from the primary source.

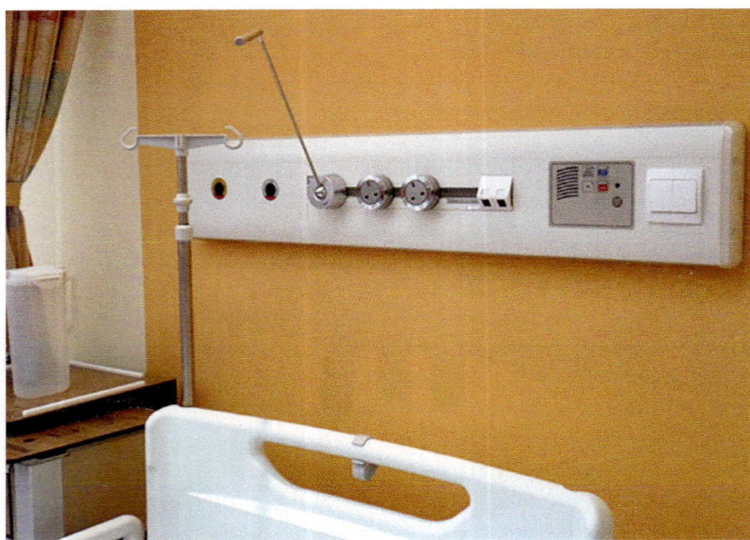

Fig. 19: Bed head panel.

Toilets

These should enable entry of wheelchairs and should have grab bars and panic buttons. They should have doors that slide or open outwards to facilitate opening in case of emergency, such as patient falling unconscious against the door. They should have two-way operable latches.

Minimum Space to Allow Resuscitation and Other Procedures

The minimum space requirement is 0.9 m between the head end and the wall and 1.2 m between the foot end and the wall. It is recommended to have minimum distance of 3.5 m between centers of two adjacent beds. These spaces are required to facilitate resuscitative procedures, end-tracheal intubation and use of radiography equipment.

Visibility of Patients

Patients should be visible from the nursing station. There should be individual rooms with full height glass walls between the room and the corridor. Curtains may be drawn over the glass walls as and when required. The need for patient privacy should be an essential design consideration.

Windows

Windows constitute an important aspect of sensory orientation and should be provided for patients to maintain visual contact with the outside world. Windows should approximately constitute 15% of floor area.

Equipment Installation

Wall or ceiling installation of equipment should be done to facilitate easy accessibility, personnel movement and necessary cleaning procedures.

Storage/Utility Area

The equipment storage areas should be conveniently located to provide easy access by staff. Alcoves should be provided for the storage and rapid retrieval of resuscitation trolleys and portable monitors/defibrillation equipment. There should be storage space for housekeeping supplies with janitor closet, sink and bedpan flushing facilities. There should also be facilities for lockable storage for controlled drugs.

Visitor Waiting Room

This should be provided outside the entry to the ICU. It should have comfortable seating arrangements along with toilet facilities. There should be an overnight room facility for relatives/friends along with areas for the storage of clean gowns and masks.

Nursing Station

The location should provide optimum visual observation of patients. There should be provision for computerized individual monitors at the bedside with facilities for automatic communication to the computer located at the nursing station. The nurses fatigue factor should also be considered while planning. U-shape or semicircular layouts minimize the nurses fatigue factor.

The other important facilities in ICU to be considered are:

- A treatment room should have provision of medical gas outlets.
- It should have provision for procedure room for conducting emergency invasive procedures. It should be designed for fluoroscopy, and have provision of medical gas outlets.
- There should be duty rooms for doctors with sleeping accommodation, bath and toilet facilities.

Briefing room adjacent to the waiting room would be helpful for doctors to talk to the relatives/friends of the patients in privacy.

- Handwashing facilities for staff should be sufficiently provided.
- Staff changing rooms and toilets should be separate for male and female staff.
- Depending on type of healthcare facility, an ICU bed may be equipped with wall-mounted dialysis unit.

LABORATORY SERVICES

It should preferably be situated on the ground floor/first floor in close proximity to the ambulatory and acute patient care areas as well as inpatient areas. The processing areas of the laboratory do not necessarily have to be accessible to patients but the collection point for specimens must be conveniently located, especially for ambulatory patients.

Space Requirements

The main determinants of space in a laboratory are the extent of automation and type of technology used in it. A standing human body requires 4 sq ft space, whereas a sitting posture requires 6 sq ft. The working space should be adequate with equipment and materials within easy reach of the worker.

Specimen Collection Area

There should be adequate specimen collection area for blood, urine and feces. There should be separate toilets for men and women with wash basins and counter tops to place the specimens.

Storage

Storage facilities include those for refrigeration, reagents and supplies, maintenance of patients' records and water purification.

Safety

There should be provision for safety, including eye-flushing devices, emergency shower and fire extinguishers.

Work Station

Work counters with space for equipment, microscopes, incubators, centrifuge, under-the-counter and overhead cabinets should be provided.

Lighting

Natural light should be advantageously utilized for providing the requisite illumination.

Floors

These should be made of materials that can be cleaned and disinfected easily. They should be acid, alkaline and salt-resistant. The use of seamless or self-leveling epoxy flooring is a desirable option. The load-bearing capacity of the floor should not be less than 500 kg/m^2. The requirement may be as high as 2,000 kg/m^2 in laboratories having heavy equipment.

Doors

Laboratory doors should not be less than 1 m wide. Some double doors of total width of 1.50 m should be recommended.

Corridors

Width of corridors is recommended to be of 2–2.5 m to facilitate movement of patients including those on wheelchairs.

OPERATION THEATER COMPLEX FOR A NEUROSCIENCES CENTER

It is desirable to have OT complex in proximity to surgical wards/ICU/postoperative ward, CSSD and blood bank.

OT Zoning

The aim of zoning is that when staff members, patients or supplies enter the OT suite, the risk factors of carrying the chances of infection with them get lesser and lesser, as they pass from the protective through clean to aseptic zone. Clean from dirty utility traffic flow within the OT suite should be segregated as best as possible.[59]

OT Lighting (Fig. 20)

The operating light should be of 1,00,000–1,40,000 lux with a minimum of 40,000 lux at the depth of an incision. The light as mentioned earlier should be shadow-less and with sufficient backup. Spare light bulbs are kept ready for prompt replacement.

Air-conditioning and Humidity in OT

Temperature in superspecialized OTs are recommended to be 18–20°C. Humidity about 50–55%. The laminar air flow is maintained and high-efficiency particulate air (HEPA) filter is recommended of 0.3–0.5 micron specification.

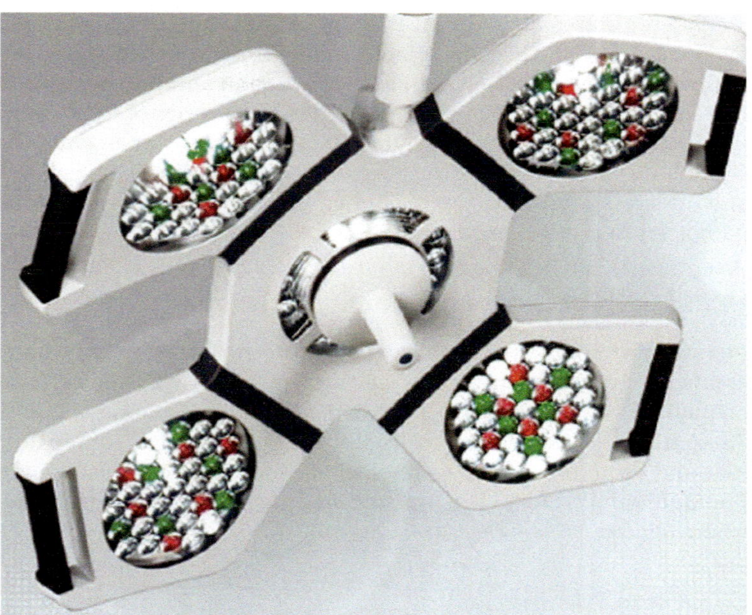

Fig. 20: Operation theater lighting.

Environmental Controls

Environmental controls are used to prevent the spread and reduce the concentration of infectious droplet nuclei in ambient air. Primary environmental controls consist of controlling the source of infection by using local exhaust ventilation (e.g. hoods, tents, or booths) and diluting and removing contaminated air by using general ventilation and secondary environmental controls consist of controlling the airflow to prevent contamination of air in areas adjacent to the source airborne infection isolation (AII) rooms and cleaning the air by using HEPA, filtration, or ultraviolet germicidal irradiation (UVGI).[60]

Maintenance HVAC Systems

Improperly maintained HVAC systems may cause symptoms associated with Sick Building Syndrome (SBS). SBS symptoms may be attributed to moisture within the HVAC systems. "Humidification systems with poor condition/maintenance are associated with significantly increased upper respiratory symptoms, eye symptoms, fatigue/difficulty concentrating, and skin symptoms.

Symptoms may be due to microbial exposures from poorly maintained ventilation systems and to greater levels of vehicular pollutants at air intakes nearer the ground level. Moisture-related HVAC components such as cooling coils and humidification systems, when poorly maintained, may be sources of contaminants that cause adverse health effects in occupants, even if we cannot yet identify or measure the causal exposures, then ultraviolet germicidal irradiation is recommended.

Ultraviolet Germicidal Irradiation

Ultraviolet germicidal irradiation (UVGI) deactivates bacteria, fungi and viruses on surfaces as well as in the air. Importantly, this protection is constant. Unlike one-time cleanings the germicidal irradiation of cooling coils continues 24 hours a day.[61]

A supplemental portable anteroom high-efficiency particulate air (PAS-HEPA) filter unit placed outside operating room suites may prevent secondary transmission of airborne microorganisms, such as *Mycobacterium tuberculosis* (*M. tuberculosis*).[61]

Filters are great for trapping microorganisms, but they do not 'kill'. Eventually filters can become colonized and act as a breeding ground for pathogens. Infected filters may be hazardous and filtration may give a false sense of security. High efficiency particulate arrestance—microbial destruction (HEPA-MD) are highly effective and remove organisms, compounds and odors. It is suggested to have a balance between UV and filtration to provide a better strategy for reducing environmental pathogens in critical care areas.[61]

Use of Current Indoor Air Quality Technologies

Photohydroionization (PHI) (Fig. 21)—hydrogen-based oxidizers are created by exposing activated oxygen molecules to a hydrated catalyst containing four unique metals and 300 nm UV light (photon energy). These friendly oxidizers are hydroperoxides, hydroxides, superoxide ions and ozonide ions. UV technology disinfects HVAC surfaces and then keeps those areas clean by continuously radiating the reservoirs where microorganisms can thrive.[61,62]

OT Design Parameters[18,63]

- Avoidance of unrelated hospital traffic flow in the area.
- Convenient functional relationship and communication with the surgical ward, ICU, CSSD, blood bank, medical imaging and laboratory services.
- Avoidance of any outdoor source of noise.
- Provision for future expansion/alterations.
- Doors should be of the sliding type with a minimum 1.2 m width in areas where patients movement is anticipated.
- Corridors should not be less than 2.85 m in width to facilitate the movement of trolley and stretchers.
- Walls and ceilings should be esthetically pleasing, nonporous, fire-resistant, water- and stain-proof, seamless, nonreflective and easy to clean.
- Floors should be smooth, non-slip, and made of impervious material that is conductive enough to dissipate static electricity but not conductive enough to endanger personnel from shock.
- Taps in the scrub room should be knee/elbow-operated or preferably electronically controlled, activated by infrared sensor.
- There should be a power backup with provision for standby generating sets.
- In operating rooms, anesthetic room(s), recovery room, holding area, the color of the walls and ceilings should be such that they do not alter the observers' perception of skin color. This will facilitate patient monitoring and management.
- An OT should have facility for high-speed autoclaves/sterilizers to meet the immediate/emergency requirements of sterilizing equipment.
- Essential pharmaceutical storage including refrigeration facilities should be available.
- There should be a waiting room with toilet facilities for the patients' attendants.

Brain Suite (Figs. 22 and 23)

Brain suite is a state-of-the-art neurosurgical operating room (OR) that fully integrates all relevant surgical and diagnostic tools, including intraoperative high-field magnetic resonance imaging (IMRI) to treat complicated neurosurgical cases.[64]

The brain suite navigation system links the real-time intraoperative images with the spatial position of the surgical instruments helping to provide the neurosurgeon with a higher level of accuracy regarding the location and amount of tissue removed. In addition, the intraoperative MRI images help neurosurgeons determine more accurately whether or not the appropriate amount of diseased tissue has been removed.[64]

The brain suite-surgical suite employs technology which provides neurosurgeons with real-time, decision-making information to treat

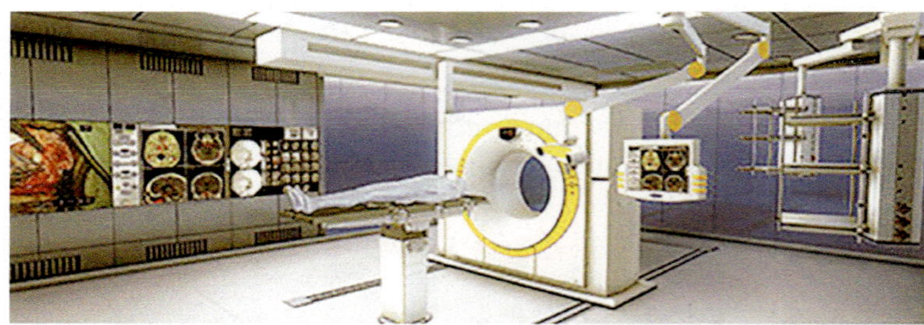

Fig. 22: Brain suite—view 1.

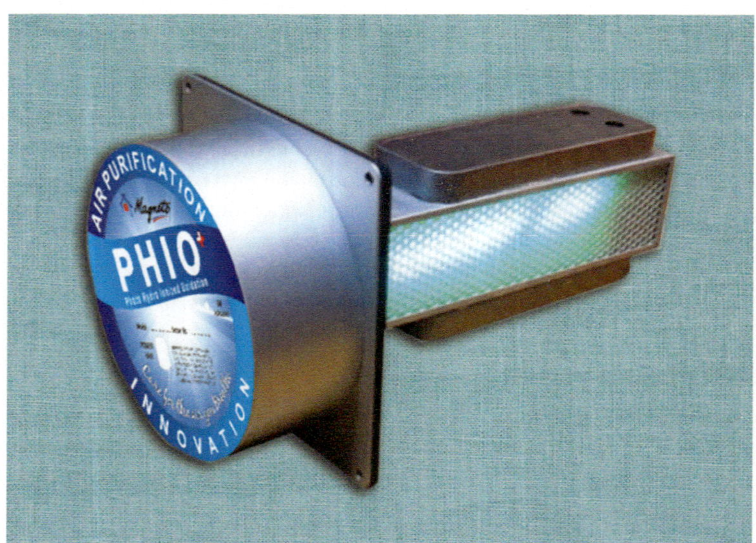

Fig. 21: Photohydroionization.

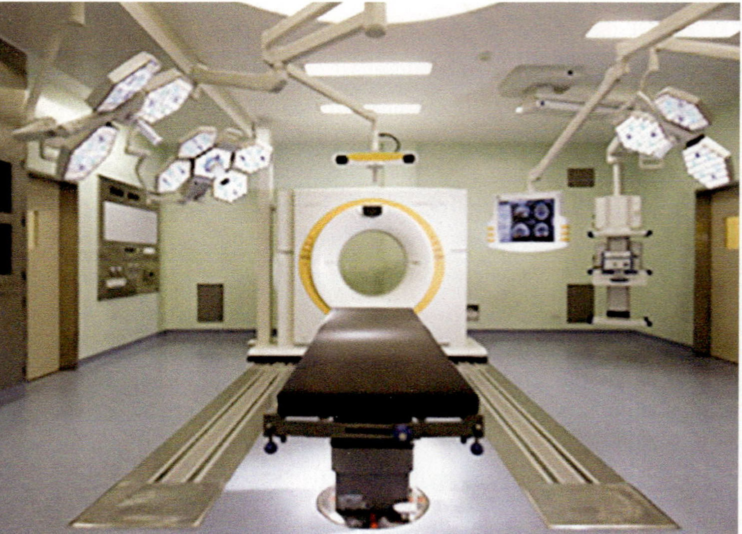

Fig. 23: Brain suite—view 2.

complicated brain tumor or other neurosurgical cases. The human brain is especially a bad place for a tumor. Surgically navigating this vulnerable terrain, completely removing tumor, and leaving without damaging key structures, only a few millimeters away, requires extraordinary precision and skill.[64]

One unique challenge of doing surgery in the brain suite is working near a powerful magnetic field. A 1. S-Tesla MRI scanner such as the one in the brain suite contains a magnet so strong that objects drawn to it can become dangerous projectiles.[64]

Surgeons, neuroanesthesiologists and others caring for patients in the brain suite must ensure that the equipment they use is compatible with the MRI or out of range of its strong magnetic field, i.e. patients are prescreened for any metallic objects or implants that might be attracted to the magnet as well.[64]

The floors of the brain suite space had to be reinforced to support the weight of the new equipment. A climate-regulated control room houses the computer equipment. All of this had to be built in an area adjacent to active operating rooms with minimal disruption and without the noise and vibration.[64]

MRI-compatible OR Design

Various new types of MRI-compatible OR design are now coming into use. The operating theater provides a large area with minimum floor obstruction by equipment bases or energy and gas lines, allowing free movement of surgeons, nurses, and support personnel. An example is the IMRIS design containing two-room configurations sited on a nominal 1,200 sq ft/25 ft × 48 ft or 112 m^2 (7.6 m × 14.6 m) floor plan area.[1,65]

Magnetic resonance imaging is safe and reliable in the surgical environment and is applicable for intraoperative guidance of neurosurgical procedures, although these procedures may have to be adapted somewhat for the MR environment. The development of navigation microscopes that can be used in the fringe magnetic field of the MR imager obviated the cumbersome and time-consuming intraoperative transport of patients and enabled microscope-based navigational support during neurosurgery in the fringe magnetic field.

OBSERVATION ROOM

This is attached to the main neurosurgical operating suite, but can be easily isolated through lead-coated sound-proof doors.[66,67]

Observation room serves multiple purposes; it is used to host the neuronavigation computer system, digital capturing and transmission system, and the electronic medical record (EMR)—media library system. Computer-based informatics programs provide comprehensive and decision-making support to the surgical care team and lead to an effective tele-collaboration with other staff members and visitors.[66,67]

The observation room could be divided into two parts—the front part accommodates the seats for the spectators and the computer-based multimedia system comprises a large screen TV, two PCs, a colored laser printer, a DVD-recorder and an audio console.[66,67]

The other half of the room is used for the neuronavigation and workstations, a rack-mounted infrastructure for the audiovisual and computer network equipment, and two cupboards for the storage of materials and personal belongings of the staff.[66,67]

In the case of three-room configurations, a magnet bay is located between the operating room and diagnostic room. The magnet bay is accessible on both sides by sliding doors. Three-room configurations can be sited on a nominal 1,850 sq ft (74 ft × 25 ft) (172 m^2/23 m × 7.5 m) floor plan area.[66,67]

Robotic Surgery

Neurosurgery was one of the first organ systems in which robotic surgery was introduced, due to the high precision that was required to localize and manipulate within the brain, and the relatively fixed landmarks of the cranial anatomy. The neurosurgical robot consists of the following components at the most basic level—robotic arm, feedback sensors, controllers which instruct the robot (end-effectors), a wireless localization system and a data-processing center (the brain).

Key design considerations for robotic surgery are adequate space for maneuverability, no current interferences, sound-proof environment, suitable lighting, and vibration-less environment.

CONCLUSION

Neurosciences center is a unique healthcare institution, not because it pertains to a unique superspecialty, but because it caters to the needs of patients who need a unique care. This care encompasses many attributes like universal design and friendly ambience, safe and free movements within the facility, high-end diagnostic aids and an error proof therapeutic environment. These characteristics demand a good and strategic planning of the facility with adequate support features.

Designs are moving forward, with/without empirical evidence, however, knowing how a space is intended to function, or a feature is expected to be used, allows for more specific evaluation of the actual impact. A neurosciences center which will have patients, who could be mentally and/or physically differently abled, should have special concern.

Designers, and planners, doctors need to work together to develop a common language and definitions to accurately describe the intent of design and this common language needs to be used to communicate the special needs and concern of these patients.[68,69]

REFERENCES

1. Apuzzo MLJ. "Architecture and Functional Design of Advanced Neurosurgical Operating Environments", Neurosurgery, 1993.
2. "Medicine: Specialized Suites", Medical and Dental Space Planning, 2015.
3. www.bioline.org.br
4. www.neuroscienceacademy.org.in
5. www.batrahospitaldelhi.org
6. www.britannica.com
7. *World Health Organization. Neurological disorders: public health challenges. Geneva; 2006.*
8. Gourie-Devi M, Guru raj G, Satishchandra P. Neuroepidemiology: Present insights and future prospects. NIMHANS J. 1999;17:423-37.
9. Bergen DC, Silberberg D. Nervous system disorders. Arch Neurol. 2002;59:1194-6.
10. Hewer RL. The epidemiology of disabling neurological conditions. Irr. Greenwood R, Banes MP, McMillan RM, Ward CD (Eds). Neurological rehabilitation. Churchill Livingstone: New York;1993. pp. 3-12.
11. Prakashi R, Gourie-Devi M. Scope of social work services in neurological setting: Initial observations. J Med Psy Social Work. 1987;1:15-20.
12. Prakashi R, Gourie-Devi M. Rehabilitation of neurologically disabled persons, implications for community participation. Rehabilitation Asia. 1988;29:8-12.
13. biomed.brown.edu
14. Aarli JA. Neurology and WHO: Challenges and issues—A report. World Neurol. 2002;17:10-1.

15. Singhal BS. Neurology in developing countries: A population perspective. Arch Neurol. 1998;55:1019-21.
16. Gourie-Devi M. Medical technologies for neurological sciences. In: Mathew L (Ed). Technology management in healthcare. Defence bioengineering and electromedical laboratory (DEBEL): Bengaluru; 1998.pp. 62-7.
17. Technology Information Forecasting and Assessment Council (TIFAC) report on healthcare, technology vision 2020. Department of Science and Technology: New Delhi; 1996.
18. mohfw.nic.in
19. Clarkson J, Inclusive Design: Design for the Whole Population, London, New York: Springer. 2003.
20. A Practical Reader in Universal Design for Learning. Cambridge, MA: Harvard Education Press, c2006.
21. Buhler, European Co-Operation Activities Promoting Design for all in Information Society Technologies—Introduction to the Special Thematic Session, Lecture Notes in Computer Science. 3118:80.
22. Bajaj. Evaluation of a Redesigned Self-checkout Station for Wheelchair Users, Assistive Technology 2006;(18):15.
23. Burgstahler S. Rebecca C. Universal Design in Higher Education: From Principles to Practice, Cambridge, MA: Harvard Education Press, 2008.
24. Catlin. Accessibility for all: A Case Study of the Access Living Headquarters, Topics in Stroke Rehabilitation. 2008;15(2), 97-102.
25. Boecker J. Highlighting High Performance: Clear view Elementary School, Hanover, Pennsylvania, www.eren.doe.gov (2004), U.S. Department of Energy Efficiency and Renewable Energy Clearinghouse (EREC) 1-800-DOE-3732.
26. Afacan Y, Erbug C. An Interdisciplinary Heuristic Evaluation Method for Universal Building Design, Applied Ergonomics. 2009;40:731-44.
27. Clokey J, Harrigan J, Mullany S, Clokey J, SL. *Video Publishing, Landsca*pe Design Series, 2004.
28. National Advisory Council on Aging (1992). Housing an aging population: Guidelines for development and design (2nd Edn.) (Electronic). Ottawa: 15. Available: www.phac-aspc.gc.ca.
29. Maher L, Rothi L, Heilman K. Praxis performance with left versus right hemisphere lesions. Neuro Rehabilitation. 1997;9:46.
30. www.fraserhealth.ca
31. Pinto MR, DeMedici S, Zlotnicki A, Bianchi A, VanSant C, Napoli C. Reduced visual acuity in elderly people: The role of ergonomics and gerontechnology. Age a*nd Ageing. 1997;26:* 339-44.
32. Kim E. Agitation, aggression and disinhibition syndromes after traumatic brain injury, Neuro Rehabilitation. 2007;17:300.
33. Murphy E. The patient room of the future: State-of-the-art care and what a view! Nursing Management. (Electronic). (2000) Available: www.nursingmanagement.com.
34. Maeshima S, Matsumoto T, Veyoshi A, Kitayama M, Nakao N, Nakai K, Itakura T. Unilateral spatial neglect associated with chronic subdural hematoma: a case report. Brain Injury. 2001;15:374–5.
35. O'Keeffe J. Crea*ting a senior-friendly phy*sical environment in our hospitals (Electronic). The Regional Geriatric Assessment Program of Ottawa. (2003) AvaiLable: www.rgapottawa.com.
36. www.partnershipsbc.ca
37. www.rgptoronto.ca
38. Mayer N, Esquenazi A, Keenan M. Assessing and treating muscle overactivity in the upper moto neuron syndrome. In: Brain Injury Medicine: Principles and Practice, Zasler N, Katz D, Zafonte R. (Eds). Demos Medical Publishing New York. 2007.pp. 615-53.
39. Hiott D, Labbate L. Anxiety disorders associated with traumatic brain injuries. Neuro Rehabilitation. 2007;17:345-55.
40. www.gov.uk
41. Shepard N, Clendaniel R, Ruckenstein M. Balance and Dizziness, In: Brain Injury Medicine: Principles and Practice. Zasler N, Katz D, Zafonte R (Eds). Demos Medical Publishing. New York, 2007.pp. 491-510.
42. Panno JM, Kolcaba K, Holder C. Acute care for elders (ACE): A holistic model for geriatric orthopaedic nursing care. Orthopaedic Nursing. 2000;19(6):53-60.
43. Ulrich R, Quan X, Zimring C, Joseph A, Choudhary R. The role of the physical environment in the hospital of the 21st century: A once-in-a-lifetime opportunity (Electronic). (2004) Available: www.healthdesign. org./research/reports/physical_environ.php
44. Schneider M, Moore C, Gajewski L, Laughlin N, Larson J, Gay C, et al. Sensory processing disorders in a nonhuman primate model: Evidence for occupational therapy practice. American Journal of Occupational Therapy. 2007;61:247-8.
45. Riggs R, Andrews K, Roberts P, Gilewski M. Visual Deficit Interventions in Adult Stroke and Brain Injury: A Systematic Review, American Journal of Physical Medicine and Rehabilitation. 2007;86:853.
46. British Columbia Health Care. Output specifications. Volume 1 Abbotsford Hospital and Cancer Center. *BC: BCHC–Partnerships British Columbia, 2003.*
47. Katz DI, Zasler N, Zafonte R. Clinical Continuum of Care and Natural History. In: Brain Injury Medicine: Principles and Practice. Zasler N, Katz D, Zafonte R, (Eds). Demos Medical Publishing. New York; 2007. pp. 3-13.
48. Jepson R, Despain K, Keller D. Unilateral neglect: assessment in nursing practice. Journal of neuroscience nursing. 2008;40. p. 142.
49. Palmer R. Acute hospital care for the elderly: Minimizing the risk of functional decline. Cleveland Clinical Journal of Medicine. 1995;62(2):117-28.
50. Wong RYM, Shaw M, Acton C, Wilbur K, McMillan M, Breurkens E, Sowden C, Trautman SM, Chan N. An interdisciplinary approach to optimize health services in a specialized acute care for elders unit. Geriatrics Today. 2003; 6:177-86.
51. Parke B, Brand P. An elder-friendly hospital: Translating a dream into reality. Nursing Leadership. 2004;17(1):32-77.
52. Jorge R, Robinson R. Mood disorders following traumatic brain injury. Neuro-Rehabilitation. 2007;17:311-24.
53. Rader J. Tornquist EM (Ed). Individualized dementia care: creative, compassionate approaches. Springer Publishing Inc. New York, NY. 1995.
54. Harmsen M, Geurts A, Fasotti L, Bevaart B. Positive behavioral disturbances in the rehabilitation phase after severe traumatic brain injury: an historic cohort study. Brain Injury. 12004;18: 787-96.
55. www.shandsliveoak.com
56. www.wbdg.org
57. www.medicalfaq.net
58. "Diagnostic Medicine", Medical and Dental Space Planning, 2015.
59. www.healthdesign.com.au
60. www.apicnyc.org
61. airborneinfection.blogspot.com
62. www.ghdonline.org
63. www.indmedica.com
64. www2.mdanderson.org
65. radiology.rsnajnls.org
66. www.athanassios.gr
67. www.imris.com
68. www.ltlmagazine.com
69. Null, "Design in Public and Commercial Environments", Universal Design Principles and Models, 2013.

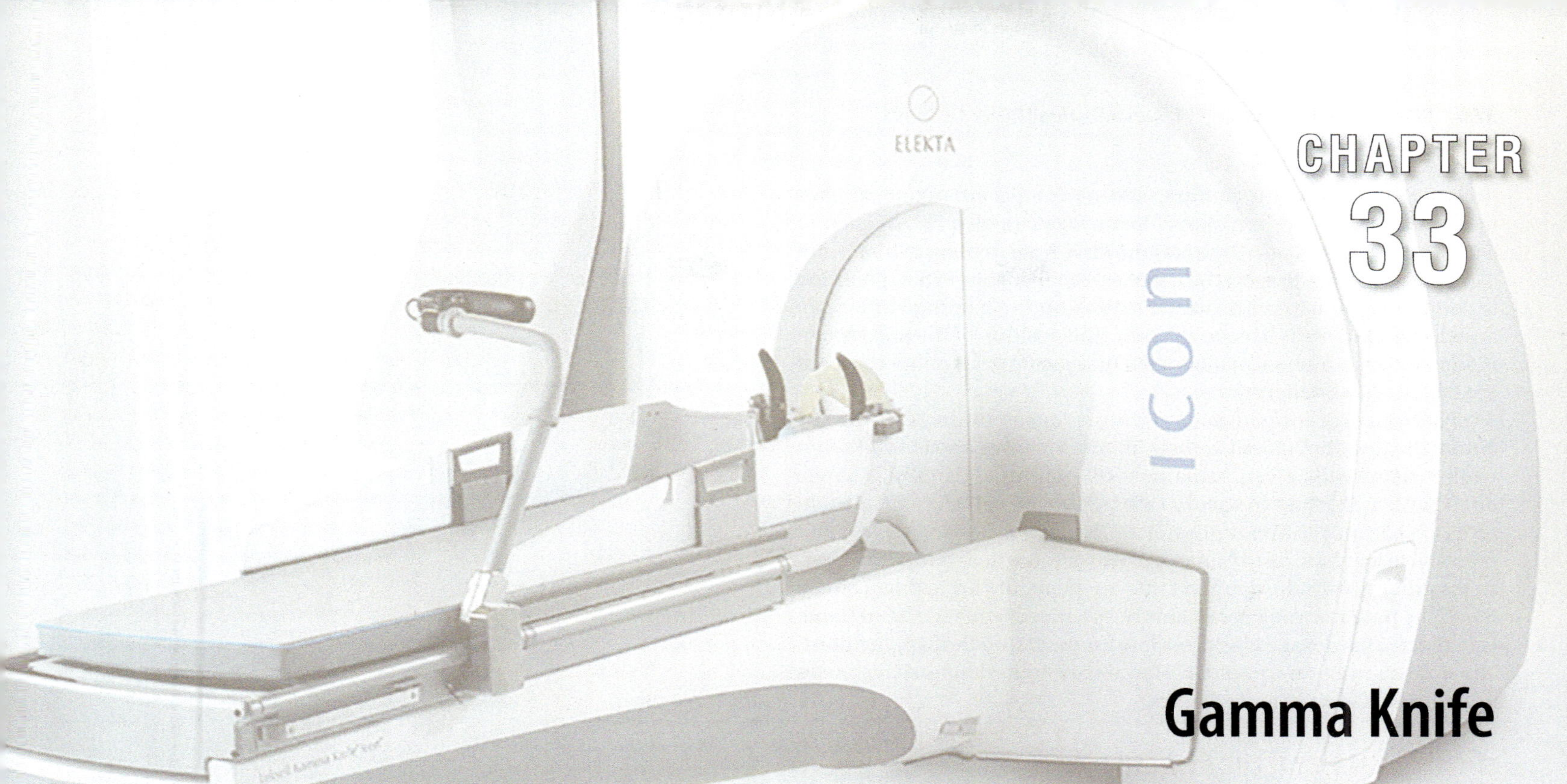

CHAPTER 33

Gamma Knife

SK Dutt, Shakti Kumar Gupta, Sunil Kant, R Chandrashekhar

INTRODUCTION

The procedure called "Stereotactic Radiosurgery" (SRS) is based on a simple concept. A series of radiation beams converge on a target from various angles. With proper planning, a high dose of radiation is given to a target, usually a tumor, with minimal dose to the surrounding tissue. Ideally, this dosage results in destruction of the tumor while sparing function of crucial organs or tissues adjacent to the treatment area, such as the optic nerve or brainstem.[1]

For nearly 100 years, this use of "cross-firing" beam techniques has evolved to allow treatment for both intracranial and extracranial sites. The most widely accepted use for SRS is still for intracranial disease.[1]

Stereotactic radiosurgery is now a standard option for many malignant and benign lesions of the brain, as well as some functional conditions. Arguably the best known SRS unit is the *Gamma Knife*.[1]

As SRS has become an accepted standard for malignant and benign conditions, the gamma knife and other SRS systems have become more affordable. Hence, the technology has expanded beyond primarily teaching hospitals into private hospitals and freestanding centers.

Stereotactic radiosurgery involves the use of an external, three-dimensional frame of reference to locate and target intracranial lesions for treatment by a large single fraction of ionizing radiation. Radiosurgery is delivered by multiple collimated and convergent beams, with rapid dose fall-off at the target boundary. This technique was originally developed for obliterating small, benign intracranial lesions, with the large dose of irradiation producing focal irreparable damage in cells within the high-dose target volume (Solberg et al. 1998). Target destruction occurs due to direct cell damage or disruption of blood supply.[2]

There are three potential methods for delivering stereotactic irradiation:[2]

- Linear accelerator (Linac)
- Gamma knife
- Charged-particle irradiation.

Fractionated stereotactic radiotherapy can also be performed using Linac and gamma knife delivery systems. This technique divides the radiation dose over multiple treatment sessions similar to conventional radiotherapy treatments. It has been proposed that fractionated dosing allows preferential repair of radiation-induced sublethal damage by normal surrounding tissue, compared with the abnormal target. This allows a differential effect to enable treatment and can be used to treat lesions located in critical areas of the brain or close to critical structures which were previously considered unsuitable for SRS.[2]

HOW GAMMA KNIFE WORKS?

Accuracy of the gamma knife is achieved by fixation of the patient's skull to the treatment table by use of a fixed head frame. A gamma knife treatment begins with placement of this head frame, usually by a neurosurgeon, on the morning of treatment. After local anesthetic is applied, four screws are used to tightly secure a rigid metal frame to the patient's skull. Once the frame is properly secured, the patient is brought to the computed tomography (CT) scanner and fixed to the scanning table in a supine position. A CT scan is acquired for treatment planning, and the patient is then released from the table and awaits treatment.[1]

The treatment planning process begins as a cooperative effort between neurosurgeon, radiation oncologist, and physicist. The crucial first step is the delineation of the target and nearby critical tissues. These structures must be outlined by hand on the planning CT scan. In many cases, the CT images alone suffice. If necessary, clearer images from and magnetic resonance imaging (MRI), done within 1–2 weeks prior to treatment, can be fused to the CT to allow more accurate contouring.[1]

When complete, radiation dose delivery is planned by placing one or more isocenters. Each isocenter represents a point at which all of the beams will converge for a certain amount of time. The result is a high radiation dose around the isocenter with a sharp falloff in the surrounding tissue. Spherical lesions require a single isocenter, while irregular shapes require multiple isocenters adjacent to one another to conform to the desired shape. Beam size can also be adjusted to achieve necessary shape—the gamma knife has circular collimators of 4, 8, 14, and 18 mm that can be used interchangeably. When planning is complete, the patient is placed supine on the gamma knife table and the head frame is fixed to the unit. The position of the head frame is adjusted with a series of dials such that the target is at the center of the beam, as defined by the plan.[1]

The most recent gamma knife unit makes these adjustments automatically. The patient is then monitored from outside the room while treatment is given, usually 30–90 minutes. Usually, a single operator is necessary to assure safe treatment delivery and patient monitoring, most often a physicist or radiation therapist. It is not practical to leave the head frame in place for more than one or two days, so treatments with the gamma knife are generally limited to a single dose. The patient typically remains hospitalized while the head frame is in place. This dosage is appropriate for most standard applications. The time allowed for treatment planning is limited but usually poses no difficulty for experienced users.[1]

GAMMA KNIFE MEDICAL APPLICATION: THE HISTORY

Development of the Gamma Knife

In the 1950s, Swedish professors Borje Larsson of the Gustaf Werner Institute, University of Uppsala, and Lars Leksell at the Karolinska Institute in Stockholm, Sweden, began to investigate combining proton beams with stereotactic (guiding) devices capable of pinpointing targets within the brain. This approach was eventually abandoned because it was complex and costly. Instead, in 1967, the researchers arranged for construction of the first gamma knife device using cobalt-60 as the energy source. Leksell termed this new surgical technique *'Stereotactic Radiosurgery'* (Figs. 1A to C). The prototype unit, used for 12 years in Sweden, was specifically designed for functional neurological surgery, that is, for treatment of patients with pain, movement disorders, and even certain behavioral disorders that were not responsive to conventional psychiatric treatment.[3]

Realizing the potential of SRS for treating brain tumors, Professor Leksell and his colleagues built a second gamma knife in 1975. It was installed at the Karolinska Institute and became an integral part of the neurosurgical service there. The third and fourth units, built in the early 1980s, were installed in Buenos Aires, Argentina, and Sheffield, England. The next two units built were at the University of Pittsburgh and the University of Virginia.[3]

The initial gamma unit design was intended for lesion generation in functional neurosurgery. Through the development of stereotactic angiography, arteriovenous malformations (AVMs) became suitable targets for stereotactic irradiation as did cranial base tumors imaged with pneumoencephalography or cisternography. In 1980s, an increasing number of patients had radiosurgery for AVMs, selected benign tumors, and small-volume malignant tumors. Today over 300,000 patients have undergone gamma knife surgery and over 35,000 per year receive the treatment.[3]

Over the past 40 years the gamma knife has evolved and each new model has become increasingly sophisticated, both in terms of the hardware as well as the radiotherapy planning software which has developed to match the explosive progress in computing over the past decades.

The current 'state of the art' model, is immeasurably better than the earliest machines and combines ease of use with incredible accuracy of radiosurgery delivery and speed of treatment, reducing the time the patient has to stay in the unit. It uses 192 shielded cobalt sources arranged around the head such that all of the beams converge at a single point. The target for treatment (AVM, tumor, etc.) is placed at the

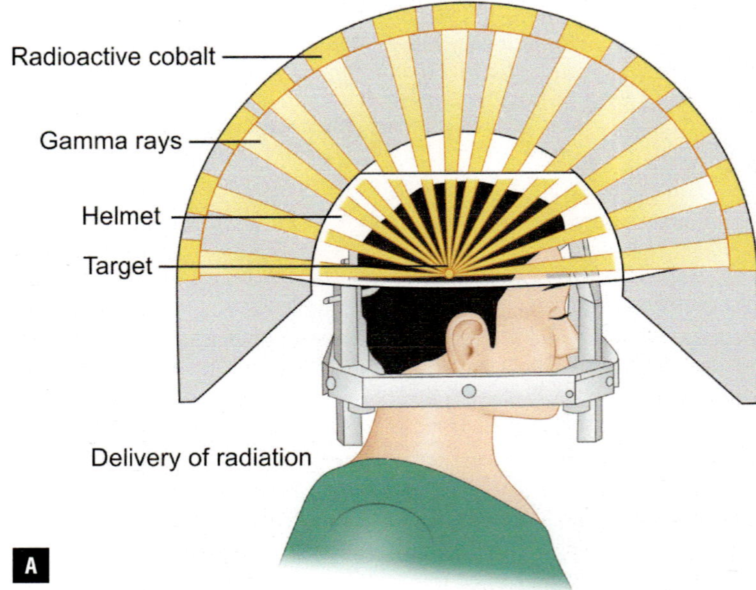

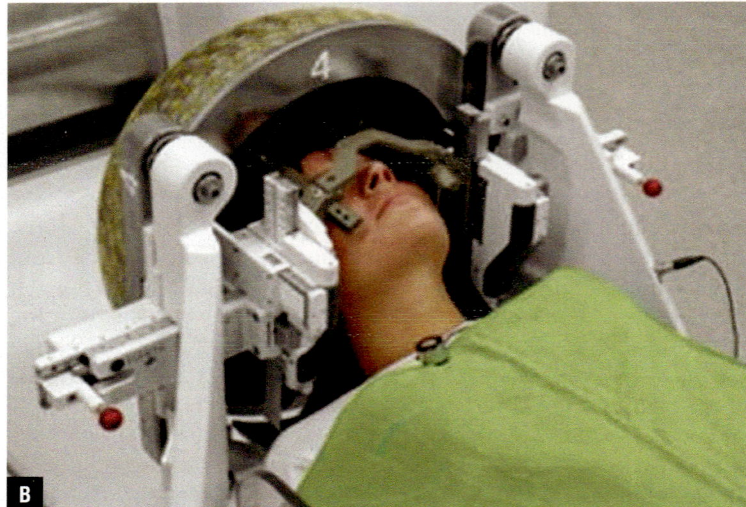

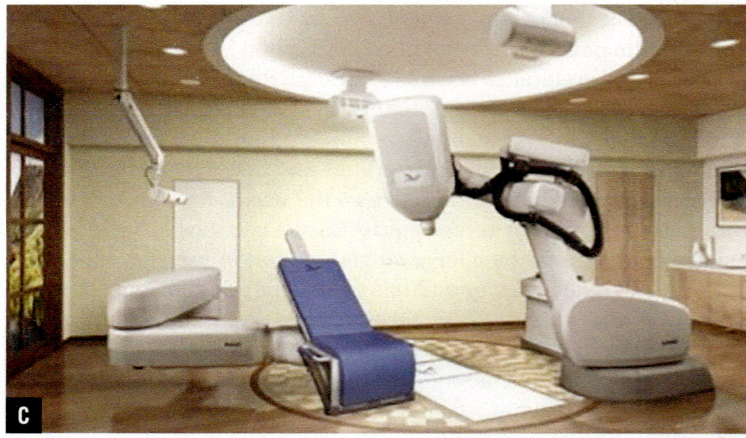

Figs. 1A to C: Stereotactic radiosurgery.

convergence point and to ensure that the whole of the target is covered with radiation, the patient's head is moved slightly between each dose, effectively 'painting' the tumor with radiotherapy.[4]

PHYSICS AND BASIC PRINCIPLES OF THE GAMMA KNIFE (FIG. 2)

The basic physics of the gamma knife has remained substantially the same since its conception. The device uses Cobalt-60 as a radiation source. Co-60 decays through beta decay to a stable isotope of nickel (Ni-60) with a half-life of 5.26 years. As a part of the decay process, one electron with an energy of up to 315 keV and two gamma rays with energies of 1.17 MeV and 1.33 MeV are emitted. It is the gamma radiation that is used to clinical effect in the gamma knife and contributes to the naming of the device.[3]

The details of the internal design of the gamma knife changes slightly among the models currently in use. Inside the gamma knife unit are an array of Co-60 sources which are aligned with a collimation system. The collimation system focuses the individual beams of gamma radiation to a very precise focus point. While an individual beam has a relatively low dose rate and causes minimal biological effect, the superposition of all beams at the focus point have a much higher dose rate (Fig. 2). The gamma knife can, therefore, target very precise areas of tissue without causing significant collateral damage to areas outside of the targeted area.[3]

In some models of the gamma knife, the beam collimation is split between an internal collimation and a removable external helmet-based collimation system. Each external collimator helmet has an array of removable tungsten collimators (one per source) with circular apertures that are used to create different diameter fields at the focus point. About 4 mm, 8 mm, 14 mm, and 18 mm collimator helmets are available. A subset of the collimators may be removed and replaced with solid tungsten "plugs" to block individual beams in cases where additional shielding is required. Modification of the isodose distribution is achieved by using combinations of isocenters using different collimators, different stereotactic locations, and differing dwell times. In the new gamma knife, the external helmet collimators have been replaced by a single internal collimation system.[3]

The gamma knife operates on the principles of stereotaxy to achieve a high level of precision in localization. A stereotactic head frame is affixed to the patient's head before the gamma knife procedure. This frame defines a reference coordinate system that allows points in the brain to be located with high precision. During imaging procedures, a system of fiducial markers is used with the frame to allow the location of all areas of interest within the images to be known relative to this stereotactic space. A computerized planning system developed for the gamma knife then allows detailed and precise dose distributions to be created that help ensure the target of interest is covered by a clinically significant dose while sparing normal brain tissue.[5]

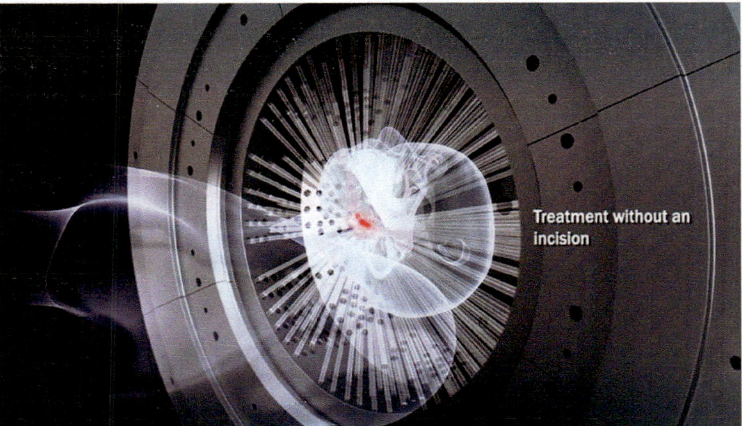

Fig. 2: Working of gamma knife.

GAMMA KNIFE PROCEDURE

A multidisciplinary team of neurological surgeons, radiation oncologists, medical physicists, radiologists, nurses, computer specialists, and physician assistants unite to provide the patient with comprehensive, advanced care before, during, and after the procedure. Patients are selected for treatment after thorough review of all prior records and imaging studies. Gamma knife radiosurgery has been described as a five-step procedure:

- Application of the stereotactic frame
- Acquisition of images (MRI/CT/DSA)
- Image transfer and registration
- Dose planning (treatment planning)
- Delivery of radiation (treatment delivery).

After admission to the hospital, the patient undergoes placement of a stereotactic frame, a mechanical guidance device, to the head. During frame placement, the patient receives a mild sedative administered in the operating room by an anesthesiologist.[3]

As such, the frame placement is pain free. Then, the patient's condition and the location and type of tumor or AVM are evaluated with advanced imaging technology, such as CT, angiography, or MRI. Next, the patient's head is placed within a large helmet-like device with small openings called "collimator ports." Radiation beams are adjusted through these ports to direct the appropriate amount of energy precisely at the target tissue.[3]

CONDITIONS TREATABLE BY GAMMA KNIFE

Currently, the gamma knife is used primarily to treat benign brain tumors, AVMs, acoustic neuromas, pituitary adenomas, craniopharyngiomas, brain metastases, other tumors of the skull base, and pineal region tumors. Selected patients with movement disorders and trigeminal neuralgia can also be treated.[3]

Common conditions for which SRS is indicated:[1]

- Neoplasms (benign/metastatic)
  - Brain metastases
  - Acoustic neuroma/vestibular schwannoma
  - Meningioma
  - Pituitary adenoma
  - Glioma/astrocytoma
  - Chordoma/chondrosarcoma
  - Craniopharyngioma
  - Hemangioblastoma
  - Ocular melanoma
  - Nasopharynx carcinoma
  - Glomus Jugulare tumors.
- Vascular disorders of the brain
  - AVMs
  - Arteriovenous fistulas (AVFs)
  - Cavernous malformations.
- Functional disorders
  - Trigeminal neuralgia
  - Obsessive compulsive disorder

- Parkinson's disease
- Epilepsy.

The common types of condition usually treated are discussed here.

Arteriovenous Malformations

These are abnormal tangles of arteries and veins that can occur in the brain. The individual affected must have born with the abnormality and may go through life without ever knowing of its presence. On occasion, they can cause epileptic seizures (fits) or may bleed leading to a blood clot forming in the brain (one type of stroke). Before the gamma knife was known to be effective for these, surgery was usually the treatment of choice, and may still be the preferred option for some AVMs. Most, however, would now consider the gamma knife to be the better option as the risks of treatment with radiosurgery are less than a standard neurosurgical operation. It should be noted; however, that radiosurgery may require more than 2 years to obliterate the malformation and cannot be used for very large AVMs (generally if greater than 3 cm in diameter). For these very large lesions, even surgery is often not recommended, as the risks of complications tend to outweigh the benefit of removal.[6]

Acoustic Neuroma

Also known as vestibular schwannoma, these are benign tumors of the nerves of balance/hearing (the vestibulocochlear nerve). They are normally very slowly growing (around 1-2 mm/year) and normally present with increasing hearing loss on the side of the tumor, coupled with noise in the ear (tinnitus) and unsteadiness. When diagnosed the options include observation with scans at intervals for small tumors, radiosurgery or surgical removal. Again, radiosurgery has become the treatment of choice for tumors under 3 cm in diameter in many centers around the world with arrest of tumor growth in more than 95% of cases. There is increasing evidence that treatment of small tumors may allow preservation of residual hearing and if this is confirmed this would make a good case to treat all small tumors before all hearing is lost on the affected side as there is no treatment that will restore hearing when lost. There is an often-quoted risk of transforming these benign tumors into cancers as a result of exposing them to radiation. Although a few cases have been documented, the overall risk is thought to be between 1:1000 and 1:10000—much less than the risk of a serious complication from surgery.[6]

Meningioma

These are also benign tumors, but these arise from the membranes surrounding the brain. When located in an easily accessible location, the treatment of choice is generally surgery as they are normally cured by removal. On occasion, perhaps if the risks of surgery are considered too great due to location, age or fitness of the patient, or if previous surgery has not been curative, radiosurgery can be used either as a primary treatment or as a addition to surgery to enhance the chance of cure. Many thousands of meningiomas have now been treated around the world with a chance of growth arrest of more than 90% in favorable cases.[6]

Pituitary Tumors

Generally these are benign tumors, sometimes these shrink in response to certain medications but generally the treatment of choice when needed is surgery. For some individuals, radiosurgery may be used instead of surgery or as an addition to surgery that has not been curative.[6]

Trigeminal Neuralgia

This type of facial pain, often described as electric shock spasms of pain in the forehead, cheek or jaw, is said to be the worst pain imaginable, on occasion leading to suicide. Drug treatment can be very effective and there are also good surgical treatments available. Radiosurgery is a relatively recent addition to the therapeutic armamentarium and can give excellent pain relief although it may take many weeks to be effective and there is a risk of later relapse.[6]

Metastatic Deposits

These are deposits of cancer that have spread to the brain from cancers elsewhere in the body— breast cancer is just one example. Traditional treatment for this is to give whole brain radiotherapy in fractions on a daily basis for 2-3 weeks. There are certain advantages to using radiosurgery for these tumors, either instead of whole brain radiotherapy or as a boost of radiation in those patients whose tumors have not responded to whole brain irradiation.[2]

CyberKnife is a recent evolution of Linac technology which involves the delivery of radiation via a robotic system. The system does not require a head frame, and unlike gamma knife and Linac-based radiosurgery, CyberKnife can more easily treat lesions in areas of the body other than the head. The system corrects for motion effects due to respiration or other patient movement in real time, and it has, therefore, been proposed that CyberKnife is more accurate than other forms of radiosurgery.[2]

Gamma Knife versus CyberKnife (Figs. 3A and B)

A fair comparison regarding CyberKnife and gamma knife must be limited to their ability to treat lesions in the head, as the latter cannot treat extracranial sites. The need for precision in SRS treatments within or adjacent to sensitive brain tissues is obvious, hence accuracy is a reasonable first point of discussion. Both the gamma knife and CyberKnife employ regularly scheduled, strict quality assurance measurements, including film, to simulate a treatment. For both, the accuracy of treatment delivery can usually be confirmed to within less than 0.5 mm. Other sources of error are unaccounted for in these measurements. The CyberKnife real-time image capture may generate an additional 0.5 mm error. The gamma knife head frame is not entirely rigid, and may account for less than 0.5 mm up to 1.7 mm inaccuracy. Regardless of these potential sources of error, most users will agree that accuracy of both units is more than adequate for treatment of appropriate intracranial lesions. Clinical efficacy is a second important point of discussion. For the numerous applications listed earlier, use of the gamma knife has been arguably the dominant resource for published literature regarding efficacy of SRS for the past 30 years. Literature specific to the newer CyberKnife is far less abundant but continues to emerge. It is fair to consider CyberKnife efficacy similar to most linear accelerator-based radiosurgery system using similar beam energies. These systems have also contributed substantially to the SRS literature for intracranial lesions, establishing their use as standard for appropriate patients. The ability to treat any body-site distinguishes CyberKnife from the gamma knife. Tomotherapy, Trilogy, Novalis, and Elekta Body Frame are other systems sharing this capability. Extracranial radiosurgery has enormous potential as a standard treatment option but is still largely an emerging application. Data, yet limited, have demonstrated promising results for certain tumors of the liver, lung and spine and for radiation resistant histologies. Results from larger published studies, including RTOG 0236, a clinical trial for early stage lung cancer, are expected

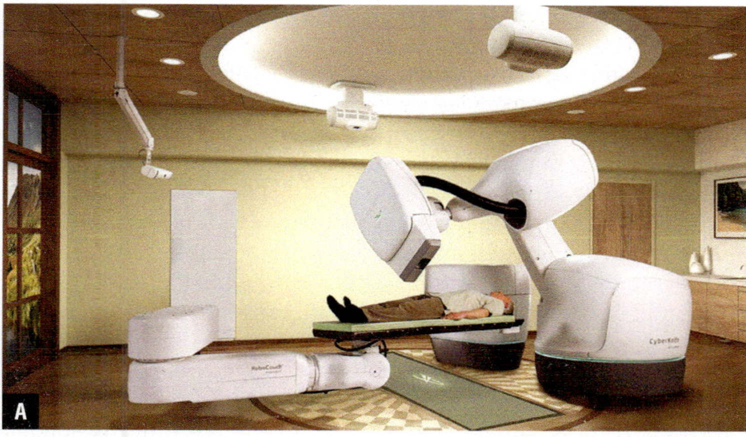

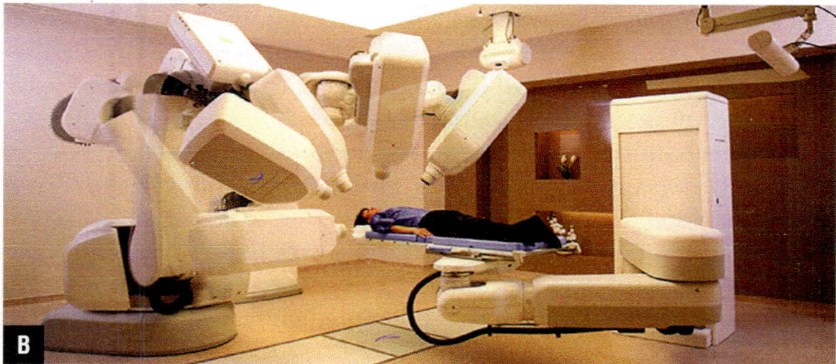

Figs. 3A and B: CyberKnife.

within a few years. Other important considerations exist. A reported but uncommon limitation of the gamma knife or any frame-based SRS system is the ability to treat peripheral brain or base-of-skull lesions. This situation can result in a collision of the frame or patient with the hardware if the target location extends beyond the treatable volume. The small size of the gamma knife collimators may be advantageous in sparing dose to critical tissues, but can create difficulty in treating lesions larger than 3–4 cm. Errors in the CyberKnife or other image-guided SRS systems may result from image resolution and registration, the quality of the planning images, and errors in couch and robot arm positioning. Cost is certainly an important consideration for any institution. Formal written estimates for the unit cost obtained from each company can vary by region but are comparable, ranging from $3.4 to $4 million dollars. It is also important to consider installation, physics, and therapist training and support, and maintenance costs for these units. Because these costs also vary by region, it is important to discuss these factors with their respective companies. The long, established history of gamma knife certainly contributed to the development of the CyberKnife and other intracranial and extracranial SRS systems. Direct, formal clinical comparisons will likely be available in the future, as more data for intracranial and extracranial applications emerge. While costly, both units are practical and effective for appropriate patients.[1]

GENERAL PLANNING CONSIDERATIONS[7]

- Gamma knife facility should be located away from high patient and/or public occupancy areas and sources of intense radiation.[7]
- Areas of source storage and handling shall be marked with radiation symbol and legend denoting the identification of active area and presence of radiation hazard. Areas of high activity and contamination shall be demarcated by physical barriers.[7]
- Walls, floor and doors of the active areas should have hard, washable, nonporous and leak-proof covering. Work surfaces should be covered with nonporous and nonreactive material.
- Ventilation system should be of once-through type with unidirectional air flow from areas of lower activity to higher activity. The exhaust from fume hoods shall be let out directly into the open after filtering.[7]
- Radiation levels at the nurse station outside the wards should not exceed 1 μSv/h.
- The following radiation monitors should be available in working condition and with recent calibration:[7]
  - Portable beta-gamma area monitor(s)
  - Contamination monitor(s) for personnel/area/surface/clothing;
  - Radioisotope calibrator.

Calibration shall be checked regularly and records maintained.

- Radiation levels around the in-house transport container shall not exceed 1 μSv/h at 5 cm from the surface. Radiation symbol shall be permanently marked on its outer surface. Means should be provided for securely locking the container.

Location

The unit should not act as a thoroughfare to other units of the healthcare facility. The floor loading weight of both equipment and shielding should be taken into consideration when locating the unit. A ground floor site may be the most suitable location but if this cannot be achieved, consider units above, below and adjoining the proposed location with regard to radiation shielding requirements, the weight of equipment and associated shielding and access for equipment and radioactive isotopes.[8]

Care should be taken to ensure that the location of the unit minimizes access by persons such as lost visitors, wandering patients from other units or those with criminal intent.[8]

Site and Layout Plan Approval

The user has to submit to Atomic Energy Regulatory Board (AERB) two copies each of the proposed layout plan, site plan, and elevation drawing of the facility indicating the floor, nature of occupancy around, above and below, if any, has to be submitted in "B3" size paper ($353 \times 500\ mm^2$) along with the application form AERB/RSD/NMF/SLA.[5]

The user has to clearly indicate the dimension of each of the rooms associated with the facility in the proposed layout plan of the gamma knife facility. When the user has to plan the laboratory, it is required that the arrangement of the various rooms associated with the facility has to follow the principle of low active area to high active area, that is, entrance of the facility should have reception/general waiting area, and at the end hot laboratory cum radiopharmacy/radioactive waste storage area is to be planned.[9]

The documents have to be submitted to the Head, Radiological Safety Division (RSD), and AERB. On scrutinizing the plans from radiologic safety point of view, necessary approval of facility is granted.[9]

Submission of Regulatory Consent Form

The user has to submit the details of the completion of the construction work as per the approved plan, installation of equipment, procurement of radiologic protection accessories, enrollment of radiation workers in personal monitoring services and availability of qualified staff as per AERB Safety Code AERB/SC/MED-IV (Rev-1 2001), shall be intimated to Head, RSD, AERB, by submitting the Regulatory Consent form no. AERB/444-NM/RC-FORM. The Radiological Safety Officer (RSO) as per the qualification mentioned in the AERB Safety Code AERB/SC/MED-IV (Rev-1 2001) has to be nominated by the employer for the NM facility by submitting the application form no. AERB/441/RSOM-II/III.[9]

Precommissioning Inspection

In this stage, the precommissioning inspection of the facility will be carried out by AERB official(s) to ensure that the construction of gamma knife facility is as per the approved plan.[9]

Approval for Commissioning/Routine Operation

On ensuring the compliance of the requirement as specified in AERB Safety Code SC/MED-IV (Rev.1. 2001) for the safe handling of radioactive material in the approved NM facility, the authorization for the procurement of radioactive material indigenously or no objection certificate (NOC) for procurement of radioactive material from abroad will be issued for the stipulated time period. The renewal for the same is done only after receipt and review of the Annual Status Report AERB/NM/Radiation Safety/02.[9]

Work Practice

In gamma knife facility, patients should be handled taking into account adequate radiation protection measures. Any unusual event that has resulted or has the potential to result in overexposure to the workers or public should be reported to the AERB. Annual Safety Status report of the facility should reach the AERB in the prescribed format at the end of each calendar year. Any change in the qualified person or design of the facility shall be reported to the AERB. Cooperation should be extended to the authorized inspectors from the AERB during inspection of the facility. Failure of compliance to radiation safety procedures may attract enforcement action by the AERB.[9]

RADIATION SAFETY CODE (FIG. 4)

Purpose

This code stipulates the radiation safety requirements in handling radioactive materials for nuclear medicine applications in order to:[7]

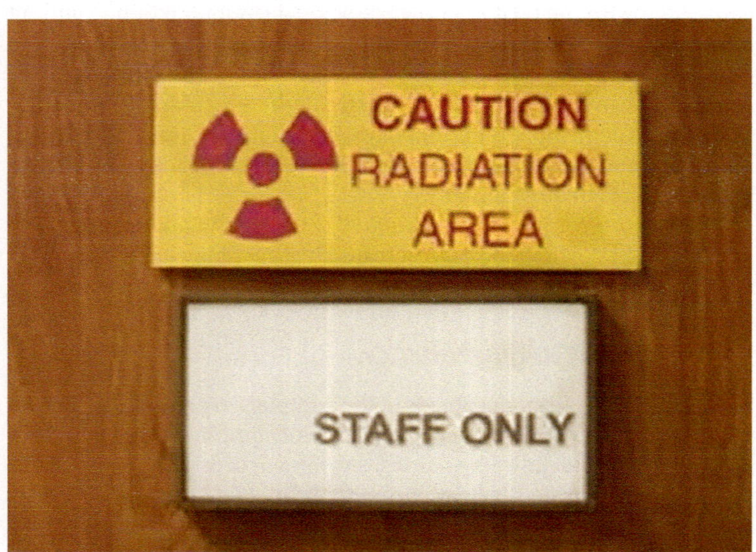

Fig. 4: Radiation safety code.

- Ensure that workers and members of the public are not exposed to radiation in excess of limits specified by the competent authority under the radiation protection rules (RPR), GSR 1601, 1971, and safety directives issued by the competent authority from time-to-time.
- Reduce such radiation exposures to levels as low as reasonably achievable (ALARA)
- Ensure safe handling, physical security of radioactive materials, patient protection and management of radioactive wastes.
- Provide for detection of hazardous situations and initiation of prompt remedial measures to mitigate consequences.

Scope

Radiation safety in handling radiation sources is governed by sections 14, 16 and 17 of the Atomic Energy Act, 1962 and the RPR, 1971, issued under the Act. The Radiation Surveillance Procedures for Medical Applications of Radiation, GSR 388, 1989 issued under RPR specify the general requirements for radiation safety of:[7]

- Persons handling radiation sources for medical applications.
- Patients who undergo medical procedures voluntarily for their health benefit.
- Persons connected with the patient either by living with him or assisting him during the medical procedure(s).
- Members of the public unrelated to medical use of radiation.

REGULATORY CONTROLS

Consent

The consent for any practice involving radiation exposure is based on a system of notification, registration, authorization, license or exemption from regulatory control as established by the competent authority.[7]

The consent is issued on the basis of a written application. The consentee should ensure that persons handling radioactive materials for nuclear medicine purposes are familiar with the mandatory provisions of the Radiation Protection Rules, 1971; Radiation Surveillance Procedures for Medical Applications of Radiation, 1989; Radiation Surveillance Procedures for Transport of Radioactive Material, 1988; Atomic Energy (Safe Disposal of Radioactive Wastes) Rules, 1987; and the safety directives issued by the competent authority from time-to-time, and other instructions of the competent authority in specific cases.[7]

The consentee should designate with the approval of the competent authority a person having qualifications to function as Radiological Safety Officer (RSO). Nuclear medicine facilities carrying out diagnostic *in vivo*/*in vitro* investigations should have an RSO of Level-II whereas facilities where therapy is also carried out should have an RSO of Level-III.[7]

Authorization from competent authority is required to procure radioactive material. The consentee shall be solely responsible for the safety and security of the radioactive material, its proper use, and the safe disposal of wastes. The consentee shall maintain an up-to-date inventory and account for decay and disposal of sources.[7]

The gamma knife facility shall not be commissioned until the competent authority approves the facility. Any change or modification to an already approved facility shall be carried out only with the prior approval/sanction of the competent authority.[7]

Transport of radioactive material in public domain shall be in accordance with the provisions of AERB/SC/TR-1.[7]

The consentee shall not take radioactive material out of the approved premises. The consentee shall not lend, gift, transfer, or sell any radioactive material and shall not receive radioactive material other than those specified in the authorization.[7]

Radioactive material shall not be disposed off without prior approval of the competent authority. The consentee shall obtain authorization, as per Rule 4 of the Atomic Energy (Safe Disposal of Radioactive Wastes) Rules, 1987, from the competent authority after submitting the prescribed application.[7]

Any person duly authorized by the competent authority may inspect the gamma knife facility, the radioactive sources available in-house, the radioisotope inventory, logbooks, records of area monitoring and contamination monitoring, instruments and devices used for the above and/or quality assurance programme, records of unusual occurrences during handling of the sources and transport of radioactive materials. If, on inspection, any evidence of noncompliance of any of the mandatory provisions is noticed, the inspector, under sections 14, 16 and 17 of the Atomic Energy Act, 1962 may:[7]

- Seal any radiation installation or any transport or conveyance carrying radioactive materials or seize any radioactive material or contaminated equipment.
- Indicate in writing to the consentee any modification aimed at providing adequate protection, and the consentee shall comply with the same.

The gamma knife facility should be decommissioned only after prior approval of the competent authority and after removing all radioactive and contaminated materials from the facility. Prior approval of the competent authority is necessary for reuse of the facility.[7]

STAFFING

A staff establishment should be developed early in the planning process in order to assess the offices, workstations and amenities that will be required. However, a unit should be large enough to ensure that the safety, security and emergency responses of staff on duty are accommodated. Sizing of the unit on this basis provides for improved operational cost effectiveness as well as compliance with security and occupational health and safety (OHS) requirements. A facility to be approved by the AERB should have the following staff/personnel.[10]

The staff establishment may include:[10]

- Medical specialists qualified in nuclear medicine including radiation oncologists.
- Neurosurgeons
- Radiologists/neuroradiologists
- Nuclear medicine registrars/residents supported by cleaners, orderlies.
- Nuclear medicine physicists
- Nuclear medicine technologists/scientists
- Radiopharmacist/s
- Nursing staff
- Administration staff.

A Radiation Safety Officer (RSO) should be appointed who may or may not be a nuclear medicine staff member.

The responsibilities that these personnel have to carry out are also given below.

RESPONSIBILITIES OF PERSONNEL

Consentee

The consentee should:[7]

- Employ adequate number of nuclear medicine physician(s), technologist(s) and an RSO.
- Provide appropriate equipment and tools to concerned persons for safe handling of radioactive material.
- Assign responsibilities to individuals in accordance with this code and establish lines of communication and authority.[7]
- Provide personnel monitoring devices to radiation workers, and ensure that they are worn as required, and also ensure that individual dose records are maintained as prescribed by the competent authority.[7]
- Provide any special personnel monitoring device, including those for internal monitoring, that may be required.[7]
- Constitute a local safety committee to review the safety of the facility in terms of operational safety, quality assurance, ethical aspects and regulatory compliance. RSO shall be a member of the committee, which shall include persons familiar with operations of the facility. Competent authority shall be informed about the committee and its work.[7]
- Report to the competent authority on any change in safety organization of the facility.
- Report any unusual occurrence, pertinent to radiological health and safety, to the competent authority within 24 hours of the event.
- Constitute a radiation protection program depending on the type of nuclear medicine facility. The program shall be submitted to the competent authority prior to obtaining regulatory consent.[7]

Nuclear Medicine Physician

- Minimum qualification
  - A degree in medicine recognized by the Medical Council of India.
  - A qualification in nuclear medicine recognized by the Medical Council of India; or an experience of at least five years in a nuclear medicine facility.
  - Authorization from the Nuclear Medicine Committee for human use of radionuclides.[7]
- Responsibilities

  The nuclear medicine physician shall:
  - Ensure the efficacy of new nuclear medicine procedures from the experience gained from previous clinical trials, animal experiments and published literature. Prior clearance from the Nuclear Medicine Committee shall be obtained for any new trial or deviation from established norms.[7]
  - Prevent any possibility of misadministration and promptly report to the consentee and the competent authority in the event of any misadministration, adverse reaction or death of a patient administered with radioactivity.[7]
  - Obtain informed consent from the patient for all nuclear medicine procedures to be performed on the patient and inform him/her on safety measures to be observed to avoid radiation exposure to the family members and others.[7]
  - Ensure that any patient hospitalized after administration of therapeutic quantity of radioactivity is kept isolated, spread of contamination prevented, and exposure of staff, other patients and public minimized.[7]
  - Instruct nursing and ancillary staff on radiation safety and precautions in nursing/management of therapy patients.[7]

Nuclear Medicine Technologist

- Minimum qualifications
  - A degree in science from a recognized university.
  - Postgraduate degree/diploma in nuclear medicine technology from a recognized institution; or an experience of five years in a recognized nuclear medicine facility.

- Responsibilities[7]
  The nuclear medicine technologist shall:
  - Ensure proper functioning of all nuclear medicine equipment, carry out periodic calibrations, quality assurance checks and maintenance.[7]
  - Ensure the purity of radiopharmaceutical, the route of administration and the accuracy of dosage before giving it to a patient and take precautions to avoid misadministration.[7]
  - Avoid spillage of radioactivity or contamination of the patient, premises, persons and material by exercising care during dispensing/administration of radioactivity.[7]
  - Report to RSO and the nuclear medicine physician of any mishap in dispensing/administration of dosage to the patient or any unusual incident.
  - Assist the RSO in maintaining records of inventory, use, waste disposal of sources and other safety matters.[7]

Radiological Safety Officer

- Minimum qualification for RSO Level-II[7]
  - A postgraduate degree in nuclear medicine from a recognized institution; or postgraduate diploma in nuclear medicine technology from a recognized institution.
  - Approval of the competent authority.
- Minimum qualification for RSO Level-III
  - A degree in science with physics as one of the subjects from a recognized university.
  - Postgraduate degree/diploma in radiological physics or equivalent recognized by the competent authority.
  - Approval of the competent authority.
- Responsibilities
  The RSO shall:
  - Advise and assist the consentee to organize a radiation protection program appropriate for the facility and ensure that staff observe safe work practices.[7]
  - Ensure safety, security and containment of radioactive sources, carry out radiation and contamination monitoring of work areas, therapy patients, patient areas, management of cadavers containing radionuclides as given in Appendix-IV, radioactive waste disposal sites and public areas, and maintain record of findings.[7]
  - Ensure that radiation monitoring instruments are kept in proper working condition and are calibrated at regular intervals.[7]
  - Establish procedures for management of emergency situations and conduct periodic drills to ensure their effectiveness.[7]
  - Report any unusual incident in writing to the consentee and take remedial measures to mitigate consequences of the incident and to prevent recurrence.[7]
  - Maintain records of the doses of workers, the inventory of sources received, used and disposed, any unusual incident, cause of such incident and remedial measures taken.[7]
  - Segregate and monitor the waste prior to interim storage or final disposal.[7]
  - Advise and assist the consentee in obtaining authorization from the competent authority for disposal of radioactive waste.
  - Advise and assist the consentee in transport of radioactive material/radioactive waste in the public domain.[7]

FUNCTIONAL AREAS

The following rooms/spaces form the main functional zones of the unit:[10]

- Reception/administration
- Outpatient waiting
- Patient holding, observation and recovery area
- Treatment areas
- Clinical support areas
- Staff offices and amenities
- Teaching and research facilities in tertiary centers.

Reception/Administration

Facilities will usually comprise:[10]

- Entry lobby and general public waiting
- Reception/enquiry desk
- Bookings office or alcove
- Administrative offices
- Clerical work area for filing, photocopying, and report typing.

Public toilets should be readily available but need not be inside the unit. If the gamma knife facility is co-located with a Medical Imaging Unit, these facilities may be shared.

Outpatient Waiting

The outpatient waiting area usually comprises:

- Separate areas for patients who may be ambulant or in wheelchairs.
- Access to toilets, shower and refreshments arranged.
- Children play area, if required.

Patient Holding, Observation and Recovery Area

An area will be required for holding of inpatients, and recovery and observation as necessary of both inpatients and outpatients. It usually comprises the following:[10]

- Dedicated inpatient entry.
- Curtained bed/trolley bays for holding, observation and recovery. The size of each bay and configuration of the overall space should permit patients to be held safely.
- A small staff base with hand basin.
- Ready access to dirty utility, linen trolley bay, sterile stock store.
- Resuscitation trolley—it is recommended it be parked in or near the viewing console.

Treatment Planning Area

All the rooms are accessed by patients and require radiation shielding as advised by consultants (Fig. 5).[10]

Clinical Support Areas

Clinical support areas usually include the following areas. However, if collocated with a medical imaging unit, some areas listed may be shared:[10]

- Viewing/reporting area
- Dirty utility room
- Disposal room
- Equipment bays

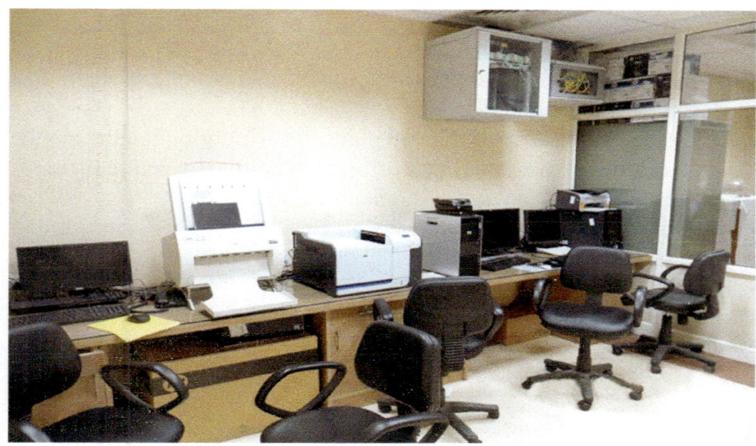

Fig. 5: Treatment planning area.

- Equipment and general stores
- Sterile stock store or clean utility room
- Print/server room.

Viewing and Reporting Area

Provide a dedicated room for viewing and reporting on scans. In determining the size of this room, consider future trends in service delivery and the need to accommodate increasing levels of technology (Figs. 6A and B).[10]

Each viewing workstation will require picture archiving and communication system (PACS) capability, image display monitors, patient information access monitors and a PC at each workstation plus shelving for resource material.

Staff Offices and Amenities

Depending on the size and location of the unit and collocation with adjoining units, staff will need access to:

- Staff room/beverage bay
- Meeting rooms and library
- Offices in accordance with staff establishment and teaching/research roles.
- Toilets, showers and lockers.

Functional Relationships Planning Access

External

- Easy, direct access for delivery of isotopes.
- Easy access to/from the inpatient units, outpatient units and staff facilities.
- Easy access for vehicles providing maintenance or delivery of large, heavy items.

Internal

Patients should have ready access to water, refreshments, toilets and shower.[10]

Parking

Patients and visitors will use the public parking facilities with access to drop-off areas and disabled parking. An identified parking area for vehicles delivering isotopes is required.[10]

Patient Amenities

The following patient amenities should be available and, where possible, should be positioned:[10]

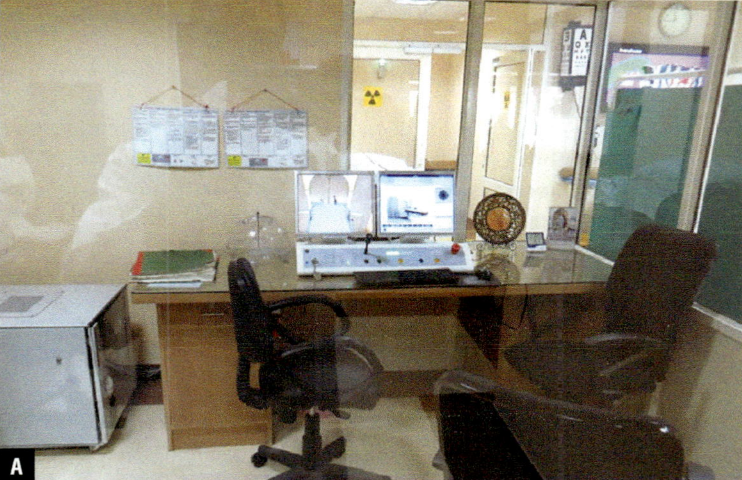

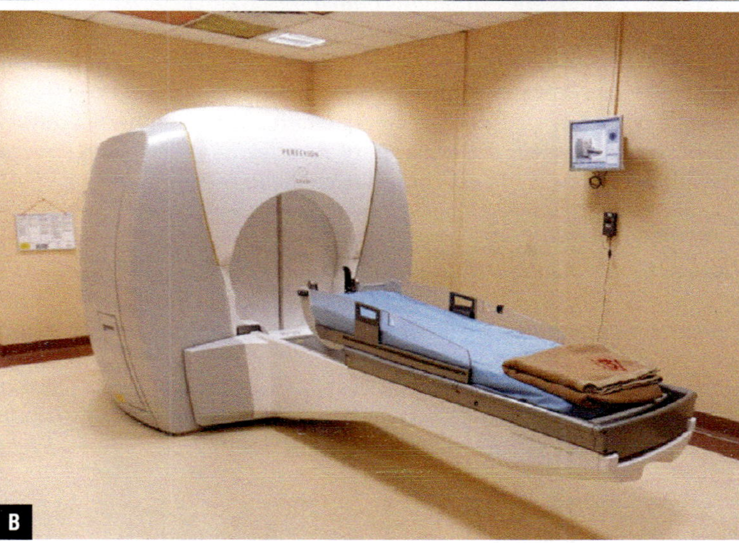

Figs. 6A and B: Viewing and reporting.

- Toilets including access toilet.
- Change cubicle/s and shower—for emergencies.

Patient Refreshments

A beverage bay or drinking fountains should be provided for patient refreshments. Many patients undergoing scanning procedures may be fasting pre-scan, may require a cup of coffee or tea to relieve headaches and nausea. Provision of refreshments should be supervised by staff.[10]

Patient Waiting

Patients should have access to drinking water and toilet facilities. It is preferable to separate outpatients from inpatients as the latter need more privacy, e.g. for bedpans, nursing care, etc. Provide separate entrances. Outpatients and their relatives need to be provided with explicit advice about the radiation safety requirements for themselves and others. Inpatients may return to their respective wards. Care should be taken if patients have to go to other areas for further tests.[10]

Patient Transport

The model of care/service plan for the unit should define whether the unit will have its own porter staff possibly shared with an adjoining unit or use a central transport department. The decision may depend on the number of inpatient studies to be undertaken. If required, facilities should comprise a small porter's base with hand basin, linen storage, portable oxygen cylinders and parking areas for trolleys and wheelchairs.[10]

Protective Apparel

Depending on unit policies, staff may need to wear a protective lead apron. Equipment bays holding the appropriate personnel protective apparel should be provided in close proximity to the scanning areas or located within the scanning rooms for ease of access and use.[10]

Radioactive Isotopes: Delivery

Gamma knife facility will receive sealed radioactive isotopes, Cobalt-60 (delivered to a licensed person) and will be required to handle and store these.[10]

Disaster Planning

Each unit will have operational plans and policies detailing the response to a range of emergency situations both internal and external. Consider the ability to effect complete lock-down and issues such as the placement of emergency alarms, the need for uninterrupted or emergency power supply (UPS) to essential clinical equipment such as scanners, electronic sensor taps and services such as emergency lighting, telephones, duress alarm systems, servers and computers. Arrangements for management of spills and radioactive exposure should be in place.[10]

Teaching and Research

The extent of teaching and research conducted in the unit will need to be ascertained to ensure that necessary offices, laboratories, and staff and student amenities are provided. All major teaching hospitals will undertake staff and student teaching, research and possibly prepare novel radiopharmaceuticals for clinical use. Units undertaking clinical trials will need to carefully assess needs in excess of routine requirements both in terms of treatment rooms and staff facilities.[10]

Infection Control

The infectious status of many patients admitted to the unit may be unknown. All body fluids should be treated as potentially infectious and standard precautions should be taken in accordance with hospital policy. Hand basins should be located in all clinical areas.[10]

Walls

Walls should be washable and easily decontaminated in the event of a radioactive spill.[10]

Finishes

Floor Finishes

Floor finishes and junctions should be impermeable and nonabsorbent in case of radiation spills.[10]

FIXTURES, FITTINGS AND EQUIPMENT

Definitions: Fixtures and Fittings

Fixtures and fittings are defined as follows:[10]

- *Fixtures:* Items that require service connection to walls, floor or ceilings (electrical, hydraulic, and mechanical) and include, but are not limited to, basins, light fittings, medical service panels.[10]
- *Fittings*: Items attached to walls, floors or ceilings that do not require service connections such as curtain and IV tracks, hooks, mirrors, blinds, joinery, pin boards, etc.[10]

General

High cost engineering areas which should receive careful consideration by design teams include:[10]

- Lighting and the impact of deep planning on lighting requirements.
- The number of sanitary fittings and the potential for reducing these by strategic location.
- Extent of the required emergency and uninterrupted power supply.
- Extent of provision of emergency doors.
- Extent of provision of essential backup systems (e.g. dual generators, chillers, boilers and dual electrical circuits).

BUILDING SERVICE REQUIREMENTS

Construction

In constructing the unit, following issues need to be addressed:[10]

- Ensure that new and existing floor structure and finishes are adequate to meet load requirements for equipment, shielding, patients, and personnel.
- Ensure that walls contain the necessary support systems for medical service panels.
- Provision should be made for cable trays, ducts or conduits in floors, walls, and ceilings as required for specialized equipment.
- The integrity of the shielding should not be compromised by ducts and penetrations.
- Ceiling height in the scanning rooms should be a minimum of 3 m.
- Ceiling mounted equipment should have properly designed rigid support structures located above the finished ceiling.
- A tiled ceiling should be considered for ease of installation, service and remodeling.

Electrical Services

A sufficient number of power outlets, both general and essential supply, including three phase outlets, are required for current and anticipated future needs. An emergency backup system for the power supply should be available for high priority equipment and illumination.[10]

Provide uninterrupted power supply (UPS) to cameras, acquisition workstations and servers to prevent data loss and/or damage during power surges or brown outs.[10]

All treatment rooms are to be body protected electrical areas. All scanning rooms require dimmable down lighting with lighting not located directly above scanning beds.[10]

Information Technology and Communication Systems

The infrastructure for the following should be considered for the present and possible future expansion:[10]

- Wireless technology
- Voice/data systems
- Video conferencing capacity
- Duress call—fixed and personal (optional)
- CCTV monitoring systems of entry points, if considered necessary and in the scanning and uptake rooms
- Infrastructure for PACS, electronic records and imaging information management system
- Server room
- Patient/nurse and emergency call systems compatible with existing hospital systems.

Mechanical Services

Additional cooling and ventilation will be required to scanning rooms and associated computer equipment rooms as the equipment is sensitive to excessive ambient heat. Additional cooling capacity should be built in to allow for future growth and technological development of scanners.[10]

General air-conditioning needs to cool equipment but not blow over partially undressed patients.

To maintain a high level of staff concentration and to minimize the possibility of accidents, the temperature of the unit should be maintained within a comfortable range not exceeding 25°C.

Smoke detectors in treatment rooms should be sensitive to radiation, i.e. photoelectric.

Medical Gases

Oxygen, suction and medical air will be required in all scanning rooms and patient bed bays.[10]

Nitrous oxide and scavenging will be required in rooms where general anesthesia may be administered, particularly in units where children are treated.[10]

Radiation Shielding

The principles of radiation safety and protection should be developed and integrated into the design and documentation of the unit from the earliest stages and it is important the design team is comprehensively briefed. A qualified radiation expert should be involved in the design.

Advice from the Radiation Safety Officer should be sought for each project. Radiation shielding will be required to a number of areas within the unit.[10]

SPACE STANDARDS AND COMPONENTS

Human Engineering

Human engineering covers those aspects of design that permit effective, appropriate, safe and dignified use by all people, including those with disabilities.[8]

Ergonomics

Design the unit so that patients, staff, visitors and maintenance personnel are not exposed to avoidable risks of injury and radiation exposure. Badly designed recurring elements, such as height, depth and design of workstations and counters, shelving and the layout of critical rooms, have a great impact on the occupational health and safety of staff as well as the welfare of patients.[10]

Consider work practices in relation to manual handling of equipment with significant weight. Manual handling requirements may be reduced by appropriate local storage.[10]

Building Elements

Building elements include walls, floors, ceilings, doors, windows and corridors.[10]

Doorways and turning circles should be sufficiently wide and high to permit the maneuvering of wheelchairs, trolleys and equipment without risk of damage or manual handling risks, and to allow ingress/egress of equipment for installation or removal.[10]

Ensure that floors are able to support the weight of equipment, and shielding, and that equipment is not located in vibration prone areas. Consider the need for shielding to floors or ceilings directly above, below or adjacent to the unit.[10]

Doors and Doorways

Doorways should be sufficiently wide and high to permit movement of bariatric patients on large hospital beds, traction beds, wheelchairs, trolleys, equipment and accompanying staff escort without risk of damage or manual handling risks. Sliding doors may be appropriate provided there is an area of wall of sufficient length. Provide the same level of shielding to vision panels in doors to treatment rooms. Doorways to scanning rooms should be flush to the floor.[10]

Radiation Shielding

Advice should be sought for each project from the Radiation Safety Officer. Radiation shielding will be required to a number of areas within the unit.[10]

General

Safety and security involves people and policies as well as physical aspects but should be built in as part of overall design and not superimposed on a completed facility. A safety audit via a risk analysis of potential hazards should be undertaken during the design process.[10]

MANAGEMENT OF MEDICAL EMERGENCIES

Management of medical emergencies will be in accordance with hospital policy. A resuscitation trolley should be located near the monitoring console room. In a very large unit, a second trolley may be required in or near the patient holding area.[10]

Management of Radioactive Substances Spills

All surfaces including floors, bench tops, walls and junctions should be impermeable and easy to clean. A decontamination kit should be stored under supervision of RSO for quick access to contain and clean up radioactive spills.[10]

Management of Radiation Emergency

Consentee shall prepare emergency preparedness plans, and such plans shall cover natural events such as fire, flood, or earthquake, in addition to potentially hazardous situations in the storage, handling, administration and transport of radioactive materials, and to persons administered with radioactive materials.[7]

Personnel shall be identified and trained in handling emergencies. Periodic drills shall be conducted to ensure effectiveness of the plans.[7]

Intervention action shall aim at limiting external exposure, intake of radioactive materials and spread of contamination. The initiation and termination of intervention shall be to maximize the averted dose.[7]

In case of spillage of radioactivity on patients, staff or public, the residual fixed contamination (beta-gamma) on the skin after decontamination shall not exceed 3.7 Bq/cm^2.[7]

Consentee shall report to the competent authority within 24 hours of the event of the following unusual occurrences which have hazardous consequences or potential to cause hazardous consequences:[7]

- Spillage of radioactive material
- Loss/theft of radioactive material
- Death of a patient administered with radioactivity
- Misadministration of radiopharmaceutical
- Adverse reaction consequent to dose administration
- Natural events like fire, floods, etc.
- Personnel overexposure.

The following details shall be reported:[7]

- Date and time of occurrence
- Radionuclide, its activity and radiopharmaceutical composition
- Brief description of the incident
- Actions taken
- Probable causes of the incident
- Steps taken for avoiding recurrence of the incident.

WASTE MANAGEMENT

General

There are several categories of waste, waste will consist of:[10]

- *Clinical waste*: Excluding sharps
- *Recyclable waste*: Usually paper and bottles/cans
- *General waste*: Any waste not included above and which is not capable of being recycled, reprocessed or re-used.

RADIOACTIVE WASTE MANAGEMENT

Waste Disposal

In India, radioactive waste management is governed by the Atomic Energy (Safe Disposal of Radioactive Wastes) Rules, 1987, GSR-125 issued under the Atomic Energy Act, 1962. Chairman, AERB is the competent authority. Implementation of the rules is primarily to ensure safety of the public and the environment.[9]

Radioactive waste needs to be managed safely because it is potentially hazardous to human health and the environment. Through good practices in the production and use of radionuclides, the amount of waste may be significantly reduced but not fully eliminated. It is important that safe waste management, in compliance with all relevant regulations is considered and planned for at the early stages of any projects involving radioactive materials. The radioactive waste in hospitals comprises different types of waste. It may be in solid, liquid, or gaseous form. The radioactive material may be mixed with different chemicals, which in itself would be hazardous or flammable. Moreover, some of the waste is mixed with biological substances, such as blood and may be infectious. Also, special precautions must be taken for disposing items, such as needles used for injection. All these aspects must be accounted for in the planning of waste treatment in a hospital. There may be certain sealed sources used for calibration of dose calibrators, survey instruments; these sources may end up as spent sources after their useful life or during the decommissioning of the department.[9]

The solid waste generated in gamma knife facility includes cover papers, gloves, contaminated items, empty vials, and syringes. The liquid waste may comprise decontamination effluents, laboratory washings, and so on.[9]

All the labels on the containers having contaminated radioactive material should be removed defaced prior to disposal. There are two main approaches to the disposal of radioactive waste. One is characterized as "dilute and disperse" and the other as "confine and contain." By the "dilute and disperse" concept, radioactive material, in aqueous or gaseous form, is released into the environment in such a way that the material is diluted and distributed over a large volume so that the final concentration of radionuclides is acceptably low. In the "confine and contain" approach, the waste is collected and converted into a form such that, when placed in a repository, it will retain the radionuclides until the activity has decayed, or at least will ensure that the leakage of radionuclide from the repository does not give rise to unacceptable concentrations anywhere in the environment. A decontamination kit should be readily available under the RSO for quick access to contain and clean up radioactive spills.[9]

Radioactive Waste Disposal: Solid

Solid radioactive waste includes all items/materials used in treatment and manufacture, e.g. laboratory glassware, pipette tips, plastic vials and trays, paper tissues, used syringes, tools, etc. Such items are to be suitably bagged, labeled and segregated, and retained in a dedicated waste holding area until designated safe for routine disposal.[10]

The radioactive waste store may be in the nuclear medicine unit or elsewhere on the campus and should be appropriately sited and shielded. It is preferable that the waste store is in the nuclear medicine unit, so consider a room at the perimeter with dual and carefully controlled access. However, if not in the unit itself, access should not compromise radiation safety principles.[10]

Storage

Provide different storage areas to cater for clinical and nonclinical supplies and equipment. These include:[10]

- Storage in the scanning rooms to reduce manual handling issues associated with movement of heavy or bulky articles such as collimators and scanning phantoms.
- Equipment bays for mobile items such as portable TVs, wheelchairs, trolleys, lifters and ultrasound scanners.
- General storage for smaller equipment items.
- Storage for office supplies.
- Storage for sterile stock and medical consumables.
- Storage for cleaning supplies.

SAFETY AND SECURITY

Occupational Health and Safety

The handling of people and equipment is a significant issue in this unit. As radiation exposure to staff can increase with time spent in close proximity to patients, it is important that the design facilitates efficient manual handling practices.

Consider work practices in relation to:[10]

- Manual handling of equipment for which significant weight is attached-bariatric patient beds, etc.
- Manual handling of patients, e.g. transfers from trolleys and exact positioning for scanning in narrow or confined spaces.
- Repair and maintenance of scanning equipment.

Manual handling requirements may be reduced by appropriate local storage locations and provision of space around equipment to allow transfers and use of manual handling equipment.

Safety

Health facility briefing and planning consider the impact of finishes, surfaces and fittings on safety. In particular, consider:[10]

- Slippery or wet floors
- Protrusions or sharp edges
- Stability and height of equipment or fittings
- Fittings which should be well above floor level and/or waterproof.
- Adequate protection for workers against infection and any other hazards—particularly radiation exposure.

REFERENCES

1. www.swmedicalcenter.com
2. www.msac.gov.au
3. med.virginia.edu
4. https://www.capitalhealth.org/
5. www.medicine.virginia.edu
6. www.totalhealth.co.uk
7. www.aerb.gov.in
8. www.healthdesign.com.au
9. www.ncbi.nlm.nih.gov
10. https://aushfg-prod-com-au.s3.amazonaws.com/HPU_B.0300_6_0.pdf

OTHER REFERENCES

- healthfacilityguidelines.com.au
- Gamma knife vs Cyber knife; S. Christopher Hoffelt, MD, Medical Director of Radiation Oncology at Southwest Washington Medical Center and Assistant Professor of Radiation Oncology at Oregon Health Sciences University in Portland, Ore.
- Stereotactic Radio surgery for Patients with Metastatic Tumors; International Radio surgery Association; May 2008.
- VA Guidelines for gamma knife Facility.

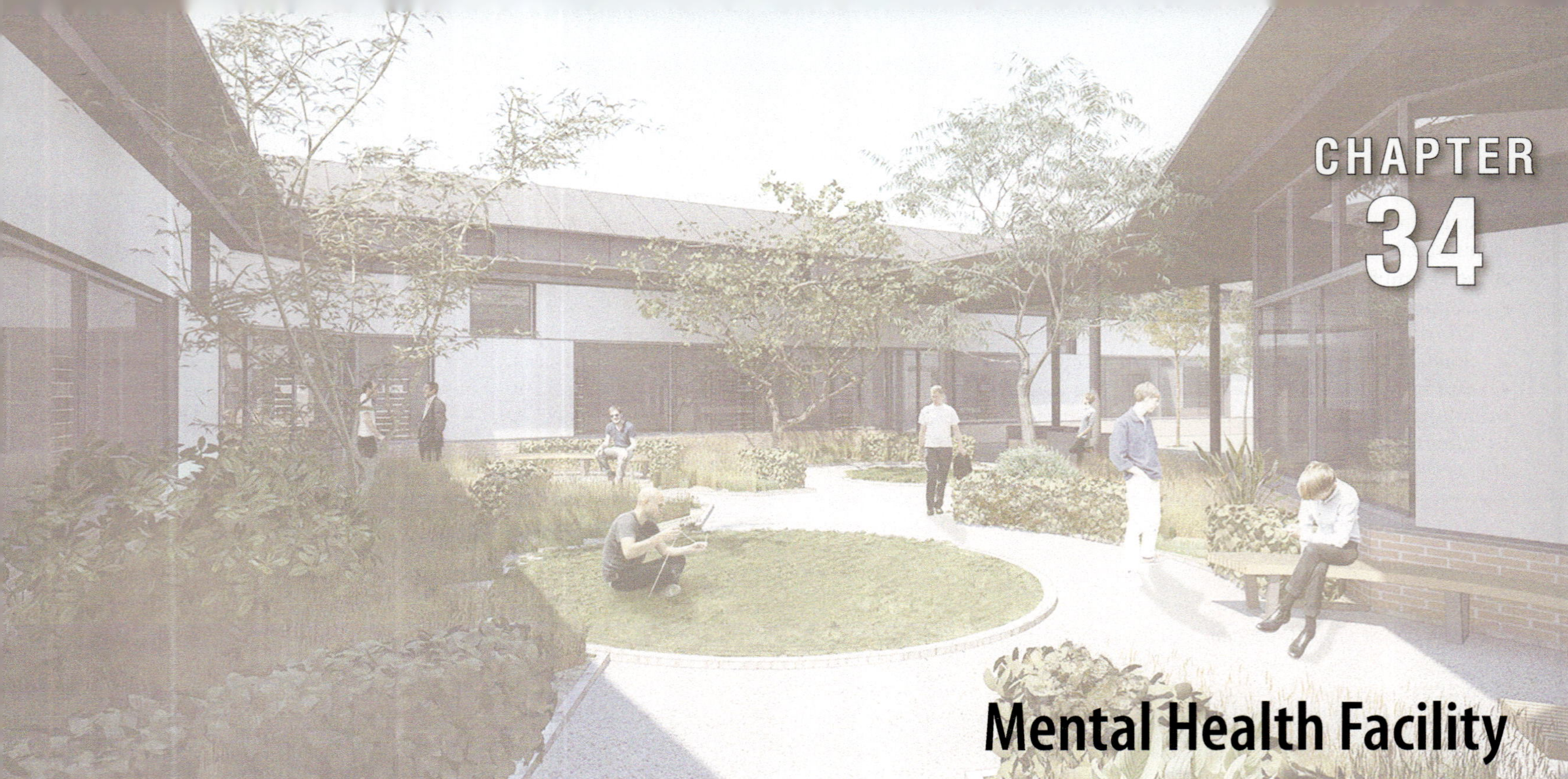

CHAPTER 34

Mental Health Facility

Laxmi Tej Wundavalli, Shakti Kumar Gupta, Sunil Kant, R Chandrashekhar

INTRODUCTION

The World Health Organization (WHO) defines mental health as a state of well-being in which the individual realizes his/her own abilities, can cope with the normal stresses of life, can work productively and is able to make a contribution to his/her community. Mental and behavioral disorders is likely to increase to 15% of the burden of diseases by 2020. The prevalence of mental disorders is higher in developed countries, but the global burden of untreated mental disease is higher in developing nations. Eighty percent of the population suffering with mental illnesses lives in low- and middle-income (LAMI) countries. The presence of mental illness not only affects the individual and his personal, social, educational and occupational life, but also his entire family to suffer from negative consequences. The mean number of psychiatric beds in the world per 10,000 population is 4.36 (Standard Deviation: 5.47). The median number of psychiatric beds per 10,000 population is 1.6 and varies from 0.33 in the South-East Asia Region to 8.7 in the European Region. Most of the psychiatric beds (65.1%) in the world are in mental hospitals.[1-4]

As per WHO in India, neuropsychiatric disorders are estimated to contribute to 11.6% of the global burden of disease. A study conducted in National Institute of Mental Health and Neurosciences (NIMHANS), Bengaluru reported that the burden of mental and behavioral disorders ranged from 9.5 to 102 per 1,000 population. In another study, the prevalence rate of mental disorders in the Indian industrial population was estimated to be 14–37%. Specifically, the suicide rate for males is 12.2 per 100,000 population and for females is 9.1 per 100,000 population. There are currently 43 mental hospitals available in the country available at the rate of 0.004% per 100,000 population. There are around 17,835 beds in mental hospitals available that cater at the rate of 1.469 per 100,000 population. The admission rate to mental hospitals is 14.52 per 100,000 population.[1,3]

NEED FOR THE CENTER

While there has been a shift from institutionalization to community-based care owing to several technical and sociopolitical events that have occurred in the world over the years, the need for mental health facilities cannot be ignored. The key issue for service planners is to determine the optimal mix of services and the level of provision of particular service delivery channels. Often, patients with severe mental disorders like major depression, schizophrenia, bipolar affective disorder, and dementia would require short-term hospitalization especially during the acute conditions. It is therefore necessary to plan for mental health facilities taking into account various factors that influence and inform persons with mental illnesses.

Psychiatric inpatient facilities present a unique set of challenges, and the solutions to designing safe facilities are often completely different from what is typically done for medical/surgical units in a general hospital. Variables that influence key components of the design of a mental health facility are low tolerance for risk and safest possible environment for patients, home-like ambience, require upgraded finishes, funding source (public or private), organizational structure (not-for-profit or for-profit), patients' average length of stay, diagnoses, disease acuity, age of patients, co-existing medical conditions, whether the patients are voluntary admissions or committed by the court. Suicide prevention and other patient and staff safety (including sexual safety) issues in psychiatric treatment units are some extremely important parameters to be understood while designing a mental health facility.[5,6]

HISTORICAL EVOLUTION OF MENTAL HEALTH FACILITIES

The planning and design aspects of mental health facilities have undergone changes based on how mental illnesses were recognized, understood, labeled and treated over the years. From the 4th century AD many public buildings such as monasteries, nunneries and churches were used for healing mentally deranged persons. In the middle ages, some hospitals began to admit persons with mental illnesses as a new type of patient.[7,8]

The concept of asylums arose with the era of industrialization. Urbanization and increased pressure for family members to be productive within the industrial era made family and parish-based models of care difficult to sustain. An institutional response was demanded by Britain's middle-class, who were increasingly driven by self-interest. The asylum, as it was understood within the nineteenth century, was a constructed environment in which architecture and landscape were carefully articulated to aid the restoration of sanity. Architecture was thus considered a therapeutic tool; one of the few remedies available for the treatment of an affliction that carried devastating consequences.[7,8]

The early asylum architecture was based on prison (Fig. 1). The evolving treatment paradigms continued to influence architecture meant for persons with mental illnesses. The introduction of moral treatment initiated independently by the French doctor, Philippe Pinel and the English Quaker, William Tuke in the eighteenth century further informed the processes of care and heralded the reform movement.

Samuel Tuke, WAF Browne and John Conolly were the three most influential men in nineteenth century asylum design. Tuke's *Description of the Retreat* (1813) was a key text in the spread of moral treatment and its corresponding architectural approach. This text became a constant guide for asylum reformers in Britain between 1813 and 1845. Browne's *What Asylums Were, Are and Ought to Be* (1837) and Conolly's *The Construction and Governance of Asylums* (1847) also followed as significant guides to asylum administration and design. The idea that asylums should be curative environments was central to the reform movement and, as a consequence, the approach to asylum design changed.[7,8]

The York Retreat in England was founded by Quakers, in 1792, for the treatment of patients from their own society of friends. The establishment of the retreat was motivated by the observation that the general treatment of insane persons was too frequently calculated to depress and degrade, rather than to awaken the slumbering reason, or correct its wild hallucinations.[7,8]

From 1843 onwards, asylum architecture began to align more closely with the principles developed at the York Retreat and shifted away from the custodial solutions that had hitherto informed this typology. Samuel Tuke's *Description of the York Retreat,* published in 1813, was a constant guide for reformers. The Retreat, therefore, was instrumental in the promotion of moral treatment in Britain. The York Retreat was the first asylum purpose built with moral treatment in mind.[7,8]

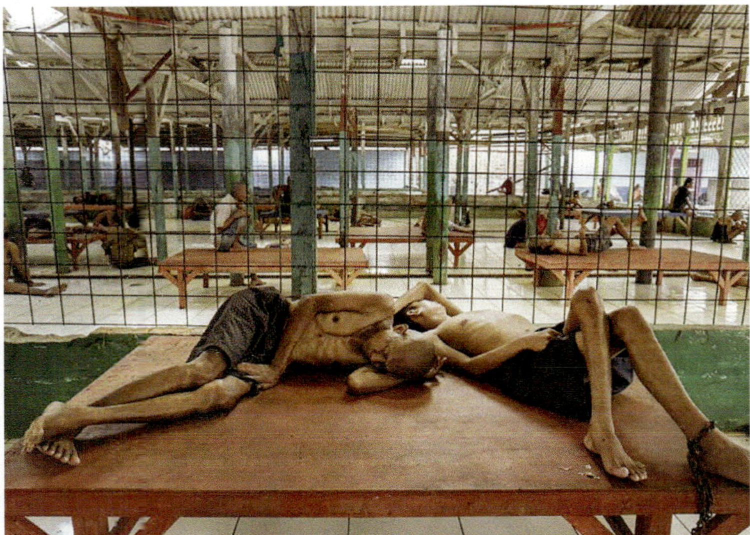

Fig. 1: Early asylum architecture was based on prison concept.

From its architecture to its domestic arrangements, the Retreat was designed to encourage the individual's own efforts to reassert his powers of self-control. York Retreat was constructed with a domestic ambience in order to mask the unpalatable necessity that the insane must be detained. The terms "deliberately domestic" and "parallel universe" have been used to describe the Retreat. Within the retreat the rituals of everyday life were preserved as closely as possible. The architecture reflected this with spaces organized to encourage patients to maintain civil habits and dining rooms increasingly mimicked the appearance of domestic settings. Pictures adorned the walls and mantelpieces, while tables were set with flower vases, napkins, cutlery and water glasses.[7,8]

It has been suggested that the asylum, its goals and functions, are inseparable from its architecture because moral management and moral architecture are synonymous.

An important aspect of treating mental illness was to remove the patient from the stresses of daily life and from the environment in which madness had developed. Rural locations were favored for asylum construction owing to their ability to 'neutralize the moral poisons of congestion and disorder' that were prevalent in cities. In the nineteenth century, cities were viewed as both morally and physically unhealthy. While rural locations enabled an array of outdoor recreations and employments, a necessary aspect of moral treatment, pastoral views, made an equally important contribution. A pleasant and tranquil outlook was believed to have a calming influence on the mind. The American landscape architect Frederick Law Olmsted, who completed designs for New York's Central Park (1858) and the Buffalo State Asylum (1872–80) believed that pastoral scenery "subconsciously exerted a calming and rejuvenating influence on the psyche."[7,8]

The first asylum to be constructed in America was the Friends Asylum, in Philadelphia, in 1817. This was the direct result of a letter of encouragement sent by Samuel Tuke to the Quaker community resident in Philadelphia.

In 1851, an American version of the asylum was beginning to emerge. Physician Thomas Storey Kirkbride (who was also a Quaker) believed that establishing a new building type was "essential" for improving rates of cure. Kirkbride collaborated on many projects with architect Samuel Sloan and created a plan known as the "linear" or "Kirkbride" plan which influenced the construction of 30 American asylum prior to 1866 and a further forty by 1890. The principal difference between the American and the British style asylum was the closed quadrangle typology of the British compared to the more open and domestic form of the American asylum symbolizing a desire to connect to the community.[7,8]

Kirkbride was a founding member of the Association of Medical Superintendents of American Institutions for the Insane (AMSAII), forerunner of the American Psychiatric Association. Through this association and in his writings, Kirkbride promoted his standardized method of asylum construction and mental health treatment, popularly known as the Kirkbride Plan, which significantly influenced the entire American asylum community during his lifetime. The building style almost immediately adopted by the AMSAII as the model for state hospitals, ensured that many state hospitals followed this building design.[7,8]

In his book, on the construction, organization and General Arrangements of Hospitals for the Insane written in 1854, Dr Thomas Kirkbride writes that choosing the site for the new institution should be done with utmost care because the site "may depend to no small extent, the future character and usefulness of the institution; for the best style of building and the most liberal organization can never fully compensate for the loss sustained by a location that deprives the patients of many valuable privileges, or subjects them to varied annoyances." The desired sites should have close access to the railroad or roads in the proximity of a moderately sized town to allow for the easy transportation of patients and goods to the facility. The land itself must offer good opportunities for landscaping as a means of creating a beautiful place in which the patients could exercise while also possessing soils capable of supporting farming as a way of promoting a more self-sustained way of life at the asylum. This land was to total no less than one hundred acres. The tasteful architectural character of the building was required so that it impressed both the patients and any visitors. The asylum building was not to house more than 250 individuals. A population any larger than 250 would sacrifice the comfort of the patients and the abilities of the staff to cure them. To prevent the noxious human exhalations from infecting other patients, physicians believed ventilation and access to fresh air was of great importance in the asylum, and this played a large part in the signature floor plan.[7-9]

Everything from ventilation needs, water access, roof material and construction, the floor plan of the infirmaries and water closets, and descriptions of the roles of the staff were laid out in the Kirkbride model. The most well-known portion to come out of his works was the floor plan, commonly referred to today as the Kirkbride plan. Contemporary usage of the term describes the particular layout of an asylum which consists of a main administration building with wards that fall back in an echelon formation, creating an obtuse V-shape, or "batwing". This layout allowed for optimal access to the landscaped views and fresh air and created a practical system for sorting the patients—the sexes were segregated to separate wings on either side of the administration building and the most disruptive patients could be placed at the far ends of the building, so as not to disturb the calmer patients toward the center.[7-9]

TYPES OF ASYLUM PLAN

Corridor Plan

Earlier asylums followed a basic corridor plan. In this plan, wards flank a central administration block on either side with a central corridor that runs through the length of the building.[9]

Pavilion Plan

This involved a cross-ventilated single ward connected to one another by perpendicular-running corridors.[9]

Radial Pavilion Plan

It is a plan laid out in a spoke-and-wheel pattern. Around the 1870s, this asylum design began to toy with the idea of breaking up the larger echelon structure.[9]

Transition Plan

This plan is a literal transition from large structures to the cottage style structures. The plan incorporated wards setback from Kirkbride-type buildings but they connected to each other via underground passageways making it appear as if the wards were separate entities.[9]

John Conolly, a leading advisor on asylum design and management, recognized, in 1830, that even the best conducted asylums would fail to benefit more than one-third of the patients they treated. For the remaining two-thirds of any asylum population the experience of confinement with other lunatics would "fix and render permanent" mental afflictions that might otherwise have been transitory. Factors such as inadequate funding, difficulties in obtaining staff and the necessity of accommodating more patients than each hospital had been constructed for exacerbated the risk of harm.[7,9]

Conolly's Ideal Features Found in the British Lunatic Asylums[10,11]

These are as follows:

- An appropriate site with some form of scenery
- An arrangement of the buildings that allowed light in and cross ventilation with no building overshadowing another or the airing courts
- A linear form to the layout
- It should accommodate no more than 360–400 inmates
- A building that offered a range of wards for classification
- Each ward should have its own attendant's rooms
- There should be open areas as opposed to day rooms for patients
- Each ward should have access to a bathroom, lavatory and water closets
- Each ward should have a wide gallery furnished as a day room with windows low enough to allow a view outside
- There should be a large recreation room
- School rooms
- Work rooms and workshops
- A prayer hall for the use of patients
- The offices should be centrally located
- There should be a means of accessing the various wards without passing through each
- Attendant's should have their own dining hall
- Accommodation should primarily be in the form of single rooms with a few dormitories.

Arguments against the Asylum Architecture

The detrimental effects to a patient's self-esteem that resulted from the strict daily routines, the forced use of collective space and the social hierarchies that accompanied asylum life were argued against the asylum architecture. It was believed that the architectural acknowledgment of confinement would adversely affect a patient's dignity and impede the curative process. Architectural elements like high walled airing courts and safety bars in stairwells which gave the "gloomy and painful" impression of iron cages were criticized to the extent of recommending erection of single storey asylum to remove the need for stairwell entirely.[7,12]

Villa System (Cottage or Colony System)

In contrast to a monolithic asylum, these hospitals consisted of detached cottages placed throughout the landscape. The key difference between this new hospital type and traditional asylums was that it could, if managed correctly, offer "maximum liberty to those best able to appreciate it". The villa hospital was intended to be run on an "open door system" where traditional, physical means of control such as high fences, locked doors and barred windows would be replaced with "humane but stringent supervision" by nurses and attendants. The physical configuration of the villa hospital facilitated open-door practices because patients with similar behavior could be grouped together and the security measures for each villa specifically tailored in response.[7,8]

Villa hospitals accommodated patients in detached pavilions of between 24 and 50 beds. This allowed for the greater classification (separation) of patients so that those deemed trustworthy were no longer subjected to the strict security concerns of those who were not. It was considered a more humane approach to institutional care because patients who demonstrated consistent behavior were no longer confined to a room, or a building, but given relative freedom within the wider boundaries of the hospital.

Many of the recommendations made by Tuke, Browne and Conolly remained relevant in the construction of villa hospitals, though the physical shape of this model resolved many of the issues encountered with traditional asylum design. Buildings of only two stories, distant from each other within the landscape, allowed easier access to sunshine, natural light and the outdoors, while the smaller scale and domestic esthetic mitigated the "perceptible confinement" present in traditional asylums. Securing a tranquil environment around each patient was also easier since dormitories were generally smaller, superintendents had more options for classification. Like their predecessors, villa hospitals were sited rurally and outdoor employment remained an important feature of the institutional routine.[7,8]

Some of the requirements set out by Tuke, Browne and Conolly either lost their relevance to mental hospital design or had become so ingrained in the planning process that they were no longer discussed. The need for elevated sites disappeared. Flat sites (facilitated by technological advances in drainage) allowed a single villa design to be replicated multiple times with minimal changes to documentation, cost or construction method and thus enabled the easy extension of these hospitals. Maintaining a close proximity to society and issues of safety were no longer discussion points in the design of new mental hospitals. The village model allows patients to exercise more responsibility and control over their experience.[7,8]

Although described as being revolutionary, these cottages segregated patients in the same way as the large linear plan buildings. Just as in the linear plan, patients housed in the cottages were segregated by sex, race, and by degree of insanity. This set up, it was believed, would allow for greater social interaction among the patients and promote a more community curative environment.[7-9]

Arguments against the Villa System

It has been suggested that the villa hospital model was created primarily as a public relations exercise, a response to early antipsychiatry sentiments exhibited by the German public. The priority was for the architecture to simply "*look free*" and thereby present an image of greater humanity in asylum care without necessarily delivering an improved patient experience.[7]

It was also suggested that the psychiatric profession utilized the typology of the asylum as a vehicle to advance their own professional standing with the development of the "villa hospital" in the late nineteenth century.[7]

MENTAL HEALTH FACILITIES IN INDIA

Perhaps the first establishment for treating the mentally ill was the one established by Surgeon George M Kenderline in Calcutta in 1787. However, it could not be granted 'official recognition' as the surgeon had been previously dismissed from service for neglect of duty. Soon after, William Dick in Calcutta established a private asylum for 'insane officers and men, and civilians of various stations' in 1788. Others in Mumbai and Chennai followed. The asylum at Chennai was ordered to be built in 1793, for 16 patients, and given a generous endowment and land, on the provision that no rent was to be paid as long as the building was devoted to public purposes. Asylums within Bengal (Murshidabad, Dacca), Madras (Chittoor, Tiruchirapalli and Masulipatnam) and the Bombay (Colaba) presidencies were set up. Prompted by this, the East India Company in 1802 ordered asylums to be built for the wandering insane in all its territories.[13]

Indian kingdoms were not very encouraging. However, Hoenigberger, a German doctor, who traveled overland and lived in Punjab, did establish a small asylum in Lahore early in the nineteenth century. This was paid for by the court at Lahore, but had been ordered by the British Commissioner. It existed for a few years, and was staffed by European doctors, but it fell into disuse once Hoenigberger returned to Europe. Most asylums were seen to be a cluster of ill-constructed and poorly maintained buildings, resembling gaols rather than asylums. Conditions within were deplorable, with indifferent staff, unwholesome food, inadequate clinical classification and care.[13]

Increasing amounts of admissions to the asylums was now causing significant overcrowding. A significant development was the establishing of the hospital for the European insane in 1918 in Ranchi. Though the most modern, its superintendent, Colonel Berkeley-Hill noted 'that those responsible for the original design were obsessed with its custodial function so as to sacrifice most, if not all, of its remedial potentialities ... it has anything but an agreeable appearance'.[13]

The asylum buildings, Professor Mapother caustically notes, 'were a permanent monument to brutal stupidity', perhaps 'guided by a PWD concept of a lunatic ... (one ward) a replica of the accommodation for tigers at the Regent's park Zoo' and some a 'desolate waste, based on the assumption that the insane are indifferent to discomfort and ugliness, and are destructive'. He rated the asylums on a grade of 'badness', with only the Asylums of Ranchi (for Europeans) in British India, and the one in Bengaluru in the Kingdom of Mysore having anything to commend them. However, he wondered at the waste of money on an asylum for Europeans, recently established by Berkeley-Hill with much triumph, 'based on a concept of race that in practice is unreal, and does not correspond to education, mode of life or any valid claim'. On the other hand, the asylum in Bengaluru, he told Sir Sikander Mirza, the *Diwan* of Mysore, was a 'monument to the vision and wisdom of all those responsible for the mental defectives in the East. The institution is almost unique among mental Hospitals in India ... it is quite evident that modern methods of diagnosis and treatment are available and freely used'.[13]

Dr Vidyasagar in the Amritsar Mental Hospital introduced one of the most remarkable innovations in mental hospital care in the early 1950s. He erected tents in the grounds, and encouraged families to live with the patients, until they recovered. He shared almost all his working hours with the patients and their families. Principles of mental health, derived from religious and medical sources, were shared. This significantly reduced the stigma of mental illness, and demonstrated the feasibility of community care.[13]

Models of psychiatric care in the last fifty years have been based on the ideal of a therapeutic milieu or community. There has been a general progression towards an open ward policy (Fig. 2). Together with major advances in psychopharmacology, this has changed the treatment and care offered in psychiatric facilities. Altered treatment has led to an area of deinstitutionalization, and the psychiatric inpatient care is now mainly designed for short-term treatment of the severely mentally ill.[13]

The Mental Healthcare Act 2017 mandates the setting up of Mental Health Authorities at National and State levels will supervise all mental health establishments develops quality and service provisions norms for such establishments. As per the Act, every person will have the right to access mental healthcare services. Such services should be of good quality, convenient, affordable and accessible.[14]

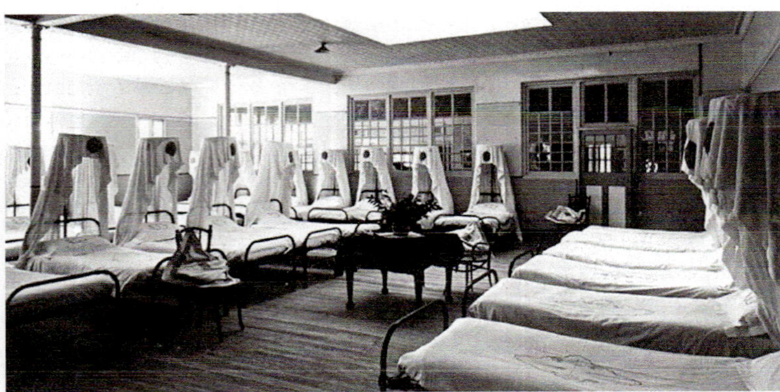

Fig. 2: Toward an open ward policy.

PLANNING AND DESIGN CONSIDERATIONS

Design Considerations Specific to a Mental Health Facility

The salutary potential of architecture is increasingly being recognized especially in facilities that provide mental health services. Though the evidence for direct impact of therapeutic design on treatment outcomes is scarce, there is evidence to suggest that architecture can influence mental health outcomes.

A mental health facility should be designed in such a way as not only to serve as a temporary home for psychiatric patients but its environment should aid recovery. Psychiatric patients, more so than general hospital patients, present a range of symptoms, illnesses and responses to the physical environment that require special attention and understanding by the designers. Patients are prone to distorted perceptual systems that make them especially vulnerable to confusing building forms and layouts, or even to a lack of tactile, acoustic, temporal, olfactory or visual stimulus. Some may have sensory processing deficits or cognitive disorders. Typical behaviors exhibited by patients include—aggression, violence towards self and/or others, destruction of their environment, an inclination to abscond and loss of capacity for self-control.[15-18]

The relationship between a patient and the environment is transactional and not fixed. The environment effectively changes according to the subject's sensory and perceptual abnormalities such as hallucinations and disorders of thought such as delusions. Perception has been defined as a complex neurochemical process that is highly reactive to the surrounding environment and yet it is the only channel for receiving new information of any sort. The act of perception itself can trigger psychotic events. The mental health facility has the responsibility of ensuring the well-being of the patient and protecting his/her sense of meaning.[18]

Comprehensibility is an important design consideration in view of the symptoms like delusions that are pathognomonic of major psychiatric disorders. The design should minimize ambiguity and maximize comprehensibility by using simple typologies, clear wayfinding/signages, and clear textures, objects and lines.

Typology of the architecture can influence symptomatology as each typology is symbolically and phenomenologically loaded. The design has to be specifically sensitive to typologies that may have negative meanings. The efficacy of healthcare design will also depend on the implicit messages it communicates to different users.

As per the stress model, any design that increases stress levels should be avoided in health design unless the stress itself can have a salutogenic effect.

A stimulating environment maintains and restores synaptic plasticity. On the other hand, a socially and materially deprived environment causes synaptic atrophy. Also, many patients have limited or atrophying cognitive abilities and skills. These aspects should be considered during the spatial design and arrangement in a therapeutic manner.

Apart from the built environment visual and physical access to natural settings like woods, garden, parks, etc. have been recognized to play a crucial role in the process of recovery as well as to therapeutically engage the patient.

The institutional character of settings directly affects a patient's wellbeing leading to unwanted and threatening behaviors. The external and internal architectural features and interior design elements should be carefully designed so as to give a residential feel without compromising on security and safety including sexual safety. It is necessary to minimize the potential for furnishings, fixtures, and equipment within the facility to be used as a weapon or anchor point for hanging care should be taken that while the design of the facility makes manageability for the staff extremely efficient, it should not take power from the patients and erode their sense of meaning. The atmosphere should support patient autonomy and spontaneity.

Overall, the facility should be client centered, with the aim of maximizing well-being which itself is an important health outcome.

TYPES OF MENTAL HEALTH FACILITIES

Psychiatric facilities include psychiatric hospitals, psychiatric and neuropsychiatric nursing units of general hospitals, facilities for the psychiatric medically infirm, geropsychiatric units, alcohol and drug addiction treatment facilities (both inpatient and outpatient), mental health clinics, day hospitals, day treatment centers, and others.[15]

Therapeutic Milieu or Environment

Therapeutic milieu is a term that is also interchangeable with patient-centered design and healing environments. A therapeutic environment can be defined as a patient care environment that helps make patients more receptive to the treatment provided by staff. Some who provide services to psychiatric patients feel the built environment where these patients receive services should resemble a "typical residential" atmosphere. Unfortunately, patients from different backgrounds may have entirely different views of what constitutes a home-like setting. A more realistic goal, then, should be to create a non-threatening environment in which patients can feel relaxed and comfortable. To achieve this, architects must work closely with hospital staff, patient groups, interior designers, and psychiatric hospital consultants.[7,8,18]

A critical consideration for securing recoveries was that a tranquil environment would be secured around all patients, yet, no clear set of principles was provided for the architectural realization of tranquility. While specific recommendations were available regarding planning configuration, surface finishes, lock types and window heights, they did not distil the relationship of these elements to the treatment delivered. Nonetheless, a number of architectural elements were relevant to the provision of tranquility, such as asylum size, the provision of private versus public space and, the size and location of dormitories and wards.[7,8,18]

Kaplan-included three components that are necessary for the restorative experience: "being away," which implies not merely entering a new setting, but instead a change that "involves a conceptual rather than a physical transformation"; an environment that is rich but that maintains coherence; and compatibility between the environment and one's own goals.[18]

Dobrohotoff and Llewellyn Jones make the following recommendations for designing the optimal physical environment:[18]

- Optimize patient and staff safety, manage patients' physical health, and design a productive ward environment.
- Ensure access to a psychiatric intensive care unit (PICU) or high dependency unit (HDU).
- Provide space—a garden, a quiet area, a seclusion suite, an activity and games room.
- Include separate bedrooms with louver-type observation panels, doors that open two ways, vandal-proof dimmer light fittings, and safe fixtures and duress alarms.
- Design an environment that is secure, structured, with minimal stimulation, non-intrusive, and supportive.
- Create a design that facilitates patient observation as well as high nurse-to-patient ratios.
- Facilitate limited use of restraints and seclusion.
- Make it possible for cognitively impaired patients to be segregated from those who are not cognitively impaired.
- Create separate male and female sections.
- Provide direct access to usable outdoor space.
- Have clear indications for the intended use of each area or room.
- Optimize the location of nurses' station to enable direct line of sight to as much area as possible.
- Ensure locked doors on secure wards.
- If possible create good external visibility and access to public transportation.

In addition, design should incorporate deinstitutionalization features such as:

- Separate living and treatment areas.
- The elimination of long echoing corridors and highly reverberant spaces.
- Residential features such as a laundry and galley kitchens.
- Reduced psychopathology among younger patients facilitated by design solutions that encouraged social interactions—ward kitchen, an open nursing station, and a dayroom module for crafts and other occupational therapy activities.

Entrance

The presence of numerous and diverse activities and services in a hospital can cause a 'sensory overload'. For this, the morphology of the environment is particularly important. It should facilitate the identification of main directions. The unitary language of the architectural elements and furnishings is important too. The user, especially the patient, should be able to perceive it as simple and cross instinctively, without being confused. So the presence of a system of way finding assumes a fundamental role, contributing to the construction of mental maps.[5]

Reception Area

There should be an identifiable reception area for greeting patients and their families in a lobby area. This should be located away from the core patient area to provide privacy. In addition to functional benefits, a reception area sends a welcoming message to users. Sufficient signage should be placed to direct patients and families to this area.[14,16]

Patient Room and Units[7,15,17-24]

For a facility to be therapeutic, it must preserve a sense of privacy and dignity, be well apportioned and maintained and maintain a sense of stability and safety. The creation and maintenance of tranquil spaces has been an area of study since many centuries. Private sleeping spaces were favored and attention was directed toward mitigating sound transmission between bedrooms. Tuke stipulated a maximum ward size of ten patients since he felt that familial relationships tended to develop in a ward of such limited size. Private space offers patients territorial control, feelings of ownership, identity, a sense of dignity and the ability to regulate social interaction, which all enhances the well-being of patients. It is also related to better adjusted behavior and better functioning. Besides, lack of comfort and personal control over the physical environment can lead to distress and helplessness. While, there is no definitive evidence that single rooms provide either clinical or safety advantages, the FGI guidelines recommend a maximum of two patients per room (except that four patients are allowed in children's units). Some studies have reported that private or semi-private space was shown to have a positive impact on social behavior. The use of the room and interactive behaviors decreases as the number of beds per room increases. Two-person rooms require more than double the space required for a one-person room. Irrespective of the number, activity type rather than mathematical density should dictate room size.[7]

The UK Royal College of Psychiatrists (1998) recommends units of ten to twelve beds to optimize clinical and financial viability. Units smaller than 6–7 beds may not be clinically or financially viable, and may limit the level of amenity/range of recreational facilities that can be provided. However in Australia, fifteen bed units are favorably reported.[14]

Children and young people may have differing needs in relation to bedroom and bathroom facilities: *young people*—privacy will be enhanced through provision of single bedrooms with en suites; *children*— where rooming-in is the preferred approach, larger bedrooms should be provided to accommodate a family member. Shared bedrooms may be appropriate in some circumstances, i.e. where a parent is not 'rooming in'.

Geriatric Patients

Bed numbers are recommended to be between 8 and 12 beds per cluster depending on local factors. Larger facilities may be more confusing for older patients and high quality care is easier to provide in small groups. Groups of eight beds have been found to be sufficiently small for the care of mobile, confused and disturbed older people. An 18–24 bed unit, consisting of multiple clusters, is considered to be efficient from a staffing and budget perspective.

Windows and Natural Daylight

Multiple windows with views of nature as an important design feature because these views can reduce psychological distress as well as recovery time. It has been stated that larger windows low to the ground have the potential to improve sensory abilities and reduce delirium and paranoia among patients. By reducing stress and fatigue, exposure to nature may facilitate recovery.[25]

Lighting

The role of natural light has been implicated in disorders like eating disorders, depression, Alzheimer's disease. It has physiological implications related to circadian rhythm, sensory stimulation, therapeutic design, and therapeutic patient rooms. The different effects of natural versus artificial lighting on patients, specifically in the areas of illuminance, uniformity, diffusion, color, and UV radiation have been found to affect human chronobiology. These play a key role in disorders like seasonal affective disorder (SAD), sleep disorders, work disruptions, etc.[16,18]

Natural circadian rhythms regulate melatonin production, which influences biochemical and hormonal body rhythms, which have the following effects upon mental health—reduced depression, decreased length of stay, improved sleep and circadian rhythm, lessened agitation, eased pain, and easier adaptation to night-shift work.[18]

Numerous clinical studies demonstrate that artificial bright light can suppress the onset of melatonin and therefore reduce depression among patients with bipolar disorder. Furthermore, there is strong evidence that exposure to bright light in the morning is more effective in reducing depression than exposure to bright light in the afternoon. In addition, the natural circadian rhythm of light regulates melatonin production, influencing biochemical and hormonal body rhythms. The body's circadian rhythms are governed by eating and regulation to natural light cycles; therefore, because eating disorder patients cannot use food to regulate the body, natural light can be a key design consideration. Morning light has also been shown to reduce agitation.[18,24]

While it has been proven that people's moods are affected by different lighting conditions, these mood changes are not consistent in every setting. Given the same lighting conditions, an individual's discomfort, preferences, expectations, and gender will determine how a given lighting condition influences their mood. These differences are essential to the design of a psychiatric hospital.[24]

Patients prefer natural light to artificial light. While some patients such as the bipolar cases benefit from bright morning light, manic-depressive patients are often highly sensitive to light and glare. In addition, antipsychotic and antidepressant medications have the side effect of heightening photosensitivity. For this reason, designers should provide plenty of options for shading and the reduction of glare, and give patients as much control as possible over their experience of natural and artificial light.

The control of light can be exercised on two levels. First, in patient rooms, blinds can be installed between panes of glass so that patients can control their own windows without risk of injury. Second, allowing lights in private rooms to be controlled by a dimmer switch rather than an on/off mechanism will allow patients more control over their experience. While such a function would require a community decision in dayroom areas, it is possible architecturally to allow patients a choice as to how much natural daylight they would like to experience; both sunny and shaded areas can be designed within the same room.[18]

Direction of the Rooms

The building's orientation needs to maximize sunlight to internal and external spaces in the unit, in particular bedrooms and activity areas. In a study conducted at the University of Milan, it was found that bipolar depressed inpatients in east-facing rooms (exposed to bright light in the morning) stayed an average of 3.67 days less in the psychiatric treatment facility than similar patients in west-facing rooms.[18]

AGITATION AND LIGHT (FIG. 3)

Morning light has also been shown to reduce agitation. It was found that when elderly patients were exposed to 2500 lux for 2 hours in the morning for two 10-day periods, their agitation was reduced. The study also demonstrated that the patients were significantly more agitated on nontreatment days.[22]

Studies have suggested connections between exposure to bright light and depression as well as the length of stay in the hospitals. Symptoms of seasonal affective disorder (SAD) and the depressive phase of bipolar disorder were diminished through exposures "between 2,500 and 10,000 lux," with the greatest benefits found in the morning rather than the evening.[16,18]

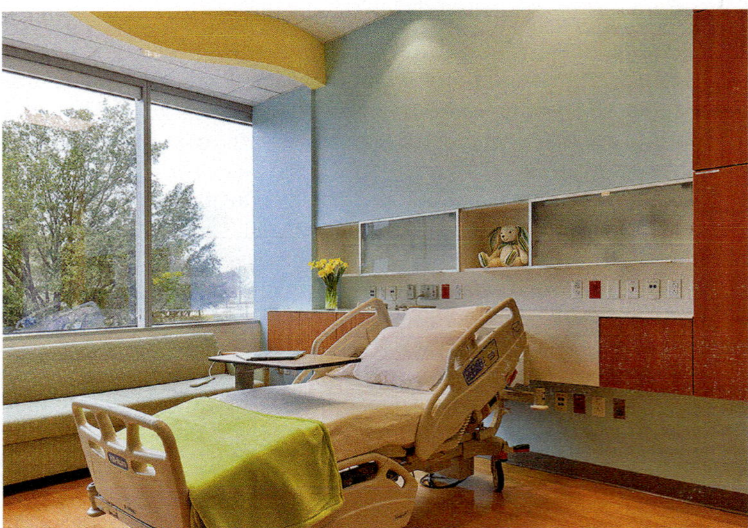

Fig. 3: Use of natural light.

Geriatric Patients and Light (Fig. 4)

The light requirements for older people may be five times higher than that of young people. Older adults take between 5 and 30 minutes to adapt to change when entering space with considerably lower light level, such as entering from outside. In a study by Brawley, the focus was on the links between Alzheimer's, therapeutic design, and sensory stimulants, saying that lighting is important for more than just vision, affecting endocrine systems and producing vitamin D, as well as other benefits already mentioned. The positive associations of daylight and routine activities outdoors with sensory stimulation and interaction with nature was seen to have a beneficial effect on patients suffering from Alzheimer's. Simultaneously, the problem of controlling indoor glare and flicker should be considered.[16,18]

Safety Issues Related to Lighting

Lighting with 2 × 4 inch fluorescent fixtures, commonly used in general hospitals, does not provide a residential feel and replacing such fixtures with round or oval vandal-resistant fixtures or vandal-resistant wall sconces can simultaneously improve safety and make a big difference in the character of a facility. Lighting must limit patient access to the bulbs, and thus to their glass and electrical contacts. Table lamps are very difficult to do well and should generally be avoided. Lighting fixtures in patient toilets and showers should be a security type with fully enclosed frames, lenses of polycarbonate or similar material, and security fasteners.[6]

General Illumination

About 2 × 2 inch (0.6 m × 0.6 m), 2 × 4 inch (0.6 m × 1.21 m) recessed fluorescent fixtures/LED lights or 9 inch diameter (228.6 mm) vandal/wet-lensed down-lights may be used with a high strength acrylic lens and flush trim anchored with tamper resistant screws.[18]

Over-bed Lighting

Wall mounted over bed lighting, especially for semi-private rooms should be installed above the bed. These fixtures should be designed so they cannot be used as an anchor point, should be securely fastened

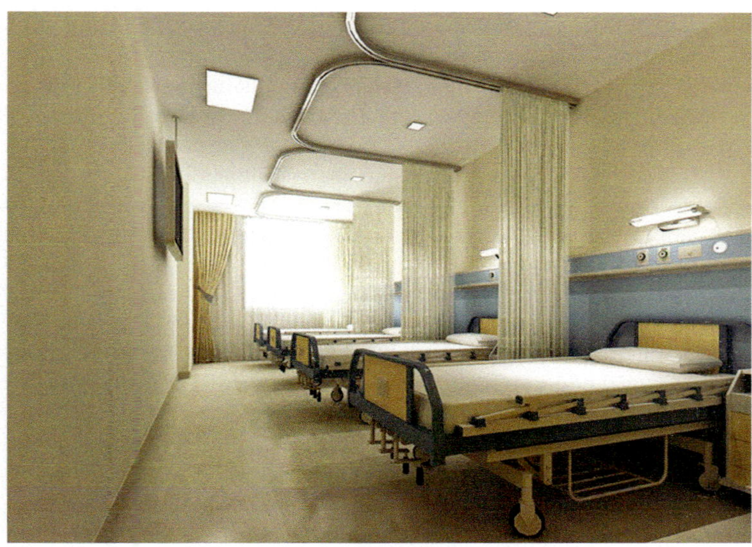

Fig. 4: Geriatric patients and light.

to the wall with tamper resistant screws and have high strength acrylic lenses. Correctional type wall mounted lights should not be used for overbed lighting.[18]

Night Lighting

Night lighting should be provided in all patient rooms and bathrooms to prevent patient falls and injury and also to allow staff to verify a patient's well being during the night without turning on additional lights.[18]

Color

The color blue has been indicated to subdue aggressive individuals and "visual monotony can contribute to physiological and emotional stress."[16,18]

Sensation and Perception

In terms of touch, Mazuch and Stephen noted the important role this can have in the recovery of patients, as surfaces help to "re-engage with the materiality of the world". They emphasized that perceptual confusion should be avoided (e.g. a wood-grain finish on a metal door would give inaccurate sensory information because a metal door will be heavier and colder than would be expected with a real wooden door). The architects noted that smell can relax muscles and aid concentration; pleasant smells help produce endorphins and can decrease heart rate. Pleasing aromas may reduce blood pressure, slow respiration, and lower pain perception levels; unpleasant odors stimulate anxiety, fear, and stress.[16,18]

Sound

Echoes, as well as repetitive sounds, should be eliminated as much as possible as this exacerbates delusional 'voices'. It must be noted that hard materials absorb less noise. Excessive noise has implications for increased heart rate, blood pressure, respiration, and blood cholesterol. Noise has been shown to inhibit the ability to learn, increase stress, reduce prosocial behavior, and increase the potential for conflict and aggressive behavior. In one study, acoustics was rated as the most significant architectural feature influencing the behavior of autistic children.[5,18]

Elements of Design not Desired in a Psychiatric Unit[6,18]

Providing general hospital elements in typical behavioral health units unnecessarily reinforces the institutional character of such facilities, may needlessly increase cost, and may actually lessen safety in the built environment. Elements, such as 2 × 4 inch fluorescent light/LED fixtures, medical gas outlets, bedpan washers, nurse call systems, light fixtures located directly over the bed to enable staff to perform medical procedures, wrist handles on faucet valves, paddle-style door hardware are not recommended in a psychiatric unit.[6,22]

Any fitting or fixture capable of supporting a consumer's weight should be avoided, unless it is an item of furniture intended to bear the consumer's/patient's weight. Fittings in this unit require a breaking strain of no more than 15 kg.[6]

In addition, fittings should be safe, durable, tamper proof and concealed where possible. They should be flush with the surfaces to which they are attached, or designed in a way that prevents attachment of anything around them.[6]

Issues of Safety in Bathrooms

According to the Joint Commission, 75% of inpatient suicides take place in the bathroom, bedroom, or closet. Bathrooms must be designed with safety in mind, and compromises in these rooms can have disastrous results.[6]

It is recommended that there should be one patient toilet room per patient room located directly accessible to the patient room without the need to enter the corridor. Some facilities are not comfortable with this requirement and prefer the staff to be able to observe when patients enter the toilet rooms.[6,17]

Patient toilets are the location of many acts of self-harm because patients are alone in them without supervision and the rooms typically have many potentially hazardous features. It is important that patient toilet room doors swing out of the room to reduce the opportunity for patients to barricade themselves in these rooms and to allow staff access in the event a patient passes out while in the toilet room. Care must be taken to avoid conflict during operation between an in-swinging patient room/corridor door and an outswinging patient toilet room door.[6,18]

Toilet room doors themselves can present numerous hazards. Several suitable products are available to use instead of standard doors. Some facilities are considering the option of leaving doors off the toilet room in single-patient rooms with no direct line of sight into the toilet room from the corridor when the corridor door is open.[6,18]

Soap dishes should be recessed and not have grab handles.

Shower Curtains

If possible, shower stalls should be designed so a shower curtain is not needed. Use of shower curtains is highly discouraged since they simultaneously provide an attachment point and a ligature in the form of the curtain. If they must be used, an aluminum track mounted flush to the ceiling with an absolute minimum of breakaway fasteners could be provided. However, the curtain can be bunched up so the holding weight of all the fasteners can be added together. The shower curtains themselves should always be made of a breathable material such as woven fabric with applied waterproofing. The shower curtain should be suspended from a recessed track with plastic clips or Velcro tabs that will allow the curtain to collapse, with less than 1.81 kg (4 lbs) of weight applied.[16-18]

Light Fixtures

Light fixtures in the patient toilets and showers should be security type with fully enclosed frames, polycarbonate or similar lenses and security fasteners.[18]

Grab Bars

It is recommended that all patient toilets have at least one ligature-resistant and suicide resistant grab bar to assist patients who are on medications that disturb their sense of equilibrium. It must be especially important that the handrail should allow full grip. There should be no space for hiding items. The most common solution to open grab bars as a hanging hazard has been to install a bar with a stainless steel plate welded to the bottom to close the opening between the bar and the wall. However, this arrangement creates an undesirable side effect where the plate meets the bottom of the bar where water can collect and create an infection control problem which can be addressed.[6,19]

Preferably, the use of horizontal grab rails in toilets and showers should be avoided. Solid, vertical rails with moulded hand grip are preferred.[6,18]

Towel Dispensers and Soap Dispensers

Towel dispensers and soap dispensers are not recommended. Hard plastic paper towel dispensers and soap dispensers can be fairly easily removed from the wall and broken to yield very sharp pieces of plastic that can be used as weapons. Towel bars should not be used. Collapsible hooks for towels should be provided.[6]

Toilet Paper Dispensers

Toilet paper dispensers can be hanging hazards, and springs from spring-loaded tubes that hold the paper can be removed or smashed and made into sharp objects. One solution is a stainless steel tube that is recessed into the wall to hold the entire roll. Some facilities object to this as an infection control issue because everyone using the roll has to handle it. Another option is a steel product that completely contains the roll of paper.[6]

Lavatory Tap/ Faucet and Valves

The lavatory tap and valves also provide attachment points. Wall-hung lavatories are losing favor because of their institutional appearance and because they provide little space for patients to set their toiletries. Solid-surface countertops with integral sinks are much more functional and residential in nature. Pipes below the countertop can be enclosed with a rather typical looking vanity cabinet (with recessed pulls and securely locked doors). Ligature-resistant valves that will give patients control of the duration of flow and temperature of the water (within limits) are preferable as these give behavioral health patients, who have so much control taken away from them, some control of their environment.[6]

Shelves

Shelves, either recessed or ligature-resistant surface-mounted units, can be provided to hold a few towels. Some object to this suggestion, saying patients will use the towels to clog the toilets. However, if they are so inclined, they can simply remove a quantity of paper towels from a typical dispenser, which also provides other hazards.[6]

Patient Showers and Bathtubs

Patient showers and bathtubs are of major concern. The obvious hazard of potential drowning plus the added risks from valves and fill spout are problematic. Patients can use showers if careful attention is given to all aspects of the design of the room, including the following:[6]

- Institutional-type shower heads have been around for a number of years and work reasonably well in this environment.
- A variety of water control valves provide ligature resistant as well as control of water temperature and duration of flow.

For remodeling work, assemblies that have stainless steel panels with the head and valve already mounted are available.

Alternative arrangements for towel storage, such as a bench or shelf, should be considered to avoid use of towel rails or hooks.

Windows and Window Coverings

Studies have shown that a lack of windows and connection to the outside world can heighten stress and depression. In the past, very heavy stainless steel screens were often installed as a safety measure. Although still used in some facilities, these screens provide a very institutional or prison-like appearance. A variety of window glazing materials that cannot be easily broken to produce sharp shards of glass and, if broken, will stay in the frame to resist egress are appropriate for use in psychiatric facilities. Tempered glass breaks into very small pieces that do not stay in the frame; laminated glass will stay in the frame but yields shards. Polycarbonate sheets satisfy both of these requirements (provided the stops are deep enough to account for the amount of deflection in large pieces). Polycarbonate may require frequent replacement if graffiti is scratched onto its surface and therefore is not recommended as it suffers from surface scratching which obscures vision. Any windows that open should be designed so that they will not allow patient escape, with locks under the control of staff. Locks should be flush with surrounding window frames and not provide a ligature point. Fixed fly screens should be attached to opening windows to prevent removal by consumers. New cyclone and bomb resistant glazing materials and films that can be applied to increase shatter resistance are also available.[6,16,18,21]

Flooring

Flooring in mental health facilities, both inpatient and outpatient, should promote a warm, bright, and healing environment. The flooring material should be secured to the floor, not easily torn or dislodged and free of tripping hazards. Floors with high glare can cause difficulty for psychotic patients and older patients and, therefore, should be avoided. Wood grain pattern sheet vinyl flooring and molding profile rubber base enhance the residential feel. Sheet vinyl flooring now comes in a range of colors and textures. The wood grain patterns in particular create a more residential feel and are strongly recommended for inpatient units. Use of wood toned vinyl flooring can significantly brighten up the area and enhance the esthetic environment. Similarly, rubber base manufactures now produce a base that simulates wood base profiles which creates a residential image without sacrificing safety.[15]

Wall/Ceiling Finishes

Basic wall finishes in the patient rooms should be painted gypsum board. At least one of the walls should have a soothing warm color accent to avoid an all neutral, institutional look. High impact panels with a wood grain texture create the appearance of wood wainscot. This is an excellent feature that can add great warmth throughout the unit and to exterior areas leading to the unit.[17]

Height of Ceilings

High ceilings have been recommended to hinder access to ceiling fixtures that can be used as anchor points for hanging.[15]

Furniture[6,17]

Soft, upholstered furniture with wood accents that is constructed to withstand severe abuse can be anchored in place to avoid stacking or throwing. Use of color, texture, and natural materials such as transparent wood finishes can provide a more residential feel. Patient room furniture should be anchored securely, with the possible exception of a desk chair (if provided). This is to reduce the possibility of patients using furniture to barricade themselves in a room or stacking or piling the furniture for other purposes. Patients have been known to throw furniture or use it to strike staff. Electric hospital beds present extreme hazards and have been used in successful suicides. Careful attention should be given to the furniture arrangement and the location of the door. Seating for staff should always be closer to the door than the patients' chairs. Although somewhat counterintuitive, this arrangement is very important so that staff always have an escape route in case a patient becomes violent. Duress alarms are also highly desirable in these rooms.

All outdoor furniture should be anchored firmly in place. This is to prevent the furniture from being moved to create barricades or stacked to allow climbing over fences, into windows or onto buildings.

Alternately, modular furniture has been suggested so that it can be converted and re-arranged. Furniture should not be located adjacent to a fence or a wall.

Furniture Location and Arrangement

Several studies suggest a relationship between furniture location and arrangement and frequency of social interaction. These studies indicated that sociopetal arrangements (seats facing one another or seats perpendicular to one another) are often preferred to sociofugal arrangements (seats parallel to one another or seating arrangements in which seats face away from one another). Simultaneously, greater distance between seating should be provided to decrease social pressure.[16]

Furniture should be sized appropriately to the child and/or young adolescent patient group and be arranged to promote positive group dynamics.[13,21]

Mirrors

Mirrors should be preferably made from safety glass or other appropriate impact-resistant and shatterproof construction; are scratch proof; and are free from distortion. Mirrors should be fully glued to a backing to prevent loose fragments of broken glass. In areas where damage to glass may be anticipated, larger pane sizes should be avoided as smaller panes are inherently stronger.[21]

Standard Patient Beds

Beds for mental health inpatients without mobility or other medical needs should consist of a heavy duty platform bed. Edges should be rounded. Provisions for restraints on the sides of the bed frame may need to be incorporated. Beds for bariatric patients should be similar but larger dimensionally. Electric hospital beds may be substituted for platform beds where appropriate for geropsychiatric patients and other patients with medical needs requiring this type of bed. All cords on this bed should be less than 12 inch (304.8 mm) in length to prevent abuse.[18]

Doors

Anti-ligature hardware should be used for patient room doors to prevent tampering or use as an anchor point. The door hinge should be continuous to prevent the hinge from being used as an anchor point.[16]

Bedroom doors should open outwards to prevent patients from blockading themselves in their bedroom. Outward opening doors should be recessed to prevent obstruction of corridors.

Bathroom Doors[15,17]

- *Door-top pressure sensitive alarm*: This option allows a standard door to be installed in inpatient rooms. A sensor either mounted on the door top or within the door frame, signals the nursing station if weight is applied to the door. This technology is evolving, and experience to date with this option has been limited.
- *Out-swinging door with sloped top*: This option utilizes a standard swinging door with the top of the door cut at a 30° angle or greater to prevent the top of the door being used as an anchor point. This modified door is not as visually appealing and home-like as a straight edge door and provides more limited privacy. The bathroom door should swing out into the patient room, the door hinge should be continuous, and the door hardware should be a lever type with no return for use as an anchor point. The door latch should release when attempted to be used as an anchor point.
- *Sliding door*: A third option for a patient bathroom door is a sliding door. This option requires the top sliding track be inset within the wall and have a receiving wall on the patient room side. A pocket door installation is not recommended. With this option, the top of the door cannot be accessed to use as an anchor point. This door also has the advantage of maintaining privacy and having visual appeal. A potential disadvantage to this option is that use of a track on the floor may present an infection control concern, though this may be effectively managed and may not present a major issue. Use without a track is not recommended, as this may provide the potential for the door to be kicked out by a patient. The sliding door option may not be appropriate for patients with limited upper body strength.

Bathroom Accessories

Mirror: Mirrors in patient bathrooms should be reflective polycarbonate with a stainless steel frame firmly anchored to the wall. No shelf should be part of this frame assembly.

Toilet paper dispenser: A safety toilet paper dispenser consisting of a soft spindle should be used in all patient bathrooms. Recessed toilet paper holders without a spindle should not be used for infection control concerns.[17]

Grab bars: As required for accessible rooms, grab bars should be fixed to the wall with a welded horizontal plate on the bottom of the bar to prevent using these bars as anchor points. Because of patient safety concerns, swinging grab bars at toilets should not be used.[17]

Clothing hooks: Clothing or towel hooks should be designed to collapse when any weight above 1.81 kg (4 lbs) is applied. Shower/Floor drains—Drains should be attached with security screws to prevent removal by patients. Paper towel Dispenser—Paper towel dispensers in patient bathrooms shall be recessed. Soap dispensers—Soap dispensers shall be wall-mounted with sloped tops to prevent this fixture from being used as an anchor point.[16]

Fire Safety

The typical code issues of lighted exit signs, fire sprinklers, fire extinguishers, and so on must be provided, even though they may contribute to a facility's institutional appearance.

However, using the door swing direction often requires provision of fire code-required recesses or alcoves in the corridor, which create observation difficulties. Corridor doors also may be required to be fire-rated and/or equipped with smoke seals and closers. Air grilles and fire sprinkler heads should be provided.[6]

Manhole Covers

All manhole covers, access panels, and area drain grates should be anchored firmly in place to prevent them being removed and used as weapons or allowing patients to enter the underground piping.

Nursing Stations

The nursing station should blend in both in scope and design with the therapeutic environment.

Nursing stations tend to be the social center of the ward. As a result of this dynamic, there are often benches or chairs nearby to provide a place for patients to sit or socialize.

The nursing station has historically been the place where the boundary between patient and caregiver is most clearly drawn. It is also a place where patient information, medication and supplies are stored. It is of the utmost concern that these spaces be secure to protect patient, confidentiality and safety.[17]

The nursing station should be open and not enclosed. Open nursing stations promote nursing staff engagement with patients and involvement on the unit. Open nursing stations send an important message that staff are accessible and often lead to reduced attention seeking behavior by patients. If necessary, laminated glass can be installed in the counter top to prevent patients from accessing the nurse work areas. This glass should be as open as much as possible to allow patients to interact with staff—typically 18 inch laminated glass above the highest counter (frameless to minimize its visual impact) is recommended in such situations. Available reports of experiences with open nursing stations do not support concerns of patient abuse of increased access to nurses.[17]

The nursing station should have direct visibility of all patient wings and activity areas. Bedroom corridors and primary patient activity areas should be directly visible from the nursing station. The primary design focus for the nursing station is to maintain patient confidentiality during significant inputting or reviewing of patient information that requires stationary computer access. The opportunity for equipment within the nursing station to be used as a weapon by the patient should be minimized by integrating computer equipment and storage area into the hardware of the nursing station. In addition large spaces behind, or adjacent to, the nursing station should be avoided, as this often serves as a place for staff to congregate rather than to be out on the floor with patients. Within the nursing station, the task chairs and keyboards should be adjustable to accommodate different staff.[17]

Heating, Ventilation, and Air-conditioning Requirements

Special consideration should be given to ventilation outlets and equipment used:—provide air grilles and diffusers that prevent the insertion of foreign objects;—provide tamper-resistant fasteners where these are exposed;—construct all convector or heating, ventilation, and air conditioning (HVAC) enclosures expressed in the room with rounded corners and with closures fastened with tamper-resistant screws;—use HVAC equipment that minimizes the need for maintenance within the room; and—vents should be fixed to the ceiling to prevent access to the roof cavity.[21]

Outdoor Courtyards and Gardens (Fig. 5)[5,15-25]

Even as early as 1712, it was noted by Joseph Addison that "delightful scenes, whether in nature, painting, or poetry, have a kindly influence on ... the mind, and not only serve to clear and brighten the imagination, but are able to disperse grief and melancholy..."

An essential component of any inpatient mental health facility should be direct, yet secure access by patients to the outdoors. Outdoor spaces should be designed with three key principles in mind:[16]

- Located within the unit to be visible by staff from the nursing station.
- Sufficiently enclosed to discourage the threat of patient elopement.
- Designed with hardscape and landscape features that do not support self-harm or assaultive behavior.

The open precincts within the hospital are necessary (i) to provide a safe outdoor environment; (ii) to provide a place for reflection; (iii) to provide a place for relaxation; (iv) to provide a place for socialization; and (v) to provide a place for people to maintain the hobby of gardening.[3]

The presence of the gardens can be one of the most positive aspects of psychiatric treatment. Curtis, Gesler, Priebe, and Hickman (2009) noted that in the post-asylum age of mental healthcare, long-term patients were known to return to the asylums in which they were housed in order to walk in the gardens because of an attachment to and their positive associations with the therapeutic benefits of such places.

In terms of actually experiencing nature, literature reports evidence of "lowered stress and muscle tension" and fewer incidences of violence. Indoor plants were also shown to be beneficial. Nature access or views have been shown to be important in helping people cope with stress and recover from mentally fatiguing experiences. Problem solving is poorer and verbal and physical aggression higher when people are deprived of nature.

The case that a lack of environmental challenge leads to a host of health-related problems, stereotypies and underdeveloped neural connections has been demonstrated in other species. An optimal amount of complexity in therapeutic settings has been suggested to engage the patients. Natural settings in contrast to built settings have

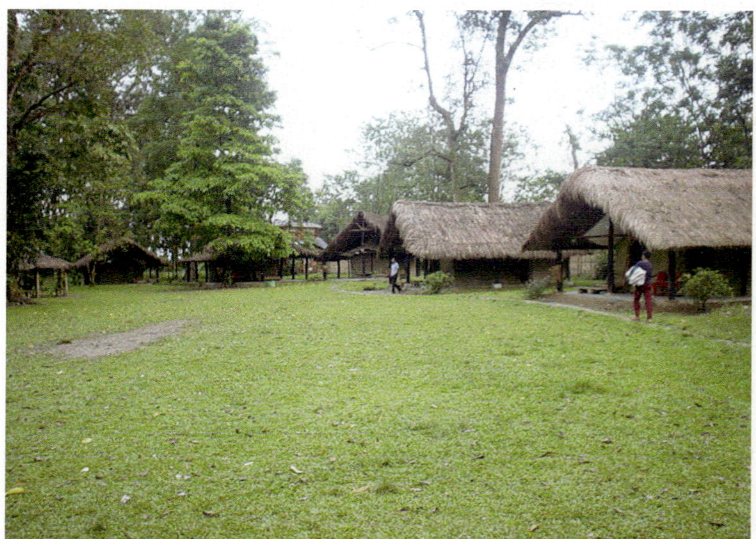

Fig. 5: Outdoor courtyard and garden.

been found to lend themselves to engagement. Engagement is a quality of the setting to maintain active interest over a period of time. The individual can easily derive a variety of experiences with qualities of the setting and can be intrigued by elements and their relationships. There are components of complexity, diversity, discovery and achievement in settings that are engaging. Patients who had access to the exterior environment valued it for its salutary effects and the environment itself was read as a place of meaning. Studies have also highlighted that a garden has its own therapeutic potential with multiple behavioral and sensory possibilities. It is suggested that there should be provision for direct access to outdoor space.

Many clinical studies demonstrate that the presence of nature and exposure to the outdoors in a healthcare setting can provide a positive distraction from many sources of stress.

It has been studied that for patients with dementia, aggressive behavior associated with a stressful experience could be diminished by playing recorded nature sounds during the event. Multiple windows with views of nature as an important design feature because these views can reduce psychological distress as well as recovery time. Larger windows low to the ground has the potential to improve sensory abilities and reduce delirium and paranoia among patients. By reducing stress and fatigue, exposure to nature may facilitate recovery.

Perimeter Security

The entire mental health facility requires a secure perimeter. A recommended height for perimeter fencing has not been established. A typical range is 2.7–4.0 m, however, fencing should not be to height as to create a prison-like environment, or to increase the possibility of falling injuries should an escape attempt be made. In determining an appropriate height, consideration will be given to the proximity of the perimeter fence to buildings, the topography of the site and consumer profile. Security is enhanced by installing curved fencing rather than having angled joins. Attention should be given to detailing roof overhangs, guttering and drain pipes, which may provide a means of escape.[21]

Sanctuary Trauma

First, evidence-based medical reasons for the cessation of seclusion and violence have now come to light. This reasoning generally revolves around the fact that a high proportion of psychiatrically hospitalized patients are themselves trauma survivors. This means that in many cases, the process of seclusion represents a reenactment of trauma which can retrigger the survivors' experience with profound helplessness and lead to retraumatization. This situation can also be described with the phenomenon known as *sanctuary trauma*, defined as "expecting a protective environment and finding only more trauma". The damaging implications of sanctuary trauma cannot be overemphasized.

Comfort Room

The comfort room is a relatively new concept which lies at the intersection of architecture and psychology. It is not a simple substitute for a seclusion room, but rather a preventative tool designed to reduce or eliminate the use of seclusion. Comfort rooms are well-furnished, visually appealing rooms for people to voluntarily enter. Their two most critical purposes are to provide a sanctuary from stress while also providing a place for people to feel and express a wider variety of emotions than they are able to on the ward.

Residential Atmosphere

A final issue in the design of a psychiatric treatment center is the concern, voiced by Michele McKinnie and others, that it is inadvisable to make the facility too home-like or comfortable for patients. It is often believed that while the facility should provide all of its services well, it should at the same time inspire patients to work diligently in their treatment so that they can leave the ward and return to their own more comfortable living situations.

Quality Measurement

The Royal College of Psychiatrists has postulated the following ten standards for adult inpatient mental healthcare in the document, *Do the right thing—how to judge a good ward. Ten standards for adult inpatient mental healthcare (Box 1).*[26-28]

Electroconvulsive Therapy Unit

Stand-alone electroconvulsive therapy (ECT) suites can provide excellent and clinically effective ECT. ECT services must be designed in a patient-focused manner that respects the need for autonomy and privacy.[22]

An ECT suite should consist of a minimum of three rooms:

- A waiting area with access to a toilet and change area. The waiting area should be quiet and separate from other clinical areas, respect patients' need for privacy, and accommodate their level of distress.
- A treatment/procedure room. The treatment room must comply with the rigorous standards for safety.
- A separate recovery area. The recovery area must comply with the rigorous standards for safety.[22]

Recovery from anesthesia should take place under appropriate supervision in a designated area. Contingency plans should exist for the safe emergency evacuation of patients from the operating suite and or recovery areas under adequate medical supervision. All areas should be linked with common doorways so that there can be a smooth movement from one area to the next before leaving the suite. The doors and corridors need to be wide enough to accommodate trolleys and hospital beds. The rooms need to be large enough to accommodate the number of people who are involved in the procedure. The size may vary dependent upon the flow of patients through the service. Services with a high volume of patient care will need more space for the treatment and recovery areas than those sites that are of low volume/occasional users.[22]

The treatment room should contain a stainless steel sink, drainer, and scrub-up basin. Space is also required for a fully equipped emergency trolley, sterile supplies, bed linen, instruments, equipment, and an area

Box 1: Standards for adult inpatient mental healthcare.[28]

- Bed occupancy rates of 85% or less
- Ward size maximum of 18 beds
- A physical environment that is fit for purpose
- The ward (must be) a therapeutic space
- Proportionate and respectful approach to risk management and safety
- Information sharing and involvement in care-planning
- A recovery-based approach: Links with the community and other agencies
- Access to psychological interventions
- Personalized care: Staffing and daily one-on-one contacts
- Providing socially and culturally sensitive care

that complies with the minimum standards for the safe and proper storage of drugs including provisions for scheduled drugs. This space should have—suitable illumination, airflow and/or air-conditioning that meet the needs for the different areas; telephone and computer facilities to aid communication; and a duress system to obtain assistance in the event of an emergency.[22]

CONCLUSION

The mental healthcare facility requires exclusive considerations in planning and designing for patient care and safety. It is essential that these are incorporated in the planning process. Existing facilities may require reengineering/retrofitting. These must be given priority.

REFERENCES

1. iapsmupuk.org
2. www.ruralneuropractice.com
3. www.who.int
4. www.ncbi.nlm.nih.gov
5. www.aia.org
6. www.fgiguidelines.org
7. researcharchive.vuw.ac.nz
8. www.kirkbridebuildings.com
9. tigerprints.clemson.edu
10. www.socialwelfarehistory.com
11. www.mdx.ac.uk
12. McLaughlan, Rebecca. "Corrupting the Asylum: The Diminishing Role of the Architect in the Design of Curative Environments for Mental Illness in New Zealand", Architectural Theory Review, 2016.
13. cscs.res.in
14. The Mental Healtcare Act 2017; Government of India.
15. www.godtsygehusbyggeri.dk
16. Connellan KM, Gaardboe DR, Due C, Reinschmidt A, Mustillo L. Stressed Spaces: Mental Health and Architecture. Health Environments Research & Design Journal; 2013.
17. www.cfm.va.gov
18. journals.sagepub.com
19. bjp.rcpsych.org
20. www.brikbase.org
21. healthfacilityguidelines.com.au
22. www.health.nsw.gov.au
23. psychservices.psychiatryonline.org
24. www.healthdesign.org
25. www.healthdesign.com.au
26. www.rcpsych.ac.uk
27. www.hawkesbay.health.nz
28. http://disabledpf.org.uk

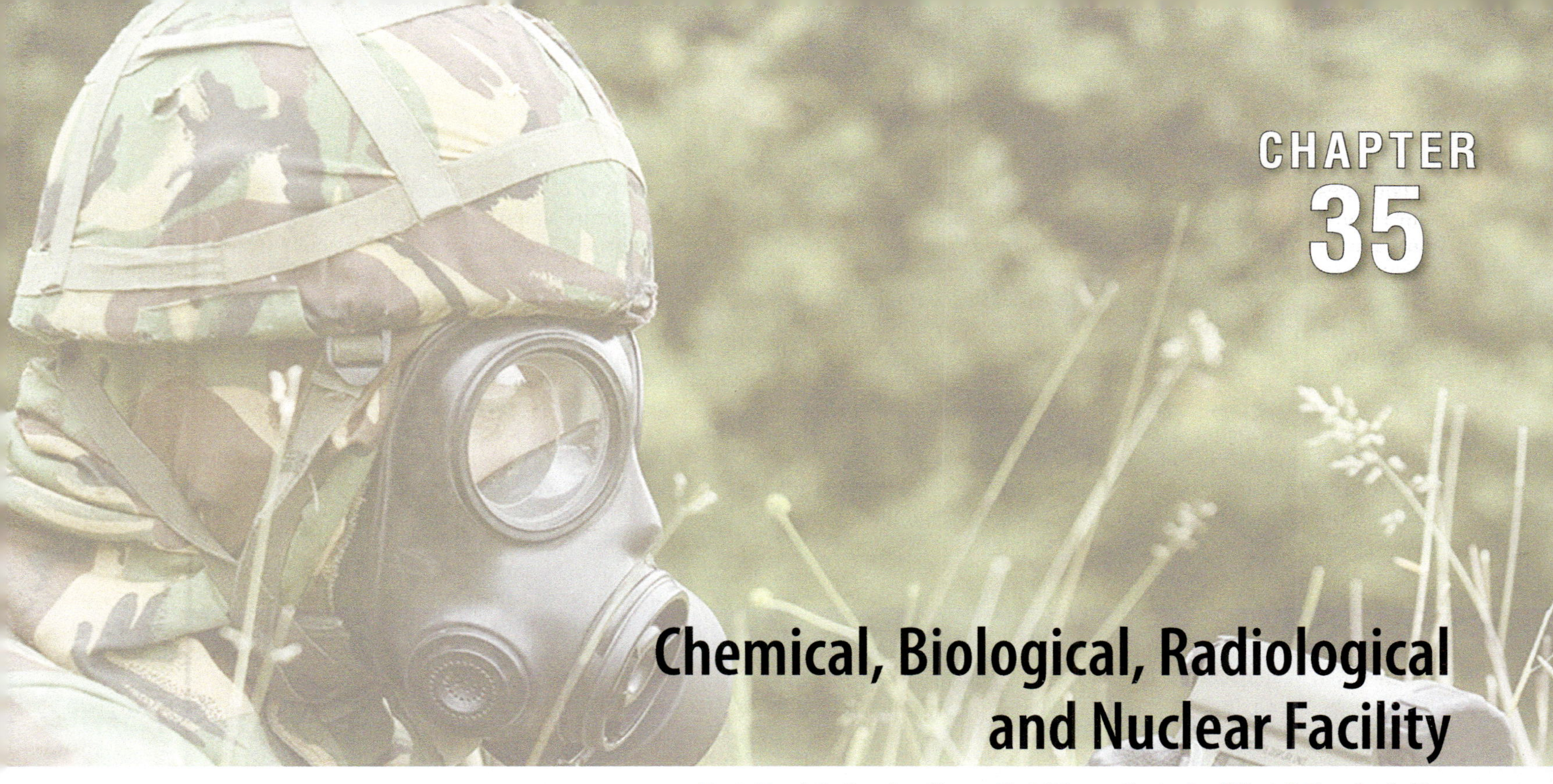

Chemical, Biological, Radiological and Nuclear Facility

Meeta Tyagi, Sudharshan Kumar, Shakti Kumar Gupta, Sunil Kant, R Chandrashekhar

INTRODUCTION

Hospitals are the most complex of *building types*. Each hospital is comprised of a wide range of services and *functional* units. These include diagnostic and treatment functions, such as clinical *laboratories*, imaging, emergency rooms, and surgery; hospitality functions, such as food service and housekeeping; and the fundamental inpatient care or bed-related functions. This diversity is reflected in the breadth and specificity of regulations, codes, and oversight that govern hospital construction and operations. The diversity of functioning is more challenging once the hospital is dealing with the situation of mass casualty.[1,2]

Hospitals play a critical role in healthcare infrastructure. Hospitals have a primary responsibility of saving lives, they also provide 24 × 7 emergency care service and hence, public perceive it as a vital resource for diagnosis, treatment and follow-up for both physical and psychological care. They are central to provide emergency care and hence, when a disaster strike the society falls back upon the hospitals to provide immediate succor in the form of emergency medical care.[3]

"Mass Casualty" refers to a combination of patient numbers and care requirements that challenge or exceed a community's ability to provide adequate patient care using day-to-day operations.[4] A mass casualty incident (MCI) in any community has the potential to quickly exhaust resources available for response. Hospital response capability is dependent on having a comprehensive emergency management plan inclusive of the worst case scenario, like an MCI, to enhance the level of readiness required to respond to a community's healthcare needs. The sudden arrival of a surge of patients presents a logistical challenge to rapidly process a large number of casualties through the system.[4,5]

As per Guidelines for Hospital Emergency Preparedness Planning an Initiative by GOI-UNDP hospital needs to calculate what constitutes a disaster or unmanageable incident and its normal capacity.[1]

TYPE OF CBRN FACILITIES

Based on the Number of Casualties

Here the categorization is based on the number of casualties coming to a hospital at a time and the ability of the hospital to cope with those casualties. Categorization will differ from hospital to hospital and depend on several factors, such as the number of doctors and nurses available and the availability of supplies and support services. Assessment of the capacity of a hospital to respond to a given emergency situation can be assessed by the following two ways:

- Hospital treatment capacity (HTC), is defined as the number of casualties that can be treated in the hospital in an hour and is usually calculated as 3% of total number of beds.
- Hospital surgical capacity (HSC) is the number of seriously injured patients that can be operated upon within a 12 hours period, i.e. HSC = Number of operation rooms × 7 × 0.25 operations/12 h.
  Thus, for a 1,000 bedded hospital, the various category of MCI are:
  - *Category 1*: Up to 30 patients belonging to a single accident or any other emergency, coming to a hospital casualty at one time.
  - *Category 2*: About 30–50 patients belonging to a single accident or any other emergency, coming to a hospital casualty at one time.
  - *Category 3*: More than 50 patients belonging to a single accident or emergency coming to the hospital casualty at one time.

Based on Type of Casualties

A universal color coding triage system is followed for this type of categorization:[6]

- *Category A (Color coding—Red)*: Patients in critical condition—include cases of polytrauma with head injuries, thoracic injuries, abdominal injuries, fractures of major bones with profuse bleeding, etc. These patients require immediate resuscitation and supportive measures. About 10% of these are beyond salvage.

- *Category B (Color coding—Yellow):* Patients in serious but not life-threatening condition—include polytrauma cases of a less serious nature, for example, fractures and crush injuries of limbs without major blood loss, facial injuries, spinal injuries, etc.
- *Category C (Color coding—Green)*—Walking wounded: These patients may have minor injuries requiring wound toileting and dressing and/or limb fractures requiring closed reduction and immobilization.

Mass casualty events may occur as a result of natural or human-caused disasters or after an act of terrorism. The boundaries between natural and man-made threats and their resulting hazards are often difficult to distinguish at the time of the incident. Initially, it may not be possible to differentiate between a deliberate attack and an accidental release, or the outbreak of an endemic/pandemic pathogen.

Chemical, Biological, Radiological and Nuclear

Chemical, biological, radiological and nuclear (CBRN) attacks are a credible threat to our society. Such attacks can cause a large number of fatalities or injuries in high-occupancy buildings (e.g. school buildings, hospitals and other critical care facilities, nursing homes, daycare centers, sports venues, theaters, and commercial buildings) and residential neighborhoods.[7,8]

The CBRN is a term that covers a distinct range of hazards which are as below:[9-11]

- *Chemical:*[11] Chemical agents are substances which are intended for use in military operations to kill, seriously injure, or incapacitate humans through their physiological impact. Chemical agents can be dispersed by explosive shells, rockets, missiles, aircraft bombs, mines, and spray devices. Also, water supplies have the potential for contamination by either water-soluble or miscible liquids or solids. Chemical agents can affect different physiological systems by entering the human body through ingestion, skin or eye absorption, and inhalation. They are categorized according to their physiological effects—nerve; blood and choking; and blistering agents. A second classification is persistent and nonpersistent agents. However classes of chemical agents are:
  - *Lethal agents*: These comprise the nerve agents, blood and choking agents, and blistering agents.
    - ◊ *Nerve agents*: These agents inhibits cholinesterase enzyme thus interfere with the nervous system and disrupt bodily functions such as breathing and muscular coordination. They may be in persistent or nonpersistent form and are cumulative in effect, so that repeated doses will produce progressively more serious effects. For example, tabun (GA), sarin (GB), soman (GD), GF and V-agent (VX).[6]
    - ◊ *Blood/cyanogen agents*: These agents prevent body tissues from utilizing oxygen in the blood and, in high concentrations, cause rapid respiratory failure. They tend to be highly nonpersistent in nature and are generally lighter than air which lessens their overall utility as they persist for only a brief time (seconds/minutes) in the immediate area of employment. Nonetheless they can represent a significant challenge to respirator filters. For example, hydrogen cyanide (AC) and cyanogen chloride (CK).[6]
    - ◊ *Choking/lung damaging agents*: These agents produce injury to the lungs and irritation of the eyes and the respiratory tract. They may also cause intractable pulmonary edema and predispose to secondary pneumonia. They are nonpersistent in form. For example, phosgene (CG), diphosgene (DP), chlorine (CL), and chloropicrin (PS).[6]
    - ◊ *Blister agents/vesicants*: These agents injure the eyes and the lungs, and burn or blister the skin. Most blister agents are persistent, however, persistency varies depending on the chemical form and environmental factors. They present a contact hazard and both local and downwind vapor hazards. They cause inflammation and, after several hours, blistering of the skin, eyes and breathing passages. Effects are cumulative, as with nerve agents. For example, sulfur mustard (H/HD) and nitrogen mustard (HN), arsenical [lewisite (L)], and phosgene oxime (CX).[6]
  - *Incapacitating agents*: These agents cause temporary disabling conditions which can be either physical or mental and can be viewed normally as nonlethal. However, in extreme concentrations or where unprotected personnel are exposed to them over extended periods, they may also cause death but this is not their primary purpose. Incapacitating agents are not, by their legal definition, considered to be chemical agents when used for law enforcement purposes, such as riot control.[6]
- *Biological*: Illnesses caused by the deliberate release of dangerous bacteria, viruses, fungi, or toxins (e.g. the plant toxin, ricin). The major classes of biological agents are:[6,10,11]
  - *Bacteria*: Bacterial agents are those that are pathogenic to humans, plants and animals either by causing infectious diseases or by producing toxins. Generally controlled by antibiotics however, bacteria can gain antibiotic resistance, either naturally or through genetic modification.
  - *Viruses*: Viruses, the simplest type of microorganisms, lack a system for their own metabolism and depend on host cells. They cause disease by damaging host cells in target organisms (humans, animals, plants). The most common viruses which may be utilized in biological warfare are smallpox, alphaviruses e.g. *venezuelan equine encephalitis* (VEE), and hemorrhagic fever viruses.
  - *Toxins*: These are harmful substances produced by living organisms (animals, plants, microbes). Features that distinguish them from chemical agents, such as VX, cyanide, or mustard, include being not man-made, nonvolatile (no vapor hazard), usually not dermally active (mycotoxins are the exception), and generally much more toxic per weight than chemical agents. This toxins considered to be among the most likely to be used are botulinum toxins, ricin, staphylococcal enterotoxin B (SEB), and T-2 mycotoxins.[6]
  - *Parasites*: These are organisms that benefit by exploiting their hosts (animal, human or plant) for food, habitat and dispersal. Parasites reproduce more quickly and in greater numbers than their hosts, and can rapidly reduce the health of the host.[6]
  - *Fungi*: These are primitive organisms that are capable of causing disease in humans. Spores of mycotoxin-producing fungi are possible antipersonnel biological weapon agents due to their stability, ease of manufacture, and ease of dissemination in aerosol form. Several species of fungi are also effective weapons against domesticated animals. Fungi can also serve as anticrop agents.[6]
- *Radiological events:* It can occur on a small scale event in hospital, laboratory or nuclear power plant with only few casualties to a large scale event following damage to nuclear plants on large scale, nuclear weapon detonation or terrorist attacks with radiological weapons. As per American National Council on Radiation Protection Report No. 138, the radiation exposure could result from radiation exposure device, radiological dispersion device like "dirty bombs" or

improvised nuclear device same as nuclear weapons. There are four main types of radiation present during the nuclear process are:[10-13]

- *Alpha particles* are charged helium nuclei. They only travel short distances (3 cm in air) and cannot penetrate the outer layers of skin. Damage is caused if ingested, inhaled or incorporated.[12]
- *Beta particles* are electrons. They can penetrate skin and will cause damage if taken internally. They will travel about 3 m in air or about 5 mm in tissue.[12]
- *Neutrons* are noncharged particles and usually only occur during the fission (nuclear) process. They are highly penetrating and, when they interact with biological tissue, are very damaging.[12]
- *Gamma/X-ray radiation* is at the high energy end of the electromagnetic spectrum. With no mass, it has a very long range and is difficult to shield against.[12]

The illness produced on radiological exposures are—Deterministic like acute radiation syndrome, burn injuries, blast injuries and stochastic-damaging DNA, causing mutations and cancers in survivors and future generation.

Toxic industrial material (TIM): It is a generic term for toxic chemical, biological and radioactive substances in solid, liquid, aerosolized, or gaseous form created for industrial, commercial, medical, or domestic purposes. Normally, such materials are retained within their planned manufacturing, storage, and transport facilities. However, their intentional or accidental release may pose a significant hazard. These are classified into:

- Toxic industrial chemical (TIC)
- Toxic industrial biological (TIB)
- Toxic industrial radiological (TIR).

Medical Response to CBRN

Medical response is a critical component of CBRN attack. One of the key components of effective planning and preparedness for the emergency medical sector is an understanding of the mechanism of injury. It is important to understand the means by which CBRN scenarios affect people and create victims who will need help from the medical system. Different types of causative agents will produce different types of victims, which will have varying effects on the medical system that is trying to care for them. The medical response for CBRN is at field level where the incident has taken place and definite clinical care at hospital level.[14]

Chemical Scenario

At Field Level

Chemical and hazardous material (Hazmat) incidents will have the highest potential for casualties requiring acute care. In a majority of scenarios involving chemical agents respiratory distress and breathing difficulty requires the most acute care. Oxygen administration, clearing of airways, assisted ventilation, and suction may be required, all of which entail manpower and logistics. A few of the threats (nerve agents and cyanides) have specific antidotes. Decontamination will be important in cases involving actual deposit of material on skin and clothing, but it is less important than airway clearing and breathing. Many types of chemicals will have latency, and signs and symptoms will not be apparent at the field level.[15]

At Hospital Level

At the clinical level in hospital, the agent and route of exposure will drive the requirement for care. The general capacity of a hospital's emergency department to handle patients is usually driven by the normal caseload of medical and trauma patients. The mechanisms of injury from chemical situations may overload a hospital's specialized capabilities. Injuries from chemicals with latency periods, such as phosgene or mustard, will provide for situations where victims may self-refer directly to a hospital emergency department when their symptoms appear. Pulmonary, eye, and skin injuries are likely to predominate in many scenarios. Blister and pulmonary (choking) agents are likely to provide a heavy burden on respiratory specialists and equipment. The amount of ventilation equipment may be the critical factor in how many patients a facility can care for in chemical scenarios. Blister agents and many industrial chemicals will cause skin and eye injuries, such as chemical burns. In an ideal situation, a CBRN/Hazmat incident will have good scene control, and all victims will be decontaminated and transported to care as clean patients. However, many people may turn-up at a hospital in a contaminated state. Therefore, it is necessary to build decontamination procedures and equipment into hospital emergency plans.[15]

Biological Scenario

At Field Level

In biological immediate signs and symptoms will not occur in casualties except for biotoxins, where the mechanism and response will be similar to that of chemical scenario.

At Hospital Level

In the biological scenario, casualties are similar to some form of routine illness in the early stages. Patients will demand hospital care once the acute symptoms of illness appear. Several of the more lethal biological agents, such as pneumonic plague, botulinum toxin, and anthrax, may require significant levels of respiratory support. Often, the mechanism of injury that produces the most lethality is respiratory distress. Others may require only general supportive measures. Some pathogens are contagious from person to person, so isolation or other measures may be needed. Diagnostic resources, such as laboratories and pathologists, may be in heavy demand. In addition, public health response is needed to contain the spread of disease in population resulting from biological agent.[15]

Radiological Scenario

At Field Level

Radiological incidents may present as acute radiation illness. Explosive dispersal of radiological materials is cause conventional injuries from blast and fragmentation. Thus radiation detection, decontamination and trauma care assumes importance for care of casualty resulting from radiation scenario.[15]

At Hospital Level

Conventional blast and fragmentation casualties may present with significant levels of radioactive material about their persons and clothing. Radiation detection at emergency department, decontamination prior to entry in hospital, treatment for burns and radiation injuries. Disposal of contaminated clothing, dead bodies and disposal of waste resulting from treatment assumes importance.[15]

The defense against CBRN events rests on five principles which are:[9]

1. Detection, identification and monitoring.
2. Information management.
3. Individual and collective physical protection.
4. Management of CBRN hazard.
5. Medical countermeasures, support and treatment.

Medical countermeasures during event of CBRN are different from the routine emergency or during natural disasters. Healthcare workers risk occupational exposures to chemical, biological, or radiological materials when a hospital receives contaminated patients, particularly during MCI.

When consistent with the functional program and disaster planning, acute care facilities with emergency services can serve as receiving, triage, and initial treatment centers in the event of infectious disease outbreaks; natural or man-made disasters; or nuclear, biological, or chemical (NBC) exposure. These facilities should have the capacity to handle a surge of patients above the current emergency department capacity and should designate specific area(s) for these functions.[16,17]

Indian Scenario

Indian subcontinent is one of the most disaster prone regions in the world. The periodicity and intensity of disasters have increased manifold in the last few decades, resulting in a large number of human casualties and huge economic losses. In many disasters, human and economic losses can be minimized by prevention, mitigation and preparedness measures. Under Section 6 of the Disaster Management Act, 2005, the National Disaster Management Authority (NDMA) has been mandated *inter alia* to issue guidelines for preparing action plans for the holistic and coordinated management of all disasters. CBRN-related guidelines have issued by NDMA for biological, chemical disaster (industrial), chemical terrorism, nuclear and radiological emergencies. At national level Indian Army is carrying out regular training on preparedness for CBRN attacks with capabilities of setting-up field hospitals for treatment of casualties and NDRF has trained its personnel's on CBRN attacks.[18-21]

National Disaster Management Authority stresses on 'all hazard' hospital disaster management (DM) plan to be prepared by hospitals which shall focus on the specialized requirement of personal protective equipment (PPE), decontamination facilities at hospitals, creation of specialized medical teams and facilities, adequate laboratory support, training of specialists, nurses, pharmacists, and paramedics including adequate knowledge of various CBRN agents their effects, and treatment protocols including awareness of specific prophylactics and antidotes.[18-21]

CBRN Facility Standards

At present for planning and designing purpose of hospitals, standards/bylaws are available for protection of hospitals against Natural Disasters and Accidents such as fires, earthquakes, floods, etc. from Model Building Bye Laws in India, Bureau of Indian Standards for building, NDMA Standards for healthcare facilities and International Building Codes 2009.[22,23]

However, these standards are for protecting the buildings against natural hazards. Guidelines on planning and designing of healthcare facilities are available in various documents including Federal Guidelines Institute publications on designing on design and construction of healthcare facilities, Unified Facility Criteria Documents by Department of Defense United States of America and Risk Management Series from Federal Emergency Management Series (FEMA-577).[24-27]

These standards are useful in designing the healthcare facilities in CBRN scenario as well but special provisions on decontamination, HVAC, specialized laboratories, exits, hot/cold zones in treatment area, disposal of dead bodies and disposal of biomedical waste in CBRN environment are needed.[14,28-30]

Armies all over the world today have guidelines for dealing with CBRN casualty near the battle field or war scenario. Guidelines on setting CBRN Decontamination Centers in field scenario near the site of incident have been published.[11,12,31]

CALCULATION OF NUMBER OF HOSPITAL BEDS FOR MITIGATION OF CBRN SCENARIO

In planning stages, the requirement of hospital beds are based on parameters like catchment area, population of the area, treatment facilities available with their bed strength, workload and hospital utilization indices but while planning for CBRN facility straightforward guidelines are not available. Calculating the number of beds required for CBRN facility are based on casualties in various presumptive scenarios and hospital surge capacity.

The Emergency Mass Casualty Assessment and Planning Scenario (EMCAPS) software by Johns Hopkins University provides estimation of casualties based on population density, various meteorological conditions and strength of CBRN agent. This software has scenario for Radiological Dirty Bombs, scenario for biological attacks, for chemical and one for improvised explosive device (IED). The limitation of this software is that it does not address the nuclear explosion scenario. In the present study, one scenario each from CBR attack was taken to note the casualties expected.

The EMCAPS was utilized to find the number of casualties anticipated in various chemical and biological scenario. The worst case scenario was utilized for calculating the number of casualties by EMCAP software. For nuclear attack scenario, the principle of most probable casualties in nuclear attack with 20 kiloton (kt) warheads, was utilized.

The assumptions made in calculation of casualties are:[5]

- Less seriously injured casualties who self-transport to the hospital typically arrive before those who are more seriously injured.
- Casualties may arrive at hospitals without having been triaged, decontaminated or receiving first aid.
- The "dual wave phenomenon" has been used to describe how casualties tend to arrive at hospitals. In no-notice events, patient flow starts suddenly, sometimes without warning, and builds rapidly.
- The first wave of casualties may include those who only require minor care. They are not in need of extrication and are able to walk; therefore they may appear within the first 15–30 minutes depending on the distance from the scene to the closest hospitals.
- The second wave may include those who require transport and may include those in emergent need of immediate care. The delay in arrival of those who are more seriously injured is due to a number of factors including the need for nonambulatory transport methods and the need for search and rescue to locate those who are unresponsive and who may require extrication.
- Approximately 50% of acute casualties may arrive at the facility within 60 minutes. About 50–80% may arrive within 90 minutes. Most arrive within 1–4 hours.
- About 80% of red tagged casualties, 50% of yellow tagged casualties and 20% of green tagged casualties are expected to reach/transported to the hospital.

Casualty arrivals will differ in biological attack. These arrivals tend to be insidious, beginning slowly but then growing exponentially within hours to days. Recognition that there are persons arriving with similar symptoms or coming from the same location is essential for taking action to accommodate the surge. Reporting data for biological outbreaks into a syndromic surveillance system assists hospitals and country health departments in monitoring trends in a number of disease syndrome categories, enhances the detection of disease outbreaks, and improves situational awareness. Reporting data may enable a timelier public health response to these events.[5]

KEY PLANNING AND DESIGNING PARAMETERS OF CBRN FACILITY

Patient Flow Through the Facility

The first step in planning and designing of a facility is to understand the movement through the facility. In CBRN event the treatment areas are divided into warm zone where the casualties are decontaminated and cold zone where casualties enter after decontamination. As per OSHA these zones in hospital are decontamination zone and post decontamination zone.[7,8] The Figure 1 provides the movement of patient through the facility. Figure 2 shows the stack diagram for the facility.

Functional Areas Essential for a CBRN Facility

Figure 1 shows the movement of patients in the hospital. Depending on the type of event casualties can arrive in a contaminated state on own or in vehicles. The vehicle carrying the contaminated casualty will also become contaminated. To achieve functional efficiency as per guidelines on the treatment of CBRN casualties following functional areas are required for a CBRN facility [9,10, mass preparedness NDMA]:

- Triage area
- Decontamination area for vehicles
- Decontamination room for patients
- Detection facilities
- Decorporation unit
- Operation theater
- Intensive care unit
- Isolation unit
- Burn unit
- Bone marrow transplant unit
- Convalescence unit
- Advanced laboratory facility
- Blood bank facility
- Radio diagnostic facility
- Mortuary/Dead body storage area.

The facility described in subsequent paragraphs does not describe the blood bank facility and radio diagnostic facility as these services will be shared by the main hospital. The other support services such as dietary, CSSD, laundry are also not mentioned.

Special Engineering Consideration

The CBRN agents have to be contained and disposed with utmost care hence, the planning parameters for engineering services will include:

- Waste water disposal from CBRN facility.
- HVAC system with positive pressure ventilation with special CBRN filters.

Disposal of Waste Water of CBRN Facility

A delay tank is to be constructed to handle waste from the contaminated patients at a place where there is no movement of public. Only authorized workers after PPE are to be allowed to control the flow of effluent, collection of samples, treating the waste water by adding various chemicals and discharging waste water from the tank to the main sewerage once it is fit for disposal. The tank has to be leak and corrosion proof and should have a smooth surface from inside. The outlet of the sewerage tank has to be much higher to avoid back flow. During a one month period, the effluent should be allowed to flow into only one tank to allowed using a set of valves provided on the pipelines leading to the tanks from the radiation wards. When this is full, the tank inlet should be closed and the effluent should be allowed to flow into the second tank. During the collection period, the radioactivity in the first tank will undergo decay, so that it can be disposed off when discharged limits are achieved. The activity level at the time of discharge into the

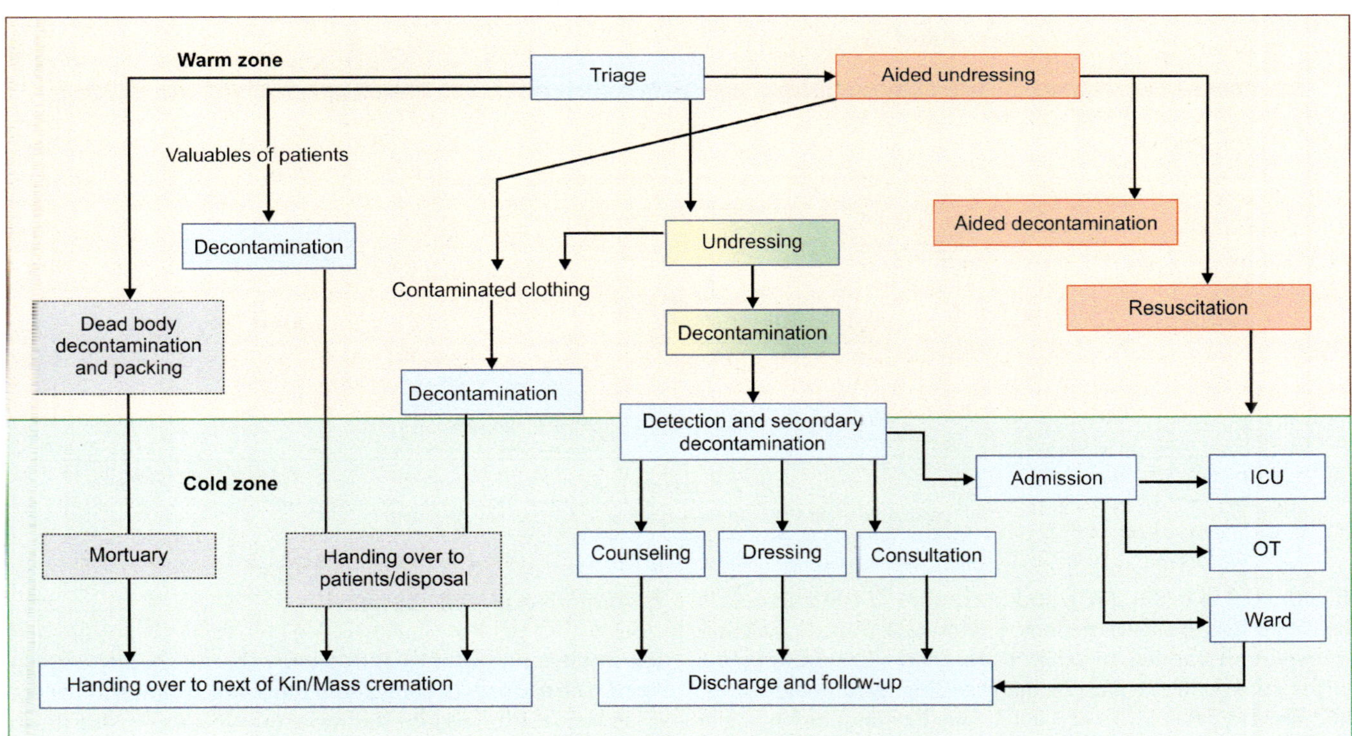

Fig. 1: Movement of patients in the hospital.

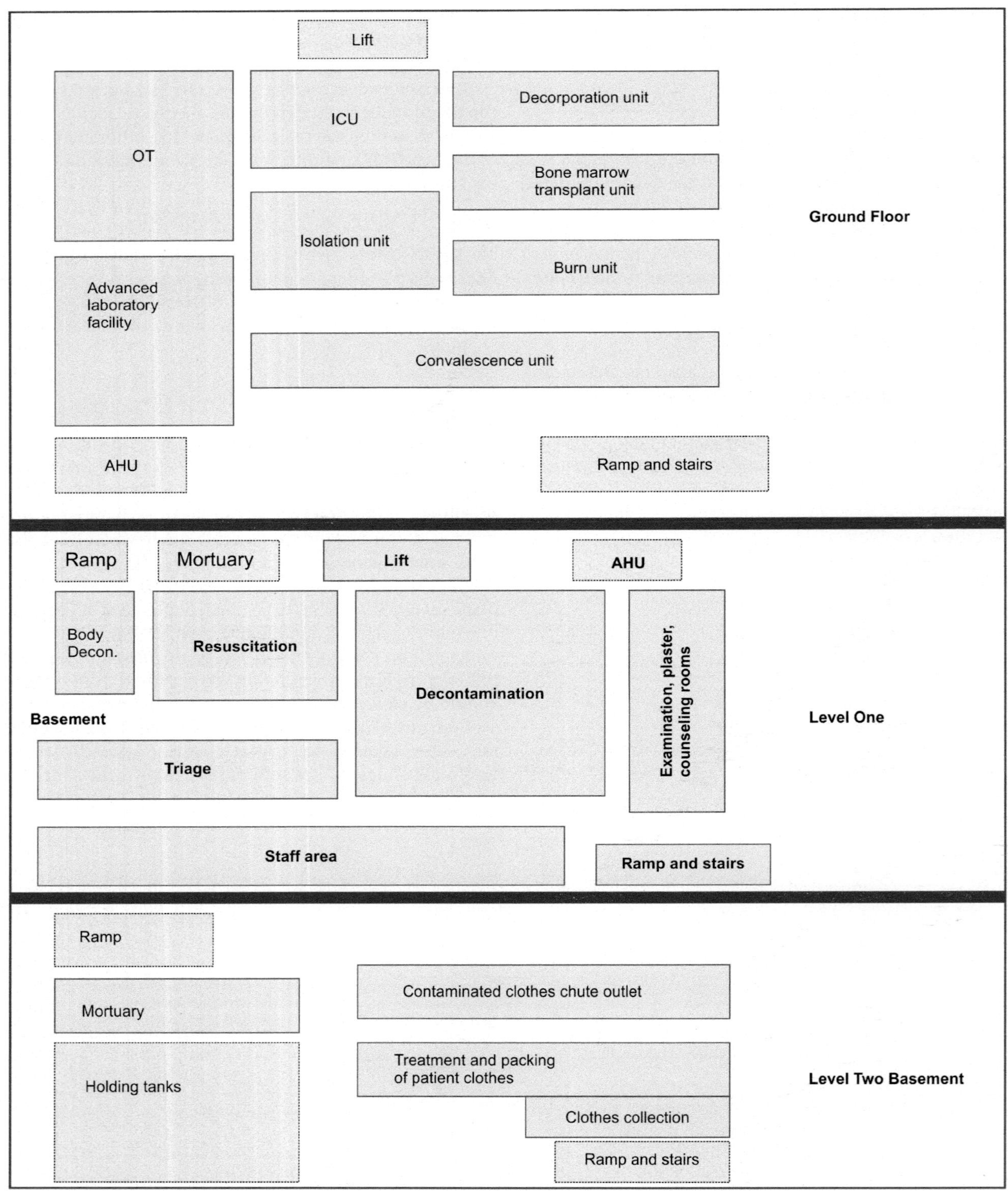

Fig. 2: Stack diagram.

(OT: operation theater; ICU: intensive care unit; AHU: air handling unit)

sewer will come down to 0.6 μCi/L and maximum of 100 microcurie can be discharged into the sewer per day. For biological attack, calcium hypochlorite solution is added. In a chemical scenario depending on the agent involves waste water is neutralized by adding various chemicals. For a 50 bed ward, 5 delay tanks of 6,000 L may be adequate. In a 100 bedded CBRN treatment facility 6 delay tanks with 10,000 L capacity will be adequate.[32,33]

Ventilation and HVAC System[34]

The whole building of a CBRN facility should classify as a Class 1 safe room. The features of such a safe room are as under:[7,34]

- Pressurization requires introducing air from outside the protective enclosure; therefore, the removal efficiency of the filters is more critical in determining the protection provided. The system must

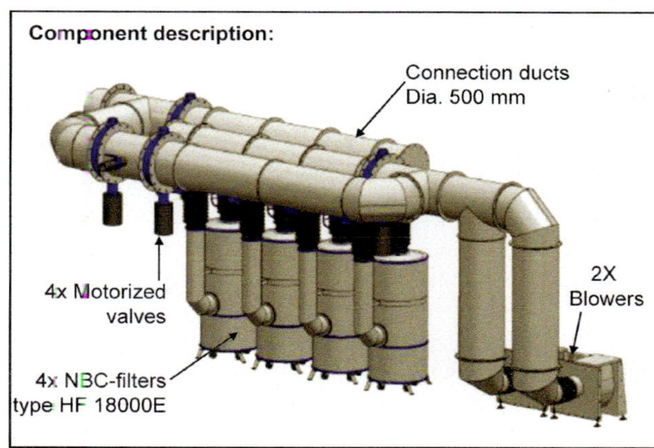

Fig. 3: CBRN filtration units and components.
(NBC: Nuclear Biological Chemical)

employ ultra-high efficiency filters, and it must allow no air to bypass the filter as it is forced into the safe room.

Filter Unit (Fig. 3)

The collective CBRN-Filtration System is designed to filter chemical, biological, radiological and nuclear contaminants.

The filter is made of two main stages. The first stage is a mechanical filter which employs a high-efficiency particulate arrestance (HEPA) media having efficiency higher than 99.995%. The HEPA filter arrests airborne particles (viruses, bacteria, radioactive fallout, etc.). The second stage is the chemical/gas filter which is made of highly porous activated carbon grains. It adsorbs the chemical agents in the gas and neutralizes them by chemical reaction with special impregnation. The filter is designed to be in standby mode for many years and is almost maintenance-free. Hence, the filter unit must have both a HEPA filter and an ultrahigh efficiency gas adsorber in series.

- The adsorber must contain carbon impregnated ASZM-TEDA or the equivalent. Carbon mesh size should be 12 × 30 or 8 ×16.
- The adsorber must have efficiency of at least 99.999% for physically adsorbed chemical agents and 99.9% for chemisorbed agents.
- The adsorber must have a total capacity of 300,000 mg/min/m^3 for physically adsorbed chemical agents.
- Bypass at the seals between the adsorber and its housing must not exceed 0.1%.
- For installation of the filter unit outside the safe room, the fan must be upstream of the filters (blow-through configuration).
- For installation inside with a duct from the wall to the filter unit, the fan must be downstream of the filters (draw-through configuration).
- If a flexible duct is used outside the shelter to convey air from the filter unit to the safe room, it must be made of a material resistant to the penetration of toxic chemicals.
- Ventilation: For Class 1 safe rooms, 15 cfm per person is the desired ventilation rate; however, the minimum ventilation rate is 5 cfm per person if that rate is adequate for pressurization.

OPERATIONS CONTROL STATION (CBRN CONTROL CONSOLE)

The control system for the CBRN facility is should be designed in such a manner that all essential function could be controlled, monitored and operated from the central control console. Its design and engineering should be unique. The main instruments developed for this system are the control panel duplicated by a computer and the display system.

Contamination Status

The red and green indicators on panel will have various inscription such as Biological Monitor, Chemical Monitor, Radiation Monitor. The red light will indicate prevalence of contamination and green lights will indicate no contamination. If contamination is due to chemical agents the respective red light will glow and likewise in biological and radiation contamination.

Contamination status of air being supplied to protected areas will also be available for NBC detectors and NBC filters. Central panel will also indicate contamination status of those persons who were contaminated and sent through the process of decontamination. No change of status takes place when contamination is down to safe limits.

System Status

System status will be indicated by different colour coding and the following operations could be controlled by the console:

- NBC ventilation system
- Door control
- Water supply
- Air curtains
- Manual override
- Differential Air Pressure.

Simulation software is also incorporated in the software to check the functionality of monitors on computer. The input for the control console will be from the NBC sensor software and this console will only function on Password and RFID Card. It is generally designed to provide both audio and visual warning of any occurrence.

Standalone or Integrated Facility

Foremost aspect of facility planning and design that needs to be considered is whether the facility would be on a standalone mode or this will be a part of a multispecialty tertiary care institution. Though a standalone facility will provide integrated care delivery system, however it needs to have all necessary support services in terms of logistics, manpower and administration involving a costly option.

The unique requirement of a CBRN facility lies is the fact that the staff, other patients (if facility is planned as a part of tertiary level hospital) do not get contaminated and the contaminants (clothing/waste water, etc.) are disposed in an effective way.

Once adequate decontamination is done and no signs of contamination are present in the patient, he can be treated in the respective department of the tertiary level hospital nearer to the CBRN facility. Moreover, in case there is no CBRN casualty, the facility can be utilized in situations of disaster or in other situations when hospital resources are overloaded. This sharing of resources will be cost effective.

Therefore, it is prudent to plan the facility linked to a tertiary level hospital. This will allow the utilization of radiodiagnostic facility, CSSD, laundry, kitchen and blood bank facility of the main hospital. Radiation injury treatment center, burn center, advanced laboratory facility, bone marrow transplant facility, operation theater, isolation facility and mortuary should be incorporated in the same building premises. The purpose of this is to minimize the possible threat of spread the contamination while performing the invasive procedures/procedures involving the body tissue and fluids. Moreover, the need of these facilities is anticipated for the treatment of a CBRN casualty.

DESIGN OF THE BUILDING

Configuration of Building[34]

Siting Consideration

Siting of shelters for nuclear protection has typically been underground, as tunnels, caves, or buried structures. The mass of the geological materials absorbs the blast energy and provides radiation shielding. Perhaps the most convenient and safest is below ground level, in a basement. Basement provide the greatest degree of protection against missiles and falling debris. It also provides shielding against gamma radiation—neutrons shielding 0.5; initial gamma shielding 0.3 and residual shielding 0.01.[7]

Building Material Consideration

Shielding potential of material plays a key role in selection when planning for shelters. Generally, the denser or heavier the material, the better shielding it offers. Concrete provides 5.6 cm (2.2 inch) shielding potential risk.[6,34]

The CBRN facility described here is with a Level 1 and Level 2 basement and a ground floor. It is located 60 m downside from the main hospital complex and residential area. It is connected to the main hospital through a covered path. It has a separate entry and exit from the main access road to hospital.

GROUND FLOOR

Decorporation Unit

This area is to provide treatment with decorporation agents to eliminate radionuclides from the body.[35] Once the decorporation is completed the patients can be shifted to the convalescence unit. Two isolation rooms are planned here to cater for the immune compromised and patients with pre-existing diseases.

The considerations for this area are as follows:

- Storage area for storing decorporation agents and basic medicines.
- A pneumatic system for sending the samples to laboratory.
- The collection of all effluents is to be done in a holding tank of 4,000 L capacity with inlet and outlet facilities into the main sewer. The internal finishing of the tank is to be of nonabsorbent and noncorrosive material. It should be built underground with one meter of earth cover on top.

Space Parameters

The space required for the decorporation room are shown in Table 1.

Operation Theater

The function of this operation theater is to provide surgical interventions to who are severely injured requiring extensive immediate surgical care. These patients may be contaminated with any of a variety of materials. Most of these materials will not constitute a significant hazard to operating room personnel.[36] In order to minimize and restrict contamination there are certain additional precautions which should be taken by the healthcare staff which are:[37]

- All personnel in the operating room area should wear masks in place at all times when potentially contaminated patients are being cared for.[37]
- Once an operating room has been used for the surgical care of nuclear accident patients, monitoring and decontamination will be necessary before it can be used for other surgical cases.[37]

Table 1: Space parameters of decorporation unit.

Sl. No.	Area	Space (m^2)
1.	Isolation room class 'P' × 2	30
2.	4 × 6 beds cubicle	216
3.	Toilet patient × 4	5 × 4
4.	Staff station	14
5.	Store-equipment + General	20 + 9
	Total	309

- All waste material will be saved in suitable containers. These must be tagged, so that they can be identified later and examined by qualified personnel from among the technical teams responsible for salvage and disposal at a nuclear accident.[37]
- When personnel remove their surgical gowns, caps, and gloves, they must be considered as contaminated also.
- All personnel must shower completely after working on such cases and must not be released from the area until after monitoring.[37]

Apart from the above mentioned functional aspects, the designing parameters of operation theater of a CBRN facility are similar to any other OT. Standards for OT should be fulfilled, viz. pressure zoning, lighting, room space, manifold, etc.[37]

Space Parameters

The space required for the OT is shown in Table 2.[23]

Intensive Care Unit

The space required for intensive care unit is shown in Table 3.[23]

Isolation Unit[37]

These rooms will house the patients who can transmit infection to others or those who are susceptible to infections. Based on the requirements, both positive pressure and negative pressure rooms are planned. A set of isolation rooms will comprise of common anteroom and four isolation rooms. Two of such sets will be with positive and two with negative pressure.

Airborne infection isolation room should have an area for hand washing, gowning, and storage of clean and soiled materials located directly outside or immediately inside the entry door to the room. The perimeter walls, ceiling, and floors, including penetrations should be sealed tightly, so that air does not infiltrate the environment from the outside or from other spaces. Each room should have self-closing devices on all room exit doors. Separate toilet, bathtub (or shower), and hand washing stations should be required for each airborne infection isolation room. Rooms should have a permanently installed visual mechanism to constantly monitor the pressure status of the room when occupied by patients with an airborne infectious disease. The mechanism should continuously monitor the direction of the airflow.

The rooms may be used for noninfectious patients when not needed for patients with airborne infectious disease.

Space Parameters[25]

The space required for isolation unit is shown in Table 4.

Burn Unit

The considerations for this area are as follows:

Table 2: Space required for the operation theatre.

Sl. No.	Area	Space (m^2)
1.	Reception	10
2.	Scrub up/gowning area	06
3.	Anesthesia induction room	15
4.	Operating room (major)	36–48
Support areas		
5.	Anesthetic room	10–15
6.	Mobile equipment bay	4
7.	Linen bay	3
8.	Janitor cupboard	2
9.	Clean-up room	12
10.	Disposal room	10
11.	Flash sterilization room	5–6
12.	Set-up room	20
13.	Store-equipment	20–40
14.	Store-sterile	20–40
15.	Store nonsterile	20–30
16.	Store-anesthesia	20
Recovery area		
17.	Patient bay	9
18.	Resuscitation trolley bay	2
19.	Clean utility	12
20.	Dirty utility	10
21.	Hand washing bay	1
22.	Staff station	6–14
Administrative staff area		
23.	Change room	10–30
24.	Office	9
25.	Store	10
26.	Toilet staff	4
27.	Shower staff	4
Total		290–386

- Relative humidity should be 80%.
- *Saline bath unit*: It is a specialized area for cleaning the burnt body of the patient. Normal saline at room temperature is utilized for cleaning. A minimum space of 4 × 4 m is required.
- As most patients will require sedation/anesthesia before the procedure, there should be provision of manifold outlets located conveniently. There should be provision of ample supply of saline, warming facility and flexible hose with pump system for directing saline under pressure whenever required. As there is a possibility of wound being contaminated with CBRN agents, therefore, the drains should lead to the holding tank.
- *Skin/amnion banking facility*: This facility is required for storage of skin and amniotic membrane which is used for dressing of burn patients. Here tissue and amniotic membrane is kept at very low/ultralow temperature. Apart from the space required for the special refrigerator, it should also have adequate circulation space. An area of 16 m^2 is considered adequate.

Space Parameters

The space required for burn unit is shown in Table 5.

Table 3: Space required for intensive care unit

Sl. No.	Area	Space (m^2)
1.	Bed bay	20 × 12
2.	Hand washing bay	01
3.	Mobile equipment bay	04
4.	Janitor closet	02
5.	Trolley bay	09
6.	Clean utility	12
7.	Dirty utility	10
8.	Disposal room	08
9.	Medication room	10–12
10.	Staff station	14–20
11.	Store for equipment	20–30
12.	General store	15–20
13.	Office clerical	12
	Toilets	
14.	For disabled	05
15.	For patients × 2	06
16.	For staff	02
17.	Bathroom	10
18.	Office	09
Total		389–412

Table 4: Space required for isolation unit

Sl. No.	Area	Space (m^2)
1.	Set of isolation × 4	
2.	Isolation room × 4	22 × 4
3.	Anteroom	16
4.	Total for 4 sets	416
5.	Staff station	14
6.	Store-general	9
Total		439

Table 5: Space required for burn unit.

Sl. No.	Area	Space (m^2)
1.	Set of isolation room class 'P' with 4 beds and anteroom	104
2.	6 bed room × 3	54 × 3
3.	Toilet patient × 3	5 × 3
4.	Saline bath unit	16
5.	Skin/amnion banking facility	16
6.	Staff station	14
7.	Store—general	9
Total		336

Bone Marrow Transplant Unit[38]

This facility will cater to the radiological and biological agent victims, who develop bone marrow depression. The specific features of patients admitted here is that they will be immunecompromised.

The special considerations of this unit are as under:[39]

- Should consist of exceptionally clean environments with HEPA filtration.

- A counter top with scrub sink and space for high-level disinfection procedures should be available outside the entrance to each patient room.
- There should be an anteroom before patient room with airflows from the anteroom, to the patient room and the corridor.
- Each bone marrow transplant patient room should be of an immunosuppressed host airborne infection isolation (protective environment/airborne infection isolation room). It should have a private toilet, which contains a water closet and a bathing facility, for the exclusive use of the patient.
- Windows should be provided so that each patient may be cognizant of the outdoor environment. Window sill height should not exceed 3 ft above the floor. All windows in the unit should be fixed sash and sealed to eliminate infiltration.
- Viewing panels should be provided in doors or walls for nursing staff observation.
- Flame-retardant curtains or other means should be provided to cover windows and viewing panels when a patient requires visual privacy.
- Glazing should be safety glass, wire glass, or tempered clear plastic to reduce hazard from accidental breakage.
- Each patient room should be provided with a nurses calling system accessible at the bed, sitting area, and patient toilet room. An emergency call system should also be provided at each patient bed and toilet room to summon additional personnel from on-call rooms, consultation rooms, and staff lounges. Facilities for administration of suction, compressed air, and oxygen should be provided at the bed.
- All surfaces floors, walls, ceilings, doors, windows, and curtains should be scrubbable.
- The flooring will be electroconductive.
- All water supplies to pass through water purification.

Space Parameters

The space required for bone marrow transplant unit is shown in Table 6.

Table 6: Space required for bone marrow transplant unit.

Sl. No.	Facility	Floor area in m^2	Constructional requirement
Protective zone			
1.	Reception	7.00	Counter terminal
2.	Shoe change	3.5	Built-in shoe rack
3.	Change room		
	Male	7.00	Built-in cupboard
	Female	7.00	Built-in cupboard
Clean zone			
4.	Doctor's room	7.00	
5.	Nurses room	7.00	Shelving
6.	Toilet	3.50	Wc, WHB
Sterile zone			
7.	Scrub up	3.50	Swan neck, elbow controlled tap
8.	Transplantation chamber	28.00	Fixed pendant, central suction, oxygen, compressed air facility
9.	4 patient room with attached toilet	88.00	Central suction, oxygen, compressed air terminal, entry through anteroom
10.	Common anteroom	16.00	
11.	Sterile store	7.00	Ample shelving
Dirty zone			
12.	Dirty utility	7.00	Sink with drain board
Total		188.00	

Convalescence Unit[38]

Five cubicles of 4 bed each is planned to cater for the patient who have completed decorporation cycle or those who need daily routine monitoring/observation. Cubicles can be marked separately for male, female and children. There should be an attached toilet and bathroom with each cubicle. The space parameters for this area is similar to general nursing unit.[24]

Space Parameters

Space required for convalescence unit is shown in Table 7.

Table 7: Space required for convalescence unit.

Sl. No.	Area	Space (m^2)
1.	4-bed cubicle × 5 204	40.8 × 5
2.	Mobile equipment bay	04
3.	Janitor closet	02
4.	Sluice room/dirty utility	10
5.	Dressing/procedure area	12–24
6.	Store for equipment	20–30
7.	General store	15–20
8.	Nursing counter	8
9.	Nurses duty room	12
10.	Room for other staff	12
	Toilets	
11.	For disabled	05
12.	For patients × 4	12
13.	For staff	02
14.	Bathroom × 2	20
Total		338–365

Advanced Laboratory Facility[39,40]

- The function of this lab is to identify the CBRN agent, to monitor the level of agent in patient, to monitor the effect of treatment. Therefore, the laboratory will have the components of clinical laboratory and forensic laboratory.
- *Chemistry section*: For examinations involving wet chemistry procedures. Wet-chemistry laboratories are spaces designed for the handling of hazardous chemicals. To mitigate these hazards, these laboratories utilize fume hoods and other specialty containment devices. This section also relies on substantial numbers of instrumentation units, such as gas chromatography (GC)/mass spectrometry (MS), Fourier transform infrared spectroscopy (FTIR), inductively coupled plasma (ICP)/mass spectrometry (MS), and other computer-driven, diagnostic instrumentation.
- *Biology and toxicology section*: For the examination of blood and urine for the presence of CBRN agents and the development of DNA profiles. The material would be infectious or highly prone to cross-contamination. Like the chemistry section, the toxicology section uses various types of gas-consuming, heat generating, noise-producing instrumentation requiring isolation and special design considerations.

- *Clinical laboratory section*: This section is planned for biochemical and hematological samples of patients. The histopathological and microbiological tests will be carried out in biological section as they are likely to be contagious.

The special considerations for laboratory for CBRN are as under:[33,41-43]

- *Laminar flow clean hoods*: Used only to protect process (not to protect operator), they are not exhausted.
- *Radioisotope hoods*: Special purpose fume hood with eap-filtered exhaust discharge. Generally uses slightly higher face velocity than conventional fume hoods (125 fpm) requires welded stainless steel exhaust duct system. Can be open or gas-tight (glove box).
- *Perchloric acid hoods*: Straight exhaust duct run (no horizontal offsets) is mandatory. Requires automatic wash down system. Discharge must be carried to the lab waste system. Requires welded stainless steel exhaust duct system.
- *Biosafety cabinets*: Either of the following classes will be required for all the sections:
  - *Class II-B2 biosafety cabinet*: (100 fpm, 100% exhausted to exterior through HEPA).
  - *Class II-B3 biosafety cabinet*: (100 fpm, 100% exhausted to exterior through HEPA), plena under negative pressure to room.
  - *Class III biosafety cabinet*: Gas-tight cabinet, supply through HEPA, exhaust through 2 HEPA.
- *Bench-top work surfaces*: Solid chemical-resistant material, such as epoxy resin, in laboratory space where fume hood or chemical-rated biological hood is installed.
- In spaces where biologically contaminated material is to be placed on work surface, it should be of stainless steel. Standard plastic laminate in nonlaboratory spaces such as offices, conference rooms, lunch room, toilet rooms, etc.
- *Laboratory floors*: Chemical-resistant sheet rubber or rubber tiles with welded seams and an integral cove base. Should be vibration-proof and high-strength flooring.
- *Laboratory walls*: Epoxy-painted concrete masonry units or gypsum wall board, bullet-resistant wall with epoxy coating at firing range.
- *Laboratory ceilings*: Nonshedding acoustical tiles, except in postamplification rooms and wash-down rooms, such as evidence drying rooms, which are epoxy-painted gypsum wallboard.
- *Nonlaboratory spaces*: Acceptable interior finish standards for offices and nonlaboratory support spaces.
- *Hands-free sinks*: At all clean sinks.
- *Clean sink areas*: Located at the entrance to every laboratory section. Used only to wash hands upon leaving a laboratory section.
- *Caustic (acid/alkali) waste plumbing*: At all epoxy resin sinks and fume hood cup sinks.
- *Bulk chemical and clandestine laboratory evidence storage rooms*: To include dilution system, neutralizing filters, or holding vessels. Exhaust system to expel both heavier- and lighter-than-air vapors. Explosion-proof electrical fixtures and chemical spill containment.
- *Biovestibules*: Locate between "clean" and "dirty" spaces, between main circulation corridor and entrance to a laboratory section that potentially contains hazardous airborne contaminants. There should be an interlock between clean and dirty spaces with air handled through differential pressurization to prevent ex-filtration of contaminated air.[41]

Space Parameters

The space required for the laboratory is shown in Table 8.[35] and the line diagram at Figure 4.

Table 8: Space required for the laboratory.

Room/Area	*Area in m²*
General area	
Reception	15
Stores (many may be required)	10
Staff change room	06
Toilets	
Patients	04
Staff (common)	04
Administrative office	12
Circulation	30%
Clinical laboratory section	
Biochemistry laboratory	15
Hematology laboratory	10–20
Toxicology and biology section	
Bench space per analyst	4.5 m
Radioimmunoassay room	12
Reagent preparation	18
Refrigerated storage	18
Mitochondrial DNA (mtDNA) room	18
Chemical section	
Bench space per analyst	4.5 m
Examination room	14
Wet blood preparation	10
Reagent preparation	18
Electrophoresis, photochromatography	18
PCR preparation room	11
PCR detection room	10

LEVEL ONE BASEMENT

Entrance: There should be separate ramp entrances for ambulances and walk in patients. The doors should be sensor based for remote activation. From the entrance of ramp positive air pressure at a gradience of 30 Pa should be maintained in order to avoid any decontamination from outside environment. Both entrances should direct the flow of patients toward the triage area.

Triage and Detection Area

Location: It should be located with barrier free entry. The entrance should naturally lead to this area. An open space of 30–40 m^2 minimum should be marked as the triage area.[23] There should be a centralized nurse station. There should be one oxygen cylinder and vacuum suction located in triage area.[24] A quick screening for the coding should be done here and the casualties to be directed to the respective earmarked areas based on the prioritization. This area differs from other mass casualty incidences triage in the following ways:

- The triage will be based on level of decontamination along with type of injury.
- Chemical and radiological detectors will be utilized to check the level of contamination.

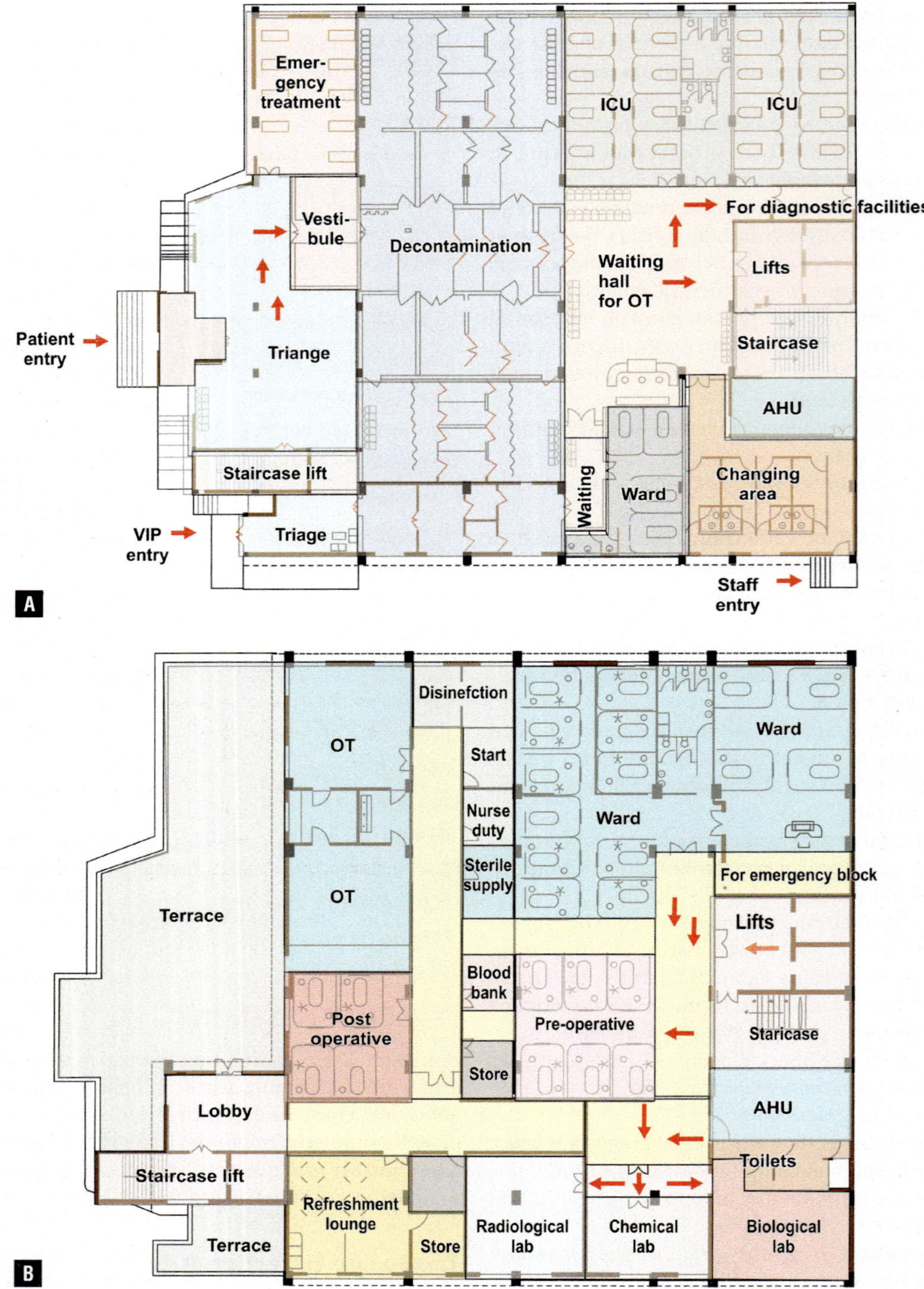

Figs. 4A and B: (A) Ground floor plan; (B) First floor plan.

- The staff present in the triage area should be using PPE's.
- Wheelchair and stretcher storage shall be provided for arriving patients. This shall be out of traffic with convenient access from entrances.

Decontamination Facility[38, 41-43]

There should be a place for undressing and earmarked space to keep contaminated clothing. There should be separate place for people requiring assistance and those not requiring assistance. The casualties requiring assistance are laying casualties and children.

The considerations for this area are as follows:

- There should be no windows or doors about the defined area or where all doors are securable from the outside and all windows are capable of being shuttered.
- Boundaries shall be defined on the paved ground surface with a yellow paint line and the word "DECON" painted within these boundaries.

- Negative airflow but drawing air within the confines of the decontamination structure; exhausted directly to the outdoors, no less than 50 ft (15.24 m) away from the decontamination site with no recirculation of air.
- This system should be defunctionalized when the decontamination structure is not in use.
- Ceiling, wall and floor finishes should be smooth, nonporous, scrubbable, nonadsorptive, nonperforated, capable of withstanding cleaning with and exposure to harsh chemicals, nonslip, and without crevices or seams.
- Floors should be self-coving to a height of 6 inches (152.4 mm)
- The surface of the floor should be self-finished and require no protective coating for maintenance.
- Water drainage must be contained and disposed of safely to ensure that it does not enter the hospital or community drainage systems. There should be a "saddle" at the floor of the door buck to prevent efflux.
- Provision for ample cold and hot water.
- Flexible water hose with pressurized water shower system.
- Specialized stretches for decontamination of lying casualty.
- Floor should be nonporous and nonskid type.
- Floor drains and contaminated water trap.
- Area for assisted decontamination must be provided with nonporous glazed tubs, 1 m × 2.2 m. The staff providing assisted decontamination shall be at all times using PPE.
- A separate overhead tank for storing decontamination solution with common pipelines with two way outlets (taps/showers).

The decontamination facility is planned as a walk through passage such that there is pressure difference of 15 Pa from undressing room to decontamination chamber, and 15 Pa from decontamination chamber to detection room. An air curtain will be installed at the exit of undressing area.

Undressing Area

- 2.2 m wide and 2.2 m long chambers—4 for assisted undressing and 10 for unassisted undressing.
- The partition of chambers will be done with prefabricated steel partitions with in-built pressurized chutes with decontaminant solution jets on either side.
- The chute will have its outlet at the basement to a double bin tank with internal porous tank to drain out the detergent solution and this will go to the holding tank.

Decontamination Area

- 2.2 m wide and 6.6 m long 4 chambers for assisted decontamination and 10 for unassisted decontamination. Two of the assisted decontamination chambers should have tubs.
- The partition of chambers should be done with prefabricated steel partitions with in-built pressurized water jets on either side.
- Each of the chamber should further have a opaque bathroom curtain partition at a distance of 2.2 m, such that each chamber has three areas separated by curtains. Such a design can accommodate three casualties in a chamber at a time.

Secondary Detection and Secondary Decontamination Room

This room should be manned by hospital staff with PPE. The staff should assist in detecting traces of any contaminants. Separate rooms for male and female should be planned. Two rooms one each for male and female 30 m^2 each should be adequate. The patients from this area if decontaminated completely, should be sent to drying and dressing room and if contaminants are detected, further decontamination should be done by the staff.

The considerations for this area are as follows:

- Flexible water hose with pressurized water shower system.
- Flexible water hose with pressurized decontamination solution.
- Staff with PPE for carrying out detection.
- Adequate space for sterile clothing storage.
- There should be at least 2 cubicles of 2.2 × 2.2 m of clear floor space for each cubicle.
- Cubicles should be separated from each other by curtains for privacy.
- A contamination detector sensor at the automated exit door which opens only if people passing by are not contaminated.

Drying and Dressing Room

Separate rooms for male and female and children should be present. Each room should have of at least 5 change cubicles of 2 m^2 each. These should be separated by curtains. There should be ample storage space (almirahs) with set of cloths of varying sizes and towel. A space of 20 m^2 will be required for each room. One male staff in male dressing and one female staff in female dressing room should be present to provide assistance if required.

Resuscitation Room

A minimum space of 30 m^2 is required for each resuscitation cubicle. The planning considerations for this area are as follows:

- Space to ensue good access (preferably 360°) to the patient.
- Adequate lighting.
- Provision for passive decontamination.
- Floor drains.
- Storage areas for supplies and medication and auto injectors.
- Pneumatic tube system for sending the samples to laboratory.
- Each cubicle, with vacuum, oxygen, and air outlets, monitoring space, and nurse call buttons.
- Cubicles should be separated from each other by curtains for privacy
- This area should include space for registration, as well as a physician/nurse work station.
- Hand washing stations one per treatment cubicle
- At least one treatment/examination room should be designated for pelvic examinations.

Consultation and Examination Room

The considerations for this area are as follows:

- Storage area for storing basic medicines and examination lights
- This area should include space for registration, discharge, and waiting, as well as a physician/nurse work station.
- Space required for each consultation room is 12 m^2
- Hand washing stations one per consultation room
- At least one examination room should be designated for pelvic examinations.

Counseling Room

The room will provide counseling to the worried well who are in fear of contamination without actual contamination. A space of 15 m^2 will be required.

Plaster Room

This area will cater to those patients who have been decontaminated and have minor injuries or simple fractures and who are expected to be discharged after plaster. The space required is 30 m^2.

The considerations for this area are as follows:

- Storage space for splints and traction equipment.
- If a sink is used for the disposal of plaster of Paris, a plaster trap shall be provided.
- This room will also house a mobile X-ray machine.

Vehicle Decontamination Area

A slightly raised platform of 100 m^2 in the open area is required for decontamination of ambulance and vehicle bringing patient from contaminated area. This area should be located 100 m away from the patient decontamination and triage site.

- There should be water hose with pressurized water system which can produce pressure of 60–120 pound/sq inch.
- Water hose with pressurized soap solution.
- Provision for hot water.
- Floor drains connected to the holding tank (each vehicle requires around 1,200 L of water).
- Staff with PPE for carrying out decontamination.

Dead Body Decontamination and Packing Area

Although in a CBRN event, only those casualties will be transported to hospitals that have fair chance of survival but still there is a likelihood of enroute death or death while resuscitation. To cater for such situations a separate room for decontamination and packing of dead bodies should be provided. After packing the bodies will be moved to storage area till its final claim/cremation. A room of 15 m^2 would be adequate. The considerations of this area are:

- There should be water hose with pressurized water system
- Water hose with pressurized soap solution
- Provision for hot water
- Floor drains connected to the holding tank
- Staff with PPE for carrying out decontamination
- Built-in cupboards for body storage bags.

Space Parameters

The total space required for the triage, decontamination of patients dead bodies and vehicles is shown in Table 9.

Table 9: Space requirements for triage and decontamination.

Sl. No.	*Area*	*Space (m^2)*
1.	Triage area	30–40
2.	Decontamination area	
	Undressing with assistance	20
	Undressing without assistance	48
	Decontamination with assistance	58
	Decontamination for unassisted	145
	Secondary detection and secondary decontamination room	30 × 2
	Drying and dressing room	20 × 2
3.	Resuscitation room	30
4.	Consultation and examination room	12 × 2
5.	Counseling room	15
6.	Plaster room	30
7.	Vehicle decontamination area	20–30
8.	Dead body decontamination and packing area	15
9.	Staff decontamination area	4
10.	Staff rest room	20–30
	Total	559–589

Table 10: Pressure gradient requirements.

Parameters	*Specifications*
Air pressure relationship to adjacent areas	
Outside to entrance of basement	Positive, + 30 Pa
Triage area	Negative, –15 Pa
Triage area to undressing room	Negative, –15 Pa
Undressing to decontamination room	Negative, –15 Pa
Decontamination to detection and secondary decontamination	Positive with air curtains
Secondary decontamination to dressing	Positive with air curtains
Dressing to other areas	Normal

Table 11: Space requirements for mortuary.

Sl. No.	*Area*	*Space (m^2)*
1.	Body storage room	42
2.	Relatives waiting room	20
3.	Staff room	12
4.	Office for documentation	12
	Total	86

Pressure Gradients

The air pressure assumes importance in a CBRN environment. The various specifications are shown in Table 10.

LEVEL TWO BASEMENT

The level two basement should house the following facilities:

- *Area for delay tanks*: The entry to this area should be restricted. The space should be adequate to hold minimum six tanks of 10,000 L capacity each. There should be space for installation of additional tanks if required.
- *Mortuary*: The mortuary planned for CBRN facility will be used only for body storage and handing over of bodies when claimed. No autopsies will be carried out as this might lead to contamination of facility.

It should have a body storage room with mortuary cabinets. There should be minimum two cabinets for holding six bodies each. Space required is 3.5 m^2/body (Table 11).

Space Parameters

Refer to Table 11.

- *Area for treatment, packing and handing over of patient clothing*: The chutes of undressing area will have its outlet here into double bin tanks with internal porous tank. There should be space of atleast two 50 kg drying machine for decontaminated clothes. Space and provision of hand held detectors.

REFERENCES

1. Robert F. C Hospital, NIKA Technologies, Inc. for VA Office of Construction and Facility Management (CFM) Revised by the WBDG Health Care Subcommittee downloaded from http://www.wbdg.org/design/hospital.php.
2. www.gcx.com
3. Guidelines for Hospital Emergency Preparedness Planning. National Disaster Management Division, Ministry of Home Affairs; Government of India North Block, New Delhi.

4. Hospita Medical Surge planning for Mass Casualty Incidents. Florida Department of Health.
5. www.doh.state.fl.us
6. www.gov.uk
7. Risk Management Series Design Guidance for Shelters and Safe Rooms providing protection to building against terrorist attacks.FEMA 453/May 2006.
8. www.wbdg.org
9. Guidance for Hospitals on Surface Decontamination of Self-Presenting Persons Potentially Exposed to Hazardous Chemical, Biological, or Radiological Substances April 2012 Scotland Government NHS Scotland downloaded from http/www.readyscotland.org/.../guidance_for_hospitals_on_the_surface_decontamination_of_self_presenting_persons_-_april_2012.pdf.
10. Allied Joint Doctrine for Chemical, Biological, Radiological and Nuclear Defence, AJP- 3.8 Edition A version 1; 2012 Published by NATO Standardization Agency.
11. SA Bland. Chemical, Biological and radiation causalities: Critical Care Consideration. JR Army Med Corps. 155(2):122-174.
12. Medical Management of Radiological Emergencies. Armed Forces Radiological Research Institute Bethesda Maryland; 2010 downloaded from http://www.afrri.usuhs.mil/outreach/infoprod.htm#guide.
13. www.fas.org
14. Dan K CBRN and HAZMAT Incidents at Major Public Events Planning and Response; John Willey and Sons Inc Publication. Hoboken, New Jersey; 2013.
15. Kaszeta. "Medical Preparedness", CBRN and Hazmat Incidents at Major Public Events Planning and Response, 2012.
16. Hospital Based First Receivers of Victims from Mass Casualty Incidents Involving the Release of Hazardous Substances December 2005, Occupational Safety and Health Administration.
17. Guidelines for Design and Construction of HealthCare facilities. The Facility guideline Institute 2001 ed Published by ASHE (American Society for Healthcare Engineering of the American Hospital Association155 North Wacker DriveChicago, IL 60606.
18. National Disaster Management Guidelines Chemical Disasters (Industrial) 2007. National Disaster Management Authority. Government of India.
19. National Disaster Management Guidelines. Management of Chemical Terrorism Disasters 2009. National Disaster Management Authority.Government of India.
20. National Disaster Management Guidelines; Management of Nuclear and Radiological Emergencies 2009. National Disaster Management Authority. Government of India.
21. National Disaster Management Guidelines; Management of Biological Disasters 2008. National Disaster Management Authority. Government of India.
22. NFPA-99, Standards for Health Care Facilities ed 2005: National Fire Protection Agency ; Washington DC USA.
23. International Building Codes 2009; International Code Council, USA.
24. Gupta S, Kant S. Modern Trends in Planning and Designing of Hospitals: Principles and Practices. Jaypee Brother Medical Publisher Pvt. Ltd. 2007.
25. Guidelines on Design and Construction of Healthcare Facilities. The Facility Guideline Institute Published by American Society of Healthcare Engineering of American Hospital Organisation; Chicago. USA; 2010.
26. Unified Facility Criteria; Design Medical Military Facilities; 2011; Department of Defense; USA downloaded from http://dod.wbdg.org
27. Risk Management Series: Design Guide for Improving Hospital Safety in Earthquakes, Floods and High winds; FEMA 577; 2007.
28. Guidance for Protecting Building Environment from Airborne Chemical, Biological and Radiological Attacks. Department of Health and Human Services, Center of Disease Control and Prevention NIOSH; April 2003.
29. Wood CM, et al. Guidelines for Handling Decedants Contaminated with Radioactive material; Department of Health and Human Services Center of disease Control and Prevention Georgia.
30. Building and Infrastructure Protection Series. Reference Manual to Mitigate Potential Terrorist Attacks Against Buildings FEMA -426/ BIPS-06/October 2011.
31. Text Book of Military Medicine, Medical Aspects of Chemical and Biological warfare: Borden Institute Walter Reed Army Medical Center. 1997 downloaded from http://www.nbc-med.org/SiteContent/HomePage/WhatsNew/MedAspects/CWBWFMelectrv699.pdf
32. www.nidm.gov.in Internet
33. Protecting waste water assets planning for decontamination waste water Publishers: National Association of clean water agencies. Downloaded from www.ncawa.org
34. mmrs.fema.gov
35. Forensic Science Laboratories: Handbook for Facility Planning, Design, Construction and Relocation; National Institute of Standards and Technology; US Department of Commerce; June 2013.
36. National Disaster Management Guidelines; Medical Preparedness and Mass Casualty Management; October 2007; National Disaster Management Authority. Government of India.
37. www.dtic.mil
38. www.fgiguidelines.org
39. www.scribd.com
40. https://www.nist.gov/publications
41. labmanager.com
42. www.pdc.arizona.edu
43. camfilfarr.info

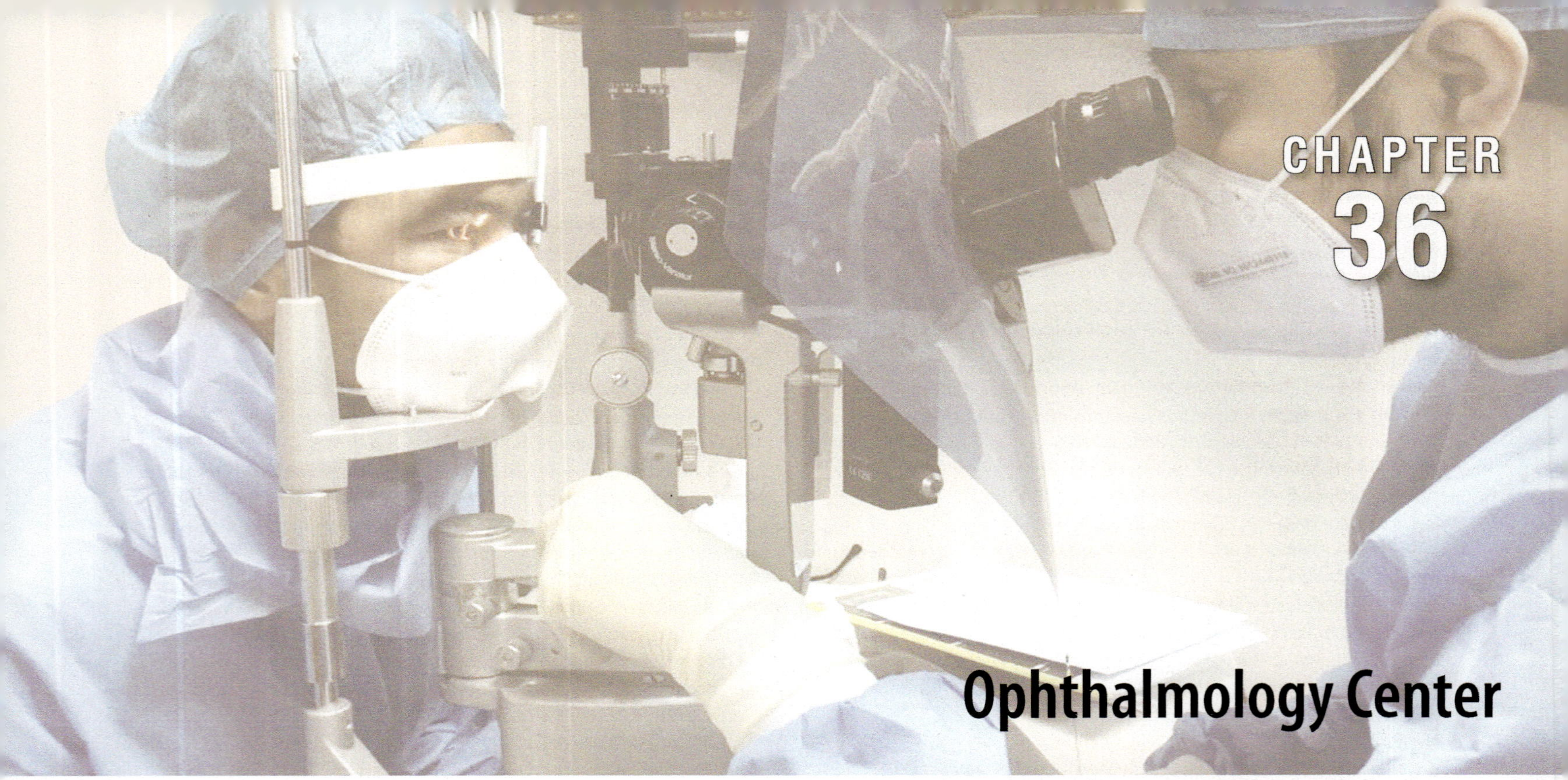

CHAPTER 36

Ophthalmology Center

Parmeshwar Kumar, Kanika Jain, Shakti Kumar Gupta, Sunil Kant, R Chandrashekhar

INTRODUCTION

Visual impairment, perhaps amongst all disabilities, leaves the patient the most debilitated, helpless and dependent. It is also a largely preventable illness. Globally, the number of people of all ages visually impaired is estimated to be 285 million, of whom 39 million are blind, with uncertainties of 10–20%. People 50 years and older represent 65% and 82% of visually impaired and blind, respectively. The major causes of visual impairment are uncorrected refractive errors (43%) followed by cataract (33%); the first cause of blindness is cataract (51%).[1]

According to a study published in Lancet in 2017, globally, of the 7.33 billion people alive in 2015, an estimated 36-0 million were blind, 216.6 million people had moderate to severe visual impairment and 188.5 million had mild visual impairment. Functional presbyopia affected an estimated 1094.7 million people aged 35 years and older, with 666.7 million being aged 50 years or older. The estimated number of blind people increased by 17.6% from 30.6 million in 1990 to 36.0 million in 2015. This change was attributable to three factors, namely an increase because of population growth (38.4%), population aging after accounting for population growth (34.6%) and reduction in age-specific prevalence (-36.7%). The number of people with moderate and severe visual impairment also increased, from 159.9 million (80% UI 68.3–270.0) in 1990 to 216.6 million in 2015.[2,3]

Blindness is a major public health problem in India and other parts of the developing world. In earlier days, trachoma was the leading cause of blindness. With socioeconomic development and increased longevity, cataract has been the leading cause of blindness since 1986. It is estimated that there are 9–12 million blind people in India, amounting to about one-fourth of the global number.[4,5]

A Brief History

The word 'eye' has its origin in Anglo-Saxon, probably from the Baltic languages, with the Friesian 'oie' the closest precursor. There is a town of Eye in Suffolk (a county in England), and eye hospitals are an Anglo-Saxon phenomenon. Their origin in the early part of the 19th century had been preceded by the recognition of the surgeon oculist as a separate entity on the 18th century medical register. After the inception of eye hospitals ophthalmology was accepted as an individual specialty.[3,6]

History of Ophthalmology as a Science

The Indian surgeon *Sushruta* wrote *Sushruta Samhita* in Sanskrit in about 800 BC which describes 76 ocular diseases (of these 51 surgical) as well as several ophthalmological surgical instruments (Fig. 1) and techniques. His description of cataract surgery was more akin to extracapsular lens extraction than to couching. Sushruta has been described as the first cataract surgeon.[7]

Medieval Islamic scientists (Fig. 2) combined theory and practice; Ibn al-Haytham (Alhazen) wrote extensively on optics and the anatomy of the eye in his *Book of Optics* (1021). Ibn al-Nafis wrote a large textbook, *The Polished Book on Experimental Ophthalmology*, and divided it

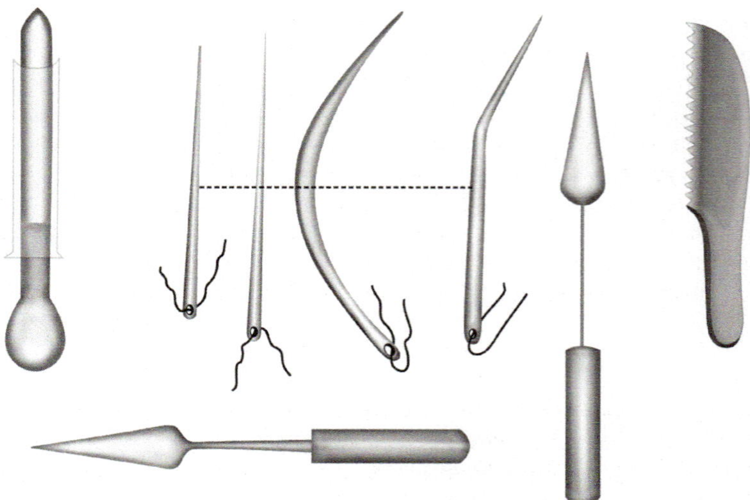

Fig. 1: Surgical Instruments used for cataract surgery by *Sushruta*.

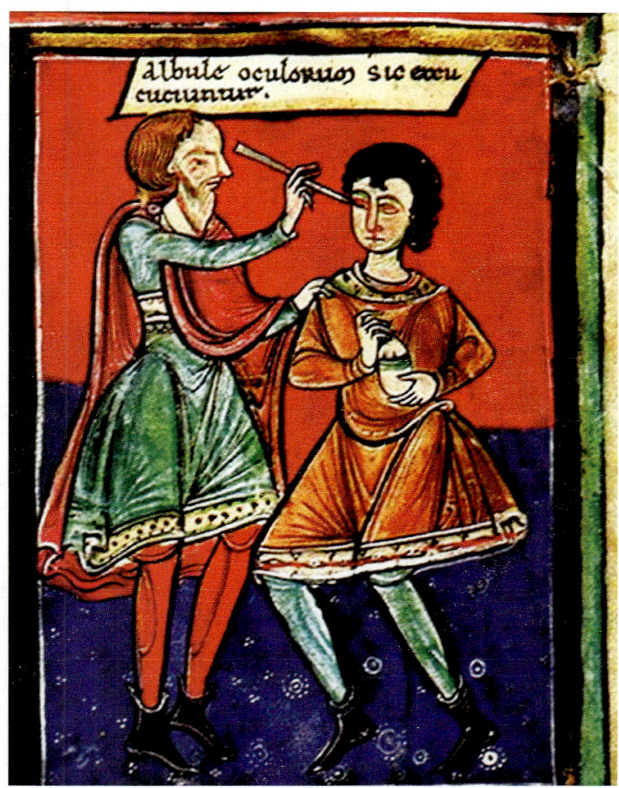

Fig. 2: Eye surgery in the middle ages.

into two parts, *Theory of Ophthalmology* and *Simple and Compounded Ophthalmic Drugs*.[7]

The first ophthalmic surgeon in Great Britain was John Freke, appointed to the position by the Governors of St Bartholomew's Hospital in 1727.[7]

Eye Hospitals[4,6]

The earliest blind asylums in Europe coincided with the crusades, in Germany at Meiningen (1173) and in France the Quinze-Vingts (1266). The latter was specifically founded to treat crusaders 'afflicted by the burning plains of Egypt and Syria.'[3,6]

Blind asylums in Dublin (1781), Liverpool (1791), Edinburgh (1793), and Bristol (1799) all preceded the establishment of eye hospitals while, in London, the Blind Asylum at St George's in the Fields, Southwark, was contemporaneous with the Royal London Hospital for Diseases of the Eye and Ear, later known as Moorfields Eye Hospital (1805) (Fig. 3).[8]

Moorfields Eye Hospital located in London, UK, it is the oldest and largest eye hospital in the world and is internationally renowned for its comprehensive clinical and research activities. The hospital is a major international tertiary care and training center in ophthalmology. Together with the UCL Institute of Ophthalmology, which is adjacent to the hospital, it forms the world's largest site for eye care and research.[8]

Dimensions

Blindness has been defined as a best corrected visual acuity of ≤6/60 (≤20/200) with both eyes open. The global prevalence of blindness is 0.7%. Though there are no reliable data on the incidence of blindness, it is estimated that the number of blind persons globally increases by about 1–2 million per year. Two-thirds or more of this blindness

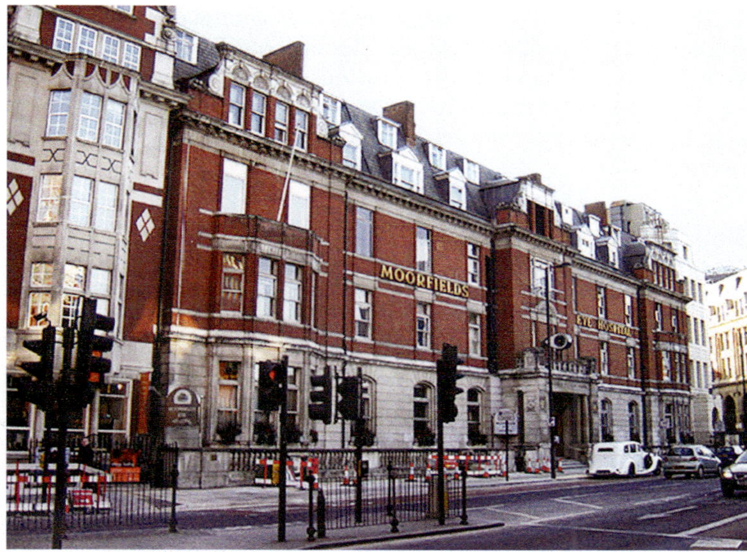

Fig. 3: Moorfields Eye Hospital (1805): Oldest eye hospital in the world.

is avoidable, in that the causes are either treatable or preventable. Programs under the global initiative, vision 2020—The Right to Sight are designed to eliminate the causes of avoidable blindness by the year 2020, and bringing to all people in need the advantage of efficient and effective eye care services.[9,10]

National Program for Control of Blindness

In 1976, India became the first country in the world to start a National Program for Control of Blindness (NPCB).

Refractory Error

The NPCB-WHO survey found that refractive errors were responsible for 7.35% of blindness. The prevalence of uncorrected, presenting, and best corrected visual acuity of 6/12 (20/40) or worse in the better eye was 6.4%, 4.9%, and 0.81%, respectively. Refractive error caused 81.7% of the visual impairment [VA ≤6/12 (≤20/40)].[9,10]

Childhood Blindness

Childhood blindness is defined as a best corrected visual acuity of less than 3/60 (20/400) in the better eye of a child aged less than 16 years. Childhood blindness contributes significantly to loss of productivity as the total number of blind years suffered by the blind child is more than those suffered by a person who becomes blind in adulthood. The prevalence of visual impairment and blindness in children varies from 0.1/1,000 in wealthy countries to about 1.1/1,000 in the poorer countries. The prevalence in India is estimated to be 0.5/1,000 children. The main causes of childhood blindness were congenital globe anomalies (25%) and retinal diseases (22.2%); optic atrophy, cataract, corneal diseases, and glaucoma were the others.[9,10]

Childhood blindness alone accounts for 28.7% of the economic burden of blindness in India. The cumulative economic loss from childhood blindness, amounts to US $ 22.2 billion.[9]

Corneal Blindness

The NPCB-WHO 1986–1989 survey done across the country reported corneal opacities to be responsible for 1.52% of the blindness. The most common cause of corneal opacities is exanthematous fever during childhood. Other causes included chemical burns, use of traditional medicines, corneal edema due to various causes, and pterygium. It is estimated that approximately 20,000 patients with corneal blindness were being added to the backlog waiting for corneal transplants each year.[9]

Glaucoma

Glaucoma is estimated to affect 12 million Indians and causes 12.8% of the blindness in the country. The prevalence of primary open-angle glaucoma (POAG), primary angle-closure glaucoma (PACG), and ocular hypertension (OHT) in the VES is 4.1, 43.2 and 30.8 per 1,000 population, respectively. If strategies to prevent 90% of the preventable blindness due to corneal disease and glaucoma were successful, 29 million blind person years would be prevented by 2020.[9,10,11]

Infrastructure and Human Resource Development

The activities of NPCB included establishment of regional institutes of ophthalmology, up-gradation of government medical colleges and district hospitals, development of mobile eye units, recruitment of adequate manpower, and provision of various ophthalmic services.[9]

Human Resource Development

The current ophthalmologist: Population ratio is estimated to be nearly 1:100,000, in rural areas it is 1 per 219,000. About 70% of the ophthalmologists are located in urban areas. There is no data on other eye-care providers in India (optometrists, ophthalmic technicians, and opticians), who primarily provide refractive services.[9]

Need for the Center[9,11-13]

Over the past 30 years, the magnitude of blindness has steadily increased, with South-East Asia carrying the greatest burden. The risk of blindness increases significantly with poverty and older age and in women. Among the elderly; visual impairment is second only to hearing disability. The three strategic components of vision 2020 program are—Controlling of causes of blindness, human resource development, and development of infrastructure and appropriate technology. One of the major limiting factors in the combat against blindness in the developing countries is the lack of appropriate infrastructure for delivery of eye care. A 10 bedded tertiary level ophthalmic center would form a vital block in the pyramid between a secondary and a center for excellence.

As per information available from various studies, there are an estimated 12 million bilaterally blind persons in India with visual acuity less than 6/60 in the better eye, of which nearly 7 million have visual acuity less than 3/60 in the better eye (presenting vision). Recent survey (1999–2001) in 15 districts of the country indicated that 8.5% of population aged 50+ years is blind (visual acuity <6/60). A survey was conducted in Delhi to assess the prevalence and causes of blindness and low vision in children aged 5–15 years. The survey indicated that 1% of children in this age group had vision <6/18 in the better eye. As already stated, the large cataract surgery deficit, the infrastructural lacunae and the large percentage of visually impaired populace (21%) residing in India, need to be addressed. Besides, it drains the nation economically as well.[1,2]

Functions of the Center

The facility should sub-serve the functions envisaged by the vision 2020 document for a tertiary level eye care center.

- 1 for 5,000 population
- 1 for 50,000 population
- 1 for 5 million population
- 1 for 0.5–1 million population.

The functions should be as follows:

- Treatment of eye problems referred from the service centers and developing an effective follow-up system.
- Surveillance of eye diseases
- Developing human resources for eye care through the training of ophthalmologists, OT personnel, ophthalmic assistants, and management training.
- Stimulation of clinical research in ophthalmology
- Developing policies and programs for advocacy of preventive ophthalmology.
- Teleconsultation facility
- To provide facilities for the training, organization and research in eye bank, including corneal grafting and tissue transplantation.
- Rehabilitation.

Components of an Ophthalmic Center

- Outpatient department (OPD)
- Inpatient areas including operation theaters
- Casualty for ophthalmological emergencies and trauma care
- Clinical departments
- Eye bank
- Research laboratories and training facilities
- Diagnostic services
- Support services
- Engineering services.

PLANNING PREMISES

The followed data has to be collated for a given area during the project planning:

- Magnitude of blindness in the given service area population.
- Estimation of the incidence of blindness in the given service area population.
- Percentage of blindness distribution for different eye diseases.
- Distribution of eye diseases in different age group.
- Surgical capacity based on infrastructure and manpower available.

Resource utilization in terms of surgery per ophthalmologist and surgery per bed per year.

SITE

The first step is to identify the area where the service is needed; a comprehensive situational analysis is done. To estimate the prevalence of blindness and assess its various causes, any of the following methodologies can be adopted:[13]

- A rapid assessment survey.
- Referring to a previous survey in the same area or in an area similar to the one in question, and extrapolating its figures to arrive at a rough estimate.

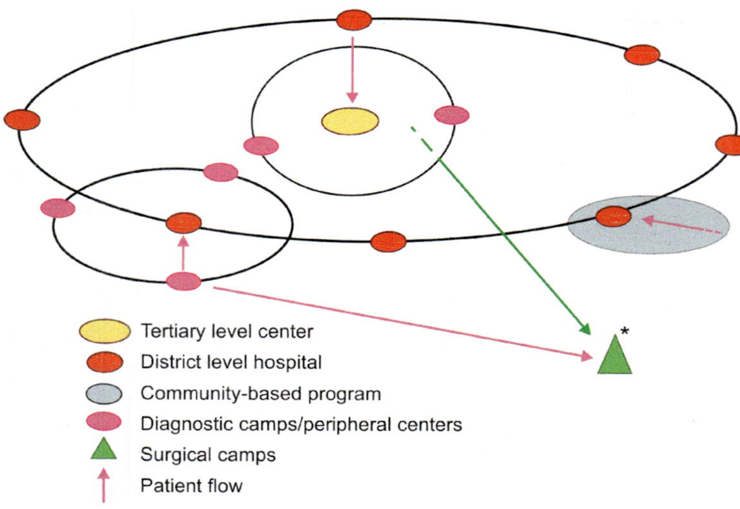

Fig. 4: Role of the center in relation to other eye care facilities and patient flow.

- Organizing a community-based eye care program like a diagnostic/screening camp or primary eye care center or vision center. This modality can also help in assessing the level of existing eye care services in the area, their quality and their acceptance in the local population.[13] This would also help in understanding of the patient flow between these facilities and their spheres of influence, and also form long-term networks of which the center becomes an integral part as depicted in Figure 4.

GENERAL PLANNING CONSIDERATIONS

Location

Location of the clinic in an area of greatest need is a prime concern. The sites that are chosen should be central to the local population. Public access is vital. Convenient access from patient parking or arrival areas is necessary; pedestrians, vehicular traffic and public transportation are other necessary factors in location. Concerns such as access to the site by staff and parking for both users and staff is very important. Most patients at ophthalmology clinics are of an older age than the average clinic patient and they are often doubly handicapped. It is therefore very important that parking be located as close as possible to the entrance. Barrier free design requirements are very explicit about handicapped spaces and access walks to the building. Clear signage with Braille configuration is essential, since visually impaired patients can easily become confused if signage is not easily discernible.[6,14]

Access

Ease of access to the center for visually impaired and wheelchair patients is critical. General eye OPD and casualty are best located on ground floor level. Directions to OPD should be very well signposted bearing in mind the need of low vision users. It is helpful to have 'drop off' parking areas close to the ophthalmic OPD and daycare facility where patients can be dropped off by relatives or ambulances.

Covered Entry

Provisions for a covered entrance at the primary access point to the eye center are required. Provide enough covered area to accommodate two vehicles, one behind the other. The width of the roadway or motorable area under the covering should be designed to accommodate an accessible van to park at the entrance while allowing a separate vehicle to pass by.[15,16]

It is not uncommon for emergency vehicles to access. Therefore, height of covered entrance is to be designed to allow clearance for large emergency vehicles. The covered entrance is also an area where visitors and patients may relax and sit. Ample space for seating and circulation should be planned near the entrance.[15,16]

Parking Areas

Space should be marked for parking for disabled, parking for ambulances and parking for the staff. While the space allocation for parking for the staff and ambulances should be as per the regular norms there should be a dedicated lot with accessible parking spaces (1.5 spaces per bed) with safe and easy access to buildings. Site roadways to and from parking areas should be capable of accommodating two-way traffic. Proper signage and direction arrows may enhance clarity of destinations and paths.[14]

SIGNAGES

Signages (Figs. 5 to 13) deserve a special focus while planning an eye care facility. Braille signage is important. 'Americans with Disabilities Act,' mandates that all signs which identify 'permanent rooms and spaces' contain a variety of special features, such as raised letters and Braille so the signs can be 'read' tactually (by feel) by blind people, in addition to being read visually by sighted persons and is being used by many other countries.

Standard Guidelines for Braille Signage

Location: To address the needs of visually impaired people, signs must be in a predictable location and have easily readable text. For people

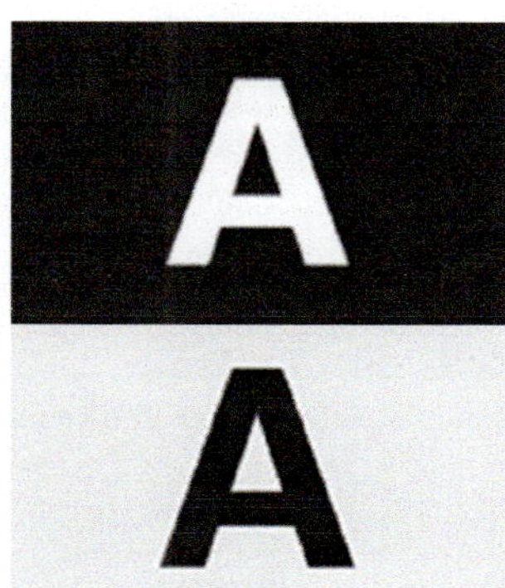

Fig. 5: Text with contrast: light against dark backdrop or vice versa.

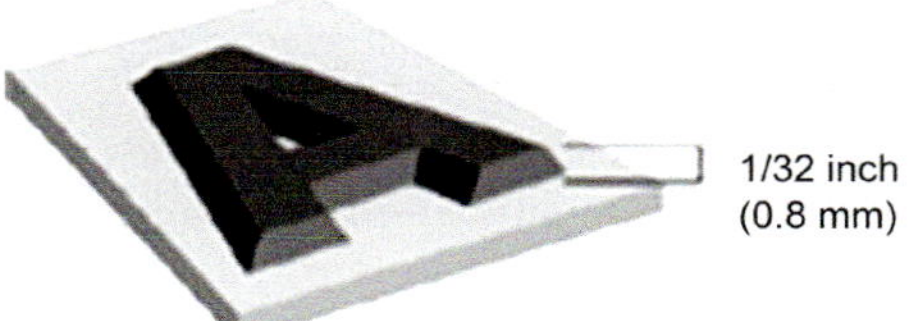

Fig. 6: Tactile text to be raised a minimum of 1/32 inch from the sign surface.

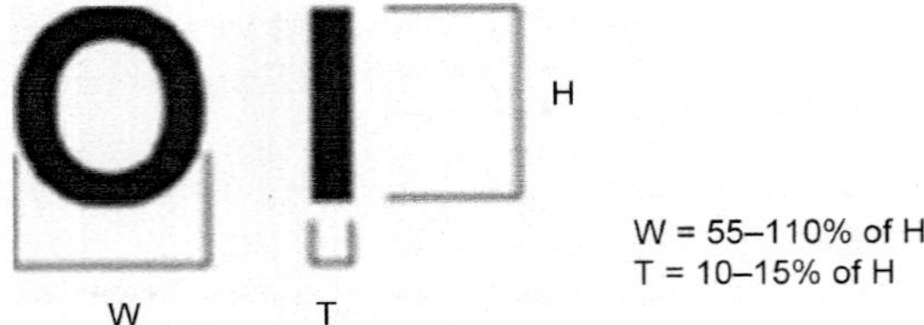

Fig. 7: Tactile text must be uppercase. Text must have a character width (based on the upper-case letter 'O') falling between 55 and 110% of the character height (based on the upper-case letter 'I').

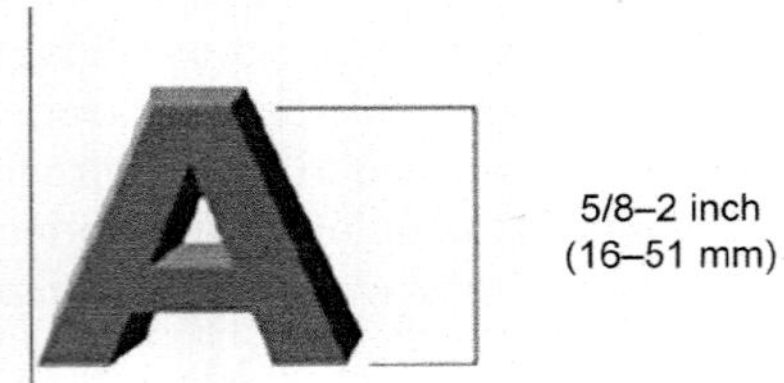

Fig. 8: For visual/tactile text, letters must be from 5/8 inch to 2 inch high.

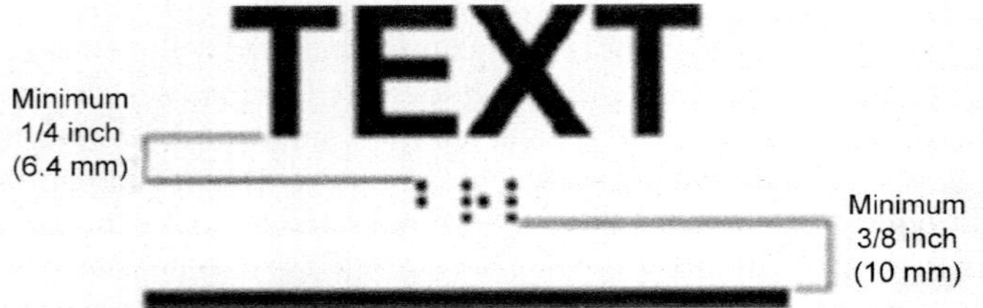

Fig. 9: Braille dots must be at least 3/8 inch from raised borders or any other raised decorative elements and a minimum of 1/4 inch from the raised text.

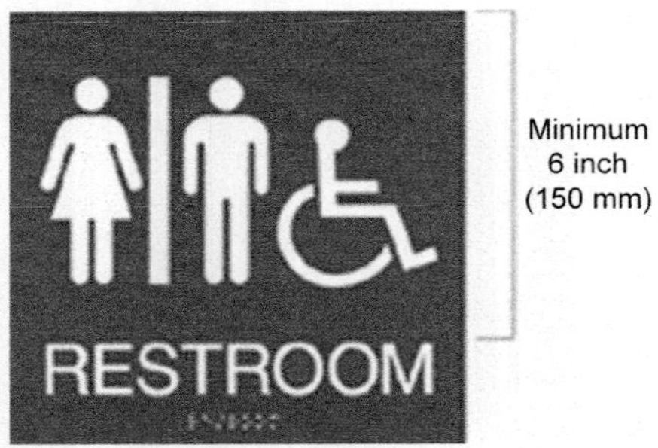

Fig. 10: Border dimension of a pictogram shall be 6 inch minimum in height.

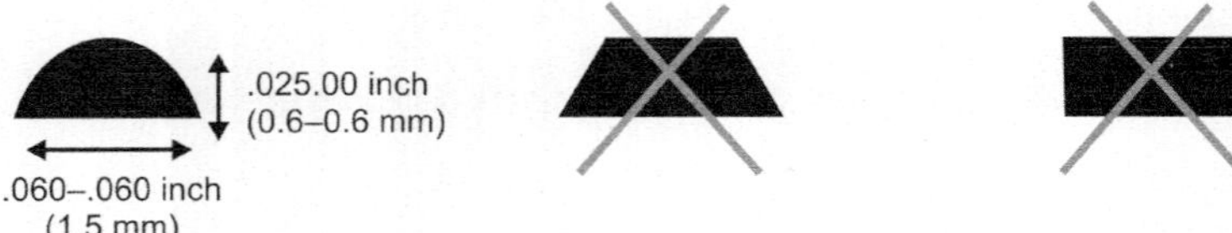

Fig. 11: Braille dots must be domed or rounded, not flat-topped, and reach a height of between 0.025 inch and 0.037 inch above the surface of the sign.

who rely on Braille, the Braille location and readability is important. For partially sighted people, the requirement, 'easy to read,' leads to specific text formatting, spacing and color requirements. Text must be in 'Sans serif' font and touching the letters on a sign allows a

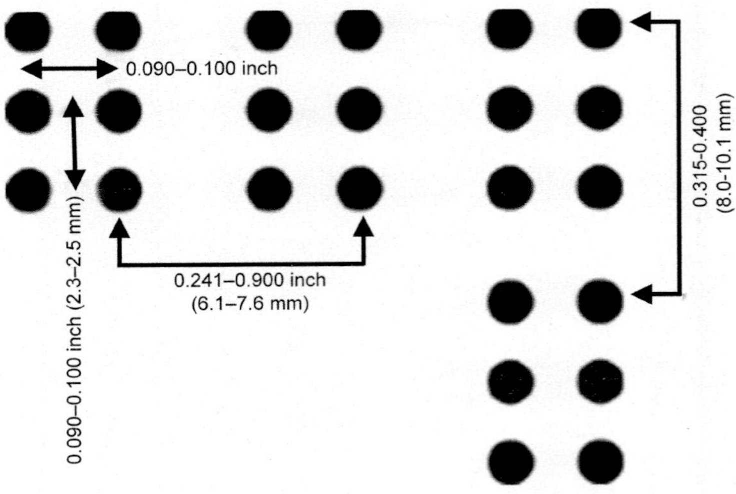

Fig. 12: The spacing between dots must fall between 0.090 inch and 0.100 inch so the patient can feel when one cell stops and the next cell begins.

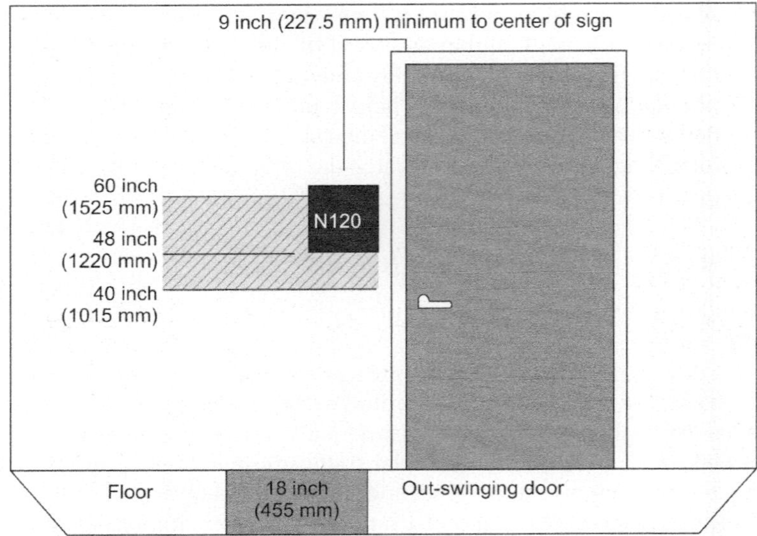

Fig. 13: Braille on the sign must be placed between 40 inch and 60 inch from the floor and mounted on the wall adjacent to the latch side of the door, center of the sign at least 9 inches from the door.

sight-impaired person to 'read' the text message using their fingertips (Fig. 13).[17]

Talking Signs System

Braille signs, even where available, do not replace the functions of print signage because they cannot be read from a distance; they have to be searched for and found before the information they contain can be used; and a majority of people who are unable to read print signs (because of visual limitations) have not learned to read Braille. The concept of remotely readable infrared signage is to level the playing field for those unable to use printed signs. For example, the Talking Signs System uses infrared transmitters placed at sign locations or on key environmental features. Transmitters send out a spoken message on a beam of infrared light. The prerecorded human speech frequency modulates a 25 KHz carrier.[18]

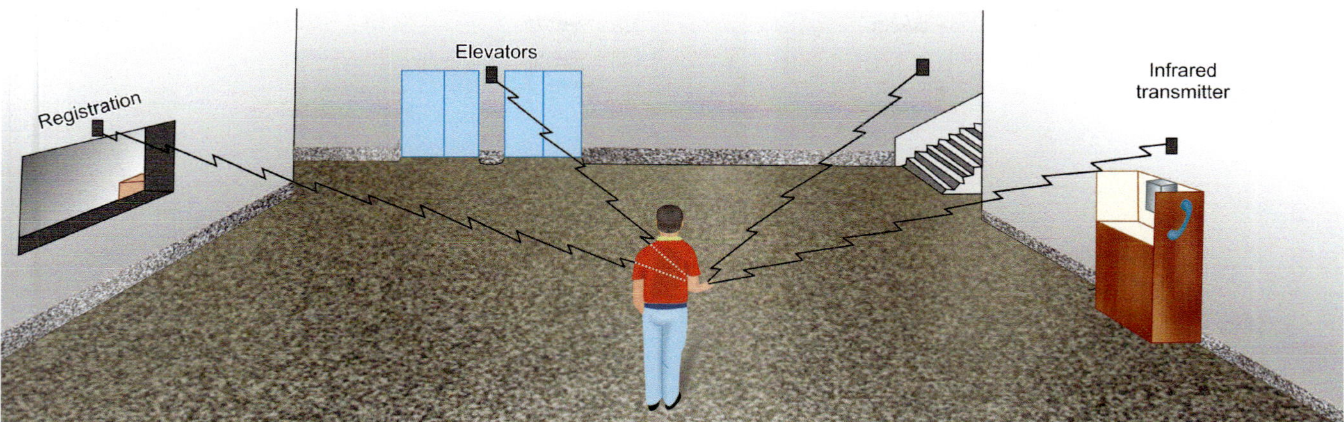

Fig. 14: Talking sign system.

The blind user carries a receiver which, when activated by a push button, translates the message back into spoken language. Users hear the digitally recorded message whenever the front of the receiver is pointed in the direction of the infrared transmitter. Adjustment of the transmitters and the LED arrays ('tuning' of the system) allows control of the maximum distance at which the talking sign message is received, the direction in which a message is transmitted, and the area the message covers.[18] This can be used by the inpatients or even outpatients in the hospital (Fig. 14).

Ramps[15]

Any part of an accessible route with a slope greater than 1:20 should be considered a ramp. The function of a ramp is to provide accessible building entrances across steep topography where a gradual incline is not possible.[14]

Requirements

- *Slope:* The maximum slope of a ramp in a new construction should be 1:12.
- *Width:* The minimum width of a curb ramp should be 36 inches (915 mm), exclusive of flared sides. However, Gupta et al. recommends a minimum width of 1200 mm.
- It is convenient to have a landing planned every 9 meters. Landing length should be a minimum of 60 inch, i.e. 5 ft - 0 inch (1524 mm) - clear. If ramps change direction at landings, the minimum landing size should be 60 in by 60 inch, i.e. 5 ft - 0 inch × 5 ft - 0 inch (1524 mm × 1524 mm).

Handrails installed on both sides and mounted at a height of 2 ft - 9 inch (838 mm) and extend 1 ft - 0 inch (304 mm) beyond beginning and end of ramp. About 4 inch (101 mm) high × 8 inch (203 mm) wide curbs on each side to prevent wheelchairs from scuffing walls or catching on railing posts. Smooth transitions between vehicular pathways and pedestrian walkways should be ensured by means of curb ramps.[14]

Walkways

The walkways provide a continuous and accessible surface free of any steps or change in levels. The surface should be slip resistant and the surface slope should be conducive for the patients movement. A minimum width sufficient for two individuals in wheelchairs to pass each other comfortably must be provided [7 ft - 0 inch (84 inch) (2133 mm)].

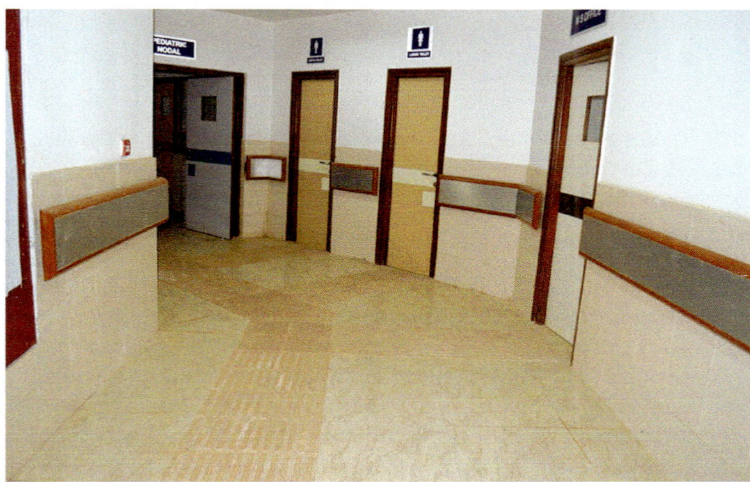

Fig. 15: Tactile strips along with the hospital floors.

Tactile strips and textured tiles (Fig. 15): These help in guiding the visually challenged throughout the hospital. Tiles can be placed over walls or before steps or lifts (Fig. 16).

Lifts/Elevators

The elevator door should facilitate the movement of beds, trolleys and multiple wheelchairs. A set of double hand rails is recommended. It is important to have Braille signages besides the lifts. The dimensions that take into both visually impaired as well as visually impaired wheelchair bound patients are:

Length	:	2400 mm
Breadth	:	1850 mm
Door opening	:	1200 mm

Doorways and Passages

Doorways to rooms should be 1500 mm wide or wider to accommodate patient beds, electric wheelchairs and other personal mobility devices. A level space should extend on either side of the doorway for facilitating opening/closing by a visually challenged person. The entrances and exits of passages should be wide enough to move to heavy machinery, beds and trolleys in and out. The corridor width should be in the range

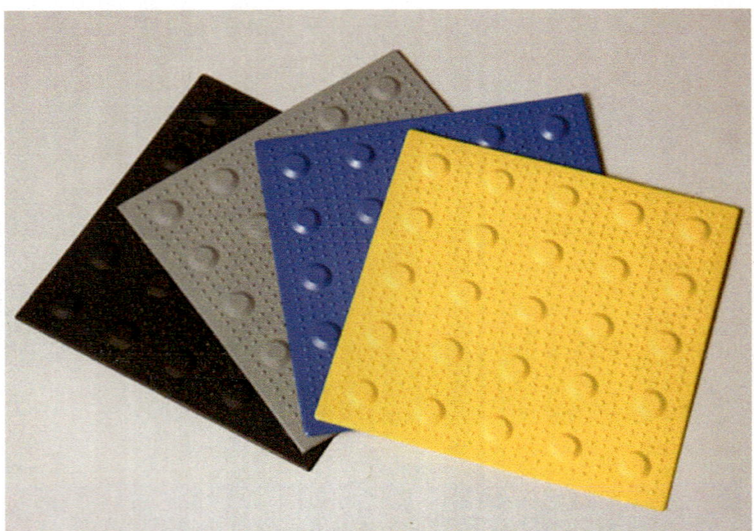

Fig. 16: Textured tiles can provide warning to the visually challenged.

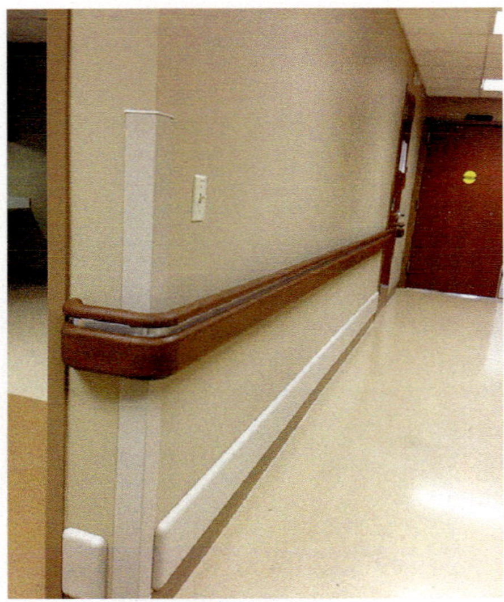

Fig. 17: Wall protection.

of 2100 mm to 2400 mm. Automatic doors as an option at doorways should be actively considered also be considered.

Wall Protection (Fig. 17)

Measures to protect the wall should be employed to reduce damage caused by wheelchairs, stretchers, and carts. A crash rail located 8 inch above the floor is beneficial, as well as one located at chair rail height. This upper bumper guard may be combined with a handrail to provide additional assistance to patients traveling along corridors. In areas that experience only cart traffic, the upper rail may be eliminated. Solid sheet products installed between the upper and lower crash rails can protect this area from dents and marks caused by rolling equipment and wheelchairs.[18,19]

Engineering Services

Water Supply

The water requirement in the hospital for is 500 L/bed/day for inpatients excluding fire-fighting needs. There shall be separate tank for water for firefighting. A 3 days reserve should be available at all times.

Electric Supply and Power Backup

The requirement of electricity is 5 kW/bed/day for as for super-specialty hospitals. This should ideally from 2–3 grids. The proper wiring and earthing should be done in accordance with the state electricity board. A suitable generator backup should be provided.

Heating, Ventilation, and Air-conditioning and Indoor and Indoor Air Quality Standards

While designing a hospital heating, ventilation and air-conditioning (HVAC) system, designers have to hold twin views of the facility—One from the functional point of view and the other from the HVAC point of view. Both views are interrelated. According to the American Society of Heating, Refrigerating, and Air-Conditioning Engineers (ASHRAE), from the functional standpoint, a typical hospital facility basically comprises seven categories of areas:[6,14]

- Surgery and critical care (operating room)
- Nursing (patient rooms, daycare facility, etc.)
- Ancillary (radiology, laboratories, etc.)
- Administration (offices)
- Diagnostic and treatment (examination room, therapy room, etc.)
- Sterilization and supply (sterilizer room, equipment storage, etc.)
- Service (kitchen, laundry, etc.).

The functional requirements dictate the HVAC requirements. The HVAC, however, views all the spaces from the point of view of—temperature and humidity, ventilation, pressure relationship with surrounding spaces, air cleanliness level, air distribution, operating hours and system reliability.[6]

The minimum air changes in the OT are 15 air changes per hour (acph) and in the wards it is 4 acph. Transfer air should not be more than 2.8 m^3/min (100 cfm) per undercut door. Care should be taken to minimize the short circuiting between supply and return/exhaust in the spaces. Corridors should not be used to supply or exhaust/return air from rooms except exfiltration/infiltration, from positive/negative pressure rooms adjacent to a corridor should be considered in balancing airflow. Corridor air may be used to ventilate toilet rooms. Seismic bracing should be provided as part of making the hospital safe from earthquakes.

Concept of Energy Recovery

Energy recovery wheel or enthalpy wheel, which can recover both sensible and latent energy, has been used for the operating theaters. The wheel, installed upstream of supply air AHU, recovers energy by allowing transfer of heat (sensible and latent) from the outdoor air to the exhaust air. To get an idea of the performance just in terms of the sensible energy, the outdoor air can be expected to cool from 32° to 26°C when passing through the wheel and transferring energy to the exhaust air (typically at about 21°C).[6,20]

Fire Safety

The building shall be constructed incorporating the fire safety features as per National Building Code 2016.

GENERAL DESIGN CONSIDERATIONS

Outpatient Department

OPD Complex

- Glaucoma clinic and ward (2nd floor)
- General OPD
- Cataract clinic and cataract ward (same floor).

The Eye Care Facility is planned with following perspectives

The broad design principles for an ophthalmology hospital are:

- Planning and designing to promote infection control and better hygiene
- Appropriate and sustainable technology
- Design to follow function
- Response to social context/community design
- Esthetic appeal with focus on green and evidence-based designing
- Hospitals safe from disasters
- Facilities development process, i.e. to allow for future growth.

The areas can be broadly divided into:

- Direct patient care units
  - Outpatient department
  - Inpatient department
  - Daycare
  - Operation theater
  - Casualty.
- Diagnostic services
  - Radiology
  - Laboratory medicine
  - Blood transfusion unit.
- Support services
  - Central sterile supply depot
  - Laundry
  - Manifold
  - HVAC
  - Dietary.
- Training and research facilities
  - Seminar room
  - Simulation room
  - Lecture theaters.
- Specialized facilities
  - Eye bank
  - Telemedicine.

Figure 18 shows 3D depicting the concept of same level specialty OPD, corresponding laboratories and wards.

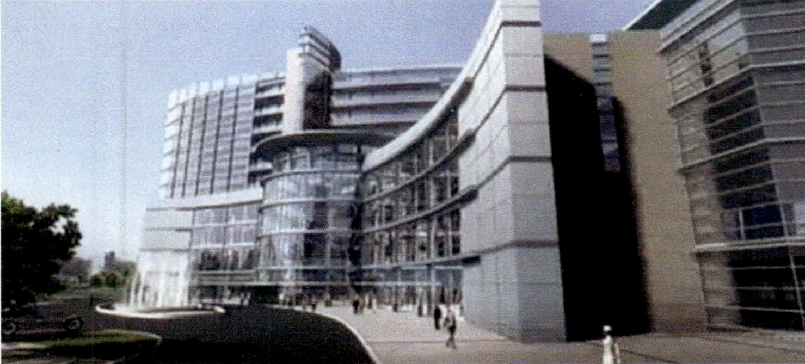

Fig. 18: A 3D view depicting the concept of same level specialty OPD, corresponding laboratories and wards.

FLOORWISE DISTRIBUTION OF AREAS

Ground Floor

- Reception
- General/screening OPD
- Radiological facility
- Casualty including emergency OT
- Pharmacy
- OPD investigation laboratories
- Value-added services including cafe, optician's clinic, ATM, information kiosk, patient assistant services.
- *Vehicles:* Ambulance services for eye bank, staff vehicles.

First Floor

- *Specialty OPD:* Cataract and lens clinic
- Cataract ward
- Community ophthalmology ward
- Special investigation laboratories (separate for inpatients and outpatients) for cataract.
- Excimer laser surgery clinic.

Second Floor

- Cornea clinic and glaucoma clinic
- Glaucoma ward and cornea ward
- Glaucoma laboratory and cornea laboratory
- Consultants' chambers (cornea and glaucoma).

Third Floor

- Pediatric ophthalmology clinic
- Pediatric wards
- Pediatric ophthalmology consultants' chambers
- Visual stimulation and play room
- Ophthalmoplasty clinic.

Fourth Floor

- Retina clinics (medical and surgical)
- Ocular oncology clinic
- Retinal laboratories
- Ward A: Medical retina and oncology
- Ward B: Surgical retina and onco surgery.

Fifth Floor

- Neuro-ophthalmology clinic
- Orthopedics and squint clinic
- Consultant's chambers
- Outpatient department and IPD laboratories (for squint and neuro-ophthalmology).

Sixth Floor

- Private wards
- Telemedicine facility
- Consultant's chambers.

Seventh Floor

- Simulation laboratory and research facility
- Community ophthalmology department
- Ocular pathology
- Ocular microbiology
- Ocular biochemistry
- Administrative offices
- Staff cafeteria.

Eighth Floor

- Operation theaters complex: GA and LA
- Daycare facility
- Eye bank
- Lecture theater.

Basement

- Medical records
- Main stores—medical, surgical, stationary and IT
- Central sterile supply department (CSSD)
- Laundry
- Manifold
- Engineering services
- Computer facility.

Stack Diagram: Ophthalmology Center

Refer to Flowchart 1.

GROUND FLOOR

Outpatient Department

Introduction and Context

The majority of adult patients attending ophthalmic OPDs are over 65 years of age. Similarly, the majority of people with sight problems are aged over 60. These large numbers of older people attending ophthalmology OPDs are added to by large numbers of diabetic individuals with or at risk of eye disease. Importantly, ophthalmology OPDs also deal with significant numbers of children.[20,21]

At present a significant proportion of both ophthalmic primary care and management of long-term care for ophthalmic chronic

Flowchart 1: Stack diagram: Opthalmology center.

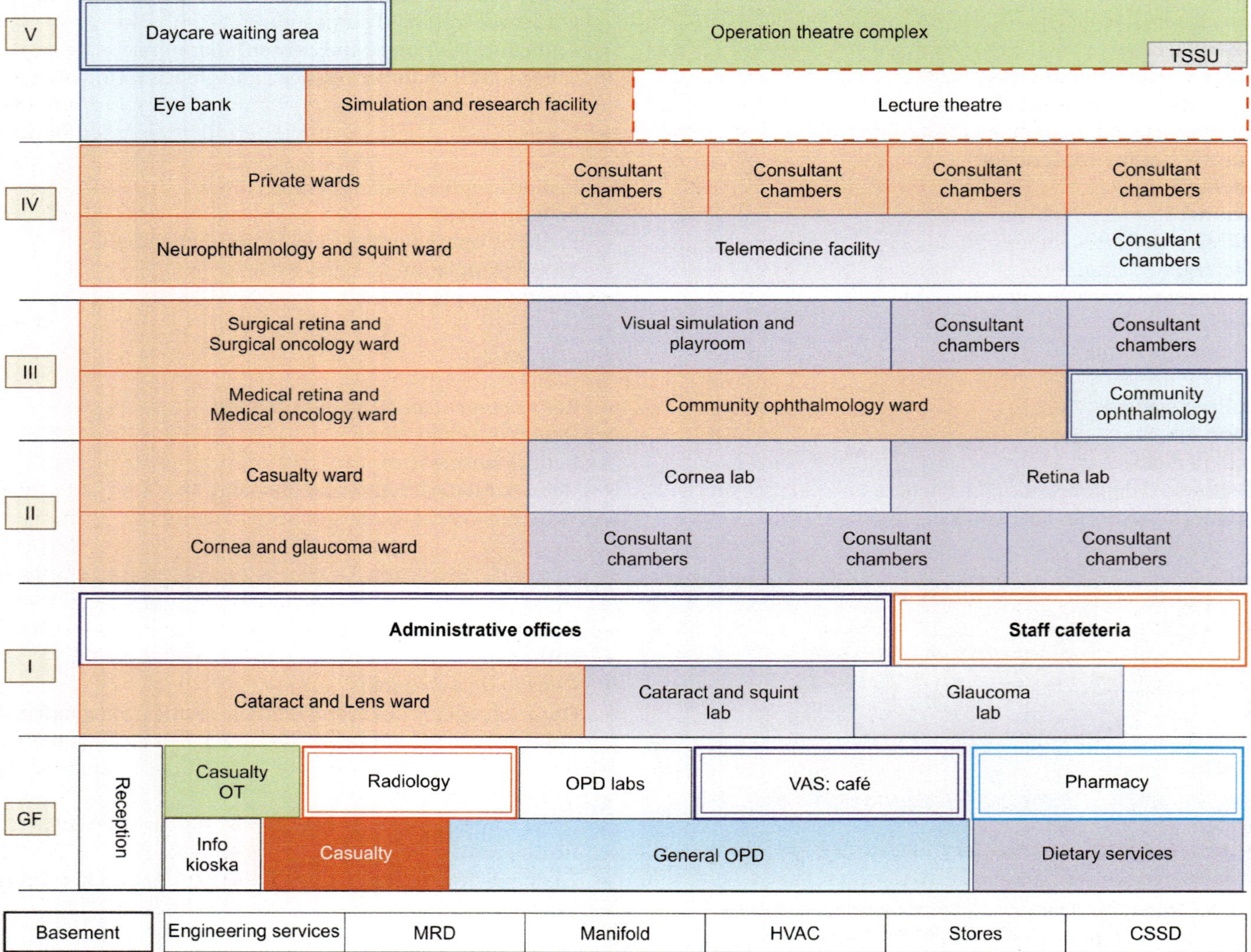

(VAS: value added services)

conditions takes place in the tertiary Hospital Eye Service in OPD. All of these factors make the ophthalmic OPD a hub of activity and underpin the importance of quality OPD architecture, layout and patient flows.[20,21]

Eye Clinic Design

The plan envisaged has the general OPD on the ground floor with specialty OPDs staggered over the floors in such a manner that OPD of the particular specialty, e.g. cataract or glaucoma clinic would be flanked by the wards of the same specialty with the joining limbs having the OPD investigative modalities.

Figure 19 illustrates an innovation that can be used. In the revolving screening OPD module, the healthcare personnel remain stationery while the patient revolves around them. This design promotes high volume OPD throughput.

The OPD area should be close to the operation theater and treatment area functionally so that patients can be progressed directly to treatment where this is appropriate, such as might be the case for intravitreal injections for acute member degeneration AMD patients. Self-contained ophthalmology units which are discrete within a hospital's design often demonstrate better patient flow.[21]

Outpatient Department Patient Pathway

It is helpful to use service improvement techniques to identify and reduce any bottlenecks in the patient flow in OPD. On arrival patients should be directed to a clearly signposted reception desk and then advised where to wait until they are called into the clinic rooms. The clinic nurse should be aware of any patients with special needs. Clinics work more efficiently if thought is given in advance to patient flows. For new patients, a patient letter vetting process can usefully include a series of initial instructions when the patient arrives in the clinic (in addition to visual acuity testing) such as:[20,21]

- Examination for afferent pupillary defect
- Field of vision examination
- Orthoptic assessment
- Refraction examination undertaken on arrival
- Instillation of mydriatic eyedrops.

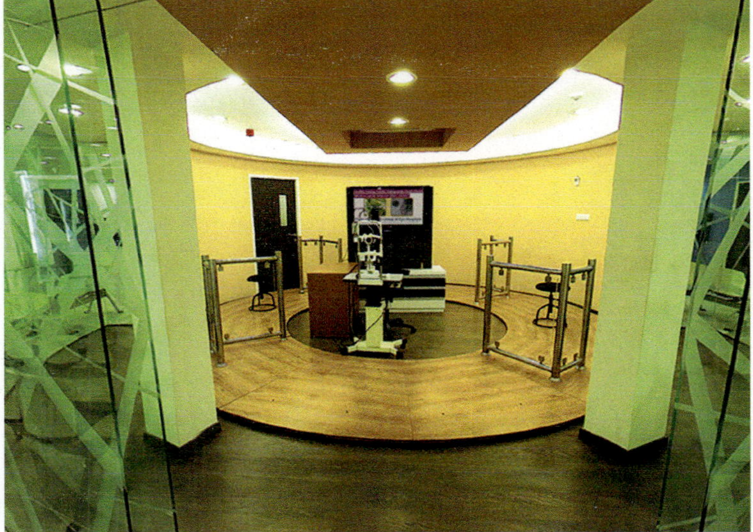

Fig. 19: Revolving screening outpatient department chamber.

RELATIONSHIP DIAGRAM

Planning and Design Considerations

- Net-to-department gross factor (NTDG) for OPD is 1.60. This number when multiplied by the programmed net square foot (NSF) area determines the departmental gross square foot.[17]
- Patient corridors should be a minimum of 8 ft wide, to accommodate wheelchairs, motorized scooters, or gurneys
- Consideration should be given to the effects of building vibration, as building vibration could interfere with the accuracy of patient testing
- Exam/treatment rooms should be designed to the specialized equipment required for eye testing. Windows to the exterior may be provided but total room darkening capability should be able to be attained. Each exam/treatment and low vision examination/training room should be provided with a hand washing sink, paper towel dispenser, and waste receptacle. The sink needs to be provided with either wrist blades or motion sensors for infection control purposes. Light dimming should be available. The rooms should be designed to accommodate the specialized equipment required for eye testing that includes special ophthalmic equipment stand arms and ability to move/glide the patient examination chair necessary for wheelchair, scooter, or gurneys patients[6,14,17]
- Interior partitions should be primarily painted gypsum wallboard on metal stud construction. Partitions around exam and treatment rooms should have sound attenuation batts between the studs[14]
- Floors in offices, exam and treatment rooms, waiting area and most other spaces should be vinyl composition tile with a 100 mm (4 inch) high resilient base.
- Toilets should have ceramic tile floors and bases[14]
- Ceilings should be lay-in acoustic ceiling tile systems
- Interior doors should be primarily 45 mm (1¾ inch) thick hollow core wood in metal frames. Hollow metal may be used where fire rating is required.[14]

Consultation Chamber

It should be possible to vary the lighting level in the chamber, preferably via a dimmer switch near the slit lamp or by remote control. Window blinds are needed to ensure darkened examination rooms and air-conditioning should thus be present throughout the department. All rooms should include an illuminated snellen visual acuity test chart although there should be provision in the eye clinic for log medicine administration record (MAR) charts and contrast sensitivity testing. For adult clinics, the 6 meters distance between patient and chart can be reduced to 3 meters by using a mirror.[20,21]

Each clinic room or workstation must be equipped with a slit lamp, tonometer, indirect ophthalmoscope as well as a reclining chair or examination couch. A portable slit lamp and tonometer should be available for occasional use.[21]

There must be adequate hand washing facilities and alcohol gel dispensers to allow clinical staff to decontaminate their hands between each patient contact. Guidance on instrument decontamination from the relevant ophthalmology guide books should be followed.

Rooms must be large enough to allow visually impaired and wheelchair patients to be transferred-use safe manual handling techniques-to the slit lamp or examination couch. Cantilever mounted slit lamps can be used to examine patients in wheelchairs as an alternative.[20,21]

Many eye units use a modular system incorporating the slit lamp along with other diagnostic equipment combined with an electrically adjustable chair, suitable for most patients. The clinician's chair must also be adjustable and provide good lumbar support.[21]

Equipment for obtaining microbiology and virology specimens from the ocular surface should be available. Equipment needed for undertaking examination of lacrimal drainage apparatus should be readily available as should any surgical equipment as needed if minor eyelid procedures, such as treatment of chalazion are undertaken in the OPD.[20,21]

Many ophthalmology OPDs may undertake some teaching of medical and or optometric students who often 'sit in' during clinic sessions. Where such teaching is undertaken video screen display of slit lamp images is helpful.[20,21]

Information Technology Compatibility

All clinic rooms should have access to the hospital's network and internet access. Such computers must have adequate quality monitors for diagnosis of patient images captured from retinal angiograms or diabetic retinal screening and optical coherence tomography (OCT) and for viewing of other digital examinations, including radiology images.[21]

Visual field testing should be undertaken in a room with appropriate lighting conditions and laser rooms should conform to regulations governing the safe use of class 4 lasers. There must be emergency resuscitation equipment available if fluorescein angiography is carried out.[21]

Examination of Children

Clinic rooms should be appropriately equipped for the examination and assessment of children. There should be a separate waiting area for children and parents/guardians.

Optometric examination rooms should have appropriate facilities for visual acuity testing and refraction and there should be a slit lamp and keratometer available for contact lens fitting.[20,21]

Clinic Waiting Areas

These should be well lit and ventilated, and with air-conditioning separate 'sub-waiting' areas are usually provided for patients who have had their visual acuities measured and are waiting to see the clinician or who are waiting for drops to dilate their pupils. Provision should be made for patients in wheelchairs.[20,21]

Public Utilities

Toilets (including facilities for the disabled)(1/8 WC and 1/16 urinal) and facilities for refreshments should be available and clearly signposted.

OPD Waiting Area

Public telephones and direct taxi lines should be available.

Treatment Room

Noncontact tonometry, BP check-up, stitch removal and minor treatment, dispensary for OPD.

Patient Information Booklets

Letters advising patients of appointment detail times and location should be printed on a high quality printer with a font size of at least 14 points. Patient information leaflets (of appropriate size and quality print) explaining common ophthalmic conditions and surgical procedures should be readily available as should information leaflets on patient support groups and access to social services. This information should also be available on audio cassettes or CDs for patients with severe visual impairment and where possible should also be available in languages other than English.[21]

OPD LABORATORIES

The tests carried out in the OPD laboratories (located in proximity to the OPD). Most patients would require refraction and dilatation. There is a need for the following facilities:

- *Ophthalmic ultrasound (Fig. 20):* This would reveal any pathological alteration of the anterior or posterior segment of the eye. It would require a separate chamber with reclining couch.
- Anterior segment laboratory/clinic with slit lamps for use by optometrists.
- Noncontact tonometry to measure the intraocular pressure
- *Autorefractometer:* To test the refraction.

DIAGNOSTIC SERVICES: RADIOLOGY

Radiology imaging services can be organized as one central department which serves casualty, outpatients, and inpatients. Thus, it is preferable to locate it in the ground floor. Core design is preferred over cluster design as this is not a full fledged department and it will reduce patient and staff travel time.

All radiology procedure rooms should be designed to accommodate patients with disabilities as well as space for the transfer of patients from a stretcher to the diagnostic equipment. PACS system can also be used.

The essential facilities are:

- Digital X-ray unit

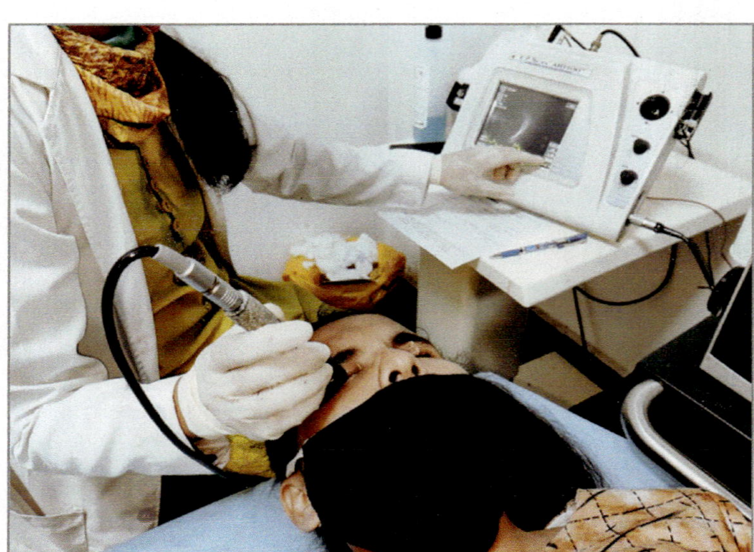

Fig. 20: Ophthalmic ultrasound.

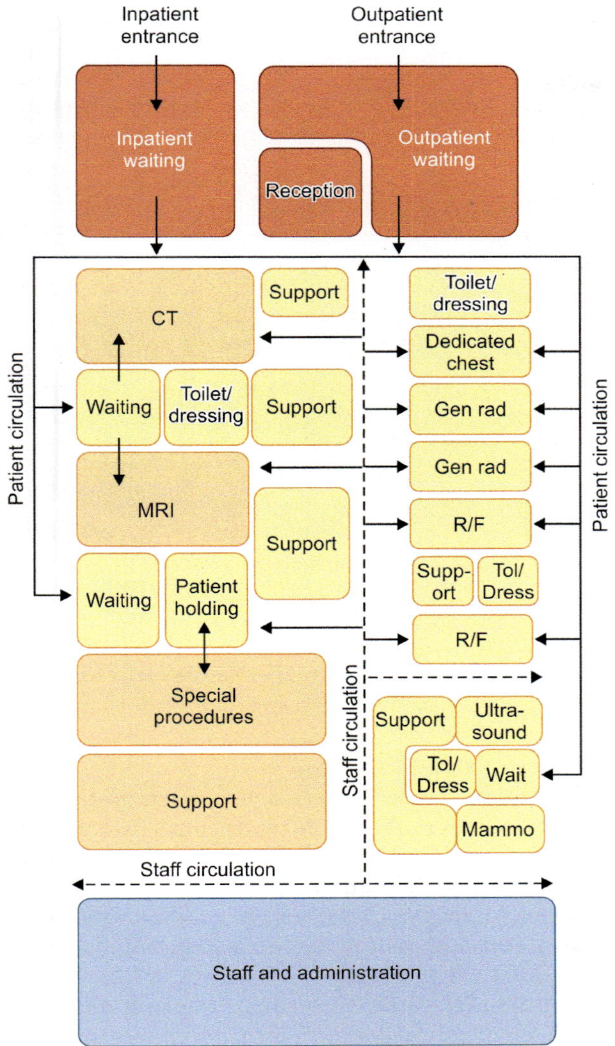

Fig. 21: Functional flow of radiological facility for the eye center.

- Ultrasonography
- Computerized tomography
- MRI.

The functional flow of radiological facility for the eye center is shown in Figure 21.

EYE CASUALTY

Ophthalmology is really a specialty of equipment and instruments and the eye casualty is no exception to the rule. The rules of accessibility such as proximity to road head, signages and patient flow as applicable as in any other casualty. However, special physical facilities and space requirements are discussed here.

Access to Emergency Department

- The directional signs to the ED would be unmistakably marked and clearly visible, day and night. Weatherproof fittings and accessories would be used in all external situations. Per 100,000 annual visits about 6 parking spaces would be provided in a nearby parking lot, or as per the local regulations.
- Space requirement the thumb rule for total special need is—a daily patient load of 100 patients requires about 1,000 m^2.

Public Area

- Stretcher, trolley, wheelchair store. A trolley, stretcher, and wheelchair store or bay would be located immediately adjacent to the entrance. Usually, a wheelchair per about 800 annual visits is needed. Stretchers would, be sturdy and provided with wheel-locks.
- Separate waiting area for emergency patients and relatives, for accompanying children a separate waiting area would be provided. A pram bay of about 6 m^2 is needed.

Administrative Area

- *Registration area:* A room of about 10 m^2 near the entrance hall equipped with a desk, chairs and telephones would serve the purpose.
- Additional area for security guards would be essential.

Clinical Areas

Facilities Required

- Examination/treatment room(s) with examination tables, examination lights, work counters, cabinets, wash basins, X-ray film illuminators, medication storage scrub station located conveniently between the observation rooms.
- Additional adjustable space for dilatation and observation.
- Equipment.
  - Slit lamp (Figs. 22 and 23)
  - Ultrasonography machine-A
  - Snellen's chart and E-chart
  - Clinical photography machine
  - Direct and indirect ophthalmoscopes
  - Flash autoclave (Fig. 24).

Slit lamp: The cornerstone of ophthalmological examination.

CASUALTY OPERATION THEATER

The location must be proximal to the casualty. The contemporary stainless steel operation theater shown in the Figure 25 offsets the

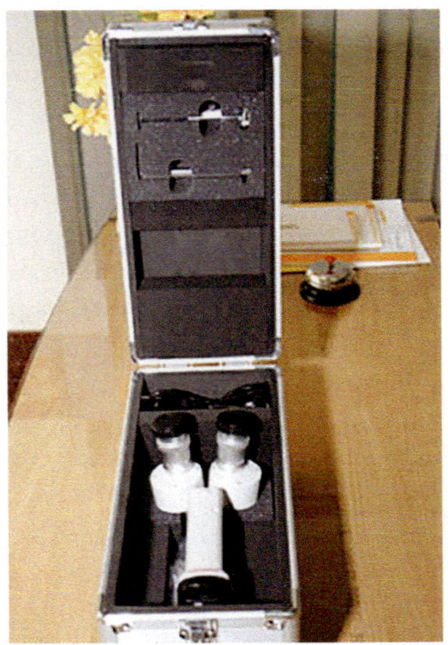

Fig. 22: A hand held slit lamp.

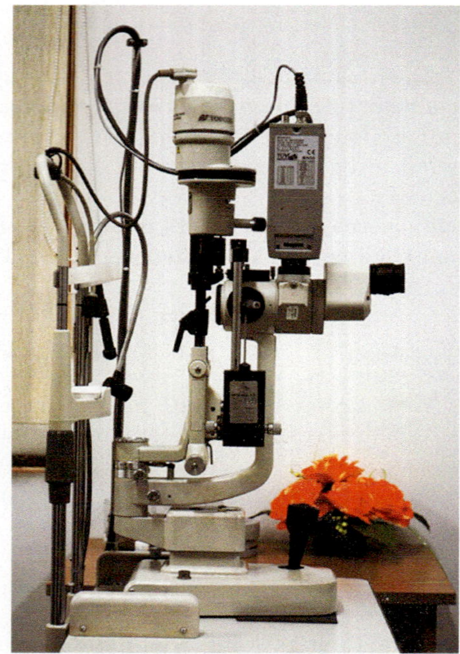

Fig. 23: A traditional slit lamp.

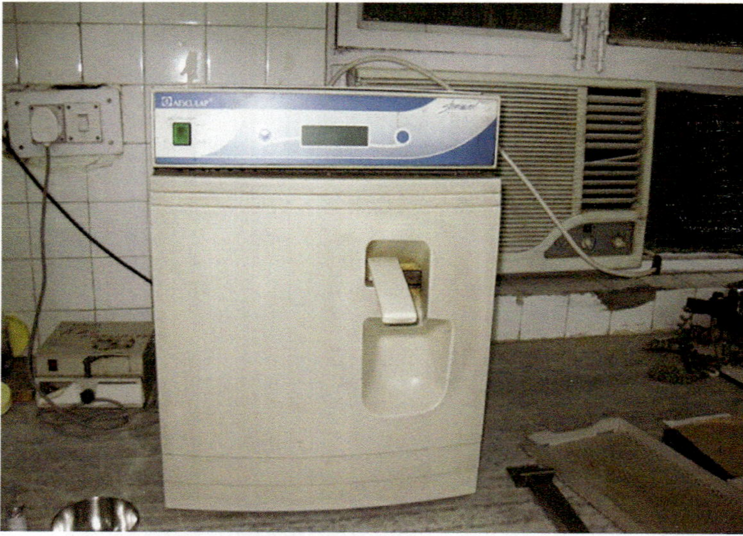

Fig. 24: Flash autoclave for sterilizing instruments in eye casualty.

disadvantage of the ground floor location of the OT and also aids in maintaining asepsis and helps in the rapid turnover. An independent waiting room with changing facilities is also important.

Besides the usual assortment of equipment for any OT, the casualty OT must have an ultrasonography machine and a pachymeter.

VALUE-ADDED SERVICES

- Patient assistance services
- Information kiosk
- Patient check-in
- Patient surveys
- Clinics, doctors surgeries
- Health information access, forms filling
- Virtual receptions.

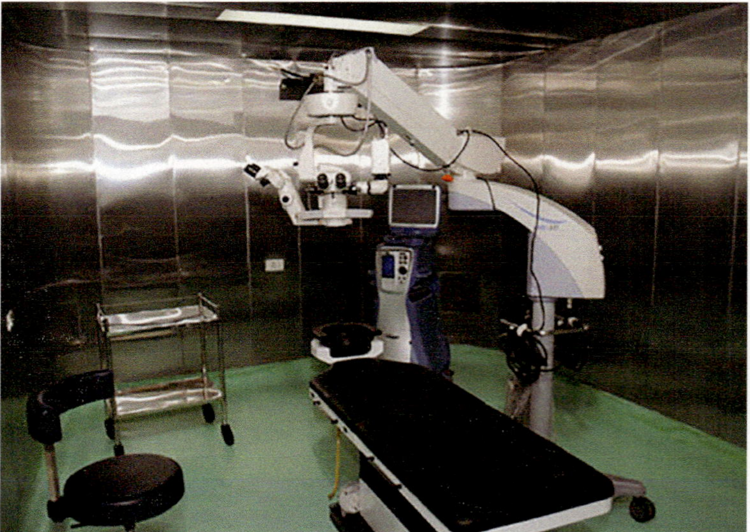

Fig. 25: Steel operating microscope.

Space Criteria: Applicable for the Relevant Floors

Reception Areas

- *Waiting area:* 100 NSF (9.3 NSM)
  - An additional 55 NSF per each projected optometry and ophthalmology exam/treatment room greater than one
  - 100 NSF provides for three standard seats, one wheelchair accessible seat and waiting space for one stretcher. 55 NSF additional allocates 25 NSF for one accessible seat and 30 NSF for two standard seats per exam room greater than one.[14,17]
- Reception 100 NSF (9.3 NSM)
  - An additional 10 NSF for each projected optometry and ophthalmology exam/treatment room greater than three[17]
  - Public toilets, 50 NSF (4.7 NSM).

Patient Areas

- Exam/treatment room, optometry 130 NSF (12.1 NSM)
  - One for each whole increment of 2,400 annual optometry clinic visit.
- Exam/treatment room, ophthalmology 130 NSF (12.1 NSM)
  - One for each whole increment of 2,100 annual ophthalmology clinic visit.
- *Waiting area, dilation*: 100 NSF (9.3 NSM)
  - One per eye clinic.
- *Visual fields room*: 120 NSF (11.2 NSM)
  - An additional room per every increment of five optometry and ophthalmology exam/treatment rooms.[17]

  Note: The visual fields room accommodates testing, evaluation, and monitoring of the visual fields of a patient who may/may not be ambulant. This room may also be used as a patient's darkroom adaptation. One room will be provided in smaller clinics and used for both manual and automated perimetry. A movable partition separating the equipment should be provided. In larger clinics, two separate rooms will be used for manual and automated perimetry.[14,17]
- *Photography room:* 150 NSF (14.0 NSM): 02 in no
- *Pretesting room:* 120 NSF (11.2 NSM).

  An additional 50 NSF if the total number of projected optometry and ophthalmology exam/treatment rooms is greater than five.[17]

Note: The Pretesting room is used by the technician to assist in the performance of preliminary testing and preparation of the patient's profile with the supervision of the optometrist or ophthalmologist. In eye clinics with greater than five optometry and ophthalmology exam/treatment rooms, space for a rotary screening center which provides visual field screening, visual acuity, autorefractor, autolensometer, autotonometer, autokeratometry, and autobiometry instruments located on a single table may be provided.[14,17]

- *Eyeglass fitting and display, and dispensing room:* 140 NSF (13.1 NSM). The eyeglass fitting and display, and dispensing room is used by the technician to assist in the fitting, adjustment, repair, and dispensing of eyeglasses. An area for the display of eyeglasses should be included.
- *Ultrasound/optical coherence tomography room:* 180 NSF (16.8 NSM).[14,17]
  Diagnostic uses of the ultrasound room are for the location of unseen intraocular foreign bodies, for retinal detachment, and for internal view when the patient's eyelid cannot be opened or the patient's eye is blocked by blood or cataracts impeding the examiner's view. The ultrasound room is provided with ultrasound equipment with diagnostic A and B modes, a calculation/computer for intraocular lens calculations, and a reclining patient chair. The optical coherence tomography room for ocular imaging may be combined within the ultrasound room space allocation.[14,17]
- *Eye procedure room:* 220 NSF (20.5 NSM) : 01 room.
  The eye procedures room is designed for any treatment that requires surgical intervention that is deemed 'an office procedure'. Procedures commonly performed in this space are chalazion excision, tarsorrhaphy, biopsy, eyelid tumors, suture external eyelid lacerations, and pterygium removal.[14,17]
- *Laser room (Figs. 26 to 28):* 130 NSF (12.1 NSM): 01 room per clinic. The laser room accommodates treatment of ocular problems including diabetic retinopathy, glaucoma, retinal detachment, occludable angles/ocular hypertension. Equipment commonly provided is laser instruments, a laser cart, a slit lamp delivery system, and safety equipment. The laser room may include more than one laser system.[14,17]
- *Electrodiagnosis room:* 150 NSF (14.0 NSM) 01 room per clinic.

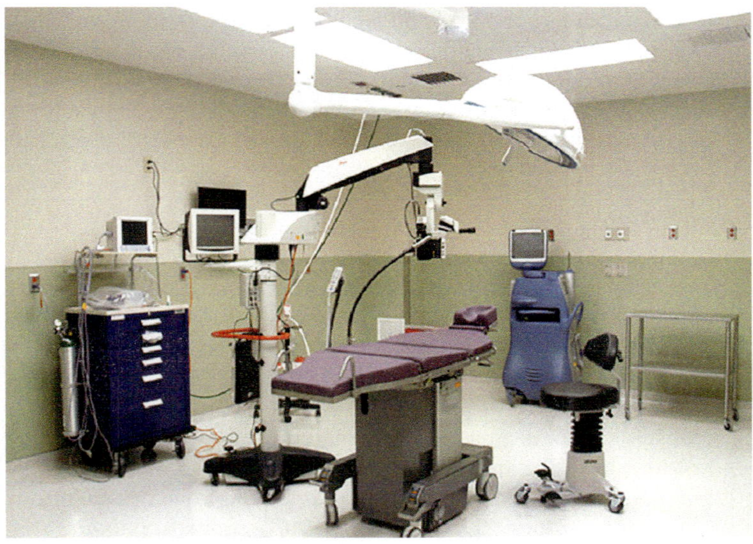

Fig. 27: Laser surgery room.

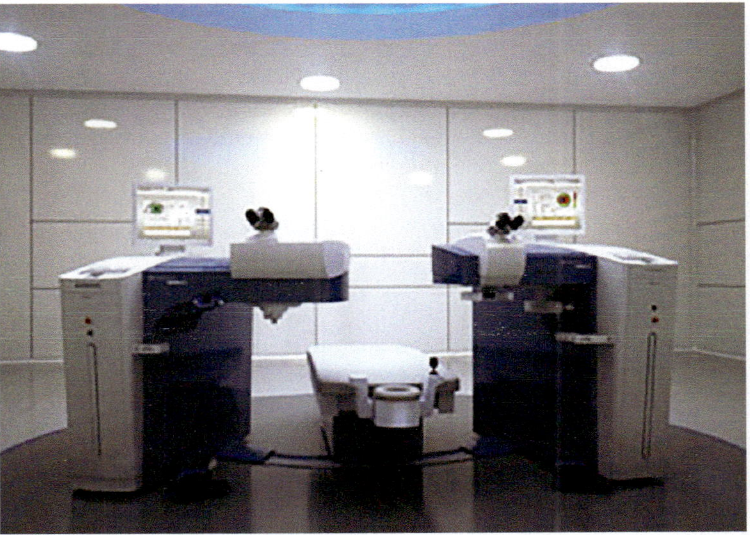

Fig. 28: Laser or bladeless LASIK surgery via the wavelight refractive suite.

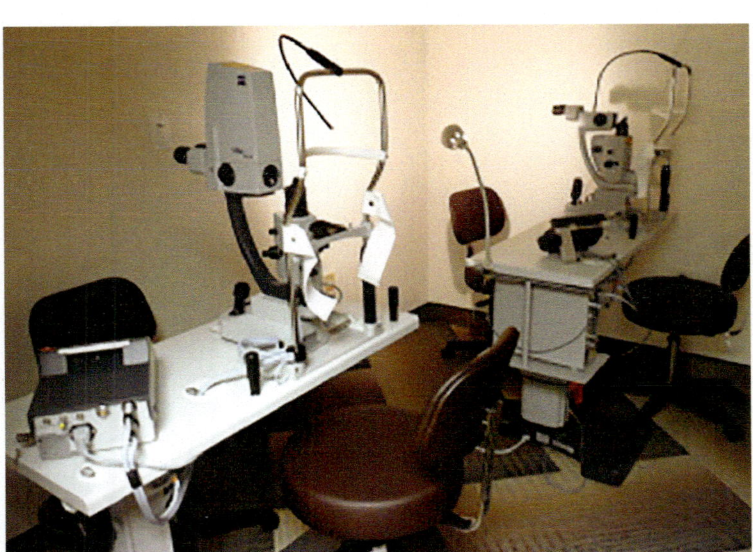

Fig. 26: Laser room.

The electrodiagnosis room accommodates visual digitized equipment for conducting electro-oculographic, electroretinographic, and visual evoked cortical potential testing of retina, optic nerve, and visual pathway functioning with analysis.[14,17]

- *Exam/training room, low vision:* 180 NSF (16.8 NSM) 01 room per clinic.
  The low vision examination/training room is used for the examination of low vision patients, storage of low vision devices, and for minor training and education for adult daily living skills[14,17]
- *Training room, low vision/polytrauma:* 400 NSF (37.2 NSM) 01 room per clinic.
  The low vision/poly: Trauma training room is used to provide vision rehabilitation care. Patient education and eye care counseling sessions are conducted so that patients can learn how to use prescribed low vision and other aids in order to perform everyday skills, activities of daily living, and to improve their overall functional independence. If advanced, victors, polytrauma rehabilitation network site or polytrauma rehabilitation center vision rehabilitation services are authorized, two rooms are recommended[14,17]

- Patient education/contact lens dispensing room 130 NSF (12.1 NSM). The patient education/contact lens dispensing room is used to educate patients about their eye diseases and vision conditions, instruct them on the proper use and instillation of eye medications, provide training in the insertion and removal of contact lenses, and dispense contact lenses.[14,17]

Support Areas

- *Clean supply room:* 80 NSF (7.4 NSM): 01 per clinic.
  The clean supply room provides storage for medical supplies used in the delivery of patient care. It should be accessible from the corridor and located near the eye procedure room.[14,17]
- *Soiled utility room:* 80 NSF (7.5 NSM): 01 per clinic.
  The soiled utility room provides an area for clean-up of equipment, utensils, and for disposal of waste material. It provides a temporary holding area for material that will be picked-up by supply, processing, and distribution (SPD). It should be accessible from the main corridor and located near the eye procedure room.[14,17]
- *Medication preparation room:* 80 NSF (7.5 NSM)
  The medication preparation room should be secured and provide storage for medication. It should be accessible only from within the staff area.[14,17]
- *Storage, equipment:* 120 NSF (11.2 NSM).
- *Storage alcove, medical equipment:* 15 NSF (1.4 NSM).
  The medical equipment storage alcove is reserved for storage of equipment, such as a crash cart, requiring monitoring by the eye clinic staff. The alcove should be located in the clinic area but out of the main traffic flow.
- *Storage alcove, wheelchair:* 40 NSF (3.8 NSM): 01 per eye clinic.[14,17]
- *Storage, eyeglass frame:* 80 NSF (7.5 NSM).

Staff and Administrative Areas[14,16,17]

- *Director:* Ophthalmology 150 NSF (14.0 NSM)
- MS office 120 NSF (11.2 NSM)
- *Office, ophthalmology senior faculty:* 120 NSF (11.2 NSM)
- *Office, faculty:* 120 NSF (11.2 NSM)
- *Office, deputy nursing superintendent (DNS) OPD:* 120 NSF (11.2 NSM)
- *Office, Clerical:* 80 NSF (7.5 NSM)
- *Office MSSO:* .120 NSF (11.2 NSM) 01 per clinic
- *Nurse work room:* 120 NSF (11.2 NSM)
- Office support equipment area 40 NSF (3.8 NSM)
- Office, patient receptionist 120 NSF (11.2 NSM)
- *Consultation/viewing room:* 175 NSF (16.3 NSM)
- The consultation/viewing room will provide staff, residents, and extern/intern students an area to review specific case information as it relates to patient examination and treatment.
- *Conference room:* 300 NSF (17.9 NSM)
- *Group counseling room:* 120 NSF (11.2 NSM)
- *Conference/classroom:* 300 NSF (27.9 NSM)
- *Library, ophthalmology/optometry:* 240 NSF (22.3 NSM).

Staff Lockers, Lounge, and Toilets[14,16,17]

The spaces below provide programming of lounge, lockers, and toilets at department/service/chapter level.

- *Lounge, staff:* 80 NSF (7.5 NSM)
- *Locker room, staff:* 80 NSF (7.5 NSM)
- *Toilet, staff:* 50 NSF (4.7 NSM).

The subsequent floor-wise discussion would only describe specialized structural requirements, while focusing on the equipment requirement.

Specialty Outpatient Departments

The stack diagram reveals the relationship shared by the respective specialized OPD with their wards and investigation modalities. The patient circulation in these OPDs shall be similar and is shown in Figures 29 and 30.

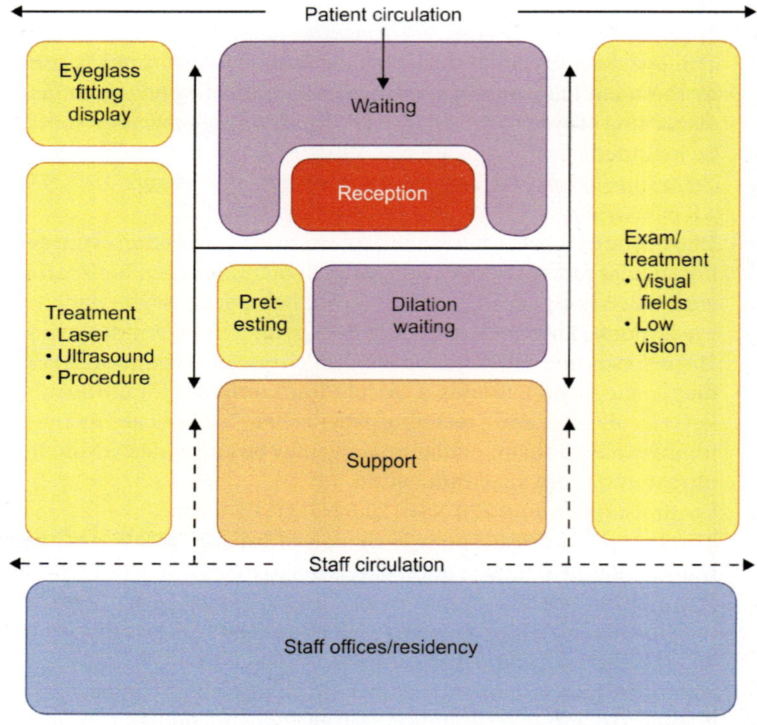

Fig. 29: Prototype patient flow in a specialty outpatient department.

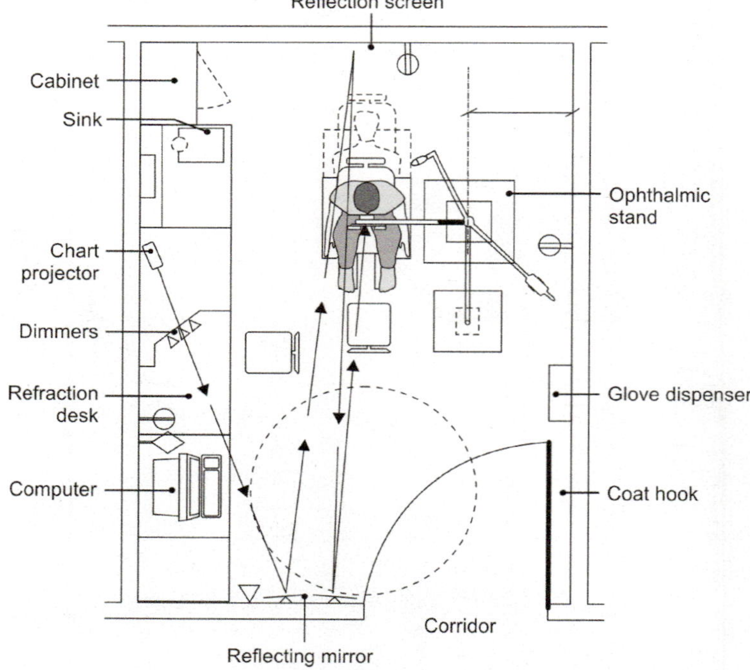

Fig. 30: Equipment and utility plan of the examination and treatment room.

PATIENT CIRCULATION IN SPECIALTY OUTPATIENT DEPARTMENT

The physical structural and design parameters of the clinics and the patient flow would be similar in all the specialty OPDs to maintain structure and functional uniformity. The unique design and equipment requirement of specialty OPDs and facilities on each floor are described along with the floor plan description.

First Floor

Facilities on this floor maybe:

- *Specialty OPD:* Cataract and lens clinic
- Cataract ward
- Community ophthalmology ward
- Special investigation laboratories (separate for inpatients and outpatients) for cataract
- Blood bank
- Excimer laser surgery clinic
- Cataract and lens clinic.

Utility Plan of the Examination and Treatment Room (Cataract and Lens Clinic) (Fig. 31)

Key design parameters

- Architecture
  - Gypsum ceiling height: 2.4 m (minimum height)
  - The flooring should be of vinyl composition.
- Lighting
  - The general ambient lighting: 500 lux
  - Task lighting: 1,000 lux
  - 600 mm × 1200 mm recessed light fixtures.
- *Power:* General 800 W (receptacle)
- Heating, ventilation, and air-conditioning.
  - Minimum percentage of outside air: 25%
  - Minimum air changes: 4 ACPH
  - Relative humidity: 50%.

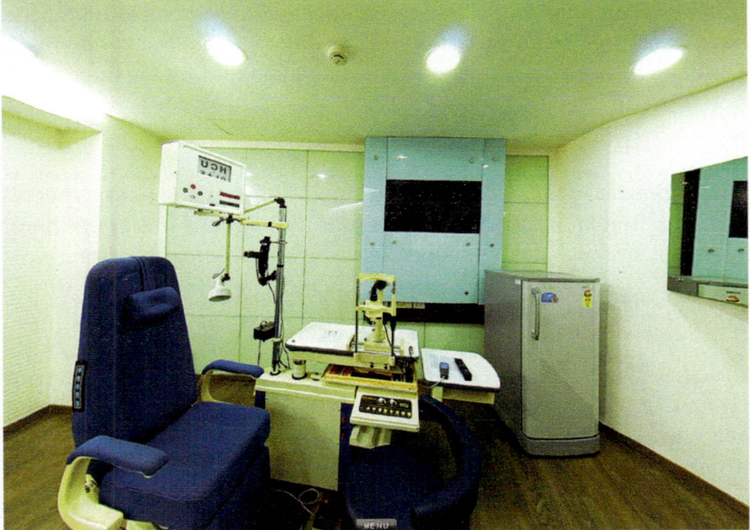

Fig. 31: Examination room in a typical eye clinic.

CATARACT/COMMUNITY OPHTHALMOLOGY WARD

Examination Room with Slit Lamp/ Nursing Station and Changing Room

Nursing Unit

Efficiency of operation, economy of space and comfort of the patients are the utmost considerations while designing a nursing unit. Since traveling within the nursing unit occupies almost one-sixth of a nurse's time, the farthest distance travelled would not be more than 25 ft to reduce nurse fatigue factor. The nursing station must be proximal to the elevator, stairway and the corridor.

Design Considerations

- The unit would be of 6 cubicles of 04 beds each (the pattern would be followed in wards except the pediatric and private rooms)
- The cubicles would have a minimum floor area of 29.722 m^2 (320 sq ft)
- There would be at least 0.37 m^2 (4 ft) of space between the beds, and sufficient space between the bed and the wall to allow the nurse and equipment to pass.
- The patient room toilet would be provided with grab bars, an emergency call button within easy reach, and a flush valve for bedpan cleaning.
- Bed would have a built-in wardrobe and the regular furniture. Doors would open outward towards the corridor with an outside lock
- The height of the window-sill would not exceed 0.91 m (3 ft) to allow the patient an outside view
- Examination and treatment room with wash basin, counter, shelf, etc.
- Clean workroom or clean holding room
- Workroom with clinical sink, worktop, waste receptacle, etc.
- Clean linen store
- Equipment storage room recessed space for storing stretchers and wheelchairs
- Staff facilities like lockers, etc. for staff's personal effects
- Pantry with sink, worktop, storage cabinets and space for temporary storage of dietary trays
- A multipurpose room for staff and patient conference, education, demonstration, etc.

Blood Bank/Blood Transfusion Unit

In planning, the design of a blood transfusion unit, the activities and flow of operation should be considered for adequate utilization of space. The functional plan of a blood transfusion service is thus based on the paths taken by the donors, the blood unit, blood samples and material:[21]

- *Donor complex*: The donor complex consists of a donor waiting area, donor registration, medical examination room with preliminary testing, blood collection area, apheresis area, donor rest room and kitchen/pantry. The flow of donors should be uniform and clearly defined to avoid unnecessary traffic in the corridors. The donor complex should be pleasant and comfortable.[21]
- *Blood storage*: Initial storage of blood (known as quarantine storage) should be in the vicinity of the place where donor blood is collected. After all the tests are performed, blood should be stored in vicinity of the issue area.[21]
- *Component preparation:* The area for blood component should be close to quarantine storage. The component laboratory should be clean, dust-free and well lit.[21]

- *Serology laboratory:* This laboratory is basically meant for red cell serology testing and donor and patient samples. A separate laboratory may be designated for antenatal and specialized serology.[21]
- *Laboratory for transfusion transmitted disease:* A separate laboratory should be designated for screening of all donor units for transfusion-transmitted diseases.
- *Issue counter:* Outside the serology laboratory a small counter should be designed for accepting blood samples and issue of blood, to avoid unnecessary and unauthorized entry of personnel in the laboratory. Besides the essential donor and laboratory complexes, the premises should have provision for quality assurance laboratory, washing room, disposal facilities, distillation room, daycare/therapeutic area, conference room, departmental library, administrative office, store and staff room.[10,21]

Second Floor

The following facilities are placed on the second floor:
- Cornea clinic and glaucoma clinic
- Glaucoma ward and cornea ward
- Glaucoma laboratory and cornea laboratory
- Consultants' chambers cornea and glaucoma
- Administrative offices.

The two most equipment intensive laboratories are the cornea and the glaucoma laboratories.

Cornea Laboratory (Fig. 32)

Equipment in the cornea laboratory:
- Confocal microscope—for imaging the different layers of the cornea to localize the pathology
- *Pachymeter:* A device used to measure the thickness of cornea
- *Orboscan machine:* Used to measure the corneal topography
- *Specular microscope:* For obtaining the endothelial cell count
- *Noncontact tonometry:* Noncontact method used to measure the intraocular pressure air puff ejected from the NCT deforms the cornea, the amount of deformation is inversely related to the IOP.

Glaucoma Laboratory

- *YAG machine (Fig. 33):* For performing YAG peripheral iridectomy and YAG capsulectomy.

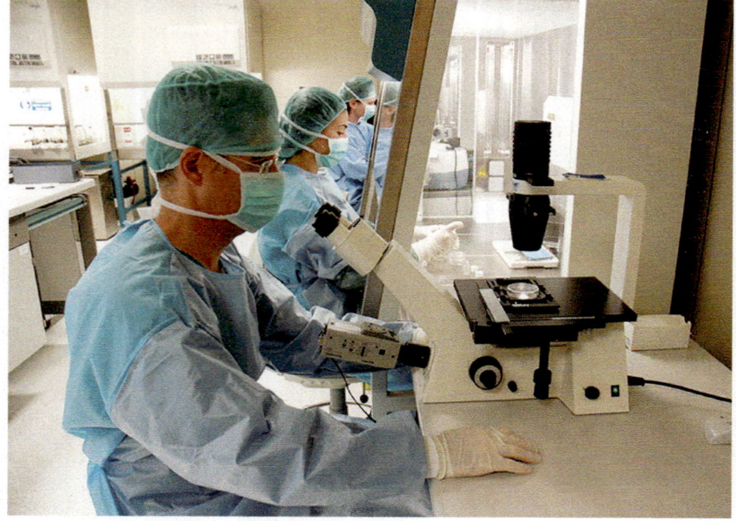

Fig. 32: Cornea laboratory.

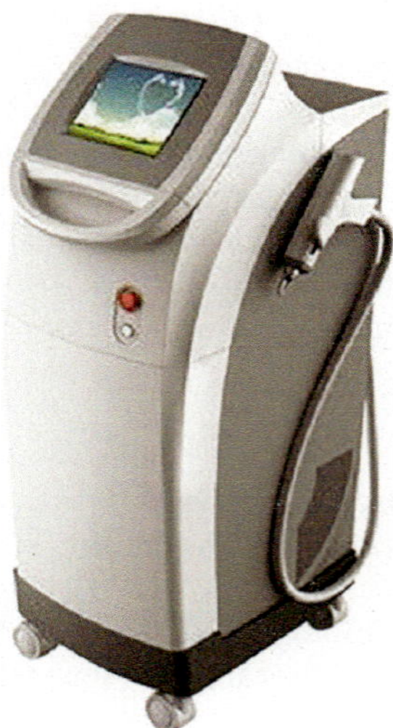

Fig. 33: YAG machine.

- *Heidelberg retinal tomogram (HRT):* Provides the tomography of the optic disk in glaucoma.
- *Scanning laser polarimetry (GDx-VCC):* Estimation of the retinal nerve fiber layer in glaucoma evaluation.
- Applanation tonometer is also used for calculating the IOL.
- The cornea and glaucoma wards also have 24 bedded wards each along the same lines as the cataract ward.
- Administrative offices already enumerated in the space criteria are located on this floor.

Third Floor

The following facilities are present on this floor:
- Pediatric ophthalmology clinic
- Pediatric wards
- Pediatric ophthalmology consultants' chambers
- Visual stimulation and play room
- Simulation lab and research facility.

Pediatric Clinic

This needs to be as lively and colorful as possible to ensure that the child is compliant and examination is done in an effective manner. Comic strips, colorful flooring and interesting lighting are important.

PEDIATRIC WARD

The pediatric ward needs to be around 20 beds to ensure special attention that kids deserve. The décor is also equally important here. Figure 34 shows an esthetically pleasing public sector hospital.

CONSULTANT'S CHAMBER

The consultant's chamber on all floors may be similar and the utility plan given in Figure 35 explains the relation between this chamber and the adjoining room for examination of patients and training of students.

Key Design Parameters

- Architecture
  - *Gypsum ceiling height:* 2.4 min (minimum) with a resilient base
  - The flooring should be of vinyl composition
  - No special equipment is required.

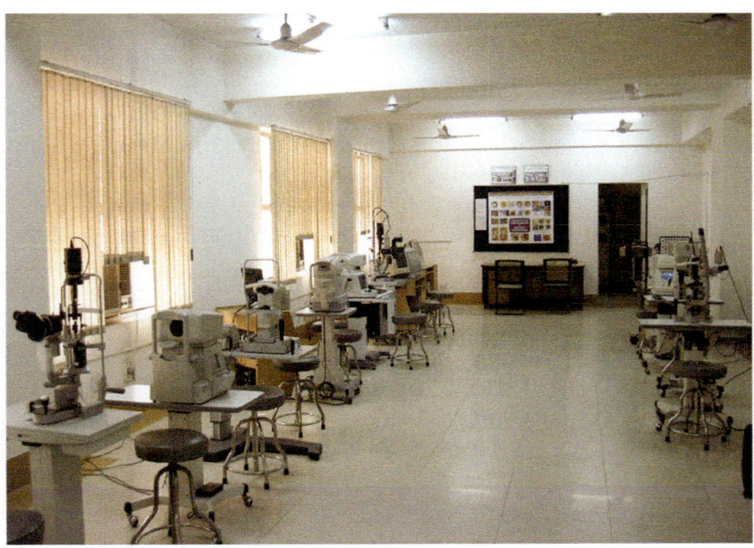

Fig. 34: Esthetically pleasing public sector hospital.

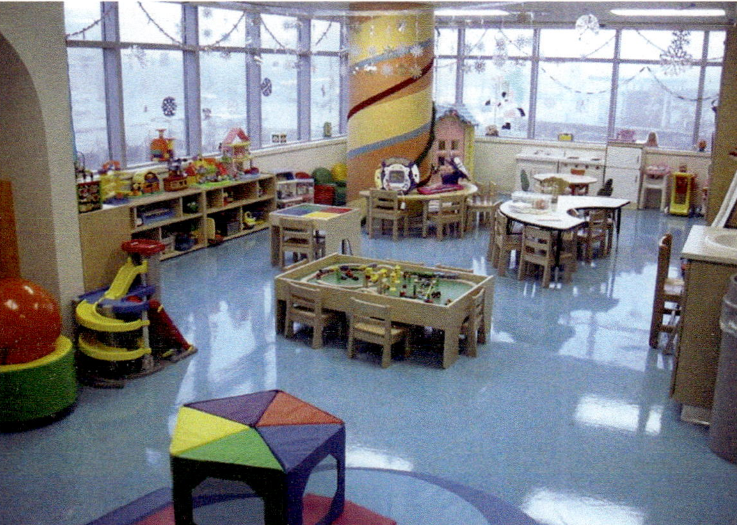

Fig. 36: A colorful playrooms with sunlight visibility.

- Lighting:
  - *The general ambient lighting:* 500 lux
  - *Task lighting:* 1,000 lux
  - 600 mm × 1200 mm recessed light fixtures
  - No special lighting required.
- *Power:* General 800 W (receptacle)
- HVAC.
  - *Minimum percentage of outside air:* 25%
  - *Minimum air changes:* 4 acph
  - *Relative humidity:* 50%.

Visual Stimulation Laboratory and Play-room

Play rooms and outdoor play areas for children must be provided. The play rooms would be in the sunny areas Figure 36. It would be furnished with low stationary tables and child sized chairs and must ensure plenty of sunlight.

VISUAL STIMULATION LABORATORY

In order to maximize vision, a young visually impaired (VI) child must have appropriate visual stimulation as well as physically interact with the visual stimulation to form the brain connections that will last a lifetime.[22]

Some of the most 'powerful' visual objects include high contrast, black and white objects including alternating black and white bars (Fig. 37), known as a grating, as well as checkerboards (Fig. 38). More complex visual objects include faces.[22] The greater differences between the light and dark areas of the object the higher the contrast and the more likely the object will provide appropriate visual stimulation.[22]

For older children, letters of the alphabet as well as numbers can also be constructed to teach the child the alphabet and numbers, accordingly. The white area should never be less than the black (tape) area or stroke width.[22]

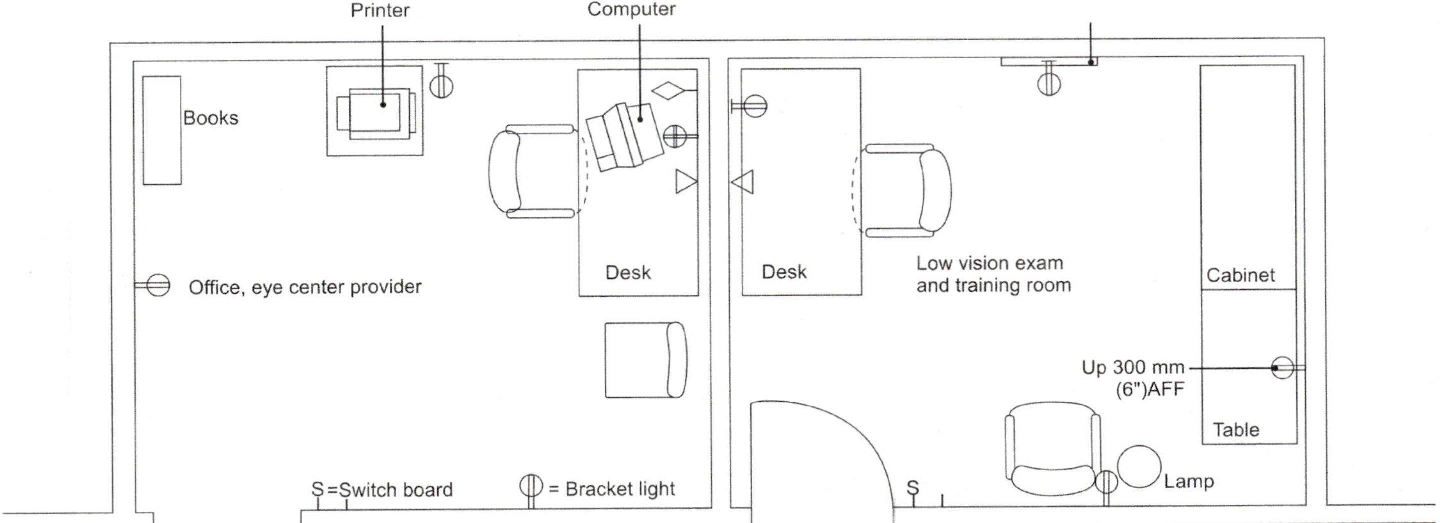

Fig. 35: Equipment and utility plan; consultant's chamber.

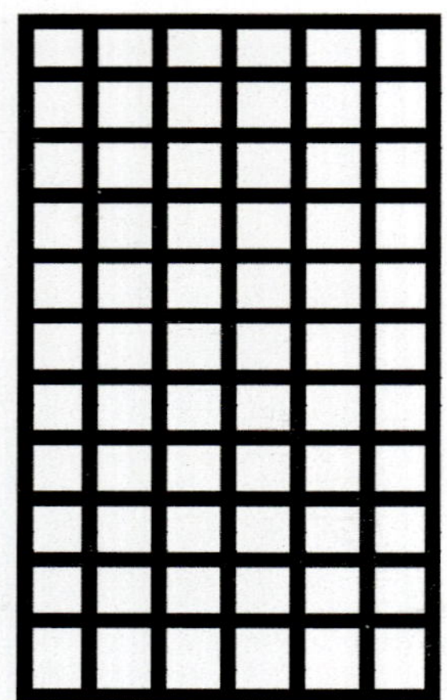

Fig. 37: Grating; a powerful visual tool.

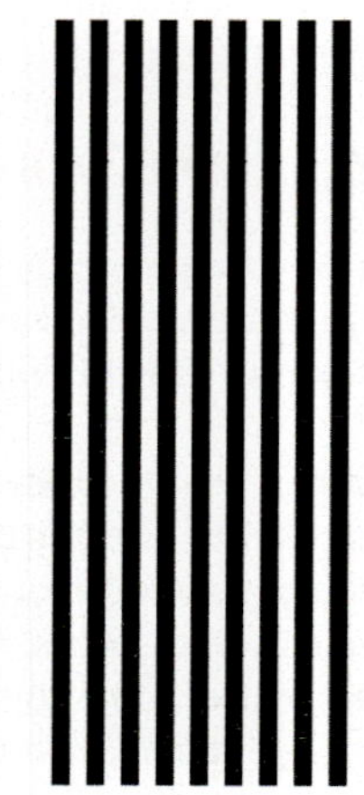

Fig. 38: Checkerboard as a visual stimulus.

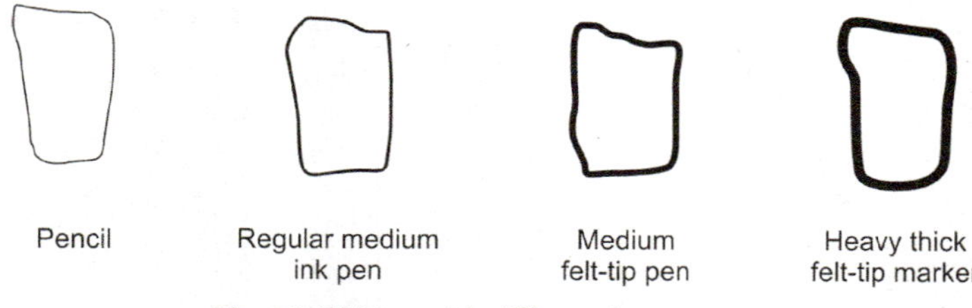

Fig. 39: Writing with different instruments.

Figure 39 illustrates simple drawings made with different writing instruments. For a VI child, the drawing made with the pencil (far left) may be difficult or impossible to see while the drawing with the medium felt-tip pen is easy to see, even though the drawings are of the same overall size.[11,22]

Fourth Floor

This floor has the retina clinics (medical and surgical), ocular oncology clinic, medical retina and oncology, surgical retina and oncosurgery. The layout of the retina clinic is shown in Figures 40 and 41.

- Fundus fluorescein angiography
- Photodynamic therapy.

Equipment for a Retina Clinic and Laboratories

- *Fundus fluorescein angiography: Intravenous fluorescein* angiography (IVFA) or fluorescent angiography is a technique for examining the circulation of the retina and choroid using a fluorescent dye and a specialized camera.
- *Optical coherence tomography:* This noninvasive technique uses a 3D volumetric or high resolution cross-sectional tomogram of the retinal fine structure with histologic-quality.
- *Nd: YAG laser (for retinal conditions):* Frequency-doubled Nd:YAG lasers (wavelength 532 nm) are used for pan-retinal photocoagulation in patients with diabetic retinopathy.

LAYOUT LASER ROOM

Ultrasound biomicroscopy (Fig. 42): This is used to assess the angle structures of the eye.

Fifth Floor

This floor has the squint and the orthoptic clinic, as well as the neuro-ophthalmic clinic as well as the respective wards. There are no special requirements in these clinics or these wards in addition to what has already been described elsewhere.

Sixth Floor

This floor comprises of the following facilities:

- Private wards
- Telemedicine facility.

Private Ward

The private ward would be 20 bedded with 10 beds on each flank each with 09 rooms of the same dimension and 01 each being deluxe room.

Teleophthalmology Facility

Teleophthalmology is a branch of telemedicine that delivers eye care through digital medical equipment and telecommunications technology. Broad-based applications of telemedicine could greatly enhance screening efforts for potentially blinding conditions such as diabetic retinopathy, macular degeneration, and glaucoma. Telemedicine could help bring subspecialty expertise to small or rural communities, or even to parts of country or even to the developed world.[22]

Scope in India

Eighty percent of India's population lives in rural areas and there is one ophthalmologist per 100,000 population, 70% of whom practice in urban area. Telemedicine offers several answers. There can be at least 50 community centers attached to one tertiary hospital center (http://www.laico.org/v2020res source/files/teleophthalmolog_in_india.PDF). In these 'Vision Centers', there are mid-level ophthalmic personnel (MLOP), who are similar to trained ophthalmic nurse practitioners. They are trained to take anterior segment and retinal images and perform intraocular pressure checks. They communicate online with a consultant ophthalmologist at the main hospital providing anterior segment and retinal images as appropriate and discuss clinical details of the patient.[23,24]

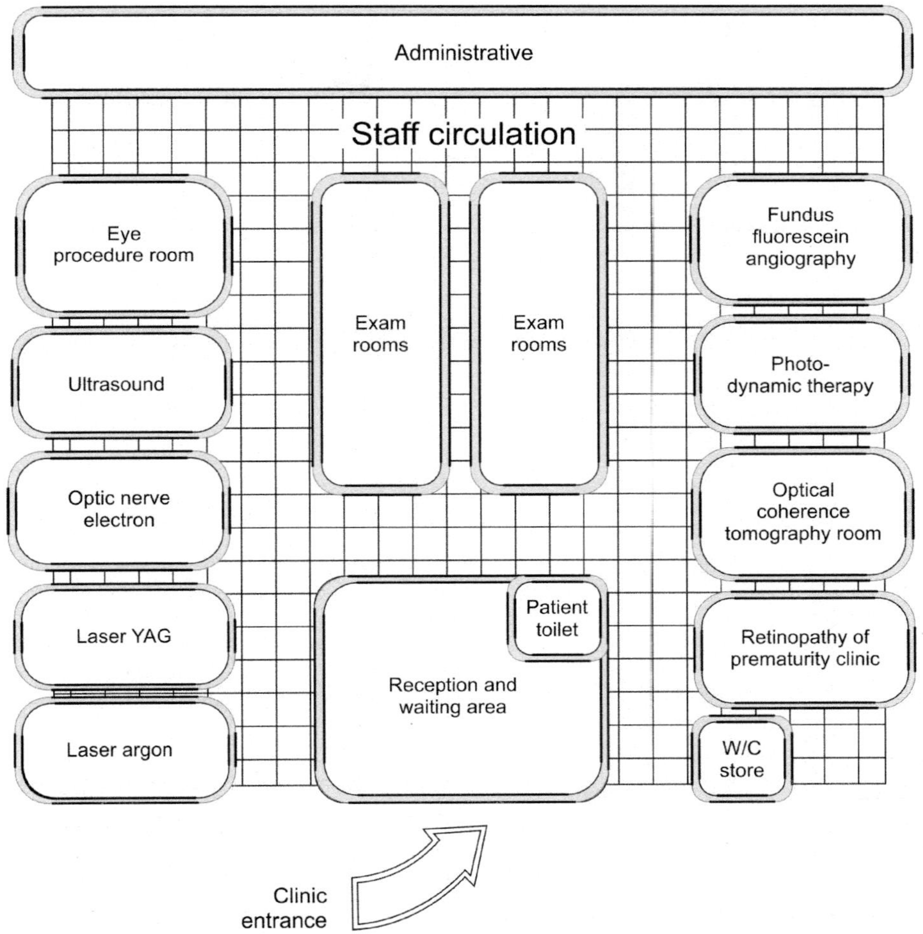

Fig. 40: Layout plan of a retina clinic.

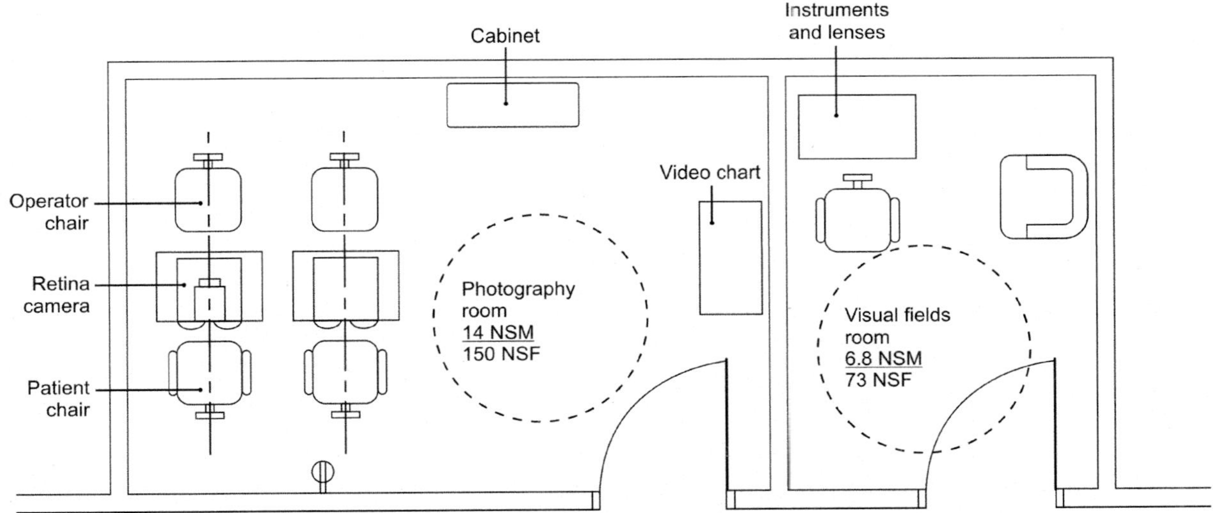

Fig. 41: Layout plan of retina laboratory.

Process Flow

Fundus photography is performed by a fundus camera, which basically consists of a specialized low power microscope with an attached camera. Teleophthalmology services can be provided primarily in two ways synchronously or asynchronously:[7]

- Synchronous teleophthalmology enables real-time interaction between participants (using standard telemedicine technologies, e.g. video-conferencing), synchronous to supervise the removal of corneal foreign bodies and for consultations[7]
- *Asynchronous teleophthalmology* in a 'store-and-forward' method, where data is captured and transmitted for review at a later time.[7]

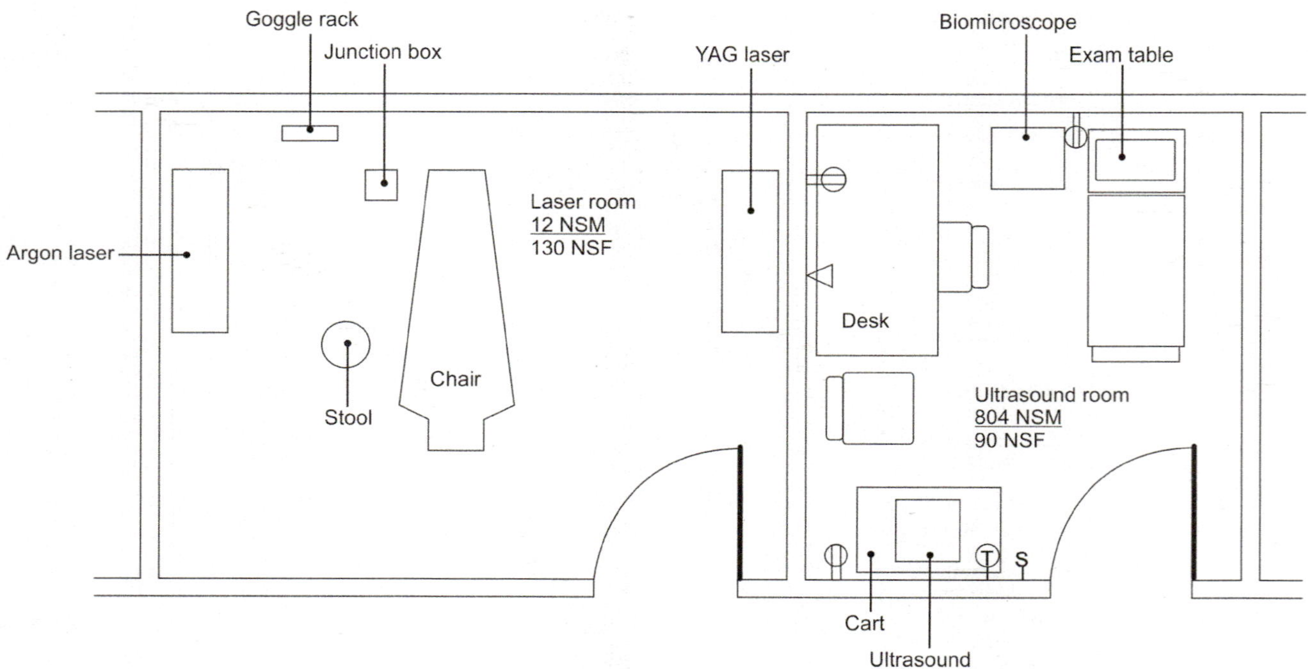

Fig. 42: Layout of laser room for diabetic retinopathy treatment.

Images of the eye can be captured noninvasively through various methods, generally by a technician or nonphysician healthcare professional.

External eye: Standard digital stills or video camera.

Anterior segment: Slit lamp connected to a camera.

Posterior segment or retina: Fundus camera.

SEVENTH FLOOR

The facilities on this floor would be:
- Simulation laboratory and research facility
- Community ophthalmology department
- Ocular pathology
- Ocular microbiology
- Ocular biochemistry
- Administrative offices
- Staff cafeteria.

SURGICAL STIMULATION AND RESEARCH FACILITY

It is imperative that laboratory planners are aware that the research facility (Fig. 43) must not be designed exclusively and permanently for any one pattern or type of research work. The focus of research is constantly changing. It should be expected that the direction of the facility's research program may change between design and activation. The design should conform to flexibility, safety, quality of environment and cost-efficiency.[14,24]

VIRTUAL REALITY ROOM CHROMATOGRAPHY DRY AND WET LABORATORIES ENTRY

Laboratory Space Planning

There are two plan options:
- The open plan.
- The closed plan. The open plan reduces construction costs (requiring fewer walls), improves square footage efficiency, and is oriented toward research teams. The closed plan allows tighter security and provides containment.[14,24]

The ophthalmology central research laboratory should be a closed one. A modular design should be conceived.

General Space Criteria

Laboratory ceilings should be set at a minimum of 2700 mm (9′-0″) from floor to ceiling with 600 × 1200 mm (2′ × 4′) acoustical tile. The finishes in laboratories must be impervious to contaminants and able to withstand washing with detergents. Laboratory floors should be of a nonslip finish. Common instrument rooms have latex mastic floors and coved bases to allow for ease of maintenance.[14]

The standard for aisles between benches or equipment is 1500 mm (5 ft - 0 inch), to allow space in which two people may work back-to-back at apparatus and a third person may pass between them. Aisles should be aligned in the direction of egress. Main corridors in laboratory neighborhoods need to be 1800 mm (6 ft - 0 inch) wide to allow enough of a turning radius for equipment entering/exiting the laboratories. A corridor wider than 1800 mm (6 ft - 0 inch) is likely to become a storage area. Partitions used within laboratories to hang casework

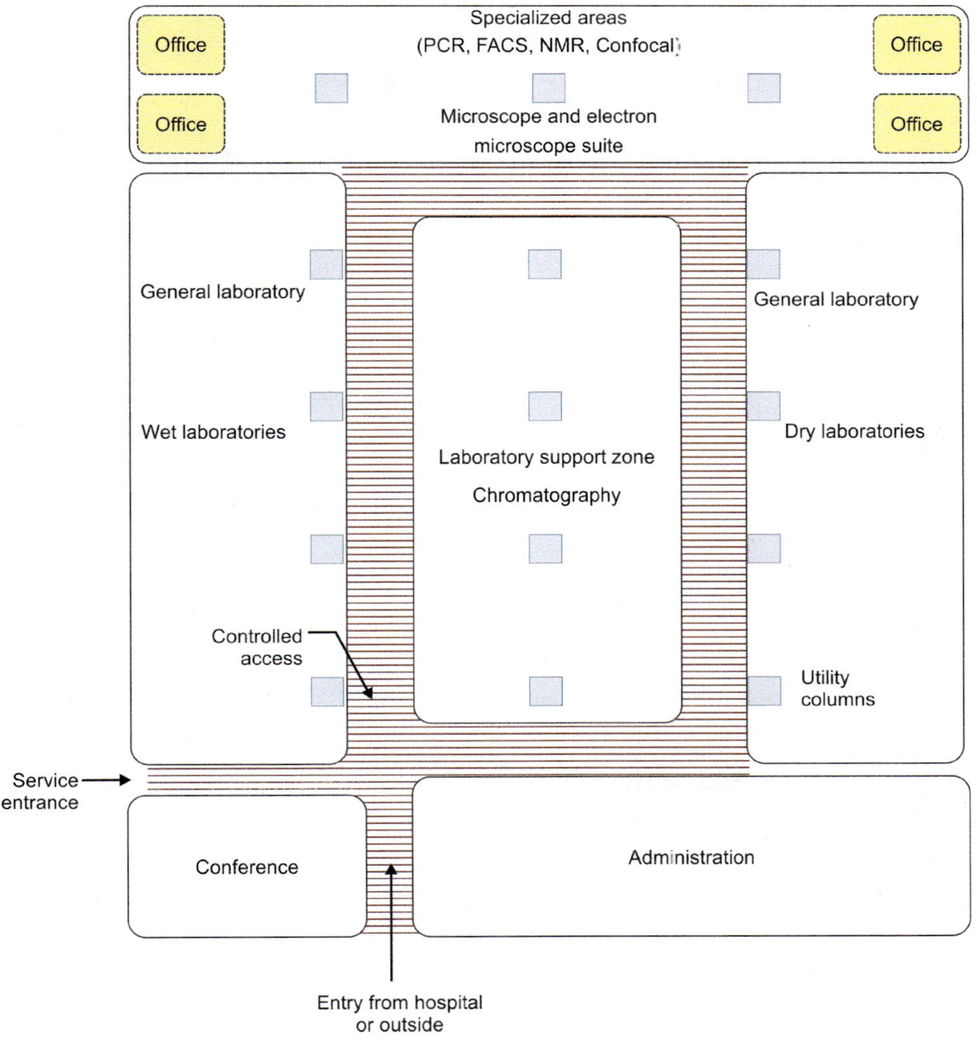

Fig. 43: Layout of a research and surgical skill laboratory.

may be replaced by free-standing cabinets and shelving. A decision to locate the disabled persons access—If a disabled researcher works in a laboratory, then all parts of the laboratory and its emergency equipment must be designed or adapted to meet the user's needs.[14]

Heating, ventilation, and air-conditioning: Laboratory, specialized, and support areas: Laboratory areas should have a dedicated air handling unit, 100% outdoor air, a minimum of 12 acph of room supply air, a negative room pressure created by exhausting 15% more air than is supplied, a room noise level not to exceed NC-45, and room conditions of 24°C , 50% RH in summer, and 22°C , 30% RH in winter.[14]

OCULAR PHARMACOLOGY

High-performance liquid chromatography (HPLC) (Fig. 44): It is a chromatographic technique used to separate a mixture of compounds in analytical chemistry and biochemistry with the purpose of identifying, quantifying or purifying the individual components of the mixture. HPLC has many uses including medical (e.g. detecting drug content in tear drops), research (e.g. separating the components of a complex biological sample, or of similar synthetic chemicals from each other), and manufacturing (e.g. during the production process of pharmaceutical and biological products.[14]

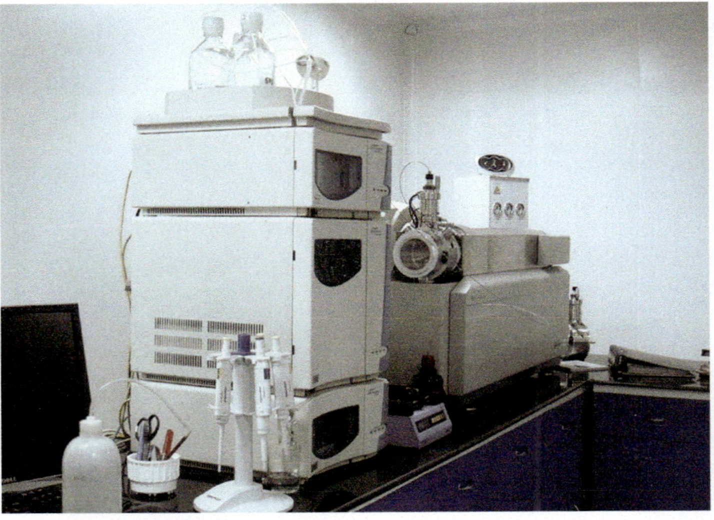

Fig. 44: High performance liquid chromatography.

In ophthalmology, this extremely important equipment can be used for all three purposes especially to develop in house R and D to assess the efficacy of a drug on the eye by using tear drop as the sample against the solvent to explore the efficacy.

OCULAR MICROBIOLOGY

The routine biochemical laboratory test notwithstanding, the ocular microbiology laboratory must also have a large research component to study the biochemical, immunological and genetic aspects of eye diseases. The focus must be on age-related senile cataract, uveitis, optic neuritis, corneal ulcer, etc. The following laboratories must be integral to the facility:

- Tissue and cell culture laboratory
- Stem cell culture facility to study molecular basis of ocular diseases, mainly ocular tumors and glaucoma.

Beside the essential equipment such as the autoanalyzer, the laboratory must have a real time PCR machine (Fig. 45).

OCULAR PATHOLOGY (FIGS. 46 AND 47)

The laboratory has the following components:

Histopathology and frozen section: Diagnostic histopathology of ocular specimens received from operation theater. In addition, frozen section-guided excision of lid tumors and frozen section for various histochemical stains.

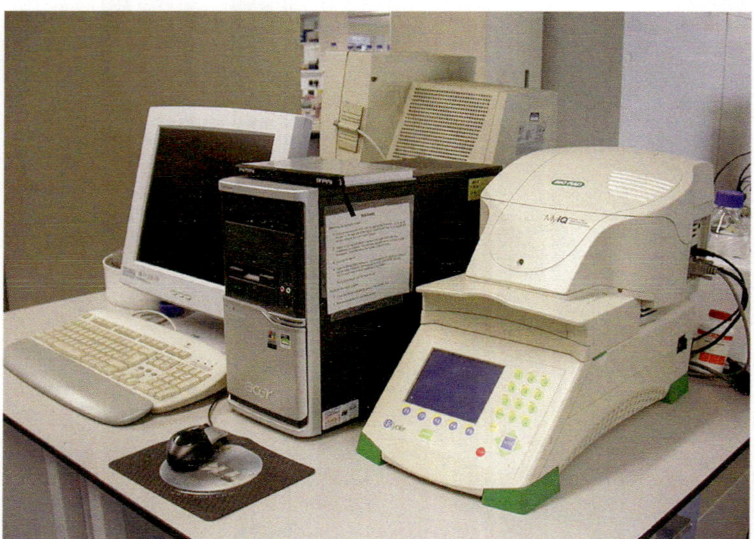

Fig. 45: Real time (RT)-polymerasechain reaction (PCR) machine.

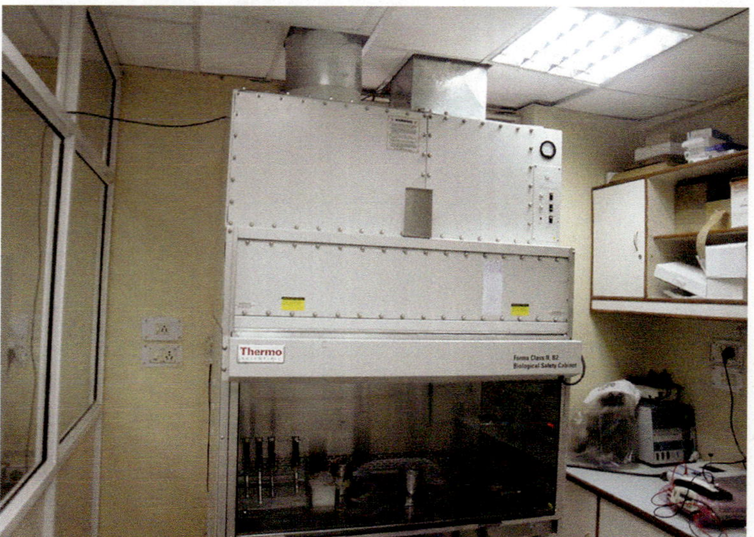

Fig. 46: A biosafety cabinet for ocular pathology research.

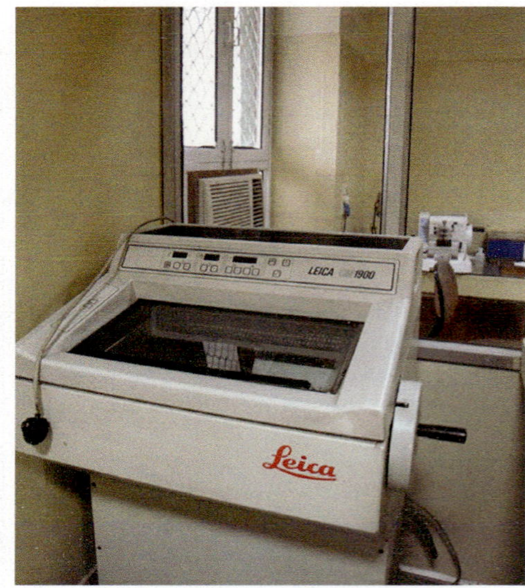

Fig. 47: A cryostat for slicing frozen specimen.

Cytopathology[23]

Impression cytology: Done for diagnosis of dry eye, corneal, conjunctival neoplasias, ulcerative eyelid lesions.

Fine needle aspiration cytology (FNAC): Done for preoperative diagnosis of palpable orbital, eyelid lesion and enlarged lymph node.[25]

Vitreous and aqueous cytology: For intraocular lymphomas and metastatic endophthalmitis.

Clinical Pathology

Hemogram: Blood investigations are done with the help of autoanalyzer.
Urine analysis: Routine examination.

Immunohistochemistry

Diagnostic and research purposes—aids in differential diagnosis of tumors and as cancer biomarkers.

Molecular Pathology Laboratory

As a part of the department of ocular pathology, this section undertakes tests based on various molecular biology tools including polymerase chain reaction (PCR), methylation specific PCR (MSP), ISH, reverse-transcriptase PCR (RT-PCR) for mRNA expression analysis, mutational analysis (collaboration) for research purposes (Fig. 48).[25]

WET Laboratory

A wet laboratory in ophthalmology is a facility where an artificial tissue eye or a goat's eye is used for practicing operating facility (Figs. 49 and 50).

VIRTUAL REALITY IN OPHTHALMOLOGY (FIG. 51)[32]

Wet-laboratory experiences are effective in modeling surgical technique, but they are limited in their availability partly as a result of their financial cost.

Today, the apprentice model carries with it the realities of an unstructured curriculum dependent upon patient flow, heavy financial costs, human costs, and unmanageable time constraints. More

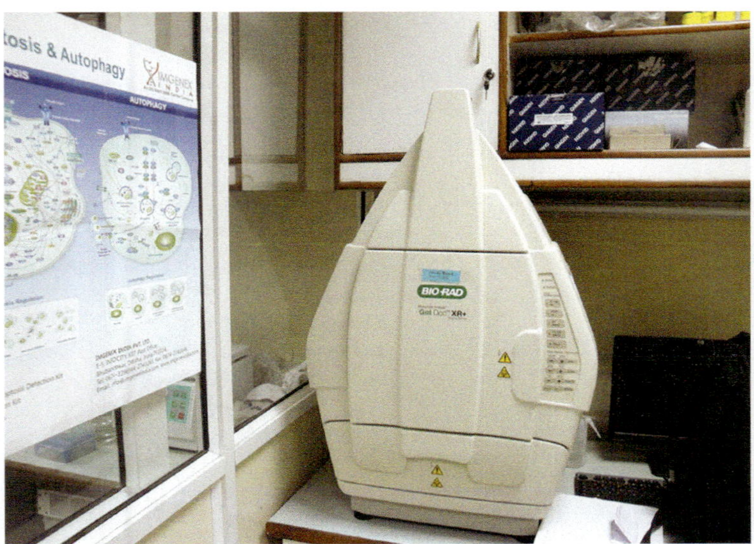

Fig. 48: Molecular pathology laboratory.

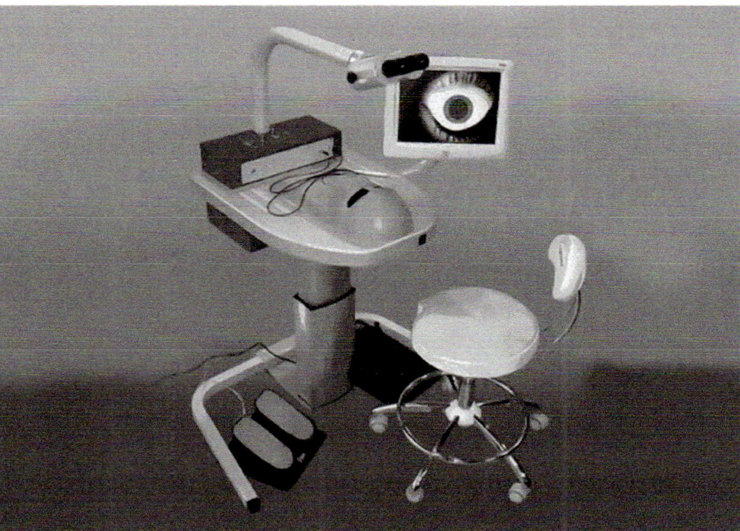

Fig. 50: Vitreoretinal and anterior segment modules.

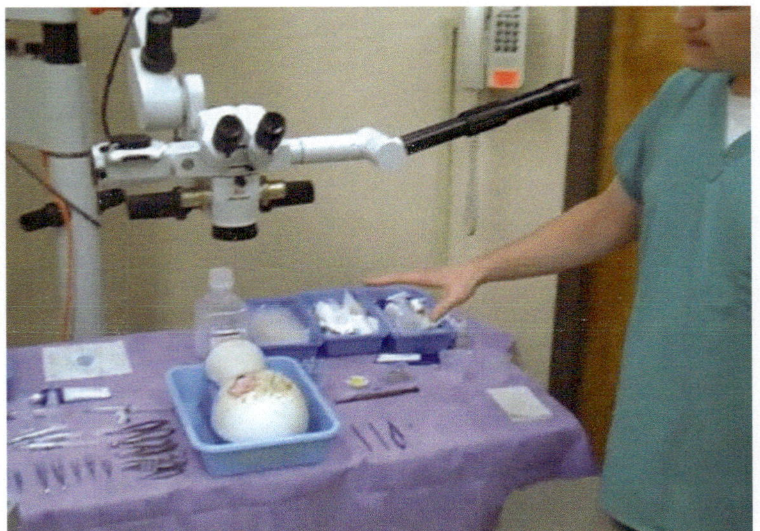

Fig. 49: Artificial operating eye. Operating microscope.

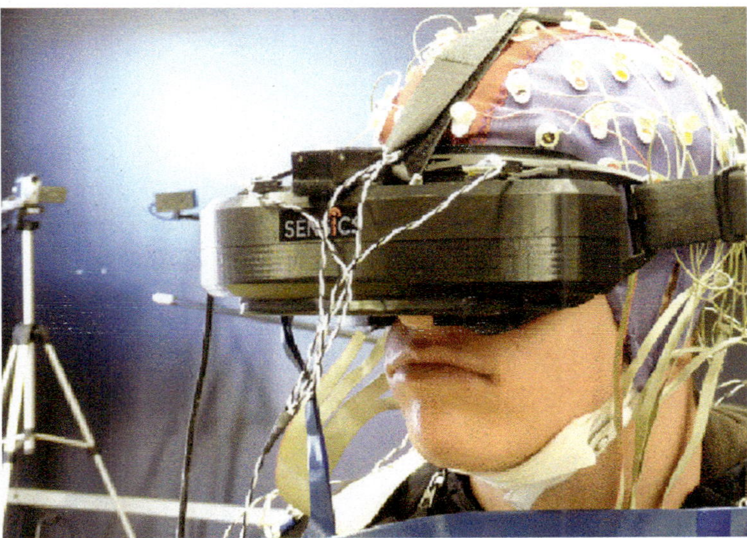

Fig. 51: Virtual reality in ophthalmology.

importantly, with patient safety being so important, we are in need of an instructional medium that will reduce surgical risk to patients, expose surgeons to surgical experience and complications.[26]

Having recognized these limitations in the apprentice method and citing the increasing demand for surgical simulation, researchers have developed many ophthalmic virtual reality surgery simulators (Fig. 52). The training systems published in the literature include retrobulbar injection, capsulorhexis cataract extraction via phacoemulsification retinal photocoagulation, and vitreoretinal surgery.

Layout (Fig. 53)

The trainee sits at the controls looking through the stereo-operating scope that peers down onto two separate images of the operating field. Each image is specific for the view from either eye, thus, providing depth-perception. The SGI graphics computer is responsible for the visual rendering of the images displayed on the monitor. The surgeon interacts with a virtual eye using a virtual surgical instrument controlled by a handheld 3D position-tracking stylus that continuously reports position and orientation to the computer. The tip of the stylus is connected to three motors that generate component force feedback in response to the tool-tissue interaction.[26]

Staff Cafeteria

The staff cafeteria should have an informal feel as well as certain privacy from patients as well as the attendants. It should be, however, be proximal to the OT so that surgeons can quickly take refreshments between cases.

Total dining NSF	:	1,812
Serving area NSF	:	1,400
Total area	:	2,250 NSF

Eighth Floor

This floor would include:
- Eye bank
- Lecture theater

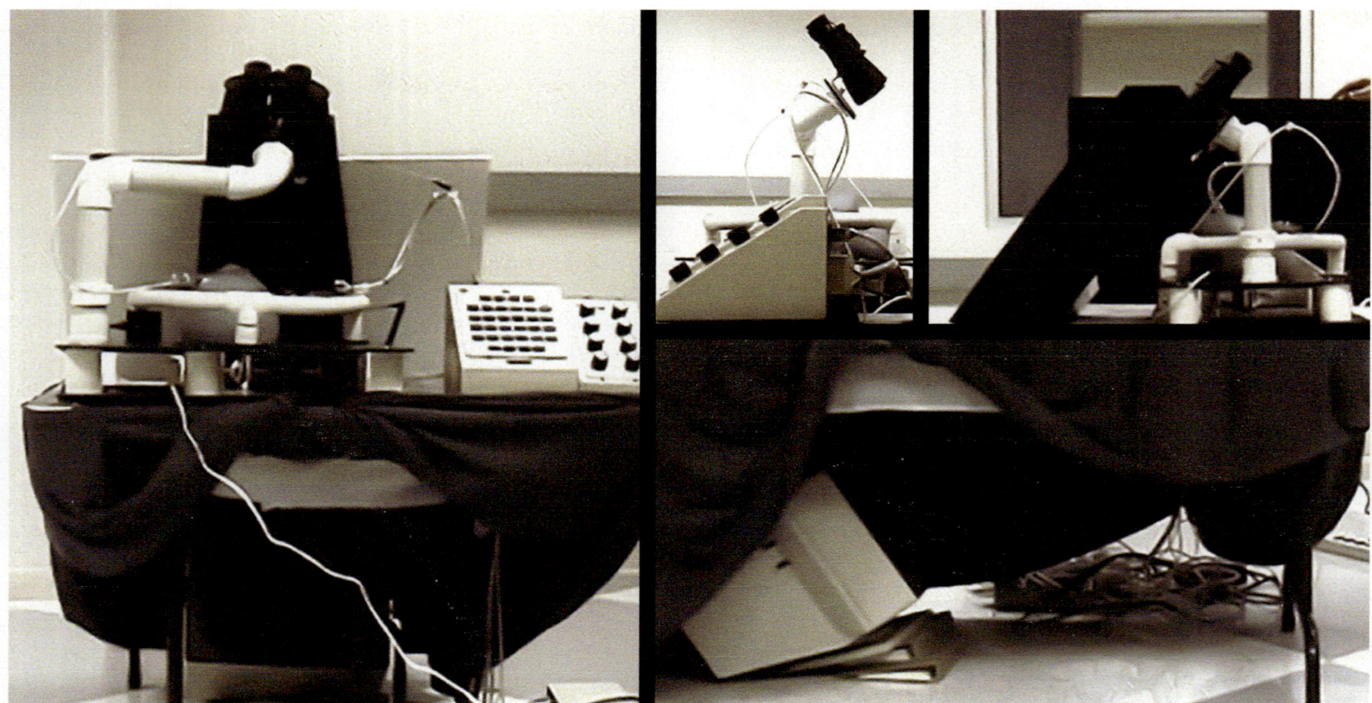

Fig. 52: Cataract surgery simulator developed in 1995 at Medical College of Georgia.

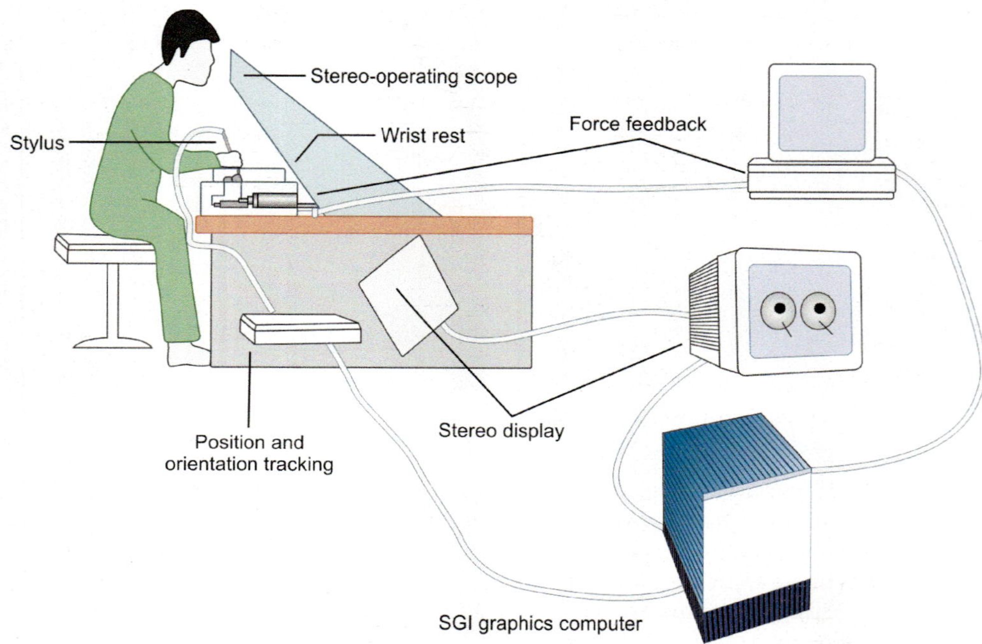

Fig. 53: Schematic of virtual reality simulator components and layout. (SGI: Silicon Graphics International)

- Daycare
- Operation theater complex.

The specialized eye bank needs to have 600 sq ft of minimum space and depending upon the proximity to tertiary level hospitals and availability of eyes, can be training center as well. The components would be as follows:

- Serology laboratory
- Tissue processing laboratory and
- Evaluation, storage and shipping laboratory.

Infrastructural Requirement for an Eye Bank

- Instrument cleaning laboratory
  - Sink for instrument wash
  - Autoclave
  - Countertop and storage of instruments and supplies.
- Serology laboratory
  - Refrigerator for sample and kit storage
  - Centrifuge and serum testing equipment like enzyme-linked immunosorbent assay (ELISA).

- Tissue processing laboratory:
  - Sterile counter for processing (biohazard cabinet)
  - Countertops.
- Evaluation, storage and shipping laboratory
  - Slit lamp and specular microscope for tissue evaluation
  - Refrigerator for storing donor tissue.

EQUIPMENT

- Refrigerator (–4° to –20°)
- Serology equipment
- Slit lamp
- Specular microscope
- Autoclave or ethylene oxide (EtO) sterilizer
- Laminar flow hood (class-II)
- AV equipment
- Lecture theater.

Standard guidelines are available in terms of acoustics, seating HVAC and safety which are to be followed while planning a lecture, details can be accessed at (*http://www.umbc.edu/oit/classroomtechnology/about_files/LH_Standard.pdf*).

- *Access:* A sufficient number of doors are to be provided for a maximum clearance time of 5 minutes for quick and efficient changeover between lectures. The front row of seats is to be at the same floor level as the adjacent entry doors for disabled persons access
- AV facilities:
  - 35 mm slide projection (side by side).

DAYCARE AND OPERATION THEATER FACILITY (FIG. 54)[18]

Some eye surgery can be performed within the outpatient clinic environment. Minor procedures, such as chalazion surgery, can be undertaken in an appropriately equipped clinic room, while other procedures, e.g. corneal suture removal, can be performed at the slit lamp.[20,21]

Some invasive procedures such as intravitreal injections can also be performed with full sterile precautions outside the operating theater environment, but the room should be equipped appropriately and approved by the hospital microbiology department.[20,21]

Decontamination and sterilization should be undertaken by an appropriate hospital sterilization and decontamination unit (HSDU). Where this is not available, disposables offer an easier alternative than local decontamination. If local decontamination and sterilization has to be undertaken, compliance with extant guidance is essential.[20,21]

Although intravenous access and cardiac monitoring is rarely needed for most minor ophthalmic operations, it is essential that staff are familiar with resuscitation procedures and equipment.[20,21]

Most eye surgery should be performed in ophthalmic theaters, ideally dedicated for ophthalmic use.

LAYOUT AND FLOW

Clustering of Accommodation[27-29]

The following accommodation should be an integral cluster with access through a single, secure entrance:

- Communications base
- Operating theaters (with associated ancillary accommodation)
- Anesthetic rooms (Equal to total no. of operating theaters)
- Patient support facilities
- Recovery unit (with associated ancillary accommodation)
- Staff support facilities
- Storage areas (equipment, bulk store)
- Disposal areas (dirty utility, disposal hold, housekeeping room).

The following accommodation could be integral or co-located with access through the main entrance or with its own secure entrance adjacent to the operating department:

- Education and training facilities
- Anesthetic department
- Administrative offices.

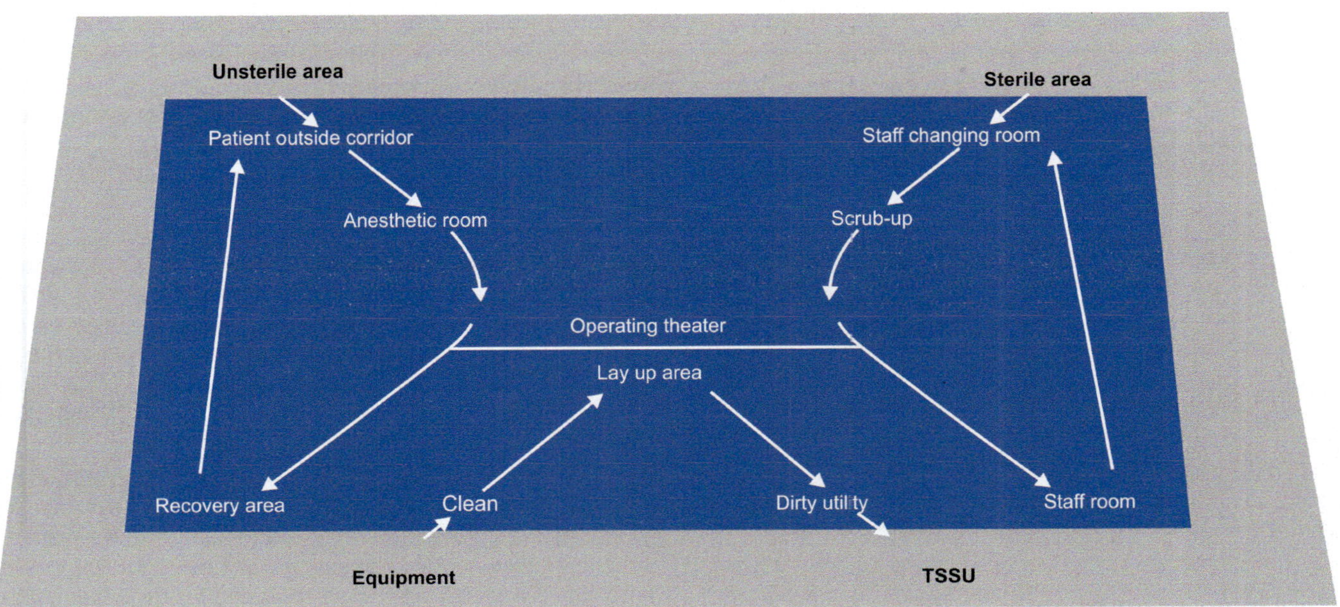

Fig. 54: Schemata diagram of facility.
(TSSU: theater sterile supply unit)

The operation theater or have the following features (Fig. 55):
- Zoning concept including sterile, clean, protective and disposal is essential
- The sterile and unsterile areas are segregated, preferably by an air lock or buffer zone or by colored lines—scrubbed staff remains in the sterile zone and the circulating staff and patients remain within the unsterile zone
- Preferably, the entrances for patients and staff should be separate
- The operating room should preferably have seamless walls and a nonporous floor (Use of marble is contraindicated).

Heating, Ventilation and Air-conditioning

Central air-conditioning of the operating room is ideal and in case where resources are not a constraint, ventilation (HVAC) system may be installed. These systems include high efficiency particulate air (HEPA) filters, maintain indoor air temperature, humidity, and odors, clean the contaminated air and minimize the risk of transmission of air-borne microorganisms. In addition, HEPA filter along with ultraviolet (UV) lights are essential.[29]

Parameter Desired Range[29]

- Temperature 20–23°C
- Relative humidity 30–60%
- Air movement—from clean to less clean areas, laminar flow
- Air changes—minimum 15 total acph

EQUIPMENT RELATIONSHIP AND LAYOUT WITHIN THE OPERATION THEATER[23] (FIG. 56)

Equipment

Operating Microscope (Fig. 57)

Essential features include co-axial illumination and foot pedal controls. The assistant's microscope should have a stereoscopic view similar to the surgeon's view.

Desirable features include:[21]
- Video camera (3 chip - or better), with recording facility (ideally digital)
- Foot pedal control of light intensity
- Yellow safety filter
- Vertically adjustable eyepieces
- A ceiling mounted microscope is desirable in a dedicated ophthalmic theater.

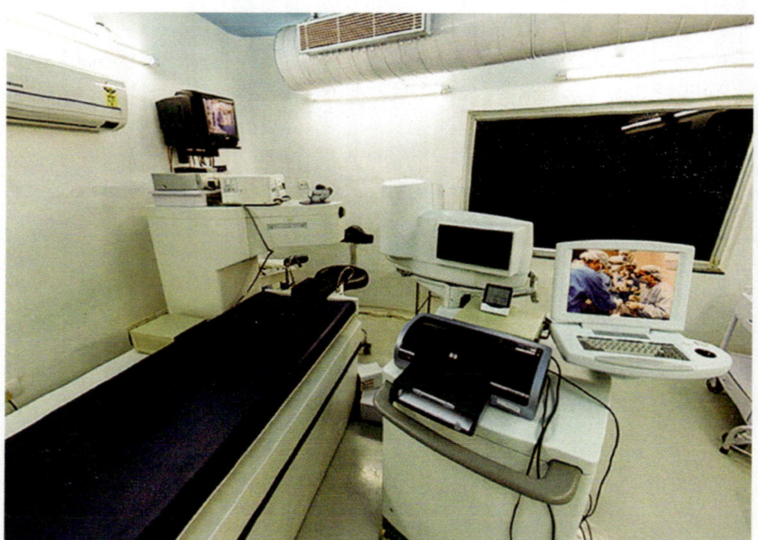

Fig. 55: A modern ophthalmology operation theater.

Operating Table/Surgery Trolley/Chair

The operating surface should be readily adjustable for height and tilt. The equipment used will depend on local arrangements, but should take into account each unit's layout and individual surgeons' ergonomic requirements.[21]

It should be possible to adjust the table for the comfort of the patients and the headrest should be adjustable both vertically and with tilt. Rapid head down tilt should be possible for general anesthesia cases.[21]

Caution should be exercised to ensure that controls cannot be inadvertently operated, particularly during surgery, especially with models with electric controls with 'memory' positions.

Phacoemulsification

Operating theaters in which cataract surgery is undertaken should be equipped with phacoemulsification machinery, which should be maintained and updated regularly.

Vitrectomy capability, for the management of complications, and a bipolar cautery system are essential. The equipment should be regularly maintained in strict compliance with manufacturers' instructions. Units relying on a single machine may consider that the potential hazards of a technical problem occurring justify the purchase of a 'backup' device.[21]

The manufacturer's requirements concerning the cleaning and sterilization of the handpieces should be followed. Single-use items such as phaco needles should not be reused.

Other Operating Equipment[21]

This should include:

Cryosurgery system, bipolar cautery, indirect ophthalmoscope:

Depending on the surgery:
- *Vitreoretinal surgery:* Vitrectomy machine, laser, gas/air/fluid exchange systems, silicone oil pump, image inverter for the operating microscope
- *Pediatric cases:* Operating gonioscopes, Perkins tonometer, laser, etc.

Miscellaneous Facilities

There should be ample provision of theater chairs/stools. For the surgeon and assistant, these should have hydraulic height adjustment. Armrests should be available as an option. There should be enough instrument trolleys to cater for the operating list. At least 3 trolleys are essential. Other equipment should include X-ray viewing via a PACS system or a light box, clock with stop-watch facility, whiteboards, video viewing and recording system (ideally digital format) and, ideally, facilities for playing recorded music.[21]

The suite should be adequately soundproofed to minimize intrusive external noise during surgery. The lighting should include high-intensity operating light units and fully variable background lighting.

The theater should have signage and blackout facilities to comply with safety guidelines for laser treatments. The power supply should be adequate for the laser equipment to be used. Facilities for recording operating details ideally should include an electronic format that will allow ready access for audit of procedures such as cataract surgery.[21]

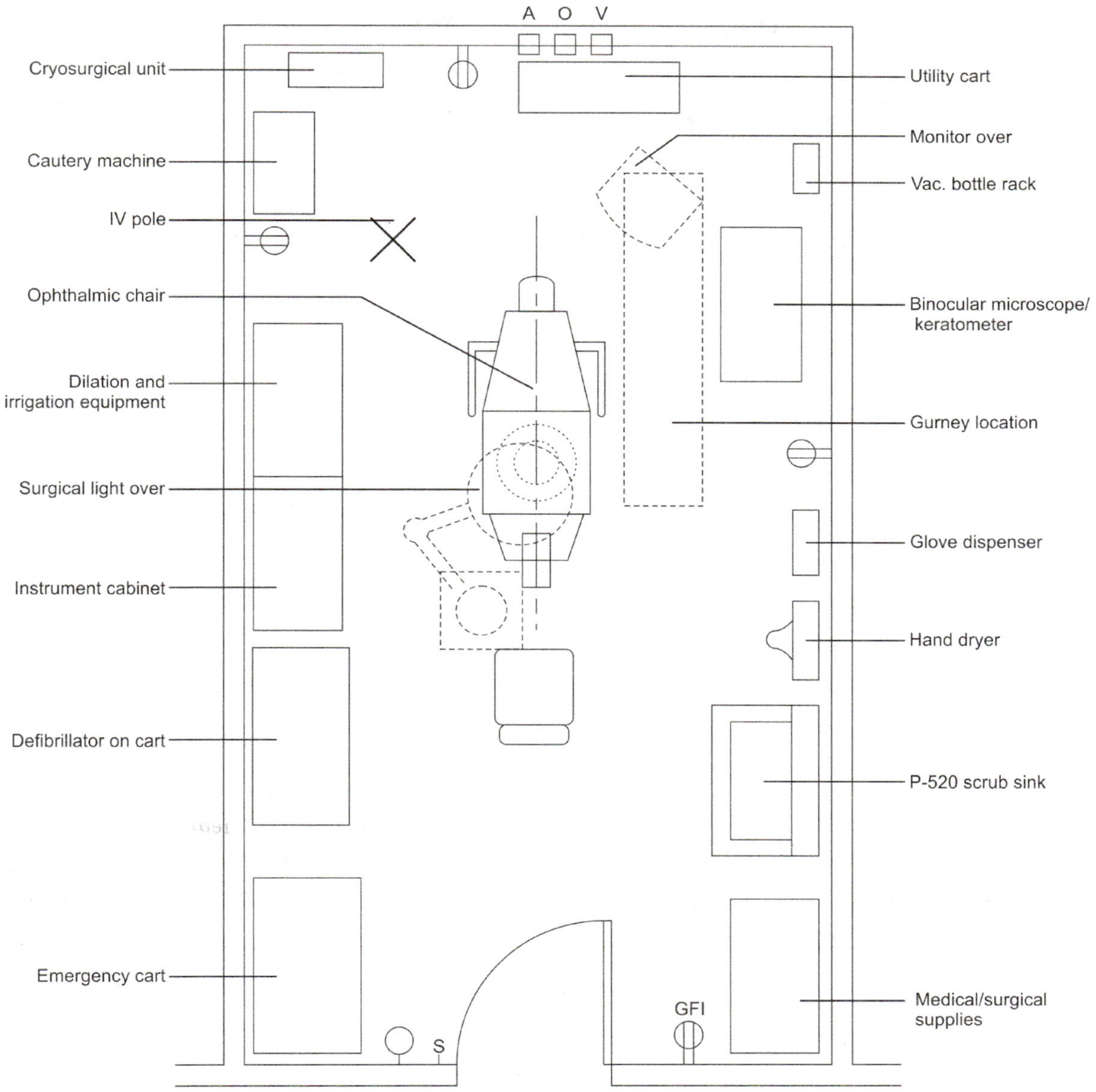

A O V
Cryosurgical unit
Utility cart
Cautery machine
Monitor over
Vac. bottle rack
IV pole
Ophthalmic chair
Binocular microscope/ keratometer
Dilation and irrigation equipment
Gurney location
Surgical light over
Glove dispenser
Instrument cabinet
Hand dryer
Defibrillator on cart
P-520 scrub sink
Emergency cart
S
GFI
Medical/surgical supplies

Fig. 56: Equipment and utility plan eye procedure room.

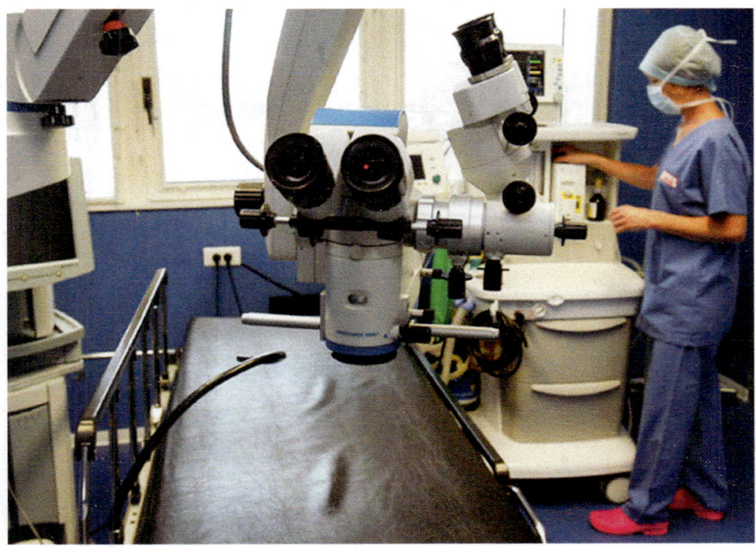

Fig. 57: Operating microscope.

Drugs and therapeutic agents: An ophthalmic theater should have provision for storage of various drugs, both anesthetic and ophthalmic.

BASEMENT

The basement may have the following facilities:
- Medical records department
- Central sterile supply department
- Manifold
- Laundry
- Hospital stores
- Engineering services
- Computer facility.

REFERENCES

1. bjo.bmj.com
2. https://www.syndicateofhospitals.org.lb/
3. www.va.gov

4. www.who.int
5. lvpei.org
6. www.ncbi.nlm.nih.gov
7. en.wikipedia.org
8. https://www.moorfields.nhs.uk/
9. www.fhs.mcmaster.ca
10. www.scribd.com
11. Thomas, R. "Present status of eye care in India", Survey of Ophthalmology, 2005.
12. medind.nic.in
13. www.cehjournal.org
14. www.wbdg.org
15. www.aios.org
16. wabenbow.com
17. www.cfm.va.gov
18. www.ski.org
19. www.entrepreneur.com
20. ishrae.in
21. www.rcophth.ac.uk
22. ohiolionseyeresearch.com
23. eyeworld.org
24. www.intechopen.com
25. www.aiims.edu
26. Khalifa YM. Virtual Reality in Ophthalmology Training, Survey of Ophthalmology, 2006.
27. www.johnsonmedical.com
28. www.sightsaversindia.in
29. www.vision2020india.org

OTHER REFERENCES

- "Action on cataracts: good practice guidance." 2000, Department of Health, PO Box 777, London SE1 6XH Tel: 08701 555455 Fax: 01623 724524 http://www.dh.gov.uk/PublicationsAndStatistics/Publications/PublicationsPolicyAndGuidance/PublicationsPolicyAndGuidanceArticle/fs/en? CONTENT_ID=4005637&chk=BbkQzd
- Architectural designs for a high Quality, large volume, sustainable cataract programme. (accessed on 12.11.12)Available at: laico.org/v2020resource/files/archdesign.pdf
- Bourne RRA, Flaxman SR, Braithwaite T, et al. Magnitude, temporal trends, and projections of the global prevalence of blindness and distance and near vision impairment: a systematic review and meta-analysis. Lancet Glob Health, 2017 Sep;5(9):e888-e897. doi: 10.1016/S2214-109X(17)30293-0. Epub 2017 Aug 2.
- Cataract Surgery Guidelines. The Royal College of Ophthalmologists. http://www.rcophth.ac.uk/scientific/publications.html
- Commission on Macroeconomic and Health: National Programme for Control of Blindness. (Accessed on 10.01.13.) Available at: http://www.who.int/macrohealth/action/Report %20of%20the%20National%20Commission.pdf
- DB 9602 Guidance on the Safe Use of Lasers in Medical and Dental Practice, MHRA 1996. BS EN 601-2-22 Published by the Medicines and Healthcare products Regulatory Agency.
- Eye clinic VA Design Guide Veterans Health Administration Washington, DC (accessed on 10.11.12) Available at: www.wbdg.org/ccb/VA/VADEGUID/eye.pdf
- Health Building Note 26—Facilities for surgical procedures. HBN NHS Estates 26 Vol. 1 ISBN: 0113224958 (October 2004).
- Michael R, Wegener A. Recent trends in eye care surgery equipment and devices. J Opt Soc Am. A 21, 2004;1388-92.
- National Programme for Control of Blindness: Standards for eye banking in India. (accessed on 02.1.13). Available at: npcb.nic.in/writereaddata/mainlinkfile/file176.pdf
- Ophthalmology Outpatient Department space planning; The royal college of ophthalmologists, UK (accessed on: 18.12.13), Available at:http://www. eyeOPD.gov.uk/StatBase/Expodata/Spreadsheets/D7399.pdf
- Radiological Services Design Guide: VA Design Guide Veterans Health Administration Washington, DC 20420, (Accessed on 03.01.13.) Available at: www.wbdg.org/ccb/VA/VADEGUID/radio.pdf

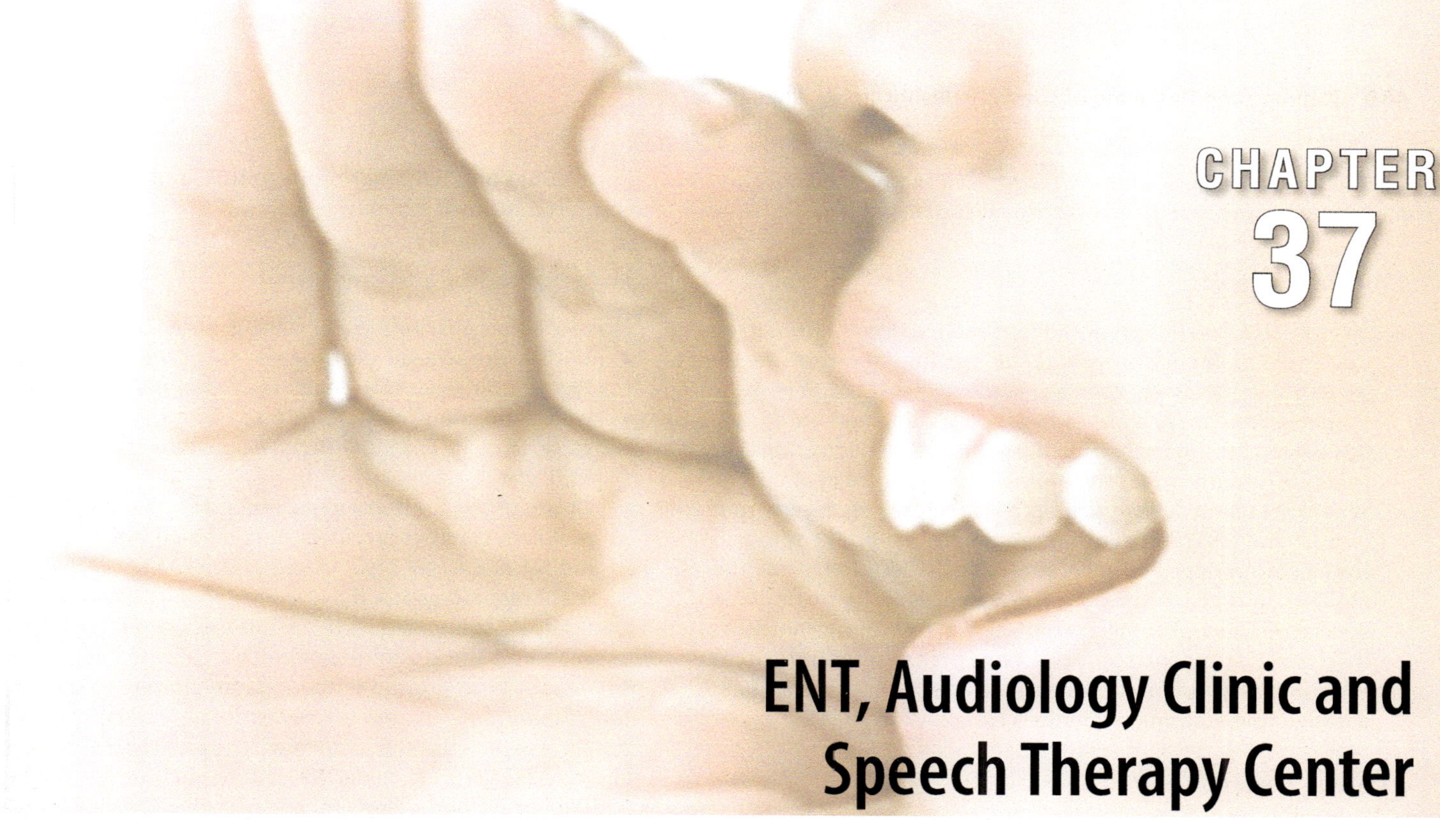

ENT, Audiology Clinic and Speech Therapy Center

Vijay Kumar Tadia, Shakti Kumar Gupta, Sunil Kant, R Chandrashekhar

INTRODUCTION

The planning and design of ear, nose and throat (ENT) and audiology clinics, and hearing aid centers is inter-dependent. These are usually located in general outpatient departments (OPDs) of hospitals, but could be located elsewhere too. ENT and audiology include complete spectrum for ENT-related ailments. Historically, all aspects of specialist care for people with ENT conditions have come within ENT services, with audiology departments providing support in diagnosis and rehabilitation. Speech therapy is also associated with the ENT clinic, providing specialized examination, visualization and analysis of vocal function and speech rehabilitation.[1,2]

GENERAL SERVICE CONSIDERATIONS

The main functions of ENT and audiology clinics are:[1]

- Specialist consultation, examination and treatment in respect of diseases and disorders of the ENT that do not require inpatient activity.
- Assessment and treatment of balance disorders and deafness.
- Following-up and monitoring the condition of patients who have received inpatient treatment.

Factors Affecting the Size of a Service[2]

One of the principal factors affecting the size of an ENT service is the number of consultants in a particular locality. The recommendation by the British Association of Otolaryngologists in 1993 for a rate of one consultant per 80,000 population, would indicate a minimum viable ENT department size of three consultants providing a service to a population of a quarter of a million.

Examination room capacity calculation is based on the following formula/parameters:

$$\frac{\text{(Operating days per year) (hours of operation per day)}}{\text{Average length of encounter (ALOE) in minutes}} \div 60 = \text{Utilization factor}$$

Average Length of Encounter

In these space criteria, an encounter is defined as a face-to-face professional contact between a patient and a consultant vested with responsibility for diagnosing, evaluating, and treating the patient's condition. The length of encounter is the time between set-up and clean-up of the exam room. The average length of encounter (ALOE) is used to capture variations in length of encounter among similar clinical encounters that will take place in an exam room.[1,2]

Utilization Factor[1,2]

This is also known as capacity utilization rate, this factor provides flexibility in the utilization of a room to account for patient delays, scheduling conflicts and equipment maintenance. A room with an 80% utilization factor provides a buffer to assume that this room would be available 20% of the time beyond the planned operational practices for this room.

Patients[1]

Outpatients attending ENT or audiology clinics:

- Are mainly ambulant
- May be of any age, with a predominance of the very young and the elderly
- Are frequently accompanied by an attendant
- May be physically handicapped
- May have a hearing or speech disability.

The environment should be responsive to the needs of children, physically handicapped and sensorily disabled people.

Children's Needs

- It is important to design outpatient services for children to ensure that scale, ambience and character are appropriately provided to them. If a separate children's OPD is not provided, it is suggested that a discrete area, with appropriate staffing and equipment, be designated for children within the adult department, or that specific times be designated for the exclusive attendance of children.[1]
- Where a separate area for children is not possible, the environment of both the ENT and audiology clinics should take into account the large number of children attending. In addition, preschool age children may also be present when a parent is in the outpatient.[1]
- Special care should be taken to ensure that children are not distressed by the sight and/or sound of patients undergoing treatment. Provision of appropriate waiting facilities is important, including a designated area where children can play.[1]

Children's ENT

- A characteristic of this specialty is that treatment for children differs significantly from that for adults.
- Ear, nose and throat medicine for children under 15 years of age is largely concerned with conditions arising from upper respiratory tract infections.[1]

Children's Audiology

While defects of hearing affect all age groups, screening services for babies and young children (age up to five years) are of great importance so that disorders can be identified early enough to avoid impairment of speech, and educational difficulties.[1]

Adult ENT and Audiology

Common conditions found in adults vary from relatively minor complaints such as sinusitis and nasal polyps to neurological disorders, different types of carcinoma and disorders of the inner and middle ear. It may be more appropriate for the assessment of the hearing of people with learning difficulties to be undertaken in children's hearing assessment centers.[1]

Accidents and Emergencies

Patients with emergency ENT problems will be seen initially in the accident and emergency department. However, it may be considered more appropriate to transfer some patients to the ENT clinic, where specialist staff and equipment are available. This is particularly so in the case of a young child with a foreign body in an ear or nose.[1]

GENERAL FUNCTIONAL AND DESIGN REQUIREMENTS

Planning and Design

Patients attending ENT and audiology clinics, particularly for the first time, may be apprehensive and every effort should be made to reassure them. The general atmosphere in the clinics should be open, pleasant and friendly; this will help both patients and staff feel at ease. Furnishings and lighting should contribute to creating a relaxed and comfortable environment.[1]

Location and Relationships

There are four possibilities for the location of an ENT clinic:[1]

- Within the overall curtilage of the general OPD of a hospital. Figure 1 illustrates key locational relationships;
- As a stand-alone clinic within a hospital;
- Close to the ENT inpatient provision, maximizing the use of skilled ENT staff;
- Close to the children's department.

An audiology clinic will normally be combined with, or in close proximity to, an ENT clinic (see Fig. 1).[1]

A hearing aid center may be located in the hospital, where it will normally be co-located with an audiology clinic.[1]

Where ENT and audiology clinics are located within the OPD, they will ideally be at ground floor level and close to the main entrance of the hospital. Separate entrances are not necessary, but patients should not have to pass through clinical areas to reach the ENT and audiology clinics. As far as practicable, the arm should be to site the clinics toward a quiet corner of the hospital away from noisy locations, such as car parks and roads, busy circulation areas, service areas and plant rooms.[1]

The ENT patients may attend the radiology department during a clinic session. The radiology department should therefore be reasonably accessible.

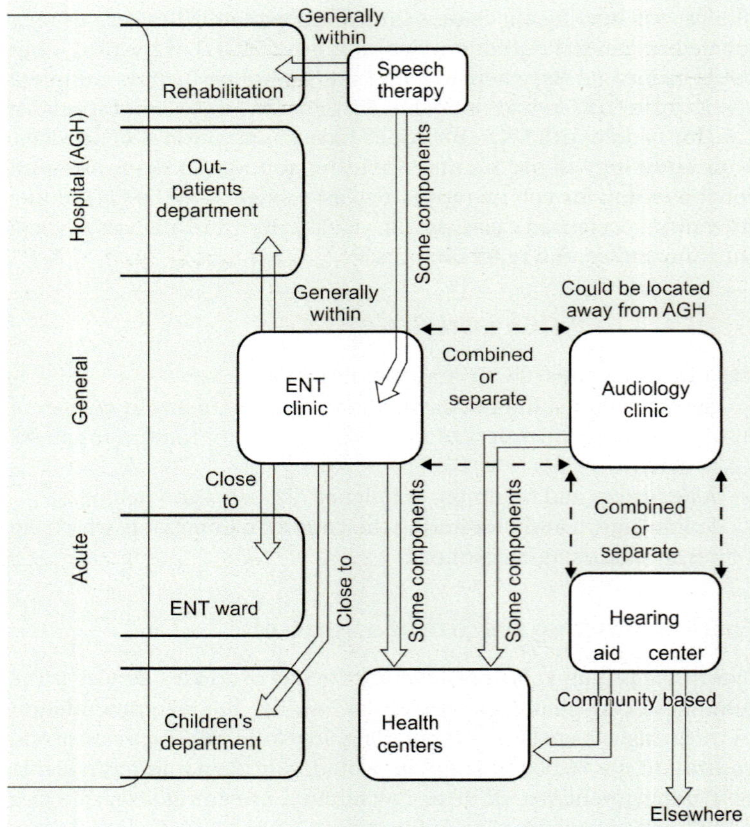

Fig. 1: Locational relationships between ENT and audiology clinics, hearing aid center and speech therapy accommodation.
(ENT: ear, nose and throat)

Patients in the accident and emergency department may need to be transferred to the ENT clinic for an emergency procedure.[1]

Accommodation in ENT and Audiology Clinics and a Hearing Aid Center (Fig. 1)[1]

Specific spaces in ENT and audiology clinics and a hearing aid center are as follows:

ENT Clinic

- Consulting/examination room
- Treatment room
- Preparation room
- Cleansing/disinfecting room recovery room
- Staff base
- Speech therapy consulting/examination/treatment room.

Audiology Clinic

- Audiometric testing area
- Vestibular function test room (Fig. 2)
- Audiology equipment store.

Hearing Aid Center

- Interview and fitting room
- Environmental devices demonstration room
- Hearing aid workshop
- Ear mould workshop.

Speech Therapy

The provision for speech therapy must also be there.

FUNCTIONAL DIAGRAM: ENT CLINIC, AUDIOLOGY AND SPEECH THERAPY

Functional diagrams show the relationship of each functional area to the whole department. In some instances, it shows important spaces within a functional area and how staff and patients may flow through the department. This diagram is not intended to serve as a "bubble diagram" that the planner/designer will create for an individual project. Size and shapes of spaces do not reflect actual configuration or square footage of spaces/rooms (Fig. 3).[1,2]

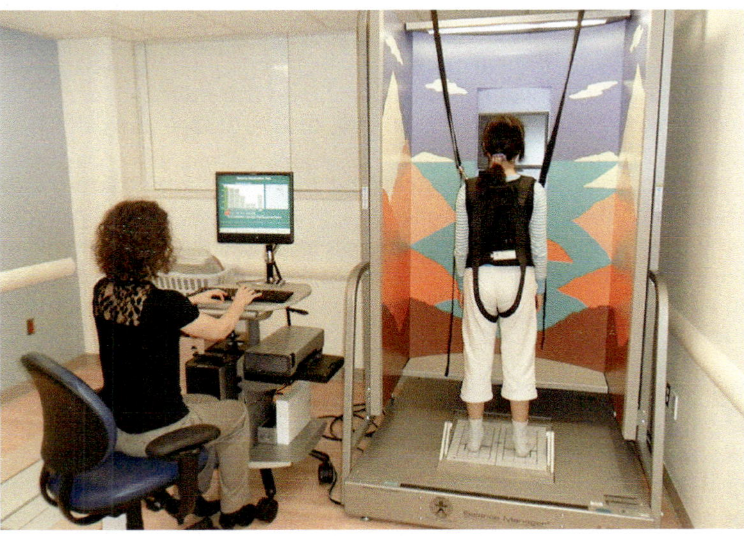

Fig. 2: Vestibular function test room.

Hard of Hearing Patients

Certain measures which may be taken to assist hard of hearing patients when attending the ENT OPD. Such measures may include adapting conventional telephones by providing, for example, volume controls and portable amplifiers, installing induction loops where appropriate, providing a visual patient call system in the reception/main waiting area, and reducing background noise.

Noise and Sound Attenuation

Ear, nose and throat and audiology clinics include a number of rooms in which low noise levels are required. Other areas, including the interview/fitting room, speech therapy consulting/examination/treatment room, and the control areas of the audiometric testing area should also be sound insulated, but to a less exacting standard (Fig. 4).[1]

The audiology booth is a specialist acoustic environment. The other rooms regarded as being sensitive to sound can be protected by a number of measures, which may include:[1]

- Constructing the enclosing partitions up to the underside of the structural slab with dense bricks or blocks, and ensuring there are no voids in the joints.
- Plastering both sides of the partition with dense fibrous plaster.
- Providing a solid door, acoustically sealed to its jambs, head and threshold.
- Packing the door frame tightly to the masonry aperture.
- Ensuring any window is double glazed with a cavity/air gap of 100 mm minimum, and is acoustically sealed.
- Providing a suspended ceiling.

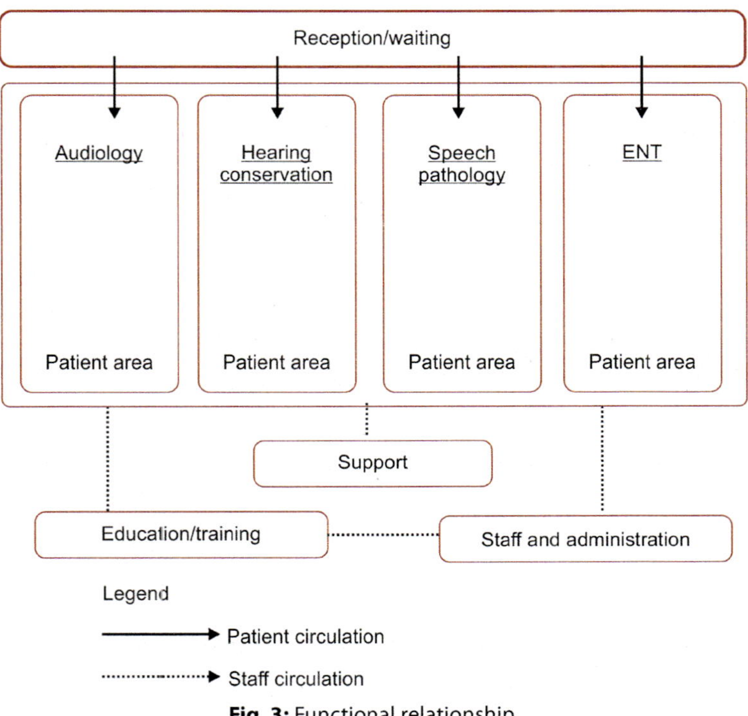

Fig. 3: Functional relationship.
(ENT: ear, nose and throat)

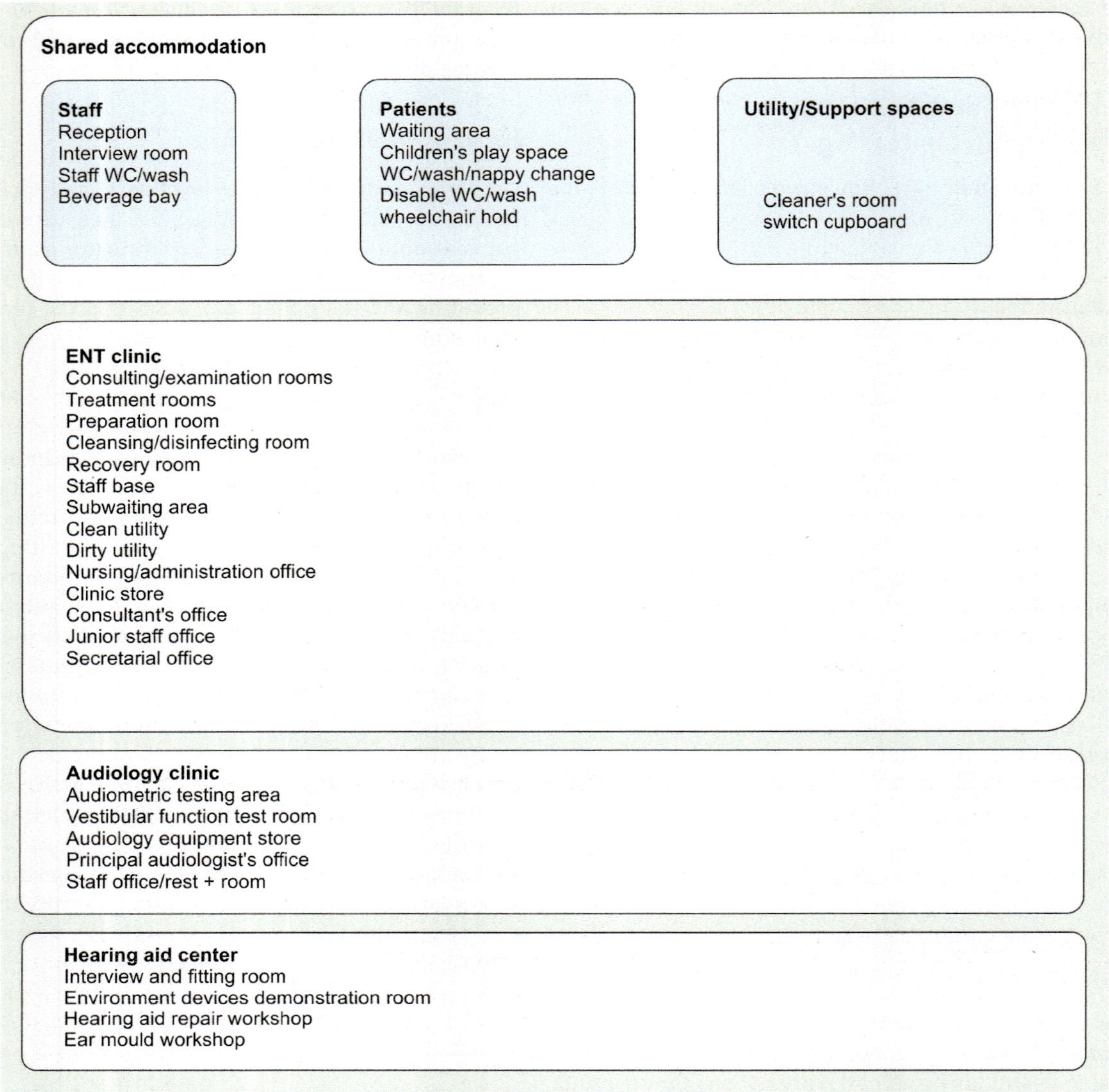

Shared accommodation

Staff	Patients	Utility/Support spaces
Reception Interview room Staff WC/wash Beverage bay	Waiting area Children's play space WC/wash/nappy change Disable WC/wash wheelchair hold	Cleaner's room switch cupboard

ENT clinic
Consulting/examination rooms
Treatment rooms
Preparation room
Cleansing/disinfecting room
Recovery room
Staff base
Subwaiting area
Clean utility
Dirty utility
Nursing/administration office
Clinic store
Consultant's office
Junior staff office
Secretarial office

Audiology clinic
Audiometric testing area
Vestibular function test room
Audiology equipment store
Principal audiologist's office
Staff office/rest + room

Hearing aid center
Interview and fitting room
Environment devices demonstration room
Hearing aid repair workshop
Ear mould workshop

Fig. 4: Functional grouping.
(ENT: ear, nose and throat; WC: water closet)

- Finishing the room with appropriate carpeting and acoustic underlay, and decorating the walls with fabric wallpapers.

SPECIFIC FUNCTIONAL AND DESIGN REQUIREMENTS[1]

Spaces Common to ENT and Audiology Clinics and a Hearing Aid Center

Reception[1]

A reception desk, dedicated to support the ENT clinic and/or audiology clinic is required where:

- Patients can be received and registered.
- Re-appointments, and appointments with other clinics, can be made.
- Health records can be held temporarily.
- Telephone(s) and visual display terminal(s) (VDT) should be used.

Some of these activities may need to be carried out discreetly.

The reception desk should be located adjacent to the waiting area and reasonably close to the consultation rooms. The receptionist should be able to observe the main waiting area and any sub-waiting spaces supporting the consultation rooms.

As most deaf and hard of hearing people rely to some extent on lip reading, it is important to ensure that the receptionist's face is in clear view. A well-lit quiet environment facilitates communication. A glass screen barrier between the receptionist and the deaf or hard of hearing must be avoided.

To assist some elderly, deaf and hard of hearing patients to know when they are being called to a clinical room, the receptionist may use a supplementary visual system. The fewer the number of patients waiting at any one time, the easier it is for a personal approach to be made in identifying and escorting a patient to a consultation room.

Waiting Area

Ideally, the main waiting area should respond to the differing needs of adults and children. It may be possible for a large waiting area to be designed with smaller seating areas in which certain patients can be grouped for example, children or those with a hearing or speech impediment. This may be achieved in a single space by arrangement of seating, different chair colors, indoor planting and the use of screening.[1]

However, arranged, the waiting area should provide a pleasant environment where patients can sit and relax prior to an appointment. It should be adjacent to, and be overseen by, the receptionist and have easy access to all clinical rooms. There should be a variety of seating and adequate space for wheelchair and pushchair users.

The size of the waiting area is affected by:[1]

- The flow of patients through the clinic
- The number of companions
- The number of wheelchair and pushchair users.

A variety of up-to-date reading material should be available. It is important to remember that for those wearing a hearing aid, any background noise is amplified and therefore sound from low-level background music or a video system may not be appropriate here.[1]

Children's Play Space

A play space should be provided for children who are patients or who are accompanying adult patients. Young children should be able to play or read in safety without disturbing adult patients.[1]

The play space should be located so that children can be easily supervised by adults in the waiting area. A cupboard or toy box should be provided for the storage of toys, books, etc.[1]

Patients' Toilets

The water closets (WCs) with hand washing and nappy changing facilities should be readily accessible from the waiting area. At least one toilet designed for wheelchair users should be provided.[1]

Wheelchair Hold

If not conveniently available elsewhere, a space for parking a single wheelchair is required.[1]

Cleaners' Room

It is assumed that domestic services staff who provide a cleaning service to the ENT and audiology clinics and hearing aid center will use the cleaners' room in the general OPD as a base, wherever possible. However, if any of the clinics are provided on a stand-alone basis, a cleaners' room will be required.[1]

ENT CLINIC[1]

A notional plan of an ENT clinic comprising six consulting/examination rooms is depicted at Appendix 1.[1]

Consultation/Examination Room

The specialized requirements associated with consulting and examining ENT outpatients include:[1]

- The examination of an ENT outpatient does not, usually, require a couch with a curtained area. An appropriate chair for the patient should therefore suffice. On the infrequent occasions that a patient needs to lie horizontally, use may be made of an ENT treatment room, where a multipurpose chair/couch is provided.
- Other requirements may include an examination light, cautery, suction, mirror heater, and the presentation of instruments.
- Project teams may wish to consider installing commercially available, purpose-designed, built-in fixtures, fittings and equipment.
- While the presence of daylight within a consulting/ examination room is commended, it should be noted that at times the room will require dimming and blackout arrangements.

TREATMENT FACILITY

The treatment facility comprises the following spaces:[1]

- Treatment rooms
- Preparation room
- Cleansing/disinfecting room
- Recovery room
- Staff base.

These spaces will be used during clinic sessions as required. The level of provision will depend upon the size of the ENT clinic and the local practice for conducting clinical investigations and treatments. Operative procedures, under general anesthesia, are not expected to be undertaken in the treatment facility.[1]

Treatment Room

Investigations and treatments not appropriate to a consultation/ examination room may be carried out in a treatment room, with the patient either supine or sitting. A multipurpose chair/couch may be considered useful.[1]

Most activities are conducted in the vicinity of the patient's head, where the clinician stands or is seated. The clinician will require a trolley for presenting instruments and equipment.[1]

Certain clinical procedures will require the use of an endoscope, flexible or rigid, with accessories. A light source for the endoscope, and suction and cautery are required. An operating microscope, wall-mounted or mobile on a stand, should be provided. A mobile microscope may be used, if required, in a consulting/examination room, but the problems presented by the transportation and storage of this bulky, yet delicate, instrument must be considered. A wall-mounted microscope requires a rigid supporting structure, otherwise vibration may occur. It should not be assumed that an existing structure is suitable.[1]

Preparation Room

The preparation room may serve as the focal point for the ENT clinic to receive trays of instruments and packs from a sterile services department. These items may be held here until required for use. The preparation room will be used to prepare trolleys and equipment for use in a treatment room or consulting/examination room. It should therefore be adjacent to the treatment rooms it supports, and easily accessible to the consulting/examination rooms.[1]

Cleaned and disinfected endoscopes may be brought to, and stored within, a cupboard constructed specifically for the safe and secure storage of delicate and expensive equipment.[1]

Cleansing/Disinfecting Room

Instruments and items of equipment which need to be reprocessed should be returned to central sterile services department (CSSD). Flexible endoscopes and accessories are delicate, easily damaged and costly to repair. Therefore, it is appropriate that such items are reprocessed in a cleansing/disinfecting room, within the ENT clinic.[1]

An awareness of the need for thorough cleansing and disinfecting of all endoscopes is recognized as an essential feature in preventing cross infection. While rigid endoscopes may routinely be cleansed and disinfected with ease, flexible endoscopes are more prone to damage and, because of the materials used in their construction, they cannot be subjected to a 134°C steam sterilization process. A number of suitable automated disinfecting systems are available. Following a rigorous manual clean, an endoscope can be attached to an automated system for a controlled, cold chemical disinfection cycle.[1]

Glutaraldehyde is currently the cold chemical disinfectant most commonly used. It is a hazardous substance, being toxic, irritant and allergenic, and extreme care must be taken to avoid inhalation and skin and eye contact.

Storage is required for appropriate personal protective clothing such as nitrile gloves, goggles, impermeable aprons and respiratory protection suitable for use when mixing and dispensing solutions of glutaraldehyde.[1]

Used instruments for return to central sterile services department can be held temporarily in the cleansing/disinfecting room whilst awaiting collection. Alternatively, and dependent on the policy agreed with the central sterile services department for reprocessing basic instruments, there may be a need to provide facilities for such items to be washed manually and sterilized using a bench-top sterilizer. If a bench-top sterilizer is provided, it should not be sited adjacent to the automated disinfecting system used for endoscopes, because the local convection currents generated by the sterilizer may adversely affect the toxic vapor extract performance of the autodisinfector.[1]

Suction bottles will also be emptied and cleansed in the cleansing/disinfecting room.

The cleansing/disinfecting room should be close to all treatment rooms.

Recovery Room

Following an investigative or treatment procedure, patients may require a short period of time to recover quietly. Easy chairs are required for patients and their companions.[1]

Staff Base

A small staff base is required to act as a focal point for the treatment area and to oversee patients awaiting treatment, patients under medication and those resting in the recovery room. Administrative tasks may also be done in the area.[1]

Subwaiting Area

A subwaiting area is required where patients who have received medication will wait prior to further treatment. Patients will be overseen by staff at the staff base.

Clean and Dirty Utilities

The clean and dirty utilities provided in the main OPD, or in an adjacent clinic, may also serve the needs of an ENT clinic. If the distances are too great to be effective, then suitably-sized dedicated clean and dirty utilities to meet the needs of the ENT treatment area may be required.[1]

Nursing/Administration Office

An office is required within the ENT clinic for routine office work, staff interviewing and discussions.[1]

Interview Room

In view of the number of hard of hearing patients attending the ENT clinic, a room where patients and relatives can be interviewed and/or counseled in privacy should be provided in a quiet location. Natural light and ventilation are desirable. Semi-easy chairs and a coffee table are required.[1]

Clinic Store

Storage for small supply items and equipment is required.

Consultants/Junior Staff/Secretarial Offices

These offices may be located within the ENT clinic or alternatively centralized with other consultants' offices, elsewhere within the hospital.[1]

AUDIOLOGY CLINIC[1] (TABLES 1 AND 2)

Patients attending the audiology clinic may do so as a result of having a clinic appointment, or they may be referred to the audiology clinic by the ENT consultant, immediately following consultation and examination.[1]

On completion of the audiological examination and test, a patient may return to be seen by the ENT consultant.

AUDIOMETRIC TESTING AREA (FIG. 5)

Soundproof accommodation, providing a controlled acoustic environment, is required where patients may be examined audiometrically. These soundproof spaces may be referred as booths. Such accommodation may comprise a single booth in one room, or a number of booths in one or more rooms. It is expected that each booth and its associated control area will be located to limit the extent of extraneous noise which may compromise the test conditions. At the same time, there is a need to ensure an acceptable working environment for staff. Natural lighting through windows and boosts to the mechanical ventilation may assist in dissipating oppressive atmospheres when the booth is in continuous use.[1]

The examinations and tests likely to be undertaken within an audiology booth include:[1]

- Pure tone threshold audiometry, air and bone
- Sound-field testing
- Impedance tests/tympanometry
- Speech audiometry, using earphones.

One of the booths must be large enough to permit sound-field testing and multioccupancy, for example, to accommodate a child and parent. Dependent on the examinations and tests being conducted, space may also be required for audiology staff and others, for example, a psychologist.[1]

The number and sizes of booths required is based on the clinic's projected workload.

Audiology Booth (Fig. 6)

The level of noise reduction required can be achieved by the use of commercially available booths or by locally constructed soundproofing measures. Due to the difficulty in achieving acceptable noise reduction levels, increasing use is being made of specialist manufacturers who supply and install purpose-built booths complete with internal

Table 1: Schedules of accommodation of audiology clinic.[1]

Activity space		1 Booth		3 Booth	
	Space area	Total area		Total area	
	m²	Qty	m²	Qty	m²
Entrance and reception			–		–
Reception	10.0	1	10.0	1	10.0
Main waiting		1	7.0	1	16.0
Childrens' play space	13.0	1	13.0	1	13.0
Water closet/Wash/Nappy change	4.5	1	4.5	1	4.5
Disabled water closet/wash type 5	4.5	1	4.5	1	4.5
Patient areas			–		–
Audiometric testing area		1	45.0	1	77.0
Vestibular function test room	17.0	1	17.0	1	17.0
Utility/support spaces			–		–
Principal audiologist's office	9.0	1	9.0	1	9.0
Staff office/rest room		1	15.0	1	30.0
Switch cupboard	2.0	1	2.0	1	2.0
Storage/supplies			–		–
Equipment store	7.0	1	7.0	1	7.0
Net total			134.0		190.0
ADD-planning provision		5%	6.7	5%	9.5
Total			140.7		199.5
ADD-engineering zone		3%	4.2	3%	6.0
ADD-circulation		25%	35.2	25%	49.9
Total			180.1		255.4
Departmental areas			180.0		255.0

Table 2: Ear, nose and throat clinic of audiology clinic.[1]

Activity space		3 C/E rooms		6 C/E rooms	
	Space area	Total area		Total area	
	m²	Qty	m²	Qty	m²
Entrance and reception			–		–
Reception desk	10.0	1	10.0	1	10.0
Waiting area		1	20.0	1	31.0
Children's play space	13.0	1	13.0	1	13.0
Water closet/Wash/Nappy change	4.5	2	9.0	3	13.5
Disabled water closet/wash type 5	4.5	1	4.5	1	4.5
Patient areas			–		–
Consultions/examination room	16.5	3	49.5	6	99.0
Treatment room	12.5	2	25.0	3	37.5
Preparation room	7.0	1	7.0	1	7.0
Recovery room	9.5	1	9.5	1	9.5
Staff base	6.0	1	6.0	1	6.0
Sub-wait		1	5.0	1	7.0
Utility/support spaces			–		–
Nursing/administration office	11.0	1	11.0	1	11.0
Cleansing/disinfecting room	7.5	1	7.5	1	7.5
Switch cupboard	2.0	1	2.0	1	2.0
Interview room	7.0	1	7.0	1	7.0
Storage/supplies			–		–
Clinic store	6.0	1	6.0	1	6.0
Net total			192.0		271.5
ADD-planning provision		5%	9.6	5%	13.6
Total			201.6		285.1
ADD-engineering zone		3%	6.0	3%	8.6
ADD-circulation		30%	60.5	30%	85.5
Total			268.1		379.1
Departmental areas			270.0		380.0

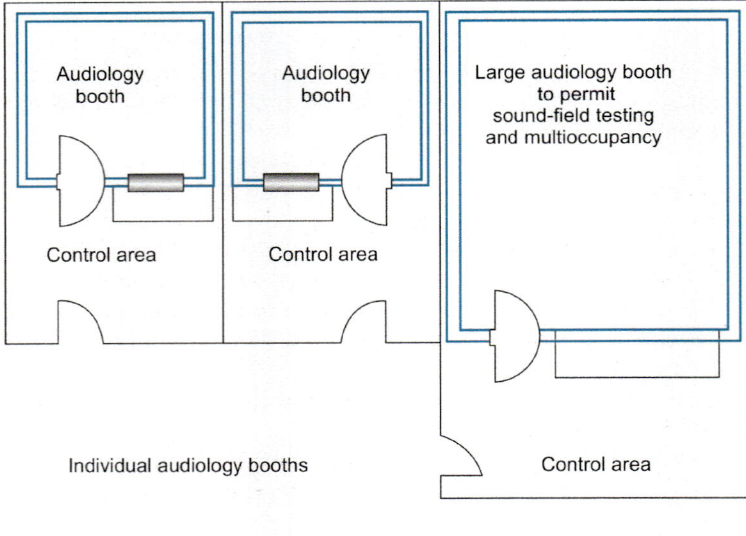

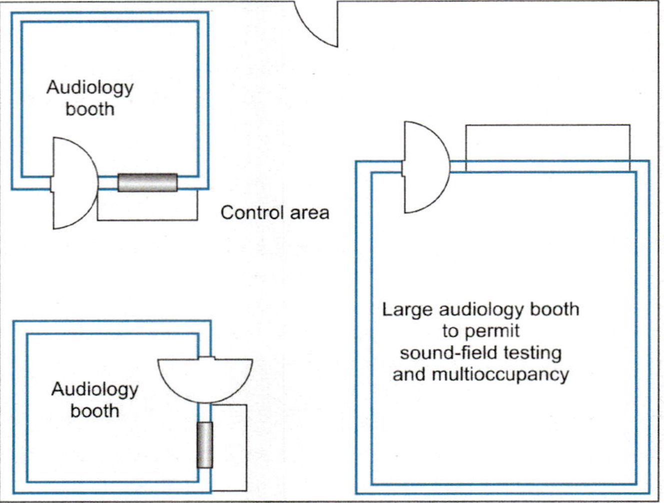

Fig. 5: Audiometric testing area; design options.

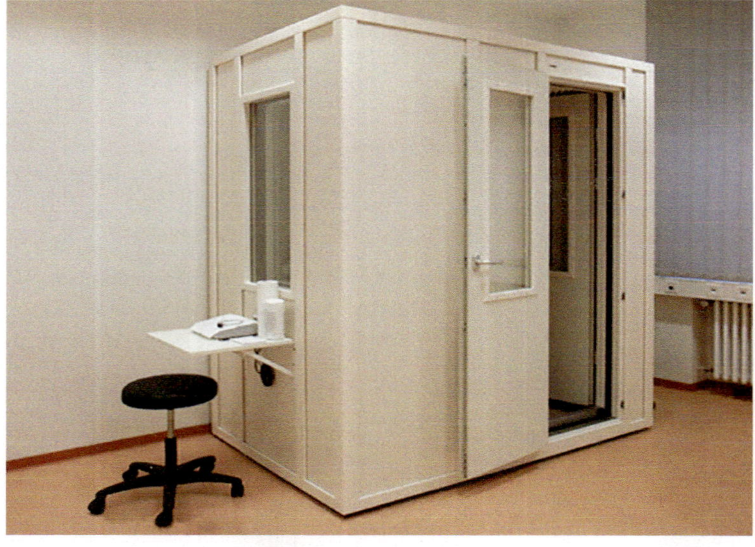

Fig. 6: Audiology booth.

finishes and decorations, electrical power, lighting, communications and mechanical ventilation and cooling.[1]

The design and construction of commercially available booths is based on the expertise of specialists, such as clinical users, acoustic engineers and research. They are designed so that they "float" within a structure and thereby eliminate structure-borne sound. Commercially available booths comprise walls which may be single or double-skin, and roof and floor which are all independent of the surrounding construction. Floors "float" on properly loaded vibration isolators. Double-skin walls are recommended to achieve sound insulation which virtually eliminates all external structure and airborne sound.

Any windows, observation panels and doors fitted to an audiology booth must not compromise the level of sound insulation provided by the booth.

Where audiology booths are installed into an existing building, the floor of the booth will be 150–200 mm above the normal floor level. A ramp, either permanent or temporary, should be provided at a slope not exceeding 8.5% to facilitate access for wheelchair users. Space will need to be allocated to allow for this. Where an audiology booth(s) is planned as part of a new building, consideration should be given to floating the booth so that its internal floor is level with the clinic floor.[1]

The doors of audiology booths, whether double (to provide an acoustic break) or single, are heavy and can be a hazard. In particular, when a door opens outwards, there is a need to protect personnel and the surrounding walls/structure, fixtures and fittings from the unexpected swing of the door.[1]

An intercom system between an audiology booth and its associated control area is required, designed and installed in a manner that preserves the acoustic integrity of the audiology booth.

Expert advice in respect of audiology booths should be sought early in the planning process.

Control Area

A desk-height worktop, with sufficient space and socket-outlets to accommodate audiometric testing equipment and controls, is required immediately outside each audiology booth. The control worktop must not touch the audiology booth. An audiologist may work at the worktop, communicating with the patient and initiating and recording the examinations and tests being undertaken.[1]

An audiology booth used for adults and older children requires a two-way observation panel between the audiology booth and the control area to enable staff to take note of all activities occurring within the booth, and for the reassurance of patients.[1]

In booths where sound-field testing is undertaken, a one-way observation panel, from control area to booth, is required. During sound-field testing, an audiologist must be able to view the actions of a child at any point within the booth.[1]

When more than one booth is located within the same room, the control area of each booth is shared, providing a less claustrophobic working environment. While the control area needs to be sound insulated, this need not be to the same level as the audiology booth.[1]

Vestibular Function Test Room

The examination and tests undertaken in a vestibular function test room (also known as a labyrinth test room) will include electronystagmography (ENG) including caloric, smooth pursuit, optokinetic, positional and others.[1]

The vestibular function test room does not require soundproofing. It should be large enough to have a patient area, and an area to hold the equipment required for the test procedures and for recording the data obtained.[1]

Total darkness is required, and as the test and recording equipment will be difficult to operate in total darkness, the patient-monitoring equipment should be screened from the patient area. Screening should eliminate any light associated with the equipment. The screening should also protect the patient's area from being light-compromised should the room door be opened, even inadvertently, during a procedure.[1]

A couch, with an adjustable head section, is needed to position the patient's head at the angles required.

The use of air caloric testing or water caloric testing are two options for the project team to consider in consultation with the clinical and technical specialists. The more recently introduced air induced nystagmus evoked by irrigating both ears, using warm and cold air, requires a specific piece of equipment. Air stimulation avoids the dangers associated with irrigating a perforated membrane with water and there are no water tanks to fill and clean. The air pump is built-in. Water caloric-induced nystagmus, evoked by irrigating both ears with warm and cold water, also requires a specific piece of equipment. More recently designed equipment provides water containers which are easy to remove and are resistant to spillage.[1]

A worktop should be provided within the vestibular function test room for the test and data recording equipment held permanently within the room. Storage drawers for electrodes, etc. will also be required. The room should have a remote control light switch. Windows and carpeting are not required.[1]

Screened Room

Traditional equipment necessary for the examination and testing for evoked potential investigations requires screening from external radio frequency interference. This has been achieved by building a radio frequency (RF) shield into the fabric to create a screened room. However, recent technical advances have enabled equipment to be produced which is less sensitive to RF interference and can also be mobile, eliminating the need for a dedicated room.[1]

Audiology Equipment Store

A small store with shelves is required for the storage of portable equipment used for audiometric testing and for holding equipment prior to dispatch for servicing or repair. The equipment being stored is expensive and the store should therefore be lockable and dedicated for use by the audiology clinic.[1]

Principal Audiologist's Office

An office is required for the principal audiologist where administrative tasks can be undertaken.[1]

Staff Office/Rest Room

An office is required for the audiology staff where administrative tasks can be carried out. The office may additionally include an informal area with beverage facilities, easy chairs and a coffee table.[1]

Hearing Aid Center

The issue, fitting and evaluation of hearing aids for babies and young children will be undertaken in the audiology clinic rather than within a hearing aid center.[1]

RECEPTION

Patients attend a hearing aid center primarily on a "drop-in" basis, without appointment and they require a discrete reception point. It should be borne in mind that all patients attending the hearing aid center will be hard of hearing.[1] Reception should be well lit and quiet.

Administrative tasks associated with the hearing aid center will usually be carried out at reception.

As the center operates on a "drop-in" basis, patients' hearing aid case notes should be readily accessible to reception staff.

WAITING AREA

If conveniently close, patients attending the hearing aid center may use the waiting area; otherwise, a small dedicated waiting area will be required.[1]

Interview and Fitting Room

In an interview and fitting room, audiologists and hearing therapists will:[1]

- Interview and counsel patients
- Undertake real ear analysis tests
- Take impressions for an ear mould
- Issue and fit a hearing aid appliance.

An audiology training amplifier should be provided.

Secure storage for a stock of hearing aid appliances, batteries and disposable items should be provided.

An interview and fitting room should provide a well-lit, quiet environment. Windows, providing natural lighting beneficial for the interviewing and counseling activities, should be capable of being darkened. The room does not need to be soundproof.[1]

When a hearing aid center is combined with an audiology clinic, the interview and fitting room should be easily accessible from the main waiting area.

Environmental Devices Demonstration Room

Bell boards, flashing lights and other environmental devices may be demonstrated, to deaf or hard of hearing persons, to help the selection of devices which compensate for individual hearing disabilities, particularly for day-to-day situations.[1]

Manufacturers of various devices are usually prepared to demonstrate to organized groups and will bring their own equipment for this purpose. A supply of electric socket outlets and a TV aerial socket, positioned above an open bench top which extends along one wall of the room, are required to facilitate the differing demonstrations.

The room should be naturally lit and ventilated, and have seating for those attending a demonstration. Supplementary lighting may be necessary during a demonstration.[1]

Hearing Aid Repair Workshop

A workshop is required for undertaking minor repairs to hearing aid appliances. An appliance requiring a major repair is likely to be returned to the manufacturer.[1]

Ear Mould Workshop

The manufacture of ear moulds may be carried out in a hearing aid center or produced commercially. In the latter case, the ear mould workshop will not be required.[1]

Where a workshop is provided as part of a hearing aid center, the dust produced by drilling, grinding and buffing tools should be removed by the use of an exhaust hood.[1]

SPEECH THERAPY[1]

Consultation/Examination/Treatment Room

A room is required sufficient in size to accommodate a therapist and patient (who may be in a wheelchair) plus a companion and/or assistant speech therapist. The room should be naturally lit and provide a relaxing atmosphere. It must be mechanically ventilated and acoustically treated, making it suitable for recording and sound-sensitive equipment. There should be storage for files, clinical materials and small assessment items. A full length mirror, either fixed or free-standing, is also required.[1]

Speech audiometry is not expected to be undertaken in this room, as the special needs for this type of procedure will be available in an audiology clinic.

MECHANICAL SERVICES

Heating

The general heating requirements for the ENT and audiology clinics and hearing aid center will be similar to those for the OPD. The accommodation will not normally be in use at night and during weekends. Notional space temperatures are shown in Appendix 2.[1]

Ventilation

An audiology booth is designed to control noise transmission and will need mechanical ventilation and cooling. The noise level in this space should comply with recommended noise spectrum. The design should ensure that extraneous conversation is not overheard via the supply and extract ducts. Particular care is therefore required in the selection, design, siting and installation of fan motors, fan silencers, dampers, supply and exhaust air ducts and grilles. Where the multioccupancy booth is used solely for children, the noise level criteria may be relaxed by up to 10 dB against the test tone frequency range.[1]

The speech therapy consultation/examination/ treatment room should also be mechanically ventilated and may need to be mechanically cooled.[1]

Notional air changes per hour are shown in Appendix 2.

Cooling plant should be designed to maintain an internal temperature of 25°C when the external ambient is 28°C.[1]

Disinfection of endoscopes with a solution of glutaraldehyde should be carried out in a cabinet which has a separate mechanical ventilation extract system to ensure compliance with the occupational exposure standard (OES). The room containing the cabinet should also be mechanically ventilated.[1]

Hot, Cold and Drinking Water Services

Hot and cold water pipe runs and drainage runs should be planned so as to minimize the risk of transmission of noise to the audiometric testing area and speech therapy consulting/examination/treatment room.[1]

Caloric Testing

Where water caloric equipment testing is preferred, a cold water supply and drainage is required. Where, however, portable air caloric testing equipment is preferred, a power supply only is needed.[1]

Piped Medical Gases and Vacuum

Piped medical vacuum may be required in each ENT treatment room.

ELECTRICAL SERVICES

Lighting

High frequency fluorescent luminaires, due to a number of advantages, may be the best choice for lighting throughout the clinics. Conventional fluorescent equipment is liable to generate noise and, if used in the audiology booths, it will be necessary to locate the inductive equipment elsewhere. LED lights are preferred.

Dimming facilities will be required for the general lighting in the consultation/examination and treatment rooms in the ENT clinic.[1]

Where sound-field testing is carried out in the multi-occupancy audiology booth, the lighting should be well- diffused, shadowless and free from glare or contrasts. Two ceiling-mounted spotlights are required, one on either side of the chair, for use as light stimuli.[1]

Small fixation lights should be fitted on the ceiling above the couch in the caloric test area in the vestibular function test room. Two other small ceiling-mounted lights for calibrating electronystagmography equipment will also be required. Notional illuminance levels are shown in Appendix 2.[1]

Power Supplies

Socket outlets and switches in the multioccupancy audiology booth should be at a height such that they cannot be reached by toddlers.[1]

Notional socket outlet requirements are shown in Appendix 2.

Telephones

Telephones should normally be of the desk pattern. The telephones in the audiometric testing area should be of the type having lamp instead of a bell signal.[1]

An acoustic hood with a payphone for the use of patients should be sited in or adjacent to the main waiting spaces unless a hospital payphone is nearby. This telephone should be of the adjustable boost receiver type and should be connected directly to the public exchange and not via the hospital exchange. It should be mounted at a height suitable for use by wheelchair patients.[1]

Clocks

Clocks should have silent movements and, in treatment areas, a sweep second-hand.[1]

Communication Circuits

Communication circuits are required between the audiology booths and their associated control area.

The microphones for the multioccupancy audiology booth where sound-field testing is carried out, are usually suspended from the ceiling.[1]

The circuits should enable recorded sounds to be reproduced from loudspeakers in the multioccupancy audiology booth and simultaneously, as required, in the associated control area. A microphone in the control area should be connected to the loudspeakers in the multioccupancy audiology booth.[1]

Microphones should be provided in the other audiology booths so that patients can communicate by loudspeaker with the audiology staff in the associated control area.[1]

Conduits between each audiology booth and its associated control area should be sealed to control the transmission of noise.[1]

Essential Complementary Accommodation (Tables 3 and 4)

Essential complementary accommodation (ECA) comprises activity spaces which are essential to the running of the ENT and audiology clinics and a hearing aid center but which, in certain circumstances, may be available in a convenient location elsewhere. The following essential accommodation may be shared:[1]

- Staff WC/wash
- Cleaners' room
- Wheelchair hold
- Clean utility
- Dirty utility
- Consultant's office
- Junior staff office
- Secretarial office.

Table 3: Essential complementary accommodation.[1]

Activity space		*5%*	*3%*	*30%*	
	Space area m²	*Planning m²*	*Engineering m²*	*Circulation m²*	*Total area m²*
Staff water closet/wash-type 1	2.5	0.1	0.1	0.8	3.0
Cleaners room	7.0	0.4	0.2	2.2	10.0
Wheelchair hold	1.5	0.1	0.0	0.5	2.0
Clean utility	7.0	0.4	0.2	2.2	10.0
Dirty utility	6.5	0.3	0.2	2.0	9.0
Consultant's office	11.0	0.6	0.3	3.5	15.0
Junior staff office	11.0	0.6	0.3	3.5	15.0
Secretarial office	9.0	0.5	0.3	2.8	13.0

Table 4: Optional accommodation and services

Activity space		*5%*	*3%*	*30%*	
	Space area m²	*Planning m²*	*Engineering m²*	*Circulation m²*	*Total area m²*
Beverage bay	6.0	0.3	0.2	1.9	8.0
Ear mould workshop	12.0	0.6	0.4	3.8	17.0
Speech therapy	–	–	–	–	–
Consulting/examination room	15.5	0.8	0.5	4.9	22.0
Speech therapy office	11.0	0.6	0.3	3.5	15.0

APPENDIX 1

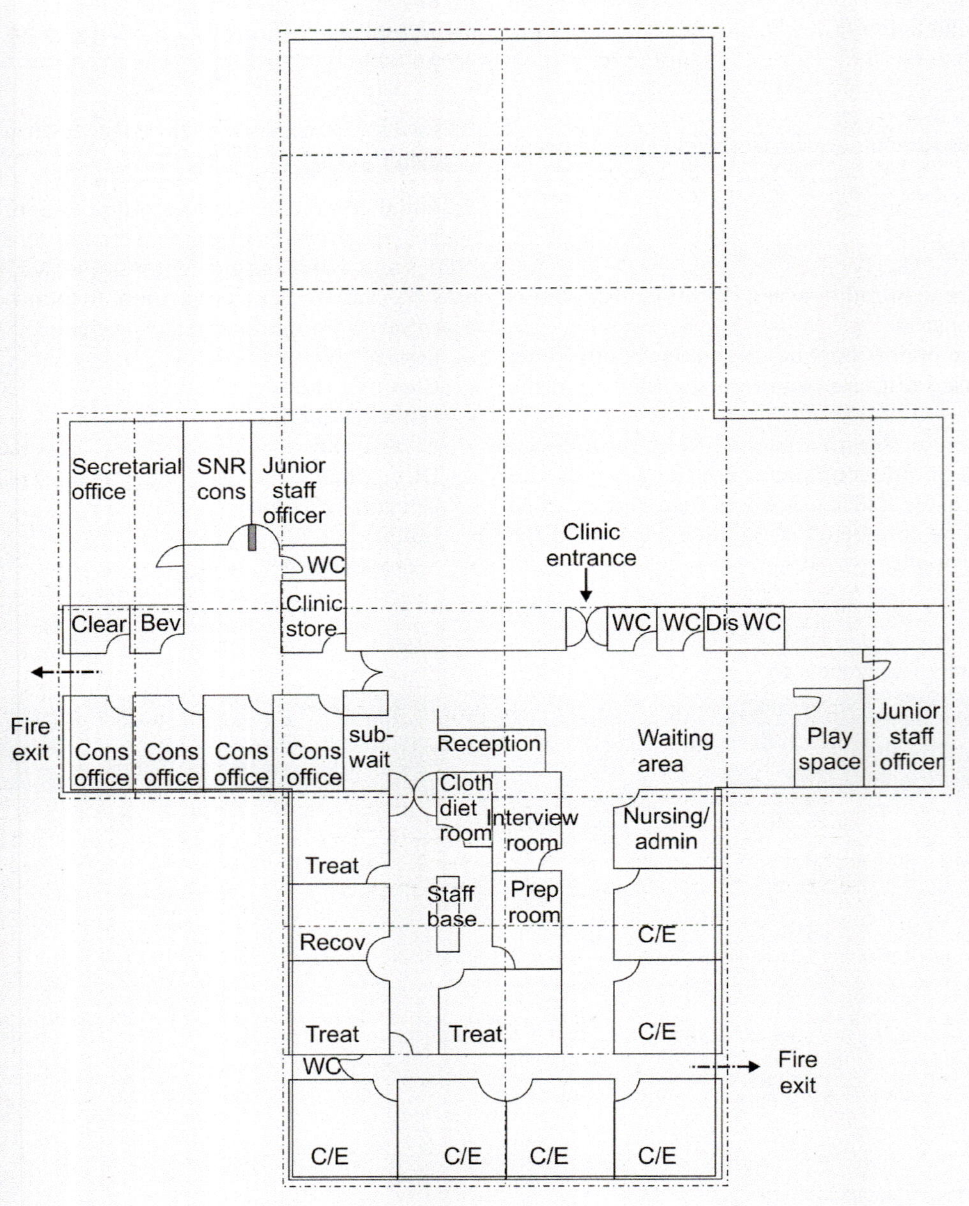

ENT clinic

(C/E: Consultation and Examination)

APPENDIX 2

Design Data[1]

The following notional air changes and design data is provided for preliminary planning. The actual figures should be determined by a detailed examination of the functional requirements and planning relationships of the spaces.

Activity space	*Temp (°C)*	*Air changes/hour*	*Illuminance (Lux)*	*Twin socket outlets*
ENT consulting/examination room	18	NV	300	3
Treatment room	18	NV	100	2
Preparation room	18	6	300	2
Cleansing and disinfecting room	18	EV	300	2
Recovery room	18	NV	100	1
Audiology booth	18	6	150	5
Control area	18	6	150	3
Vestibular function test room	18	6	100	4
Interview and fitting room	18	NV	100	2
Hearing aid repair workshop	18	NV	300	2
Ear mould workshop	18	EV	300	2
Speech therapy consulting/examination/treatment room	18	6	100	3

(ENT: ear, nose and throat; EV: extract ventilation; NV: natural ventilation)

REFERENCES

1. www.wales.nhs.uk
2. www.wbdg.org

OTHER REFERENCES

- Health building note 12 supplement 3 Out-patients department Supplement 3—ENT and audiology clinics, hearing aid centers 1994.
- Minimum requirements for otolaryngology departments in NHS hospitals. The British Association of Otolaryngologists, 1993.
- McCormick B. Paediatric audiology: 0–5 years. Whurr Publishers, 2nd edition, 1993. ISBN 1897635257.
- DoD Space Planning Criteria, Chapter 310: Audiology, Hearing conservation, Speech-language pathology and ENT Clinic July 28, 2015.

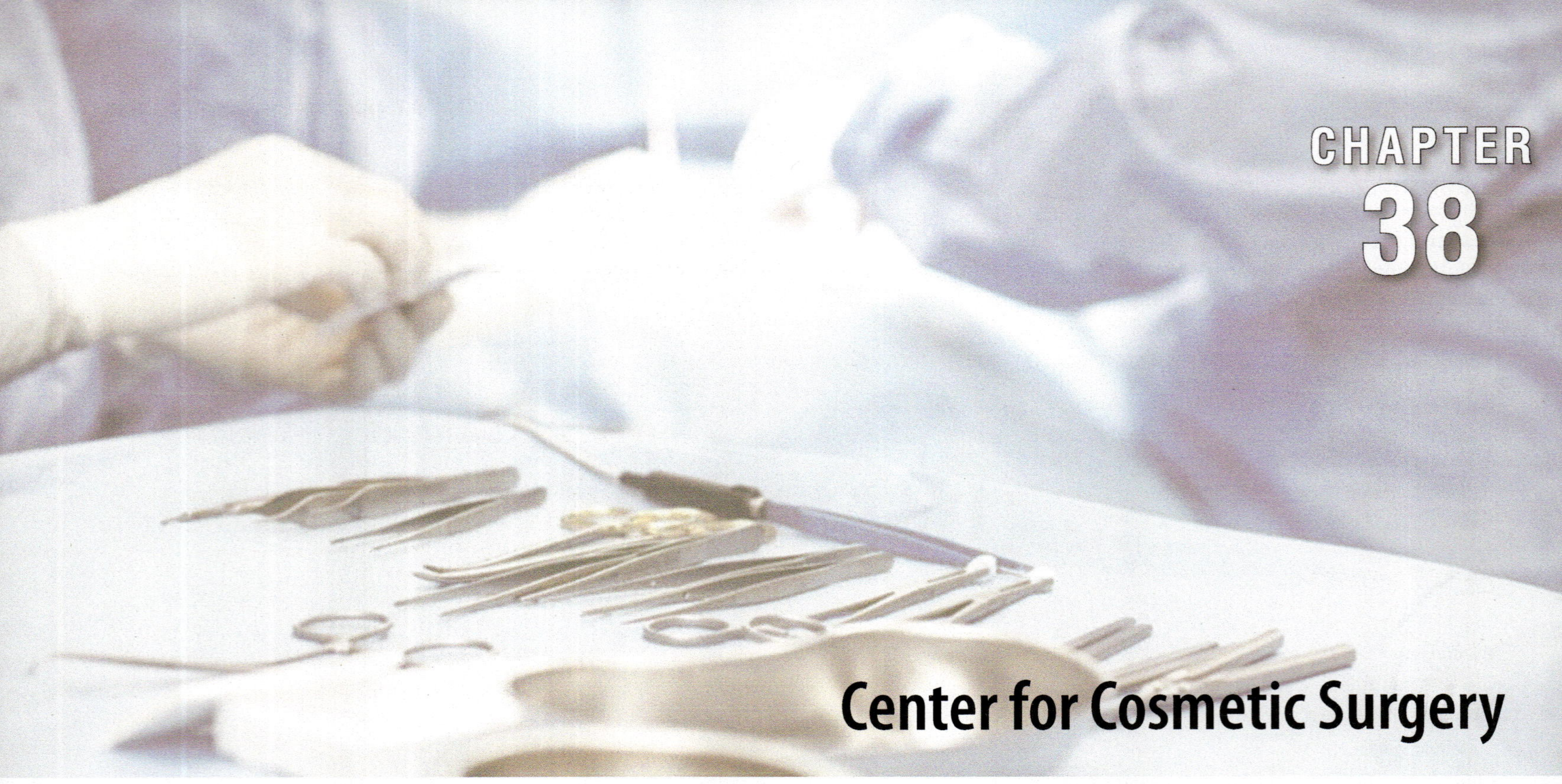

CHAPTER 38

Center for Cosmetic Surgery

Sanjeev Sood, Shakti Kumar Gupta, Sunil Kant, R Chandrashekhar

INTRODUCTION

Cosmetic (or esthetic) surgery is a subspecialty of plastic or reconstructive surgery, which is concerned with the correction or restoration of form and function. While famous for cosmetic surgery, plastic surgery also includes a variety of fields such as craniofacial surgery, hand surgery, burn surgery, microsurgery, and reconstructive surgery. The word "plastic" derives from the Greek 'plastikos' meaning to mould or to shape.[1]

Cosmetic surgery is mostly performed as an elective procedure, and is carried out sometime after the diagnosis has been made and when best suited for the condition of the patient and the hospital. Cosmetic surgery is performed on parts of the body with the purpose of improving a person's appearance and/or removing signs of aging. Studies prove that this type of surgery plays an important role in individual's self-esteem because by making changes to the body it contributes not only to the patient's physical appearance but also to the mental health of the patient. In certain cases, the cosmetic surgery may have to be performed following plastic surgery in a quest to further improve patients overall body image, say following breast reconstruction.[2]

The cosmetic procedures (surgical or nonsurgical) may be performed by a plastic and reconstructive surgeon, esthetician or a dermatologist. A cosmetic center may function as a standalone unit or as a part of hospital complex. Several cosmetic surgery procedures can be performed as a daycare procedure, where the patient is discharged to the home same day.

FUNCTIONS AND SCOPE OF SERVICES

Cosmetic surgery includes both invasive and noninvasive procedures.

Various procedures and services include—breast augmentation, breast lift surgery, ear repairs, tummy tuck/abdominoplasty, facelift surgery/rhytidectomy, liposuction procedure, brow lift, facial implant (chin, cheek, jaw), wrinkle filling, lip augmentation, hair restoration surgery, buttock/thigh lift, liposuction, etc.[3]

Skin enhancement services include—trifractional light therapy, photorejuvenation, skin tightening, vascular, pigment and lesion treatment; light therapy, microdermabrasion microlaser peel, profractional, silk peel; injections for Botox cosmetic, excessive perspiration (hyperhidrosis); chemical peels—minimizing the appearance of acne, chicken pox, and other scars as well as wrinkles (depending on concentration and type of agent used, except for deep furrows), solar lentigines (age spots, freckles), and photo damage in general. Chemical peels commonly involve carbolic acid (Phenol) , tri-chloroacetic acid (TCA), glycolic acid (AHA), or salicylic acid (BHA) as the active agent; dermal fillers for lips, cheeks and facial lines.[2,4]

LOCATION

Standalone cosmetic surgery centers are usually located in urban areas where there is high demand for such cosmetic repair or enhancement procedures catering to youth and people from media or film industry.

LAYOUT AND SPACE REQUIREMENTS

A cosmetic center needs to cater for following spaces:

- *General area*:
  - Doctors office—200 sq ft—should be equipped with sanitizer bottle, magnifying glass, skin scope, hair scope, face wipes, hand mirror, examination lamp, a mini fridge to store Botox, fillers.
  - Reception (Fig. 1) and patient registration counter—600 sq ft—should have telephone lines, LCD TV for promotional films and offer, sand packages deals, air-conditioning, comfortable seating, soft music, aroma air fresheners, promotional flyers, magazines, tissue papers and paintings.
  - Waiting room—200 sq ft—for patient's relatives

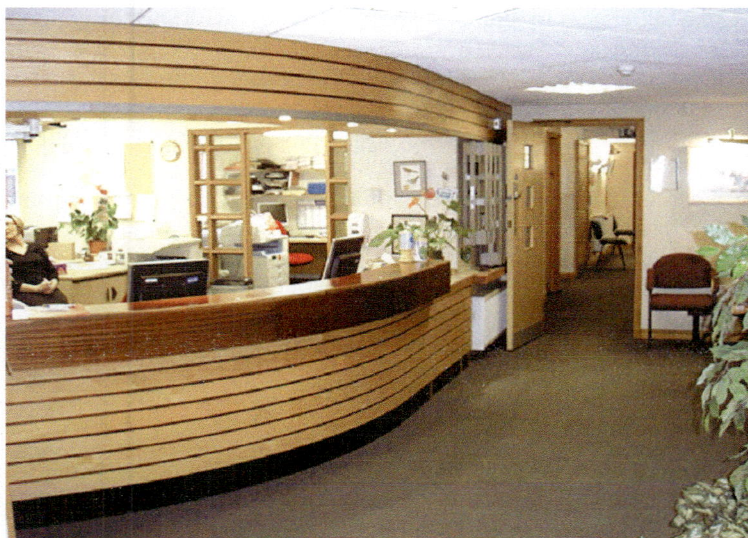

Fig. 1: Reception area.

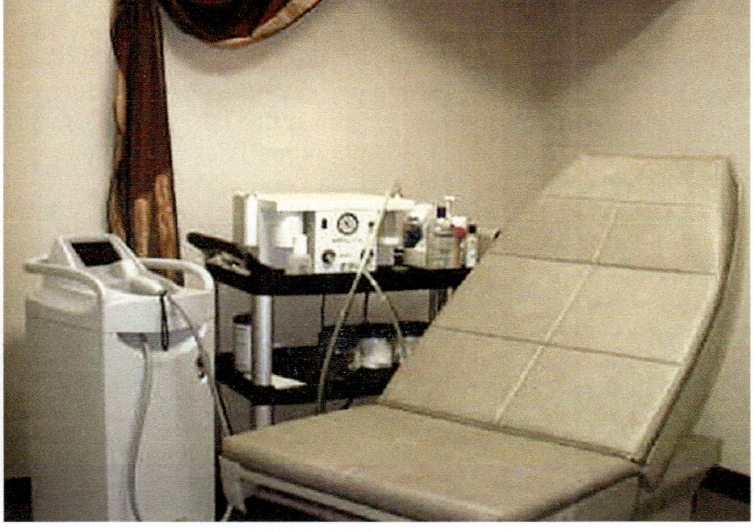

Fig. 3: Laser room.

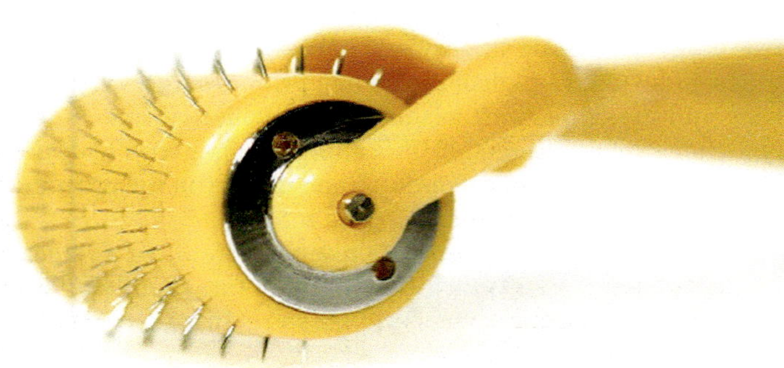

Fig. 2: Dermarollers.

- Changing room, grooming cum and resting room for staff—100 sq ft
- Pantry—100 sq ft
- Rest rooms—100 sq ft.

- *Protective zone*: It provides facilities such as:
  - Minor— operation theatre (OT) 200 sq ft—to perform procedures like radio frequency (RF), Botox, fillers, dermaroller, (Fig. 2) mesotherapy for skin and hair.
  - Preanesthesia room—100 sq ft
  - Peel room—100 sq ft
  - Laser room—150 sq ft (Fig. 3)
  - Store room—100 sq ft
  - Autoclave/TSSU—100 sq ft
  - Trolley bay—50 sq ft
  - Control area of electricity
  - Room for three-dimensional (3D) imaging system and software—100 sq ft.
- *Clean zone*: It provides facilities such as:
  - Preoperating room
  - Recovery room
  - Theater work room
  - X-ray unit with dark room
  - Sisters work room
  - Staff work room
  - Anesthesia station.
- *Sterile zone*: This zone has facilities such as:
  - General OT:[5]
    - ◊ OT size: Standard OT size of 20 ft × 20 ft × 10 ft (height below the false ceiling level is considered)
    - ◊ Equipment load: Standard equipment load of 5–7 kW considered per OT
    - ◊ Ambient temperature and humidity at each location to be considered while designing the system.
  - Scrub station
  - Anesthesia room—100 sq ft
  - Instant instrumental sterilization
  - Instrument trolley area.
- *Disposal zone*: This zone provides facilities like:
  - Dirty washroom
  - Disposal corridor
  - Janitor's cupboard.

UNIQUE DESIGN FEATURES

A cosmetic center should have good esthetic ambience and tastefully done up interiors. Other design feature pertain to requirements of heating, ventilating and air conditioning (HVAC) and lighting system for OT, as discussed below.

HVAC SYSTEMS—REQUIREMENTS FOR GENERAL OT

Air Change per Hour

Minimum total air changes should be 25 based on international guidelines although the same will vary with biological load and the location. The fresh air component of the air change is required to be minimum 4 air changes out of total minimum 25 air changes.[5]

Air Velocity

The vertical down flow of air coming out of the diffusers should be able to carry bacteria carrying particle load away from the operating table. The airflow needs to be unidirectional and downwards on the OT table.[5]

Positive Pressure

There is a requirement to maintain positive pressure differential between OT and adjoining areas to prevent outside air entry into OT. The minimum positive pressure recommended is 15 Pa (0.05 inches of water as per ISO 14644 clean room standard).[5]

Air Handling in the OT Including Air Quantity

Air is supplied through high-efficiency particulate arrestance (HEPA) filters in the air handling unit (AHU). The minimum size of the air supply area should be 6 ft × 4 ft to cover the entire OT table and surgical team. The minimum supply air volume to the OT (in CFM) should be compliant with the desired minimum air change.[5]

Temperature and Humidity

The temperature should be maintained at 21°C ± 3°C inside the OT all the time with corresponding relative humidity between 40–60%. Though the ideal RH is considered to be 55%. Appropriate devices to monitor and display these conditions inside the OT may be installed.[5]

Air Filtration

The AHU must be an air purification unit and air filtration unit. There must be two sets of washable flange type pre-filters of capacity 10 microns and 5 microns with aluminum/SS 304 frame within the AHU. The necessary service panels to be provided for servicing the filters, motors and blowers. HEPA filters of efficiency 99.97% down to 0.3 microns or higher efficiency may be provided in the AHU.[5]

LIGHTING

A modern medical supply unit not only delivers light, but also all the necessary media with connections for electricity, medical gases, nurse call systems, and data transfer–everything from a single conduit. Background illumination is furnished by ceiling lights which should be evenly distributed throughout the room. The anesthesiologist must have sufficient light, to adequately evaluate the patient's skin color for icterus, cyanosis, pallor, or erythema. Lighting, both natural and artificial, should be of an appropriate illumination. There is a complete range available with 100% white light for conventional surgery and 5% green light for microinvasive surgery to RGB color light control for operations, when the patient is conscious.[6]

To minimize eye fatigue, the ratio of intensity of general room lighting to that of the surgical suite should not exceed 1:3. This contrast should be maintained in corridors and scrub areas, as well as in the room itself, so that the surgeon has photopic vision (light adapted) before entering the sterile zone. Color and hue of the lights should be consistent.[6,7]

The LED OT light delivers a brightness that usually occurs at noon on a sunny summer day, i.e. 100,000–160,000 lux with a color temperature of 4,700 K that corresponds closely to color temperature of standard daylight (5,500 K). The color rendering index is approximately, greater than 95 and for the entire dimming area.

The overhead operating light must fulfill the following essential requirements:[6,7]

- Provide an intense light, within a range of 50,000–125,000 lux, into the incision without glare on the surface. The light may be equipped with an intensity control rheostat.
- Provide a circular light pattern and focus appropriately for the size of the incision. The fixture should provide focused depth by refracting light to illuminate both the body cavity and the general operating field.
- Decrease shadow multiple light sources and/or reflectors decrease shadows.
- Produces a blue-white color and appears as close to daylight as possible.
- Be freely adjustable to any position or angle by having vertical and horizontal range of motion.
- Should enable easy cleaning.
- Should be aerodynamically designed to facilitate laminar airflow.
- Generate minimal heat. Halogen bulbs generate less heat than other types.

SPECIAL EQUIPMENT

The facility requires specialized equipment including RF machine (Fig. 4), Laser machine (Fig. 5), Skin scope (Fig. 6), Galvanic and Microcurrent machines (Figs. 7 and 8).

3D Imaging System and Software

The modern day cosmetic surgery clinic uses the advanced 3D imaging system to provide patients with the most complete education possible regarding their plastic surgery procedures. Using this system, a three-dimensional photograph of the patient prior to surgery is taken. Then, using software simulation tools, 3D representations of how patient could look after surgery is created. This allows the patient the opportunity to preview various surgical options, and decide on the procedure that best suits your personal goals.[4]

The 3D camera captures a 3D photograph of the subject. Using multiple cameras, it takes a number of pictures simultaneously from several different points of view. This is used to build a 3D virtual model of the subject.[4]

The 3D photograph is processed by software to display the virtual model on a computer monitor. It can be rotated on the screen and viewed from almost any angle. The software then allows surgeon to apply simulation tools that change the size, shape and position of patient's breasts or any other part to achieve the desired appearance. Once patient is satisfied with the results, surgeon develops a surgical plan based on the changes patient has made.[4]

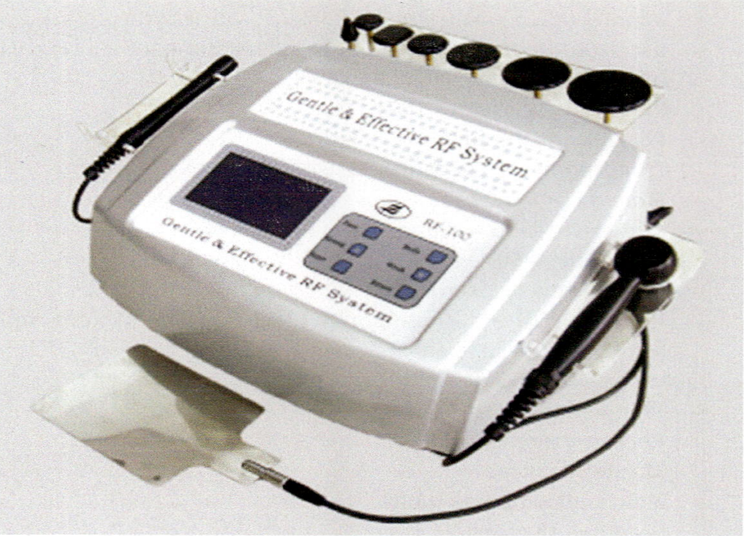

Fig. 4: Radio frequency machine.

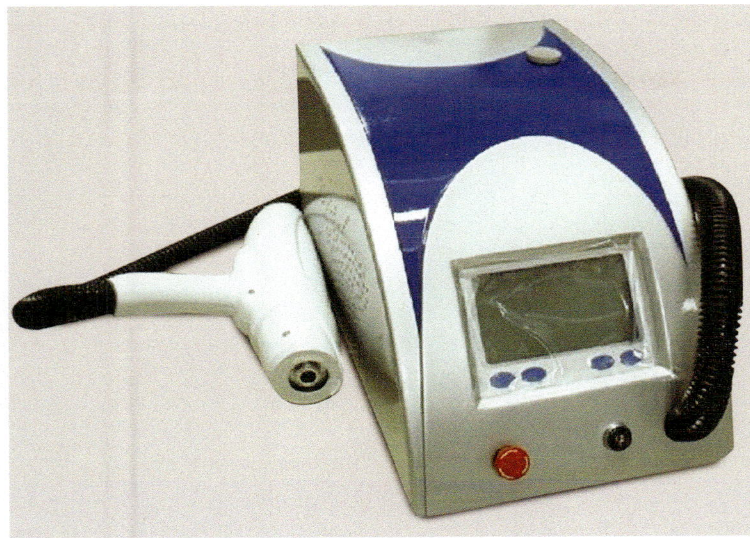

Fig. 5: Laser machine: Nd:YAG.

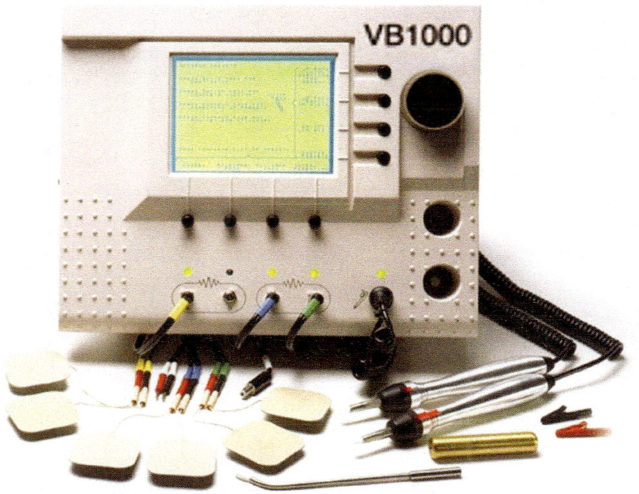

Fig. 8 : Microcurrent machine.

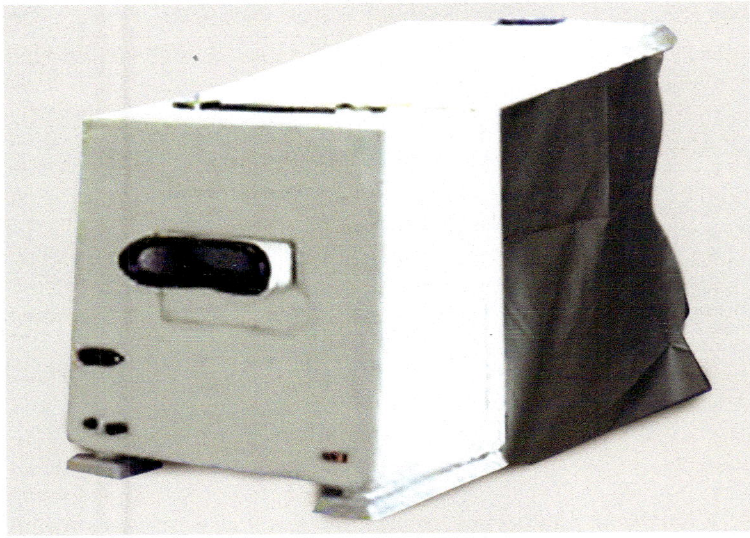

Fig. 6: Skin scope.

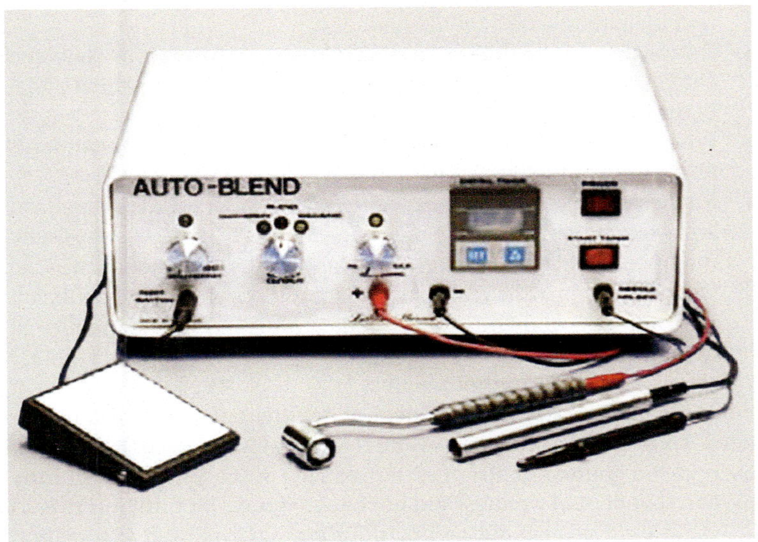

Fig. 7: Galvanic machine.

Radio Frequency Machine

A cosmetic RF machine utilizes RF waves in administration of medesthetic treatments such as skin blemish removal (mostly facial), skin rejuvenation or unwanted hair reduction [when combined with Intense Pulse Light (IPL) or Laser technologies].

Since RF radiation may be used in conjunction with other types of technologies in order to heighten affectiveness of hair reduction treatments and skin rejuvenation therapies leading aesthetic machine manufacturers have began to incorporate more than just one technology into their more advanced models of cosmetic machinery.

LASER MACHINE: Nd: YAG

A long-pulsed, 1064 nm is required for hair epilation along with safety goggles, shaving foam, cold compress, ice-cubes and razors.

There should established program for inspection, testing and maintenance and calibration of equipment in a cosmetic surgical center.

CONCLUSION

Cosmetic surgery is mostly performed as an elective and daycare procedure to enhance appearance or restore form or function. This is an important surgical modality to improve patients overall confidence and mental health. The scope of specialty includes range of services and procedures that need modern operation theater facilities, biomedical equipment and advanced imaging and other technologies.

REFERENCES

1. www.wikidoc.org
2. en.wikipedia.org
3. www.superstarplasticsurgery.org
4. drshenker.com
5. agorameditechnic.com
6. www.indmecica.com
7. www.medvarsity.com

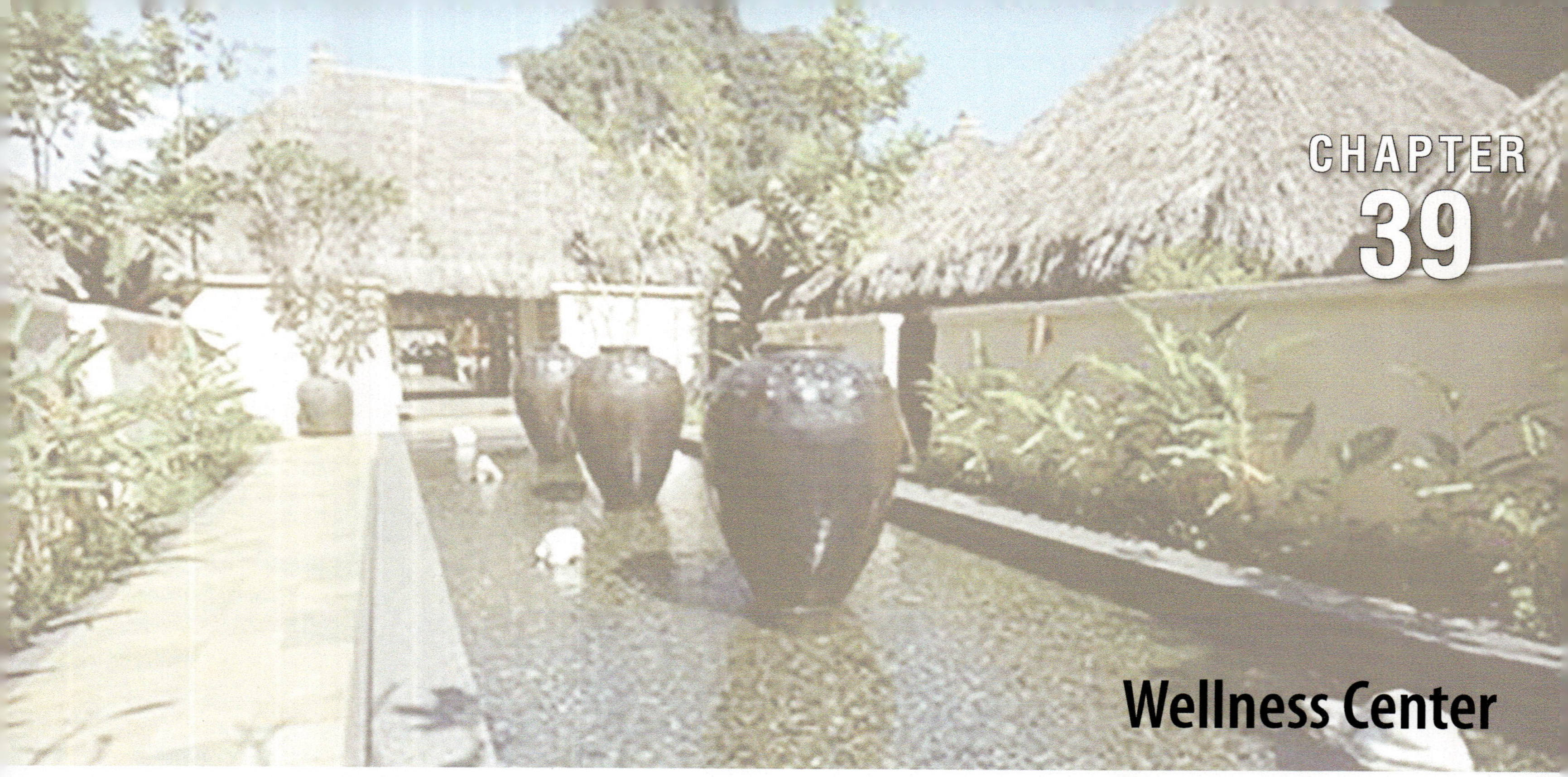

CHAPTER 39

Wellness Center

Shalini Kumar Bhalla, Shakti Kumar Gupta, Sunil Kant, R Chandrashekhar

INTRODUCTION

Defining Wellness

According to the World Health Organization (WHO), health is defined as—"A state of optimal well-being, not merely the absence of disease and infirmity." These dimensions of well-being include physical, mental, emotional, environmental, spiritual, and social components. This integrated perspective of optimal well-being recognizes the importance on each dimension as well as their gestalt.

An individual's well-being and vitality is greater than the sum of his/her parts. Although this concept has been around since Hippocrates, it seems to have been lost with the rise of conventional medicine and its reliance on specialization, technology, and separating the disease from the person.[1]

Need of Wellness Centers

Paradoxically, where on one end, with the turn of the century morbidity seems to be on the rise and disease trends seem to be changing due to a change in the basic life-style patterns, yet at the turn of the road into this new century, some dynamic elements in just about all cultures have combined to produce a change in the way, we live and maintain our health. A new sense of spiritual awareness, personal responsibility, and empowerment, supported by evolution in the world of business and technology, an awareness of what is truly important in life, and a return to basic values have all led to this moment in time where we want to take our health in our hands and are beginning to understand that responsible behavior can promote wellness well into old age (Flowchart 1).

Flowchart 1: Need for wellness centers.

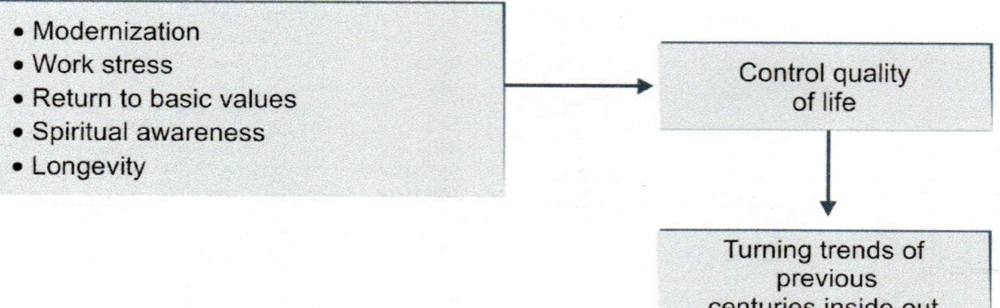

MEDICAL WELLNESS

Medical wellness is an approach for delivering healthcare that considers the multiple influences on a person's health. Accordingly, there are multiple options for treating and preventing disease. Further medical wellness provides:[1]

- A balanced, appropriate application of wellness practices within the clinical setting that are based on evidence-based practices.[3]
- Promotes a cross-disciplinary approach to patient care, based on informed consent and decision support between the practitioner and the patient.
- Establishes a foundation for dialogue and collaboration between conventional and complementary practices with the primary goal of promoting optimal health and well-being.
- Promotes the development and application of professional standards for wellness practices across clinical practices.
- Medical wellness integrates healthcare providers through medical and wellness practitioners working together. Whether it is a physician, therapist, allied health professional or wellness practitioner, medical wellness can provide real solutions for today's changing healthcare environment. Aptly it is said, "Medical wellness" is the practice of health and medical care relating to wellness outcomes. Figure 1 shows the dimensions of wellness.[3]

Wellness is generally used to mean a healthy balance of the mind-body-spirit that results in an overall feeling of well-being. It has been used in the context of alternative medicine since the 1950s, but the modern concept of wellness did not become popular until the 1970s.[2]

Wellness was also defined by the National Wellness Association (Singapore) as an "active process of becoming aware of and making choices toward a more successful existence". Wellness is a view of health that emphasizes the state of the entire being (hence-body-mind-spirit) and its ongoing development.

Medical wellness is the practice of health and medical care relating to *wellness outcomes*. The more specific definition of medical wellness is an approach to delivering healthcare that considers multiple influences on a person's health and consequently multiple modalities for treating and preventing disease as well as promoting optimal well-being. *It is often viewed as the integration of wellness practices and programs within a clinical environment.*[1]

ENVIRONMENT AND MEDICINE (FLOWCHART 2)

Hippocrates of Kos wrote of the therapeutic qualities of seawater, mentioning, its healing effects on the injured hands of the fishermen. Sea water not only restricted infection, but patients also found it gave them relief from pain.

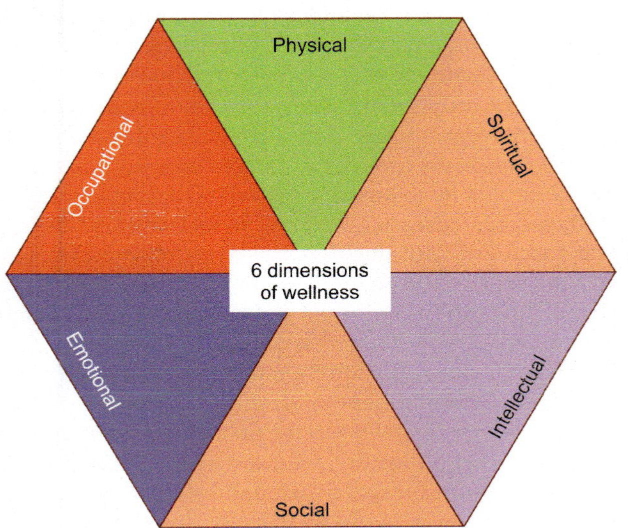

Fig. 1: Hexagon of wellness.

Flowchart 2: Environment and medicine.

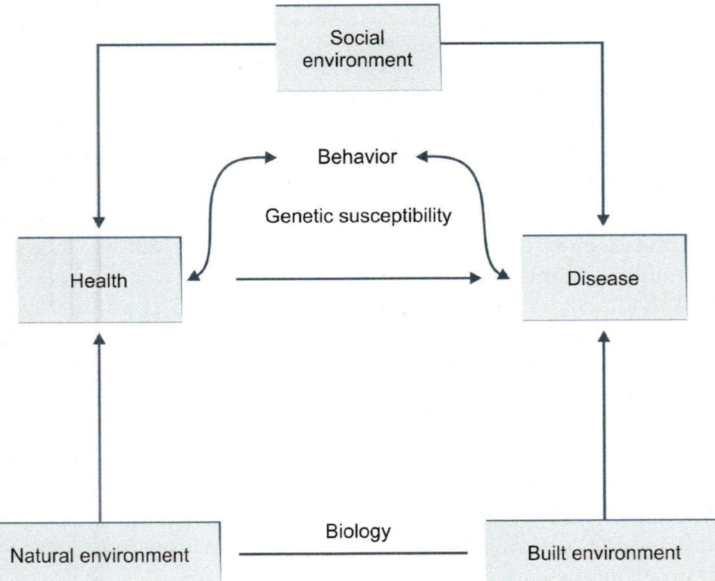

The Royal Mineral Water Hospital in Bath, England, founded in 1738, was in part the product of the efforts of men central to the remarkable growth of the spa town of Bath as a resort in the 18th century the architect John Wood the Elder, his patron Ralph Allen, and Beau Nash. The hospital was founded to provide charity care for ill people attracted to the spa town of Bath by the healing properties of mineral springs. Enlarged in 1793, the hospital was expanded further in 1860 by a second building project.

In the fourth century BC, Hippocrates, the father of Western Medicine, prophetically wrote; "Human health cannot be treated separately from the natural environment."

The natural, social and build environment and their complex inter-relationships, affect human health. Together, they comprise environmental health. According to WHO, environmental health is "the study of direct pathological effects on health of chemical, physical and biological agents and the effects of the broad physical and social environment on human health."[2]

THERAPEUTIC SPA MOVEMENT (FIG. 2)

As hospitals focused on medical education and technology, the resort spa movement in Europe and in the United States continued to focus on nature as a therapeutic modality. Dedicated to the notion of reconnecting highly stressed individuals in the industrial economy to their bodies and health, these typologies emerged in the private sector as the most powerful and potent connection to disease prevention.

Initially, these buildings included tuberculosis sanatoriums. Alvar Aalto's sanatorium in Paimio, Finland (1929–1933), a surviving example of early twentieth-century hospital building retains a strong connection between nature and healing (Fig. 3).

FEW APPLICABLE DEFINITIONS

Day Spa (Fig. 4)

A day spa is a business establishment which people visit for professionally administered personal care treatments such as massages and facials.

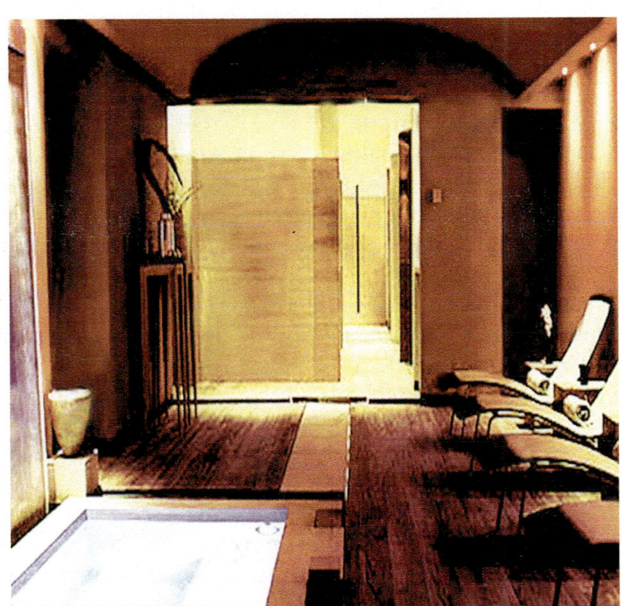

Fig. 2: Facility of the therapeutic SPA movement.

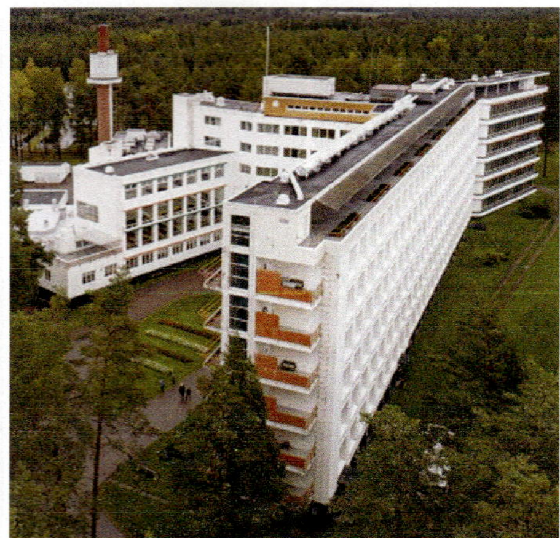

Fig. 3: Arial view of Paimio, Tuberculosis Sanatorium, Finland.

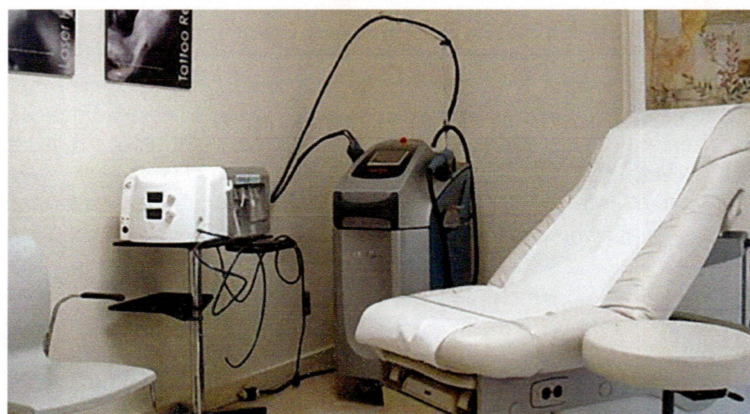

Fig. 5: Medical spas.

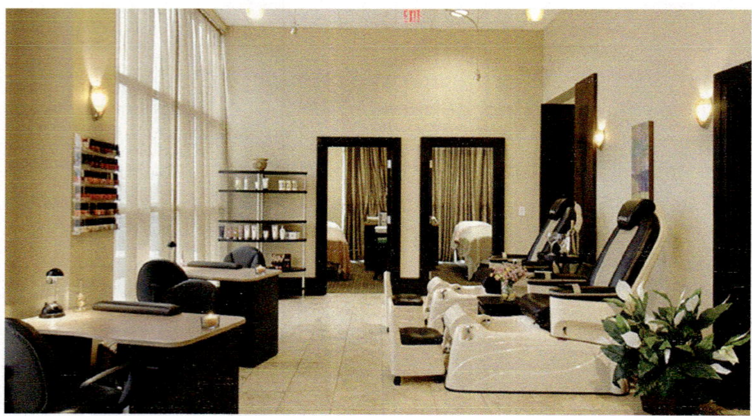

Fig. 4: Day spa.

It is similar to a beauty salon in that it is only visited for the duration of the treatment. Day spas sited in airport terminals are often called airport spas, which also offer services for hair and nails. In contrast, a destination spa offers the same services in a hotel setting where people reside for one or more days.[3,4]

Medical Spas (Fig. 5)[5]

A medical spa or med spa is a day spa that operates under the supervision of a licensed healthcare professional, such as a medical doctor. Medical spas may offer additional treatments that can only be administered by licensed medical practitioners. Additional treatments offered depend upon the scope of practice of the licensed practitioner and may include:[3]

- Laser and intense pulsed light procedures
- Medical microdermabrasions
- Photo-facials
- Botox and Restylane injections
- Medical peels.

Evolution of Wellness Centers

The evolution of wellness centers began with Ken Cooper's Cooper Aerobic Center, Houston, Texas, in the early 1970s and with the new emphasis on diet as it related to health pioneered by Nathan Pritikin. Up to this point in time, with the exception of healthful eating programs set-up within the Adventist Hospital Systems, hospitals were serving food that was nutritionally unsound for the most part and, in some cases, with a high content of substances now considered taboo.[5,6]

Academic medical centers across the nation took small steps in the right direction; the results of the now classic Framingham Heart Study at Massachusetts were among the first to relate cardiovascular disease to risk factors. This study revolutionized medicine by postulating that there were controllable, changeable behaviors that could influence the risk of cardiovascular disease. High cholesterol levels and the ingestion of high fat diet, along with smoking, lack of exercise, and stress, were among the factors considered in the study. Here was a turning point in the history of self-responsibility and self-care—changing habits could result in avoiding a heart attack.[5,6]

In 1982, the Riverside Health System in Newport News, Virginia, began one of the first wellness programs and projects. In Melrose Park, Illinois, Gottlieb Hospital was the first in the USA to create a free standing wellness center facility, followed by the Sports Med Center for Fitness, suburban Chicago, developed by a group of orthopedic physicians who created a 55,000 sq ft center. In 1991, the Galter Life Center, also in suburban Chicago, built the first free standing urban center in the United States.

PLANNING A WELLNESS CENTER

The Planning Process

The starting point for an organization's decision to build a wellness center is the organization's strategic plan. The strategic plan is the framework within which the evaluation and implementation take place; it defines the broad criteria according to which feasibility will be determined.

If, for example, a strategic plan has an objective of achieving a 15% rate of return on program investment, then one factor in financial feasibility is defined.

The strategic filter, the fabric of criteria created to measure program additions, is typically composed of an organizational assessment and a plan development section. The organizational assessment attempts to describe the current state of the organization thinks it should be at some point in the future and how it plans to get there.

Management considerations include those administrative, legal, and other operational issues that require resolution during the evaluation phase. The test for deciding whether a management issue should be included in the evaluation phase is whether the issue influences the feasibility of the wellness center program.

Technological considerations are those that pertain to what will be included in the clinical program of the wellness center design and how the movement of certain clinical programs will affect the technological requirements of the system. These issues are especially important for the more technologically intense clinical programs, such as outpatient surgery and imaging that may be included in the wellness center program.

For example, if outpatient surgery and imaging will be included in the program, a rough estimate of equipment costs should be made. It will also be important to consider exercise equipment and larger amenities such as swimming pools. Fitting these requirements into the overall budget for equipment is the first step.

THE INDIAN SCENARIO

Wellness in India

The Indian systems of medicine have age old acceptance in the communities in India and in most places they form the first-line of treatment in case of common ailments.

Of these, Ayurveda is the most ancient medical system with an impressive record of safety and efficacy. Siddha, Unani and Homeopathy are rationally recognized systems of medicine and have been integrated into the national health delivery system.

India enjoys the distinction of having the largest network of traditional healthcare, which are fully functional with a network of registered practitioners, research institutions and licensed pharmacies.

Department of Indian Systems of Medicine and Homeopathy (ISM&H) was created in March, 1995 and renamed as Department of Ayurveda, Yoga and Naturopathy, Unani, Siddha and Homeopathy (AYUSH) in November, 2003 with a view to providing focused attention to development of Education and Research in Ayurveda, Yoga and Naturopathy, Unani, Siddha and Homeopathy systems.

- All these complementary medicine branches focus nature cures, yoga, meditation, herbal treatments, massages, water therapy, air therapy, fire therapy and space therapy. Also included are mud therapy, acupressure, magnotherapy, chromotherapy and many others. The system of AYUSH works under the Central Department of Health and Family Welfare and has four research councils:[8]
  i. Central Council for Research in Ayurveda and Shiddha (CCRAS)
  ii. Central Council for Research in Unani Medicine (CCRUM)
  iii. Central Council for Research in Homoeopathy (CCRH)
  iv. Central Council for Research in Yoga and Naturopathy (CCRYN)

The AYUSH (Fig. 6) is also mainstreamed under the National Rural Health Mission (NRHM) with several provisions for its healthcare delivery. The system of traditional medicine in our country falls within the wellness component as well. Now AYUSH functions as an independent Ministry.

Due to the upcoming trend of wellness in our country the National Accreditation Board of Hospitals and Healthcare Providers has framed standards for wellness centers as well, clearly stating the trends to come.

Definition of wellness [as per National Accreditation Board of Hospitals (NABH) and Healthcare Providers draft standards for Wellness Centers, India] is—"Wellness is a state of a healthy balance of the mind and body that results in overall well-being. "Wellness has different facets, each one equally vital to the pursuit of healthy life.

The dimensions of wellness are:[7]

- Intellectual
- Social
- Spiritual
- Emotional
- Physical
- Occupational.

1. *Intellectual wellness:* The intellectual facet includes stimulating mental activities, expanding our knowledge and skills, sharing information with others, and participating in intellectual and cultural activities.[7]
2. *Social wellness:* The social facet emphasizes contributions to our human and physical environments, interdependence with others and nature, and the pursuit of harmony.[7]
3. *Spiritual wellness:* The spiritual facet involves the pursuit of meaning and purpose in human existence, and the development of a deep appreciation for life and natural forces that exist in the universe.[7]
4. *Emotional wellness:* The emotional facet emphasizes an awareness and acceptance of our feelings and behavior, a positive attitude about ourselves, a realistic assessment of our limitations, effective stress management, the pursuit of satisfying relationships, and the development of autonomy.[7]
5. *Physical wellness:* The physical facet encourages regular physical activity for cardiovascular flexibility and strength, knowledge about food, nutrition, and medical care, cosmetic care and the discouraging of tobacco, drugs, and immoderate use of alcohol. Physical wellness also encourages exploration of different medical delivery systems coming together for well-being of individual.[7]
6. *Occupational wellness:* The occupational facet involves choosing work which is personally satisfying and enriching, and the development of a positive attitude about our occupation and life plan.[7]

Any organization involved in delivering services which will facilitate customers to achieve anyone or combination of the six facets of wellness stated above is called as wellness center (NABH Standards, India).

All the above should be focused on achieving quality of life.

In the Indian scenario, the concept of wellness centers currently focus more on ayurveda/spa-like concept, and so, the design tenet. Trends are, however, changing even in the Indian market. Some development profiles in the Indian scenario shown in Figures 7 and 8.

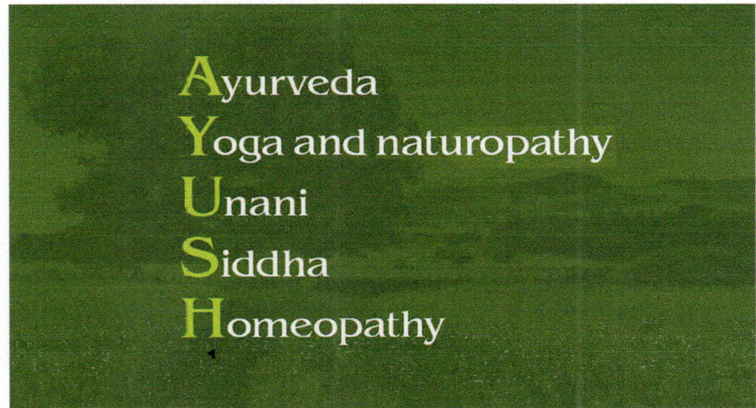

Fig. 6: AYUSH.

Wellness Center Programming Issues

There are several issues concerned with setting up wellness centers. They have been briefly tabulated in Table 1.

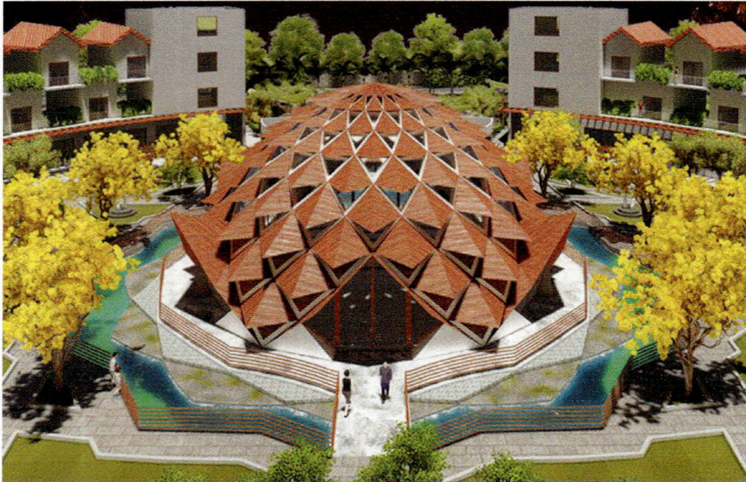

Fig. 7: The Pine Wellness Centre, DTTC, Delhi.

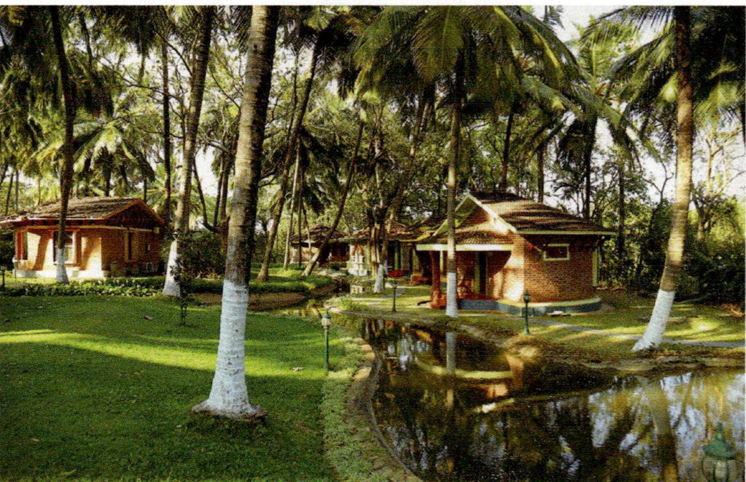

Fig. 8: Kairali Ayurvedic Healing Village.

Table 1: Issue question facility implications.

Management structure	• What will the ownership of the wellness center be? • How will ownership affect management and operation? What future programs are planned?	• Owners control program mix. Managers may have objectives that are different from those of owners. Identify future programs to ensure flexibility of space
Clinical program	• Which programs will move from the hospital to the wellness center (e.g. cardiopulmonary, physical therapy)? • Which physicians are likely to relocate to the wellness center or to share space there?	• Identify specialized requirements associated with each clinical program • Are dedicated physician offices required?
Fitness program	• What are the goals of the program? What are groups will be served? • Will the age demographics change over time? • How will clinical rehabilitation and fitness exercise machinery be selected? Will rehab patients be separated from fitness clients? • Will there be a separate area for obese patients?	• Will phasing for future development be included? • Adult/senior/children fitness facility balance. Daycare, children's lockers, fitness areas • Will more adult or senior-oriented programs be required in the future than there are now? • Are separate areas required for rehab and fitness equipment? • May be combined with others
Education program	• Will classes be mostly small or large? • Will there be cooking classes?	• Space accommodations range from 5 to 7 persons through auditorium size • Fume hoods, additional mechanical requirements
Spa program	• What level of spa services will be included?	• Sauna, steam, whirlpool, therapeutic massage, Vichy showers, and salon services
Common area program	• Will a retail program be included? • What type of food service is desired?	• Pro shop, salon, library or bookstore, nutritional supplement sales, juice bar, snack bar, cafe, cafeteria, full service restaurant

DESIGNING THE WELLNESS FACILITIES

An environment can be powerful medicine. We are affected everyday by the choices made by others as to the ease, joy, and comfort we feel in our travel through spaces.

Whatever the concepts of wellness one may adapt, common rules apply to all whether it be a clinical/spa/ fitness/resort setting. The basics of these are documented below.

Increasing Control through Design

A basic objective of wellness center design is to give patients a sense of control within the environment. To this end, the following elements should be incorporated into any design plan:

- Privacy
- Good lighting and color planning
- Comfortable seating for patients and family members
- Visual access to the outside environment
- Good visual cues and signage
- Predictability
- Reasonable sound levels
- Control of room temperature (in appropriate areas)
- Access to rest rooms, water fountains
- Parking access.

Everything in the environment of a wellness center must be designed to be clear. The path of the person moving through the spaces for a course of therapy or to examination, imaging, or treatment rooms should be rational, not full of surprises.

Predictability and the ability of the patient to feel psychologically and physically comfortable are keys to good wellness center design. These conditions are also important for the fitness participant. Not everyone who works out is in top condition. Therefore, it is important that a person who comes to the wellness center for fitness services can move easily from front desk check in, to locker room, to exercise area, and back again especially if that person is pressed for time.

In order to address the future needs of the wellness center facility with two major business lines that have unpredictable futures—healthcare and fitness—flexibility is the only rational approach. Flexibility should be built into the design to accommodate any future requirements of the environment.

Design Tenets

The intricate design of well-ordered spaces for both major uses—the clinical and fitness functions (Fig. 9)—can be done well if some primary tenets are adhered to, as discussed in the following paragraphs:

- *Signage:* Way-finding systems should be extremely clear. The rhythm of spaces should follow a clear logic, and the visitors, patient, or member should be clued accordingly.
- *Professional appearance:* Clinical functions should be designed in such a way as to communicate professionalism, without appearing coldly clinical. A hospital-like, clinical design would be in appropriate for examination rooms, mammography suites, and similar rooms. The aim is to create a clinical function room that offers little confusion to the patient about the professional treatment he/she can expect.
- *Engineering systems:* Engineering considerations should be taken into account early in the design process. Indoor relative humidity of 50–60% in a pool area is challenging to maintain and may require the design of a special air handling unit or units to supply constant air volumes to various spaces. Humidity control in a building that houses both fitness and clinical functions may be difficult to achieve. Failure to address these issues at the outset, however, can result in creating an environment for medical technology that is not consistent with good engineering practice, as well as missing the mark in the design of fitness spaces, which are likely to be high-humidity. Another engineering issue is maintenance of air changes so as to refresh the environment, without allowing chlorine odors to invade common spaces (Patients receiving medical treatment, especially cancer patients, are sensitive to such odors).
- *Acoustics and basic zoning considerations:* It is of critical importance to zone clinical functions away from fitness functions so as to maintain good acoustical control. Within the pool area, the design should include baffles or other devices to reduce the echo effect. Not only is sound reduction important from an esthetic standpoint, but also important from the standpoint of communication. Arthritis patients who are receiving aquatherapy must be able to hear the instructor. And because many arthritis sufferers are elderly, acoustics become even more important.
- *Age separation and integration:* Wellness center patients and members represent a great cross-section of ages and sexes. The idea of the wellness center as community center has great promise. At the same time, segregation of certain sub-functions should be considered. Caregiver locker rooms can be a vital necessity. Similarly, family locker rooms can be necessary too. Men and women with young children should have space to change the children without interfering with adult patients and members. Areas zoned for adults and families, and a more private area for caregivers, is the ideal arrangement.
- *Other accommodations:* All areas of the wellness center should be handicapped accessible. The professional standard of care should include extra handrails worked sensitively into the design of corridors and large gathering spaces, along with the creation of frequent areas of rest. There should be a natural rhythm of stopping points for patients and members throughout the facility, with water foundations available. Communication devices of some type are also important, such as telephones with a nurse call system. Wellness centers typically include telemetry in their designs, particularly around the running tack. A patient/member monitoring system can be even more comprehensive.
- *Site location, access, and design:* The wellness center should offer specially designated parking for members and patients, adequate handicapped parking, well-lighted spaces, and good signage. If at all possible, the drop-off area should be canopied, as should a pedestrian link to the parking area. A wellness center should not be located close to magnetic fields generated by power plants and high voltage electricity transmission lines.

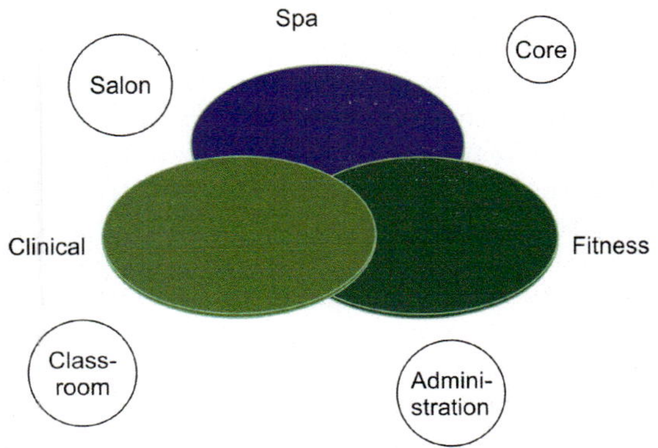

Fig. 9: Inter-relation of spa, clinical and fitness component of wellness.

Green Design

Symbolically and practically, it is of primary important that a wellness center be designed with materials that protect health and that it encourages, by example, this way of incorporating healthy design into the mainstream of the community.[5]

In the past few years, there have been sporadic gestures toward design of "healthy buildings." Sick buildings are those whose users complain of ailments ranging from chronic headache and fatigue to more serious asthmatic conditions. These buildings suffer from either bad design (sealing the building envelope, so tightly as to allow no infiltration of air and so causing a series of problems that result from lack of air movement) or the specification of unhealthful materials or a combination of such factors. Additional ailments produced by exposure to the chemicals in these materials range from flu-like symptoms to joint pain and brain dysfunction—dizziness, confusion, inability to concentrate.

Materials that are harmful range from the obviously dangerous and carcinogenic—urea foam formaldehyde, asbestos, lead paint-to-furniture manufactured with chemicals that release unhealthful vapors, to certain paints that produce odors while drying.

Natural light is best, but for activities taking place in the wellness center after the sun has set, the next best lighting type is full-spectrum light. The incorporation of full-spectrum lighting, whenever possible, is encouraged for both ambient and task lighting. People suffering from seasonal affective disorder, attention deficit disorder, or attention deficit hyperactivity disorder are subtly disturbed by lack of light and by the glare of fluorescent light (Figs. 10 and 11).

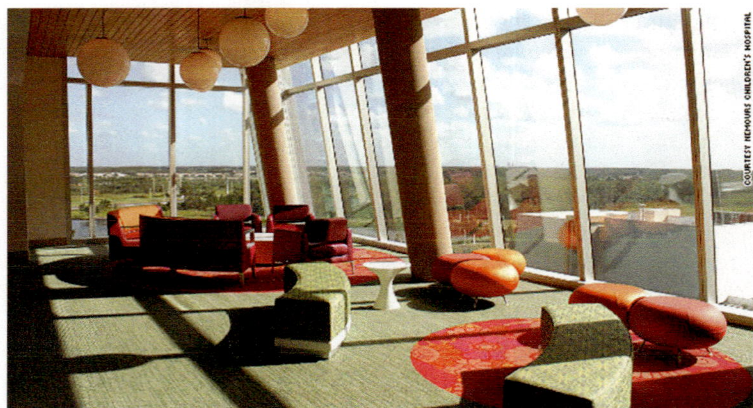

Fig. 10: Natural light is best.

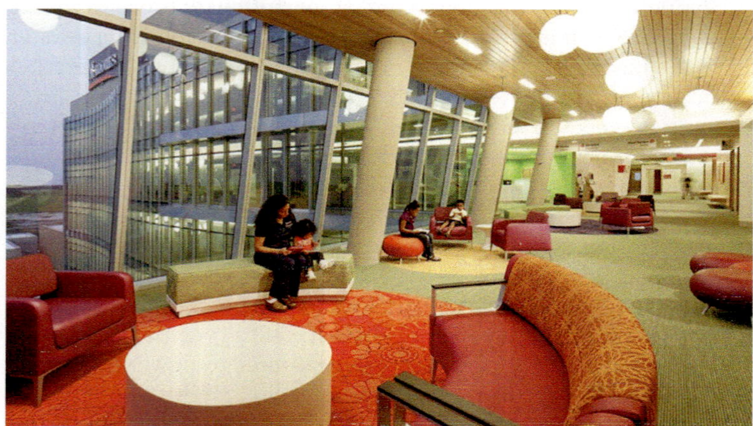

Fig. 11: Full-spectrum light.

Critical Adjacencies

As noted earlier, the primary zoning for functional areas at the wellness center fits into two major categories, *clinical and fitness*. The separation of these areas is a design response to the logic of the anticipated activities in each.

Pool areas and garden areas should be visible (Fig. 12), if possible, from other areas in the wellness complex in order to bring a sense of aliveness and fun, rest and respite from the hard work of everyday life. These areas often serve as magnets and focal points for people, lighting the often serious nature of the clinical experience and providing some visual relief. If pool areas are totally enclosed, with minimal exposure to the outdoors, less sunlight, and less able to suggest the natural environment beyond, then we are less enthusiastic about relating the building spaces to the pool as a focal point.

If the pool area is a focal point, it should be designed to project the image of a resort/spa environment rather than of a high school gym, even though it may indeed include lap spaces and areas specially designated for aquatherapy.

The more therapeutic areas, such as aquatherapy (Fig. 13), should be located beyond the less utilitarian areas, so that patients can realize the benefits of this therapy without being vulnerable to the gaze of every passing visitor. In all cases, where a rehabilitation patient is working under the guidance of a medical professional in a space adjacent to a fitness activity space, the goal is for the patient to have a view outward toward the fitness area while maintaining a measure of personal privacy.

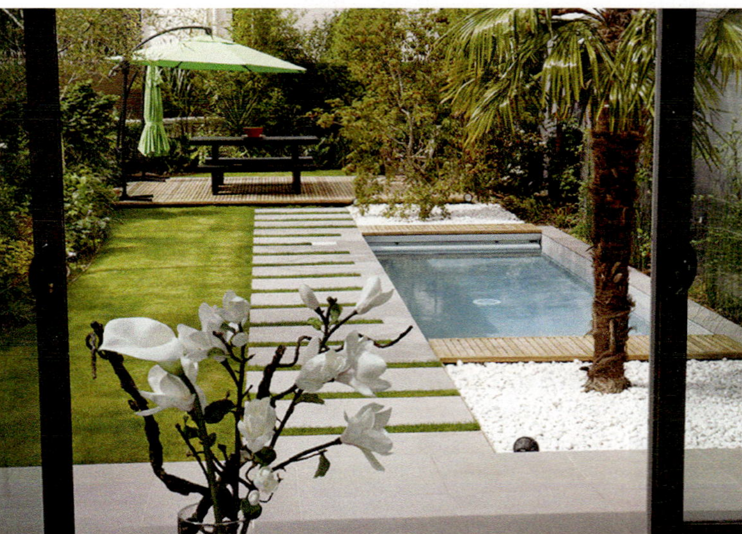

Fig. 12: Pool areas and garden areas.

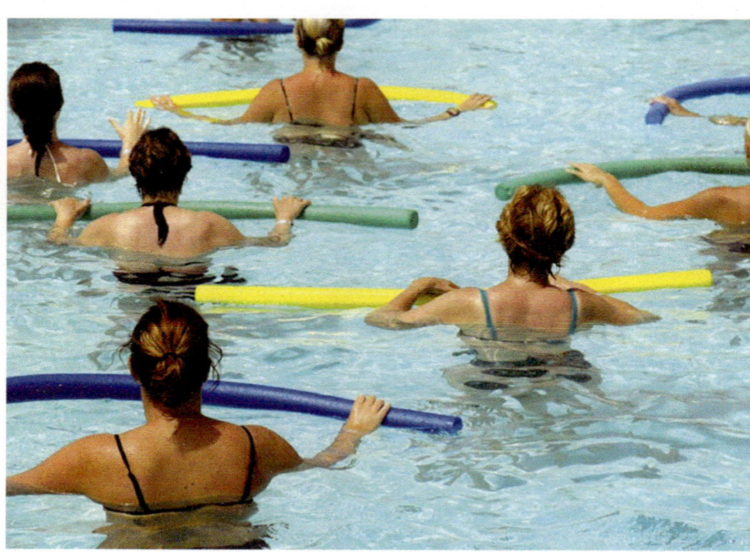

Fig. 13: Aquatherapy.

The design goal to be achieved here is a sense of balance and control for the patient, a sense of being special. The patient is indeed special and should not have to compete with fitness members for weight machine time. Likewise, a fitness member should have the sense that he/she is in a luxurious high-tech environment where the emphasis is on prevention and wellness, rather than in a rehabilitation facility.

Rehabilitation patients should share locker rooms with the fitness members, because a further delineation would border on social engineering. The option for caregiver locker room, spaces that include a handicapped-accessible water closet, sink, and lockers, should always be available.

Similarly, handicapped accessibility in all areas of a wellness center, including weight training areas, is of utmost importance. There are specially designed weight training machines for people with disabilities, and these should be included in the design of the weight training areas. The design must take care to work out the dimensional radius needed to maintain the proper angle of approach to these machines. Also, the designer must give some thought to how a wheelchair-bound person can make the transition from one type of flooring, typically carpeting or conditioned wood flooring, to the dense rubber-tire like flooring typically used in weight machine areas.

Aligned with this challenge is the need to find a way for a disabled person to access pool areas for general swimming or aquatherapy lessons. Wellness centers frequently include a handicap ramp that brings swimmers down from deck level to pool level—this presents a special design challenge. Lifts (Fig. 14) are an expensive alternative, but their use can realize a tremendous gain in terms of pool space. More pool space can typically be devoted to the actual therapy itself instead of being used by a cumbersome solution to access.

Another design challenge is whirlpool and hot tub design. The therapeutic effect of hot water has long been known and arthritic as well as disabled people deserve to have this therapy. Unfortunately, most spa and hot tub designers have not considered how to make them available to everyone, but accessibility should be of vital concern in the design of the wellness center pool and spa areas.

Decking materials in these wet areas can be a danger for everyone. The usual choice in most instances is either to leave raw concrete or to invest in ceramic. Moisture-resistant grout will surely accompany a good tile installation and will increase durability and discourage the growth of mold. Efficient dehumidification systems and attentive mechanical engineering design can ensure a comfortable and safety environment.

Pool and spa areas should naturally be close to locker rooms and toilet rooms. A small transitional corridor is about the maximum amount of space desirable from the locker room area to the pool area. There are many reasons for this; chief among them is privacy. Locker rooms should always be located near pool areas.

Similarly, when the spa area includes more than the whirlpool and sauna spaces typically associated with pool areas, when the concept of the spa is broadened to include other therapies involving the use of water, such as Vichy rooms, eucalyptus steam rooms, constitutional hydrotherapy (an alternative medicine therapy that involves the application of hot and cold compresses in alternation), cold friction rubs (an alternative therapy that involved the application of ice water packs after preparing the patient with steam, sauna, immersion baths, and hot sprays), these wet areas should be located near the spa/sauna/pool/locker room functions.

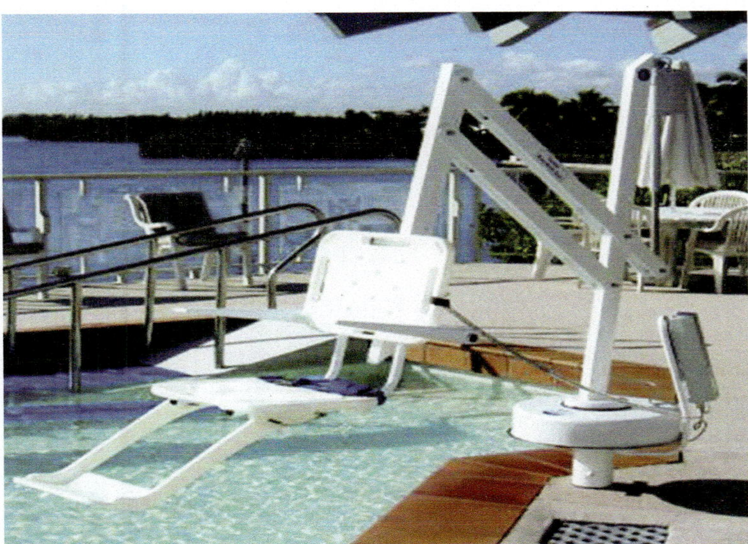

Fig. 14: Splash pool lift.

As spa areas are broadened to include areas for self-care they should also be located adjacent to one another. Self-care areas may include massage rooms, acupuncture therapy rooms, and the more cosmetic functions—hairdressing salon, facial rooms, and manicure and pedicure rooms. In the more mature wellness center facilities around the USA, these spa areas are being expanded and some of them are having difficulty in retrofitting administrative spaces to include expanded spa functions. Since administrative functions have almost never been located next to locker rooms or pool areas, there is some challenge in reengineering these spaces to perform reasonably well, to be appealing and functional for the user, without complicating the transition from the spa area back to the locker room. If an administrative space does become a spa, however, the relative cost of this expansion is extremely high. Thus, the basic design caveat for all medically related facilities is borne out once again—designs should be flexible. If engineering systems are built with the potential for future change, the overall design of the facility will benefit.

Similarly, the structural grid should be built with the same logic, and plenum space should be adequate for the future reconfiguration of the various areas. There is always the possibility in a facility of this kind that more intense (an increase in equipment means larger space requirements) technological equipment for medical procedures may be located in the wellness center.

If trends reverse or take a different course, the nature of the wellness center may shift and, in doing so, it value in terms of real estate remains in its ability to convert to a smaller or different set of functions. Unduly large or over designed wellness centers are as much an absurdity as unduly small and underdesigned centers with little or no thought built into the program for future expansion.

The clinical function/examination rooms, diagnostic rooms, treatment room, and separate administration area within a wellness center should serve as the clinical component's own discrete environment, which can allow for the possibility of a "demising walls" so as to separate zones for purposes of separating the ownership and/or financing of different areas of the center. Such flexibility is key to the financial success of a wellness center. Similarly, the retail and food service functions, services that are included in approximately half of all wellness centers built today in the United States, should be designed to be functionally discrete (although they should not project the image). The retail function may include an area for sales of sports clothing similar to that in a golf club pro shop, a limited range of sports equipment, sports drinks and food supplements, reading material, tapes and CDs small electronic equipment items, a scaled-down version drugstore inventory, basic necessities, some cosmetics, child care items, and similar items.

Ideally, upon entering and proceeding through a wellness center, a person should get a clear idea of where everything is. Spatially, this means drawing the user to a central location, a reception area where he/she will be able to check in, check appointment times, receive passes and locker keys for the locker areas, allow the clinical receptionist to know that the patient has arrived and direct that person to the appropriate area.

WELLNESS CENTER DESIGN GUIDELINES

Clinical Space

Architectural prescriptive standards for wellness centers have yet not been formulated in our country. In designing the clinical component of a wellness center project, there are certain rules of thumb that apply to the design of any clinical space. The American Institute of Architects

(AIA) Guidelines for Construction of Hospital and Medical Facilities is an excellent guide to the design and development of all medical and medically related facilities as:

- Space for files, records, administrative activities
- Hand washing facilities within the therapy unit
- Space and equipment for carrying out therapy
- Convenient facility access usable by disabled individuals
- Lockers for storing patient's personal effects
- Dressing facilities/shower facilities
- Storage for supplies and equipment.

The AIA Guidelines clearly state that each outpatient facility must ensure patient dignity, as well as audible and visual privacy, during interviews, examinations, treatment, and recovery. Clean storage and soiled utility spaces/soiled holding rooms spaces, must also be addressed in complementary therapy and spa function spaces.

Waiting Area

The reception area in the front, or central to the front desk, is often a place where people gather and meet. It should be generously sized, so that conversations between members are not within hearing distance of the front desk.

There may be instances in which there are multiple gathering spaces, defined perhaps by the intersection of corridors. Like family waiting areas in acute care hospitals or living room clusters in hospitality areas, these smaller, more intimate spaces can be made esthetically appealing as areas that have no other purpose than to allow people to rest, relax and talk.

Spaces for Children

In the West, there is an increasing trend to include areas for children in wellness centers. Primarily such spaces are drop-off-daycare centers for parents who have come to work out. Although there is nothing wrong with this necessary function, some patients are asking for expanded programs and the children themselves are interested to exercise.

Locker Rooms

Locker room design is driven by the number of lockers to be integrated into the designer, the proposed relationship of locker room to the shower and toilet areas, and the relationship of these spaces to other wet areas—the pool, spa, and salon—of the wellness center.

Critical to the design of locker rooms in a wellness center facility is the primary decision that must be made, whether to include separate family locker rooms, and/or caregiver locker/dressing rooms in the overall design. The criteria for solving this design issue will be predicated on the market feasibility study and the market projections and demand analysis. The wellness center building committee has to decide at the outset what sort of facility it wants to develop, what people will use the center with what frequency, and at what times of day certain areas will be most active.

A rule of thumb suggested by locker manufacturers is to estimate the largest number of members. This allows for the swing factor, which means members coming and going before and after peak times. Using the by system of planning a locker room space is a good starting point. This involves the creation of a four-foot-wide circulation aisle at the end of each bay (a row of lockers with seats in between). Dry shoe traffic and wet shoe traffic should be separated at opposites of the locker room space. Fixed benches are typically used in the center of each bay configuration.

The distance between the face of the locker and the bench should be a minimum of 3 ft, more if this space is also used as a traffic aisle. Locker rooms may be carpeted with high wear loop carpeting or tiled with vinyl or ceramic tiles.

Shower areas adjacent to locker rooms should have built-in dressing areas, separated for privacy with a curtain for each area. Paying attention to the issue of privacy for members and patients alike is critical to the success of the wellness center design.

In both women's and men's locker rooms, if there are no separate family locker rooms, the center should provide an area to accommodate parents changing children, including infants. Although child care areas may or may not be provided, more than likely some parents will have occasion to take care of children while at the center.

Dressing, makeup, and grooming areas are also important design considerations. Spaces for these activities need not include a sink, but should contain generous counter space and good lighting.

Lockers are available in metal, laminate, and wood. Wood is the most expensive and is often selected for use in high-end country clubs.

Pool and Spas

Whirlpool spas (Fig. 15) are used for hydrotherapeutic massage, muscle relaxation, stress reduction, and pain relief. A whirlpool spa may be constructed of ceramic tile, concrete with a treated finish, or one of the many prefabricated system available on the market today.

Decisions must be made regarding the size and configuration of the whirlpool bath itself, the shell (in the case of the prefabricated whirlpool), the type of water jets and their configuration and the seating arrangement. Special foot wells can be selected that focus water jet pressure on the feet. Spas should be designed to be barrier free.

Swim spas are larger than relaxation spas and have no area for seating—combination units are available. Floatation therapy spas are also available on the market. These spas, designed to provide mental and physical relaxation through spa floatation, typically have 1,000 pounds of Epsom salts added to the water and are soundproof and lightproof.

Muscle stresses are relieved by the positioning of 'cluster' jets toward the lower back. Other types of jets available are 'power massage,' 'standard,' and 'mini.' Each jet type has a different function; many can be used effectively in combination with others.

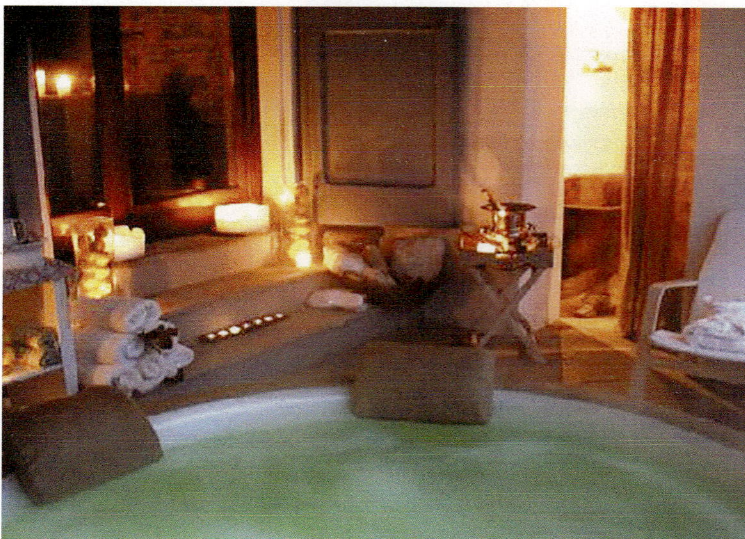

Fig. 15: Whirlpool spa.

High-volume pumps power the jets, enabling them to produce the high pressure needed to create the intended effect. The size of a whirlpool spa pump relates to the number of jets it can supply not the degree of pressure it can maintain.

Whirlpool spas, like pools, must be well-designed, with appropriate filtering and water purification systems.

Pools

Typically, wellness centers include in their initial design a 25 m pool for laps (Figs. 16 and 17). Larger centers separate aquatherapy areas from the lap pool by actually enclosing the therapy pool in a separate room.

Planning criteria for pools are a primary consideration for wellness center design. Lap pools generally follow standards requiring that the overall length be 25 m as a minimum, in keeping with interscholastic and intercollegiate requirements.

Lanes in lap pools are usually 2 m wide, and the recommended pool deck area is 3 m wide. Removable floating lane dividers are available.

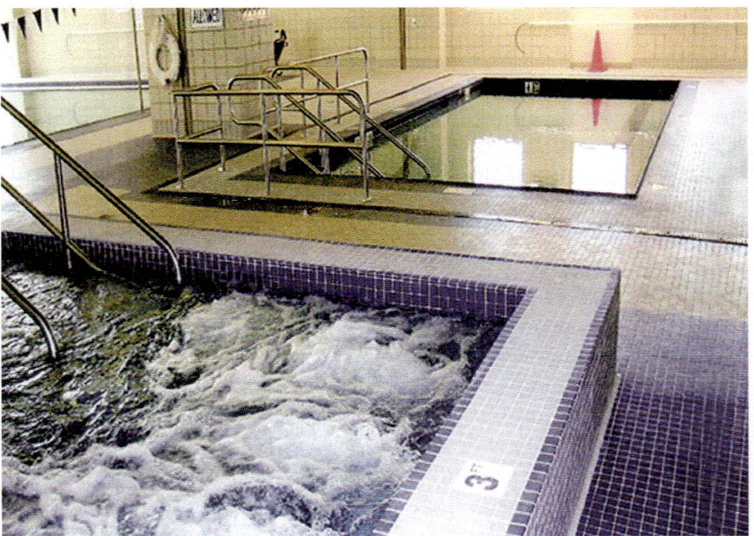

Fig. 16: Therapeutic whirlpool at Stamford Hospital, USA.

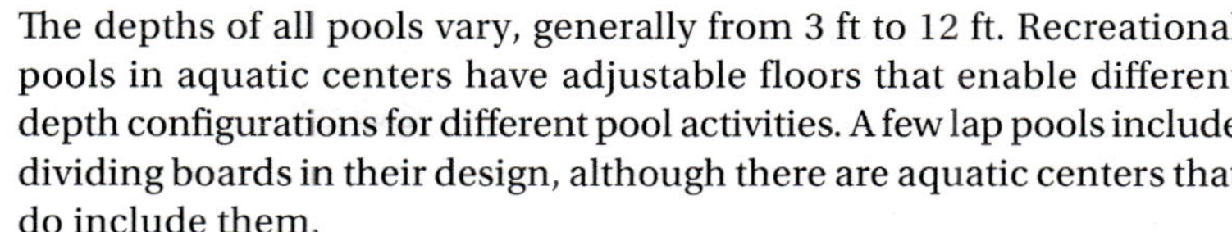

The depths of all pools vary, generally from 3 ft to 12 ft. Recreational pools in aquatic centers have adjustable floors that enable different depth configurations for different pool activities. A few lap pools include dividing boards in their design, although there are aquatic centers that do include them.

Warm water therapy pools can vary in size, depending on the planning criteria of the center. Handicapped accessibility is important in all pool areas. Perimeter gutter systems should be used for water and wave control. Sufficient deck space should be included at poolside, first for reasons of safety, and second because these areas, like waiting areas and lounges, frequently become gathering places for groups of people. Poolside relaxation areas, both indoor and outdoor terraces, present a respite from the bustling activity areas and the serious clinical and therapeutic components of a wellness center. The introduction of nature at poolside is a wonderful way to provide visual relief from the hard edges of the swimming pool environment.

Pool and Spa Heaters

Pool and spas must be heated. There are several choices offered by manufacturers today. A heat pump, which transfers heat from the outside air to the pool water, is used mainly in outdoor applications. A gas heater heats water from the pool, which is then returned to the pool (gas heaters tend to heat pools rapidly). There are also electric pool heaters, which have the advantage of being compact, and oil heaters, which use diesel fuel.

Saunas

Sauna (Fig. 18) rooms can be built from scratch or assembled from kits that offer precut parts in many standard sizes up to 12 by 12 ft with 7-foot ceilings, which is the maximum recommended height. Sauna rooms are typically built from Western red cedar or spruce and include cedar benches with back rests and head rests, walls lights and thermometers, and heaters with guard rills. Sauna heaters often include two-stage thermostats that provide consistent, comfortable heat. High air flow reduces the time it takes to bring the sauna room temperature to the desired level for bathing.

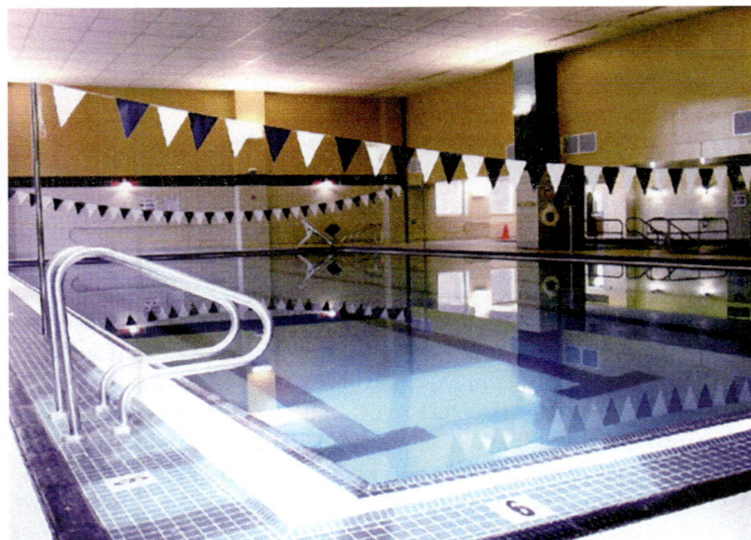

Fig. 17: Pool at Health and Fitness Institute, Stamford Regional Hospital, USA.

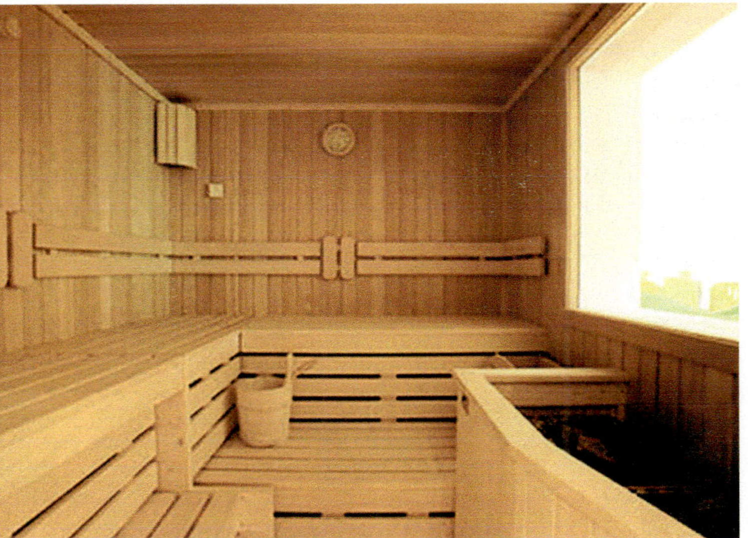

Fig. 18: Sauna.

Steam (Figs. 19A and B)

Steam baths are not always included in the design of a wellness centers, but appear to be typical in the design of the larger centers. Steam baths require generator units that are sized appropriately for the number of cubic ft of air that is being conditioned. Safety requires that the steam heads and controls do not heat in excess of 125°, in order to reduce the risk of burning. Controls can be located both insides and outside the steam bath.

Because of the hot, moist environment, the growth of mold is difficult to control in steam bath areas. It is important to be aware of the threat to public health inherent in the creation and maintenance of any environment where of any environment where people come in contact with standing water, humidity, and other people.

Some spas use ozone as an agent for water treatment. Ozone effectively kills bacteria, fungi, yeast, and molds on contract. Other water treatments include chlorine or bromine. The wellness center operator/manager should have experience in the selection of these systems and their advantages and disadvantages. Bromine, like chlorine, is a chemical used to sanitize and disinfect. Bromine will not oxidize the water or remove ammonia or nitrogen compounds. Bromine products are often sold in a two-part system that includes an oxidizing agent. An ozone generator can provide just this balance to bromine. Cautions in regard to specifying a bromine system include allergies in sensitive individuals and the compromising of plastic, vinyl, acrylic, aluminum, and other metals. Bromine can also bleach colored plaster in pools and spas and pool and spa area.

Gardens

The wellness center design should take every opportunity to bring nature indoors. Using natural light, natural materials, and producing, through skilled design, a rhythm that encourages and uplifts people is the goal.

Meditation Room and Chapel

Nearly all wellness center in the USA, have considered allotting some space to a meditation room or chapel (Fig. 20). The space allotted is typically not large, for the most part in the 120 sq ft range. What is important is that the meditation room is designed to be a place of quite repose. Soft colors and substantial sound attenuation are suggested.

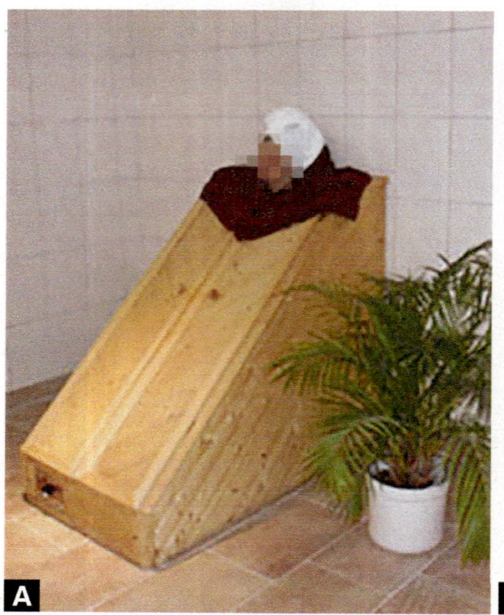

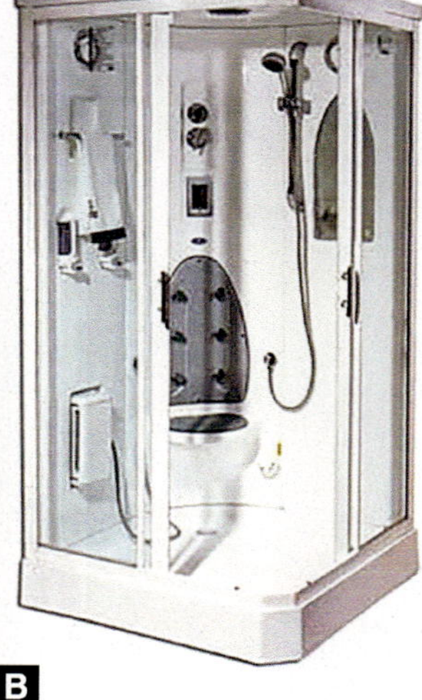

Fig. 19: (A) Steam bath; (B) Steam.

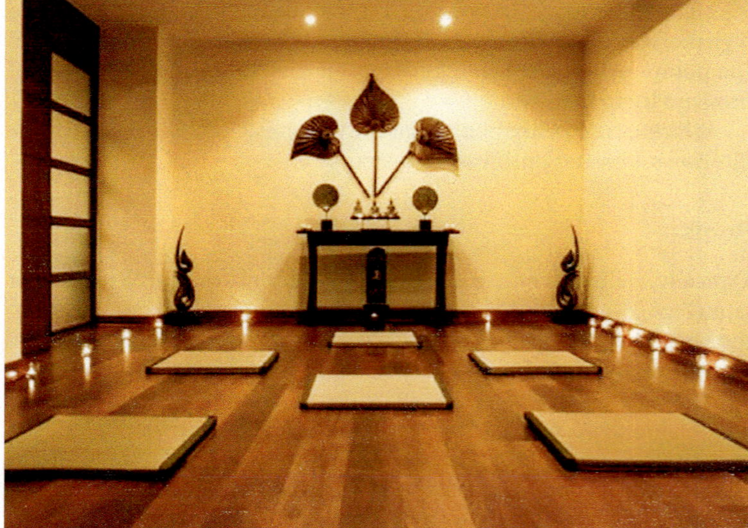

Fig. 20: Meditation room and chapel.

Laundry

Most wellness center executives see towels as a necessary amenity. This then, implies that towel storage, laundering and perhaps locker key distribution might all be located in the same space.

Wellness centers often combine the front reception/control desk with locker key sales and distribution, as well as towel distribution. Sometimes, in an attempt to reduce the number of staff allocated for these functions, the laundry facility is adjacent to this area. The danger here is that such an arrangement may put off a sophisticated clientele made-up of patients and members.

The laundry function must be carefully considered and designed appropriately in regard to the needs of the user. A wellness center will require commercial laundry equipment. Laundry facilities are often operated by maintenance staff and located close to wet areas. Members and patients should have a clear idea of where to pick-up towels before they venture to the pool, spa, salon area, or therapy area. The locker room is perhaps the most logical location for soiled towel receptacles.

A rule of thumb in designing laundry facilities for a wellness center is to calculate the total membership, ascertain the maximum number of members and patients coming through the center on a day when the center will have the most traffic, and designate two towels per member to develop a number to discuss with the manufacturer or distributor of the commercial washers and dryers.

The noise of these machines, even with the appropriate use of concrete pads and sound-dampening strategies is high. Thus, they should be located in an area that is not close to therapy meditation rooms, food service, or offices.

Lobby

The lobby and entrance area is the primary control area for a wellness center. All initial transactions—checking in, visiting, getting directions, and meeting people—take place in this most important common area. Design logic dictates that this area providing primary visual control of the main entrance and presiding over the wellness center functions, be an important and well-designed area.

The lobby desk should be large enough to accommodate two or more people working comfortably at the same time. It should also be large enough to allow each person to have private conversations with members, patients, and staff. The lobby desk is probably where communications functions will be centered. If possible, the lobby should include a waiting area sufficient to allow for the gathering of small groups. Comfortable seating, good lighting, desktop telephones, and adequate sound control should be the minimum design requirements. Clear signage, enough light, and good air circulation should set the stage in the lobby/waiting and main control desk area for a positive introduction to the space.

Near the lobby area should be a toilet room adjacent to the core areas. Stairways and elevators should be easily accessible and visible from the lobby. Quite often a space near the lobby area can be used for member testing. If such a space is located in this area, it should be private.

Administration

Adjacent to the lobby area should be a small administration area, with a reception desk/secretarial area and two or three offices, depending on the program and size of the facility. These areas should have good lighting and acoustical control. If possible, some visual contact with the lobby is suggested, but this is by no means a hard-and-fast rule.

Similarly, administrative staff members need a certain degree of privacy with which to conduct the efficient flow of business activity. Marketing or presale areas may also be located here.

Offices for the fitness manager, accountant, and center director, as well as a staff lounge, may also be included in this zone. Smaller centers, those with areas in the 35,000 sq ft range, will probably require two small administrative offices and a reception area. Another option is to be design the employee lounge near other backhouse areas such as Laundry storage, janitor's closet, and staff rest room areas.

Clinical areas should be acoustically and visually separated from fitness areas and from the lobby. Visual cues in the design of the space should lead the user effortlessly to where he/she wants to go, but can be supplemented with well-designed signage. The clinical area should have its own receptionist, office, examination and treatment rooms, laboratory (if it is included in the program), cardiopulmonary testing, records, and physical therapy/occupational therapy area.

Combined use areas, such as fitness areas used in rehabilitation, should be carefully thought out. If a wellness center has therapy facilities in the main fitness area, planners will have to make decisions early in the program as to how this can gracefully be done. By no means should it appear that "patients" are hidden from "members" on the other hand, the need for privacy during a rehabilitative procedure dictates that the design architect be sensitive to this need, so as to avoid putting people on display.

If the wellness center is small, with an overall area in the 35,000 sq ft range, the weight training area should be close to the locker rooms and pool areas. The design logic should follow the intent of the clinical program as well as the fitness program.

Color

The use of color in environmental design is one of the most important considerations. The effect of color on human emotion is far more powerful than generally assumed. The emotional and physical effects of color are uniquely interwoven. Color heals and color can be used to relax or excite, to stimulate conversation, or create a quieting effect. Color sends a message to the human psyche, which, through recent advances in science and technology, is becoming quantifiable.[13]

Similarly, at the other end of the age spectrum, children are stimulated, to a greater degree than adults by the use of bright colors. This means that in environments where the user profile cuts across age barriers, the architect must take this range into account in selecting colors for the design of well necessary center spaces.

As a general rule of thumb, one should avoid pastels that are at the muddy end of the range of hues. Brightness is encouraged in most spaces, as long as glare is prevented. Light colors reflect light and dark colors absorb light. Light sources reinforce certain colors, and the type of light greatly affects this phenomenon. Warm light, such as incandescent, affects colors differently than cool light like that emitted by fluorescent lights.[8]

The use of natural daylight and full-spectrum light should be encouraged in the design of wellness centers. Full spectrum light mimics natural daylight. The typical lighting level for an office space is 500 lumens lm/m^2. Natural daylight provides approximately 100 times more.

Artwork

The inclusion of artwork (Fig. 21) in the design of a wellness center is most welcome. Artwork has been incorporated in healthcare centers around the world. Art therapy is a bonafide therapy.

An art therapy room should be approximately 12 by 15 ft as a minimum, but an employee-lounge type area (with sinks and storage) might be used in the evenings for art therapy classes, as well as regular classroom space.

Storage and Disposal

In any wellness center, storage as a component of the overall design must be addressed with singular focus.

The design of the clinical component will have to address thoughtfully how soiled materials are to be disposed of. It may be required that staffing and operational issue for collection of biomedical and nonbiomedical waste be considered early in the design process, so that adequate space is programmed into it.

Clean supplies will need their own space in the clinical area. This storage will be in addition to shelves and cabinets already included in the design of equipment storage and require a separate closet or room. A sterilizing system must be included. In some cases, a service that delivers resealed packs may be used.

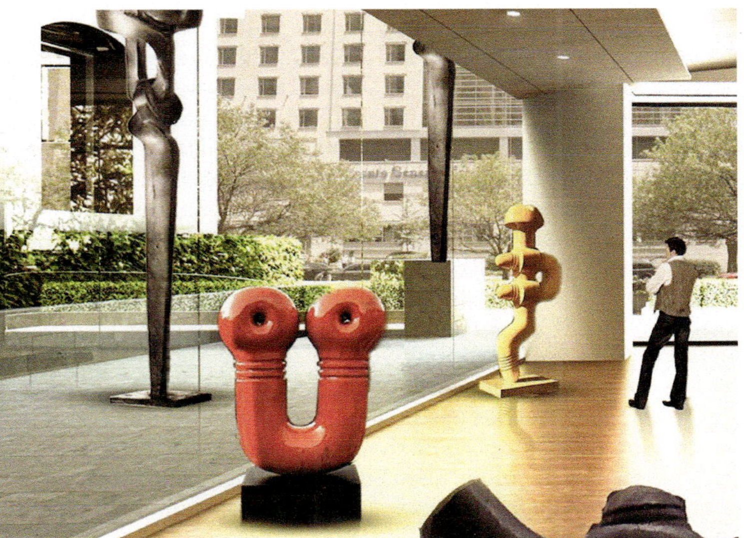

Fig. 21: Artwork.

Amenities

Unique amenities borrowed from the hospitality design industry may find their way, if appropriate, into the wellness center design. Examples are shops, cafes, juice bars. A bulletin/message board for members is also a welcoming addition.

Air Handling

The AIA Guidelines require the design of facilities that comprise a clinical component to include consideration of recognized requisites such as variable air volume systems, load shedding, programmed controls for unoccupied period (nights and week-ends), and the use of natural ventilation, site and climatic conditions permitting.

The guidelines also suggest that controls for air handling equipment be designed with an economize cycle in order to use outside air for heating and cooling. Care must be taken to avoid the possibility of large temperature differentials, high velocity supply, excessive noise, and air stagnation. To maintain asepsis controls, airflow supply and exhaust should generally by be controlled to ensure movement from clean to less clean areas.

Lighting

Natural daylight is the most desirable lights, because it includes the full spectrum of available light on the planet. The next desirable types of light are artificial full-spectrum light, which mimics natural light and is often used in light therapy treatments, and low-voltage halogen light.

If possible, fluorescent light should be avoided. LED lights to be prefered. The economy achieved with fluorescent lighting is usually not worthwhile, in as much as it can wash out the carefully selected colors of a specially designed environment.

Spa areas should have lighting that is controlled by a dimmer switch. Areas for massage and certain other body therapies facial rooms, and rooms for other beauty treatments, herbal wraps, and so forth, demand a quiet environment. Lighting levels in the waiting areas in clinical offices should be low and warm. Mammography waiting and dressing rooms are often designed with high-quality fixtures and low lighting. Lighting for different areas will vary accordingly.

Acoustics

Active noise technology (a system utilized for dampening sound) uses computes to generate sound waves in a certain sequence that meets or counters, the sound waves being generated from a particular source. In the USA, this technique is becoming more widely available. Traditionally, sound baffles used for pool areas have been successful in improving the acoustical environment. Excessive reverberation is common in these large areas with hard surfaces. At times, it makes communication difficult, especially for older people. Lack of speech intelligibility and poor acoustics make for an uncomfortable atmosphere and pose potential safety problems. A general rule of thumb is that reverberation time should be less than 2 seconds for 1,000 cubic ft of space for a person to hear speech comfortably. These panels, typically 30 inch × 10 ft are made of 2 inch fiberglass attached to aluminum framing members.

Laundry areas are noisy and should be located away from the central registration and reception area. A 6–8 inch concrete pad to top of the floor surface for the washer extractor should be a requirement. Certain steps can be taken to design quieter HVAC systems also, and this is highly recommended. For any area of a wellness center, the quieter it is, the better.

Music can be introduced in the outdoor setting, as background to conversation or rest. This, of course, must not be an intrusive level, but can enhance the overall experience of the environments if well chosen.

Interior Finishes and Materials (Fig. 22)

The best available materials to be specified for a wellness center may well be those designed for general healthcare facilities. Certainly clinical and clinical/integrative areas will benefit from the inclusion of chemical resistant laminates where appropriate bacteria-resistant carpeting, durable vinyl flooring, and ceramic tile with mold-resistant grout. Inert materials should be selected when possible, for the simple reason, that they tend to be less likely to trigger allergic reactions in sensitive individuals.

Wall Coverings

Wall coverings are an alternative to paint in wellness center buildings. Antimicrobial backing should always be specified. Vinyl wall coverings selected should be no glare types.

Carpeting

When properly selected, installed, and maintained, carpeting can perform well in a wellness center. Carpeting should be selected with care. It should meet the standards set for healthcare settings and should be utilized only if considered very essential. This consideration is important for several reasons, chiefly the materials' durability and their ability to reject the growth of mold and bacteria. However, this varies according to the climactic conditions, viz. hot and dry climatic conditions may well hail carpeting as a disaster in their set-up.

Healthcare grade carpeting is typically made-up of nylon fibers, polypropylene, and wool. Polypropylene does not perform well in

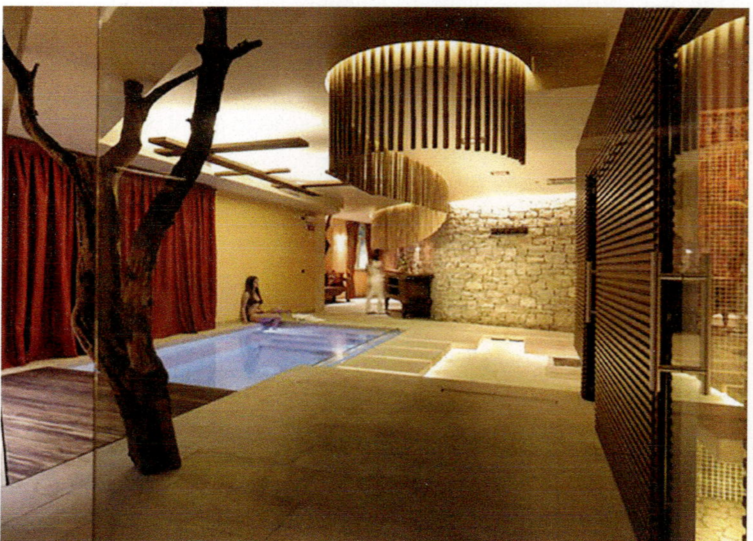

Fig. 22: Interior finishes and materials.

high-traffic areas. Nylon is less expensive than wool and has the properties needed—strength, color, and so on. Good backing materials for carpeting are critical to its integrity. Solution-dyed carpeting, which is colored through the extrusion process, is more resistant to bleach than yarn-dyed carpeting. Chlorinated bleaching products will impair the integrity of carpeting and are not recommended for use in areas that are close to wet areas of the fitness or spa functions that use a chlorine-based water purification system.

Carpeting may be an option in areas that are appropriate, particularly lobbies, waiting areas, libraries, some locker room areas, offices, some examination and treatment rooms, certain core areas, and retail and food service/restaurant areas. Carpeting for healthcare uses, as well as synthetic or vinyl backing and adhesive, can be specified to be antimicrobial.

The best carpets available today incorporate the backing as part of a permanent bond to the yarn itself. The arrangement creates a moisture barrier that makes the carpet impenetrable to stains. Stains cannot become embedded in the backing, as so often happens in areas of heavy use.

Carpets are, by their nature, glare resistant, and today they are static resistant as well. The reduction in noise level and in potential slipping should be considered when making this important material selection.

Resilient Floor

Resilient flooring is made of sheet vinyl, vinyl tile, rubber tile, or sheet rubber. Homogeneous sheet vinyl is second only to rubber flooring and solid vinyl tile in its ability to withstand traffic in high-use areas. Inlaid vinyl tile and vinyl composition tile can be used for healthcare as well as fitness area uses and can be customized to reinforce a design theme throughout the wellness facility. Laboratory areas in particulars require special vinyl flooring to resist the spills of chemicals. Marmoleum is a linseed oil-based floor material successfully used in hospitals and other healthcare settings.

Many vinyl floors are glare resistant, which helps the comfort level and mobility of patients, particularly older patients. Vinyl can be chemically bonded or heat welded to seal out bacteria and moisture that cause the growth of mold and mildew, which is especially important in the healthcare environment.

Tile

Ceramic tiles flooring is the selection of choice of owners and operators of many wellness centers today, especially for wet areas.

Textiles

Textiles included in the design of wellness centers are those fabrics used in lobbies, waiting areas, libraries, restaurants, retails areas, and other areas when they are appropriate to the design intent. Flame-resistant fabrics are designed to have great longevity and do not break down chemically in the cleaning process, which can produce allergic reactions.

Ceilings

In large activity areas, such as pool areas and basketball/volleyball courts, a painted, exposed roof structure with an accompanying array of HVAC ducts, sometimes brightly painted, seems the prudent choice. Clinical areas will most likely use suspended acoustical tile for similar reasons.

Paint

Wall coverings in different areas of the wellness center are selected according to the nature of the space and the design intent. Within a healthcare setting, it is recommended that the safest materials be selected. In choosing paint, recommended is the selection of a nontoxic paint—at the least, a latex water-based paint. Plant based paints are the ideal.

WELLNESS CENTER DESIGN STANDARDS

The goal of wellness center design should be to maintain the best and highest standard of care, reflective of those clinical and fitness components that makeup the basic elements of this new building type.

In the Western world and commonly in the USA, applicable sciences from Sports Medicine can be applied with the help of technical experts wherever there is a sports component to the wellness center. Together these standards, along with the country's national building codes, may form the basic framework for the design and development of quality environments to support the delivery of healthcare and the pursuit of wellness.

Stated in Annexure I are the space and design standards developed by the AIA for healthcare facilities for wellness.

They have been divided into four parts:

- Part I—Clinical area
- Part II—Fitness area
- Part III—Spa area
- Part IV—Common

Any and all standards that relate to the design and functioning of ambulatory care facilities apply to those clinical areas that are included in the wellness center design. The guidelines are not intended to be authoritative and it is unlikely that any single wellness center would include all the features listed in these guidelines. Nonetheless, they can serve as a starting point for the programmer and designer even in the Indian scenario.

Stated by AIA are also Environmental Guidelines (Annexure II). These give lighting, temperature, acoustic, humidity and air exchanges standards for Clinical (Part I) and Common (Part IV) areas.

AYUSHMAN BHARAT - HEALTH AND WELLNESS CENTRES[9]

The National Health Policy, 2017 recommended strengthening the delivery of primary healthcare, through establishment of "Health and Wellness Centers" as the platform to deliver comprehensive primary healthcare and called for a commitment of two thirds of the health budget to primary healthcare.

The Report of the Primary Health Care Task Force, Ministry of Health and Family Welfare, Government of India while reiterating that primary healthcare is the only affordable and effective path for India to Universal Health Coverage, also provided valuable insights into structure and processes in health systems to enable Comprehensive Primary Health Care (CPHC).

Ayushman Bharat or "Healthy India" national initiative was launched as recommended by the National Health Policy 2017, to achieve the vision of Universal Health Coverage (UHC).

Ayushman Bharat is an attempt to move from sectoral and segmented approach of health service delivery to a comprehensive need-based healthcare service. Ayushman Bharat aims to undertake path-breaking interventions to holistically address health (covering prevention, promotion and ambulatory care), at primary, secondary and tertiary level.

Ayushman Bharat adopts a continuum of care approach, comprising of two inter-related components, which are:

- Establishment of Health and Wellness Centers
- Pradhan Mantri Jan Arogya Yojana (PM-JAY)

Health and Wellness Centers (HWCs)

In February 2018, the Government of India announced the creation of 1,50,000 Health and Wellness Centers (HWCs) by transforming existing Sub-centers and Primary Health Centers as the base pillar of Ayushman Bharat. These centers would deliver Comprehensive Primary Health Care (CPHC) bringing healthcare closer to the homes of people covering both maternal and child health services and noncommunicable diseases, including free essential drugs and diagnostic services.

Health and Wellness Centers, are envisaged to deliver and expanded range of services to address the primary healthcare needs of the entire population in their area, expanding access, universality and equity close to the community. The emphasis of health promotion and prevention is designed to bring focus on keeping people healthy by engaging and empowering individuals and communities to choose healthy behaviors and make changes that reduce the risk of developing chronic diseases and morbidities.

The delivery of Universal Comprehensive Primary Health Care, through HWCs will increase the health system responsiveness to people by bringing services closer to the communities and being able to address the needs of most marginalized, through Primary Health Care and Wellness Centers.

Defining HWCs

To ensure delivery of CPHC services, existing sub-centers covering a population of 3000–5000 would be converted to Health and Wellness Centers, with the principle being "time to care" to be no more than 30 minutes. Primary Health Centers in rural and urban areas would also be converted to HWC. Such care could also be provided/complemented through outreach services, mobile medical units, camps, home and community-based care, but the principle should be a seamless continuum of care that ensures the principles of equity, universality and no financial hardships.

Expanded Services

The HWC would deliver an expanded range of services. These services would be delivered at both SHCs and in the PHCs, which are transformed as HWCs. The level of complexity of care of services delivered at the PHC would be higher than at the sub-health center level and this would be indicated in the care pathways and standard treatment guidelines that will be issued periodically.

CONCLUSION

Services that are required for the purpose of a Wellness Center have been depicted in Figure 23.

Depending on the success of the wellness center, optional services may be added or essential services may be replicated.

The areas required for the clinical, fitness, spa and common areas, as per AIA guidelines are:

Clinical (Part I):	9,530 sq ft (885 m^2)
Fitness (Part II):	30,250 sq ft (2,811 m^2)
Spa (Part III):	700 sq ft (65 m^2)
Common Areas (Part IV):	6,560 sq ft (610 m^2)
Total	47,040 sq ft (4,370 m^2)

Concluding thus, disciplinary isolation and specialization, along with sociopolitical and economic choices, encourage the sprawling medical-industrial complex to focus on the most proximate causes of disease and disability, reducing resources for preventive efforts that could address the complex inter-relationships across and within levels of ecological organization. Neither medicine nor public health gives much coherent attention to the status of, or its impact on, the larger ecological systems on which people's health depends.

Today's changing healthcare environment requires an integrative approach to medical care. Increasing medical costs threaten the economic vitality of healthcare options and limit the choices for both providers and patients. Many people are striving for optimal health and wellness. They realize medical science can prolong their lives, but they also want to live well and be healthy throughout their entire lives.[1] A well-designed wellness program and facility can fulfill people's requirement.

The very concept of wellness center speaks to people on a very basic level. Going to a wellness center instead of a "sickness center" has more than a superficial impact on a person/s being. The ability of people to focus on elements of life that are not about illness, even when they are ill, has a great positive impact.

Hospitals, as places symbolic of important moments in a person's life, are associated in people's memories with unsettling events, anxiety, and often emotional turning points. This is what will change in the next century. Beyond the bricks and mortar, financial analyses and marketing, lies the symbolic nature of the wellness center. It will be a center of healing rather than illness, a place where new memories and associations begin.

The idea that healing, although positive, is also trying and demands great discipline—hours of physiotherapy, for example, will be modified, shifted, changed with the building of wellness centers. Recreation, relaxation, spa amenities and places to rest or meet friends, places to learn about health or share in the fellowship community; these are the new images of wellness centers. A true benefit of the wellness center is the patient's ability to connect both consciously and subconsciously, healing with fun, recreation, fellowship, and beauty of the environment and of an enhanced self.[6] Never before have buildings been created to heal the sick on physical, mental, emotional and spiritual levels.

Large hospitals that have grown over the years, attempting to organize themselves with signage, quite often miss the mark. As a result patients are left frazzled negotiating the environment. In contrast, a wellness center a building type that is manageable in size, quite often free standing and in most cases entirely new, offers an opportunity to do something wonderful in design (Fig. 24).

People in weakened physical condition, such as those requiring cardiac rehabilitation, physical therapy, occupational therapy or oncology therapy, need to trust the environment they are entering. As practitioners in any physical therapies will attest, ease of movement is the key. These patients should not experience additional stress in terms of figuring out where they are, where they should park, where to find public utilities, how to register, pay the bill and where to wait.

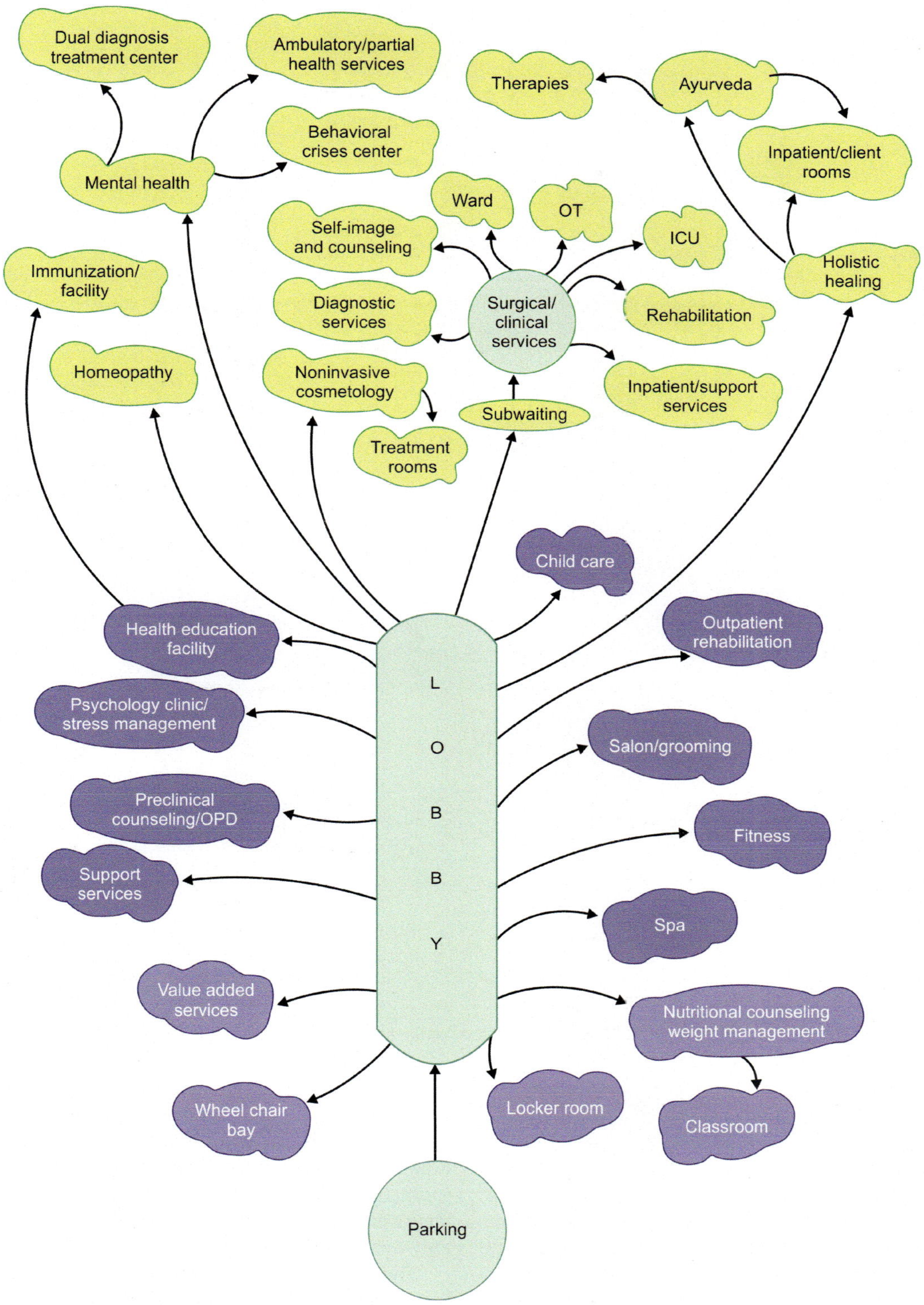

Dual diagnosis treatment center
Ambulatory/partial health services
Therapies
Ayurveda
Behavioral crises center
Inpatient/client rooms
Mental health
Ward
OT
Self-image and counseling
ICU
Holistic healing
Immunization/ facility
Diagnostic services
Surgical/ clinical services
Rehabilitation
Homeopathy
Noninvasive cosmetology
Inpatient/support services
Subwaiting
Treatment rooms
Child care
Health education facility
Outpatient rehabilitation
L O B B Y
Psychology clinic/ stress management
Salon/grooming
Preclinical counseling/OPD
Fitness
Support services
Spa
Value added services
Nutritional counseling weight management
Wheel chair bay
Locker room
Classroom
Parking

Fig. 23: Facilities of a wellness center.
(OT: operation theater; ICU: intensive care unit; OPD: outpatient department)

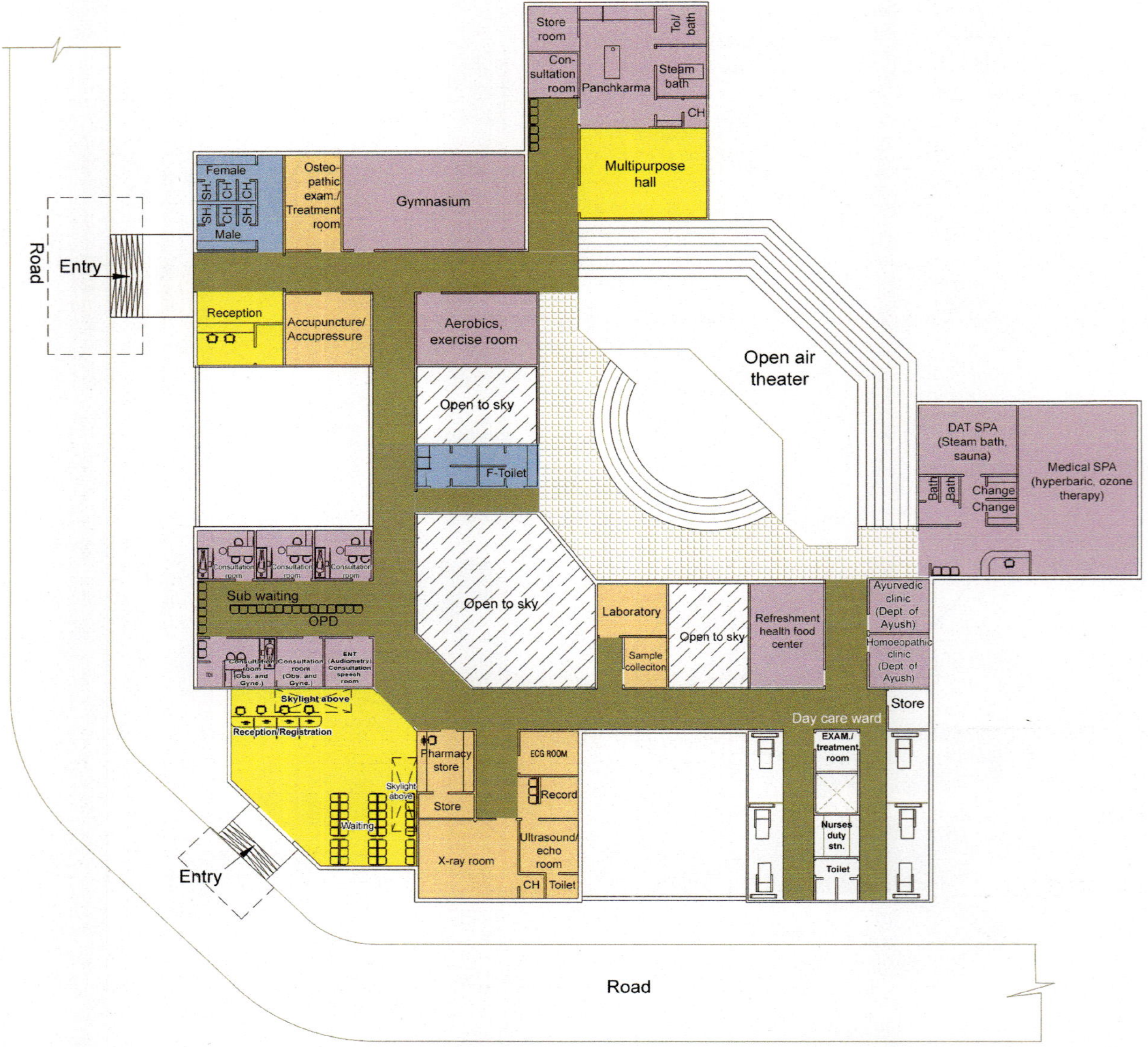

Fig. 24: Layout of wellness center

Planning and designing tenet for wellness centers, in letter and spirit, in our country, is currently limited around the concept of Ayurveda and treatments in a spa/resort type setting. However, with globalization, increasing awareness and demand of patient/customer, healthcare provider set-ups can be planned and designed around the wellness concept. Although the private hospitals may impart a certain environment to their spaces to draw clients, this concept should and can be incorporated in the public sector hospitals as well, at all levels healthcare delivery. An immunization center at PHC level can be made to look more inviting with better lighting, green design, facades, seating, public utilities and space planning just as much as a pediatric ward in a tertiary public sector hospital can be made child friendly with paintings, child friendly furniture, feeding rooms for nursing mothers, etc. In such surroundings, the patient feels well not only clinically, but also socially, spiritually, emotionally and occupationally as well.

The concept of a wellness center is the most positive, nurturing, life-affirming building type ever to evolve in the history of healthcare facilities design. The opportunity to provide people with a social center that will affect their lives in such a positive way is at the heart of this idea. It completes the continuum of care. It is indeed a perfect marriage of esthetics and clinical design.

Annexure I

The AIA Guidelines Wellness Center Space Requirements by Room

Part I: Clinical space							
Room	**Area (sq ft)**	**Remarks**	**Information systems**				
			LAN	**Phone**	**TV**	**Audio**	**Nurse call bell**
Rehabilitation medicine							
Treatment	100	Treatments tables, medical air, oxygen, vacuum. Lavatory with gooseneck inlet and wrist blades, nurse call voice and data	×	×	×	×	×
Presurgical testing	130		×	×	×	×	×
General surgery	450	Area is clear floor space; does not include built-in cabins, minimum floor area is 400 sq ft in new work, 360 sq ft in renovation	×	×	×	×	×
Recovery	130		×	×	×	×	×
Nurses station	120	2 desk-hight workstations 42 in countertop visual control of patient waiting	×	×	×	×	×
Patient waiting	260		×	×	×	×	×
Examination	100		×	×	×	×	×
Laboratory	130		×	×	×	×	×
Clerical	160	Voice and data files, visual control of patient waiting	×	×	×	×	×
Occupational therapy	450	Mat table, standing table, wheelchair table, sink, gooseneck and wrist blades	×	×	×	×	×
Activities of daily living, toilet/bath	90	Toilet, sink, tub door lock	×	×		×	×
Activieis of daily living, kitchen	150		×	×		×	×
Prosthetics/cast	150	Steel sink w/gooseneck inlet and wristblades plaster trap	×	×		×	×
Audiology office and examining	120	Audiology testing equipment provide sound attenuation	×	×		×	×
Conference room	1,200	4 panel film illuminator	×	×	×	×	
Telemedicine	160		×	×	×	×	×
Apothecary	250		×	×		×	×
Cardiopulmonary therapy							
Soiled workroom	150	Hot water and drain for pasteurizer and washer floor drain respirator stainless steel counter w/double integral sink, drainboards, backslash, and marine edge		×		×	
Clean workroom/ equipment storage	380			×		×	
Respiratory therapy/ patient waiting	210			×	×	×	
Respiratory waiting reception	150		×	×		×	×
Respiratory therapy/stress	120	Cardiopulmonary	×	×		×	×

Part II: Fitness							
Room	**Area (sq ft)**	**Remarks**	**Information systems**				
			LAN	**Phone**	**TV**	**Audio**	**Nurse call bell**
Aerobic exercise							
Exercise romm	1,500	Operable partition		×	×	×	×
Storage	80						
Fencing	750	2 pistes at 2 m × 14 m, plus 1 m at each end		×	×	×	×
Fitness							
Track	5,000	1/2 mile, resilient surface, continuous banked corners windows and access to exterior running area		×	×	×	×
Equipment exercise	3,400		×	×	×	×	×
Fitness testing	180		×	×	×	×	×
Weight training	400		×	×	×	×	×
Resistance training	250		×	×	×	×	×
Men's lockers/shower			×	×	×	×	×

Contd...

Contd...

Part II: Fitness							
Room	**Area (sq ft)**	**Remarks**	**Information systems**				
			LAN	**Phone**	**TV**	**Audio**	**Nurse call bell**
Locker room	840	120 lockers 1 private cubicle 2 soiled towel carts 100 inch coat rod			×	×	×
Lavatories/grooming	120	4 lavatories continuous counter top w/mirror above outlets at the rate of 3 ft on center		×		×	×
Shower	300	1 handicapped stall w/curtains				×	×
Toilets	300						×
Storage	40						
Integrative medicine							
Hydrotherapy	100	2 sinks, refrigerator				×	×
Whirlpool room	100	2 sinks				×	×
Chelation therapy	100	May share space with H_2O_2 therapy 2 sinks					
Artificial sun therapy	160	UVA lamps, control room (50 sq ft)				×	×
Oxygen therapy	230	Medical gases, 2 sinks				×	×
Hydrogen peroxides therapy	100	May share space with O_2 therapy 2 sinks				×	×
Hyperthermia	220	• Include diathermy, ultrasound, radiant heating • Extracorporeal heating, 2 sinks, hot tub, ultrasound equipment				×	×
Nutritional counseling	100		×	×	×	×	×
Meditation room/chapel	100						
Acupuncture	150	1 sink	×			×	×
Massage	150	1 sink	×			×	×
Naturopathic examination room	100	1 sink	×	×		×	×
Osteopathic physician examination room	100	1 sink	×	×		×	×
Environmental medicine physician's room	100	1 sink	×	×		×	×
Chiropractic examination room	150	1 sink	×	×		×	×
General clinical functions							
Conference room	150		×	×	×	×	
Staff lounge	190		×	×	×	×	
Staff locker room	100			×		×	
Staff toilet	50					×	
Office	100		×	×	×	×	
Total area for clinical	9,530						
Pool	3,500	25-yd-6-line pool		×		×	×
Pool deck	1,780	7 ft around pool					
Basketaball court							
	4,700	Collegiate size add 3 ft (min) to 10 ft (preferred) unobstructed space on all sides		×		×	×
Racquetball/handball							
	800	20 ft ceiling				×	×
Tennis courts							
	2,800	12 ft clearance on sides 21 ft clearance at ends		×		×	×

Contd...

Contd...

Part II: Fitness							
Room	**Area (sq ft)**	**Remarks**	**Information systems**				
			LAN	**Phone**	**TV**	**Audio**	**Nurse call bell**
Climbing wall							
	180	2 climbing stations at the rate of 9 ft × 10 ft each				×	×
Total area for clinical space (sq ft)	30,250						

Part III: Spa							
Room	**Area (sq ft)**	**Remarks**	**Information systems**				
			LAN	**Phone**	**TV**	**Audio**	**Nurse call bell**
Massage	120 (min)	Include 2 sinks 30 inch × 72 inch massage tables		×		×	×
Sauna	80	8 ft ceiling					
Whirlpool	40						
Salon							
Facial room	80	1 sink		×			
Manicure/pedicure	80	1 sink		×			
Hair salon	200	2 sinks for hair washing		×			
Vichy shower	100	Multiple spray heads		×			
Total area for clinical space (sq ft)	700						

Part IV: Common areas							
Room	**Area (sq ft)**	**Remarks**	**Information systems**				
			LAN	**Phone**	**TV**	**Audio**	**Nurse call bell**
Offices	600	5 at the rate of 120 sq ft	×	×		×	
Secretary	150		×	×		×	
Waiting	150	3 chairs and table	×	×	×	×	×
Classroom	750	Multipurpose seating for 25	×	×	×	×	×
Workroom	120	Photocopy, storage, work table	×	×		×	
Coatroom	10						
Storage	60						
Toilets	80					×	×
Entry/reception	250	Reception desk, sin in, key storage for locker room	×	×	×	×	×
Child care	400		×	×	×	×	×
Retail	150		×	×	×	×	×
Lounge	280	Casual seating for 63 vending machines		×	×	×	×
Locker room	600	50 lockers 1 private cubicle 2 soiled towel cart		×		×	×
Lavatories	120	4 lavatories continuous countertop w/mirror above outlets at the rate of 3 ft on center				×	×
Shower	280	1 handicapped stall W/curtain					×
Toilet	280	1 sink				×	×
Storage	40	1 sink		×			
Women's lockers shower							
Locker room	600	50 lockers		×		×	×
Lavatories/grooming	200	12 lavatories				×	×

Annexure II

The AIA Wellness Center Environmental Requirements by Room

Part I: Clinical space						
Room light	***Level (foot candles)***	***Temperature (degree F)***	***Acoustic guidelines***		***Humidity (%)***	***Air exchanges***
			STC rating	***Measured reverberation times(s)***		
Treatment	50–100	68–72	60	0.8–1.4	60 or less	6
Presurgery testing	50–100	68–72	60	0.8–1.4	60 or less	6
Operating room	50–100	68–72	60	0.8–1.4	60 or less	15
Recovery	50	69–72	60	0.8–1.4	60 or less	15

Part IV: Common areas						
Room light	***Level (foot candles)***	***Temperature (degree F)***	***Acoustic guidelines***		***Humidity (%)***	***Air exchanges***
			STC rating	***Measured reverberation times(s)***		
Locker room	50	72–78	45–50	0.8–1.4	60 or less	3
Lavatories/grooming	50	72–78	45–50	0.8–1.4	60 or less	3
Shower	50	72–78	45–50	0.8–1.4	60 or less	3
Toilets	50	72–78	45–50	0.8–1.4	60 or less	3
Storage		72–78	45–50	0.8–1.4	60 or less	3
Family lockers/showers						
Locker room	50	72–78	45–50	0.8–1.4	60 or less	3
Offices	40- 60	72–78	45–50	0.8–1.4	60 or less	3
Lavatories/groom	50	72–78	45–50	0.8–1.4	60 or less	3
Shower	50	72–78	45–50	0.8–1.4	60 or less	3
Storage	50	72–78	45–50	0.8–1.4	60 or less	3
Laundry	50	72–78	45–50	0.8 –1.4	60 or less	3

REFERENCES

1. www.medicalwellnessassociation.com
2. www.rmi.org
3. en.wikipedia.org
4. www.majestic-springs.com
5. info.aia.org
6. www.brikbase.org
7. www.cabrini.edu
8. scholarworks.montana.edu
9. https://ab-hwc.nhp.gov.in

OTHER REFERENCES

- Heart Transformation Wellness Center.com
- http://www.keralaayurvedichealthcare.com/ayurveda/ayurveda_resort_i ndia.htm
- http://www.uncwellness.com
- Medical wellness association journal, Spring; 2007;4(1).
- Moore J. Medical Wellness Journal 3, Executive Director International Health, Racquet and Sportsclub Association (IHRSA).
- NABH Standards for Wellness Centers.
- Guenther R, Vittori G. Sustainable Healthcare Architecture.
- The Fourth Factor—A historical perspective on architecture and medicine. By John Michael Currie, AIA, FRSH. The American Institute of Architects, Academy of Architecture for Health.
- www.chennai.apollohospitals.com
- www.kairali.com
- www.treatment-centers.net/treatment-directory/florida.html
- www.wikepdia.com
- "Designing a Wellness Center: Integrated Health Programming"; Journal of Medical Wellness Association; Volume 4, No. 1, 2003:(4)1.
- "Wellness Centers: Guidebook for Design Professionals: John Whaley Gallup" 1999. By John Whaley Group, USA.

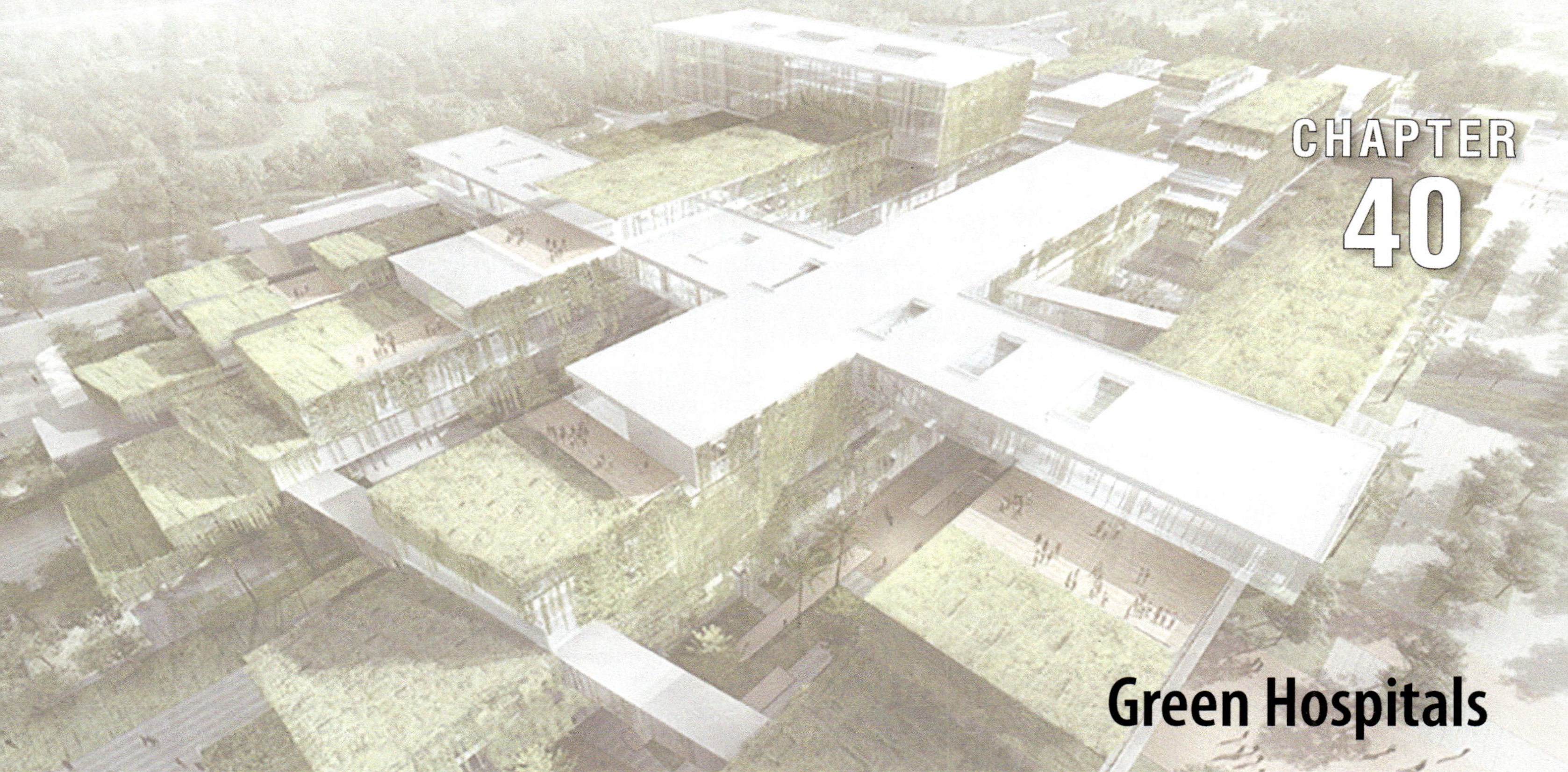

Green Hospitals

Vijay Kumar Tadia, Dibakar Rakshit, Biplab Kumar, Shakti Kumar Gupta, Sunil Kant, R Chandrashekhar

INTRODUCTION

A hospital is an institution which helps in recovering and providing relief to the sick and the injured. In order to build an appropriate facility, there is a requirement of enormous resources including financial. Hospitals consume huge amount of water and electricity. They also generate huge quantities of biodegradable, nonbiodegradable and infectious wastes further leading to a plethora of other problems, leading to pollution of both the built environment as well as the natural environment. In fact, construction of a hospital itself not only consumes water and electricity but also pollutes the environment.

A green hospital attempts to minimize the impact that it has on the health and environment throughout its lifecycle, i.e. right from building design and construction to practice and operations.

CONSERVATION AND PREVENTION

While healthcare generally focuses on curing and treatment, prevention is also an integral principle of healthcare. It is always advisable to prevent disease from occurring rather than to treat the disease after it has occurred. A green hospital tries to go a step further by not only trying to prevent pollution and wastage of resources, but also attempts to conserve the resources that are available while designing, constructing, operating and maintaining a hospital.

> Sometimes, there can be a misconception that by only providing green cover and huge lawns, a hospital can be termed as green hospital. In fact providing huge lawns is going to use huge quantity of water for its upkeep and maintenance and also results in wastage of irrigation water due to evaporation when lawns are exposed to the sun. This goes against the principle of conservation and prevention.

The American Society of Healthcare Engineering was the first organization to publish guidance statement for constructing a Green Healthcare Facility in January 2002. In its principles, it states that building design and construction practice can be shaped to protect health at three scales:[1]

- Protecting the immediate health of building occupants.
- Protecting the health of the surrounding community.
- Protecting the health of the global community and natural resources.

Some of the salient features of green hospitals are:

- Minimal disturbance to landscape and site condition during and after construction.
- Following highest health and safety standards for the construction workers.
- Use of non-toxic, recycled and environmental friendly building materials.
- Efficient use of water and water recycling.
- Use of energy efficient and eco-friendly equipment.
- Indoor air quality for human safety and comfort.
- Effective controls and building management systems.
- Use of renewable energy.
- Efficient segregation and disposal of wastes.

To certify a building or hospital as green, rating systems have been developed. Rating systems evaluate the design, construction, operation and maintenance on various parameters. The evaluation parameters are mainly grouped into:[2]

- Location and transportation
- Sustainable sites
- Water efficiency
- Energy and atmosphere
- Materials and resources
- Indoor and environmental quality.

Box 1: Brief history of green building rating systems.

The Green Building movement started in the 1990s with the creation of Building Research Establishment's Environmental Assessment Method (BREEAM), the first green building rating system in the U.K. Rick Fedrizzi, David Gottfried and Mike Italiano established the United States Green Building Council (USGBC) in 1993. The pilot green building rating system, Leadership in Energy and Environmental Design (LEED) for New Construction (LEED-NC) v1.0 was released in 1998. Since the pilot version, several updates have taken place leading to LEED NCv2.0 in 2000, LEED NCv2.2 in 2005, and LEED 2009 (previously named LEEDv3) in 2009 and culminating to the present LEEDv4 released in November 2013. LEED covers five major categories: New Construction; Core and Shell; Schools; Retail—New Construction and Major Renovations and Healthcare. Apart from these, there are LEED systems for commercial interiors, existing buildings—operations and maintenance, neighborhood development and homes.

Several countries have introduced their own Green Building Rating Systems. Some of them are BEAM in Hong Kong, European Union, EFTA member states, EU candidates, as well as the Persian Gulf, Comprehensive Assessment System for Building Environmental Efficiency (CASBEE) in Japan, Green Mark Scheme in Singapore, Green Star in Australia, New Zealand and South Africa, Pearl Rating System for Estidama in UAE. IGBC and GRIHA in india.

Green Building Movement in India started in 2001 with the establishment of Indian Green Building Council (IGBC) by Confederation of Indian Industry (CII). The Energy Resources Institute (TERI) developed Green Rating for Integrated Habitat Assessment (GRIHA) in 2005. IGBC has also released rating systems suited for India (Box 1).

The Indian Parliament has also passed The Energy Conservation Act, 2001 which led to the formation of Bureau of Energy Efficiency (BEE) under Ministry of Power in March 2002. BEE launched Energy Conservation Building Code (ECBC) in 2007 and is one of the reference standard for GRIHA and IGBC rating systems.

India presently has IGBC, LEED USGBC, GRIHA and Excellence in Design for Greater Efficiencies (EDGE) and BEE star rating systems for buildings. However, at present only LEED USGBC has a separate category for Healthcare. GRIHA also has a rating system for large developments which can be used in the certification of hospitals having a site area of at least 50 hectares (125 acres). However IGBC has exclusive healthcare facility rating system.

The following would give a brief overview of the various parameters involved in construction of a green hospital and by implementing them, the project can achieve certification under any of the rating systems as desired by the project owner. It may be noted that some of the parameters mentioned below are mandatory and individual rating system may be referred to for finding those mandatory criteria.

LOCATION AND TRANSPORTATION

Site should be selected in such a manner that it conforms to the development plan/master plan/Urban development plans formulation and implementation (UDPFI) guidelines. It should also not be located within the minimum distances as mandated by the provisions of ecosensitive zone regulations, coastal zone regulations, heritage area site regulations, water bodies (no construction is permitted within 30 m of any water body), various hazard prone area regulations, and others if the site falls under any such area.

If a brownfield is available, it could be reclaimed and remediated using strategies such as pump-and-treat, bioreactors, land farming, *in situ* remediation, etc. United States Environmental Protection Agency (EPA) remediation guidelines could be used for rigorous remediation. However, remediation methods such as incinerating the material or dumping the contaminated material off-site should be avoided as they have negative impact on the environment.

Sometimes remediation of a brownfield could prove to be costly. A decision should be taken on whether it is feasible to remediate the brownfield or locate another site.

It should be seen that at least basic services are located within walking distance from main entrance of project. Basic services include, but are not limited to: Bank; Place of worship; Convenience grocery; Daycare; Cleaners; Fire station; Beauty; Hardware; Laundry; Library; Medical/dental; Senior care facility; Park; Pharmacy; Post office; Restaurant; School; Supermarket; Theater; Community center; Fitness center; Museum; Hotel; Prosthetic and other medical devices store; Gift shop; and Other supportive healthcare services.[1]

With metro rail upcoming in many cities in India, the site could be planned to be within 500 m of an existing, or planned metro station. However, if metro stations are not planned in vicinity, the site should at least be located within 400 m of two or more different public or campus/contract bus lines and usable by building occupants.

Within the campus or outside, electric vehicles could be used for transportation. The electric vehicle should be able to cater to at least 5% of the building occupants (excluding visitors). Alternatively, Compressed Natural Gas (CNG) powered vehicles could also be used. Additionally, dedicated parking area which are easily accessible to the building entrance should be allocated for such vehicles and charging facilities should be provided within the parking area of the site for electric vehicles. One CNG filling station should be located within 5 km distance from the projects' campus entrance.

SUSTAINABLE SITES

A site survey should be carried out before start of construction. The survey should give information on topography, hydrology, climate, vegetation, soil etc. Wherever, the site allows, hospital should be so designed as to preserve at least 15% of the existing natural topography and vegetation. If there are existing fully grown trees within the project site, they must either be preserved or transplanted. It should be seen that Ministry of Environment and Forest (MoEF) guidelines are followed.

Passive design strategies should be adopted by the architect to design the hospital. Passive design strategies include but not limited to (1) reducing solar heat gain during peak summer by using trees, (2) locating service zones and corridors on the west side, (3) reduce solar insolation by massing of the building/campus, (4) favorable orientation of the building. The design should consider flexibility and ease of future adaptation.

Urban heat island effect results in the temperature of built-up areas being significantly higher than temperatures of nearby rural areas. To minimize this effect, it is suggested to rather provide shades using trees (within 5 years of occupancy) or use paving materials with a Solar Reflectance Index (SRI) of at least 29 or use open grid pavement system for 50% of the site hardscape (including roads, sidewalks, courtyards, and parking lots).

The building design should incorporate design measures for Universal Accessibility as recommended in NBC of India 2016.

A minimum of 50% of parking spaces should also be placed under cover (defined as underground, under deck, under roof, or under a building). Any roof used to shade or cover parking must have an SRI of at least 29.[1]

Roofing materials should have a SRI equal to or greater than the 78 for a minimum of 75% of the roof surface in case of low sloped roof (≤2:12). In case of high sloped roof (>2:12) the SRI should be greater than 29. Paint coatings with high SRI values are available and they can be used to fulfil this clause.

In India, we are now witnessing urban flooding, rapid runoff of rainwater and contamination of water streams due to runoff. High imperviousness on site leads to these problems, and also reduces urban rainwater recharge. Storm water plan and best management practices must be implemented on site to ensure not only quantity but also quality of the discharge. The net imperviousness factor of site should meet the National Building Code (NBC) of India 2016 norms.

To reduce outdoor light pollution, exterior lighting should be designed in a way that the light fixtures emit no more than 5% of total initial designed fixture lumens at an angle of 90° or higher from nadir (straight down). The lighting power density which is obtained by dividing lighting power by area (unit is W/m^2 or W/sq ft) should be reduced by at least 30% as compared to values mentioned in the ASHRAE Standard 90.1-2010, Section 9.4.3. Additionally, luminous efficacy of the lamps should be at least 75 lm/W.

One of the aims of healthcare facility design should be to provide places of respite connected to natural environment so that a healing environment exists for the patients and/or residents, staff, family members, and visitors inhabiting these buildings. Outdoor places of respite of at least 5% of the net usable program area should be provided out which at least 2% should be exclusively dedicated to the staff. Additionally, exterior courtyard, terrace or balcony are to be provided with a minimum area of 5 sq ft/patient served for 75% of all inpatients and 75% of qualifying outpatients with clinical length of stay greater than 4 hours.[1]

CONSTRUCTION MANAGEMENT

A construction and waste management plan should be developed before start of construction and should be adhered to during construction. A contract should be established with a local recycler for recycling waste generated during construction. The plan should list the recyclable items that are expected to be generated. Typical recyclable waste include plastic, metal, paper, wooden packing material, paint cans, empty cement bags, glass, etc. During construction period, separate designated area on site should be provided for recyclable and hazardous waste. Logs should be maintained for all the above materials. A description of as to where the material will be taken and how the recycling facility will process the material should also be provided.

During construction, the soil becomes lose due to the removal of stabilizing material such as vegetation and disturbance of stabilized existing grade, resulting in loss of topsoil and its deposition in undesirable places. A soil erosion and sedimentation control plan should be prepared, prior to construction, and should be applied effectively. Some of the measures that could be undertaken are temporary and permanent seeding, mulching, earth dikes, silt fencing, sediment traps and sediment basins. Top soil should generally be preserved till postconstruction and be used for landscaping purposes.[3]

To reduce the air and water pollution occurring during construction, the measures that should be implemented are:

- Barricading the boundary of the construction area with rigid covers at least 3 m high.
- Ensuring vehicles entering or exiting the construction site have a dedicated wheel washing facility.
- Covering fine aggregate and excavated earth on site with plastic/geotextile sheets.
- Water sprinkling on fine aggregate (sand) and excavated earth.
- Providing chimneys with their outlet facing away from the site to all diesel generators on site.

Additionally, clauses mentioned in 'During Construction Indoor Air Quality Management Guidelines' of National Building Code (NBC) of India, Part 7 - Constructional Practices and Safety should be followed.

The amount of water being used during construction can be reduced by using gunny bags, additives and ponding for curing.

A safe, healthy and hygienic working and living conditions for construction workers working in the project should be ensured. Contract document of the project management group should mandatorily mention the guidelines explicitly and routine checks should be carried out to ensure that contractors do not violate the norms. 'Constructional Practices and safety guidelines' of NBC of India 2016, Constructional Practices and Safety should be followed. The guidelines provided in 'The Building and other Construction Workers Act, 1996 and Rules, 1998' should be adhered to. Some of the measures include but not limited to providing adequate housing, sanitary facilities, first-aid and emergency facilities, adequate drinking water facilities, protective gear and safety harness, daycare/crèche facility for workers' children.

WATER EFFICIENCY

To reduce the water consumption within the building, low flow fixtures should be used. For the taps, aerators can be used. Wash basins could also have sensor based taps which will automatically stop the flow of water after a pre-set time. For the water closets, dual flush systems should be used (for example 3/6 L). Sensor-based urinals should be installed. Technical datasheets for all the fixtures should be obtained for submission to the rating authority.

To reduce the irrigation water demand, turf and lawn area should be kept at a minimum. Instead drought tolerant and native species should be planned by the landscape architect. Highly efficient irrigation systems like drip irrigation, timer-based controllers for valves, soil moisture sensors, central shut-off valve, pressure regulating devices, etc. go a long way in optimizing the requirement of water.

Many cities today are experiencing a drop in underground water table. Dynamic data regarding the water table can be obtained from India Water Resources Information System (WRIS) Geographic Information System (WebGIS) based on this data, it should be seen if rain water harvesting should be taken up. Few cities have made it mandatory to include the provision of rain water harvesting in any new buildings that are coming up. The rainwater harvesting system should be able to capture at least 'one-day rainfall' runoff volume from roof and non-roof areas.

Hospitals generate large quantity of waste water which can then be treated on site to be reused for flushing, landscaping and cooling tower makeup. The water treated on site should conform to the norms prescribed by Central (or) State Pollution Control Board. However, additional treatment could be required for cooling tower makeup water to obtain the desired amount of total dissolved solids (TDS) (Fig. 1).

Water sub-metering should be done by installing separate water meters for irrigation, indoor plumbing fixtures and fittings, domestic hot water, municipal water supply, treated waste water consumption and any other major source of water consumption. The water meters can be connected to the Building Management System (BMS) for effective water management.

ENERGY AND ATMOSPHERE

Electricity bills form a significant amount of running costs of any hospitals. Lighting and air-conditioning and equipment form a major component of the total electricity bills. The construction material of walls and roof, type of glass, type of light fixture, occupants and equipment's have an impact on the air-conditioning load. By implementing energy efficiency measures like selecting better wall material like AAC Autoclave Aerated Concrete (ACC) Block instead of clay bricks, providing overdeck insulation on the roof, selecting Double Glazed Unit (DGU) glass, the

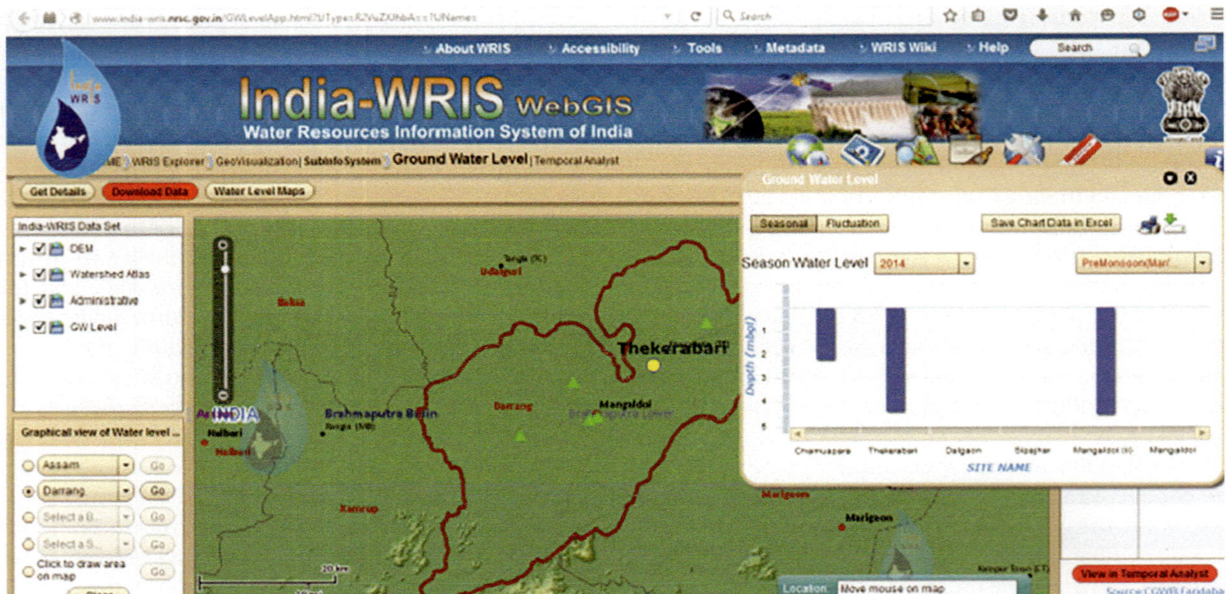

Fig. 1: Ground water level as shown on India WRIS WebGIS.

solar heat gain into the building could be reduced significantly. While to comply with some of the rating systems a prescriptive approach could be followed, a true picture of the electricity consumption and costs can be obtained only by carrying out whole building energy simulation before the start of construction. Simulation is carried out by creating building models on specialized software like eQUEST, IES VE, Design Builder, Energy Plus, etc. and inputting various parameters like construction material details, occupancy levels and profile, lighting levels and profile of use, detailed inputs of air-conditioning systems, etc. The software then gives out hourly electricity consumption based on the location and climate data. By obtaining this information, a costing analysis can be done to calculate the payback periods of energy efficiency measures and the measures which have low payback periods can then be selected (Fig. 2).

To reduce the dependence on grid purchased electricity (more than 50% of which is generated by burning coal in India), on site renewable energy systems should be installed. The capacity of the renewable energy systems could be tailor-made as per the requirement of individual rating systems, however it is suggested that at least 3% of the annual energy requirement is met by the renewable energy systems.

Energy metering and reporting both consumption (in kWh) and demand (in kW) should mandatorily be part of the building management system. Reporting should be carried out for grid supplied electricity, on-site renewable energy systems, backup power generator and for individual buildings. Apart from this, sub-reporting should be carried out for AHU, cooling tower, chillers (BTU meters) in case of centralized air-conditioning plant, indoor and outdoor lighting and any other individual energy end use that could represent 10% or more of the total annual consumption of the building. The data collected should be stored for at least 36 months and should be accessible remotely. Automatic Power Factor correction system should also be mandatorily installed. Demand response programs could be additionally installed for a dynamic load allocation on real time basis.

Preoccupancy commissioning should be carried out by a third party for mechanical, electrical, plumbing and renewable energy systems. A commissioning plan should be developed and observations should be recorded. Operation and Maintenance (O&M) manuals should be in place and specific clauses should be included in the contract document of the systems supplier for providing training to the core facility/service group responsible for the O & M of the building systems after installation. The commissioning authority must review contractor submittals, and review O & M details. Postoccupancy review after at least 10 months should be carried out.[1,2]

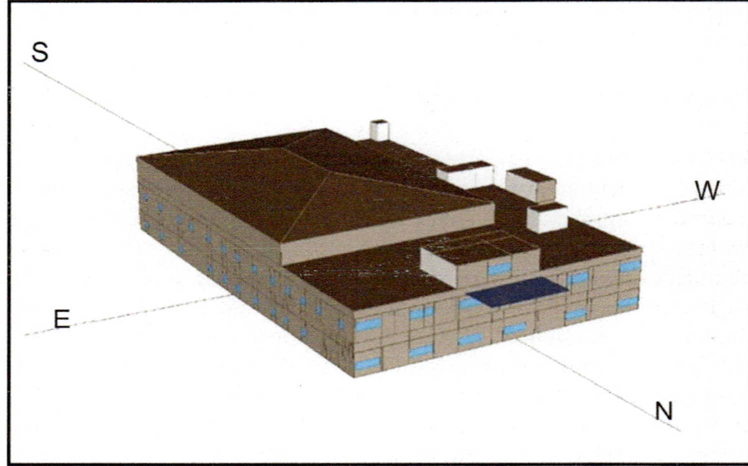

Fig. 2: 3D model in eQUEST.

MATERIALS AND RESOURCES

To reduce the embodied energy of building structure, low-energy techniques and energy efficient technologies not based on the utilization of fly ash could be used for both structural and nonstructural infill wall application. Low energy technologies for structural applications include but not limited to prestressed slab, extruded structural clay joist and filler slab, hollow floor/roof slabs, filler slabs or burned clay filler pots with RCC structure, micro concrete roofing, precast hollow plank roofing, zipbloc system, composite columns, reinforced grouted brick masonry, stone masonry, precast stone blocks, light-weight concrete blocks over dense concrete blocks, etc. Nonstructural application include but not limited to infill wall system using traditional mud walling system, stabilized adobe walling, compressed earth blocks, hollow perforated/modular bricks, interlocking bricks, traditional stone masonry, precast non-load-bearing concrete blocks, finished concrete blocks, light weight concrete blocks, over dense concrete blocks, precast brick panels, composite ferrocement walling, interlocking concrete blocks, rat trap masonry, and so on.[3]

It is also suggested that BIS recommended wastes (such as fly ash, blast furnace slag, etc.), having properties similar to conventional construction materials are used for building construction. By using them in the building structure, it helps in the diversion of these wastes away from landfills. Fly ash can be utilized in cement used in structural concrete and as well as in Ordinary Portland Cement (OPC) used for plastering walls and roof.

Certain materials that are selected for use can have either Ozone Depletion Potential (ODP) or both ODP and Global Warming Potential (GWP). It is recommended that if insulation is used in building it should be free of Chloro-Fluoro-Carbon (CFC) and Hydro-Chloro-Fluoro-Carbon (HCFC). The refrigerants being used in air-conditioning systems should be free of CFCs. Some common refrigerants which are now commonly used and are free of CFCs are R-124a and R-410A. For low temperature applications R-404A and R-507A are being used. Ammonia is a natural refrigerant having zero ODP and GWP. Fire suppression systems and fire extinguishers installed in the building should be free of halon.

It should be seen that the use of persistent, bio-accumulative, and toxic (PBT) chemicals like mercury, lead, cadmium and copper is minimized. Generally, thermometers, thermostats and switching devices, dental wastes (such as scrap amalgam, chair side traps, and separator wastes) contain mercury. Amalgam separation devices that meet or exceed the ISO-11143 standard should be used in dental care facilities. High-intensity discharge (HID) lamps should not be used within any interior spaces. If circumstances and cost permit, then fluorescent lamps should not be specified by the electrical consultant and instead LED lamps should be included. LED lamps also reduce the cooling load of air-conditioning system. However, if any functional requirement needs fluorescent lamps, then T-8 or better lamps should be specified. Information should be obtained from the manufacturer on the maximum mercury content in these lamps and should not exceed that mentioned in USGBC LEED. For pipes, pipe fittings, plumbing fittings, and faucets transferring potable water for human consumption, it should be seen that the weighted average lead content of the wetted surface area of not more than 0.25% lead is adhered to. The solders and flux used for connecting the above pipes should have 0.2% or less lead content. Interior and exterior paints should also be lead free. Electrical wire and cable with lead content less than 300 parts per million. However, lead used for radiation shielding and copper used for MRI shielding are exempt.[1,2]

To reduce the energy used up in transportation of materials, at least 25% of the total building materials (by cost) used in the building should be sourced from manufacturers within 400 km of the building site. However, assembly of building materials shall not be considered for this valuation. For example, if the project location is New Delhi and AAC blocks used for the project are manufactured in Hisar, the cost of AAC blocks shall be counted in this calculation. The steel used in the project is manufactured in Jamshedpur shall not be considered as Jamshedpur is more than 400 km away from New Delhi.

To further reduce the requirement of new materials, the project could consider using salvaged, reused or refurbished materials ensuring that the cost of these materials is at least 2.5% of the total cost of building materials. For example, door wooden frame material salvaged from another site is used to construct the legs of a staff table.

When wood-based materials are used, it should be seen that the wood used is rapidly renewable like bamboo or is certified by Forest Stewardship Council (FSC). It should be written in the contract document that Chain of Custody (COC) number should be provided. However, it might be tough to obtain the COC number in India and hence it might be better to use less number of wood-based materials.

Materials chosen for manufacture should have some amount of recycled content and these materials should constitute at least 10% of the total building materials by cost. Even common materials used like steel and glass have certain amount of recycled content in them. Certificates should be obtained from manufacturers indicating the location of manufacture of the product, the distance from the project site and the percentage of recycled content used for the manufacturing of the product.

Postconstruction, multicolored dustbins should be provided to building occupants to effectively segregate waste generated at source. Further dedicated storage spaces for these wastes should be provided within site or within the building. Contract should be in place with local recycler to safely recycle wastes like metal, paper, plastic, glass, etc. Facility could also be provided to treat all organic wastes on site. Various guidelines enlisted in Bio-Medical Waste Management Rules, 2016 must be adhered to.

INDOOR ENVIRONMENTAL QUALITY

For air-conditioned spaces, the minimum fresh air volume as mandated by American Society of Heating Refrigerating and Air-conditioning Engineers (ASHRAE) Standard 62.1-2010, Sections 4–7, Ventilation for Acceptable Indoor Air Quality (with errata), or NBC of India-2016 or ASHRAE Standard 170-2008, Section 7 has to be provided. Monitoring should be carried out using BMS. An alarm must alert staff whenever the outdoor airflow value varies by 15% or more from the outdoor airflow setpoint. Additionally, the fresh air being provided can be treated for Particulate Matter 10 microns (PM 10), Ozone and CO to attain levels as desired in the CPCB National Ambient Air Quality Standard.

The CO_2, temperature and relative humidity of the occupied spaces or at Air Handling Units (AHUs) for the air-conditioned spaces should be monitored centrally using BMS. Additionally, it is to be demonstrated that thermal comfort is being achieved as per the requirements of NBC of India 2016 or ASHRAE Standard 55-2010.

The paints, coatings, adhesives and sealants should not exceed the volatile organic compound (VOC) limit as specified in different rating systems. Composite wood and Agri-fiber materials used in the building should be free of added urea-formaldehyde resins.

IGBC

To sensitise various forms of built environment, CII established the Indian Green Building Council (IGBC) in 2001. IGBC, is a consensus driven not-for-profit Council, represents the building industry, consisting of more than 1,923 committed members. The Council encourages, builders, developers, owners, architects, doctors, consultants and several other stakeholders to embrace green, thereby contributing to the National goals on sustainability.

The Green Building Movement in India has been spearheaded by IGBC since 2001, by creating awareness amongst the stakeholders. The Council's activities have enabled a market transformation with regard to green building materials and technologies.

IGBC continuously works to provide tools that facilitate the adoption of green building practices in India. The development of IGBC Green Healthcare rating system® is another important step in this direction.

It addresses green features under the following categories:

- Indoor Environmental Quality
- Sanitization & Hygiene
- Energy Efficiency
- Water Conservation
- Site Selection and Planning
- Building Materials and Resources
- Innovation in Design Process

GRIHA

Green Rating for Integrated Habitat Assessment rating system (Version 3) consists of 34 criteria categorized under various sections such as site selection and site planning, Conservation and Efficient Utilization of Resources, Building Operation and Maintenance, and Innovation points.[4]

Registration

- A project has to be registered with IGBC/GRIHA Council through website by filling in the registration form online.
- Registration should preferably be done at beginning of a project, as several issues need to be addressed at the pre-design stage.
- The registration process includes access to the essential information related to rating.

Documentation[4]

The evaluation system covers interdisciplinary areas. Submissions required for meeting any particular criterion are elaborated in specific sections.

All documents (in soft version) related to the attempted (criteria should be submitted along with the application (preconstruction stage). Only the attempted criteria will be reviewed.

Evaluation[4]

The project documentation is evaluated online and rated in a three-tier process. After online submission of documents, the preliminary evaluation is done by team of professionals and experts from IGBC/GRIHA Secretariat, IGBC/GRIHA Council. Documentation should be complete in all respects for all attempted criteria. Any attempted criteria with incomplete documentation is not be evaluated. The documentation formats are provided online for each criterion. Online calculators provided for specific criteria need to be filled in and submitted.

The IGBC/GRIHA Council team first reviews compliance of the project with the mandatory criteria and reject the project in the event of noncompliance with such criteria.

The IGBC/GRIHA Council team will then evaluate the optional criteria and estimate the total number of achievable points.

The evaluation summary report is sent to members of the evaluation committee for IGBC/GRIHA comprising of renowned sector experts from landscape architecture, lighting and HVAC design, renewable energy, water and waste management, and building materials. The evaluation committee members will vet the points estimated by the technical team. The evaluation committee will then independently review the documents for the award of points. The evaluation committee may use the evaluation summary report submitted by the technical team as a guiding document. The evaluation committee will award provisional points and also comment on specific criteria, if need be. The evaluation report will be sent to the project proponent to review the same and, if desired, take steps to increase the score. The report will elaborate on the results of the evaluation committee along with its comments. The report will provide comments on each criteria and an overall comment on the entire report. The client will be given 1 month's time to resubmit the document with necessary modifications/additions. The resubmitted document will comprise only of the additional documents/information desired in the evaluation report. The resubmitted documents will again be put through the vetting process described above. The evaluation committee will then award the final score. The final score will be presented to The Advisory Committee comprising eminent personalities and renowned professionals in the field for approval and award of rating. The rating will be valid for a period of five years from the date of commissioning of the building. IGBC/GRIHA Council reserves the right to undertake a random audit of any criteria for which points have been awarded.[4,5]

Certification Fee[4]

The registration cum rating fee is subject to review and modification every year. The exact fees can be obtained online and is calculated upon the built-up area excluding basement for parking.
The fee includes

- Cost of IGBC/GRIHA documents and templates
- Third party evaluator fees
- Professional time for one-day training workshop for all consultants involved in the project
- IGBC/GRIHA Secretariat costs for documents collection, assimilation, valuation and submission.

The fee does not include

- Third party postoccupancy (at the operational stage) audit by BEE certified energy auditor/agency
- Travel by flight and accommodation arrangements for 2 IGBC/GRIHA Council officials for training workshop and minimum 3 site visits shall be arranged by project proponent
- Government taxes as applicable to be paid on the registration fee
- Handholding/facilitation/consultancy necessary for rating.

It may be noted that award of the rating is subject to fulfillment of all requirements as elaborated in IGBC/GRIHA document.

IGBC/GRIHA is a 100-point system consisting of some core points, which are mandatory, while the rest are optional.

Different levels of certification (silver to platinum) are awarded based on the number of points earned. The minimum points required for certification is 50 (Table 1).

After construction and prior to occupancy, an indoor air quality testing could be carried out to test for the concentration of formaldehyde, PM10, Total VOC, 4-Phenylcyclohexene and CO.

Individual lighting controls could be provided for at least 90% of individual occupant spaces in staff areas. For at least 90% of patient positions, lighting controls are to be provided such that the controls are readily accessible from the patient's bed. In multioccupant patient spaces, the controls must be individual lighting controls. In private rooms, exterior window shades, blinds, or curtain controls should be provided such that the controls are readily accessible from the patient's bed. Exceptions include in-patient critical care, pediatric, and psychiatric patient rooms. For all shared multioccupant spaces,

Table 1: GRIHA rating system.

Points achieved	*IGBC rating*	*GRIHA rating*
50–60	Certified	*
61–70	Silver	**
71–80	Gold	***
81–90	Platinum	****
91–100	Platinum	*****

Table 2: Minimum compliant perimeter area, by floor plate area as per USGBC LEED.

Floor plate area		*Perimeter area*	
(sq ft)	*(m²)*	*(sq ft)*	*(m²)*
Up to 15,000	Up to 1,400	7,348	682
20,000	1,800	8,785	816
25,000	2,300	10,087	937
30,000	2,800	11,292	1,049
35,000	3,300	12,425	1,154
40,000	3,700	13,500	1,254
45,000	4,200	14,528	1,349
50,000 and larger	4,600 and larger	15,516	1,441

multizone control systems are to be provided such that occupants can adjust the lighting to meet group needs and preferences, with at least three lighting levels or scenes (on, off, mid-level). Mid-level is 30 % and 70% of the maximum illumination level (not including daylight contributions).[2]

The Window to Wall Ratio (WWR) and Skylight to Roof Ratio (SRR) should not exceed 60% and 5% respectively and the SHGC/Weighted Façade average SHGC of all the fenestrations should mandatorily meet the SHGC requirement of ECBC-2007. A solar path analysis for all windows could also be carried out using specialized simulation software like Ecotect or IES to ensure that the window is completely shaded for the duration between 10:00 AM on 1st April to 15:00 PM on 30th September.

Excluding the inpatient units, the building floor plates should be configured in such a way that the floor area within 15 ft (4.5 m) of the perimeter exceeds the perimeter area as specified in Table 2 extracted from USGBC LEED.

Daylight simulation should be carried out for the entire building to obtain illuminance levels for inpatient units and perimeter area. The levels should then be checked with the requirement of individual rating systems.

Additionally, the following could be practised:[1]

- Scrubbers and filters for boilers and diesel generators are to be provided.
- Diesel fuels low in sulfur content should be used.
- Air quality abatement equipment should be provided for all equipment that burns fossil fuels.
- Biodiesel fuels could be used in lieu of fossil fuels.
- To eliminate biohazard from cooling water, a ground-cooled heat exchanger could be substituted for the cooling tower.

CONCLUSION

Healthcare industry is booming in India. It is high time that we construct green hospitals keeping in mind the ecological sustainability and other benefits. While an attempt has been made here to provide a gist of the requirements of a green hospital taking care of various rating systems available in India, the reader is encouraged to refer to individual rating systems and their reference guides for detailed technical information on achieving the rating.

REFERENCES

1. www.mintie.com
2. www.fbb.h–da.de
3. hareda.gov.in
4 www.IGBC.in
5. GRIHA Council, The Energy and Resources Institute; 2015; GRIHA V – 2015 Abridged Document.

OTHER REFERENCES

- Robin G, Gail V; Sustainable Healthcare Architecture; John Wiley & Sons; 2008.
- Stephanie V; 2014; Green Building Standards and Certification Systems; Retrieved from https://www.wbdg.org/resources/gbs.php
- Wikipedia; Green Building; Retrieved from https://en.wikipedia.org/wiki/Green_building
- Green Guide for Health Care Version 2.2; 2007; American Society for Healthcare Engineering.
- USGBC; USGBC History; Retrieved from http://in.usgbc.org/about/history
- IGBC; 2012; Technical Bulletin: Green Hospitals.
- USGBC; 2013; LEED Reference Guide for Building Design and Construction v4
- IGBC; 2015; IGBC Green New Buildings rating system® Abridged Reference Guide (with Addendum 4.0).
- Ministry of New and Renewable Energy, Government of India, The Energy and Resources Institute; 2011; GRIHA Manual Volume 2,3,4; TERI Press.
- Central Water Commission (CWC), Ministry of Water Resources, Govt. of India and Indian Space Research Organization (ISRO), Department of Space, Govt. of India; Web Enabled Water Resources Information System in the Country; Retrieved from http://www.india-wris.nrsc.gov.in/wris.html
- Bureau of Energy Efficiency; 2009; Energy Conservation Building Code 2007 Revised Version June 2009.

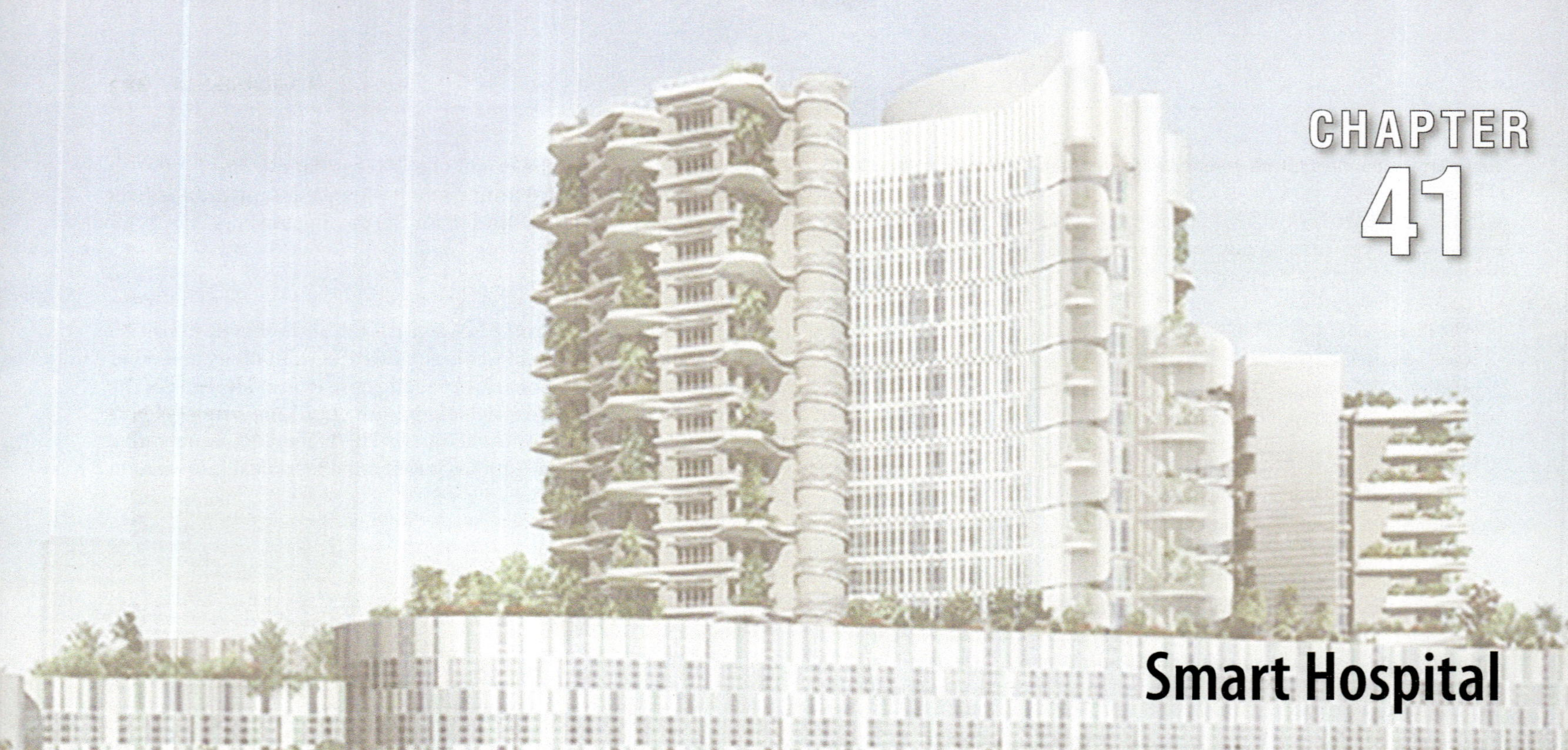

Smart Hospital

Mohd Kausar, Vijay Kumar Tadia, Shakti Kumar Gupta, Sunil Kant, R Chandrashekhar

INTRODUCTION

In 2014, more than half of the world (54%) became urban although it is only around 31% in India today.[1,2] Globally, one million people are moving into cities every week. In India alone, every minute, 30 country dwellers move permanently to a city.[3] '100 Smart Cities' programme aims to help create rapidly developing satellite cities and major urban centers that are magnets of foreign investment and jobs and symbols of efficiency, speed and scale.[4]

DEFINITION OF A SMART CITY

Smart cities provide core infrastructure, use information and communication technologies (ICT) to be more intelligent and efficient in the use of resources, resulting in cost and energy savings, improved service delivery and quality of life, clean and sustainable environment with reduced environmental footprint—all supporting innovation and the low-carbon economy with application of 'Smart' Solutions.[2,4]

Broader elements to be incorporated into a smart city include smart energy, smart environment, smart transportation, smart IT and communications, smart health, smart education, smart building and smart governance.[4,5]

With emerging developments one should include incorporation of artificial intelligence (AI). Use of natural gas from landfills to power the city's garbage trucks, bike sharing program, integrated solar panels, storage batteries, and energy efficient appliances all connected to a smart grid, virtual power plant from electric vehicles and use of radio-frequency identification (RFID) technology are flagships of the top ten smart cities of the world (Vienna, Toronto, Paris, New York, London, Tokyo, Berlin, Copenhagen, Hong Kong and Barcelona).[6]

TARGETS FOR HEALTHCARE FACILITIES IN INDIAN SMART CITIES

The targets for healthcare facilities in Indian smart cities are as follows:[3,4]

- Availability of telemedicine facilities to 100% residents
- 30 minutes emergency response time
- 1 dispensary/15,000 residents
- Nursing home, child, welfare and maternity, center—25–30 beds/ 0.1 mn population
- Intermediate hospital (Category B)—80 beds/0.1 mn population
- Intermediate hospital (Category A)—200 beds/0.1 mn population
- Multispeciality hospital—200 beds/0.1 mn population
- Specialty hospital—200 beds/0.1 mn population
- General hospital—500 beds/0.1 mn population
- 1 diagnostic center/50,000 residents
- 1 veterinary hospital/0.5 mn residents
- 1 dispensary for pet/0.1 mn residents
- *Higher education*: 1 paramedical institute/1 mn population; 1 veterinary institute

DEFINITION OF A SMART HOSPITAL

It is a type of hospital that is able to share the domain's knowledge with same or other domain and fulfill the requirement of the ubiquitous and pervasive computing environment.[7,8]

OBJECTIVES OF SMART HOSPITAL[2,4,8-11]

- *Patient-centered objectives:* To facilitate and improve patient care, satisfaction, safety, and experience.
- *Staff-centered objectives:* To facilitate and improve staff satisfaction, productivity and efficiency.
- *Hospital-centered objectives:* To facilitate and improve resource utilization, efficiency, and financial performance.
- *System-centered objectives:* To embrace and integrate with local community, public health initiatives to improve patient health and safety through more integrated population-based approach to healthcare delivery and preventive medicine.
- *Innovation-centered objectives:* To encourage, facilitate and lead the development of innovations in healthcare delivery, hospital process redesign, efficiency, and financial performance.

Similar to the smart cities, smart hospitals should rate high on:

- Innovations
- Sustainability
- Use of information technology and high end technology, a network of sensors, cameras, wireless devices and data centers.
- Digital governance
- Quality of life, adequate water supply
- Sanitation including solid waste management
- Fast delivery of services
- Efficient use of resources, alternate source of energy like solar, waste water recycling, rain water harvesting
- Energy savings, smart metering, energy efficient street lighting
- Low-carbon economy
- Smart closed-loop thinking
- The other elements of a smart hospital project are pedestrian friendly pathways, encouragement to non-motorized transport (e.g. walking and cycling), intelligent traffic management, non-vehicle streets/ zones, smart parking, innovative use of open spaces, encroachment-free public areas, and ensuring safety of citizens especially children, women and elderly.

KEY FEATURES OF SMART HOSPITAL

- Interoperable systems—people, systems and processes are connected and work together seamlessly to ensure effective sharing of data, to support seamless integration of diagnostic, treatment, and management; and business decisions. It is imperative to deliver the right information and resources at the right time to the point of care.[8]
- People, equipment, technology to be mobile. Mobile health strategy to focus on narrowing the point of care.
- *Digital information:* Information is stored in discrete and structured formats (as opposed to scanned print records), so that it is available for reporting and analysis.[8]
- *Unified communication:* Integration of audio, video, and data to allow for seamless and secure communication between patients and their caregivers, families, staff, and external healthcare providers and consultants.[8]
- High speed, reliable networking, identification technologies, sensor networks and embedded systems to interconnect the services of the facility, and provide the core infrastructure for the smart hospital, and for all future innovation projects.[8]
- *Automated systems:* Automation technologies to improve interoperability, safety, availability, efficiencies, increase productivity and, more importantly, contribute to an improved patient care experience.[8]

INTERNET OF THINGS

Through the use of internet of things (IOT), smart hospital can implement the application system based on digital environment and people can fast and accurately obtain the relevant service information.[10]

The IOT can realize diagnosis informatization, management standardization and scientific decision. At the same time, through the integration and fusion of application service, it can realize information acquisition, sharing and service in hospital, so as to promote the implementation process in smart diagnosis, smart treatment, smart management, smart decision and smart service.[10-12]

From ecologically friendly buildings, RFID and real-time location services, to smart rooms and systems that monitor, control, and adapt for energy efficiency, automated guided vehicles, there is an abundance of developments being rolled out to the market as smart solutions with flexibility to allow for the rapidly changing future.[12,13]

UBIQUITOUS COMPUTING

Ubiquitous computing (ubicomp) is a post-desktop model of human-computer interaction in which information processing has been thoroughly integrated into everyday objects and activities. In the course of ordinary activities, someone "using" ubiquitous computing engages many computational devices and systems simultaneously, and may not necessarily even be aware that they are doing so. This model is usually considered an advancement from the desktop paradigm.[7,14,15]

To respond to a technologically driven environment of care, to prepare for its evolution in the future, and to create greater efficiencies in both business and clinical processes organizations must consider bolstering the patient experience both inside their facilities and out through a keen focus on connectivity, communication, and secure access, exchange and analysis of information.[16-18] Use of sophisticated technologies is not an added value but a requirement.[19,20]

Smart hospitals have technologies ranging from interactive media to medical simulation to Web-based doctor/patient interactions, provide patients a digital portal for secure, 24-hour access to electronic medical records, scheduling, billing, registration, and educational materials from any connected device.[13,18,19]

ADVANTAGES OF SMART HOSPITAL[21-23]

- It provides a beneficial strategy for the better education and training simulation among the healthcare professionals.
- It ensures the higher levels of competence, confidence and critical thinking skills. It helps to manage the complex and changing healthcare system.
- It also supports the faculty for developing and evaluating new educational models, modalities, and teaching-learning strategies at no risk to patients.
- It also helps to integrate the better combination of ICT technologies, product and services.

The key solution of the smart hospital is online identification of all patients, doctors, nurses, staff, medical equipment, medications, blood bags, surgical tools, blankets, sheets, hospital rooms, etc.

BASIC HOSPITAL DESIGN PRINCIPLES

Design of a hospital is culture dependent—four basic design principles.[24,25]

1. Functional efficiency
   - Open design
   - Complex program in a clear structure
   - Abundance of air and light
   - Minimize walking distances
   - Combining units to reduce costs.
2. Flexibility
   - People oriented hospitals versus functional efficiency
   - Industrial construction with smart grids
   - Interchangeable rooms or units in an open configuration
   - Industrial modular assembly systems.
3. People oriented
   - Create pleasant atmosphere for all users
   - Human-friendly healing environments.

4. Well-being
   - Use of advanced and assistive technologies
   - Medical care combined with natural healing practices and holistic medicine.

The design principles should address the human needs with a multidisciplinary approach by healthcare planners/designers/engineers, clinical and technological scientist and consultants/constructors for affordable, sustainable and future proof solutions.[24,26]

Access

Located near public transit (bus and rail) stations, the campus could be designed in a way that best takes advantage of those access points and create a building scale that embrace the community at a pedestrian level while also providing direct access to neighboring buildings.[13,27]

WAY FINDING AND MOVEMENT

Simple moves with minimal turns and movement all along the edge of the building permitting orientation to the outside, intuitive wayfinding through transitions in ceiling color (different for staff and public areas) as well as architectural changes at key moments that indicate a destination area can be adopted as smart solutions.[27,28]

Adaptability

Beds that are not just acuity adaptable but standardized—from ICU to med/surg to labor and delivery, allowing them to be easily reassigned based on need. C-section rooms and ORs were built to similar standards, augmenting the building's total invasive surgery space with the ability to flex either use when necessary. ED Level 1 trauma rooms can be built with OR capabilities.[13,27,28]

Future Expansion/Usage

The building's ground level offstage area designed with 16-foot corridors to support a push system for carts and supplies today and a fully robotic transport system later, and floor loads built to support a higher weight for heavier magnets in MRIs or other larger pieces of equipment down the road.[13]

Technology

The building to include plenty of fiberoptic cable but planned to become wireless later, and technology closets are designed to hold one or two server racks today but with a generous amount of square footage to add more.[1,13,27,28]

In patient rooms, headwalls use modular systems where panels can be taken out and technology added, and the footwall features casework that houses a monitor for patient entertainment that can also be used with a Web camera for virtual consultations or eICU observation.[13]

Access to data and information will enable users to become "connected" anywhere/anytime from points such as kiosks situated throughout the hospital or on mobile devices anywhere in the building, leveraging the widespread wireless network.[13]

Up-to-date capability of PDAs, smartphones, and other portable devices at the opening of the hospital in order to provide peak functionality for staff to ensure maximum productivity.[1]

Up-to-date room information identified on flat panel monitors outside rooms, ensuring that patient confidentiality and privacy is maintained.[13]

Within the rooms, patients use integrated bedside terminals (IBTs) to control room lighting, window shades, and temperature—all at arm's length from their beds. Further capabilities of the IBTs allow patients to communicate verbally and, when needed, visually with their primary clinicians, optimizing efficiencies and enabling timely communication when it matters most.[13,27,28]

Communication and automation technologies (ICAT) fundamentally integrated with facility planning and design; innovations include:[13,26,27]

- Portable computers and interoperable equipment, including RFID-based "smart bed" technology, automatically records and transmits vital signs such as a patient's heart rate, temperature and blood pressure to secure electronic health records.
- High-level communication devices instantly deliver laboratory test results allowing caregivers to act upon the results more quickly and accurately.
- Bar coding and RFID labeling of prescription medications ensures the right patient receives the right dose of the right drug at the right time.
- Robotic delivery systems or automated-guided vehicles (AGVs) automate supply distribution.
- Pneumatic systems automate soiled linen and waste collection.
- Equipment labeling reduces staff time wasted tracking misplaced equipment.[15]
- Digital signs direct patients, their families, and visitors within the facility. Kiosks enable patients to check-in and receive information including post-treatment instructions in 50 different languages.[15]

SUSTAINABLE HIGHLIGHTS OF THE SMART HOSPITAL

- Design elements that respond to climate conditions, including prevailing winds, site orientation, seasonal sun paths and precipitation, surface water drainage and solar gain;[13,16]
- Integrated, sustainable landscape elements such as pastoral gardens, patios and a piazza, all featuring native and drought resistant plants;[13]
- Enhanced lighting strategies, improved outdoor views and maximized daylighting capture for interior spaces;
- A traffic demand management strategy, to promote alternative means of access to the site: bike lockers, enhanced public transportation access, carpooling and ride sharing, etc.;[13]
- Greenroofs (50% of roofs will be green) to help manage storm water, reduce the heat island effect, improve air quality, and beautify the views from inpatient rooms. Non-green roof areas will be painted white to help reduce building heat gains;[13,16]
- Highly efficient plumbing fixtures, including low-flow toilets, faucets, and showers. The fixtures will decrease indoor water use by 35%;[13]
- Diverting 75% of construction waste from the landfill;
- Low-emission materials for adhesives and sealants, paints and coatings, and carpets.[13]

Decentralized "Portals-of-Care" planning streamlines the ambulatory patient experience. The Portals-of-Care concept assigns each clinic its own distinct space and entrance. The clinics act as individual neighborhoods, preventing patients and visitors from walking through endless corridors to reach a destination. Once inside the appropriate clinic, visitors can access all areas of the building via the main concourse, which acts as the boulevard and connective tissue of the greater facility. Humber River Regional Hospital is the first hospital in Ontario to use the "Portals-of-Care" model at the Ambulatory Care Units.[13,15]

ENVIRONMENT OF CARE[13,25,29,30]

Advanced, Web-enabled building automation system (BAS) technology/ Building Energy Management System (BMS or BEMS).

Independent building systems can now be automated, monitored, and controlled remotely using facilities BAS capabilities including major systems in multiple buildings or even on multiple campuses from a single, central location. The BAS is also a tool in conducting an energy or critical systems audit, gathering information about the hospital's energy use and the performance of key building systems. Audits can help identify and prioritize potential energy conservation measures.

Energy reporting software lets users collect, analyze, and compare energy-consumption data across multiple buildings, units, or floors and over periods of time, provide industry benchmarks for comparable buildings.

State-of-the-art financial analysis tools include sophisticated rate engines that enable users to continuously compare actual energy consumption to historical usage rates and budgeted amounts. Software also can help allocate energy costs to various users.

Intuitive digital dashboards provide hospital staff with the ability to view, monitor, record, trend, and report data from multiple locations in real time. Dashboards can be customized to meet the user's specific requirements, including setting up alarms that automatically report environmental and system anomalies and exceptions, enabling staff members to take action before a serious problem or system failure can occur.

Using sophisticated sensors, BAS software continuously monitors and adjusts heating, ventilating, and air conditioning systems, and sounds an alert when anomalies are detected so the facilities team and medical staff can address problems before they can affect patient care. The BAS also is the centerpiece of a knowledge-based high-performance building maintenance approach, which uses condition monitoring, fault detection and diagnostics, and other advanced technologies to enable facilities teams to predict and address potential equipment problems.

Energy conservation measures can reduce costs, improve efficiency, and enhance patient care and organization's reputation in the community, improving employee morale, and attracting the best available affiliated physicians and employees.

Focus should be on lifecycle costs and savings and not just first costs.

NATURE

A smart hospital respects like orientation, wind, sun position, access and view to nature, water and landscape and air. Use of natural ventilation, (like stack ventilation by creation of atrium with glazed roof top instead of only a patio), mechanical or a hybrid model depending on the need based on ventilation studies may be done.[25,26,29]

SMART HOSPITAL BASED ON INTERNET OF THINGS

Key Technologies

- *Internet technology*: Internet network is basic precondition of IOT in order to communicate with any person and object at any time and place.
- *RFID technology:* It is a kind of noncontact automatic identification technology for objects or articles through the use of noncontact reading and writing devices.[10,29-33]

  It can be classified into three categories; passive RFID, active RFID, and semi passive RFID. All RFID systems contain three basic components. The first is the RFID tag is attached to an asset or item, contains information about it and also may incorporate sensors. The second component is the RFID interrogator (also called reader), which communicates with (also called interrogating) the RFID tags. The third component is the backend system, which links the RFID interrogators to a centralized database. The centralized database contains additional information, such as price, for each RFID tagged item. Generally speaking, a RFID system is composed of one or more reader (s) and several RFID tags. Communication between RFID tag and reader takes use of electromagnetic induction method, so direct contact is not needed.[10]
- *Sensor network technology:* Sensor networks consist of sensing nodes communicating in a wireless multihop fashion. Usually nodes report the results of their sensing to a small number (in most cases, only one) of special nodes called sinks. Usage of sensor networks has been proposed in several application scenarios, such as environmental monitoring, e-health, intelligent transportation systems, military, and industrial plant monitoring.[10,29-33]
- Wireless communication technologies mainly include bluetooth, Wi-Fi (wireless fidelity), UWB (untrawideband), Zigbee, IrDA (Infrared Data Association). In IOT, information is transmitted through these.[10]
- Embedded technology is software and hardware that is embedded in a large device or system.
- Architecture of smart hospitals (Fig. 1)[10,29-33]
  - Perception layer[10]
    - ◊ Data collection layer is to identify hospital networking nodes, *perceiving and acquiring related data,* such as identity information about doctor and nurse, identity information and medical information about patient, basic information and location information about pharmaceuticals, medical equipment and medical waste, physiological information and location information about inpatient, the environment information around hospital and so on.
    - ◊ Access layer is to transmit the data acquired from sublayer and access it to the backbone network, namely global object-conjunction network. There is a variety of access ways, such as by mobile network, by wireless network, by fixed network, by cable TV network.
  - Network layer[10]
    - ◊ Network transmission platform the backbone of hospital network, having real-time, barrier-free and high-reliable transmission of information perceived by perception layer, using technology of Ethernet, mobile communication, machine to machine (M2M) and so on.
    - ◊ Application platform to implement the integration of various data, including description of unified data, unified data warehouse, technology of data middleware, and on this basis to constitute a service platform to provide an open interface for the various services of application layer,[34] so that the third party can develop various applications on this platform for medical staff, patients and other personnel to use.
  - Application layer[10]
    - ◊ Hospital informatization application for outpatient management, hospital management, medical technology (inspection, examination, radiology, pathology, physical therapy and so on) management, drug management, equipment and material management, medical management, financial management and so on.
    - ◊ Management decision and application is the senior application, such as disease analysis (onset time, geographical distribution and treatment cost of various diseases), patients analysis (regional distribution, age distribution, proportion of free medical service and visiting time of patients), clinic

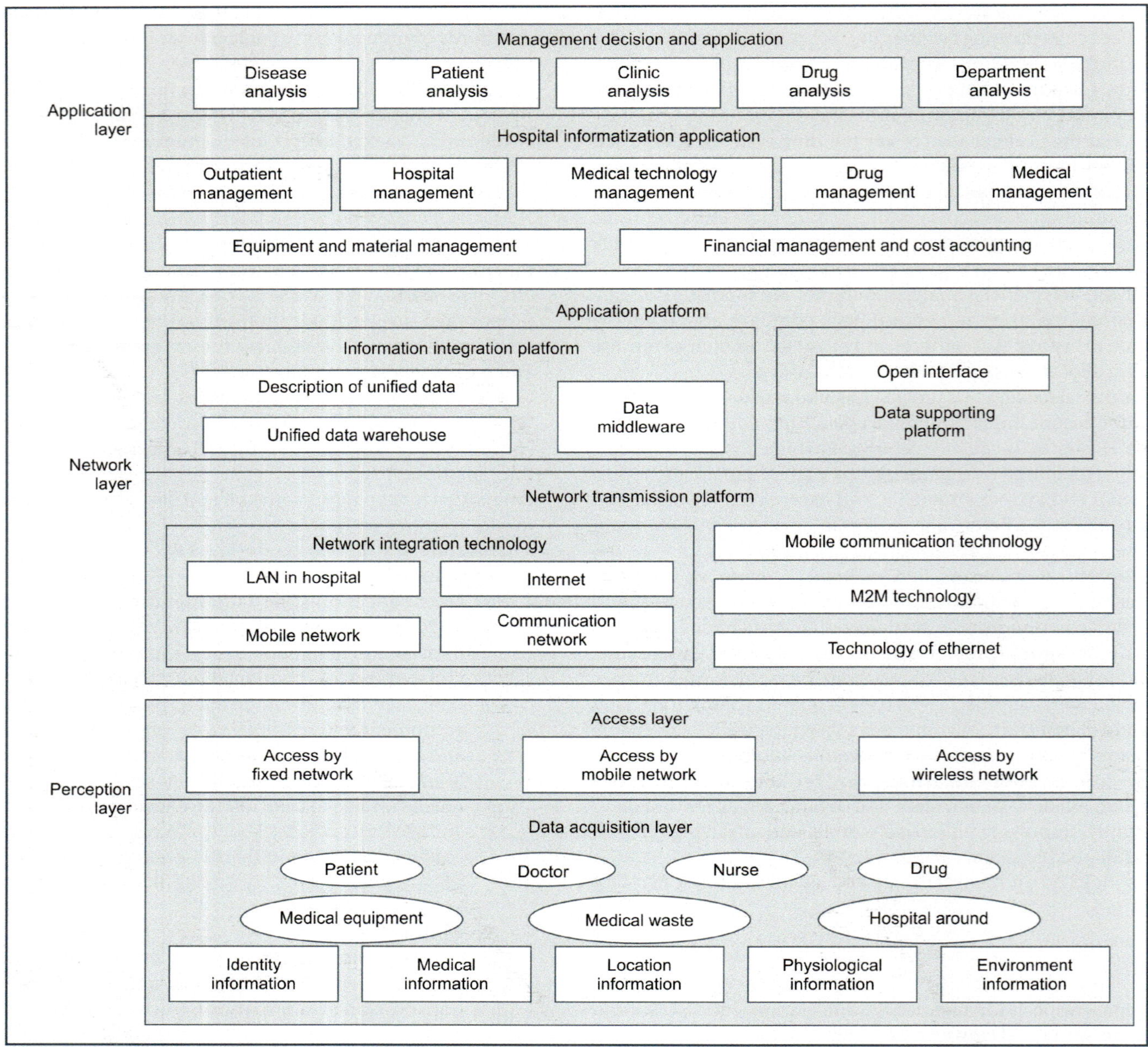

Fig. 1: Architecture of smart hospital.[10]

analysis (outpatients visits, inpatients visits and doctor visits in each time quantum), drug analysis (amount, quantity of consumption and profits of various drugs), department analysis (cost for diagnosis and treatment of every department in different periods) and so on.

- Key technique and contents of smart hospitals[10]
  - Compilation of information specification and standard
  - Construction of unified network supporting platform
  - Construction of shared data (base) platform and uniform identity authentication platform
  - Construction of integrated information service portal platform
  - Construction of embedded mobile electronic medical record application platform
- Application scheme of smart hospitals (Fig. 2)
  - Logic structure
  - Application framework
  - Network support environment.

GREENERY

Cooling effects of greenery may be utilized. A green façade changes the interaction between the building and the environment and also reduces outside temperature and inside creates a healthy environment.[25] Idea of "hospital in a park," with creation of linear parks, gardens, and views and sightlines from within the building back out onto the campus.[13]

CHECK-IN KIOSKS[13,16,19]

- Offer a convenient, on-site method of interface that patients can use to access a self-service system.
- For patients who have completed online appointment registration can simply scan their phone or a printout for identification and check in by using the kiosk barcode check-in feature.
- Can include a patient-flow management system that will track room availability and ultimately reduce wait time.

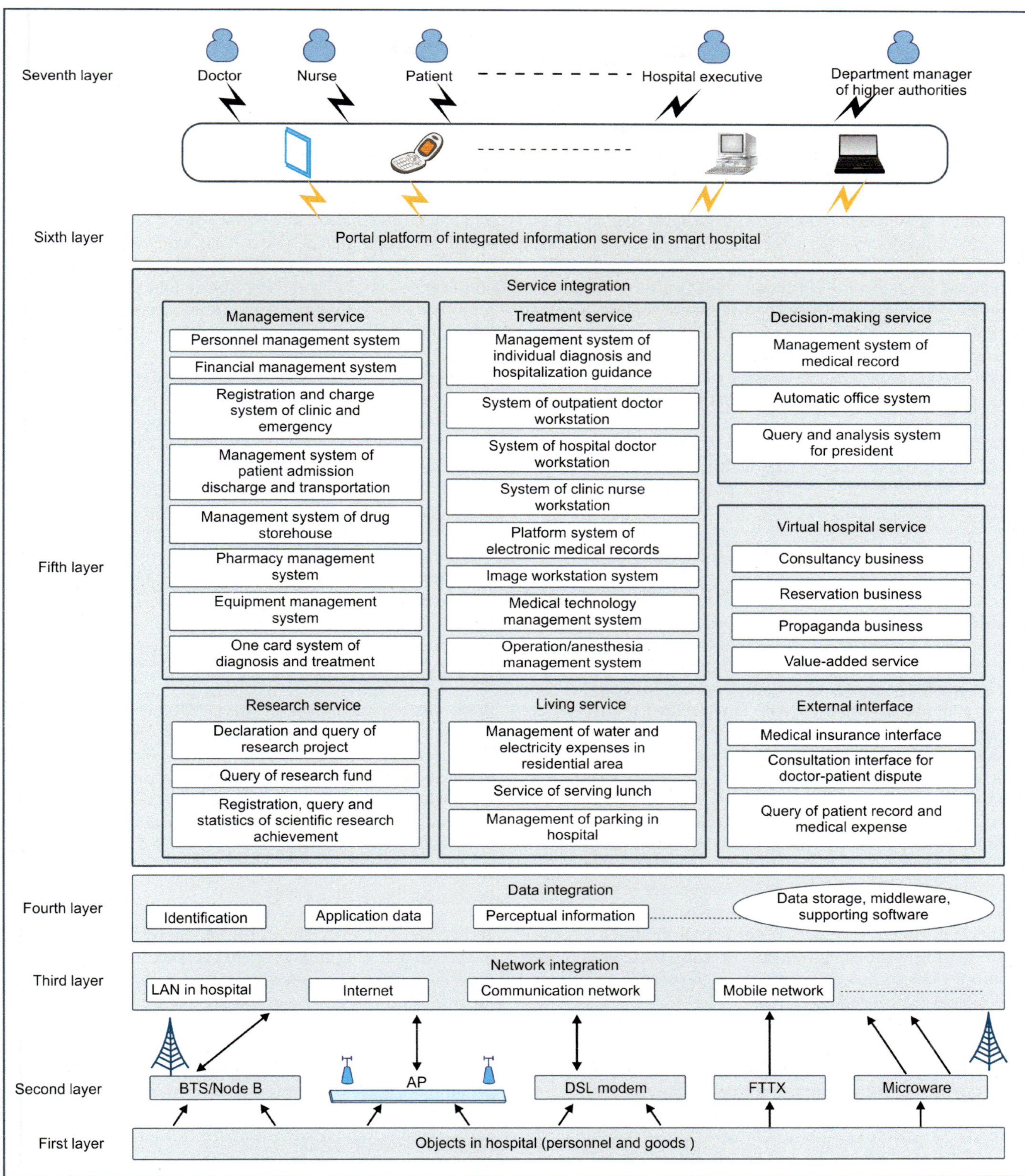

Fig. 2: Application framework of smart hospital.[10]

(LAN: local area network; FTTX: fiber in the loop; DSL: digital subscriber line; AP: access point)

CONNECTIVE FURNITURE

Today, many patients and family members sitting in waiting rooms use personal mobile devices for entertainment, to review and update personal health information, or to make payments and arrange future appointments.[13,16,19]

Institutions must accommodate this constant interaction via mobile technology—and find ways to utilize the connectivity to their advantage.[13]

When some patients experience slow (or no) Internet access and have insufficient access to outlets for charging personal devices, it causes some frustration within the waiting area.[13,16,19]

By enhancing waiting rooms with connective furniture—augmented with outlets for charging—and a robust Wi-Fi system, patients and their families can experience a new level of comfort and convenience not typically associated with healthcare facilities.[13]

Connectivity should be considered at the very beginning of a project and utilized as a planning resource to help direct the program and, ultimately, the design.

Multiple seating clusters incorporating bariatric seating in a casual and comfortable lounge-like waiting environment that's coordinated with floor outlets to provide power connections can be envisaged.[13,16,19]

HYBRID EXAM/CONSULT MODULES[13,16-19,21]

As technology allows healthcare designers to add or expand options for diagnostic, clinical, and customer services, technology also allows the opportunity to rethink standard spaces to create a streamlined, optimized environment. For instance, careful planning can allow for flexibility between departments; the development of exam/consult modules can eliminate assigned, or physician-specified, rooms, creating overlap between different clinical spaces. This overlap allows the use of a digital scheduling system to flex between available rooms, thus optimizing usage and reducing wait times.

Hybrid exam/consult rooms—interconnecting the adult and pediatric clinical spaces—are designed to increase patient comfort and personalize doctor-patient interaction. Organized into a patient zone and a healthcare provider zone, the system eliminates the need to move a patient to an office with the physical barrier of a formalized desk for the physician. Instead, a "P-top" work surface organizes the doctor, patient, and family members around a wall-mounted screen for information sharing, while caregivers can chart on a portable computer docked on the work surface, allowing them to face the patient and simultaneously enter information.

Staff also has the ability to select specific information to shift onto the patient-doctor shared screen. Connection to the patient's personal folder on the patient portal allows the doctor to easily drop in instructional videos, documents, or other important information that the patient can access later.

EDUCATION ZONES

Education zones dispersed throughout clinical areas can introduce patients to the use of devices that monitor their condition, teaching them how to interpret and utilize real-time device-generated information. As in diabetes care, research, and education, this manifests in technology training rooms and insulin pump education rooms specifically designed to introduce patients to new technologies available to help them as they live with their disease.[16,19,30]

Home scales and glucose monitors connected to the patient portal will update patient records daily and alert doctors of any important issues. Likewise, the information collected from the monitors is well-documented in order to keep the option of retro analysis available to patients and doctors.[16,19,30]

TELEMEDICINE

Current technology enables doctors and patients to connect remotely and share information in a variety of ways, through two-way video, email, smart phones, wireless tools, and more. All classrooms and conference rooms at facility are designed with interactive video conference capability, giving physicians the opportunity to work remotely with patients or provide information to family members, while both callers view the same information on their individual screens.[16,19,30]

These same building resources can be used to enhance a patient consultation by connecting remotely with a specialist at an affiliate institution or by allowing a family member to conference-in on an education session. Additionally, devices that upload information to the patient's records allow the healthcare provider to monitor a patient's progress between visits and can provide an early indication of any alarming developments and conditions.[16,19,30]

However, planning for telemedicine must go beyond current uses to anticipate future applications, such as traveling nurses connecting to doctors in real-time or "robot doctor" specialists incorporated into care facilities.[16,19,30]

ELECTRONIC MEDICAL RECORDS SCANNING ROOM

While electronic medical records (EMR) become the standard, some healthcare facilities are still in transition. Large room with space for EMR scanning equipment and the storage of medical records while this transition is considered. When the scanning is complete, the room is designed to be repurposed. Scanning equipment and files will be removed and replaced with conference furniture and systems to support telemedicine.[16,19,30]

INTERACTIVE FEATURES

Technology can entertain and stimulate while it educates—a critical tool in the planning and design of pediatric healthcare environments, especially. Offering a specialty area for pediatric diabetes, to capture the attention of young patients through an interactive wall in the pediatric waiting area. The overall goal of the installation is to promote movement, an important prevention method for pediatric diabetes patients, through custom-designed interactive games that will be simultaneously entertaining and educational.[13,30]

FUTURE FORWARD

The rapid advancement and pervasive influence of technology has created the opportunity to re-imagine the delivery of healthcare. As designers, we are tasked with the challenge of integrating known technology that will enhance the patient experience in current time while strategizing future technological advancements and possibilities. Our insights, resourcefulness, and ability to visualize physical space with emerging technology will help shape the future patient experience and care model.[1,16,19]

RADIO-FREQUENCY IDENTIFICATION TECHNOLOGIES FOR SMART HOSPITALS[10,11,15,35-41]

Radio-frequency identification is a method for remotely storing and retrieving data using devices called RFID tags or transponders.

The RFID tag is a small object, such as an adhesive sticker, that can be attached to or incorporated into a product. RFID tags are composed of an antenna connected to an electronic chip. These chips transform the energy of radiofrequency queries from an RFID reader or transceiver to respond by sending back information they enclose. Finally, a computer hosting a specific RFID application or middleware pilots the reader and processes the data it sends.

The RFID has great characteristics:

- It is possible to scan tags in motion; and
- Since radio waves can pass through most solid objects, the tags do not need to be in direct line of sight of the RFID reader.

Uses of RFID

- *Patient identification:* Patients admitted to the hospital are given an RFID-based wristband resembling a watch with a passive RFID chip in it. This chip stores a unique patient ID number and some relevant medical information such as the patient's blood type, in order to speed treatment. To ensure patient privacy and to avoid that medical records are improperly disclosed, further medical data are not stored on the devices but are rather stored in a secure database that links the unique patient's ID with its data.

  The caregiver uses a handheld computer with an RFID interrogator (an RFID-enabled PDA) to read the data encoded on the patients ID bracelets. Over a wireless LAN connection, the hospital staff can access the patient's encrypted confidential medical history as well as treatment record and can obtain information on which drugs and what dosages the patients will require.

  Patients will also be able to check their own records by scanning their wristbands using information terminals.
- *Blood tracking:* Each bag of blood at the hospital gets a self-adhesive RFID label. This chip has memory for storing a unique identification number and information on the contained blood type. These numbers are also saved in a secure database containing details about the blood's origin, its designated purpose and, once dispended, its recipient. When a nurse wants to prepare a blood transfusion, she uses a reader-equipped PDA to read the data encoded on the blood bag's RFID chip and on the patient ID bracelet. The data from the patient and the bag must match before the blood can be used. With this solution the overall process of managing blood bags is eased and less time-consuming. Moreover the risk of patients receiving the wrong type of blood is minimized.
- *Smart operating theaters:* In the smart hospital the patients get a RFID-tagged wristband containing relevant information and a digital picture of them. The photograph allows the clinical team to easily confirm they have the right patient, and the electronic record ensures they perform the correct procedure. If the wrong patients enter the operating room, the medical staff is automatically and instantly warned of the mismatch.

  Thus radio tagging makes the operating theater safer and more efficient. Moreover, the risk of litigation resulting from surgery mistakes and the costs they generated should be significantly reduced.
- Anticounterfeiting
- *Tracking equipment, patients, staff and documents:* It is worth noting that, according to a small survey conducted such losses are not so infrequent and may sometimes have bad consequences, both in terms of costs and patients safety. Several documents tracking applications have already been successfully deployed. Most of them lead to a positive ROI (Return on Investment) such as saving man-hours.

  Furthermore, using an asset tracking application within the infrastructure deployed for our smart hospital gives us the possibility to locate and trace staff members as well as patients efficiently. This can help improving the workflow of doctors, nurses and other caregivers. It can also help to locate them in real-time which is especially worthy for huge buildings such as hospitals.

  Additionally, being able to trace all the tagged equipment introduces an efficient and accurate inventory system. Again, a number of corporates have already successfully introduced RFID systems for real-time inventories. The most often cited positive effects are the reduction of assets loss. As an example Metro Group, the world's third-largest retailer, reported a improvement of about 18% in goods loss thanks to the RFID technology. Besides, tagging and tracking equipment offers many other use cases such as finer maintenance scheduling, usage statistics of equipment, placement optimization and fast localization of important material.
- *Avoiding theft of medical equipment:* The producers of medical equipment should embed the tags at the factory (on demand or as a standard), or the hospital should have the ability to tag its assets with hard-to-remove electronic identifiers.

  Wheelchairs are expensive, and technology to keep track of them would be helpful for all medical personnel at a given hospital.

DIGITAL HOSPITALS

More efficient digital hospitals have the potential to drive greater efficiency, improve quality of care and provide access for more people than ever before.[17,18]

Digital hospitals provide faster and safer throughput of patients, creating more capacity through process efficiencies, while containing costs.[17,18]

New hospitals take an average of three to 5 years to build, while existing hospitals that are retrofitted with the prerequisite pervasive, medical-grade networks and multi-modal digital communications can take as long as 5–10 years to completely modernize.

REDUCING ENERGY COSTS IN SMART HOSPITALS[9,25,42-50]

Occupancy sensors for both HVAC and lighting controls all over the building (low-hanging fruit). Temporary occupancy controls to the occupants saves energy and involves them in the energy reduction process.

Lighting

Converting operating rooms, parking ramps and other exterior lighting to LED lighting. Also since LEDs last longer, less time and money on maintenance. Reduce lighting power density. Put day lighting sensors in applicable perimeter zones.

Computer-based building control system to manage constant monitoring, built-in redundancy and a warning system.

Extensive electrical submeter monitoring system that communicates directly with the building automation system.

Zoning

Divide the area into zones with separate controls for cooling/heating as hospital buildings frequently have areas with different time and temperature requirements such as in waiting areas or individual private rooms. A thermostatic radiator valve (TRV) can provide efficient temperature control in areas, which have different usage patterns, such as treatment and consulting rooms.[44,47]

Keep the Heat in

Install automatic doors or a draught lobby, particularly in frequently used building entrances. Where possible, the two sets of doors should have automatic control to increase ease of access and help keep heat in.[44,47]

Upgrade Controls

A compensator is a form of control for heating systems that automatically regulates the cooling/heating temperature based on the weather. An optimum start controller learns how quickly the building reaches the desired temperature and brings the cooling/heating on at the optimum time prior to building occupancy, again depending on the weather.[44]

Maintain System Components

Annual review and replacing parts as necessary reduces the energy consumptions.

Variable speed drives (VSDs) can help to reduce costs by enabling the output speed of the fans to match requirements at different times of the day.[44]

Water Saving Devices[47]

The largest area for potential savings is through the installation of water-conserving devices such as:

- Tap restrictors—these provide equal flow at a number of taps in a washroom and can reduce water flow by 15%.
- Push taps—these only operate when pressed, turn off after a brief time period and are ideal for areas where taps may be left running.
- Shower regulators and water-efficient shower heads— these decrease the volume of water coming out of a tap or shower and can reduce water flow by 20%.
- Infrared controllers—these provide water only when required, switch off automatically and can save between 5% and 15% of water per tap per year.

Switching in Parallel[44]

Wiring the lights so that those closer to the windows can be switched off, while the rest remain on with separate controls enables staff and patients to make the most of natural daylight.

Consider combined heat and power (CHP) or cogeneration systems, which might be viable for many sites (if reliable gas supply is available) that incorporate a laundry.

At a power station, the heat generated when electricity is produced has to be dissipated via cooling towers. With CHP, the heat is recovered on-site, and used for space heating and hot water. This means that overall, the process is more efficient, so less fuel is used.

Heat water recovery sources include incinerator, laundry dryer exhaust, solar water heater, and water recycling.

Motors and Drives

Considerable energy savings can be achieved by good system design to minimize the motor load. A small increase in duct or pipe size can significantly reduce system losses and thus greatly reduce the fan or pump power required. Low-loss motors, variable-speed controls and effective control can realize substantial savings up to 50%.[44] A variable frequency drive can save energy in the chilled water pumping system by controlling the speed of the chiller pump as per the pressure required.[7] More efficient pumps, high efficiency chillers, boilers and water heaters lead to energy savings.

Install More Insulation

Large amount of heat can enter the building through an uninsulated roof, which increase the energy consumption for cooling the space below the roof. Insulating roof (opaque exterior and fenestration) and unfilled external cavity walls is an effective and inexpensive way of saving energy. Energy Conservation Building Code (Ministry of Power, 2007) prescribes U-factor for roof and opaque walls of hospitals (Table 1).[44]

Requirements for energy efficiency in external parts of the building, the building envelope, are generally set based on resistance to heat transparency through a unit of the construction, R-values, or a value for the heat transparency through a unit by a specific temperature, a U-factor or a U-value.[23] In cold climates, low U-values or high R-values prevent heat from escaping from buildings, and in hot climates they

Table 1: Recommendations to achieve energy savings.[19,43]

	Item	*Component*	*Recommendation*
Envelope	Roofs	Insulation entirely above deck	R-25 ci to R-35 ci, depending on climate zone
		SRI	Climate zone 1-3: 78, all other comply with Standard 90.1-2004
	Walls	Steel-framed	R-13 + R-7.5 ci to R-13 + R-21.6 ci, depending on climate zone
	Slabs	Unheated	Comply with Standard 90.1
	Air barrier	Infiltration	0.05 cfm/ft^2 of exterior wall and roof area
	Vertical fenestration	Total fenestration to gross wall area	40% max
		Thermal transmittance	U-0.20 to U-0.43, depending on climate zone
		SHGC—all types and orientations	SHGC-0.26 to SHGC-0.40, depending on climate zone
		Visible light transmittance	VLT-0.63 to VLT-0.69, depending on climate zone
		Exterior sun control (S, E, W only)	Projection factor of 0.5

Contd...

Contd...

	Item	Component	Recommendation
Lighting		Whole building interior LPD	0.88 W/ft^2
	Interior lighting	Occupancy sensors	Installed in applicable zones
		Daylighting	400 lux continuous dimming in applicable perimeter zones
	Exterior lighting	Whole building exterior LPD	2.5 W/ft^2 of exterior first floor façade perimeter
Operating Suite HVAC		Water-cooled chiller	Variable speed, centrifugal, 7.0 COP, 44.0°F outlet temperature
	Central air handling	Cooling tower	Open tower, variable speed cooling tower fan
		Gas boiler	90% efficient condensing boiler, outdoor air temperature reset
	System	Pumps	Variable speed, 80% efficient
		Air-side economizer	Differential enthalpy controlled
		Water loop heat pump cooling efficiency	4.5 COP (15.4 EER) at 86°F
		Water loop heat pump heating efficiency	5.0 COP (17.1 EER) at 68°F
		Water loop heat pump fans	55% efficient, 0.30 inch. WC pressure drop
		Condenser loop water-cooled chiller	Variable speed, centrifugal, 7.0 COP, 86.0°F outlet temperature
HVAC	Water loop heat pump/dedicated outdoor air system	Condenser loop cooling tower	Open tower, variable speed cooling tower fan
		Condenser loop gas boiler	90% efficient condensing boiler, 68.0°F outlet temperature
		Condenser loop economizer	Counterflow waterside economizer
		Condenser loop pumps	Variable speed, 80% efficient
		Dedicated outdoor air system fans	2.0 inch WC reduction over baseline central air handling system
		Dedicated outdoor air system boiler	90% efficient condensing boiler, outdoor air reset
		Dedicated outdoor air system chiller	Variable speed, centrifugal, 7.0 COP, 44.0°F outlet temperature
		Dedicated outdoor air system pumps	Variable speed, 80% efficient, 60 ft WC

(HVAC: heating, ventilation, and air conditioning; SHGC: solar heat gain coefficient; LPD: lighting power density; COP: coefficient of performance; EER: energy efficiency ratio)

prevent heat from entering buildings. U-values or U-factors will typically be given in W/m^2/°C or as Btu/sq ft/°F.[46]

Windows

Methods to improve the efficiency of windows or other glass areas include increasing the layers of glazing to double- or triple-glazing, coating the glass, or filling the space between glass plates with an inert gas or a vacuum to reduce heat transfer. Window frames that position the glass and separate panes also offer the potential for thermal efficiency improvement.[46]

Replacement of butterfly valves by ball/gate valves to control flow of water and routine maintenance could save up to 20% of the energy consumption in pumps operations in the cooling towers.

Regular Check of Building Dampness

Repair of split down-pipes, faulty gutters and leaky roof tiles as soon as an issue becomes apparent must be done.

REFERENCES

1. Ministry of Urban Development (MoUD) G of I. Draft Concept Note on Smart City Scheme [Internet]. 2014 [cited 2015 Oct 2]. Available from: http://india.smartcitiescouncil.com/system/tdf/india/public_resources/Concept-Note-on-Smart-City-Scheme_0.pdf?file=1&type=node&id=2229.
2. Ministry of Urban Development (MoUD) G of I. Smart Cities. Mission Statement and Guidelines [Internet]. 2015 [cited 2015 Oct 2]. Available from: http://smartcities.gov.in/upload/uploadfiles/files/SmartCityGuidelines(1).pdf
3. UK Trade & Investment. India's Smart Cities Programme. The UK offer to build together [Internet]. 2015 [cited 2015 Oct 2]. Available from: *https://www.gov.uk/government/uploads/system/uploads/attachment_data/file/460151/UKTI_-_The_UK_offer_to_build_together__1_.pdf.*
4. www.gov.uk
5. smartcommutepaa.ca
6. The Top 10 Smart Cities On The Planet | Co.Exist | ideas + impact [Internet]. [cited 2015 Oct 2]. Available from: *https://www.fastcompany.com/90186037/the-top-10-smart-cities-on-the-planet*
7. Weiser A. Some computer science issues in ubiquitous computing. Communications of the ACM - Special issue on computer augmented environments: back to the real world. New York, NY, USA; 1993. pp.75–84.
8. Smart Hospital Vision [Internet]. Available from: *http://mackenziehealth.ca/ioht.php?id 598.*
9. Leigh B, Welniak S, Wood A. Energy Efficiency in Historic Residences : A Case Study. 2010;(May). Available from: *http://www.keralaenergy.gov.in/seminars/Hospital/CASE STUDY Suresh BABU.pdf.*
10. Yu L, Lu Y, Zhu X. Smart Hospital based on Internet of Things. J Networks [Internet]. 2012;7(10):1654–61. Available from: *https://pdfs.semanticscholar.org/9ee5/6096afa6ca1c28fac41ce3577ada09b6a2a3.pdf?_ga=2.80211031.194417448.1579774868-631540672.1579774868*
11. Shandi M. Keeping Pace With the Smart Hospitals. Healthcare design [Internet]. 2012 [cited 2015 Oct 2]; Available from: *http://www.healthcaredesignmagazine.com/blogs/shandi-matambanadzo/keeping-pace-smart-hospitals.*
12. www.healthcaredesignmagazine.com
13. Shandi M. Technology-Enhanced Care [Internet]. Healthcare design. 2012 [cited 2015 Oct 2]. Available from: *http://www.healthcaredesignmagazine.com/article/technology-enhanced-care.*
14. dl.acm.org

15. dbpedia.org
16. Evan W. Best of 2014: How to Design A "Smart" Hospital [Internet]. [cited 2015 Oct 1]. Available from: *https://www.himss.eu/sites/himsseu/files/education/whitepapers/IBM%20Digital%20Hospital%20Evolution%20GBW03203-USEN-00.pdf*
17. Services IGB. The digital hospital evolution [Internet]. [cited 2015 Oct 1]. Available from: *https://www.ibm.com/smarterplanet/global/files/whitepaper_-_the_digital_hospital_evolution.pdf*
18. www.himss.eu
19. www.gsifundraising.com
20. Röcker C, Ziefle M, Holzinger A. From Computer Innovation to Human Integration: Current Trends and Challenges for Pervasive HealthTechnologies. In: Holzinger A, Ziefle M, Röcker C (Eds) Pervasive Health. Springer London; 2014. pp.1-17.
21. Magdy SA. Improve Of Healthcare Systems for Smart Hospitals Based on UML and Semantic Web Technology. Greener J Internet, Informatics Commun Syst [Internet]. 2013 [cited 2015 Oct 1];1(2):044–54. Available from: *http://www.gjournals.org/JIICS/JIISC PDF/2013/April/Magdy.pdf.*
22. citeseerx.ist.psu.edu
23. www.eajournals.org
24. www.designhealth.com
25. United States Agency for International Development & Beurea of Energy Efficiency. Energy Efficiency in Hospitals - Best Practice Guide [Internet]. 2009 [cited 2015 Oct 3]. Available from: https://www.keralaenergy.gov.in/files/Energy_Efficiency_in_Hospitals-_Best_Practice_Guide.pdf
26. Stephane Vermeulen. Affordable "Smart Hospitals" For China and the Asia Pacific Market. Design and Health International Symposium Session 3: Innovation in Global Healthcare Infrastructure [Internet]. Beijing; 2014 [cited 2015 Oct 1].
27. Silvis, Jennifer Kovacs. "Colossus of CARE", Healthcare Design, 2015. Publications
28. Jennifer Kovacs Silvis. Colossus of Care: New Parkland Hospital. Healthcare design. 2015;
29. Jennifer S. Using energy reporting software to optimize the environment of care [Internet]. Healthcare design. 2011 [cited 2015 Oct 2]. Available from: https://www.healthcaredesignmagazine.com/architecture/using-energy-reporting-software-optimize-environment-care/
30. Guicheng shen BL. Research on Application of Internet of Things in Electronic commerce. Third International Symposium on Electronic Commerce and Security; 2010. pp. 13-6.
31. Beam, Jim. "Using energy reporting software to optimize the environment of care", Healthcare Design/15417905, 20110901 Publications.
32. Wen H. "RFID, EPC and Things of Internet", RFID Technology and Application; 2009. pp.17-20.
33. Luigi A, Antonio L, Giacomo M, "The Internet of Things; A survey", Computer Networks; 2010. pp. 2787-2805.
34. Zhu H, Yang L, Zhu Q. Survey on the internet of things [J], Journal of Nanjing University of Posts and Telecommunications (Natural Science). 2011;31(1): 1-9.
35. Zhang S, Ding E, Xu Z, Hua G. Part III of lecture of internet of things and sensor mine— characteristics and key technologies of sensor mine internet of things [J], Industry and Mine Automation; 2010. pp. 117-121.
36. Fuhrer P and DG. Building a Smart Hospital using RFID technologies [Internet]. [cited 2015 Oct 1]. Available from: *http://www.vs.inf.ethz.ch/publ/papers/dguinard_06_smartHospital.pdf.*
37. www.vs.inf.ethz.ch
38. www.gmipsoft.com
39. Dominique G. Radio Frequency IDentification: Evaluation of the Technology Supporting the Development of an Assets Tracking Application [Internet]. University of Fribourg, Switzerland; 2005 [cited 2015 Oct 1]. Available from: *http://diuf.unifr.ch/drupal/sites/diuf.unifr.ch.drupal.softeng/files/projects/rfidlocator/download/report_rfid_guinard_unifr.pdf.*
40. Swedberg C. RFID in Healthcare. RFID J [Internet]. 2005 [cited 2015 Oct 1]; Available from: *http://www.rfidjournal.com/articles/pdf?1486.*
41. Dyke H. Study: RFID in hospitals shows ROI promise - Boston Business Journal. Bost Bus J [Internet]. 2004 [cited 2015 Oct 1]; Available from: *https://www.bizjournals.com/boston/blog/mass-high-tech/2004/12/study-rfid-in-hospitals-shows-roi-promise.html*
42. *XcelEnergy. Case study minnesota, Smart Strategy: Regions Hospital Sustainability Team Slashes $1.17 Million in Energy Costs [Internet]. [cited 2015 Oct 2]. Available from: https://www.xcelenergy.com/staticfiles/xe/Marketing/Files/MN-Bus-Cooling-Regions-Hospital-Case-Study.pdf.*
43. Eric B, Daniel S, Andrew P, Shanti P. Large Hospital 50% Energy Savings: Technical Support Document [Internet]. Colorado; 2010 [cited 2015 Oct 3]. Available from: *http://www.nrel.gov/docs/fy10osti/47867.pdf.*
44. Trust C. Hospitals-Healthy budgets through energy efficiency [Internet]. 2010 [cited 2015 Oct 3]. Available from: *https://www.carbontrust.com/media/39216/ctv024_hospitals.pdf.*
45. Laustsen J. Energy Efficiency Requirements in Building Codes, Energy Efficiency Policies for New Buildings. Buildings [Internet]. 2008;(March):1–85. Available from: *http://www.iea.org/g8/2008/Building_Codes.pdf.*
46. business.responsiblebynature.com
47. http://emtindia.net/
48. old.caba.org
49. www.pu-europe.eu
50. www.carbontrust.com

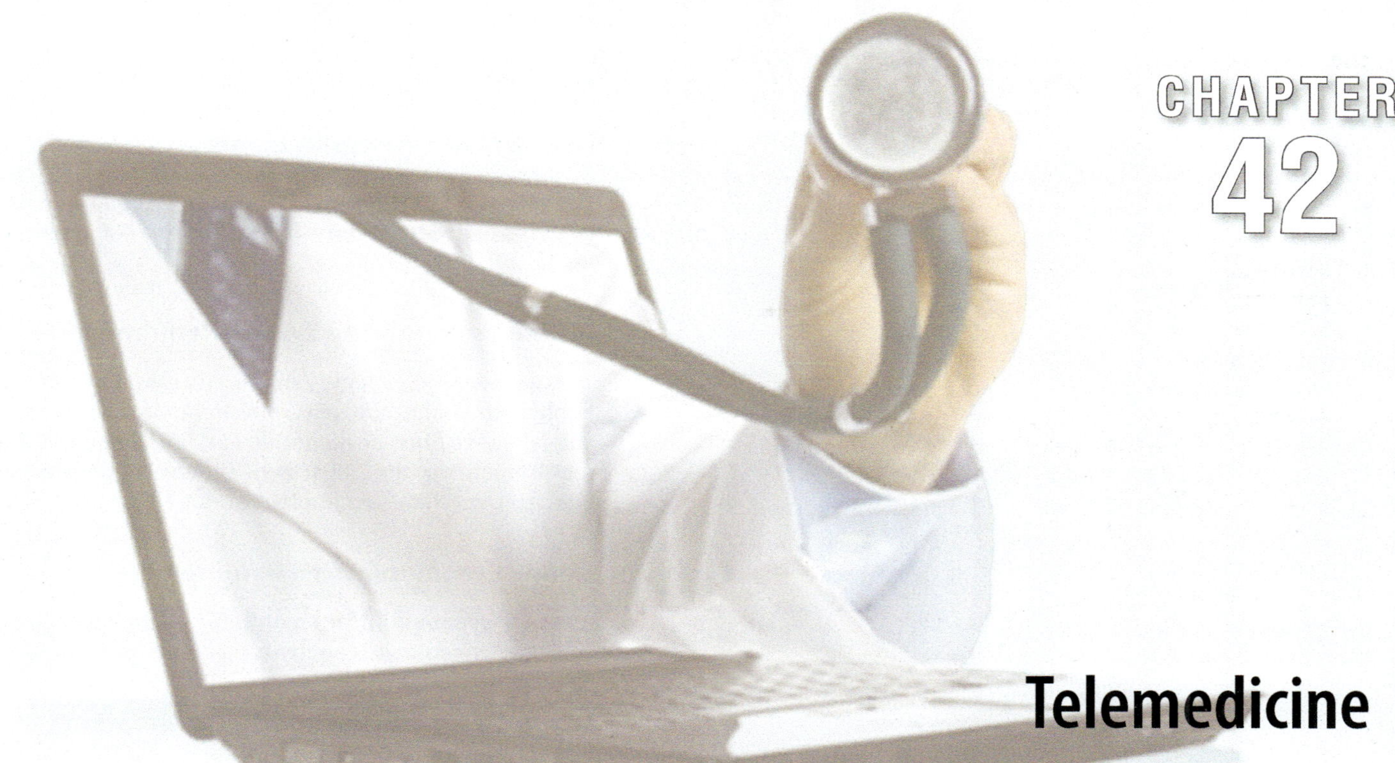

CHAPTER 42

Telemedicine

Rajiv Kumar Pathni, Shakti Kumar Gupta, Sunil Kant, R Chandrashekhar

INTRODUCTION

The importance of access to healthcare in the contemporary world cannot be over-emphasized where this is also a *sine qua non* for economic advancement. Information and communication technologies (ICT) are being increasingly used in the healthcare domain to treat or prevent health problems. Among them is telemedicine (TM), with its extensive potential of new applications aiming to modify the future of healthcare.

Telemedicine is a procedure for extending medical care to patients from a distance using ICT.

The biggest advantage of TM is that it can make healthcare more accessible to the people who are deprived of it because of various barriers—terrain, time, finance or nonavailability of specialties. It has the potential to multiply the reach of healthcare to extend specialist medical services to the "unreached" in rural and remote areas. TM can offer numerous economic and qualitative benefits to patients, physicians, healthcare providers and the community at large.

DEFINITION

The word 'Telemedicine' is made up by the combination of the Greek word "Tele" meaning distance and the Latin word "mederi" meaning to heal; the word "telemedicine" literally translates as, "distance healing".

The World Health Organization (WHO) defines TM as:

"The delivery of healthcare services, where distance is a critical factor, by all healthcare professionals using ICT for the exchange of valid information for diagnosis, treatment and prevention of disease and injuries, research and evaluation, and for the continuing education of healthcare providers, all in the interests of advancing the health of individuals and their communities".[1]

UTILIZATION OF TELEMEDICINE SERVICES

Telemedicine can be applied to almost any medical discipline. So we can have tele-nephrology, tele-neurology, tele-pediatrics, tele-ophthalmology, tele-dentistry, tele-surgery, and so on.

Telemedicine services can be utilized basically in four types of practices:

- Tele-consultation (Figs. 1 and 2).
- Tele-education (Fig. 3).
- Tele-monitoring or telemetry.
- Telesurgery.

The TM services may be provided in three time frames (Box 1).

PLANNING CONSIDERATIONS

Each institution has unique requirements and must determine whether TM can be used effectively in its particular situation. It is important to proceed in a step-wise manner while planning TM services in a healthcare set-up (Flowchart 1).

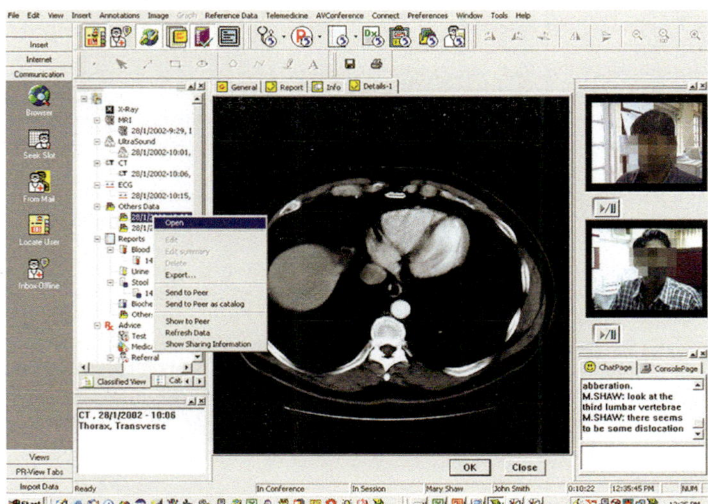

Fig. 1: Real time teleconsultation with a peripheral hospital.

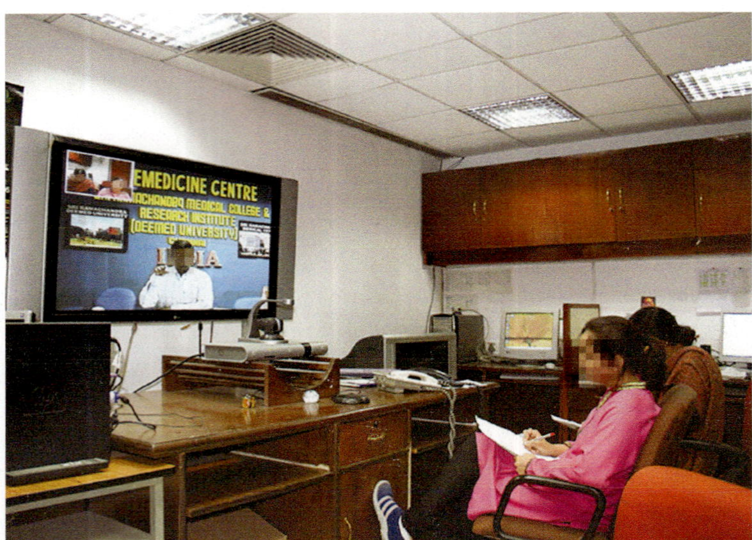

Fig. 2: Telemedicine session.

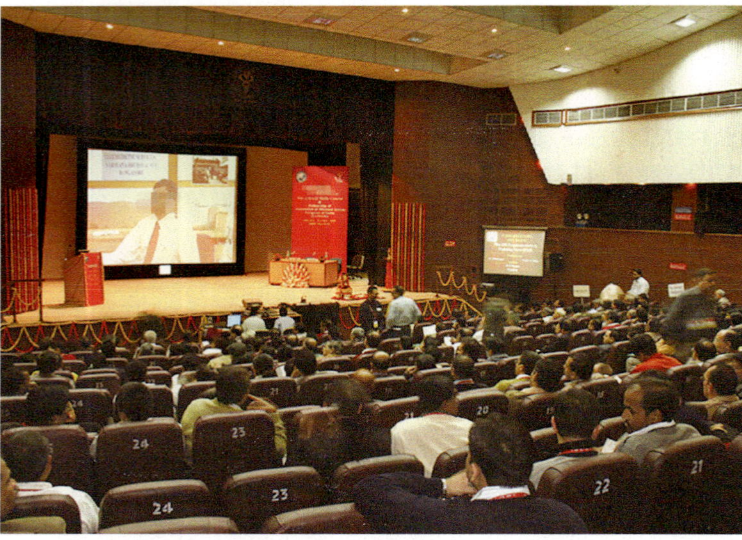

Fig. 3: Tele education: Clinical demonstration during conference using TM.

Box 1: Types of telemedicine.

Telemedicine (TM) services can be provided in three ways:

- *Real-time (synchronous or online mode):* This technology is useful for the transmission of medical image and data as it is being acquired, e.g. video conferencing with attached medical equipments. The system is completely interactive and is especially useful in emergency medical situations
- *Store and forward (asynchronous or offline mode):* In this form of TM, patient's medical data/information (text, audio, images and video) are acquired and forwarded to an expert at another location for his opinion. This technology is less expensive and well suited when a diagnosis may be made in the next 24–48 hours and sent back. It is particularly useful for diagnostic and interpretative services in radiology, pathology and dermatology
- *Collaborative:* This method involves real-time collaboration between the medical practitioner at the remote end and the specialist at hospital on the data that is shared between them. This advanced mechanism allows one side to synchronize its view with that of the other side and also allows one side to interact with data being viewed on the other side

Define Medical Requirements

Before planning a TM system the medical requirements must be stated in terms of TM. One must know how the TM system will be used in the hospital.

Define Telemedicine System Requirements

Telemedicine technology is unique and must be carefully evaluated and implemented. The hardware, software, and system features that are most cost-effective must be identified and implemented. The performance requirements of the TM system should be determined after careful analysis of available technology.

Define Communication Requirements

A variety of communication options are available, and these must be evaluated for cost and capability based on the services to be provided.[2]

Define Telemedicine Space Requirements

Space must be identified and, if necessary, modified to meet the needs of TM. Plans for hospital requirements and necessary modifications must be made and implemented. Personnel must be recruited and trained for the TM operation.

Determining Cost-benefit[2]

In the final analysis, cost is an important factor. Though it has been demonstrated that TM can improve services, a full cost evaluation is necessary during the planning process in order to determine its cost-effectiveness. An ideal or model TM system—one with all the "bells and whistles"—is not necessary to realize significant cost savings. A simple video teleconferencing system is adequate for many TM consultations. Store-and-forward is a good and cost-effective technology, especially for diagnostic requirements or nonemergency implement.

Interoperability, scalability and reliability of the TM network must be assured before it is set-up.

Key Planning and Design Parameters

The TM set-up has to be planned as per its role. Accordingly there are two types of set-ups

1. *Tele-specialist Center (TSC):* Where the specialist is located.
2. *Tele-consulting Center (TCC):* Where the patient is located.

A TM facility at a primary health center (PHC) would be set-up as a TCC whereas that at a secondary or tertiary care Hospital would be set-up as a TSC.

The essential difference between the set-ups is that the TCC would need peripheral clinical devices to capture patient related information whereas the TSC would only need equipment to view and store this information. Thus, the requirements of physical infrastructure, medical equipments and other hardware will depend on the role of the TM facility.

Layout of a TM center, as recommended by ISRO, is placed at Figure 4.

- *Location*: Although TM has no specific requirements as far as location is concerned, the room should be, if possible, located in that part of the hospital which has less traffic and is less noisy.

Flowchart 1: Planning considerations for implementing a telemedicine system.

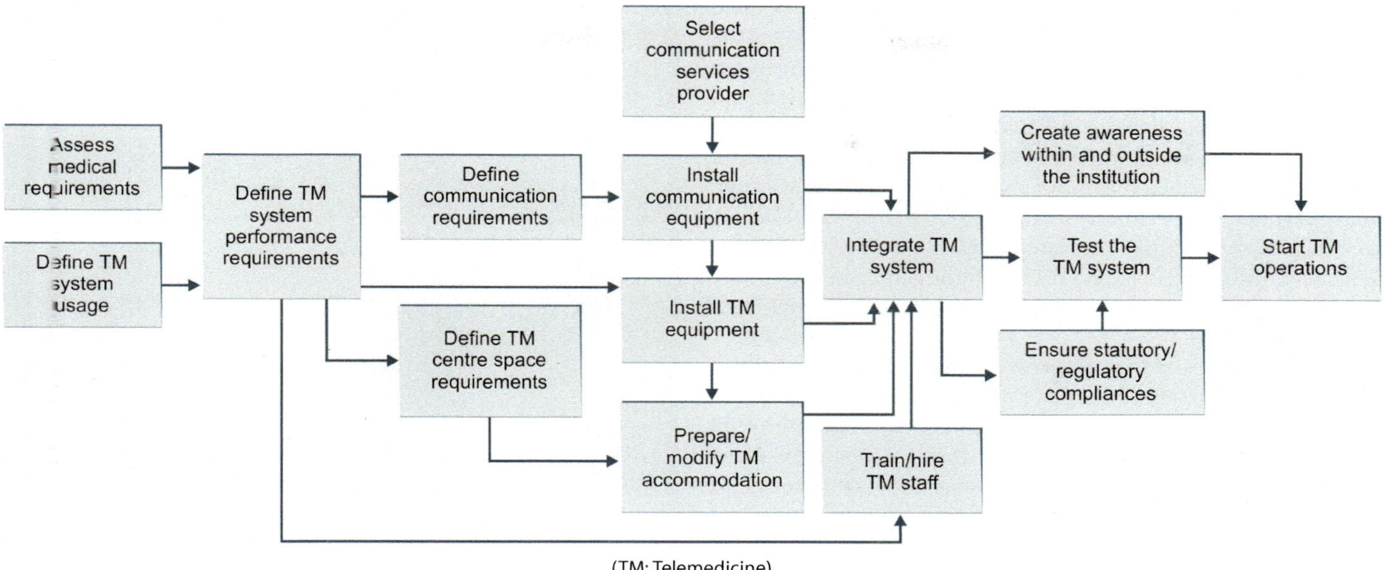

(TM: Telemedicine)

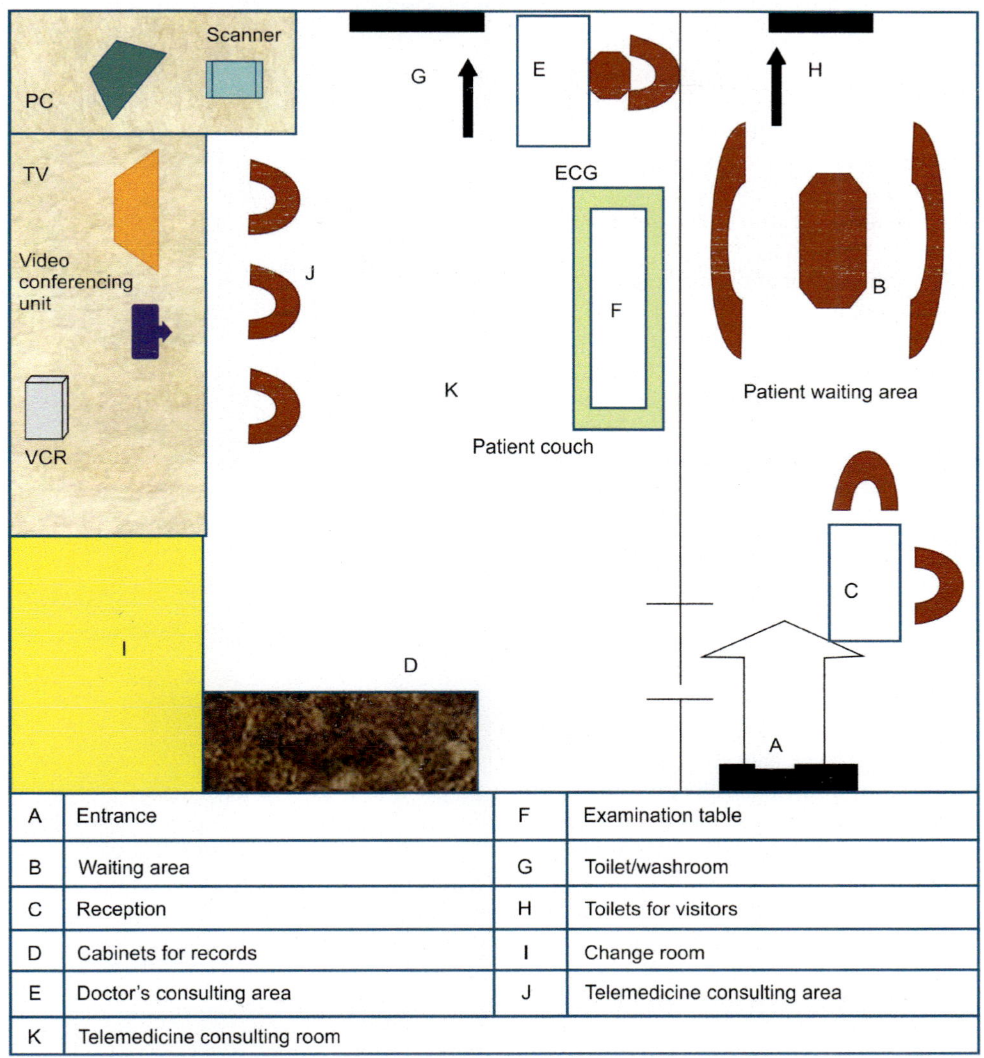

A	Entrance	F	Examination table
B	Waiting area	G	Toilet/washroom
C	Reception	H	Toilets for visitors
D	Cabinets for records	I	Change room
E	Doctor's consulting area	J	Telemedicine consulting area
K	Telemedicine consulting room		

Fig. 4: Layout of a telemedicine center.

- *Room area*: The TM room should have at least 250–450 sq ft carpet area. The actual area required would depend upon the medical equipment that is being planned to be interfaced with the TM set-up.
- The TM room should be sufficiently big to accommodate placement of two computers with 17 inch monitors each, a printer, and connectivity [very small aperture terminal (VSAT) indoor] equipment rack and few chairs. TM room at patient end should be slightly bigger to accommodate medical diagnosis equipment viz. X-ray scanner, pathological microscope, a bed for taking electrocardiogram (ECG). If the video conferencing equipment is also used for continuing medical education, then a bigger room may be required depending on the number of participants and also to accommodate a bigger TV, say 29 inch.[2,3]
- *TSC/TCC Room*: TSC room (Doctor's end) should be at least 12 × 20 ft and TCC room (Patient's End) at least 15 × 30 ft. If the patient side room also has an intensive care unit, then minimum space required for the room is 1500 sq ft. In case of Medical College hospitals, a standard class room size of at least 30 × 50 ft is required with good provision for placement of audio/video system as a virtual classroom.[2,3]
- *Environmental control*: Room temperature should be maintained between 18–25°C, preferably using a split air-conditioner for less background noise during video conferencing.
- *Electrical requirements*: Room should have electrical outlets for connecting various equipment and a very good earthing pit. Five 15 amp sockets for uninterruptible power supply (UPS) and five 5 amp sockets for other diagnostic equipment are advised, with proper arrangement of the power supply during emergency.[4]
- The UPS should be at least of 3 KVA capacity depending on the equipment load.
- *Acoustics*: Sound absorbing panels, for noise free environment during video conferencing.
- *Curtains and walls*: Should be light blue or gray, to give appropriate contrast/view for video-conferencing
- *Flooring*: Room should have good flooring, preferably vinyl or ceramic floor, to reduce noise.
- *Lighting*: Room should have good illumination, to get good picture quality for video conferencing.[2,3]
- *Antenna*: Wherever VSAT is used, antenna size is 1.8 m in diameter for remote end and 3.8 m for specialty end and weight is 500–2000 kg. Ideally the antenna should be located at the top of the building and should be within a distance of 40 m (cable length) from the TM room.[2,3]

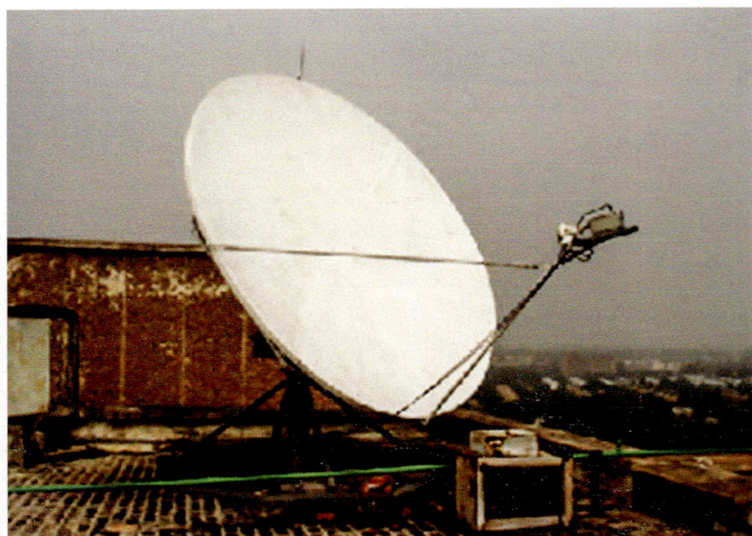

Fig. 5: A 3.8 m Very Small Aperture Terminal antenna (VSAT).

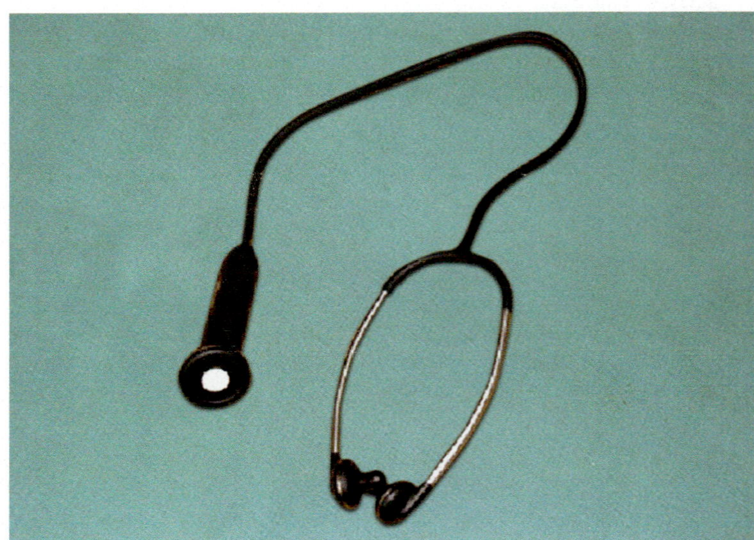

Fig. 6: Electronic stethoscope.

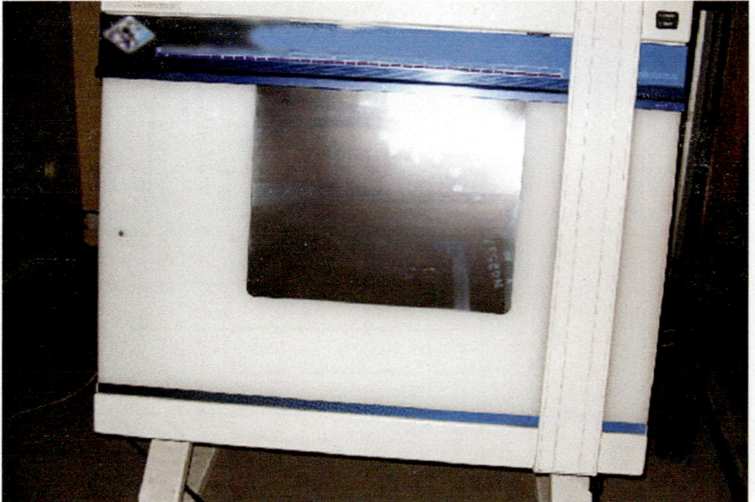

Fig. 7: X-ray digitizer.

EQUIPMENT REQUIRED FOR TELEMEDICINE FACILITY[3]

A wide range of different devices can be used in TM Figure 5 to 7. Essential requirement are devices which can capture and manipulate data so that it transmitted over a communications channel. These equipment can be used in a particular set-up in any combination, according to the availability of the technology and instruments and the requirements of the TM system.

Telemedicine Platform

The hardware platform in most of the TM systems consists of a *personal computer*. The platform can be customised as per the application—mobile, hand held (for wards, ER), fixed - (TM center, home use). The hardware platform can be a laptop or tablet computer, or even a dedicated box (set-top-box) with a processor. The system should support the interfaces as required by the various planned clinical and non-clinical devices.[4]

Clinical Devices

The clinical devices to be interfaced or integrated with the TM system should conform to the minimum parameters (performance specifications for the statutory safety. In addition, all the clinical devices should preferably provide interface to the PC with appropriate software to collect, display, transform and save data provided by the device.[5]

Specialized Medical Equipment

- *Radiology*: DICOM compliant equipment
- *Dermatology*: High resolution digital camera
- *Cardiology*: Digital ECG
- Electronic stethoscope
- Microscope adapter
- Endoscope adapter
- Otoscope adapter.

Almost any conventional equipment can be modified to adopt a digital interface and, hence, be linked to a TM system. Each specialty will need its own specific peripheral equipment. High end Tele-surgery equipment may even include Robotic arms. But the system will be built around the computer and its software.

Video Conferencing Units

Video conferencing units are offered in several distinct configurations with the TM systems. They all consist of a video camera and microphone along with appropriate software. The costs vary according to the capabilities of the equipment. All, except the most basic systems, would incorporate a PTZ (Pan-Tilt-Zoom) video camera which can be remotely controlled from the specialist end to provide views of the subject from any angle and at a desired magnification. A very high resolution camera is usually required to get effective diagnosis in dermatology consultations.[5]

Recommended Standards for Video Conferencing Units[3]

- *Video codec*: H 263, H 263+, H 264
- *Audio codec*: G 711, G 72×
- *Conferencing*: ITU-T, H 32×
- *Frame rate*: 15~25 fps
- *Video output*: Minimum 1 color composite CCIR, PAL-B
- *Signaling*: H 221, H 230, H 231, H 242
- *Data rates*: 64 kbps and above.

Communication Hardware

Connectivity is required to enable the transmission/exchange of diagnostic data/images between TM systems.[4]

Recommended Standards for Communication Hardware

- *PSTN/POTS*: V.34, 33 Kbps and above
- *ISDN*: BRI, 64 Kbps and above
- *LAN/Wi-Fi*: IEEE 802.x, 10 Mbps and above
- *GSM/GPRS/CDMA*: Serial/USB, 9.6 Kbps and above
- *ADSL/Broadband*: Ethernet/USB, 256 kbps and above
- Satellite communication.

Operating System

Several choices of operating systems (OS) are currently available for a PC—different versions of UNIX, LINUX, Windows, Android, iOS etc. The OS should support the minimum platform requirement prescribed by the intended TM system.

Telemedicine Software

The followings functionalities are desirable in the TM software:[4]

- Acquisition of patient-related information
- Storage of the patient information
- Display of patient information
- Transmission of the patient information over a communication link
- Adherence to data-formats, data-exchange standards and security standards.

The following additional capabilities may also be provided:

- Scheduling of doctor appointments
- Capturing of images/document from a scanner/camera
- Capturing of audio/video and other data from the output of the medical equipment and conversion to DICOM
- Conversion from DICOM to non-DICOM formats.

Telemedicine Standards

For exchange of clinical information and diagnostic data like X-ray, CT, ultrasound, etc. between disparate TM systems, the communication should take place using DICOM. For messaging between TM systems HL7 is the recommended standard.[5]

Digital Imaging and Communications in Medicine (DICOM): It is a standard in the field of medical informatics for exchanging digital information between medical imaging equipment (such as radiological imaging) and other systems, ensuring interoperability. Distinct from various general-purpose graphical formats, DICOM file offers a very good, diagnostic quality of the image.

Health Level 7 (HL-7): It is a protocol for electronic data exchange between healthcare institutions, particularly hospitals and between different computer systems within hospitals. It defines the format and the content of the messages that applications must use when exchanging data.

PROTOCOLS FOR TELECONSULTATION

The technical working group for TM standardization (Ministry of Communications and Information Technology) has recommended seven different protocols for Teleconsultations in India.[4]

Protocol 1

The protocol given below is of the store and forward type whereby the patient information is first transmitted and the expert opinion is given later.[4]

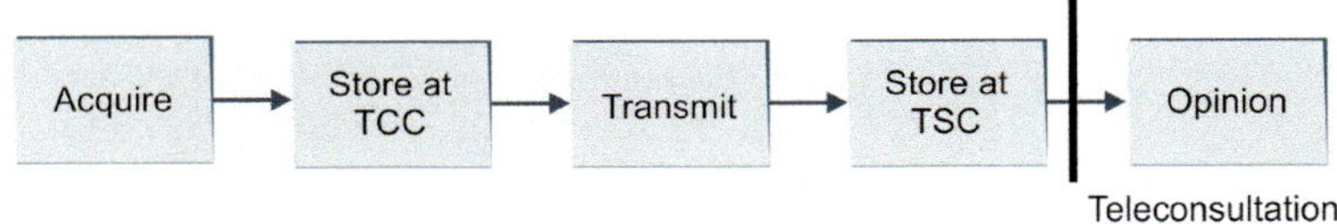

Protocol 2

The protocol given below is of the store and forward type but the transmission of the patient information is done during the Teleconsultation and the specialist gives his expert opinion.[4]

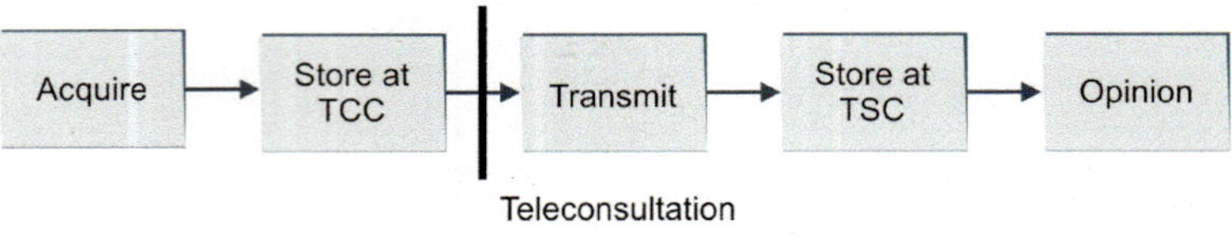

Protocol 3

The protocol given below is a combination of store and real time where the patient information is not stored at the TCC but is straightaway transmitted to the TSC where it is stored and then the Teleconsultation takes place and the expert opinion is given.[4]

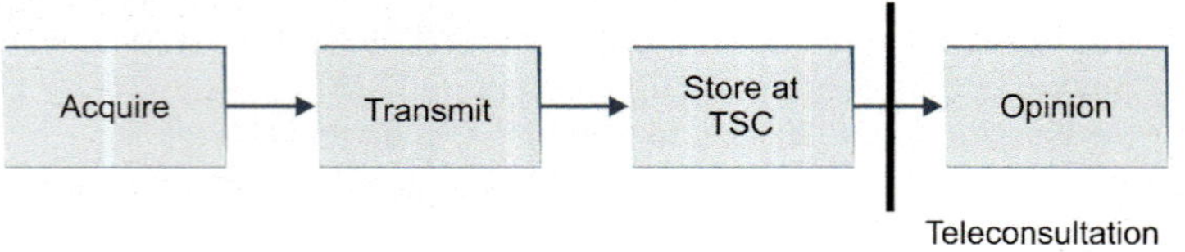

Protocol 4

The protocol given below is real time where the patient information is acquired, transmitted to the TSC during the Teleconsultation and then the expert opinion is given. In this TM process, the workflow begins only during the Teleconsultation. All the necessary functions like the acquisition of patient information, transmitting to the TSC, storing at the TSC and the expert opinion is during the time of Teleconsultation. The patient's live images (CT scan, Doppler, ultrasound, etc.) are being transmitted on a real time basis.[4]

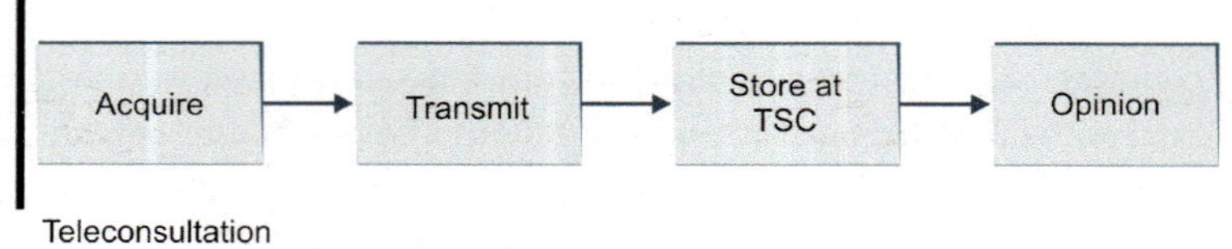

(TSC: tele specialist center; TCC: teleconsulting center)

Protocol 5

The protocol given below is real time where the patient information is acquired, stored, transmitted to the TSC and stored at TSC during the Teleconsultation and then the expert opinion is given. In this TM process, the workflow begins only during the Teleconsultation. All the necessary functions like the acquisition of patient information, storing of patient information at TCC, transmitting to the TSC, storing at the TSC and the expert opinion is during the time of Teleconsultation. The patient's live images (CT scan, Doppler, ultrasound, etc.) are being transmitted on a real time basis.[4]

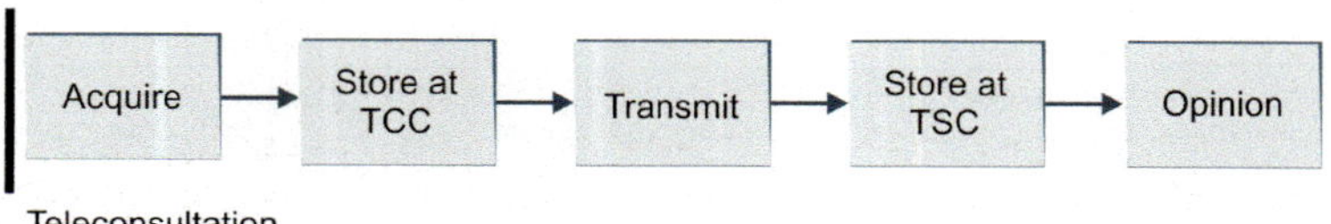

Protocol 6

The protocol given below is real time where the patient information is acquired, stored, transmitted to the TSC during the Teleconsultation and then the expert opinion is given. In this TM process, the workflow begins only during the Teleconsultation. All the necessary functions like the acquisition of patient information, storing of patient information at TCC, transmitting to the TSC and the expert opinion is during the time of Teleconsultation. The patient's live images (CT scan, Doppler, ultrasound, etc.) are being transmitted on a real time basis.[4]

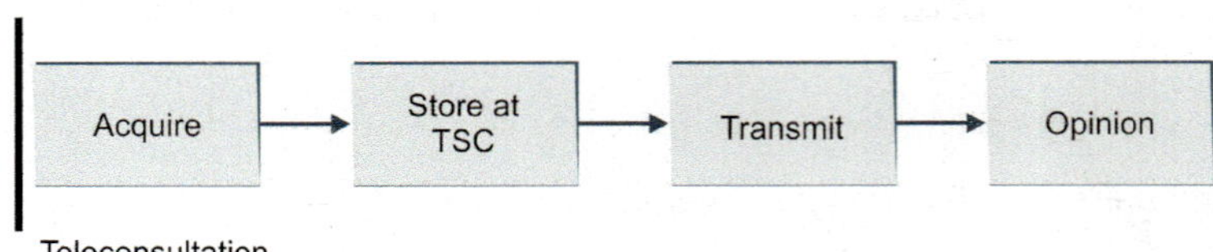

Protocol 7

The protocol given below is store and forward but the Teleconsultation commences after the acquisition of the patient information at the TCC and the storage at TCC, transmissions done during the Teleconsultation and finally the expert opinion is given.

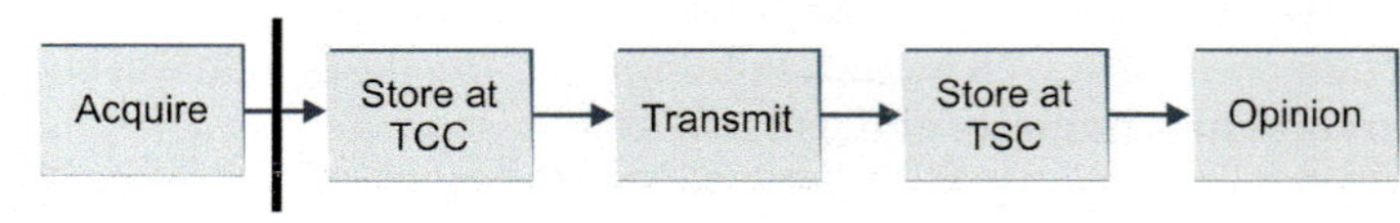

SPECIAL ATTENTION: PRACTICE OF TELEMEDICINE

As the practice of TM is fundamentally an integration of 'the practice of medicine' with 'information & communication technology', all the existing laws relating to both 'medicine' and 'IT' would *pari passu* apply to TM. This would include principles of medical ethics, including professional norms for protecting patient rights, privacy and confidentiality and digital security of patient data. It is also incumbent on the practitioners of TM to maintain the complete digital trail and documentation of consultation including the log / record of interaction, patient records & reports, prescriptions, etc. just as required for in-person consultations.

Telemedicine Practice Guidelines, 2020, issued by the Ministry of Health and Family Welfare (available on the website https://www.mohfw.gov.in) provide detailed guidelines for practice of TM in India.[5]

CONCLUSION

Telemedicine has the potential to revolutionize the practice of medicine through its reach, the potential for long-term savings by eliminating some hospital referrals, prolonged hospital stay and by reducing transportation costs. The use of appropriate technology can help bridge the gaps to reach the "unreached", i.e. the rural masses.

REFERENCES

1. www.ilntoday.com
2. www.ukhfws.org
3. laico.org
4. https://meity.gov.in/
5. https://www.mohfw.gov.in

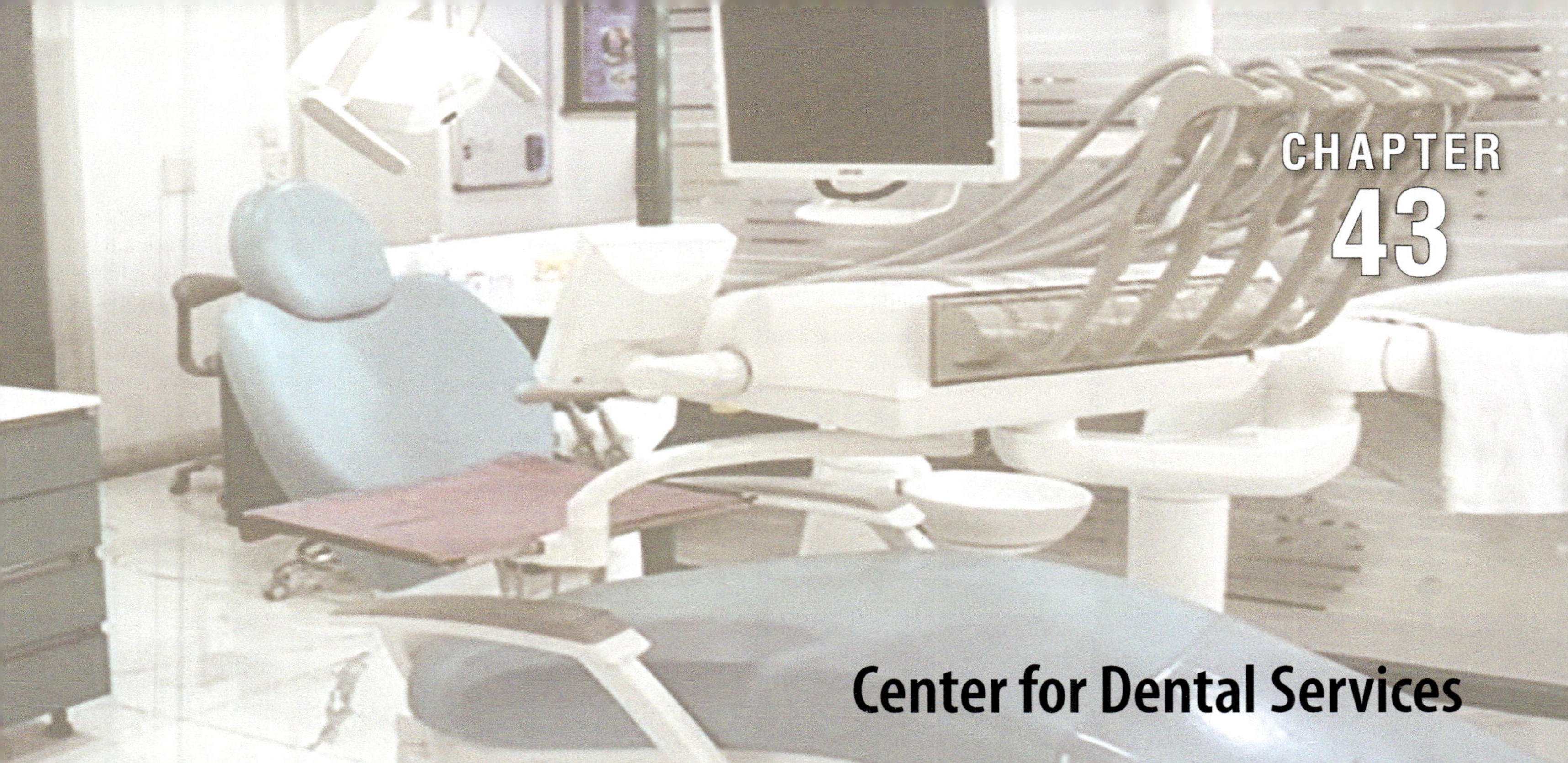

Center for Dental Services

Pawan K Singh, Balakrishan Jayan, Shakti Kumar Gupta, Sunil Kant, R Chandrashekhar

INTRODUCTION

Establishing a multispecialty dental services requires careful planning in order to ensure optimum functionality with respect to patient care and ergonomics. Myriad of problems may be overcome by proper planning. A multispecialty dental clinic is a setting with examination, treatment services with respect to all clinical dental specialties for various age groups factoring any kind of medical condition. They are proposed to be integral to a hospital-based facility. A hospital-based multispecialty dental clinic should have more than one dental operatory/chair and their layout with support services can vary. The dental facility in a hospital setting should cater to out-patient services and inpatient access to hospital-based units.

PLANNING ASSUMPTIONS

Infrastructure planning for a dental treatment facility in a hospital setting would depend on the kind of dental treatment services planned. If the facility is envisaged to provide only emergency and essential services for outpatient and in-patients of the hospital, half of dental chair/operatory may be planned with support areas like reception, waiting area, staff room, wash rooms, lab, dental radiology. In such a facility the treatment procedures that may be imparted would include dental extractions, fillings/restorations, root canal treatment, denture repairs, abscess drainage, scaling, etc. most of them listed are general dentistry services. The staffing requirement would be one/two graduate dental surgeons, dental hygienist, dental assistant, housekeeper and a clinical staff. A sample layout is represented vide Figures 1A and B.

Specialty dental center in a superspecialty hospital setting—dental surgeons do not work in isolation. They have to work closely with other medical and surgical specialists for the larger benefit of the patients. Oral health is organic to general health and wellbeing of the individual. Specialty dental center should have the capacity to deliver the following:

- General dentistry services
- Contemporary orthodontic care including surgical orthodontics, cleft orthodontics, dental sleep medicine.
- *Oral and maxillofacial care*: Procedures which can be executed under local anesthesia would be performed in the specialty dental center integral to the superspecialty hospital. Maxillofacial surgery can be performed in operation theater integral to the hospital. The intensive care unit (ICU) of the hospital can be leveraged for the patients. A dedicated 5% of the inpatient beds should be ear marked for the maxillofacial cases. The nursing support and ICU care should be provided from the hospital resources.

  The capacity of the maxillofacial team of the hospital should be to optimally manage:
  - Dental and maxillofacial trauma
  - Severe odontogenic infections
  - Odontogenic nonodontogenic cysts and tumors affecting the maxillofacial region
  - Orthognathic surgery
  - Pediatric maxillofacial cases including cleft surgeries
  - Cranioplasties
  - Access osteotomies to facilitate neurosurgeon and ENT surgeon
  - Maxillofacial implantology.
- Periodontics, periodontal plastic surgeries and dental implantology
- Dental and maxillofacial prosthesis
- Conservative dentistry and endodontics.

The layout for a specialty dental center in a superspecialty hospital can be multiple dental chairs/operatories with dedicated staff managing each of them or it can be three or more chairs with visiting specialists depending on the workload. It is always desirable to have dedicated full time specialists in the field of oral and maxillofacial surgery, periodontology and implantology, conservative dentistry and endodontics and orthodontics to facilitate prompt consultations among specialists and to facilitate the much desirable interdisciplinary approach to practice of contemporary clinical dentistry.

Each specialty is to be equipped with equipment pertaining to the specialty in addition to common equipments. Dental practice involves usage of biomaterials for restorative procedures, prosthesis, orthodontic bonding and various synthetic bone graft materials.

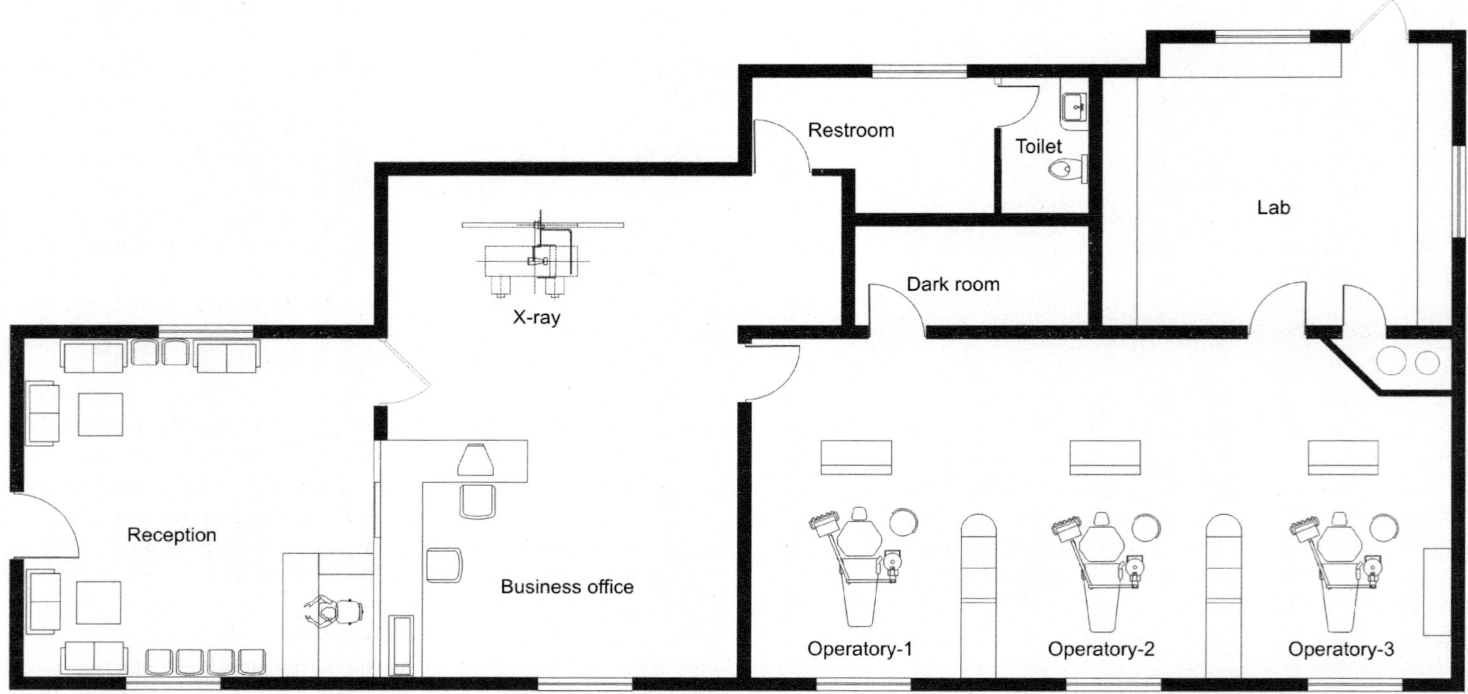

Fig. 1A: Sample layout of dental department in a hospital with 3 chairs (open layout).

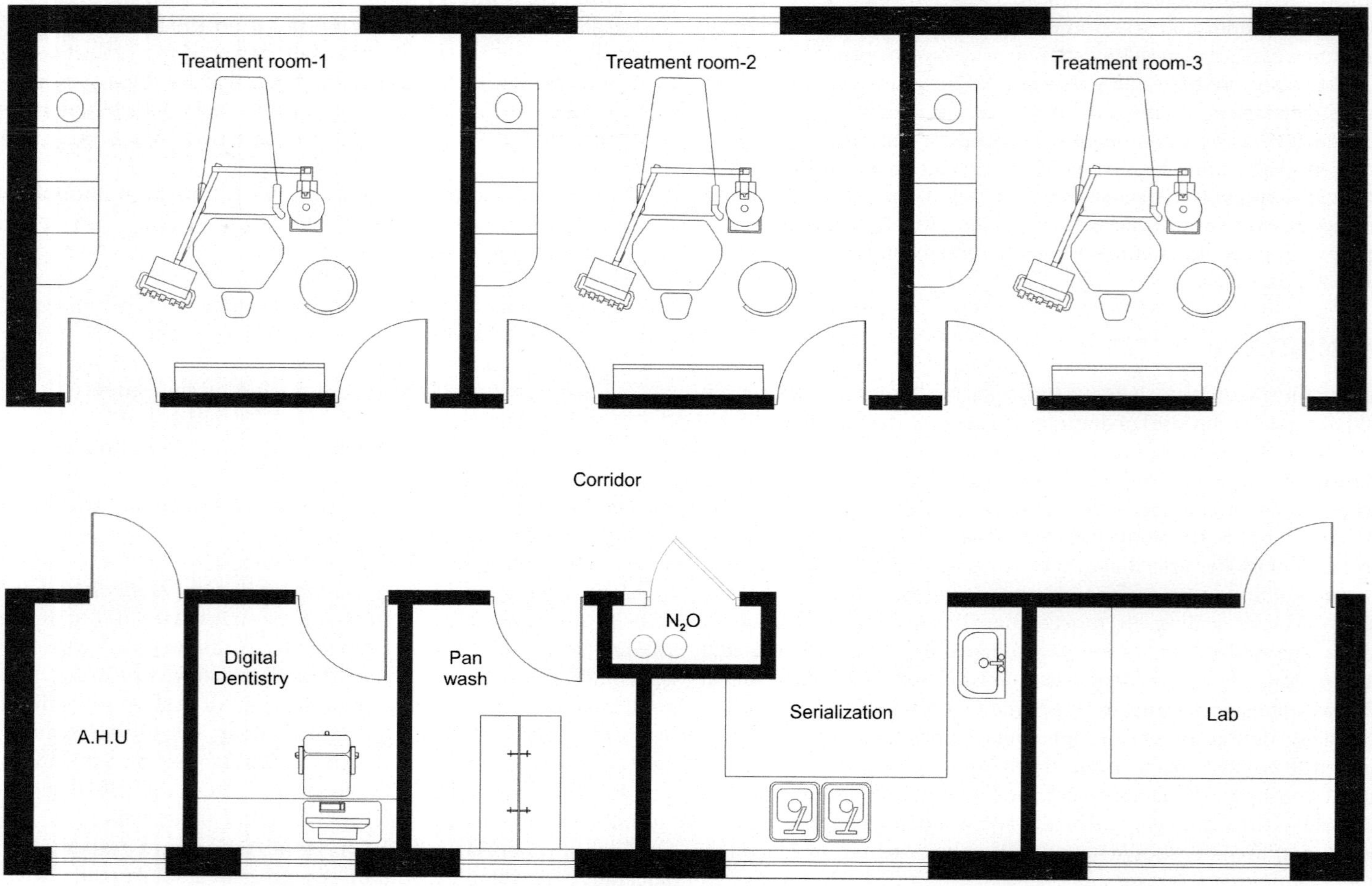

Fig. 1B: Sample layout of dental department in a hospital with 3 chairs (closed layout).

The layout of the specialty dental clinic may be a open layout in a large room divided by modular cabinetry (open concept) or each operatory can be housed in a separate room (closed concept). There are advantages and disadvantages of each design. The major issues are as follows:[1]

- Walls offer more patient privacy.
- Walls reduce noise level in the clinic, which is important when treating young children.
- Operatories with walls are slightly less expensive as less cabinetry is needed.
- Walls do not allow the sharing of X-ray which increases the cost of equipment if the ability to take X-rays is provided to each operatory (a pass through for the X-ray head can be done but you lose privacy and noise control).
- Walls decrease mobility between operatories which can decrease efficiency.

The planners can consider premanufactured cabinetry or cabinetry can be custom-build. Some sample layouts for multiple chair specialty dental clinic is represented vide Figures 2 to 5. These figures are just for an idea of basic appreciation, however various modifications can be considered depending on the other requirements. Photographs of dental operatory in rooms (enclosed concept) and open layout in large rooms (open concept) is represented vide Figures 6 to 8. A single closed surgery can be integrated with open layout to leverage the advantages of both.

The ibid fixed facility in a superspecialty hospital may have four forms of construction:[1]

- *Conventional*: All constructions take place on site.
- *Modular*: The building is fabricated at a plant and pieces are shipped on the site and joined together on the foundation.

  Modular construction is when a building is constructed off site and shipped from construction site (factory) to a location where it is used. Before shipment of the building, the foundation for it is laid and all utilities are run to site. The manufacturer then completes building on the site. If such a methodology is finalized, the manufacturer is given all specifications of the dental equipment, including brands of the equipment, so that the structure can be built to accommodate the selected equipment.[1]
- *Addition to existing structures*: Space is added to a building to allow for clinic expansion.
- *Renovation of an existing structure*: When considering renovation, it is important to keep in mind that there are a lot of utilities with specific locations in the dental clinic. This will require at least a crawl space to run the wiring and pipes that are needed for the dental unit. If the building is of concrete slab, trenches will have to be cut on the floor or false floor will have to be planned. A false floor for dental clinics is best as it gives easy access to utility lines in the event of repairs.[2]

Multispecialty dental clinic should be designed in such a way that, accessibility to people with disabilities is factored.[1]

Ergonomics is an important consideration when planning and designing a dental clinic. Ergonomics is the study of the problems of people adjusting to their environment, especially the science that seeks to adapt work or working conditions to suit the worker. Dental professionals are prone to work-related musculoskeletal injuries involving neck, shoulder, wrist, elbow, hand and lower back. If the dental clinic is designed correctly, including the lighting, the risk of these work-related injuries can be minimized.[1]

Nuances of Dental Operatory Layout[1]

The specialty dental clinic layout must be based on the type of dental chair and equipment brand selected for the clinic. It would be prudent to seek the inputs of the dental supply company or the dental original equipment manufactures (OEM) from whom the dental equipment is going to be purchased.

The operatory design must be followed to the inch during the construction phase with all utilities placed to the indicated locations otherwise efficacy may be affected. Construction oversight by a dental supply company or a person experienced in dental clinic/office construction would be beneficial to ensure equipment compatibility with design and optimizing functionality.

Administrators and hospital planners must be familiar with following terminologies when considering a specialty dental clinic in a superspecialty hospital:

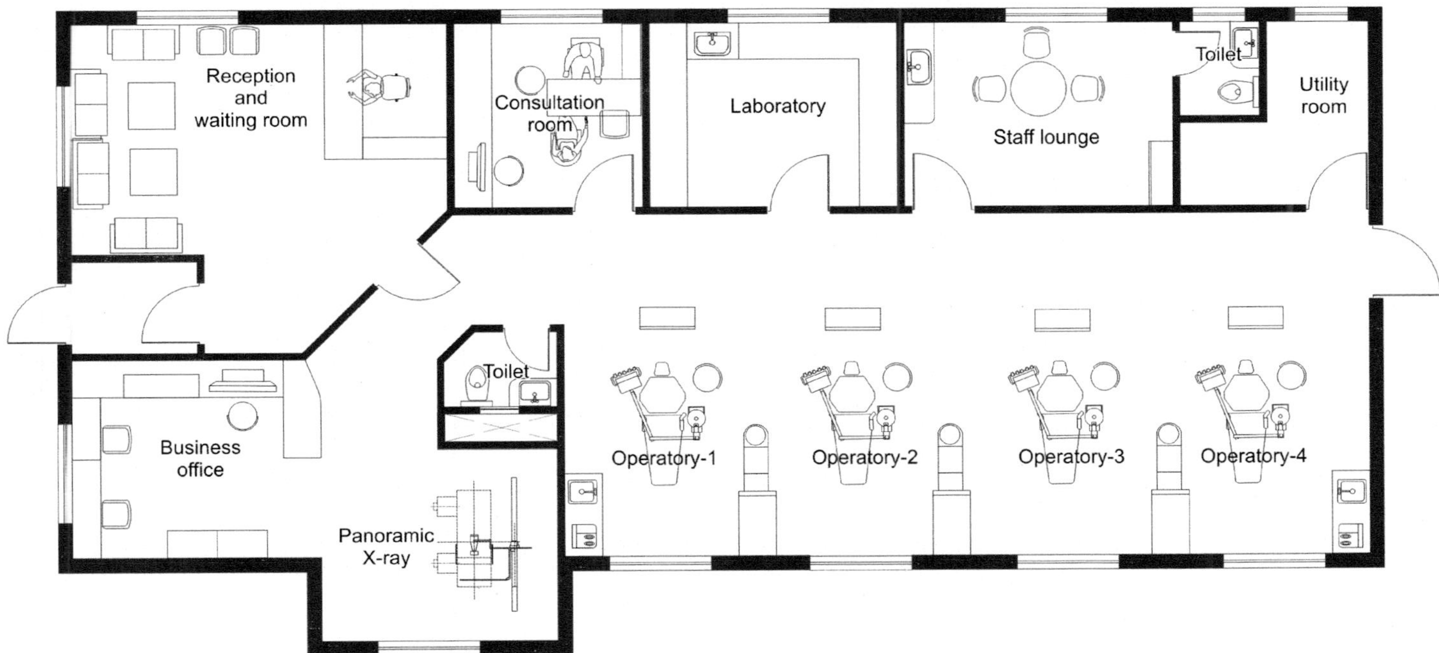

Fig. 2: Sample layout of dental department in a hospital with 4 chairs (open layout).

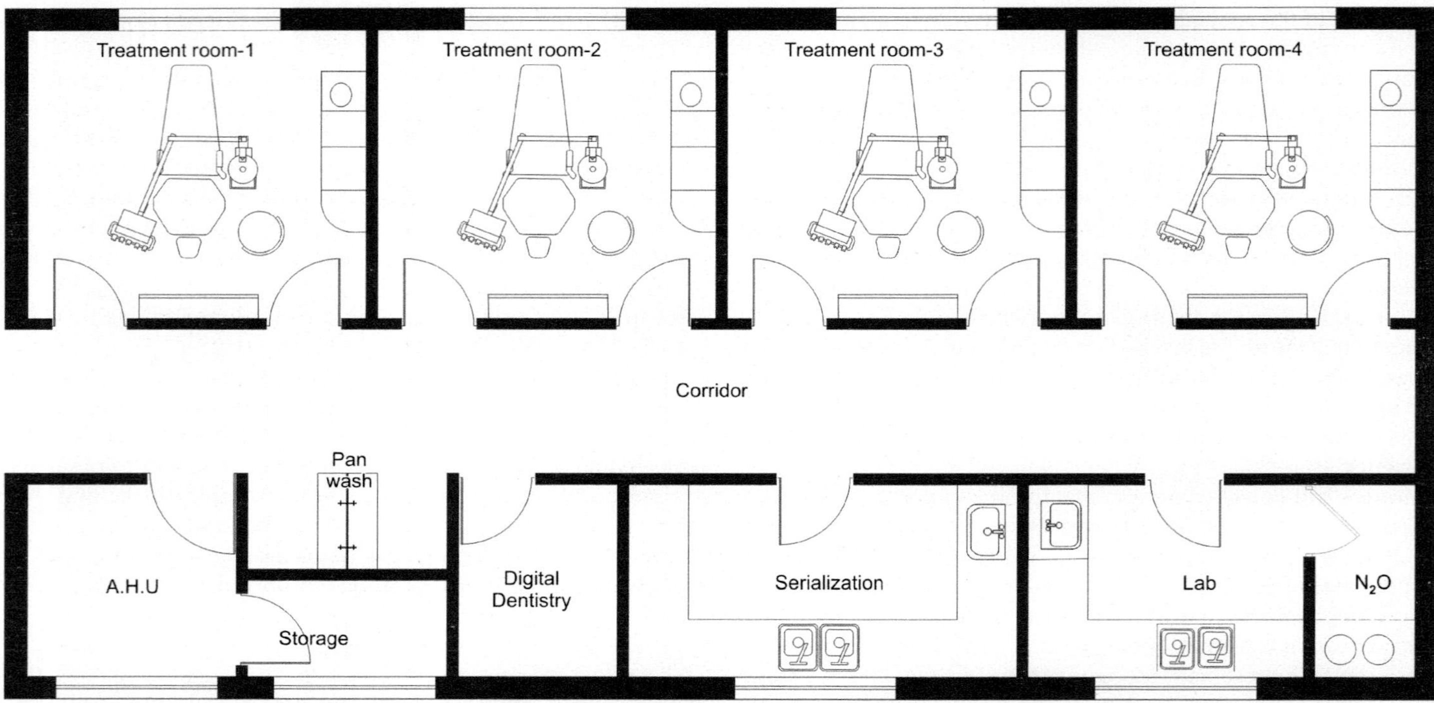

Fig. 3: Sample layout of dental department in a hospital with 4 chairs (closed layout).

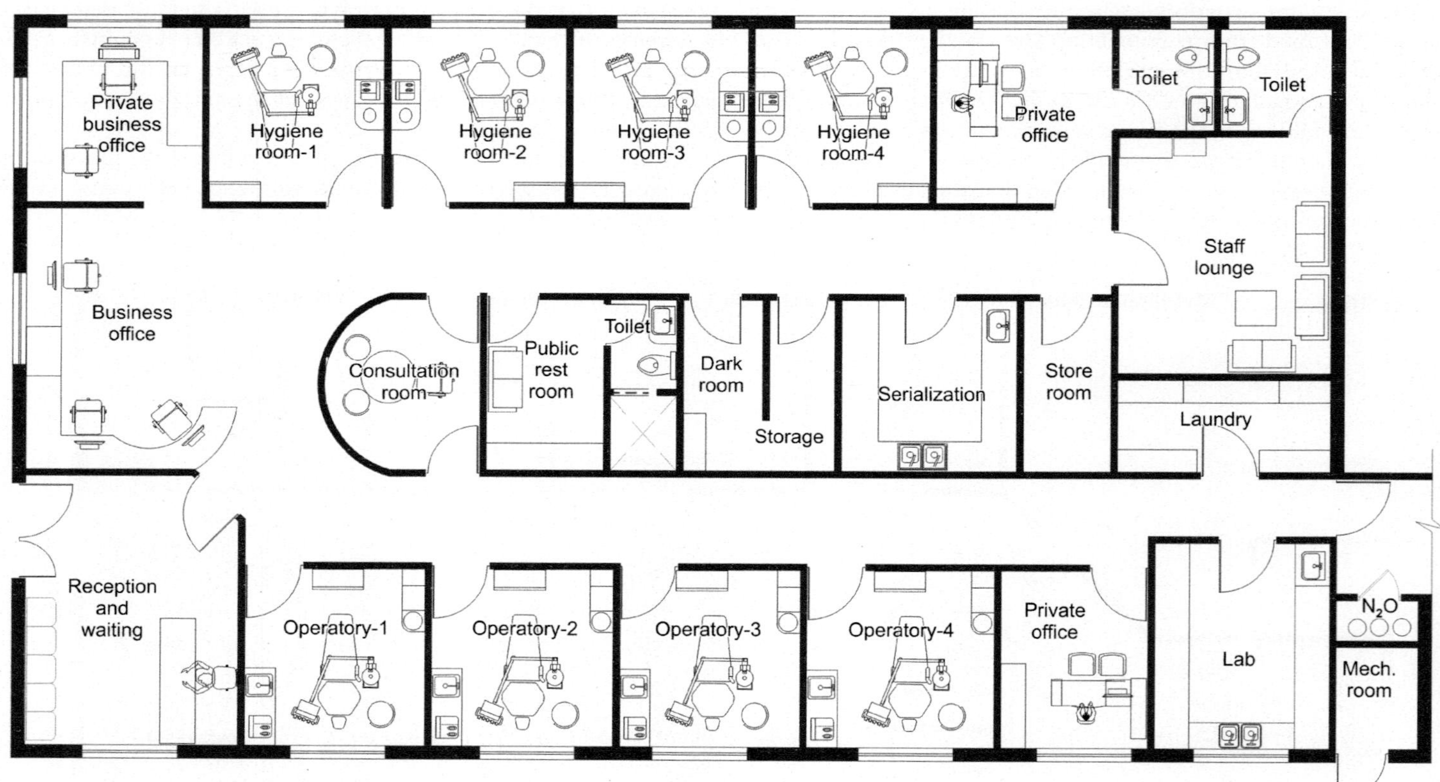

Fig. 4: Sample layout of dental department in a hospital with 8 chairs (closed layout).

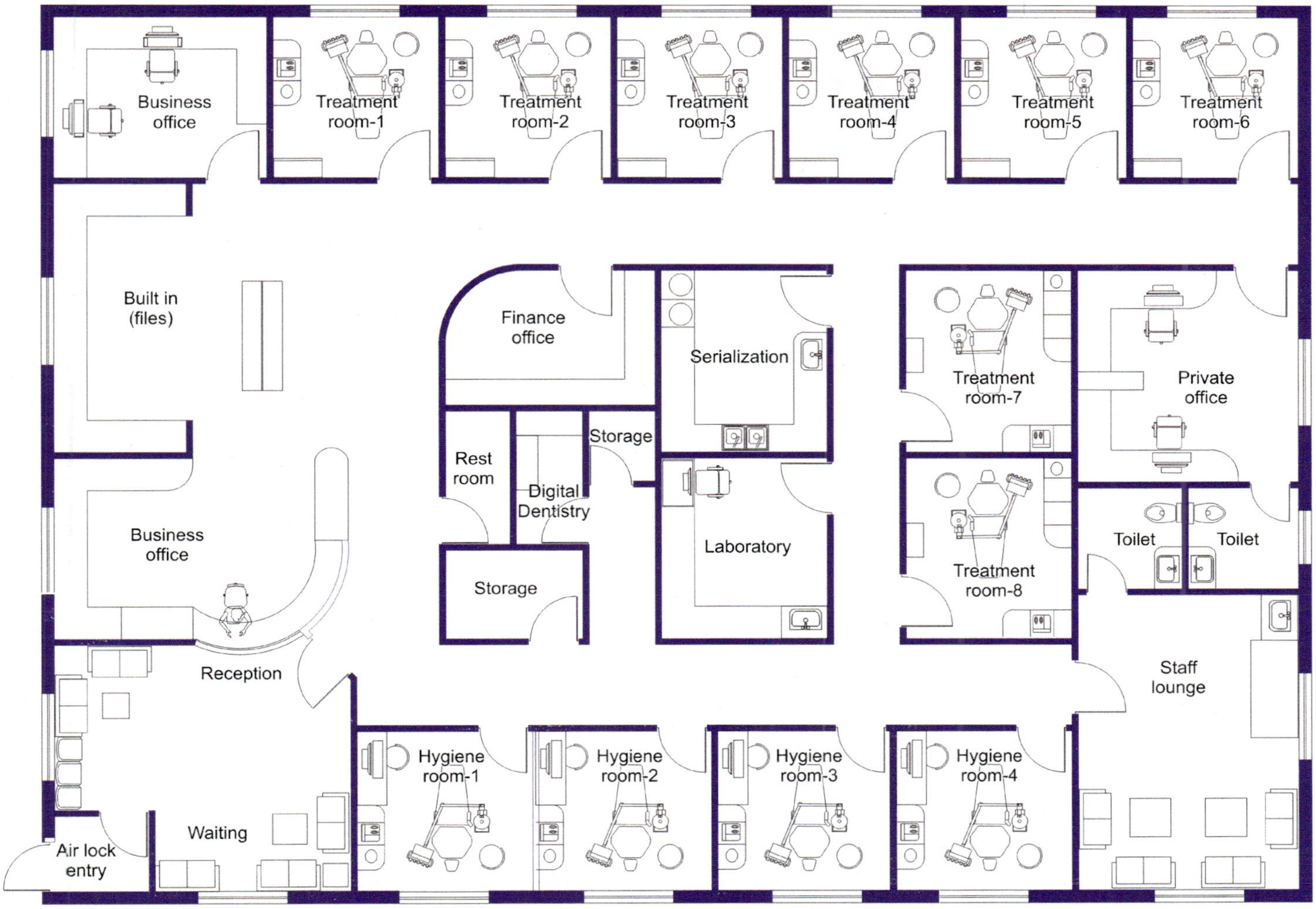

Business office
Treatment room-1
Treatment room-2
Treatment room-3
Treatment room-4
Treatment room-5
Treatment room-6
Built in (files)
Finance office
Serialization
Treatment room-7
Private office
Rest room
Digital Dentistry
Storage
Laboratory
Business office
Toilet
Toilet
Treatment room-8
Storage
Reception
Staff lounge
Hygiene room-1
Hygiene room-2
Hygiene room-3
Hygiene room-4
Waiting
Air lock entry

Fig. 5: Sample layout of dental department in a hospital with 12 chairs (closed layout).

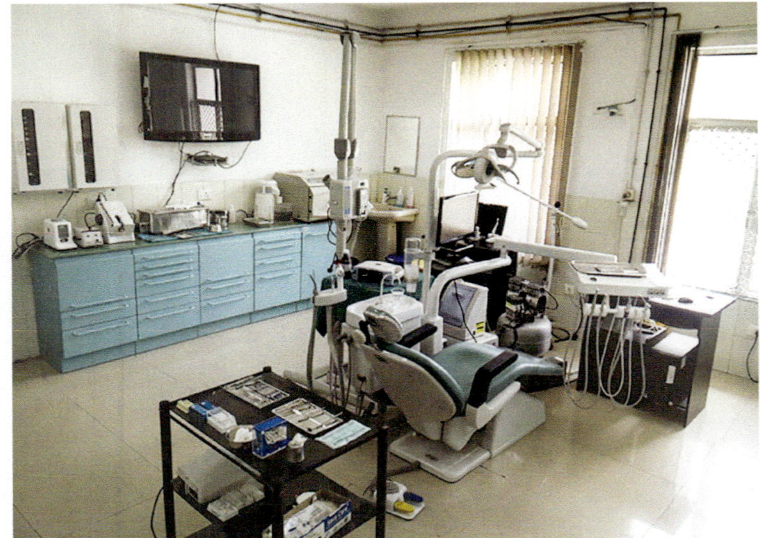

Fig. 6: A Compact dental surgery (closed layout).

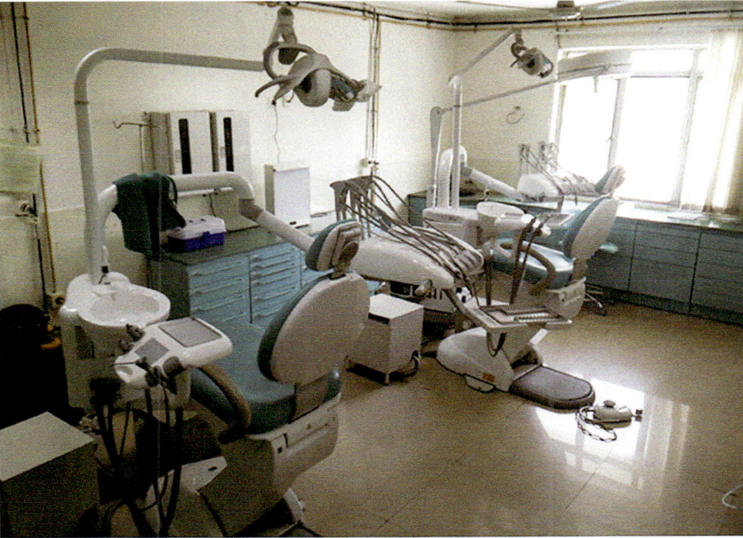

Fig. 7: Two compact dental surgical units housed in a room (open layout—ideal for training).

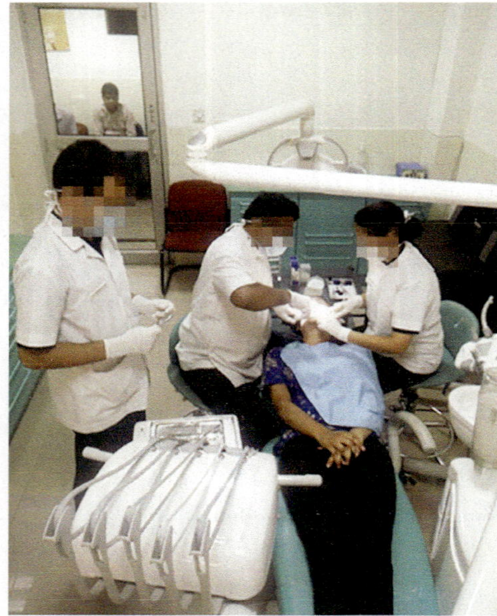

Fig. 8: Six-handed dentistry being practiced in a dental surgery (closed layout).

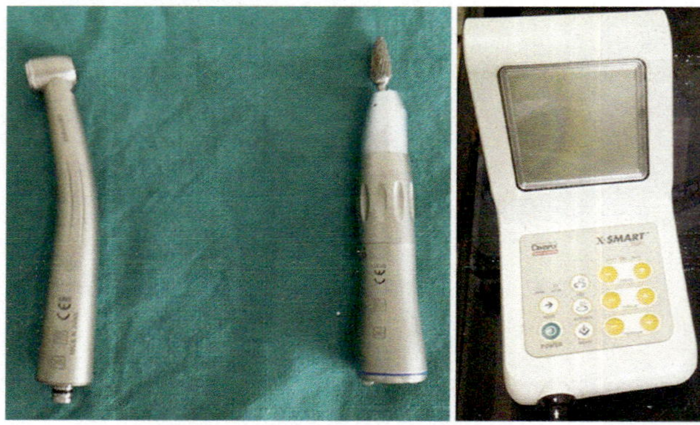

Fig. 9: Dental handpieces are one of the crucial equipment for quality care.

- *Chair*:[1] The adjustable seat in which the patient receives treatment. Dental chair is hydraulically or electrically operated by foot controls or touch key pads. They can be positioned at every possible angle from fully upright to fully reclined. The major functioning of the chair is to seat the patient, so that the dental specialist is comfortable, unobstructed access to the oral cavity from all angles. In dental terminology the dental surgeon, dental hygienist and dental assistants sit on the stools. "Chairs" refer strictly to dental clinics.
- *Delivery unit*:[1] Refers to powered instruments used by dental surgeons. The instruments (handpieces) are attached to movable platforms by flexible tubes containing air, water, fiberoptic and electric lines. It is also called control units. The control unit can be located at the side, at the rear or mounted on dental chair itself.
- *Handpiece*: An air powered or electrically powered rotary instrument used by dental surgeon for cutting and polishing operations. Handpieces are fitted with a wide range of tips and are available in high and low speeds depending on the requirement of the job (Fig. 9).[1]
- *Junction box*: The termination point for all the utilities (compressed air, fresh water, electricity, central vacuum system and drains) needed to operate dental equipment in the treatment room.[1]
- *Operatory*: It is the dental treatment room. The basic dental operatory contains dental chair, stools for dental surgeon/assistants and work surfaces for surgeon and assistant and a wall mounted X-ray. A PC is integral to contemporary dental clinic which can be mounted on the support arch of the chair for data entry and radiovisiography (RVG) (dental X-ray) viewing (Fig. 10).[1]

The dental clinic facility layout design should support effective and efficient provisioning of specialty oral health services. The following outcomes merit consideration:[2,3]

- Capacity to comply with relevant laws, bylaws and standards.
- Safe, hygienic building
- Capacity to achieve accreditation to an appropriate level.
- Innovative, stimulating responsive environment for patients and staff.
- Flexibility for future change
- Maximum energy efficiency
- Accessibility to disabled persons
- Capacity to support the development and retention of high quality staff to meet the needs of the patient.

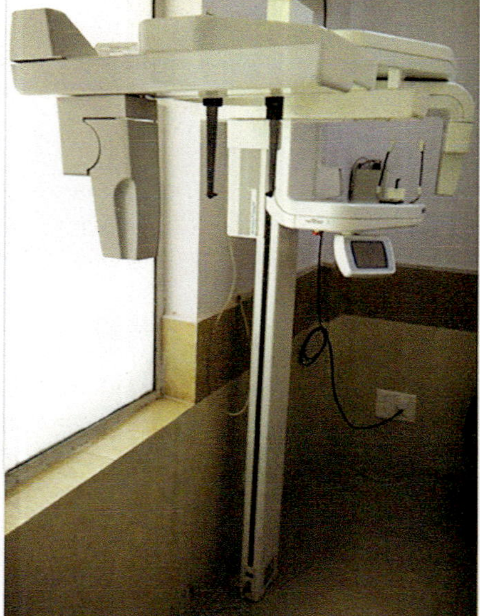

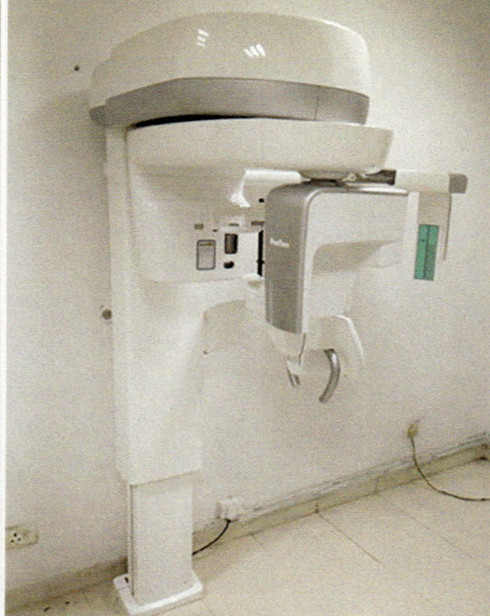

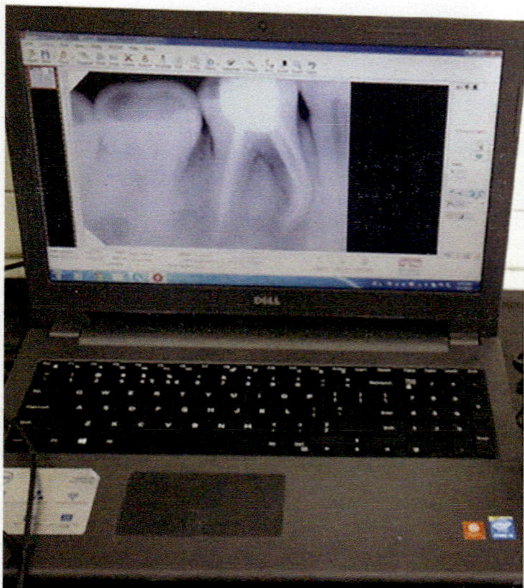

Fig. 10: Ortho pantomogram (OPG), dental cone-beam computed tomography (CBCT) and radio-visiography (RVG) are essential imaging facilities for contemporary standard of care.

Dental and Maxillofacial Imaging

Digital dental radiography is the most suitable and crucial for contemporary dental practice. The imaging facility should include orthopantomography, cephalograms and dental CBCT (Cone-beam computed tomography). The later is crucial for practice of dental implantology, airway imaging, assessing maxillofacial traumas and surgical impactions. The facility should be housed in a room as per specifications of AERB.

SUPPORT AREAS FOR A SPECIALTY DENTAL CENTER

Support areas are integral to any specialty dental clinic for efficiency, comfort and functionality.

- One of the key support areas is the common area for the reception/front desk operations (Fig. 11), waiting and washroom facilities for patients, support areas for staff (staff room, tea and coffee machine facilities and washroom facilities). The waiting area should facilitate waiting of two and half times the number of chairs. This is a rough guideline.
- *Plant room/dental manifold room*: The manifold room should be located at a distance from the specialty dental clinic. The manifold room normally houses the central compressor for compressed air and vacuum. A five horsepower (HP) compressor for 2–3 chair facility and 10–15 HP for more than six chair facility is recommended. A filtration and reverse osmosis facility to treat the waste liquid collected by central vacuum is desirable prior to final disposal. The biodental waste collection area can be integrated with manifold room or can be colocated.
- *Instrument processing and sterilization*: Central sterilization facility with multiple table top autoclaves and instrument processing facility (cleaning, drying, packing, sterilization) can be housed in a dedicated closed room.
- *Stores*: Facility of storing dental biomaterials, hand instruments and expendables should be factored in the infrastructure.
- *Linen store*. The requirement and type will depend on the type of the dental facility.
- *X-ray processing*: Contemporary dental and maxillofacial imaging is more towards digital images, so a processing room is not mandatory however, has to be factored if radiographs are manually processed or may leverage the facilities of the radiology department of the hospital.
- *Dental laboratory*: Dental laboratory service is a specialized service requiring an infrastructure to have acrylic work, metal casting, ceramic processing, CAD-CAM, etc. It would not be prudent to have the same in a hospital setting as the lab support can be outsourced to empaneled labs and moreover, it may not be cost-effective to house a dedicated lab due to huge overheads and committed manpower. However, lab support for repair of dentures, appliances, model making must be factored in the layout.

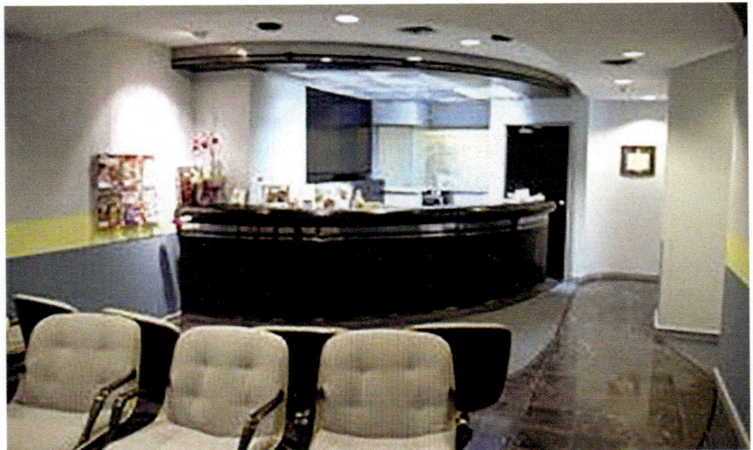

Fig. 11: Reception and waiting.

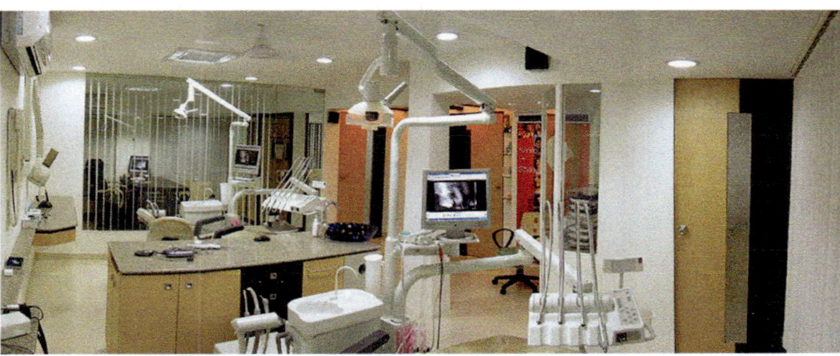

Fig. 12: Component of dental center cosmetic.

Information Technology

Dental charting and treatment data is a vital record for treatment planning, quality control and assurance, legal and forensic document. The multichair specialty dental clinic should adopt one of the contemporary dental management software. The reception, store, dental radiology and all the clinics should be connected by local area network (LAN) and integrated to main server of the hospital. RVG and digital radiology should be considered for easy transfer and storage of images. One of the basic administrative functions of dental patient care is scheduling of patients. The front desk must have the capacity to optimize scheduling of patients to different specialty and operatory depending on the laid out norms and dental chair productivity laid out by the management.

Medical Emergency and Patient Recovery Room

A dedicated room with emergency tray, oxygen delivery, hospital bed, oxygen concentrator, pulse oximetry should be factored to cater to medical emergencies in the dental practice.

Dental surgeons are completely integrated to their work environment/operatory. To treat patients, dental surgeons require a dental chair with extensive instruments and equipment. The electrical and plumbing services are crucial to facilitate water source at the dental chair, compressed chair, suction, water lines and electrical power. The compressor and suction pump create phenomenal amount of noise which is not desirable in a clinical setting; hence have to be kept away. The room configurations are crucial, hence architect dental surgeons and hospital administrators should collaborate to plan the premises.

CONCLUSION

A modern dental center has evolved as a multifaceted, complex and a multidisciplinary facility including cosmetic dimensions (Fig. 12). It is essential that synergy between the infrastructure and processes is done to optimise the available resources.

REFERENCES

1. www.dentalclinicmanual.com
2. www.healthfacilityguidelines.com.au
3. www.moh.gov.ae

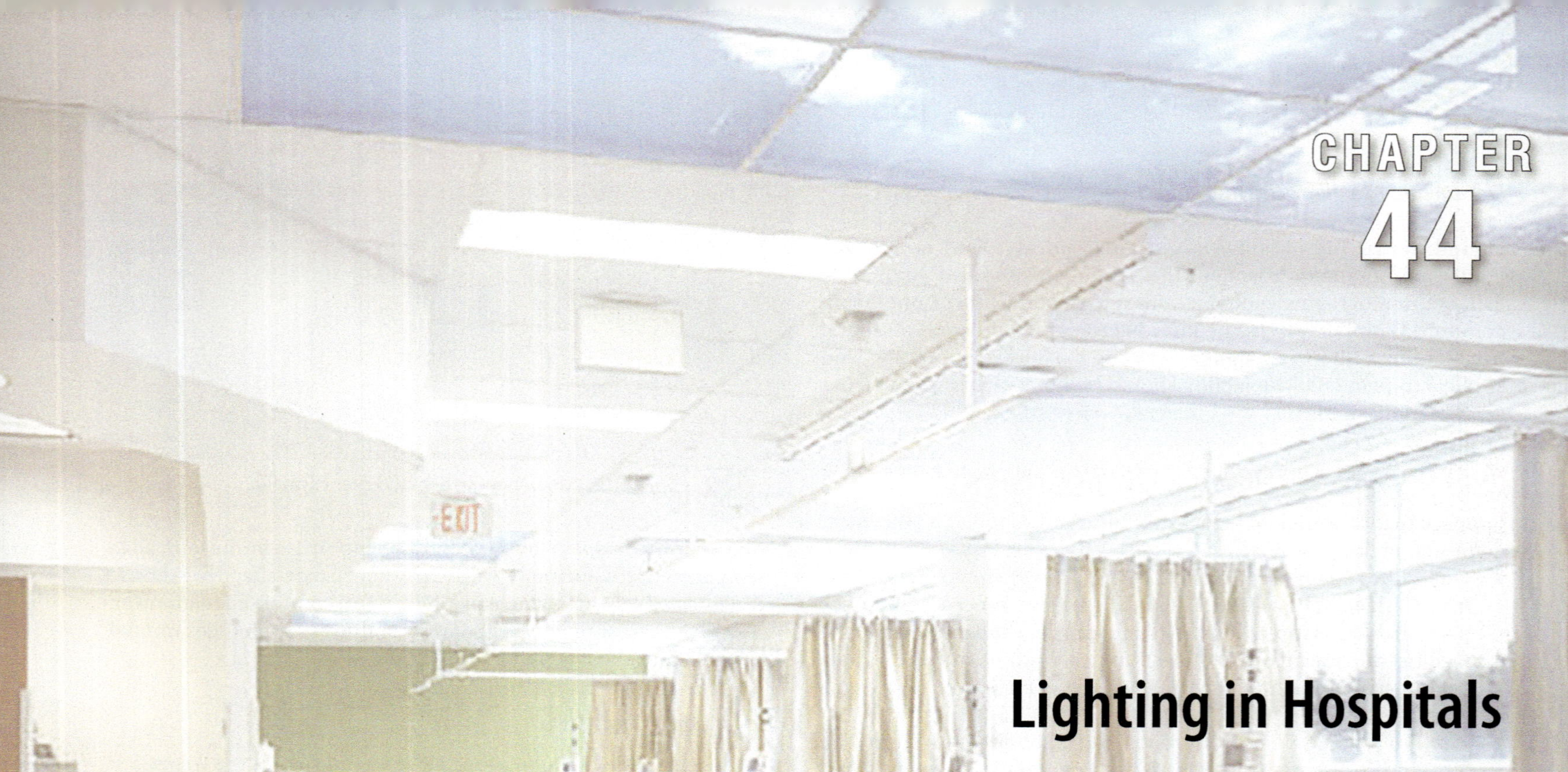

Lighting in Hospitals

Neeraj Garg, Sunil Kant, Shakti Kumar Gupta, R Chandrashekhar

INTRODUCTION

Lighting is of critical importance in hospitals. An adequate level of lighting is essential for clinical, diagnostic and other processes in hospitals. Lighting also has an important impact on operational cost of the hospital. Carefully designed lighting can transform the appearance of a space, making it attractive, welcoming and either restful or stimulating depending on the effect created. It can enhance the architectural appearance of the space and contribute to orientation and way finding.[1,2]

Every modern hospital consists of many components serving diverse functions. They may be patient caring areas or nonmedical areas, like offices, kitchens, laundries and libraries and may be lighted in the same way as those found in industry or commerce. There are also many specialized interiors, like operation theaters (OTs), clinics, treatment rooms and wards, where special lighting techniques and fittings will be required to achieve the desired standard of lighting, hygiene, electrical safety, reliability and ease of maintenance.[2,3]

Provision of a good lighting system calls for coordination from the initial stages among the various parties concerned, namely, the architect, the medical consultant and the illumination engineer. Therefore, it is essential that information regarding lighting should be exchanged between the parties from the stage of planning to installation.[2]

COMMONLY USED TERMINOLOGY IN LIGHTING (FIGS. 1 AND 2)

- *Lumen (lm):* SI unit of luminous flux. It is the unit of total light output from a light source. Typical indoor lamps have light output ranging from 50 lm to 10,000 lm.[3]
- *Lux (lx):* SI unit of illuminance. Illuminance produced on a surface of area 1 m^2 by a luminous flux of 1 lm uniformly distributed over that surface.
  lux = 1 lm/m^2
- *Luminaries:* A complete lighting unit consisting of a lamp or lamps together with the housing designed to distribute the light, position and protect the lamps, and connect the lamps to the power supply.[4]
- *Lumen/Watt ratio:* Amount of light emitted per wattage of electricity consumed by a light source. Light-emitting diode (LED) lights have high lumen/watt ratio as compared to other sources of light.
- *Glare index:* The unified glare rating (UGR) as a quantitative measure of glare. There are computer- based formulas to calculate the glare index. Recommended glare indices are given in Table 1 and 1A.
  Thus, the glare index is directly proportional to luminance of the luminary and size of the luminary and inversely proportional to background luminance and position index of the luminary.
- *Compact fluorescent lamps:* The new rare earth activated phosphor technology has led to the development of a growing variety of single ended lamps known as compact fluorescent lamps (CFLs). The lamps were originally designed to be interchangeable with conventional 25–100 W incandescent lamps, but now this lamp type includes sizes and colors to replace conventional fluorescent lamps in smaller luminaires.[3]
- *Light-emitting diodes:* LEDs are semiconductor diodes, which are electronic devices that permit current to flow in only one direction. The diode is formed by bringing two slightly different materials together to form p-n junction. In a p-n junction, the 'p' type contains excess positive charge , while the 'n' type contains excess negative charge. When a forward voltage is applied to the semiconducting element forming the p-n junction, electrons move from the 'n' area toward the 'p' area and holes move toward the 'n' area. Near the junction, the electrons and holes combine. As this occurs, energy is released in the form of light that is emitted by the LED. Illuminance produced by 5 W of LED is comparable to 15 W CFL. Thus from energy conservation point of view, LEDs are more energy efficient as compared to CFLs.[5]
- *Incandescent lamps:* An incandescent light globe is an electric light with a wire filament heated to a high temperature, by passing an electric current through it, until it glows with visible light.

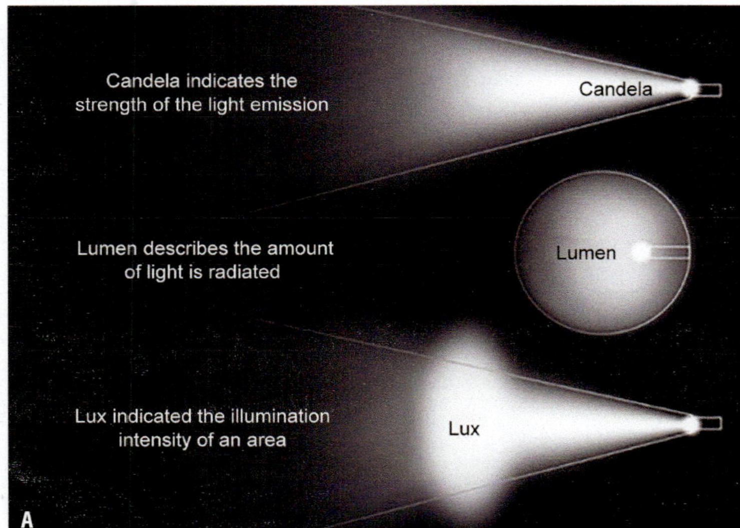

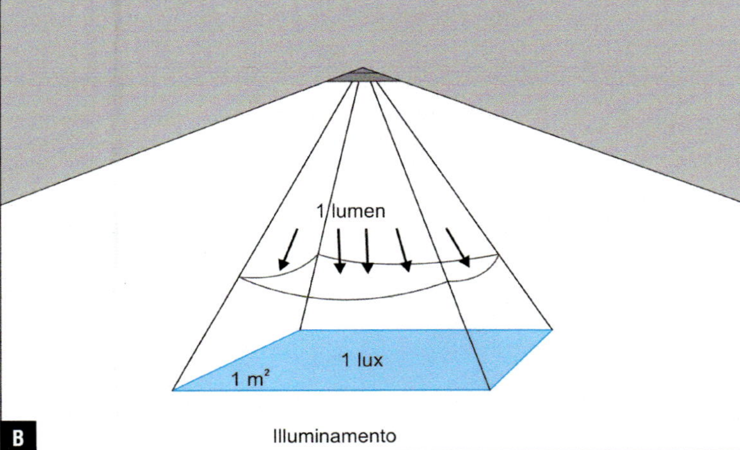

Fig. 1: Lumen versus lux.

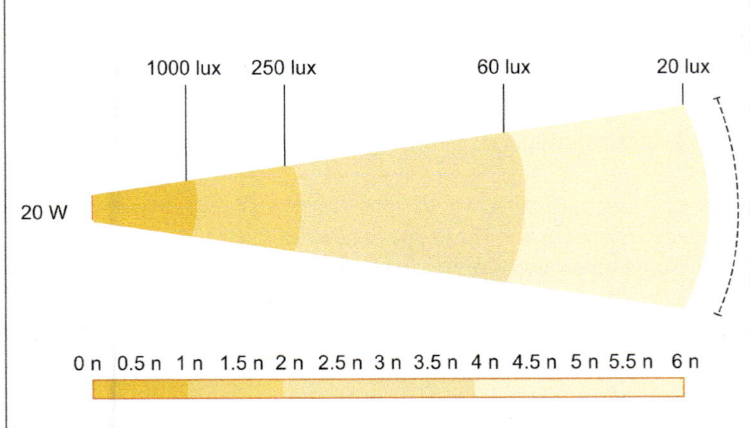

Fig. 2: Measuring lux.

Table 1: Illuminance in OT at different levels.

Sl. No.	Area	Illuminance
1.	At the source of light	100,000 lux
2.	At the body surface	40,000 lux
3.	At depth of an incision	8,000 lux

Table 1A: Recommended illumination values and glare index.

Sl. No.	Classification	Illumination (lux)	Glare index
1.	Reception and waiting room	150	22
2.	Wards (a) General (b) Beds (c) ICU bed	 100 150 400 (for examination)	 13 19 19
3.	Operating theaters (a) General (b) Tables (c) Site of incision (d) Scrub room (e) Instrument room (f) Anesthesia room	 1500 10,000–50,000 120,000 750 500 300	 10 19 19 19 19 19
4.	Laboratories	500	19
5.	Radiology departments	300	19
6.	Outpatient departments	150	16
7.	Stairs	150	25
8.	Dispensaries	300	19
9.	Morgue	300	19
10.	Autopsy area	750	19
11.	CSSD : Work area : Processed stores	500 300	19 19
12.	Corridors : Day : Night	200 100	22 22
13.	Dietary : General : Tray assembly area	300 500	22 19
14.	Emergency: General Emergency: Treatment / Examination	500 1500	19 19
15.	Laundry	300	25
16.	Pharmacy	750	19
17.	Radiotherapy	200	22
18.	Stores	200	22
19.	Toilets	300	22
20.	Department of ophthalmology general lighting	300 lux	20
21.	External eye examination	1000 lux	20
22.	Vision testing and color vision	500 lux	15
23.	Perimetry (for field of vision)	10 lux	Nil
24.	Delivery suit	750–1000 lux	22
25.	Physiotherapy	100 lux	15
26.	Manifold room	200 lux	20
27.	MI room	300 lux	22
28.	Training/seminar room	300 lux	22
29.	Medical store	300 lux	22

DAYLIGHTING AND ARTIFICIAL LIGHTING IN HOSPITALS

Daylighting in Hospitals (Fig. 3)

Windows and daylight give a building a variety and interest that can rarely be achieved in any other way. The main benefits are:[6]

- Contact with the outside world, especially a view out.
- Natural light from the sky, which people tend to prefer to electric lighting in most situations and which is therapeutic and invigorating.[6]

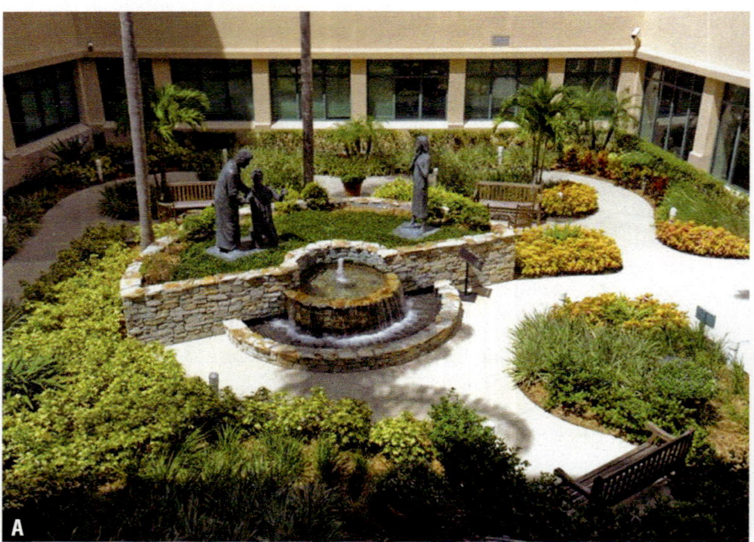

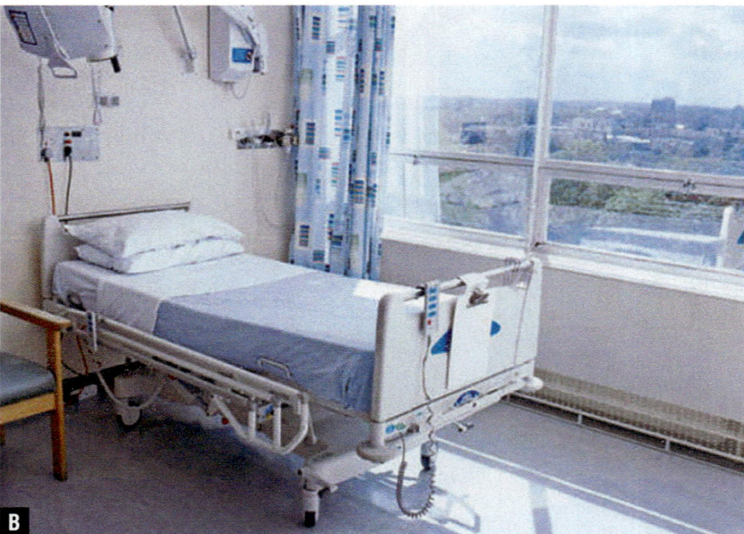

Fig. 3: View out and sunlight in various areas of the hospital.

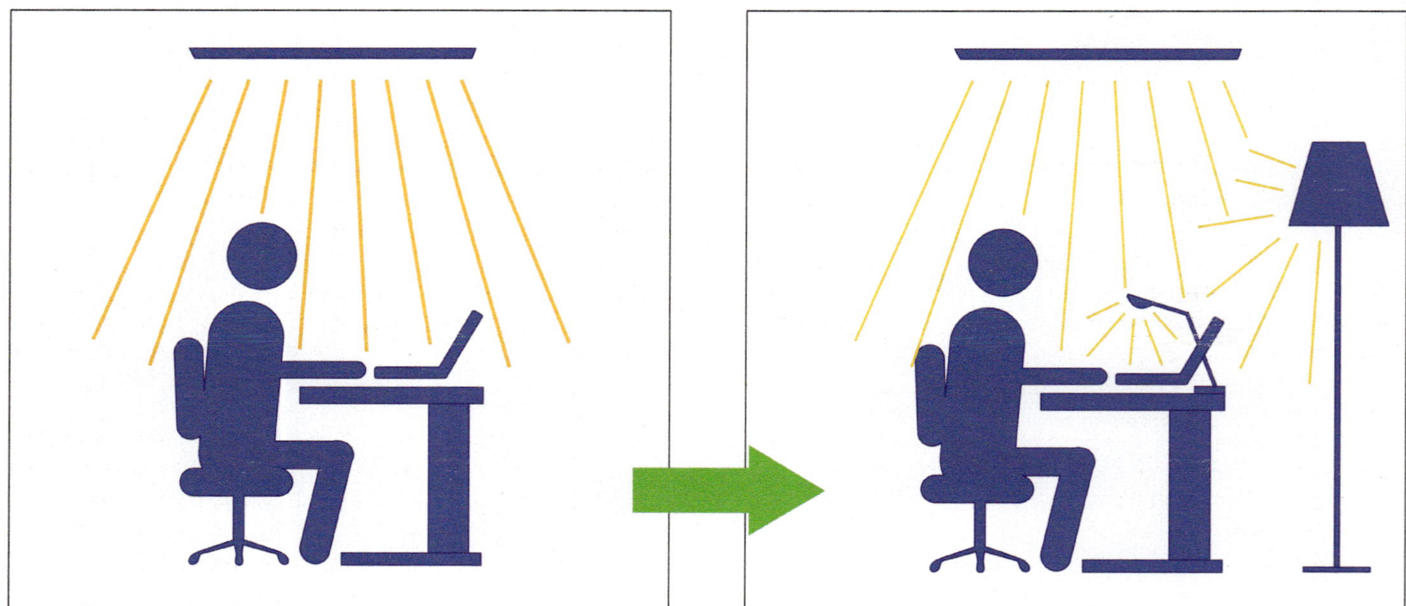

Fig. 4: Task illumination should be provided by light focussing on the specific target area rather than high intensity light over complete work area.

Artificial Lighting in Hospitals

Lighting design covers a range of issues, such as:

- *Task illumination (Fig. 4):* The person should be able to see and move around safely and carry out tasks which may be simple or complex. In planning lighting for tasks, the first issue is to understand the nature of the tasks and to some extent the visual ability of the people concerned.
  If lighting is to enable patients to read and the patients are elderly with perhaps poor sight, then a higher level of illuminance will usually be necessary than if the patients are teenagers. There can be visual benefits to highlighting the task as it helps the person to focus on the work and improves visibility. There will be energy-saving benefits by not lighting the whole room to the same level unless absolutely necessary. The designer must decide on what is required.[6]
- *Lighting appearance:* The lit appearance of the interior not only plays an important part in improving the decor but also has a functional role in reducing the level of anxiety among patients.
- *Architectural integration:* With the design and the physical elements of the building, and particularly with daylight where it is available.[6]
- *Energy efficiency:* Energy efficiency has a direct influence on running costs. Energy efficiency in lighting is measured in terms of the light provided and the energy it consumes. The light provided by a lamp is measured in lumens. The energy it consumes is measured in watts, which includes not just the lamp wattage, but the energy consumed by any ancillary circuitry that is necessary to operate the lamp. A lamp's energy-efficiency rating, or efficacy, is described in lumens per watt.[6]
  Most hospital applications will use fluorescent lamps of either the linear or compact versions (CFL), or LEDs. The lighting installation

needs to be designed to not only provide the lighting required, but also control it to the best effect.[6]

- *Lighting maintenance:* If a lighting installation is not properly maintained, it will deteriorate to the point where it ceases to provide the visual conditions required. Accumulation of dust on the light-emitting and transmitting surfaces of luminaries will mean that light is obstructed and it will cease to perform as intended; thus, energy and money will be wasted. All lighting equipment will need to be cleaned regularly and at least once a year, but in some cases for purposes of hygiene this may need to be more frequent. To enable this to happen with the minimum of difficulty, it should be possible to reach the lighting equipment easily and safely, thus should be installed accordingly.[6]
- *Lighting costs:* Including capital cost and the lifetime operational cost. Like any other hospital building services, lighting has costs attached to it. The total capital cost of the electric lighting installation will be little as compared with the cost of other building services and even smaller when compared with the total cost of the building.[6]

LIGHTING REQUIREMENTS IN DIFFERENT HOSPITAL AREAS

- Different areas of the hospital will have a wide variety of lighting requirements permanent supplementary artificial lighting of interiors as described in IS 3646 (Part 1) may be useful in hospitals, not only in wards to provide good overall lighting of the appropriate quality, but also in laboratories, service and ancillary rooms where a controlled level of working illumination is desirable and in administration offices where the lighting problems are similar to office lighting elsewhere.[3,6]
- The accommodation can be divided into five main groups:
  - *General (public) areas* consist of entrances, reception area, lobbies, waiting areas and offices.
  - *Rooms occupied by the patients,* for example, wards, dayspaces for the sick and visiting rooms.
  - *Special rooms,* for example, OTs, recovery rooms, diagnostic centers, laboratories and examination rooms.[3,6]
  - *Service areas,* for example, kitchen and dining rooms, sterilizing rooms, laundry and maintenance rooms.
  - *Circulation areas* include corridors, lifts, staircases and escalators.

Lighting of the General Areas

Entrance Areas (200 lux)

- Patients, visitors and staff in the hospital typically start their hospital visits at these places. A high quality environment including lighting will instil-confidence, giving an impression of quality of care, whereas absence will have a negative impact.
- Illuminance levels in foyers should be carefully graduated. Near to the entrance, light levels need to be high so that the foyer looks welcoming from the outside and so that people can adapt on entering from the bright outdoors. Different lighting levels can also be a guide to pinpoint main routes from the entrance to other areas or facilities.[3,6]
- Focusing of the lights over walls can make the foyer look bright and cheerful. Too much down-lighting should be avoided since the aim is to light vertical surfaces including signs and people's faces. Where the foyer may be continuously lit, energy-efficient fluorescent or discharge sources should be used. At night, lower illuminances are needed to make the foyer cheerful, so lighting controls should be provided with dimming, step switching or programmable scene-setting. Emergency exit lighting is also required.[3,6]

Reception Area (300 lux) (Figs. 5A and B)

Once inside, visitors have to find their way about; this usually means a direct line of sight to the reception desk. The reception desk is the first point of contact in the hospital. It should contrast clearly with its surroundings. This means that the receptionist and the reception area need to be the brightest part of the visual field.[3,6]

Atria (100 lux) (Figs. 6A and B)

- Generally, the atrium will be well daylit. Patches of sunlight can add welcome liveliness, but too much sun produces excessive heat gains. Sometimes atria contain the reception or other working areas. A canopy enclosing these areas will control high daylight levels and make it easier to see any computer screens.[3,6]
- Appropriate lighting controls are particularly important in atria, because without proper control there can be very high daylight levels yet all the electric lighting may still be in use. Some form of daylight-linked lighting control involving either photoelectric switching or photoelectric dimming is often appropriate.[3,6]

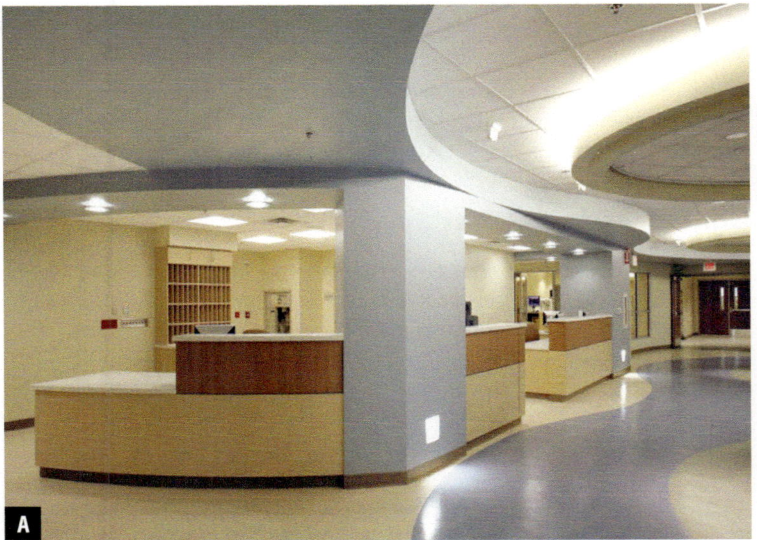

A

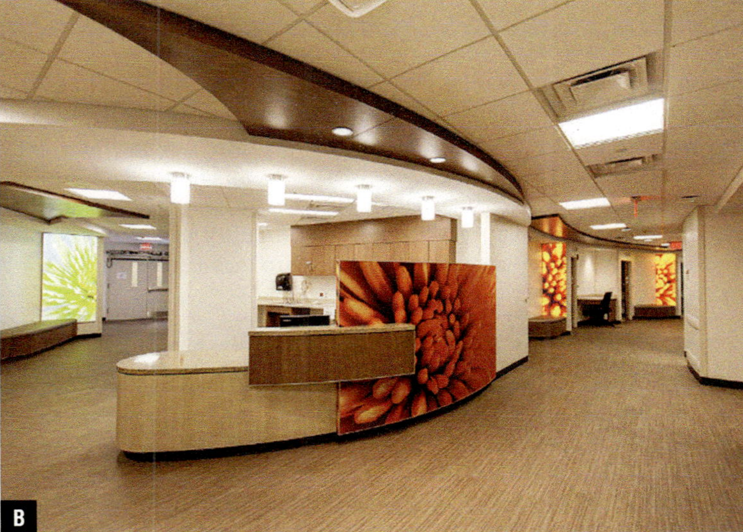

B

Fig. 5 : Hospital reception and registration.

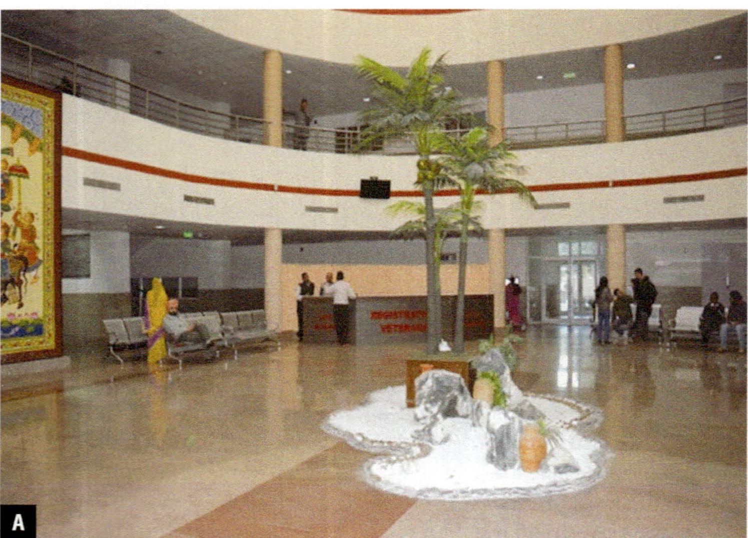

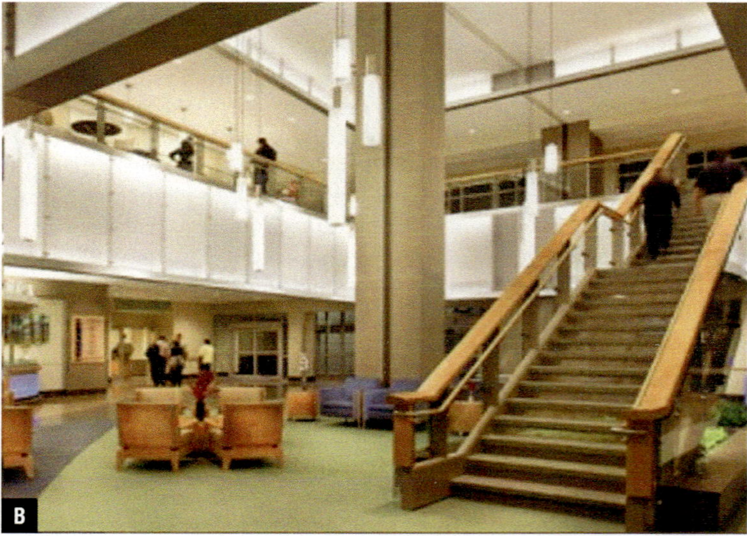

Fig. 6: Hospital atrium.

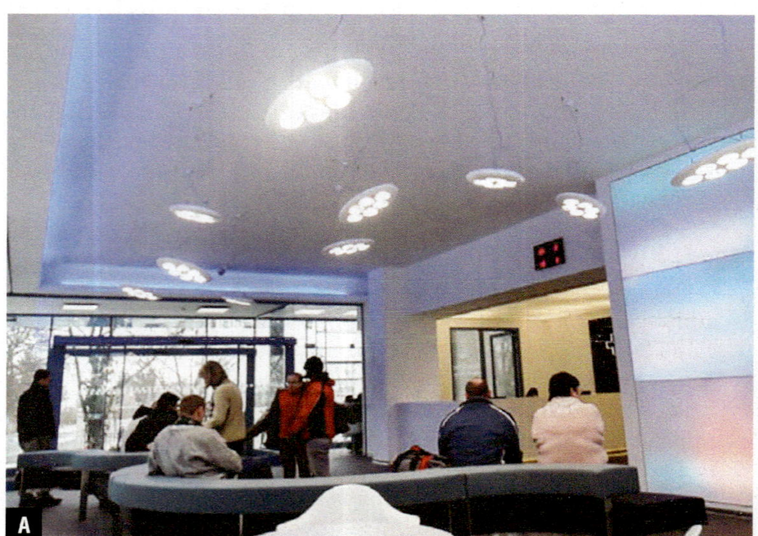

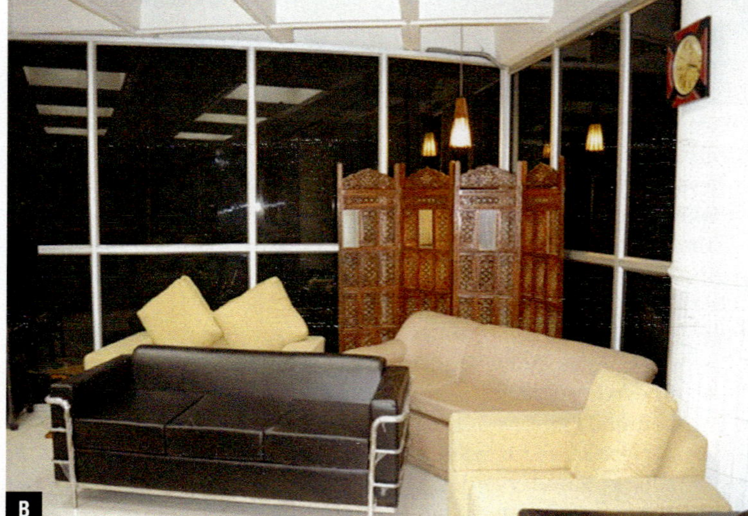

Fig. 7: Waiting areas.

Waiting Areas/ Visitors Room (200 lux) (Figs. 7A and B)

People often like to read while they are waiting; therefore, at least 200 lux illuminance should be provided for this purpose, more if predominantly elderly people use the waiting area. Ceiling luminaires can be supplemented by wall-mounted lighting to add brightness to room surfaces and give a domestic-type feel to the space. Consider time-switching to ensure lighting is switched off outside occupied hours, coupled with photoelectric controls to make use of daylighting where it is available.[3,6]

Toilets (200 lux) (Figs. 8A and B)

Compact fluorescent lamps are the ideal source for toilets because of their low wattage and size. Illuminance level of 200 lux is recommended for toilets. They need to be positioned carefully to allow light down into cubicles. One or two luminaries should be placed near the mirrors to light people's faces adequately. There should be day and night signages for the toilets indicating male and female toilets.[6]

Exit Signages (5 lux) (Figs. 9A and B)

Well lit **EXIT** signages with power backup should be installed on all the Exit points of the Hospital. It should be ensured that these signages are clearly visible from a distance and placed in the direct sight of vision.

Lighting of the Patients' Rooms/Wards

The lighting of patients' rooms is of great importance and has to satisfy the needs of the patients' as well as those of the medical and nursing staff. Moreover, the total lighting effect should be such as to contribute to the general decor and should be free of glare to the recumbent patient.[6]

Lighting for the Wards (Figs. 10 to 13)

- For the patients in the wards the lighting should create a comfortable and pleasant atmosphere. During the day, the floor should receive an average illuminance of 150 lux to ensure safe movement, but at night this should be considerably reduced. Electric lighting can be

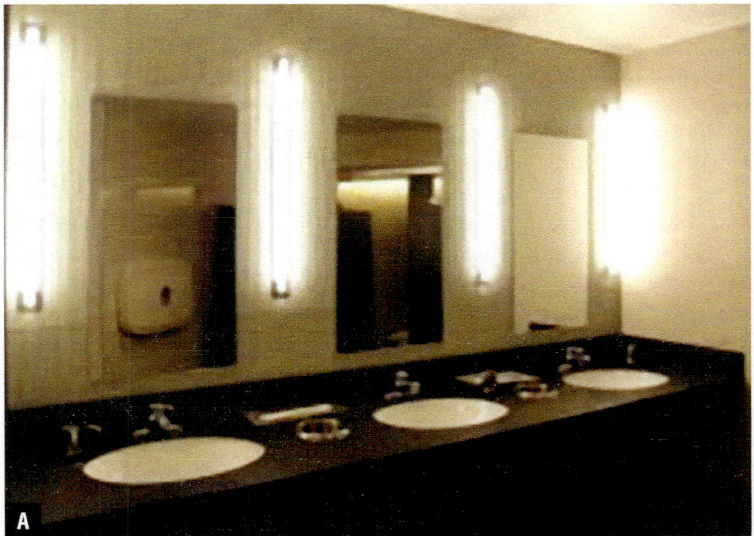

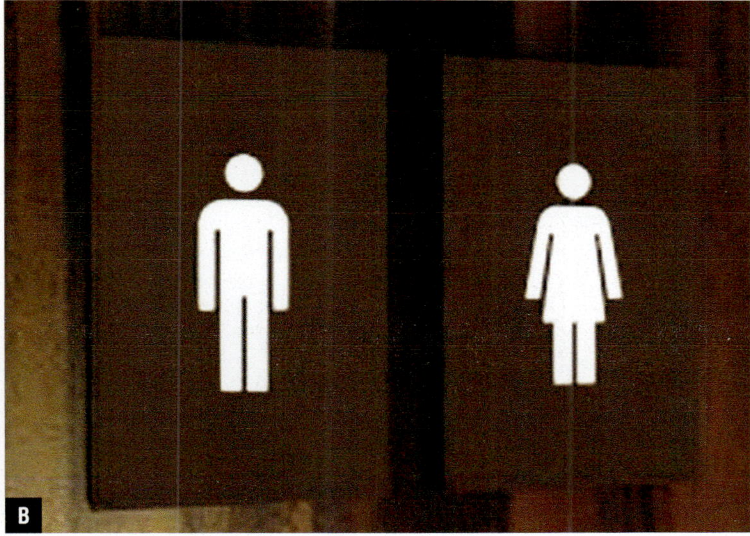

Fig. 8: Lighting in toilet with illuminated signages.

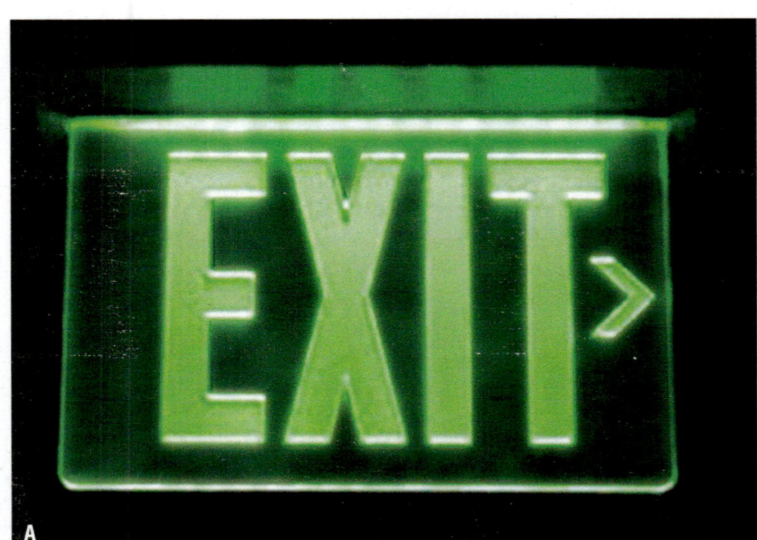

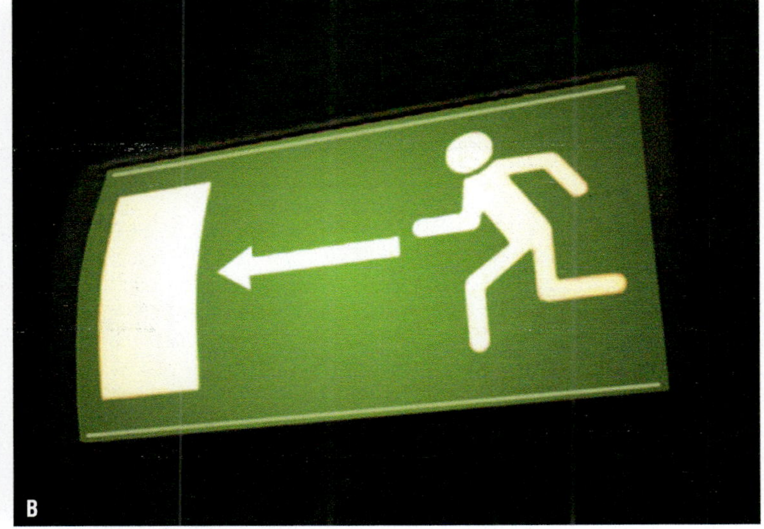

Fig. 9: Exit signages.

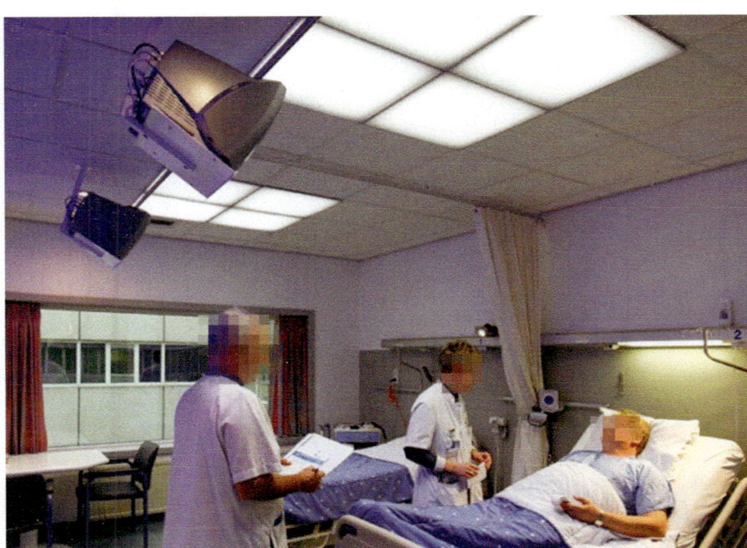

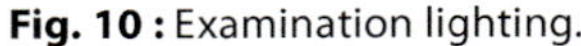

Fig. 10 : Examination lighting.

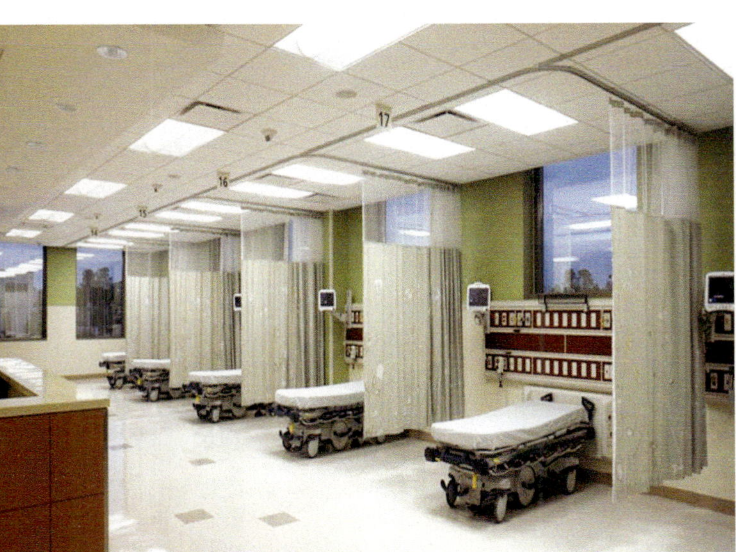

Fig. 11: General lighting.

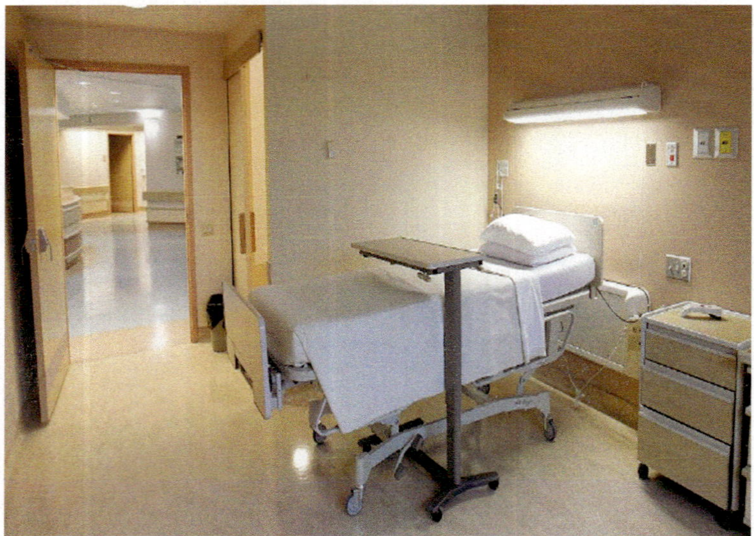

Fig. 12: Reading light.

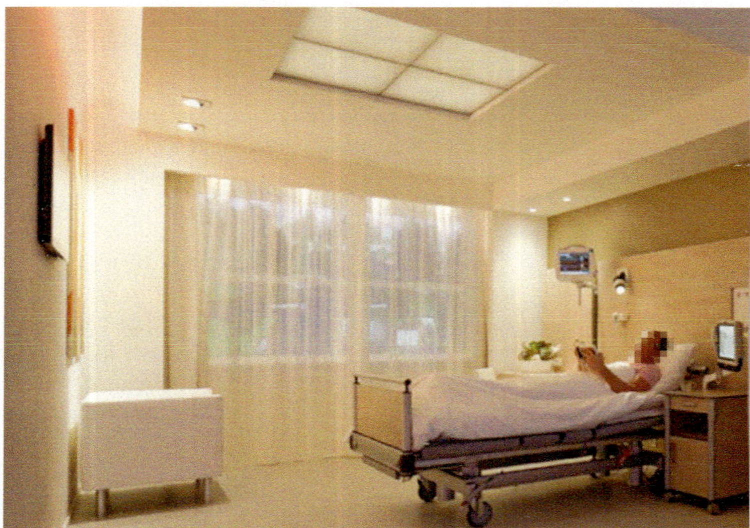

Fig. 13: Night lighting.

wall- or ceiling-mounted using fluorescent lamps, but they need to be carefully positioned, and of a limited brightness, to avoid discomfort to patients, particularly those being transported whilst lying on a trolley. The luminaries need to be selected and positioned so that at least some of the walls appear bright.[3,6]

- Apart from general lighting, individual patients should be provided with additional lighting for any occasional reading or other handiwork that they may choose to do. This should be in the form of bed head lights which can be switched on or off by the patients themselves.[3]
- It may also become necessary under certain emergencies to examine the patient in the ward itself for which an additional examination light capable of achieving 500–1000 lux may be provided.[3,6]
- The lighting installation in a ward, therefore, calls for:
  - General lighting; (100 lux)
  - Reading lamps; (200–300 lux)
  - Examination lighting; (500–750 lux) and
  - Night lighting; (5 lux).

Lighting for the Medical and Nursing Staff (200–300 lux) (Figs. 14A and B)

- This area is the hub of the ward unit; as it is a combination of reception desk for patients and visitors, office area, call center and location for visiting medical staff, it needs to be visually prominent, particularly during the day.[3,6]
- This lighting is mainly utilitarian for the staff in the sense that it should be adequate to enable them to carry out their routine tasks. There needs to be an adequate amount of light on the faces of the nursing staff manning the desk. This means using luminaries with some side illumination. Also projecting light onto the side or back wall can be helpful in making the area visually prominent. Office tasks can be illuminated using downlighters over the desk area—these can provide the required task illuminance of 300 lux. At night, the lighting levels need to be reduced.[3,6]

Installation

In wards 3 m high and greater, it will usually be possible to suspend luminaries from the ceiling, but in wards of less than 2.5 m in height, ceiling or surface mounted luminaries are recommended (Figs. 15A and B).

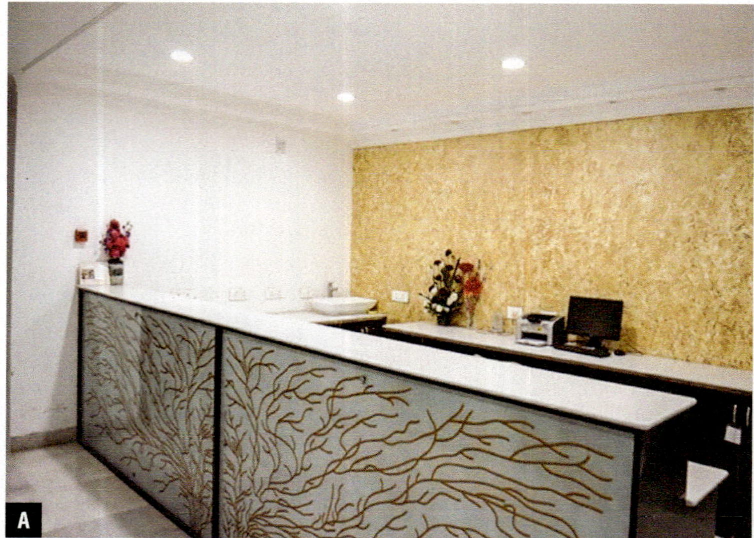

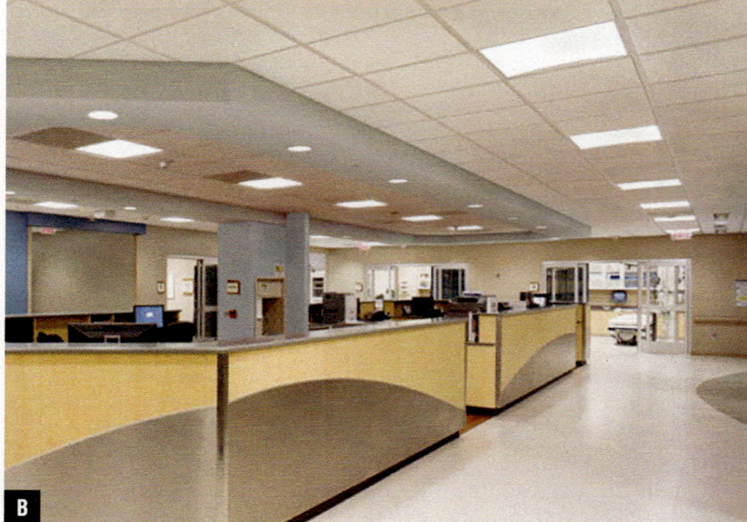

Fig. 14: Lighting for medical and nursing staff.

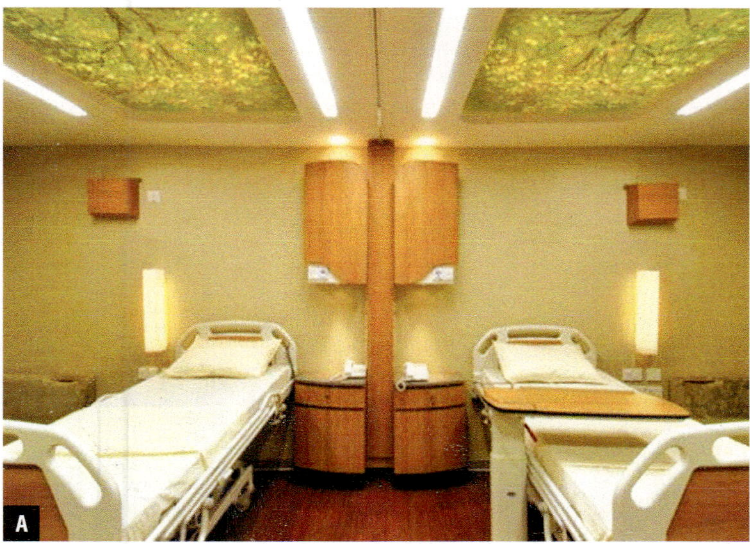

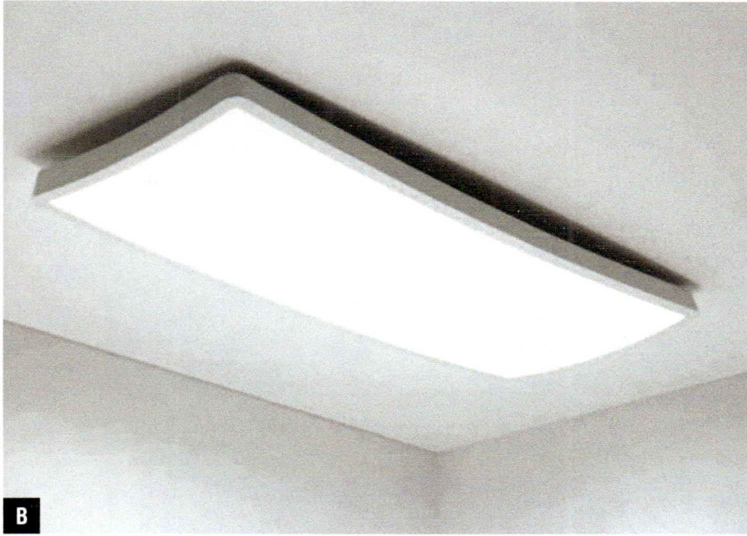

Fig. 15: Ceiling mounted luminaries.

Lighting of Special Rooms

Operation Theater (8000–100,000 lux) (Figs. 16 and 17)

The visual requirement in the theater is the detailed examination of tissue, organs and instruments at the site of the operation. The required illuminance ranges between 10,000 lux and 50,000 lux. Each lighting fitting should be capable of separate switching, to enable the individual requirements for special operations to be met.

Operation Theater Table

Highest level of illuminance is required over OT table (Table 1).

Operation table lighting equipment can be of two different types. The OT lights can be either adjustable luminaires, containing one or more tungsten filament lamps, with cantilever suspension from the ceiling, operated locally by the surgeon, or the second type with a number of sealed and adjustable projectors installed in the ceiling of the theater and located outside so as to direct their light through a transparent ceiling. They are operated by remote control and thus require skilled manipulation.[6]

Other Rooms (300–400 lux)

The general lighting throughout the OT suite including recovery rooms, laboratories, plaster rooms, endoscopy rooms and anesthetic rooms, should be similar in type to that of the theater. The recovery room requirements are similar to those for the general wards, but provision should be made for connecting an examination lamp and separate switching should allow the illuminance over each bed to be raised to 400 lux.[6]

Anesthetic Room (300 lux)

In view of the close association of this room with the theater proper, a general illumination of 300 lux is recommended with provision for a spotlight (which can be either fixed or portable).[6]

Recovery Room and Intensive Care Units (400 lux)

General lighting should be installed as in a normal ward with a separate system to raise the illumination level up to 400 lux for each bed independently. This should be provided over an area of 3 m × 2 m centered on the bed and the luminaries designs should be such as to limit the spread on adjacent beds.[6]

Luminaries

Luminaries should meet the requirements of hygiene and should be totally enclosed to provide adequate mechanical protection to the lamp and to prevent hot particles falling into the danger zone in the event of lamp breakage.[6]

Light Sources

In general, the operating table lighting fittings employ tungsten lamps and produce a very high level of illumination, with very good color rendering properties, but it is not advisable to use filament lighting for the general lighting of the theater because of the additional heat output that would be produced by this form of lighting. It is more practical to use fluorescent light sources which inherently have low heat output yet with the added advantage that they can produce good color rendering for medical purposes.[6]

The color rendering properties of the light sources should be the same as those used for the general lighting of the theater. Color rendering of skin and tissue is a critical aspect of hospital lighting and primary light sources should have an emission spectrum that provides clinically acceptable color rendering.[6]

Standby lighting

Failure of the electric supply or lamps during an operation may have serious consequences and it is necessary therefore to provide a permanent, reliable and safe emergency lighting system for the OT, anesthetic room, sterilizing sink and recovery rooms.[6]

Department of Radiodiagnosis (Figs. 18A and B)

In the screening room due to the necessity of maintaining low brightness levels, normally incandescent lamps of ruby red glass bulbs or fluorescent lamps with red fluorescent powder are used. Red is chosen because this color of light has only little effect on the state of adaptation of the eye. In the viewing room where the radiographs are studied and assessed, artificial lighting is used in the viewing boxes. Use of fluorescent lamps of about 8–10 W is recommended.

For the general lighting required for the cleaning of the rooms, for setting up the apparatus, etc, an illumination of 100 lux is provided in all these rooms.[6]

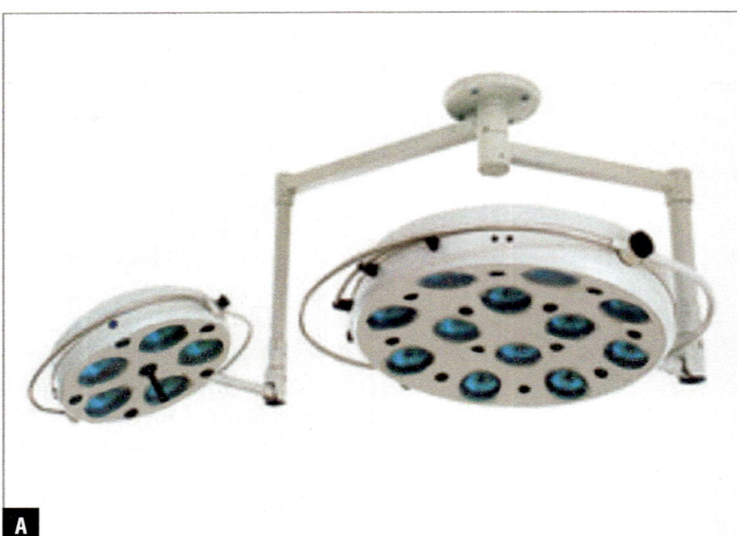

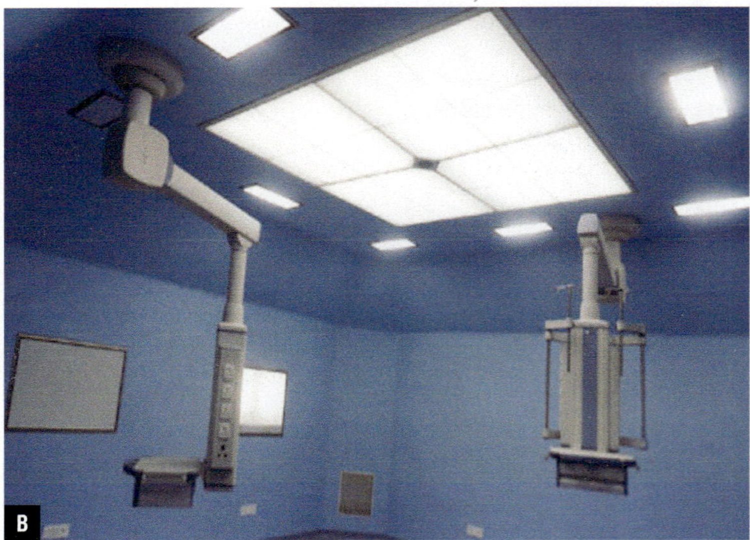

Fig. 16: Lights in operation theater.

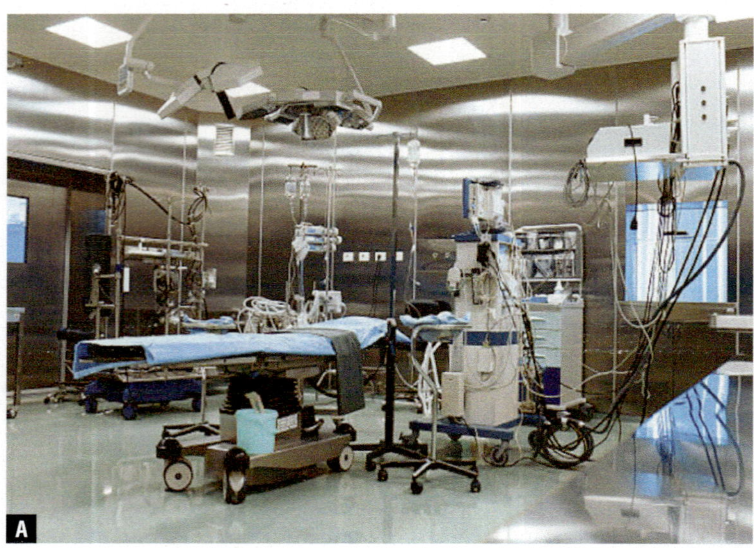

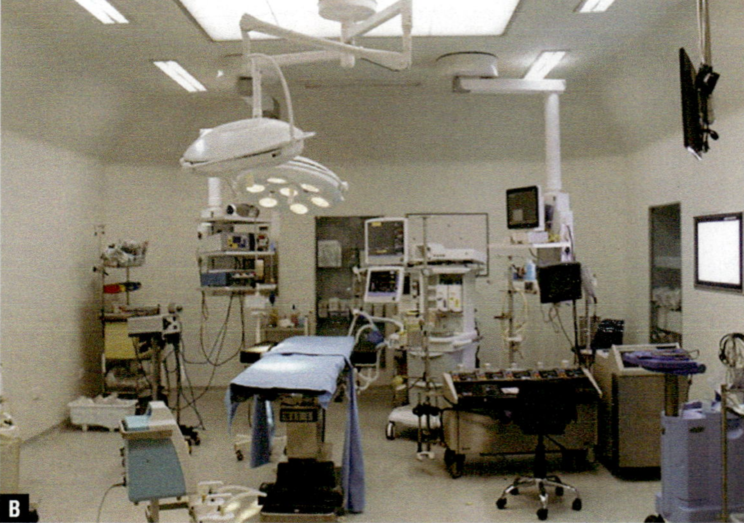

Fig. 17: Lighting in operation theater.

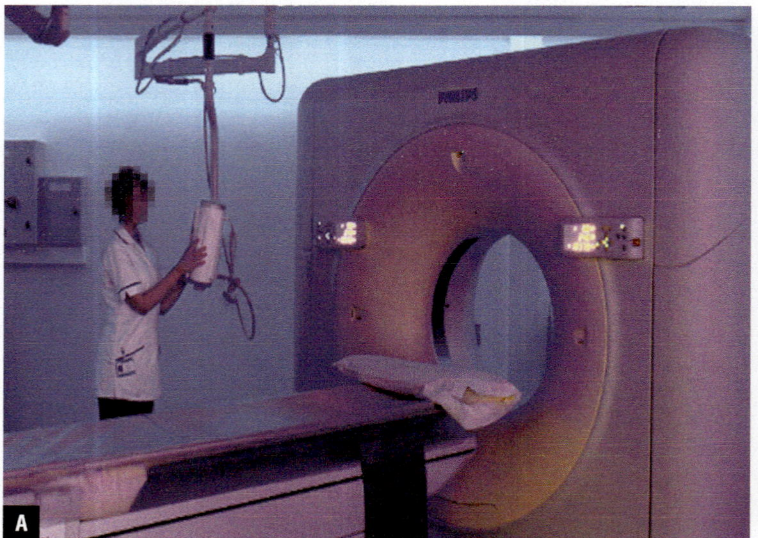

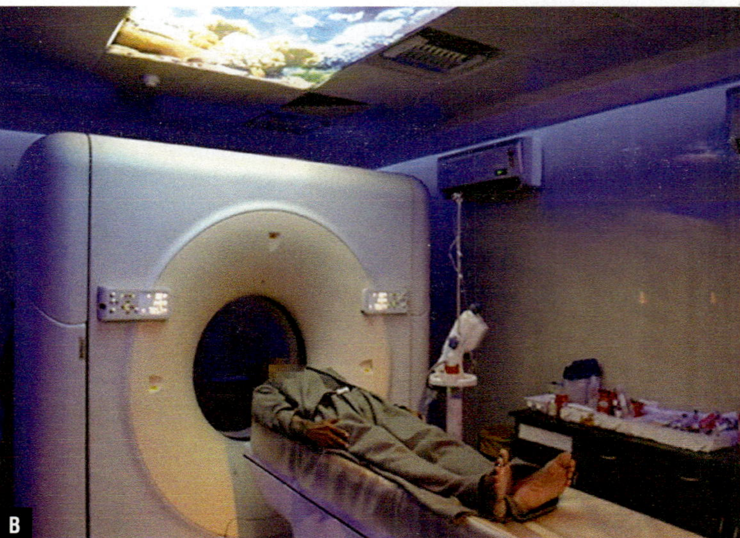

Fig. 18: Lighting in magnetic resonance imaging.

Physiotherapy Department

Special lighting applicable to this department should have the following average illumination levels at 0.8 m above the floor:

- Gymnasium 100 lux
- Hydrotherapy 100 lux.

Department of Ophthalmology

Eye examination has special lighting requirement (Table 2).

Delivery Suit

Examination lights with an illumination of 750–1000 lux should be provided on each obstetric table. General illumination of the delivery suit should be 500 lux.

Other Treatment and Service Rooms (200 lux)

The lighting of other treatment rooms does not present any special problem. A normal general illumination of 200 lux will serve the purpose. The lighting of service rooms, such as offices, laboratories, kitchens and laundries, can be tackled in the same way as corresponding interiors in other buildings.[6]

Manifold Room

Though the requirement of general lighting in manifold is same as other service rooms, but few considerations are required to ensure accuracy in reading the pressure gaze. Any error in reading correct pressure can have catastrophic effects, thus it should be ensured that there is sufficient lighting in manifold rooms especially where the pressure gaze are installed.

Table 2: Recommended luminance for different functions in eye department.

Sl. No.	*Purpose*	*Illuminance*
1.	General lighting	300 lux
2.	External eye examination	1000 lux
3.	Vision testing and color vision	500 lux
4.	Perimetry (for field of vision)	10 lux

Mortuary

Lighting requirement for body storage room is same as other service rooms, i.e. 200 lux. Autopsy room higher levels of illumination are required, i.e. 500 lux. The illumination required over autopsy table should be of 1000–1200 lux.

Central Sterile Supply Department and Laundry

The general illumination required in laundry and central sterile supply department (CSSD) is 200 lux with special provision of focus lights on the control panels of laundry and CSSD equipment.

Training /Seminar Room: 300 lux

General illumination in training/seminar room should be 300 lux. The lights should be ceiling mounted with downward focusing on the tables for task illumination as well as general illumination. Provision for dimming the lights through central console should be provided.

Medical Stores: 300 lux

General illumination in medical stores should be 300 lux. The lights should be ceiling mounted with downward focusing on the shelves for task illumination as well as general illumination.

Corridor Lighting (100–200 lux) (Figs. 19A and B)

Corridors in a hospital serve a more important function than in many other buildings because they act as transitional areas between the wards and the service rooms and between the naturally lit and artificially lit rooms.[6] Generally two types of layouts are followed for corridors.

Corridors should be lit brightly but they do not require high levels of horizontal illuminance nor do they require high illuminance uniformity. There is currently a trend to use downlighting, either ordinary office luminaires or small, circular down lighters for corridors. However, some down lighting luminaires can produce a gloomy sensation, and also down lighters do not light faces well. Downlighters can be glaring and disturbing to recumbent patients on trolleys. Both problems can be alleviated by the use of wall-mounted uplighters to lighten the vertical surfaces of the circulation space.[6]

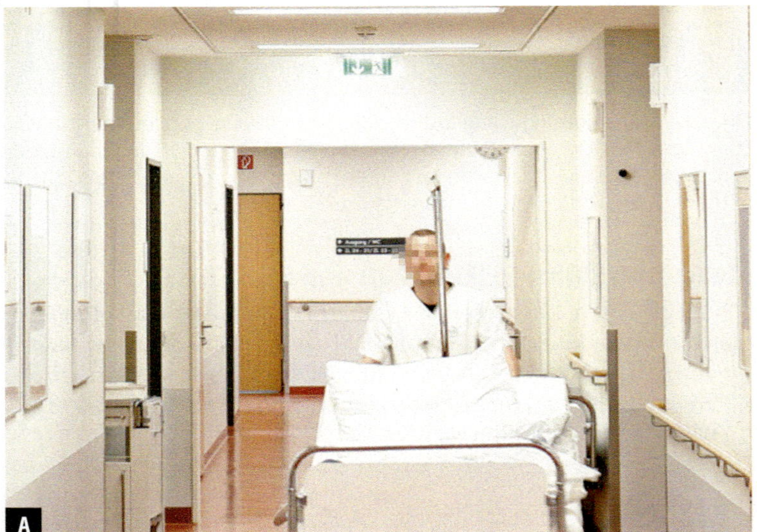
A

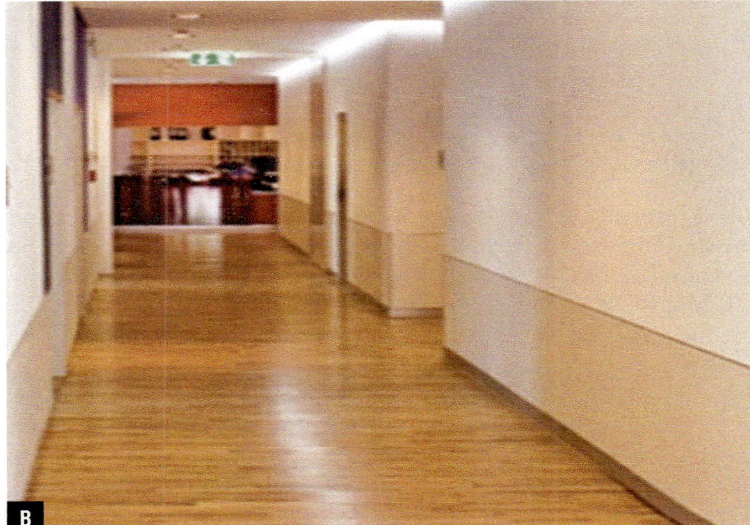
B

Fig. 19: Lighting in corridor.

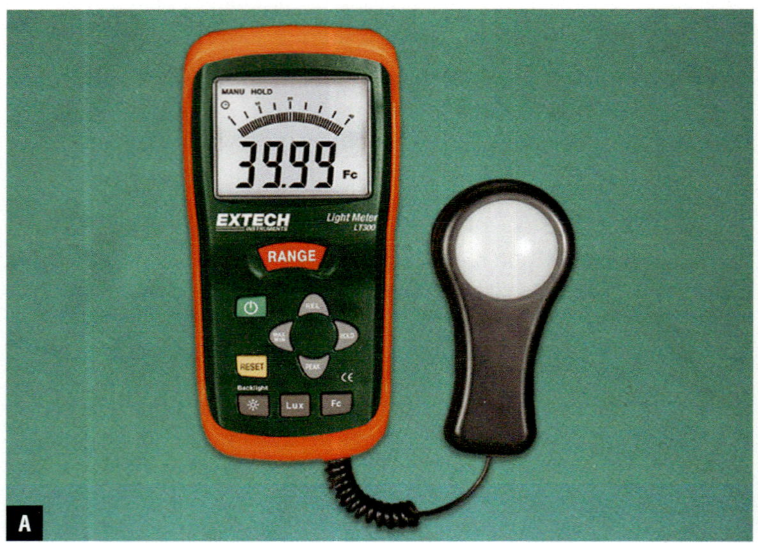

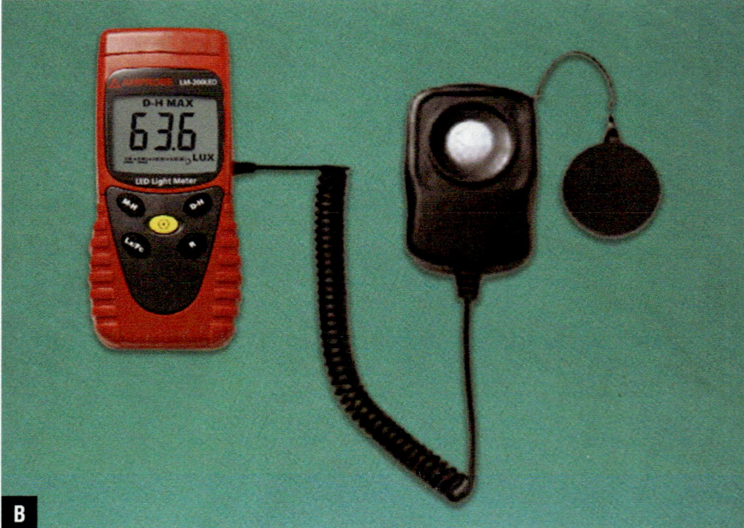

Fig. 20: Light meter to measure illuminance in lux.

Other Common Areas

Stairs and Escalators (100 lux)

Stairs should be lit well to provide a contrast between the treads and risers. Colored, contrasting nosings or illuminated or luminous nosings (tread edges) can help safety. Bright luminaires or windows should not be located in the normal line of sight of people descending the staircase. These could cause glare and lead to an accident.[6]

Lifts (100 lux)

Lighting should make the lift seem bright and open; this can be done by illuminating the walls and ceiling. Control panels should be well-lit and care taken to design fully accessible signage, control buttons and instructions. Contrast on buttons and floor-level numerals as well as conventional tactile markings such as Braille are required. Avoid narrow down lighting as it will make the lift look confined and gloomy. The interior should be bright but not too bright as this will impede adaptation to lighting outside the lift. Contrast should be used for the external and internal lift buttons.[6]

RECOMMENDED ILLUMINATION VALUES AND GLARE INDEX

Impact of Lighting on Healthcare Workers

Good color and lighting design in hospitals can facilitate the work of the staff and even make their work easier, practically, psychologically and emotionally. Vision is at its best when there is ample light on the task and when a number of conditions are fulfilled:[6]

- The overall surround must be neither too bright nor too dim.
- Glare sources, whether direct or indirect, are eliminated.
- Walls and floors should have a reasonable range of brightness levels.
- Excessive contrast is not visible in the immediate background to any task.

Insufficient illumination, glare or excessive differences of brightness within the field of view can cause considerable discomfort to those who have to perform a task which requires visual concentration.

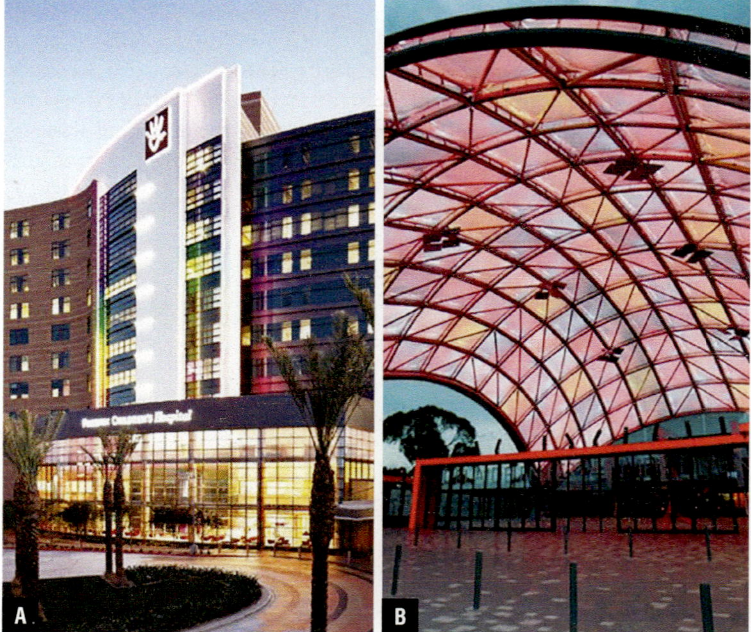

Fig. 21: Façade lighting using indirect lights. (A) Phoenix Children's Hospital: Using lighting to enhance 3D outline of the building without altering the interior lighting; (B) Adelaide Entertainment Center: Using lighting to enhance 3D shape of the building and quality of the material used.

Measuring Lighting (Figs. 20A and B)

It is useful to have a light meter available to diagnose lighting problems. Meters need not be expensive, but should have the following capabilities:[6]

- The meter should be designed to measure illuminances in lux.
- The meter should be properly calibrated by the manufacturers. It will need recalibrating very few years.

Façade Lighting

Refer Figures 21A and B.

Layout of Reception Lights

Refer Figure 22.

Corridor Lighting (Fig. 23)

Horizontally placed tubular LED lights or fluorescent lights (CFL/Tube lights) placed at a distance of 3 m all along the corridor.

Examination Room: Layout of Lights

Refer Figure 24.

Patient Room: Layout of Lights

Refer Figure 25.

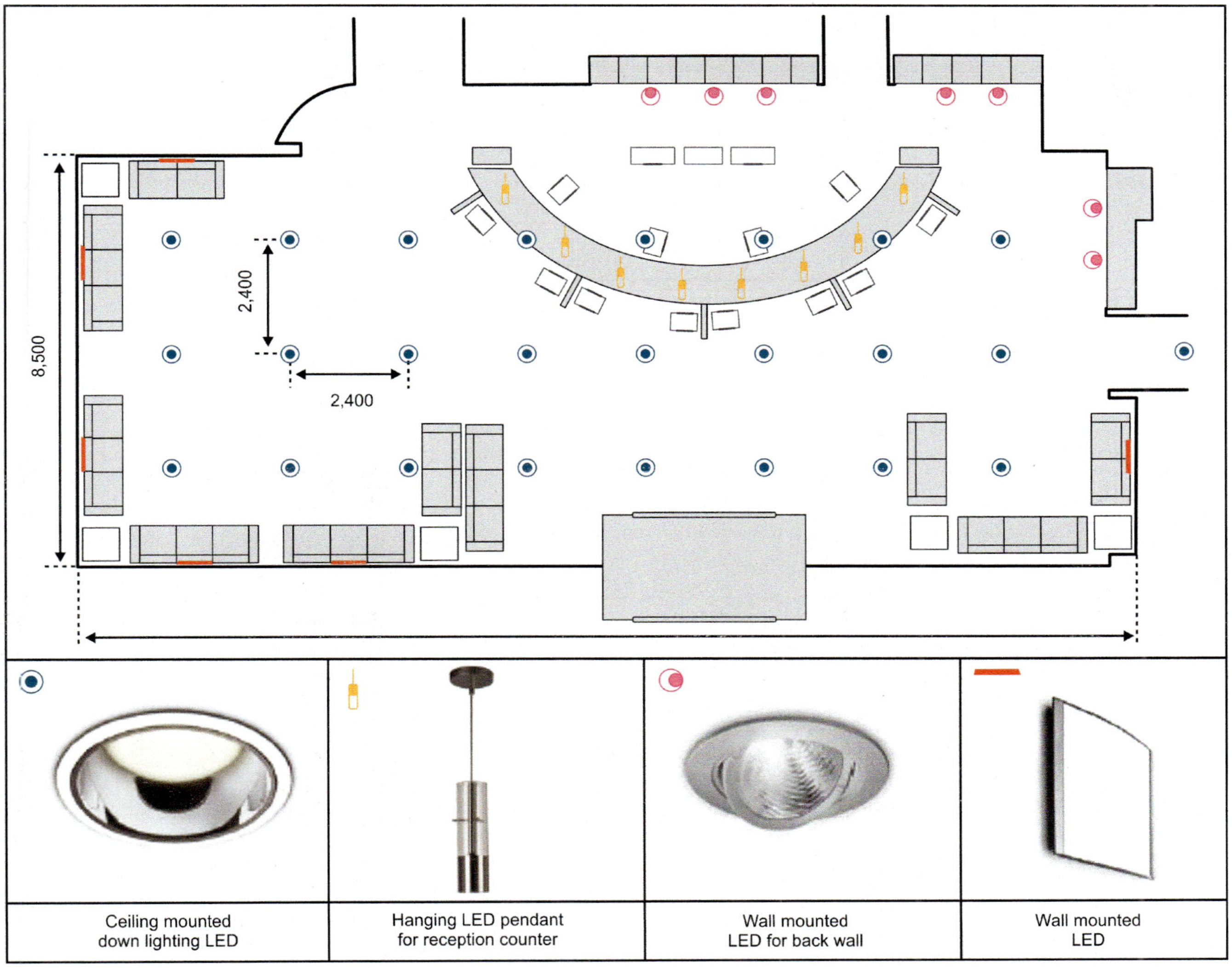

2,400
2,400
8,500

Ceiling mounted down lighting LED	Hanging LED pendant for reception counter	Wall mounted LED for back wall	Wall mounted LED

Fig. 22: Layout of reception showing the light arrangements and sitting.

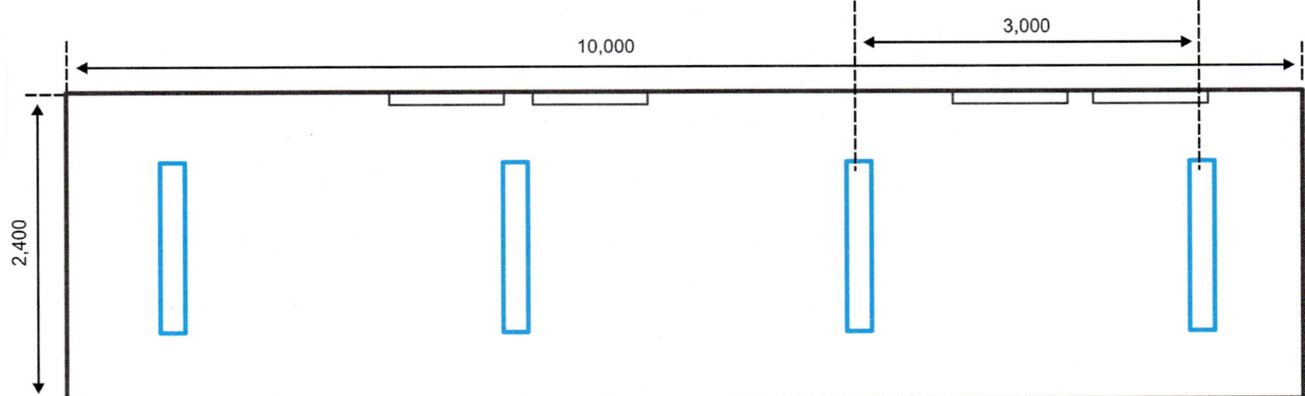

Fig. 23: Layout of lighting arrangement in corridor.

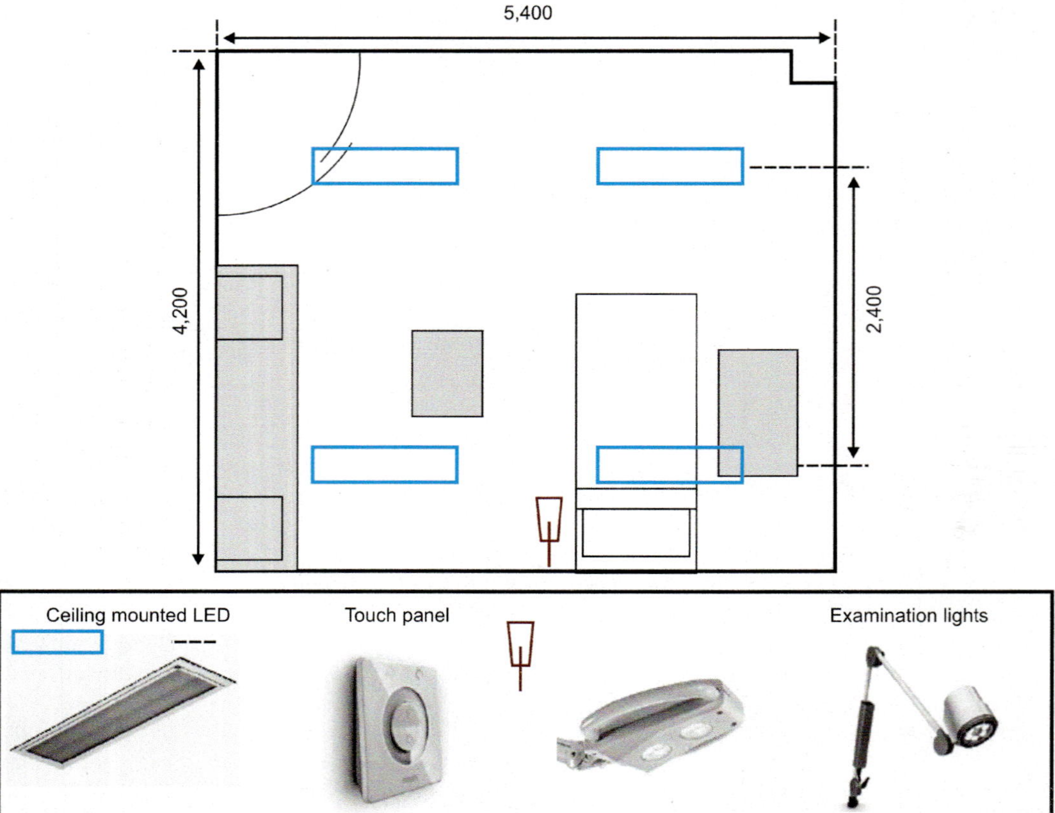

Fig. 24: Examination room lighting arrangements.

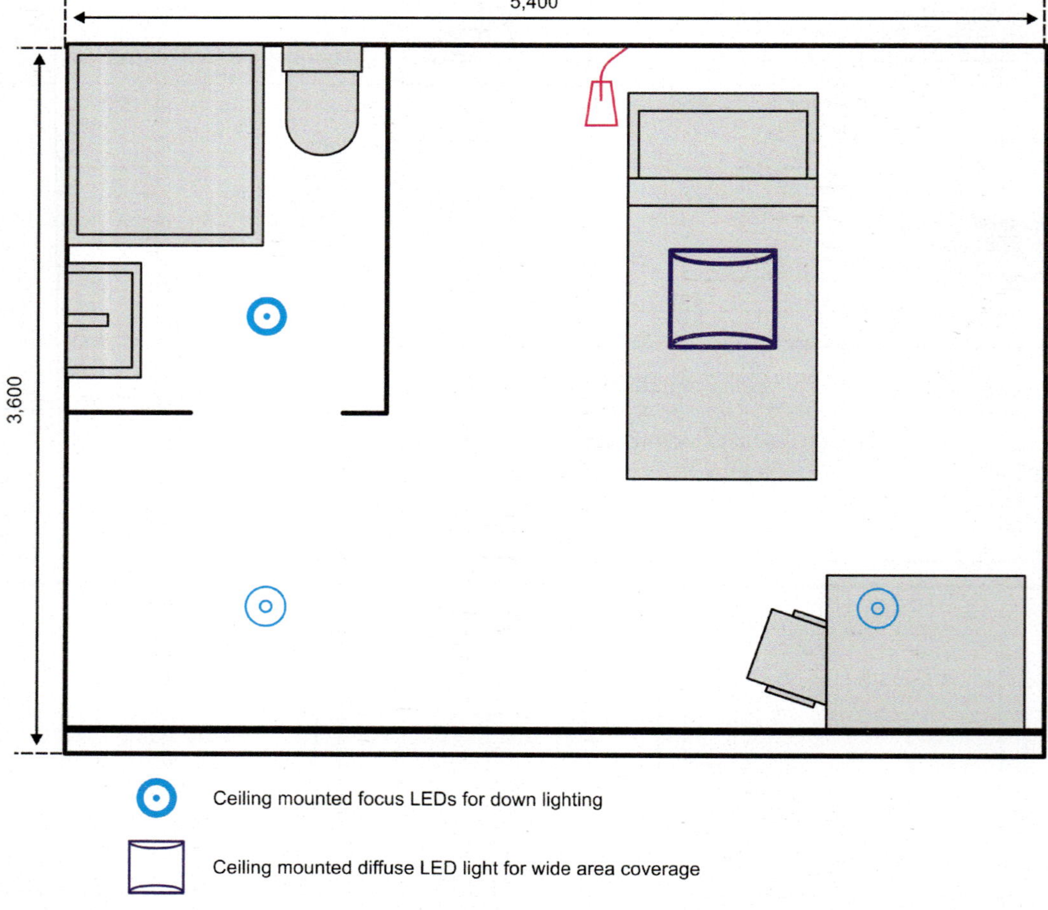

Fig. 25: Lighting arrangements in patient's room.

LIGHTING REQUIREMENT FOR SPECIAL CATEGORY OF PATIENT

Older People and the Visually Impaired

Older people form an important and growing subset of the hospital population. They have particular visual and nonvisual requirements that make good lighting and color design important. Visually impaired and older people like to feel comfortable and in control. Feeling in control includes knowing where they are and where they are going. Visually impaired people feel more confident if they can identify the location of doors. Strong contrast between objects and obstacles as well as text in signage is required. The use of color for way finding or orientation should be boosted by careful illumination to provide adequate guidance and safety.[6,7]

Persons with Psychiatric Ailments

Exposure to outdoor daylight is a key factor in determining the phase of the circadian rhythm. By controlling the circadian system, light—both natural and artificial—impacts many health outcomes among patients and staff in hospitals such as depression, sleep, circadian rest-activity rhythms, as well as length of stay in the hospital.

Other Disabled People

Other categories of disabled people have special requirements for sensitive lighting and color design:

- Wheelchair users need lighting on low level controls. Signage should be clearly lit when viewed from wheelchair level. Places where people transfer to or from a wheelchair may need extra lighting. The positions of glazed surfaces should be checked for adverse reflections and glare. These may occur where pictures and windows are at the wrong angle or level for wheelchair users and not obvious to the fully mobile.[6]

Young Patients

- The very young also have particular requirements from a lighting and color design scheme. Newborn babies, especially those born prematurely, are particularly susceptible to bright light, which can cause stress and also retinal damage. They need a recognizable pattern of night and day, however, to help them develop diurnal rhythms and normal sleep patterns. Older children may find a hospital stay stressful. Good color design can make the hospital appear less institutional and a more pleasant and stimulating place to be in.[6]

RENEWABLE ENERGY SOLUTIONS

Renewable energy is defined as electricity produced from solar, wind, geothermal, biogas, biomass, and low-impact small hydroelectric sources.

Types of Renewable Energy (Figs. 26A and B)

Solar[7]

Solar energy is energy derived from the sun. Solar energy is converted into electricity using one of two formats, photovoltaic (PV) cell, or solar power plants.[8]

Wind

Wind power utilizes moving air to turn a wind turbine which then turns an electric generator which generates electricity.

Geothermal

Geothermal energy utilizes the heat created in the center of the earth to create steam or hot water that is then utilized to generate electricity.

Biomass

Biomass is a renewable energy source because we can always grow more trees and crops, and waste will always exist. Some examples of biomass fuels are wood, crops, manure, and some garbage. When burned, the chemical energy in biomass is released as heat.[8]

Solar Powered Hospitals[9]

Hospitals need to constantly consume a high amount of electricity to power lifesaving medical equipment and keep medical and surgical services running 24 hours a day. The overall number and the cost of solar panels that should be installed in a hospital will depend on the size of the hospital and the amount of electricity needed to power

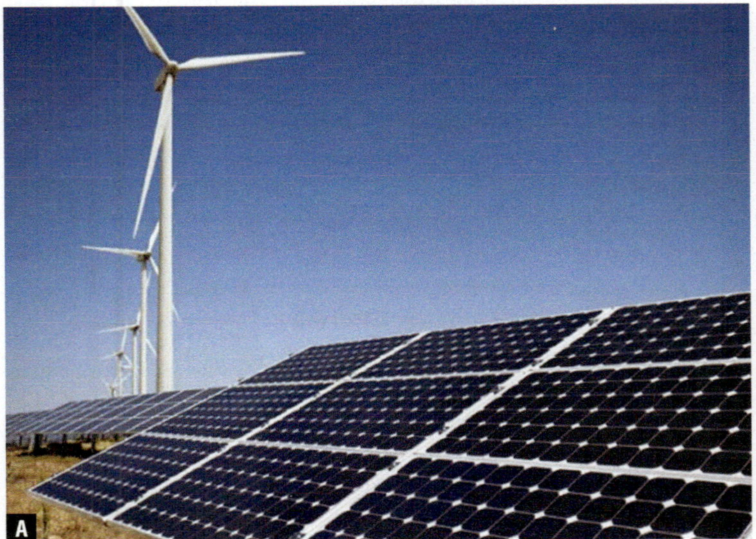

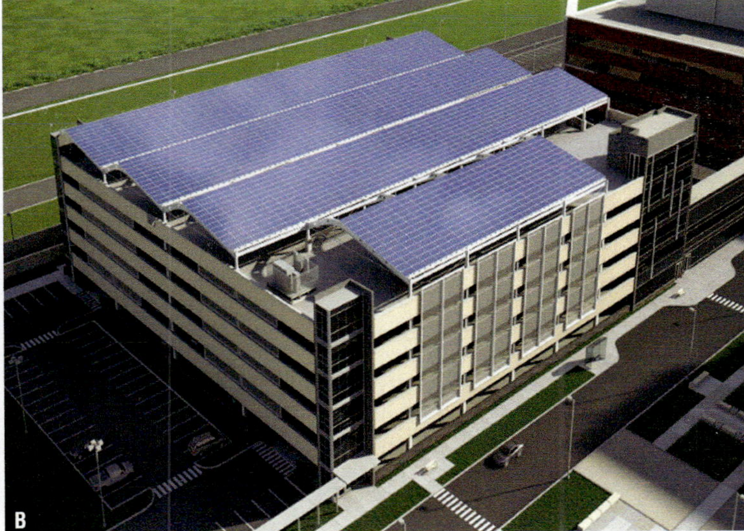

Fig. 26: Renewable sources of energy in the hospitals.

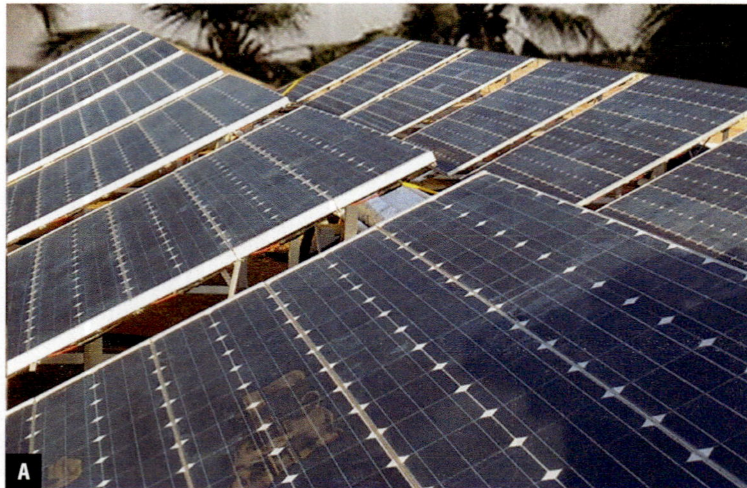

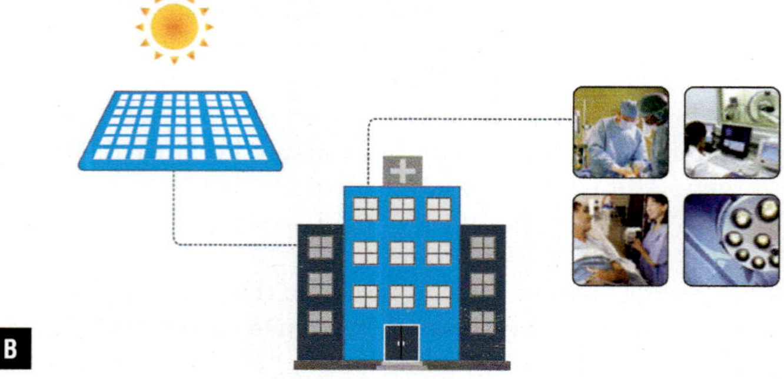

Fig. 27: Solar PV panels and their use in generating power in hospitals.

the hospitals machinery, lighting and heating. It is not advisable to consider an off-grid installation with a hospital as uninterrupted power is a basic requirement for medical emergencies and surgical operations.[10]

Benefits of Using Solar in Hospitals (Figs. 27A and B)

Hospitals that utilize solar PV panels will be able to save some money every year since they will be reducing costs on their energy bills. A hospital that generates excess electricity may sell the excess amount to their local grid via feed-in tariffs and earn cash toward providing better services.[10]

Clean and Reliable Electricity for Hospitals[9]

With solar power plants the hospital can reduce their energy bills by 80%. In addition, the hospital will benefit from carbon credits on the generated units. Solar power can be synchronized with grid electricity so as to get an uninterrupted supply of electricity.[10]

ENERGY CONSERVATION[4,11,12]

Energy Conservation Building Code

The energy conservation building code ECBC was developed by bureau of energy efficiency (BEE) in year 2009 with an aim to provide minimum requirements for energy efficiency designs and construction of buildings and their systems. ECBC compliant building can use 40–60% less energy than conventional building.

This code is applicable to buildings with more than 100 kW of connected load and more than 1000 m^2 of conditioned area. The provisions of the code apply to:

- *Building envelops:* It includes roof/ceiling, walls, glass panels, etc., which separates a covered areas of the building from open areas.
- Heating ventilation and air-conditioning system (HVAC).
- Interior and exterior lighting.
- Water heating.
- Electrical installations like transformers and electric motors.

Mandatory Requirements for Lighting

The mandatory requirements for lighting mostly related to interior and exterior lighting controls. Several different approaches can be used to control electric lighting.

- *Scheduling control:* Use a time scheduling device to control lighting systems according to predetermined schedules.[11]
- *Occupancy sensing:* Control lights in response to the presence of people in the space.
- *Day lighting:* Switch or dim electric lights in response to the presence or absence of daylight illumination in the space.[11]

Lighting

Lighting is a sector with great energy saving potential. At the places that have to be lightened 24 hours a day, high performance lamps can be used. Besides, some type of lamps that are placed outdoors, consume lot of reactive load; as a result their performance is reduced. This issue can be addressed with the local use of capacitors for power factor correction. These could result in a 50% reduction in energy consumption.[13]

Heating Ventilation and Air-conditioning System

Heating ventilation and air-conditioning system consumes considerable amount of energy in the hospitals. integrated building management systems (IBMS) with sensors should be installed for automatic climate control, including relative humidity, for optimum electricity consumption.

Low Cost Measures[13]

- Minimization of exterior lighting and use of timers.
- Modification and optimization of the arrangement of lightning devices in the area.
- Use of local lighting proportional with the type of activity in the area.
- Replacement of lamps of low luminous efficiency (e.g. glow) with more efficient lamps (e.g. compact electronic lamps of fluorescence or energy saving lamps).
- Installation of covers with light reflectors in old nakedly or with plastic cover lightning equipment for optimization of light distribution in the area.
- Control of lighting with local switches, timers, dimmers and sensors of motion.

Integrated Building Management Systems

- Integrated BMS is the key to 'intelligent buildings', equipped with a variety of monitoring devices and control systems, both automated and manned. Together they help regulate a long array of building services and utilities. The term *Building Management Systems* encompasses a wide variety of technologies which include energy management systems and building controls.

- Their function is to control, monitor and optimize building services, such as *heating, ventilation, air-conditioning, lighting, alarm systems* and certain *electrical appliances*.

Intelligent networking of information and communication technology as well as medical and building technology meets users requirements for more ease and comfort. In addition, hospital operators can save energy and therefore costs with integration, and the processes in the hospital become faster and safer.

RECENT TRENDS IN HOSPITAL LIGHTING[14,15]

Latest concepts in hospital lighting that are followed in modern day hospitals:

- Harvesting of day lights.
- Maximum use of LEDs.
- Dimming and scheduling of lights.

LEDs

Lighting has been rocked by the growing use of LEDs. Studies comparing traditional fluorescent lighting to LED illumination in healthcare facilities indicate that LEDs offer an effective strategy for energy savings with fixtures rated to operate for 50,000 or more hours. Other benefits include reduced maintenance because of the longer life of LEDs and disposal costs, and smaller physical size, offering flexibility in its use should the activities in the illuminated area be changed. LEDs can be dimmed through a control system that is installed with the fixtures, if more or less light output is required.[14]

Latest Types of Lights

Down Lights (Figs. 28A and B)

Type of LED lights which can be fixed on ceiling and used for task illumination. They are usually placed in reception counters and focuses light downwards over the working plane.

Ceiling Mounted LED Lights (Figs. 29A and B)

Fixed on ceiling for general illumination of the area. These lights are used in wards, outpatient departments (OPDs), corridors and various other clinical and service areas of the hospital.

Examination Lights (Figs. 30A and B)

High lumen/watt LED lights fixed on the wall near the head end of the examination couch in examination rooms in OPD. These lights can

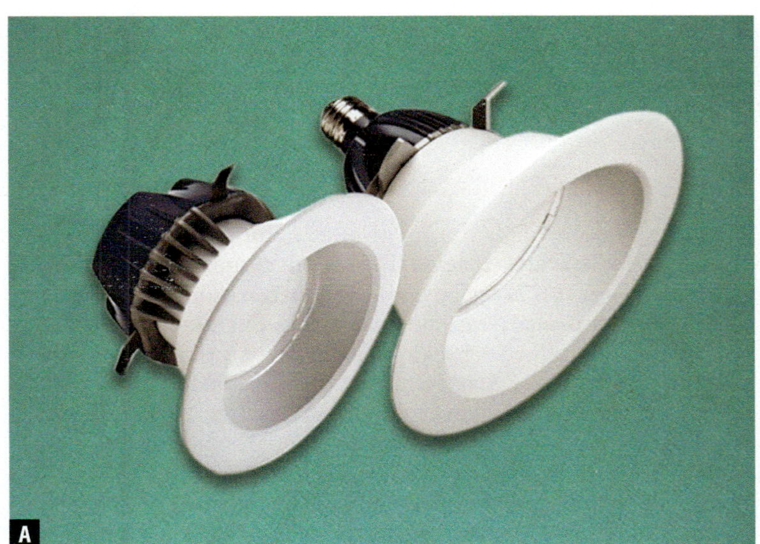

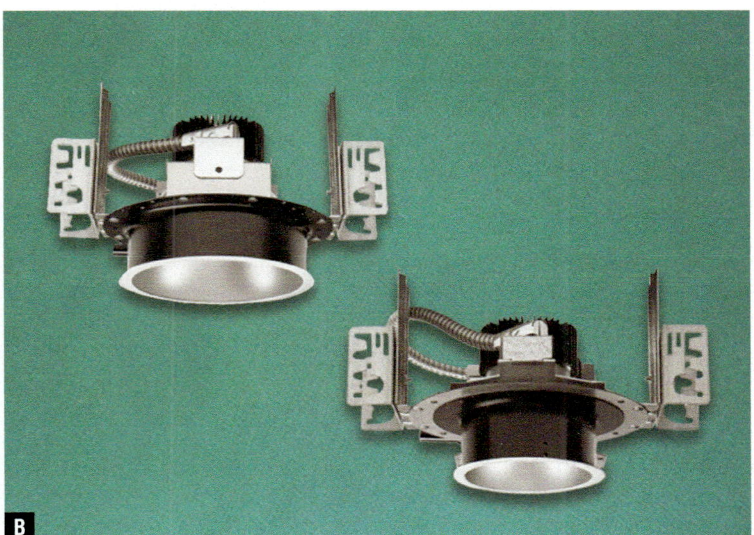

Fig. 28: Down lights.

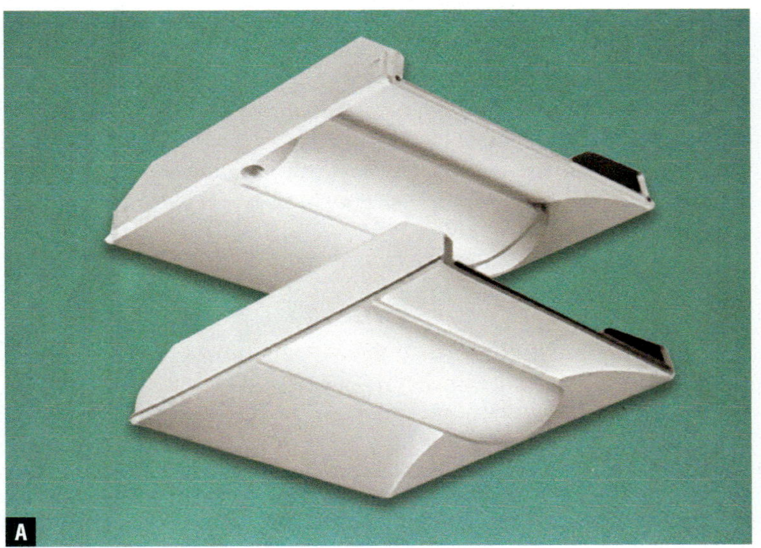

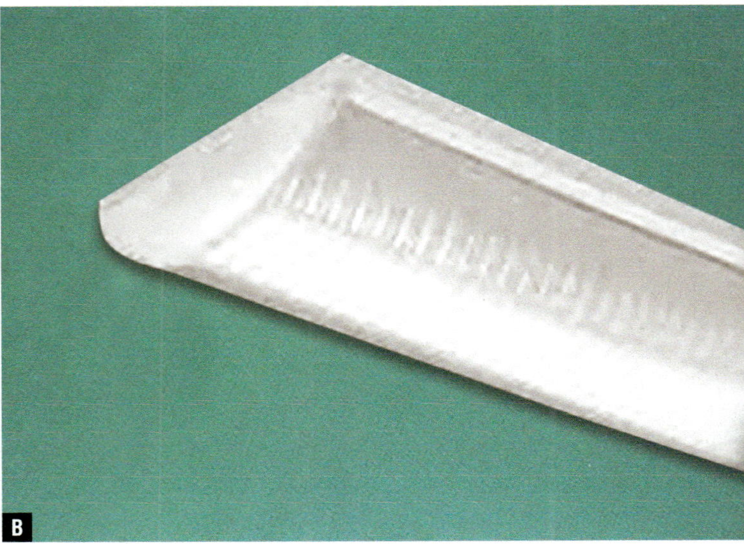

Fig. 29: Ceiling mounted LED lights.

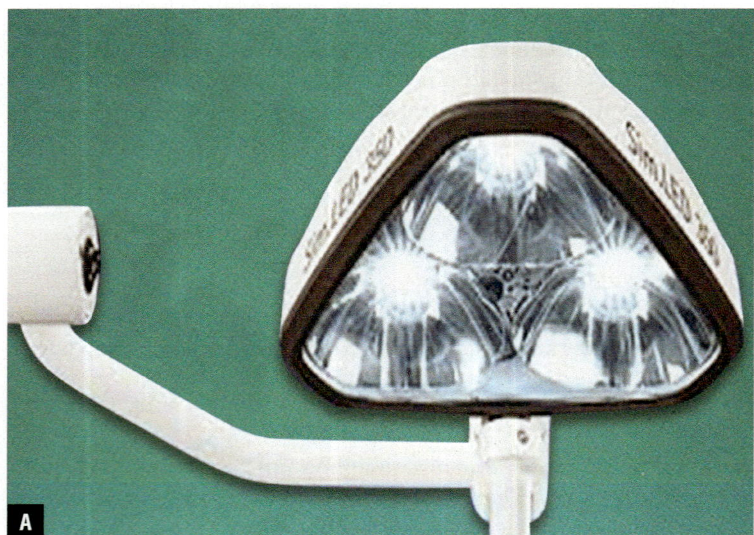

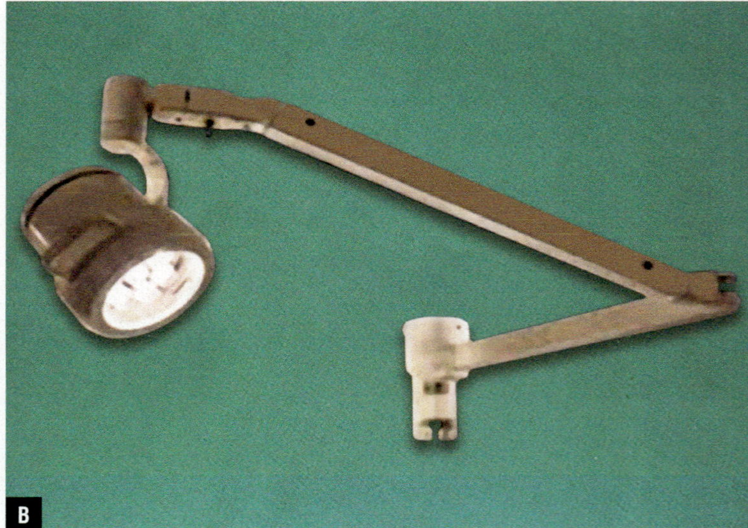

Fig. 30: Examination lights.

also be placed in the treatment room in wards. These lights help the medical and nursing staff in detail medical examination and treatment/ procedure.

Reading Lights (Figs. 31A to C)

These lights are fixed on the wall toward the head end of the patient beds in wards. These lights aid in reading especially during night hours without disturbing other patients.

Mobile Light Source (Figs. 32A and B)

Mobile light source with high lumen/watt ratio. These lights are used in wards and OPDs for examination and carrying out a procedure. These lights are highly effective as well as cost-efficient because same light can be moved to different beds, without placing individual lights for examination.

LED Tube Lights (Fig. 33)

Cost-efficient LED lights with high lumen/watt ratio. These lights are used for general illumination in wards, OPD, corridors, waiting areas, etc.

LED Luminaries (Figs. 34A to C)

Different LED luminaries with varying lumen/watt ratio as well as different wattage for general illumination.

LED Lights for Outer Areas (Fig. 35)

These are long life, high wattage and high lumen/watt ratio lights used for general illumination of outer areas like parking and roads. These lights have sturdy outer-case made of steel or PVC for better protection of luminaries in all weather.

Light Pipes (Figs. 36 and 37)

The system is essentially a pipe that sticks out of a building's roof and reflects sunlight directly into an interior room. It is more energy efficient than skylight since less energy escapes from the interior due to less surface area.[15]

LIGHTING ON GENERATORS

When utility power fails during or after natural or human created disasters, hospitals are expected to carry out certain critical functions for life safety systems. Standby power should be equipped to switch on automatically, activated by an automatic transfer switch that transfers the load from the utility feed to backup generators without intervention of a human operator. There must be sufficient onsite fuel to run the backup generators for specified length of time. In addition, the emergency source of power is allowed to supply power to optional standby loads as long as the emergency source has the capacity to supply.[16]

Emergency backup should be able to provide power for systems, the operation of which is "essential for safety to human life." It is intended to provide reliable power to critical devices and equipment. In hospitals, emergency power serves task illumination and receptacles in specialized care areas including emergency rooms, coronary units, intensive care units, OTs and postoperative recovery rooms, blood and tissue banks, telephone exchange, and nurses' call systems. Emergency power is required to activate within 10 seconds of the loss of power. The wiring must be independent of normal power, in separate raceways (Table 3).[16]

It should be ensured that all lifesaving equipment like ventilators, defibrillators, oxygen concentrators, etc. are on power backup to provide uninterrupted power supply.

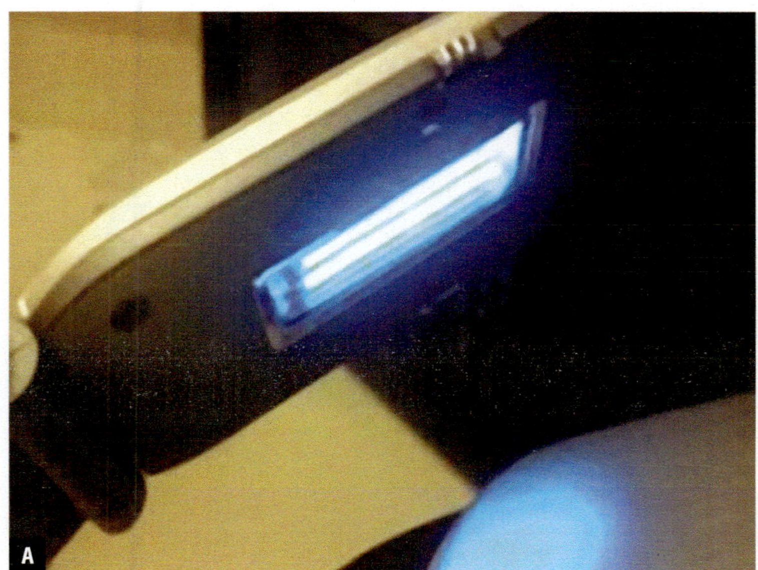

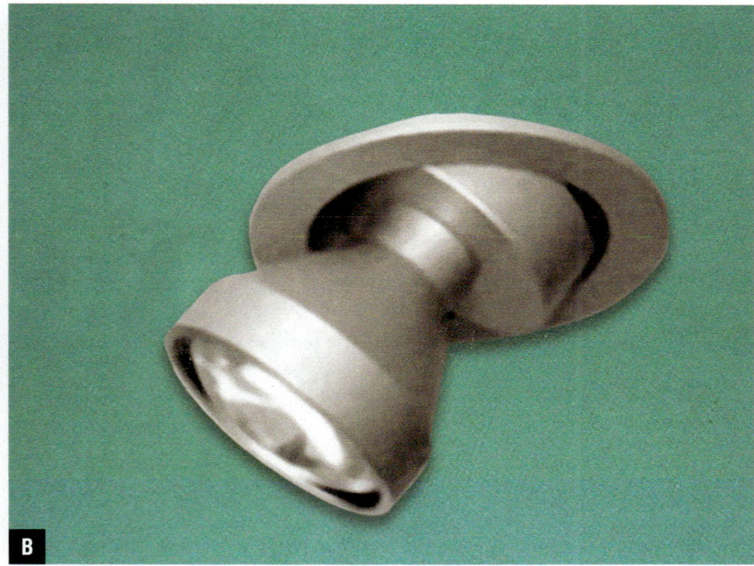

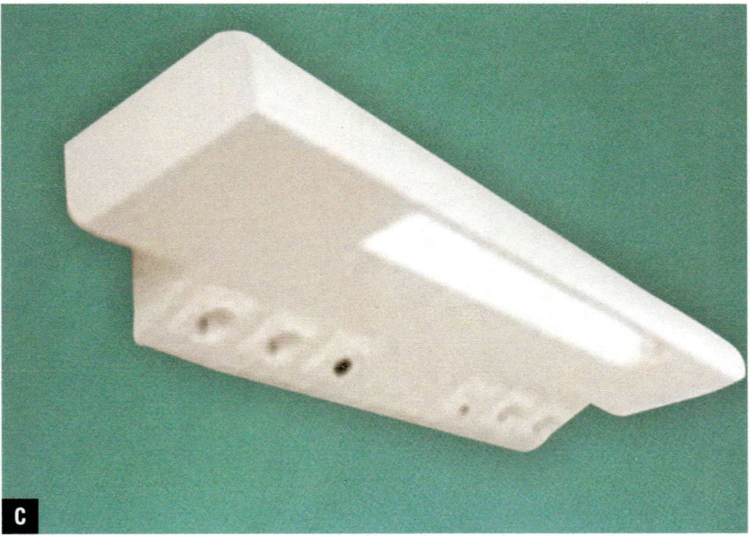

Fig. 31: Reading lights.

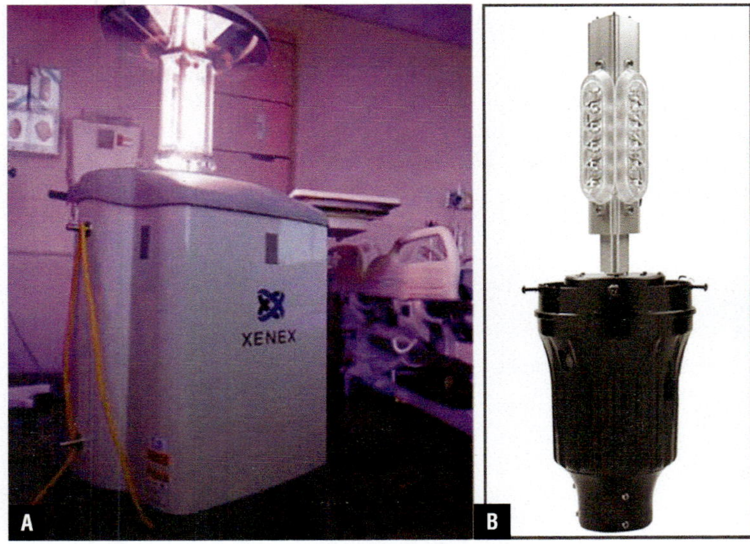

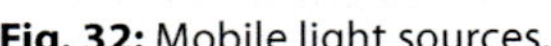

Fig. 32: Mobile light sources.

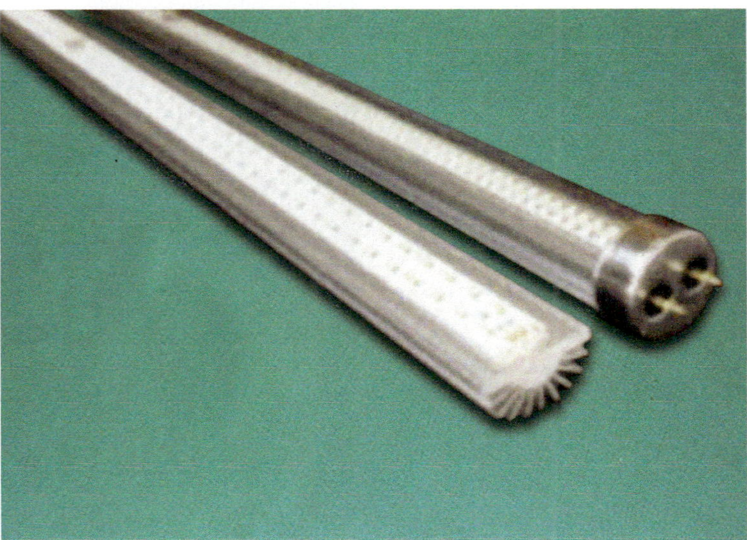

Fig. 33: LED tube lights.

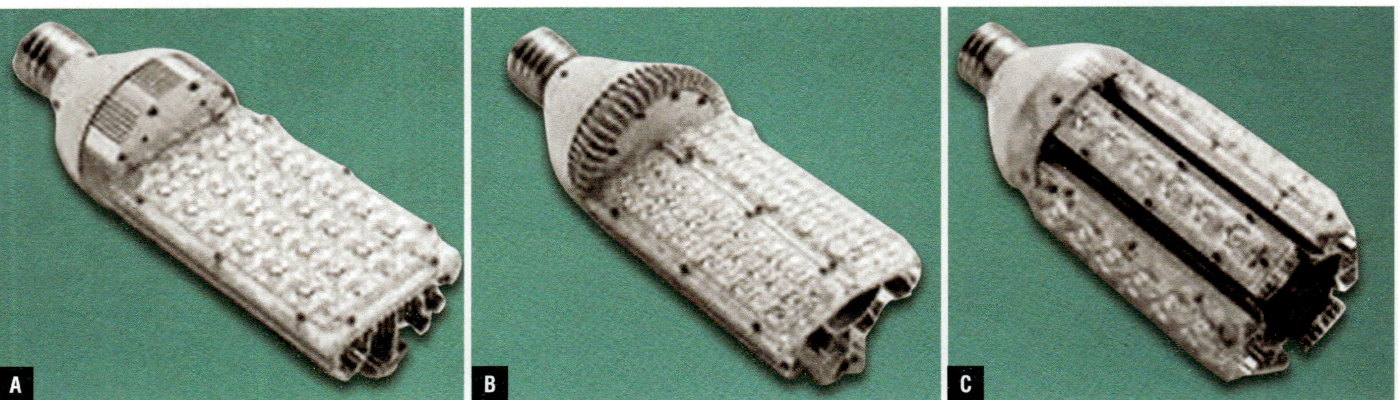

Fig. 34: Various types of LED luminaries.

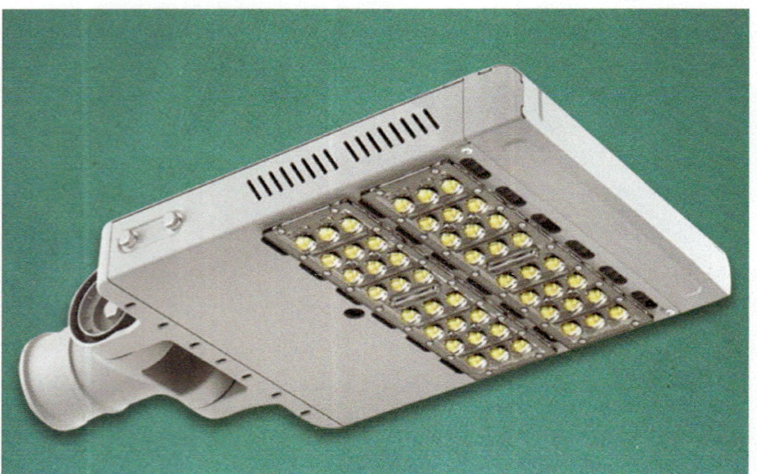

Fig. 35: LED light for outer areas.

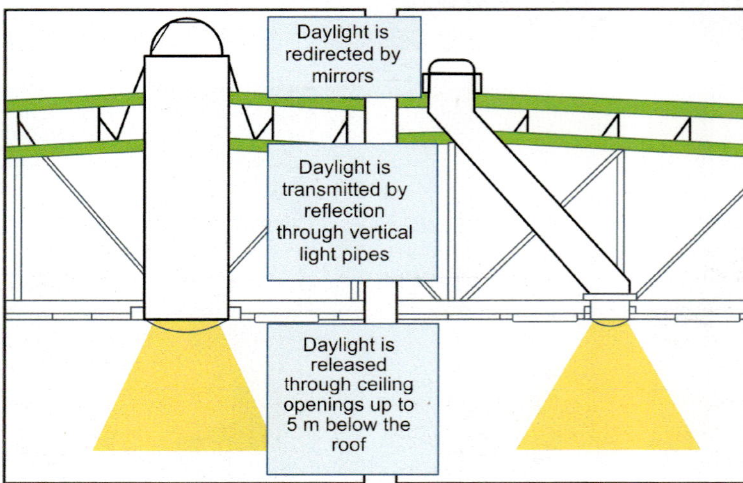

Fig. 36: Principle of light pipes.

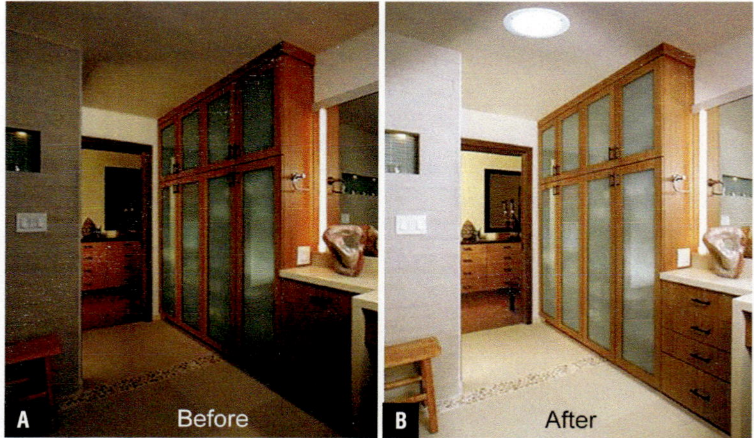

Fig. 37: Illumination of building interiors using light pipes.

Table 3: Areas required to be on power backup.

Sl. No.	Hospital area	Areas required on power backup
1.	OT	Complete area including all equipment
2.	ICU/Delivery suits/postoperative and critical care wards	Complete area including all equipment
3.	Emergency/casualty/OPD	Complete area including all equipment
4.	Wards	Examination lights on beds and treatment rooms, all lifesaving equipment, nurses workstation and 50% of lights for general illumination
5.	Lifts/exit signages	100%
6.	Fire control center	Complete area including all equipment
7.	Manifold room, CSSD, kitchen and mortuary	Complete area including all equipment
8.	Blood bank	Complete area including all equipment
9.	Radiodiagnosis	Complete area including all equipment
10.	Laboratory	Complete area including all equipment
11.	Corridors	50% of lights
12.	Other service areas	50% of lights
13.	Office areas	50% of lights and at least 50% of the computers and printers
14.	Medical/QM stores	All the deep freezers and 50% lights

CONCLUSION

In hospitals, a properly-designed visual environment, with the appropriate use of color and lighting, will have important benefits. It can make the hospital experience more pleasant for a wide range of users from the elderly to the very young. Studies have shown improved patient recovery rates, linked to aspects such as window provision and appropriate lighting. This in turn boosts overall hospital productivity and staff retention in environments which are uplifting.[6]

REFERENCES

1. www.scopemed.org
2. www.msjonline.org
3. archive.org
4. www.beeindia.in
5. www.coolight.com.hk
6. www.brikbase.org
7. healthdesign.org
8. practicegreenhealth.org
9. www.ijetmas.com
10. www.theecoexperts.co.uk
11. keralaenergy.gov.in
12. voltas.com
13. ec.europa.eu
14. www.healthcaredesignmagazine.com
15. www.bca.gov.sg
16. www.facilitymanagement.com

OTHER REFERENCES

- Electrical requirements for health care facilities review guide for: hospitals nursing facilities clinics office of state wide health planning and development facilities. Development Division (www.oshpd.ca.gov): Los Angeles, CA 90012 (USA).
- Energy Conservation Building Code (ECBC) User guide developed by Bureau of Energy Efficiency (BEE) in 2009.
- Healthcare application guide: Designing people-centric hospitals using Philips lighting solutions.
- IS 4347: Code of practice for hospital lighting in India.
- IS standard 2440:1975 Indian Standard: Guide for Day-lighting of Buildings.
- Lighting and color for hospital design R&D Report B(01)02 yr 2004 Status In Wales (UK).
- Lighting for Elderly Patients and Dementia wards: Apollo lighting.
- National Lighting Code (USA) Article 517: Specific requirements for Healthcare facilities.
- National Lighting Code 2010 of India.
- Eric E. R. Requirement for lighting levels, Pacific Northwest National Laboratory (USA). Publication 2001.
- Journal of Alternative & Complementary Medicine, March 2015.

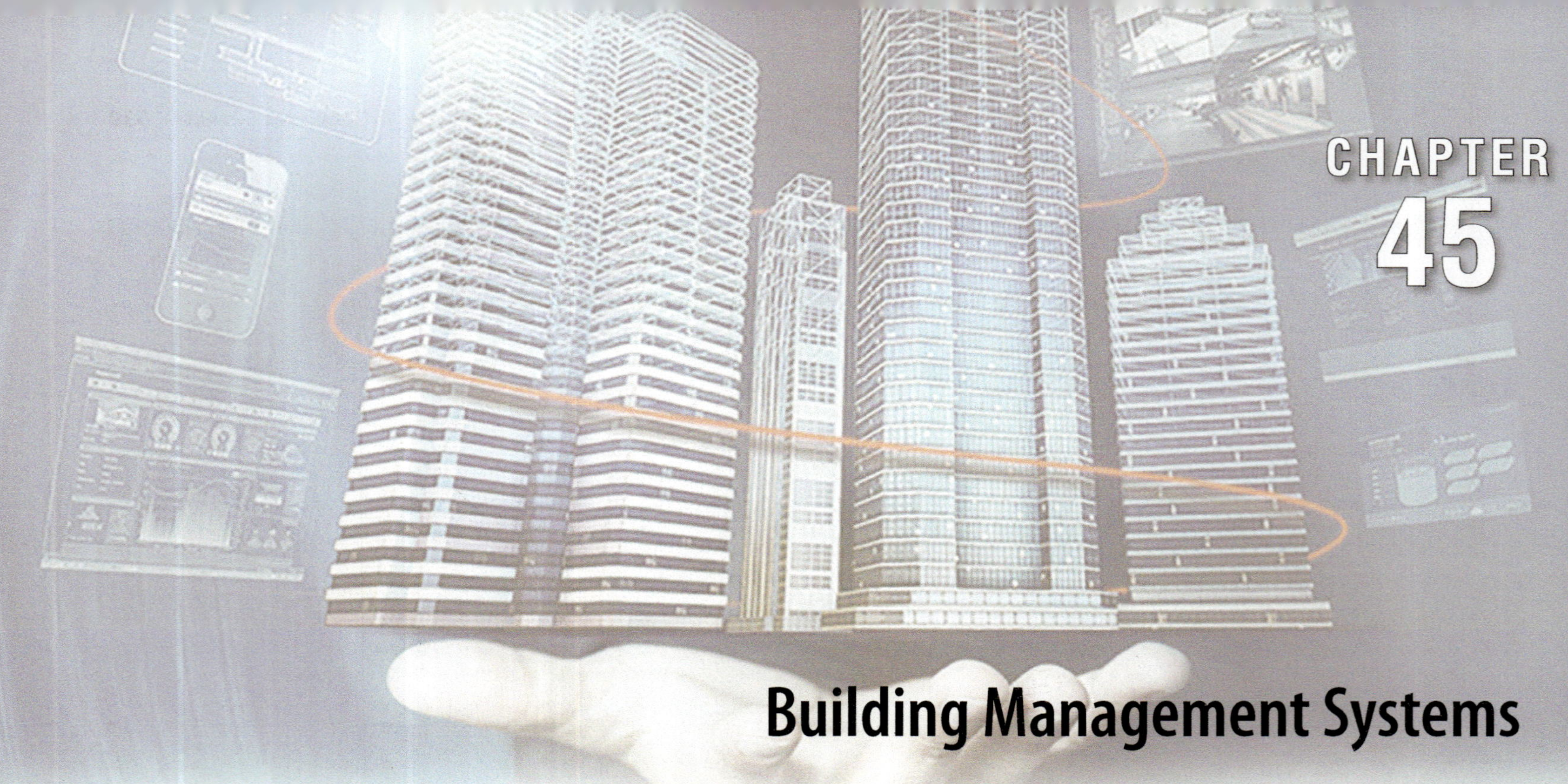

Building Management Systems

Vijay Kumar Tadia, Shrish Kumar, Shakti Kumar Gupta, Sunil Kant, R Chandrashekhar

INTRODUCTION

Building management systems (BMS) have come a long way since their introduction in the early 1970s. Modern systems cost less, are faster and more reliable, offer more features, have a more user-friendly interface and are easier to learn and use. They have been installed successfully in facilities of all sizes and types, making them practically an essential requirement to the successful management of operating costs.

Building management systems [also called building automation system (BAS)] are used in buildings for automatic monitoring and control of services such as lighting, plumbing, fire services, heating and air-conditioning systems. The term refers to a system that uses sensors, controls and activators. All these use an electronic digital processor to implement control algorithms and have the capability of communicating with other controls. The BMS term covers all control elements, including hardware, controllers, any linking network and central controllers. Generally, a control system consists of three basic elements—a sensor, a controller and a controlled device. The organization of these various control elements into a comprehensive BMS is termed the system architecture. Each component in this architecture is connected with each other via a communication system. The communications network is characterized by two essential parts:

- Physical medium—that transports the signals, e.g. wire, optical fiber, radio.
- Protocol—a set of common language rules for the communication signals.

A BMS is most common in a large building. Its core function is to manage the environment within the building and to control temperature, carbon dioxide levels and humidity within a building. As a core function in most BMS systems, it controls heating and cooling, manages the systems that distribute this air throughout the building (for example by operating fans or opening/closing dampers), and then locally controls the mixture of heating and cooling to achieve the desired room temperature. A secondary function sometimes is to monitor the level of human-generated CO_2, mixing in outside air with waste air to increase the amount of oxygen while also minimizing heat/cooling losses. Systems linked to a BMS typically represent 40% of a building's energy usage; if lighting is included, this number approaches 70%. Building management systems are a critical component to managing energy demand. Intelligent building management systems (IBMSs) are linked to access control of the Building or other security systems such as closed-circuit television (CCTV) and motion detectors. Fire alarm systems and elevators are also sometimes linked to a BMS, for example, if a fire is detected then the system could shut off dampers in the ventilation system to stop smoke spreading and send all the elevators to the ground floor and park them to prevent people from using them in the event of a fire.

Building management systems have been employed for as long as commercial buildings have existed, whether this be through manpower loading coal into coal fired boilers or opening water pipe valves manually with the use of a handle so to enable heated water to flow through a radiator circuit. However, "BMS" as a phrase, is relatively new, the concept being introduced in the early 1970s (the terms BAS, and EMS-energy management system are also used); the phrase has only really existed since the introduction of complex electronic devices that are capable of retaining data for the purposes of managing services such as power, lighting, heating and so on. It was the advent of the "modem", or "modulator-demodulator" which allowed analog signals to be digitized so that they could be communicated over long distances with a high degree of accuracy that spurred the development and deployment of modern BMSs. The Powers 570 was an example of such a system. Developed and marketed by Powers Regulator Company (later purchased by Siemens), it was deployed into the market in May 1970, as the model number suggests.

Before the modern, computer-controlled BMS came into being, various electromechanical systems were in use to control buildings. Many facilities management offices had panels consisting of manual switches or more commonly, lights showing the status of various items of plant, allowing building maintenance staff to react if something failed. Some of these systems also include an audible alarm. Advancements in signal communications technology have allowed the migration of early pneumatic and "home run" hard wired systems, to modems communicating on a single twisted pair cable, to ultrafast IP based communication on "broadband" or "fiber optic" cable.

NEED FOR BUILDING MANAGEMENT SYSTEMS IN HOSPITALS

All buildings have some form of mechanical and electrical services in order to provide the facilities necessary for maintaining a comfortable working environment. These services have to be controlled by some means to ensure, for example, that there is adequate hot water for sinks, that the hot water in the radiators is sufficient to keep an occupied space warm, that heating with ventilation and possibly cooling is provided to ensure comfort conditions wherever, irrespective of the number of occupants or individual preferences.[1]

Basic controls take the form of manual switching, time clocks or temperature switches that provide the on and off signals for enabling pumps, fans or valves, etc. The purpose of a BMS is to automate and take control of these operations in the most efficient way possible for the occupiers/business, within the constraints of the installed plant.[2]

Healthcare is one of the fastest growing sectors in India; the healthcare spending is set to increase in the coming years. Hospitals are an inseparable part of the healthcare delivery system. In most hospitals, continuous operations and the latest equipment require uninterrupted power supply for suitable functioning. IBMS can help in rational use of energy in hospitals. As per the Ministry of Power, Government of India, there is a huge potential of energy savings in hospitals and healthcare institutions. Energy Audit studies conducted across different sectors including hospitals indicate huge energy saving potential.[2]

It has been observed that if energy conservation measures are adopted and coupled with enabling architectural design to harness natural light and ventilation, it should be possible to bring about a reduction of 10% in electricity consumption.[2]

Energy Facts in Healthcare Facilities Today

The producer price index for fuels, related products, and power clearly illustrates the trend for increasing prices. High energy prices are forecast to continue due to limited supply and refining capacity, a tense global political climate, and brisk worldwide demand for fossil fuel. Healthcare-related research figures from the program indicate that energy consumption per sq ft in hospitals is much higher than many other types of buildings, primarily due to 24 × 7 hours of operation and demanding requirements for air filtration and air exchange. However, just because hospitals run 24 × 7 it does not mean there are fewer opportunities to save energy.[2]

What Drives High Energy Use at Healthcare Facilities?[3]

- High efficiency particulate air (HEPA) filtration is required to prevent the spread of disease (nosocomial infection) in the ventilation system. HEPA filters that achieve 99.7% efficiency place greater electric demand on fans for proper air circulation.[3]
- Stringent indoor air quality (IAQ) levels must be maintained, especially in operating rooms (OR), emergency rooms (ER), intensive care units (ICU), and laboratories. These rooms require 20–30 air changes per hour.[3]
- Certain types of rooms have special heating, ventilation, and air-conditioning (hvac) pressurization requirements. ORs, ERs, and ICUs, generally run over-pressure for protective isolation from airborne infection. Quarantine rooms require negative pressure (and UV lights) for infectious isolation and the control of diseases.[3]
- IAQ must be strictly regulated for temperature, humidity, and quality. This increases the need for proper heating, cooling, and fresh air intake.
- Domestic hot water must be heated to 130°F to kill legionella bacteria. Thereafter the water temperature has to be lowered to 105°F before use.[3]
- Some rooms require climate control set at 60°F to accommodate the adhesive cement used for orthopedics, which tend to set too quickly in warmer temperatures.[3]
- Laundry facilities and kitchens can consume 10–15% of the building's energy, increasing the need to more closely monitor hours of peak demand from these source.[3]
- Hospitals require that power be provided at 100% uptime for patient care and liability concerns. Backup generators contribute to increased operating costs, or cogeneration [combined heat and power, or (CHP)] investment may be necessary.[3]

Hospitals have unique and intensive energy use requirements. In addition to the need for lighting and heating 24 hours a day, hospitals demand extensive energy for ventilation, equipment, sterilization, laundry and food preparation.[4]

Every year, US hospitals spend an average of $1.67/sq ft in electricity costs, and another 48 cents/sq ft on natural gas. Lighting (25%) and HVAC (45%) are the largest parts of a typical hospital's energy bill. Both areas present opportunities for significant savings. For example, regular evaluations and tune-ups to the HVAC system (costing 4–20 cents/sq ft) have been proven to cut those costs by 10–15%. This translates into roughly $34,000/year in savings for a 100,000 sq ft facility.[4]

Energy savings have the potential to dramatically impact a hospital's budget.[4]

FUNCTIONING OF BUILDING MANAGEMENT SYSTEMS

The BMS is a standalone computer system that can calculate the preset requirements of the building and control the connected plant to meet those needs. Its inputs, such as temperature sensors and outputs, such as on/off signals are connected into outstations around the building. Programs within these outstations use this information to decide the necessary level of applied control. The outstations are linked together and information can be passed from one to another. In addition, a modem is also connected to the system to allow remote access.[1]

The level of control via the BMS is dependent upon the information received from its sensors and the way in which its programs tell it to respond to that information. In addition to offering a precise degree of control to its environment, it can be made to alarm on conditions that cannot meet specification or warn of individual items of plant failure.[1]

Occupancy times for different areas are programmed into the BMS such that the plant is brought on and off to meet the occupier requirements. These times are often under optimum start control. This means that the cooling plant is enabled, at a varying predetermined time, to ensure that the cooled space is at the set desired temperature for the start of the day. The BMS therefore, based on the outside air temperature the space temperature and the building structure, determines the plant start time (Figs. 1 and 2).[1]

BENEFITS OF BUILDING MANAGEMENT SYSTEMS

It is necessary to remember that the benefits of a modern BMS are enjoyed vigorously by different users involved with the building. These

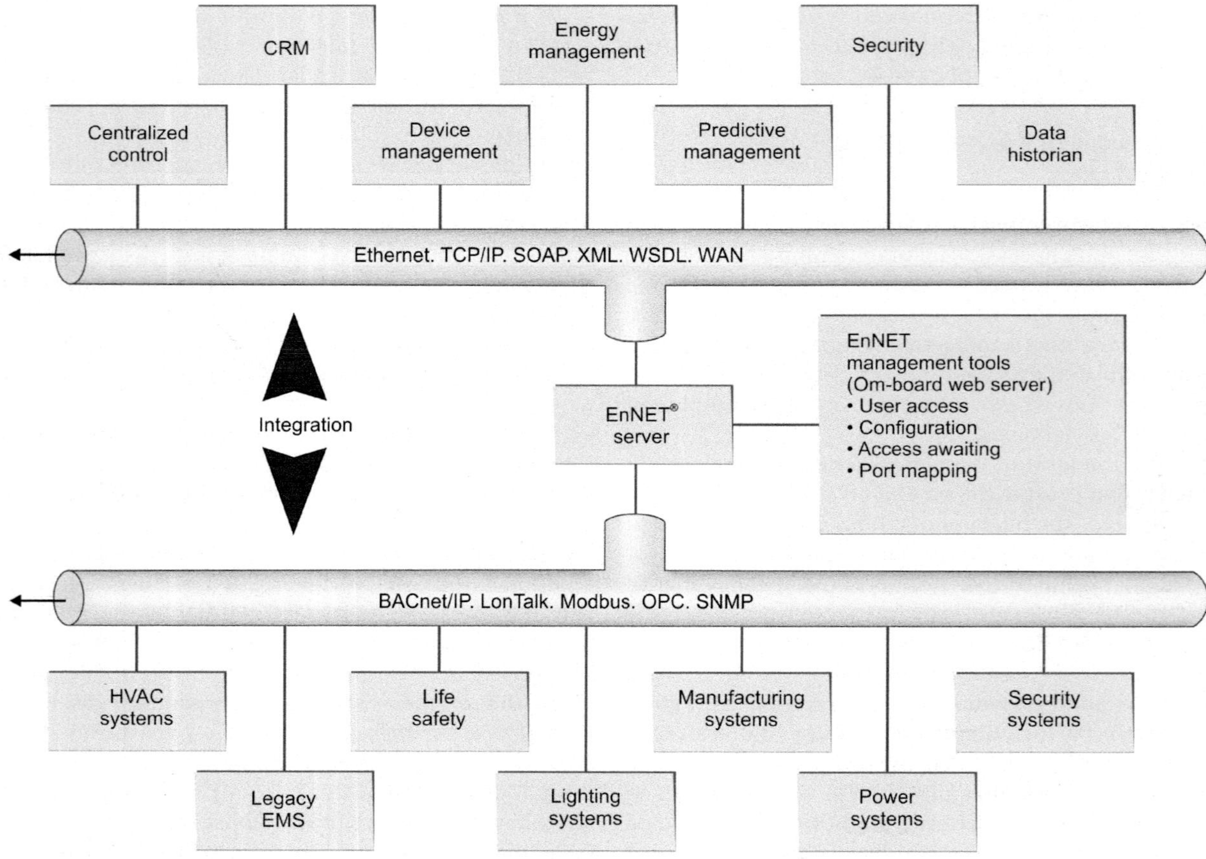

Fig. 1: Functioning network.

(TCP/IP: transmission control protocol/internet protocol; SOAP: simple object access protocol; XML: extensible markup language; WSDL: web services description language; WAN: wide area network; OPC: open platform communications; SNMP: Simple Network Management Protocol; CRM: customer relationship management)

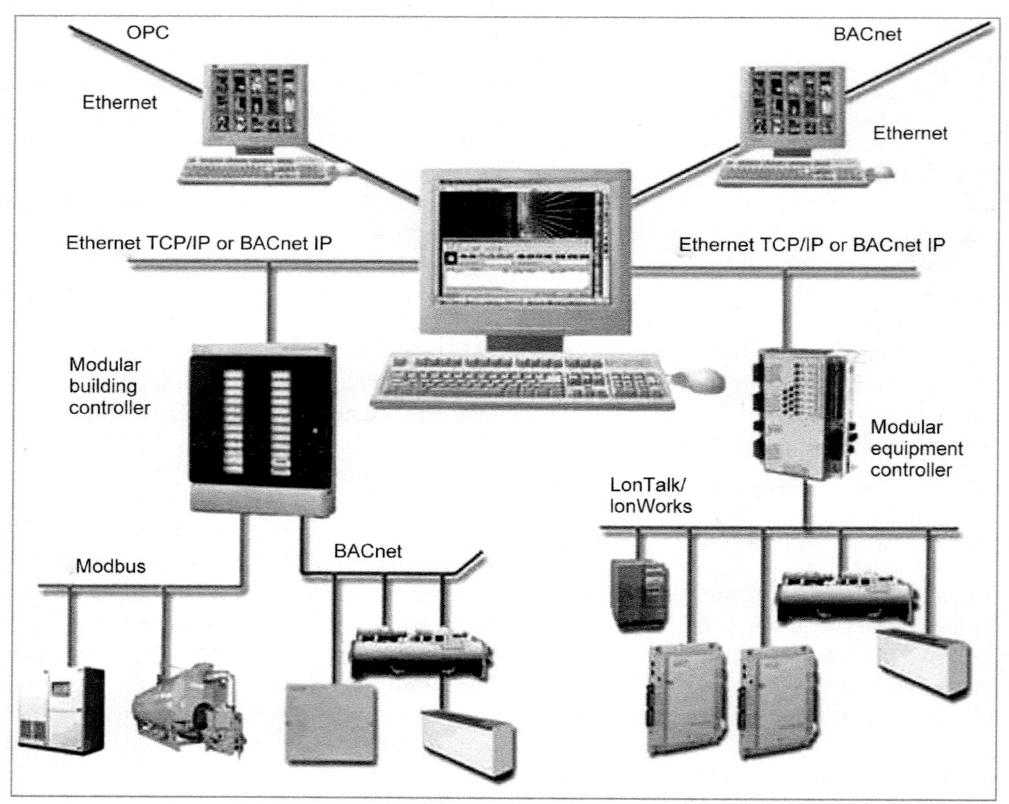

Fig. 2: System integration.

(TCP/IP: transmission control protocol/internet protocol; OPC: open platform communications)

benefits will only be obtained if the system is properly specified, installed, commissioned, operated and maintained. List of some benefits that can be achieved with an effective modern BMS.

Building Owner

- Higher rental value
- Flexibility on change of building use
- Individual tenant billing for services.

Facilities Manager

- Central or remote control and monitoring of building operations
- Low operating cost
- Efficient use of building resources and services
- High productivity
- Rapid alarm indication and fault diagnosis
- Good plant schematics and documentation.

Building Tenant/Occupants

- Effective monitoring and targeting of energy consumption
- Good control of internal comfort conditions
- Possibility of individual room control
- Increased staff productivity
- Improved plant reliability and life
- Effective response to HVAC related complaints
- Maintenance companies
- Ease of information availability problem diagnostics
- Computerized maintenance scheduling
- Effective use of maintenance staff
- Early detection of problems
- More satisfied occupants.

CHOOSING THE RIGHT BMS

Buying and installing a BMS is a significant investment. Systems are complex and expensive, and installation can cause disruptions to operations. Facility managers can take several steps to ensure that the BMS they buy is the best system for their facility needs. These considerations are discussed briefly below.[5]

BMS Capabilities

The ability of BMS to control energy cost and to modify the operation of equipment from remote locations reduces energy waste and labor costs, while improving tenant comfort. Also, integrating building functions and operations in one system is one of the most important features of today's automation systems.

Selecting a System

The selection process of a BMS should be considered in view of the following factors:

- Supplier reputation in similar projects
- How long the system has been on the market.
- Training package provided by the supplier to the operation and maintenance staff.
- Supplier after sale technical support and supplier guarantee of spare parts availability for a reasonable future period.

System Limitations

Building management system are not the cure-all for operations and maintenance problems. While they can help make operations more efficient, they cannot overcome operational shortcomings, such as lack of preventive and planned maintenance.

Identifying Automation Needs

Building management system can identify the shortcomings of the existing operations. Typical deficiencies that motivate facility managers to consider installing a new BAS include:

- High energy use
- Low maintenance productivity
- Unorganized maintenance activities
- Inability to adapt building systems to changing occupant requirements
- Lack of coordination among various building systems.

System Ability to Adopt Future Trends

Selected BMS should be capable of accommodating future trends in the industry easily, so that facility managers in the future can adopt new features into their systems without very high expenditure. It is simply the ability of upgrading systems.

DEFINITION AND OBJECTIVES OF ENERGY MANAGEMENT

The fundamental goal of energy management is to produce goods and provide services with the least cost and least environmental effect. The term energy management means many things to many people. One definition of energy management is:[5,6]

"The judicious and effective use of energy to maximize profits (minimize costs) and enhance competitive positions".[5]

Another comprehensive definition is:

"The strategy of adjusting and optimizing energy, using systems and procedures so as to reduce energy requirements per unit of output while holding constant or reducing total costs of producing the output from these systems".[5]

The objective of energy management is to achieve and maintain optimum energy procurement and utilization, throughout the organization and:[5]

- To minimize energy costs/waste without affecting production and quality
- To minimize environmental effects.

System Integration

The system provider should furnish and install a fully integrated BMS, incorporating distributed control techniques and standard open communication networks. The system should be implemented as an integrated, open solution, which enables service center connectivity through standard building operating system (BOS) interface (Fig. 3). The integrated systems should include controls and monitoring of the whole building (BMS and Security) and each room/apartment whenever applicable.[7,8]

Integrated building management and security systems should include the following subsystems:

- BMS/building automation (cooling/heating control, ventilation control, pumps, etc.)

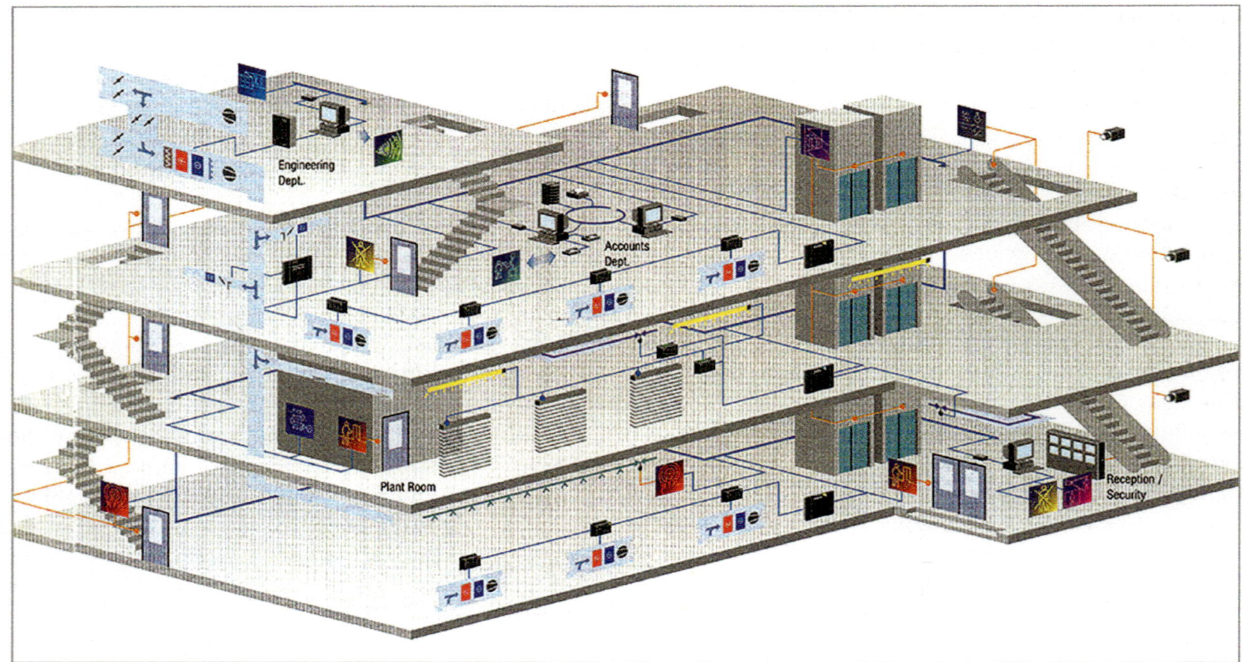

Fig. 3: Integrated building management system.

- Lighting control of common areas
- Consumption metering of water, electricity, cooling (heating) energy and gas
- Access control system for common areas
- Intruder alarm system for common areas
- Video monitoring system for common areas
- Fire alarm system
- Central battery system
- Basement carbon monoxide monitoring system.

Whenever applicable, Room Controls should include the following subsystems:[7,8]

- Room temperature controls
- Lighting controls, dimming groups
- Lighting controls, on/off groups
- Controlled sockets, enabled/disabled
- Curtain controls (optional)
- Water consumption metering (optional)
- Electricity consumption metering (optional)
- Cooling energy consumption metering (optional).

User Interfaces

Systems should be accessed through the BOS. System must have two main user interface types—professional user interface and occupant user interface.[7,8]

Professional User Interface

The system should enable a client based user interface for professional usage and for central monitoring of systems (service center usage). The professional user interface should allow for at least of the following:[7,8]

- Alarm monitoring and alarm handling by multiple operators
- Intruder alarms
- Fire alarms
- Alarms from electrical and mechanical systems
- System maintenance alarms
- Video monitoring
- Remote diagnostics, energy optimization and trending
- Setpoint adjustment
- Control optimization
- Peak load management
- Trending
- Remote diagnostics of system/devices
- Preventive maintenance
- Consumption reports for energy management and billing
- Logs and reporting
- User profile and role management
- Access rights management.

The professional user interface should be implemented as a client application, which includes an automatically adapting tree structure of the building, building's parts, individual spaces, different systems and parts of systems. The tree structure can be used for navigation through the system. All systems connected to BOS can be accessed through the same graphical user interface. The client software can be installed to unlimited number of remote computers or laptops. The client software should allow for remote internet usage of several sites using the same client.[7,8]

The professional user interface should show system views, floor plan views, trend view, alarm view and event log view per building and system layer. Any alarm should be shown in red color in both graphical views and tree structure. Each alarm message should include shortcut to relevant graphical system and floor plan view.[7,8]

Occupant User Interface

Subsystems in, e.g. meeting rooms, hotel rooms or residences should be usable through a graphical browser-based occupant user interface, using touch screen panel PC's, tablet PC's, IPTV, home computers, laptops, PDA's and mobile phones. The user interface should comply with requirements defined in the system architecture. The browser-based occupant User interface should be generated automatically using the structure of the building defined in the building information model. The browser-based user interface should utilize latest web technologies, such as AJAX. The user interfaces should provide easy access to frequently needed functionality, such as lighting controls, temperature set point modifications, alarms, and configuration of scenes and modes of the space. The same user interface functionality should be usable through any device with a browser. The browser-based occupant user interface should allow for at least the following actions:[7,8]

- Changing the mode of the space
- Modifying the mode settings of the controlled devices
- Changing the set points
- Modifying the control settings (e.g. dimming level)
- Manual controls
- Door controls
- Camera views
- Alarm list browsing.

SYSTEM ARCHITECTURE

The system should be implemented as an integrated, open solution, which enables service center connectivity through standard building operating system interface. The system architecture should consist of four levels:[7,8]

- Service level
- Management level
- Control level
- Field level.

The system should be completely modular in structure and freely expandable at any stage. Each level of the system should operate independently of the next level up as specified in the system architecture. For example, control level should operate independently without support from management level. The system should be fully consistent with the latest industry standards. To enable efficient functional system integration and to provide maximum flexibility and to respond to changes in the building use, the system offered should support the use of LonWorks, Modbus, M-bus, Ethernet TCP/IP and internet communication technologies.[7,8]

Service Level

Service level should allow the systems to be connected without additional software to one or several service center(s), for providing centralized remote monitoring, alarm and fault detection of connected building management and security systems. The service center should be capable of accessing remotely the systems through a standard interface through the BOS platform. The standard connectivity should enable providing advanced maintenance and security services, such as security alarm monitoring, maintenance alarm monitoring, remote diagnostics, main user capability, remote control and optimization of all systems, energy optimization, trending and reporting services. The service center should support connectivity of multiple sites in multioperator environment. Predefined alarms from connected sites, e.g. intruder alarms, dirty filter notifications or leakage alarms, for example, should appear in the alarm list with a specified priority. Alarms should be stored in the central database. Remote diagnostics of site systems and devices should enable proactive maintenance of technical systems, energy optimization and efficient management of the infrastructure. Centralized monitoring of all connected sites with main user capability should enable, e.g. set point changes, manual controls and camera controls by using the remote connection.[7,8]

Management Level

Management level should provide a uniform view to all systems through the open BOS platform. All the systems—controls of cooling, ventilation and lighting, consumption measurements, access controls, intruder alarms, fire alarms and NVR/DVR systems—should be integrated with the BOS using device drivers. The BOS should offer at least the following common services to be used by all connected systems:

- Alarms
- Historical trending
- Logs and reporting
- User profile and role management.

To ensure fault-tolerant system functionality, the management layer should not be responsible for any controls. The critical control functionality is taken care of by the intelligence on the control layer. The management layer should provide standard connectivity through the BOS platform with the service level, with capability to support very advanced maintenance and security services. The BOS software should also be capable of acting as a gateway between systems conveying messages, for example, from IP or Modbus devices to LON devices and vice versa.

The BOS should collect trends from defined points, collect and forward alarms from the systems. The BOS should enable efficient management of user rights. The BOS should be capable of forwarding alarms to mobile phones using SMS, local alarm printers or to service center. It should be possible to browse the alarm history for reporting and statistical purposes. The BOS should include a structured XML object model of the building, its parts and spaces, its connected systems, system parts and effect areas of each system. The XML object model should comply with COBA XML schema. The BOS should include an open interface for other applications to interact with the connected systems. Communication method between BOS and client applications should include at least Java Messaging Service (JMS). No other primary interfaces are recommended. Web interfaces should be used for lightweight clients, e.g. automatically generated browser-based user interfaces in residences for Panel PC‘s, PDA‘s or IPTV.

The network technology should be based on the IT standards, such as TCP/IP, and be compatible with latest LAN/WAN technology. The operating system of the BOS server should be Linux. The BOS should be capable of supporting current and future building management protocols through implementation of network interface drivers. The BOS should be capable of current and future systems and devices through implementation of device drivers.[7,8]

Control Level

The control level should consist of a distributed network of smart controllers, which communicate to each other using a commonly known field bus as specified herein. Connectivity toward management level should utilize standard TCP/IP protocol. The controllers should include all the intelligence of the system. All communication should be event-based, real-time peer-to-peer communication. All controllers should be capable of operating autonomously independently of management layer.[7,8]

For example, all systems react to alarms on the control layer without interference from upper layers. Each automation controller should be capable of handling several different systems in parallel through flexible distribution of I/O points. Automation controllers should function as autonomous units and form an intelligent system by communicating in real time over the free topology (FTT-10) local operating network (LON) using standard network variables types (SNVT). Security controllers should utilize RS-485 connection between the network controller and the interface panels.[7,8]

Field Level

The field level should consist of industry standard sensors and actuators, industry standard (wiegand) card readers and IP cameras. Field level is specified per system.

Building management and security systems, including building automation, lighting controls, consumption measurements, access control, intruder alarms, video monitoring, fire alarms, central battery system and home automation, should be integrated using the BOS as the integration platform, which should provide functionality as described in the system architecture.[7,8]

BUILDING AUTOMATION[6]

Building automation includes control and monitoring of cooling/heating system, ventilation system, pumps, tanks, lifts, etc. All mechanical and electrical systems should be monitored and controlled by smart control nodes connected to LON. BAS should be integrated with lighting controls, security systems and fire alarm system as specified in the system architecture. Building automation should be connected to the central user interface through the BOS.[7,8]

Distribution of Intelligence

The intelligence of the automation systems should be distributed into smart control nodes, which are connected to control network (LON). Smart control nodes must be commonly used during past 10 years in large scale commercial facilities, such as offices, business centers or hotels. It should be possible to integrate the systems on control level without interference of management level, according to system architecture. Communication between smart control nodes should be peer-to-peer communication via a free topology LON with the SNVT. All communication should be event-based. Nodes should be intelligent modules, capable of operating autonomously independently of management level. For example, all systems must be able to react to alarms on the control level without interference from upper levels.[7,8]

Usage of Input/Output Points

Each node should have about 10 input/output (I/O) points to achieve maximum reliability and flexibility. Each node should be capable of handling several different systems in parallel through flexible distribution of I/O points. The I/O points of the control nodes should be as follows:[7,8]

- DI: Digital indication, from potential free contact
- DO: Digital control, open collector
- AI: Analog input, standard measurements 0–10 VDC, PT1000 or Ni1000-LG.
- AO: Analog control, 0–10 VDC or 20 mA

The control nodes should include PID controllers and ON/OFF (thermostat) functions for implementing the control loops used in engineering system process controls. Logical functions should be implemented using configurable software objects in the control nodes.

Field devices are connected to control nodes using the common industry standards:

- PT-1,000 for temperature
- 0–10 V for other sensors and actuators
- Potential free contacts for ON/OFF indications and push buttons—24 V relays for ON/OFF controls
- Impulses for consumption measurements.

To guarantee openness, flexibility and cost-efficient maintenance of the integrated systems, the field devices should not include independent control logic. Control nodes are placed to the nearest electric cabin, side of air handling units (AHUs) or in separate cabins when adequate. All systems should use the same control network cabling, which uses free topology to maximize flexibility for future modifications and to minimize the need for cables. Electrical design should utilize star topology for controlled loads to maximize flexibility for changes.

General Purpose Controllers

General purpose controllers should be freely configurable to achieve maximum reliability and flexibility and to meet the sequence of operation and future modifications. Configuration should be done with a graphical system configuration tool, which should be compatible with the building operating system. The tool should produce BOS compatible XML document about all integrated systems, which can be used as such to run the BOS.[7,8]

Special Purpose Controllers

Special purpose controllers should be used as autonomous controllers in rooms, zones and fan coil units (FCU). Each special purpose controller alone should be capable of controlling temperature, air quality (CO_2) and lighting in the room or zone. Special purpose controllers should communicate on LON bus.[7,8]

It should be possible for the FCU controller to automatically change the FCU motor speed based on temperature deviation. The FCU controller should regulate the cooling valve to meet the desired temperature conditions. FCU controllers should communicate on LON bus and should be integrated with BMS system to enable energy optimization and reporting.[7,8]

LIGHTING CONTROLS[6]

Lighting of common areas of the building should be controlled by smart control nodes, which should be connected to LON field bus. Lighting controls should be implemented as part of the integrated. Lighting groups in the common areas are on/off controlled (and/or dimmed) as follows:

- Using local push buttons (on/off, on/off/up/down, lighting scenes)—On occupancy
- Based on illumination level (dusk)
- Time schedules

Lighting controls are integrated with building automation and security systems and connected to the central user interface through BOS.

CONSUMPTION METERING

Consumptions of water, electricity, gas and cooling energy should be measured in each area/apartment. Water and electricity meters should be equipped with impulse outputs. Impulse outputs are connected to smart control nodes, which are connected to LON. BTU meters should be connected direct to control network. All consumptions should be trended into BOS‘s database for generating regular consumption reports. Different type of reports have to be generated for professional users and occupants. Occupant reports must be easy to understand and they must increase environmental awareness according to LEED and other green building initiatives.

ACCESS CONTROL AND INTRUDER ALARMS[6]

Access control system should be integrated with building automation, lighting controls and other security systems using the BOS as the integration platform. Access control should be implemented with proximity readers, control nodes, electronic keys and electronic locks. Users can be classified so that they have access only to the spaces they are allowed to enter according to programmed time schedules. The access control system is connected to BOS for full control and reporting, and integrated into the central user interface. Intruder alarm system should include perimeter protection and indoor surveillance. Monitored doors and windows should be equipped with magnetic contacts. Movement detectors used in indoor surveillance should be sensitive enough for presence detection of a single person, so that they can also be used for lighting controls and air-conditioning controls. Intruder alarms are seamlessly integrated on software level to access control, CCTV/DVR/NVR, lighting control and building automation. Granted access disarms the alarm zones automatically. In case of burglary the system gives an alarm, which is relayed through BOS to service center and/or to specified mobile phones.

Network Controllers

Network controllers should connect access control and intruder alarm system with management level using an open interface utilizing TCP/IP protocol. Network controllers should connect with up to 32 interface panels using RS-485 bus. The door/reader interface panels should operate also autonomously with no connection to a network controller. Network controllers should buffer the offline transactions from interface panels when connection to the BOS server is down and send the transactions when the connection is restored. The network Controller should enable access control database. The memory of the Network Controller should be easily expandable. Each access group should have a schedule-based access to defined door groups. The network controllers should be able to communicate with each other to create large-scale area control solutions with independent control logics. Area control solutions should be expandable using TCP/IP network to include door/reader interface panels located under several network controllers. Network controller should have local inputs for tamper and battery failure for indications and alarms.

Interface Panels

The selection of interface panels should include at least door/reader interface panel, input monitor interface panel and output control interface panel. The interface panels should connect with network controllers using RS-485 bus. Door/reader interface panels should have two reader interfaces utilizing standard Wiegand protocol. Depending on application, the panel can be configured to control two sets of separate doors with a reader and an exit button, or one door with two-side readers (entry/exit).

In addition to the two reader interfaces, the door/reader interface panels should have the following inputs and outputs—door monitor input, exit button input, strike relay output, auxiliary relay output. Door/reader interface panels should be capable of indicating door forced and door held alarms also locally by using the internal beeper of the reader. Interface panels should have local inputs for tamper and battery failure for indications and alarms. The input monitoring interface panel should be used to interface, e.g. magnetic contacts and motion detectors to indicate alarm events. The input monitoring interface panel should include 16 supervised alarm inputs and 2 relay outputs. Output control interface panel should be used mainly to control lifts. The output control interface panel should have 12 relay outputs and 2 supervised alarm inputs. It should be possible to create complex I/O linking and rules between network controllers and interface panels.

Readers

The system should support a variety of readers using standard Wiegand protocol, including plain readers, keypad readers, long-range readers and biometric readers. Readers should be based on 125 kHz proximity technology or 13.56 MHz contactless smart card technology, e.g. Mifare or iCLASS. The system should support a variety of credentials, including but not limited to for example, traditional proximity cards and tags.

VIDEO MONITORING

Video monitoring should be implemented with digital video recording (DVR) or a fully IP based network video recording (NVR) system. The video monitoring system should be integrated to BOS server so that the system should start recording video stream upon triggering from intruder alarm system, access control, CCTV or any other system integrated to BMS. The video monitoring system should support both analog and IP cameras. The system should preferably run on Linux operating system. Usage can be done both via video monitoring system's own user interface client and the integrated user interface of the BOS. In addition to the software-based user interface, it should be possible to additionally expand the operator workstation with hardware-based keypad and joystick interfaced with the system.[6]

FIRE ALARMS

Fire alarm system should be integrated with BMS for monitoring. Fire alarm system can be integrated either by:

- Using potential free contacts of fire alarm panels connected to control modules, or
- Using system driver which gives alarm information on individual sensor level to BOS. In both cases alarm are relayed to BOS and shown in the integrated graphical user interfaces. Ventilation is shut down in the area concerned.[8]

THE STANDARD APPROACH: BUILDING MANAGEMENT SYSTEMS CAN HELP IN CONFORMING TO IEC 60364-7-710 STANDARDS

Scope

International standards, in particular International Electrotechnical Commission (IEC) 60364-7-710 (from which most national standards are derived) focus primarily on safety, in particular the protection against indirect contact. In terms of availability of supply and overall reliability in medical locations, IEC standards only require the distribution system to facilitate the automatic change-over from the distribution network to the emergency power supply which feeds essential loads. The standard suggests a classification scheme for medical locations which is based on their intended purpose.[9]

Classification of Medical Locations

Medical locations are classified by IEC according to the use of—applied parts. An applied part is a piece of electrical equipment that is brought into physical contact with the patient, or might come into contact with the patient, or needs to be touched by the patient. The classification is as follows:[9]

- Group 0: Medical locations without applied parts.
- Group 1: Medical locations where applied parts are used externally invasively to any part of the body, except for the locations described in group 2.
- Group 2: Medical locations where applied parts are used in applications such as intracardiac procedures, operating theaters and vital treatments where discontinuity of the supply can cause danger to life. In order to determine the classification of a particular medical location, the medical staff must indicate which medical procedures will take place within that location.

System Earthing and Safety Requirements

In each medical location of group 1 and group 2, supplementary equipotential bonding conductors must be installed and connected to the equipotential bonding bus bar for the purpose of equalizing potential differences between protective conductors and extraneous conductive parts located in the—patient environment.

The TN-C system is not allowed in medical locations and medical buildings downstream of the main distribution board. In group 2 locations, the IT earthing arrangement must be used for circuits supplying medical electrical equipment and systems intended for life support, surgical applications and other electrical equipment located in the—patient environment.[9]

Emergency Supply

Regarding the continuity of supply in medical locations, secure power supplies are classified on the basis of changeover time required by the service they supervise:

- Power supplies with a changeover period less than or equal to 0.5 second—secure power supply which is capable of maintaining operating theater table lights and other essential luminaires, e.g. endoscopes, for a minimum period of 3 hours and with a changeover period not exceeding 0.5 second.[9]
- Power supplies with a changeover period less than or equal to 15 seconds—secure power supply for equipment which must be connected within 15 seconds for a minimum period of 24 hours, when the voltage of one or more line conductors at the main distribution board for the critical services has decreased by more than 10% of the nominal value of supply voltage for a duration greater than 3 seconds.[9]
- Power supplies with a changeover period greater than 15 seconds—used for equipment required for the maintenance of hospital services, which may be connected either automatically or manually for a minimum period of 24 hours. This includes, for example, sterilization equipment, air-conditioning, heating and ventilation systems.[9]

Equipment Requirements

IEC requires that in the event of a mains power failure, a minimum illuminance level must be provided from a secure supply within a changeover period not exceeding 15 seconds in the following locations:[9]

- Escape routes
- Rooms in which essential services are provided
- Rooms of group 1 and 2 medical locations

Services other than lighting which require a secure supply within a changeover period not exceeding 15 seconds include fire protection systems and medical electrical equipment used in group 2 medical locations. Such equipment needs to be identified by responsible staff. The standard also provides a table listing the secure power supply requirements for different medical locations. It is important to note that a definitive list of medical locations showing their assigned groups is impracticable, as the use of locations differs between countries and even within a country.[9]

Verification

IEC 60364-7-710 defines the following tests to be carried out for locations belonging to group 1 and 2:[9]

- Functional test of insulation on monitoring devices of medical IT systems
- Verification of equipotential bonding
- Verification of secure power service
- Measurement of leakage current of medical IT transformers in no-load condition

These tests are in addition to the requirements of IEC 60364-6-61 (a standard which defines tests and verifications to be performed on installations prior to commissioning or to recommissioning after a modification or repair). Periodic checks on secure power services are recommended at the following intervals:[9]

- **Services with batteries:** Monthly/15 min capacity test
- **Services with combustion engines:** Monthly/until rated running temperature is achieved; 12 months for—endurance run.[9]

MISCELLANEOUS[10]

One of the aims of healthcare facility design should be to provide places of respite connected to natural environment so that a healing environment exists for the patients and/or residents, staff, family members, and visitors inhabiting these buildings. Outdoor places of respite of at least 5% of the net usable program area should be provided out which at least 2% should be exclusively dedicated to the staff. Additionally, exterior courtyard, terrace or balcony are to be provided with a minimum area of 5 sq ft/patient served for 75% of all inpatients and 75% of qualifying outpatients with clinical length of stay greater than 4 hours.

The Window to Wall Ratio (WWR) and Skylight to Roof Ratio (SRR) should not exceed 60% and 5% respectively and the Solar Heat Gain Coefficient (SHGC)/Weighted Façade average SHGC of all the fenestrations should mandatorily meet the SHGC requirement of Energy Conservation Building Code (ECBC)-2007. A solar path analysis for all windows could also be carried out using specialized simulation software like Ecotect or IES to ensure that the window is completely shaded for the duration between 10:00 AM on 1st April and 15:00 PM on 30th September.

To reduce outdoor light pollution, exterior lighting should be designed in a way that the light fixtures emit no more than 5% of total initial designed fixture lumens at an angle of 90° or higher from nadir (straight down). The lighting power density which is obtained by dividing lighting power by area (unit is W/m^2 or W/sq ft) should be reduced by at least 30% as compared to values mentioned in the ASHRAE Standard 90.1-2010, Section 9.4.3. Additionally, luminous efficacy of the lamps should be at least 75 lm/W. Additionally, automatic lighting controls should be placed for controlling all outdoor lighting.

Energy metering and reporting both consumption (in kWh) and demand (in kW) should be mandatorily be part of the BMS. Reporting should be carried out for grid supplied electricity, on-site renewable energy systems, backup power generator and for individual buildings. Apart from this, sub-reporting should be carried out for AHU, cooling tower, chillers (BTU meters) in case of centralized air-conditioning plant, indoor and outdoor lighting and any other individual energy end use that could represent 10% or more of the total annual consumption of the building. The data collected should be stored for at least 36 months and should be accessible remotely. Automatic power factor correction system should also be mandatorily installed. Demand response programs could be additionally installed for a dynamic load allocation on real time basis.

Preoccupancy commissioning should be carried out by a third party to for mechanical, electrical, plumbing and renewable energy systems. A commissioning plan should be developed and observations should be recorded. Operation and Maintenance (O&M) manuals should be in place and specific clauses should be included in the contract document of the systems supplier for providing training to the core facility/service group responsible for the O&M of the building systems after installation. The commissioning authority must review contractor submittals, and review O&M details. Postoccupancy review after at least 10 months should be carried out.

For air-conditioned spaces, the minimum fresh air volume as mandated by American Society of Heating, Refrigerating and Air-conditioning Engineers (ASHRAE) Standard 62.1-2010, Sections 4-7, Ventilation for Acceptable Indoor Air Quality (with errata), or NBC of India-2005 or ASHRAE Standard 170-2008, Section 7 has to be provided. Monitoring should be carried out using BMS. An alarm must alert staff whenever the outdoor airflow value varies by 15% or more from the outdoor airflow setpoint. Additionally, the fresh air being provided can be treated for Particulate Matter 10 microns (PM 10), Ozone and CO to attain levels as desired in the CPCB National Ambient Air Quality Standard.

The CO_2, temperature and relative humidity of the occupied spaces or at AHUs for the air conditioned spaces should be monitored centrally using BMS. Additionally, it is to be demonstrated that thermal comfort is being achieved as per the requirements of NBC of India 2005 or ASHRAE Standard 55-2010.

REFERENCES

1. secutronic.com.sa
2. www.hosmac.com
3. www.controlservices.com
4. www.cee1.org
5. keralaenergy.gov.in
6. www.ijirset.com
7. excellentfiresafety.com
8. www.lonix.com
9. www.socomec.de
10. www.mintie.com

OTHER REFERENCES

- Cleaner production—energy efficiency manual for GERIAP, UNEP, Bangkok prepared by. Consortium for Energy Efficiency, Inc. 617-589-3949 www.cee1.org.
- Energy management handbook, John Wiley and Sons - 2013 Wayne C. Turner.
- Guide to energy management, Cape Hart, Turner and Kennedy.
- www.bis.gov.uk/assets/bispartners/foresight/docs/energy/energy%20final/ward%20papersection%2010.pdf.
- www.climateworks.org/download/an-overview-of-indian-energy-trends-low-carbon-growthand-development-challenges.
- www.dhbvn.com/main/new/electricityconservationtips.pdf.
- www.energyusernews.com/.
- www.fireprosystems.com/solutions/bms.htm.
- www.iklimnet.com/expert_hvac/building_control.html.
- www.lonix.com/specifications/IBMS_specification.pdf.
- www.schneider-electric.co.in/india/en/products-services/buildings/intelligentbui dings/building-management-system.page.
- www.schneider-electric.com.
- www.spectralservices.net/services_ibms.html.
- www.squidoo.com/-building-management-system-in-india
- www.sustainable buildings.org/wiki/index.php/Building_Management_Systems_(BMS).

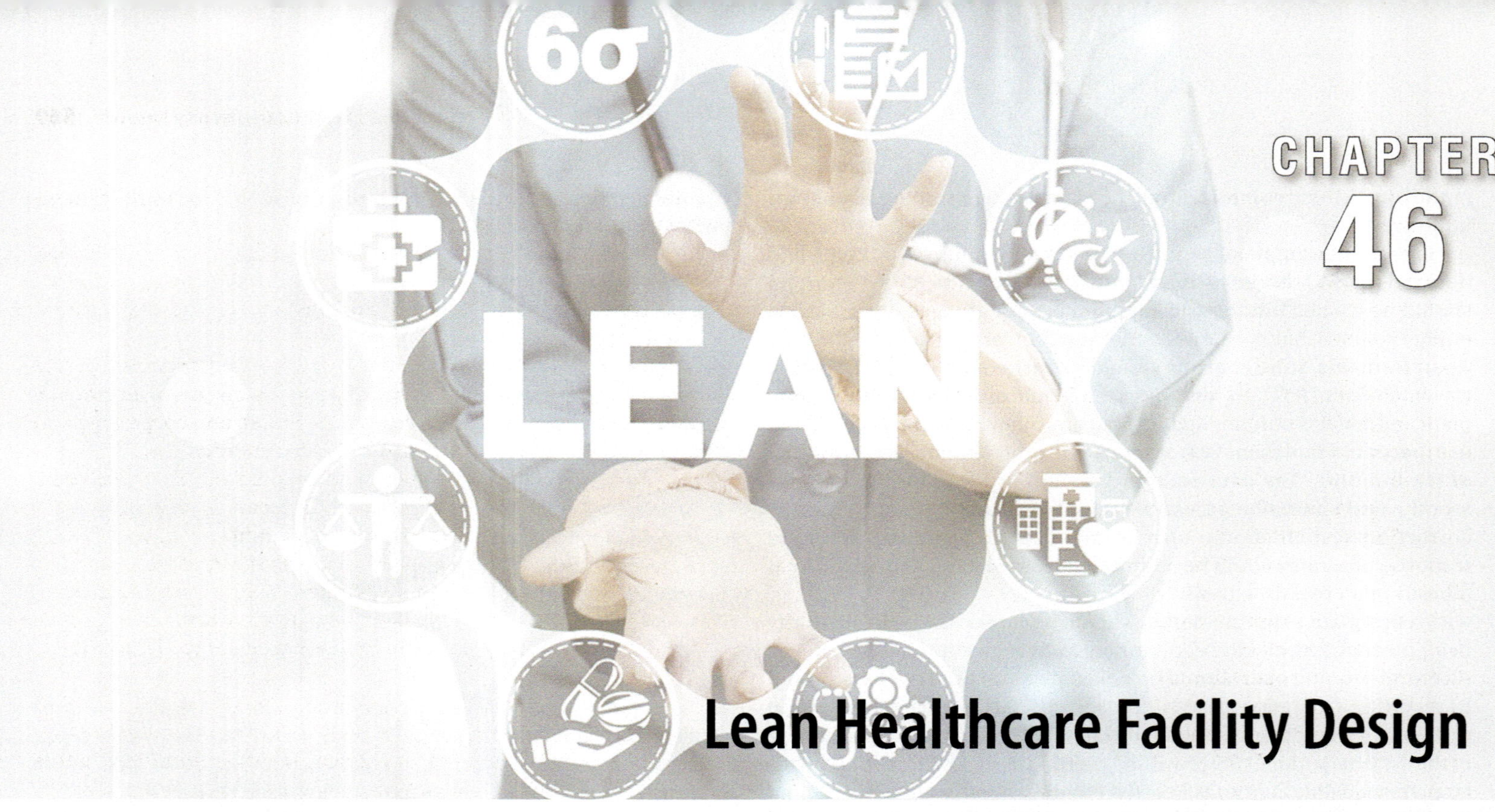

CHAPTER 46

Lean Healthcare Facility Design

Vijay Kumar Tadia, Shakti Kumar Gupta, Sunil Kant, R Chandrashekhar

"Architecture today is not seen as an important part of the healthcare delivery system...But architecture is an unexpected point of leverage for intervening in the current situation...and can play a pivotal role in the strategy for breaking free from the present mess."

—Architect David F Chambers, *Efficient Healthcare: Overcoming Broken Paradigms*

"In most people's vocabularies, design means veneer. But to me nothing could be further from the meaning of design. Design is the fundamental soul of a man made creation that ends up expressing itself in successive outer layers".

—Steve Jobs

Lean Healthcare Facility Design brings forth new meaning to the 19th Century American architect *Louis Sullivan's* heuristic that *form must follow function.* Just as Sullivan applied this thinking to skyscrapers, lean design takes into account the critical reasons for permitting function to govern structure in the design of hospitals. The perfection of its processes often requires transformation of the space in which care is given. Lean thinking contribute to both of these. In fact, no project should be considered "Shovel ready" without embracing and applying lean principles.[1,2]

When we build new hospitals without adequate collaboration among every affected person, right from the start, we literally cast in concrete certain forms of waste and insufficiency, that will have to be worked around until the next big remodeling project, which may only make things worse. Rather than building a new hospital that imports the old systems and problems, it may be imperative to re-examine the hospital design. How can a building foster continuous improvement? How can we design it to be flexible and useful well into the future? How can we do more with less inputs?

"What is Lean—Led Design? It is a systematic approach to healthcare architectural design that focus on defining developing, and integrating safe, efficient, waste free operational processes in order to create the most supportive, patient focused, physical environment possible".[3]

—Naida Grunden, Charles Hagood in Lean Led Hospital Design

Lean: Simply stated, lean is a structured way of continuously exploring and solving problems to eliminate waste in systems. The objective is to deliver value to patients. The two faces of lean are process design and facility design. Though complementary yet the lean process improvement is different from lean hospital design.

The components of lean are:

- *People*: Lean value and respect people. Patients are the recipients of the services, partners in care and the reason for the hospitals existence.
- *Process*: Lean provides a common sense, pragmatic approach to transforming processes, which is rooted in scientific method of the way in which things get done. The main focus is on elimination of waste.
- *Design*: Process transformation can be supported and accelerated through efficient design of buildings, facilities, equipment and technology.[4]

TRADITIONAL ARCHITECTURAL DESIGN VERSUS LEAN DESIGN[3]

The comparison between traditional architectural design and lean design is described in Table 1.

Table 1: Comparison between traditional architectural design and lean design.

Traditional architectural design	Lean-led design
Focus: Design	Focus: Pull value of customer/patient
Start: Functional and space program	Start: Observation at point of work
User groups (staff leaders within a department or service)	Multidisciplinary teams (cross-hierarchy) use value stream maps to analyze processes
Each user group gives feedback to designers without "the bigger picture"	Multidisciplinary consensus-bases, future-state processes drive floor plan development
Floor plans accommodate the way the hospital currently works. Anticipated process improvements remain unidentified	Floor plans validate the value stream, optimize future improvements

To build a lean hospital, lean process improvement must precede lean architectural design. It is possible to begin lean process transformation at the same time as architecture project begins. However, lean architectural design proceeds farther and faster and produces best results when the hospital has already made a significant progress with lean process improvement.

Lean design can consolidate processes and travel, increase workspace organization, and lead to another unexpected benefit, decrease in the number of sq ft area required. Lean design can be built in an environment that promotes continuous improvement efficiency, safety and better flow of information, supplies and service to patients.[3]

Lean process transformation is about continuous improvement and lean design can create an environment that can continuously improve too. Before the design ever begins, the people (users) in the organization must determine how they want to design their work. *The paradigm shifts with lean design in that users define the ideal workflows and architects are design team members who take the process information and transform it into a design. They are not the project leads but team members.* Lean led architectural design can begin as a way to remove physical barriers in the work flow. Lean design promotes culture to build only if it creates value. Every rupee and every resource that goes into new hospital building must be justified. Often it is believed that more space will solve the process related problems but only a systematic and deliberate approach of lean thinking does so. Process improvements will produce results that have implications for the use of space, facilities, and equipment.

LEAN HEALTHCARE FACILITY DESIGN: THE CHALLENGE AND THE PURPOSE

The Challenge

Healthcare facility architects and designers have worked diligently to understand the work of the end users and queried staff for input and suggestions. However, at times the staff has not always been prepared to look at their work with an eye for improving the processes to best design. Consequently, hospitals and other patient treatment facilities have been designed with good intentions, but the physical space does not exactly meet the needs of patients, visitors, staff, or providers. Ultimately, the space may not support the systems of work or patient flows economically, safely or efficiently. The end results are either resource consuming workarounds created by staff or expensive remodels of new spaces.

Traditionally, staff input to the designers is based on "the way we have always done it". Opportunities for improving the work and creating a space to support the improved work can be missed. The challenge for healthcare administrators and staff is to think differently about how we deliver care and how we do our work. This allows clinical collaboration with the architects to incorporate an improved vision for care into the design.

The challenge is to design a long lasting, flexible facilities that will support the improved vision for care delivery.

The Purpose

Based on these challenges, healthcare organizations and architecture firms are incorporating lean thinking into the planning and design of new buildings. The purpose of lean for facility design is to enhance preparation for new or remodel construction using lean methods to improve the delivery of care and eliminate waste. This is only effective if the people who do the work are engaged in the analysis of their workflow and collaborate with the design team.[5]

Integrating lean in the facility design process can result in these positive outcomes:

- An improved work environment that is patient-centered, flexible, efficient and affordable.
- Optimized patient flow and workflow to create operational efficiencies.
- Design plans that include space that is not over-built to accommodate ineffective processes, hence reducing the overall cost of the project.
- A vision for the future that is clearly developed and communicated with staff, providers, patients, and the community.

These outcomes are accomplished by incorporating the same basic principles used in any lean improvement project:

- Focus on what is "value added" for the patient.
- Relentless elimination of "waste" (non value added work).
- Understand how work currently happens before trying to fix it.
- All redesign is done by the people who do the work.
- Every change must move the organization closer to ideal care.

What is "Value" for the Patient?

Value is created when a good or service delivered to the patient is something for which the patient(s) would be willing to pay.

Patients are willing to pay for the correct medicines, delivered correctly and on time; for the correct diagnosis and medical services delivered without waste or error; for proper treatment, timely discharge, and so on.

Anything that does not add value—such as nurses hunting for supplies or calling the lab repeatedly for results, or patients waiting in the hallway or contracting hospital-acquired infections—is to be designed out of work. *In lean-led design, the objective is, as much as possible, to design a facility that paves the way for non-value-added activities to be removed from the processes and systems and hence out of the building.*

Types of Waste[5]

- Waiting
- Over-processing
- Motion/travel
- Inventory
- Defects
- Overproduction
- Confusion.

By using a lean perspective to analyze processes staff is able to identify sources of waste and redesign their work to be safer and more efficient. This analysis can be applied to all processes including staff and provider workflow, patient flow, supply flow, medication flow, etc. These systems will be significantly affected by the design of the physical space.

As with any lean work, continuous improvement is key. The lean design journey facilitates change at many levels starting with process improvement and problem solving in the existing space. Teams are able to test, stabilize, and optimize redesigned processes prior to the move into the new space. The move (supported by the rigor applied during the design phase) allows for the next levels of improvements that were not feasible in the old space. The journey continues as teams analyze and improve their processes in the new environments.

The goal is simple—redesign the processes and reduce waste. The design of the physical space is done with the intent to support the improved flows of work. This is very different from the traditional model of designing the physical space and then creating workarounds for the processes to fit the space."[5]

FRAMEWORK FOR USING LEAN IN FACILITY DESIGN

While using lean approach to facility design, there are a few prerequisites to make the most of the staff and design team effort. Clarification of the following must be made beforehand to start lean activities:

- Scope of the lean work (i.e. organization-wide, single building, or department).
- Guiding principles that must be kept at the forefront through all decisions.
- Anticipated metrics of improvement.
- Prioritization of "hot spots" and concerns by administration and design team.
- Clear assignment of lean leadership and reporting responsibilities.

Current State Analysis, Future State Development, Testing and Layout Design[1-5]

Lean is a process improvement methodology that allows one to:

- Analyze "current state" processes and flow.
- Identify opportunities for improvement.
- Develop an improved "future state".
- Articulate a plan with accountability for achieving the "future state".
- Measure the results of the improvements.
- Continuously improve the outcomes with refined iterations.

The goal of lean facility design is to incorporate these methods into the preparation for design of a new build or a remodel project. Using lean thinking along with process analysis, development, and improvement during the design phases allow for the creation of physical space that supports improved processes of work.

Current state process analysis

↓

Future state process development

↓

Future state testing and layout design

Phase 1: Current State Process Analysis

- Defining the work, reviewing the guiding principles, insuring the right players are engaged.
- Observation, data collection and analysis, interviews, utilization studies.
- Analysis of current processes using value stream mapping and "spaghetti diagrams".
- Identification of opportunities for improvement and sources of waste.

Phase 2: Future State Process Development

- Development of "Criteria for Future State" to use as evaluation criteria for all processes and/or physical space options.
- Brainstorming new ways to do work and deliver care with a focus on innovation and patient-centered design (improvement of existing processes as well as development of new services lines).
- Development and analysis of options for future state processes using bubble/adjacency diagrams and future state value stream maps.
- Establishment of implementation plans for process improvement needed to move from current state to future state.

Phase 3: Future State Testing and Layout Design

- Overview of footprint and space program.
- Testing future state processes in layout using 2D "gaming activities" or full scale mockups.
- *Analysis of key flows*: Patient, visitors, staff, providers, supplies, equipment, medication, information.
- Evaluation of layout options against "Criteria for Future State".
- Refinement of layouts and future state flows based upon above analysis.

3P/2P Methodology and Charrettes[1]

In the lean manufacturing world "3P" (Production Preparation Process) is a method for product and production design (i.e. designing a production process and production space layout for a particular product). Actually it would be sanguine if we call it "2P" in healthcare, i.e. preparation and process as there is no concept of production *per se*. The goal is to develop a process or product that meets patient requirements in the "least waste way". It is not difficult to make the intellectual leap to using 3P/2P in facility design and process improvements, particularly in healthcare where the activities of "producing" and "preparing" services for patients depends heavily on a well-tuned "process".

This activity is typically accomplished by conducting a multi-day "3P/2P event" in which a team rapidly creates and tests potential designs. The goal is to optimize flow and value to the patient. The team focuses on the processes and space related to one service line or department and is comprised of cross functional members essential to the work. During a 3P/2P event the team undertakes the following activities:

- Use lean tools and methods to "design out" waste from the start.
- Brainstorm alternative ways to meet patient needs using different processes/flows.
- Test and analyze each alternative.
- Evaluate each alternative against defined criteria.

Even though 3P is a lean method from manufacturing, the translation to healthcare is simple (2P). A team is designing a new space (not a product) but is still analyzing process and determining how to best meet the patient's needs. The team develops options for the design, tests them via 2D models or mockups, and evaluates the design options against determined criteria.

The lean methodology 3P/2P, combined with the common architectural practice of a charrettes is a successful way to guide users and design team representatives through problem solving and design solutions. Common charrette techniques are applied during the test and analyze activity of the 3P/2P event. Subgroups are challenged to brainstorm several alternatives to process flows and test different associated space layouts. The rigor applied during charrettes allows for breakthrough solutions and collaboration amongst the team members.

Charrette

Any collaborative session in which a group of designers drafts a solution to a design problem. Each subgroup presents its work to the full group as material for future dialogue. Such charrettes serve as a way of quickly generating a design solution while integrating the aptitudes and interests of a diverse group of peoples.

Layout development and testing is often done using a design practice known as "gaming" with 2D pieces of the new space (Fig. 1).

Multidisciplinary Team of Staff and Design Team Representatives

Multidisciplinary teams that include design team and user representatives are essential to maximize the value from the lean design activities. These cross-functional groups work collaboratively throughout all the key phases described above. The teams specific to each work area provides a powerful coalition of ideas, innovations and problem-solving.

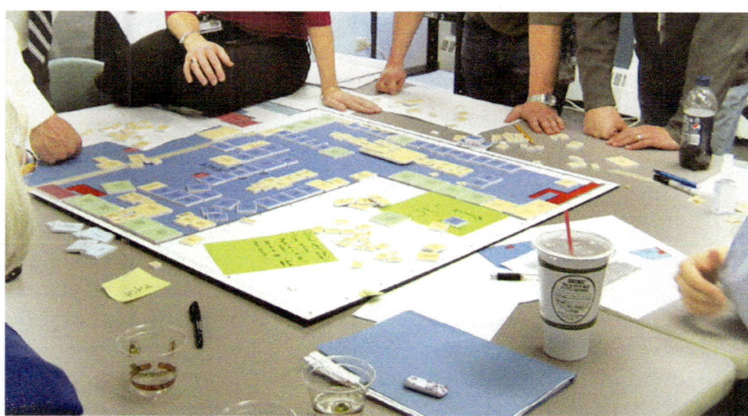

Fig. 1: Gaming.

A sample team member list for a typical nursing unit is below. The exact composition is dependent upon prioritization of process and design focus. Some team members may be "ad hoc" and pulled in as needed.

- Staff nurse
- In-charge nurse
- Physician
- Housekeeper
- Nursing administrator
- Pharmacy
- Materials management
- IT or clinical informatics
- Facilities department
- Architect
- Medical planner
- Interior designer
- Patient/family representative.

As with all lean activities, it is critical to engage the staff who are affected by the improvement and design work. The people who deliver the services are viewed as the resident experts; therefore, they are vital in the redesign. The list of the "people who do the work" should include clinical caregivers as well as support services. Housekeepers and pharmacists are just as critical as physicians and managers in determining how to improve flow and design the work environment. Clinical and administrative leadership provide the overarching direction for changes in the delivery of care, but the team in the 3P event collectively develops the "future state" to realize that vision.

It is important for design team representatives to be fully involved in all phases of the lean work and analysis. It is an advantage to understand the challenges in the current state to avoid replication of broken processes and ineffective space. The design team is not expected to tell the staff how to do their work, but having them participate in the analysis and discussion provides a valuable perspective of the vision for the new work environment. Understanding management and the clinical staff's expectations for the operations allows the design team to create a better functioning space.

Preparation for Schematic Design

The easy answer for when this framework of 3P events should be incorporated into the design process is "the earlier the better". It becomes very difficult for staff to redesign how they do their work if the functional program is set and drawings for their new space have been drafted.

The optimal time to conduct the 3P events is prior to schematic design. Hence, the 3P events most often occur before or during programming. The outcomes of this lean work may result in modifications to the functional program. Therefore, it is very important to be clear on the boundaries related to changing the program (Fig. 2).

The timing of the three phases can vary, depending on the overall project timeline and availability of human resources. 3P/2P events are often done during consecutive days. But the work can be configured over multiple weeks to align with finalization of the space program and beginning of schematic design.

To maximize the opportunities, lean thinking should be incorporated throughout the entire design process. From master planning (identifying potential expansions of services) to design development (determining where the hand sanitizer should be mounted) lean concepts should be integrated into every decision.

LEAN CONCEPTS USED IN FACILITY DESIGN

Initially it is better to introduce the lean principles to facility designer followed by conducting lean activities during the design process. Following are some of the specific lean concepts and methods that can be used to improve flow and create space that supports the new processes.

Improving Flow of Work

Spaghetti diagrams and value stream maps are used to analyze and improve flow of work activities. These tools allow teams to look for opportunities to remove waste, workarounds, rework and roadblocks that impede flow. The goal of all process redesign is to move toward an ideal state—*continuous flow of value-added work.*

There is a commonly used set of key flows to analyze and test, frequently called the "7 flows of healthcare":

- Patient and family
- Staff
- Provider
- Medicine
- Supplies

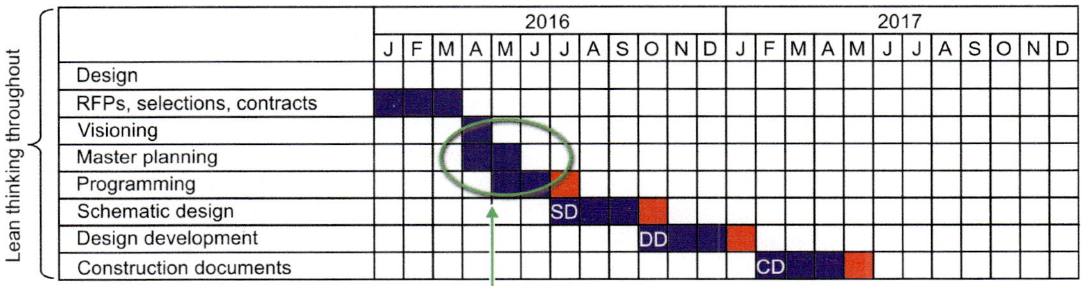

Fig. 2: Timeline.

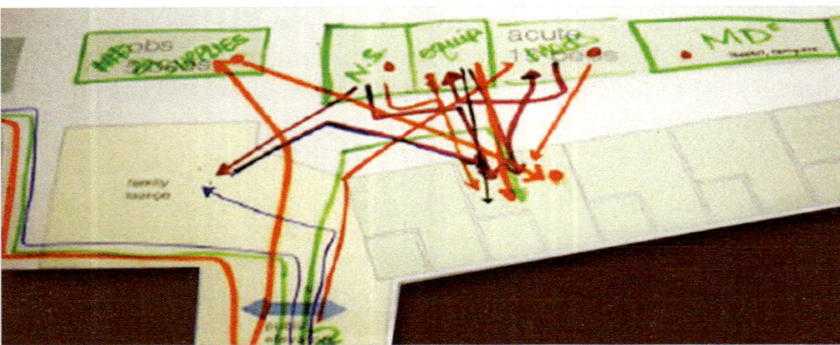

Fig. 3: Layout.

- Equipment
- Information.

As different layouts and adjacencies are considered teams should test the 7 flows to evaluate layout options. Figure 3 shows the initial round for a medical surgical unit layout with each of the 7 flows indicated by a different color.

Ideally teams would first create processes that occur with continuous flow and then design a work environment to support the new systems. This lean process development informs the design by identifying key adjacencies based on continuous flow.

Value Stream Mapping

Evaluation of processes using *value stream maps* is critical in predesign as a useful method to analyze and redesign the flow and activities of work that will occur in the new space.

A *current state value stream map* allows one to visualize the activities that are adding value (from the perspective of the patient) and recognize sources of waste. The act of creating a future state map for key processes forces participants to come to agreement on the operations going forward. The improved process, drawn as a future state map, is an image that is easy to interpret and modify as refinements are recognized.

A driver of the future state processes is the "criteria for future state". These criteria, determined by the team, are standards that reflect organizational goals for the new space. The "criteria for future state" are specific to a service line and are used as an evaluation tool for all processes and/or physical space options. Example criteria include: flexible space, privacy for patients, and family spaces. A solid list of "criteria for future state" provides a common vision for the future; something that is often lacking in traditional predesign work.

Spaghetti Diagrams (Figs. 4A to C)

A spaghetti diagram is a simple tool common in both lean and architectural practice. These diagrams can be incorporated in the current state process analysis phase and again in the future state testing and layout design phase.

When used in the current state analysis, spaghetti diagrams identify opportunities for improvement related to layout, supply/equipment locations, workflow, sequence of process steps, staff assignments, etc.

PATIENT ARRIVAL

During the testing phase, spaghetti diagrams help evaluate how the future state process is translated in the proposed new space. Figures 4B and 4C depict Spaghetti diagrams.

The colored string represents different patient flows. The team is able to compare the distance and number of trips for each patient type to evaluate the different configurations.

STANDARDIZING SYSTEMS AND SPACES[2]

Standardization of space (by size and layout) in the design of patient rooms, workstations, procedural suites, etc makes cross training and floating personnel interdepartmentally a safer and more efficient practice. Universal patient room design gives the ability to adapt levels of care in the room and can decrease transfers of patients when their acuity levels change.

With standardization comes flexibility and efficiency. The goal with truly flexible spaces is adaptability to fluctuating volumes, patient types, acuity, or procedures. This flexibility allows for efficiency of valuable resources—space, staff, and/or time.

The key to making the space function optimally is to ensure the processes work effectively. During the future state development phase teams redesigned patient flow and staffing. Later in the design process a multidisciplinary team objectively analyzed the different uses of the room and designed it to meet all essential functions. It is critical to clearly operationalize how the space will work through clarifying future state processes.

Standardization reduces complexity, which is important when flexibility is needed, as is the case for increasing surge capacity. Importantly, standardization is a key strategy in human factors design as a means to reduce the risk of error and improve quality. Human factors design (Ergonomics) focuses on improving the human-system interface by designing better systems and processes. For hospitals, standardization of patient rooms, treatment rooms, equipment and care processes, reduces reliance on short-term memory. In room design, standardizing details such as the location of bed controls, light switches, and even, which cupboards store latex gloves, for instance, are important considerations for optimizing the human-system interface.[2]

The lengthy cycle of design and construction is often overtaken by the rapid cycle of innovation in medicine and technology. As a result, some buildings are partially obsolete when they open, and nearly every healthcare structure will be obsolete in some way before it has completed its useful life. Design for flexibility is a way to reduce the inconvenience and cost of these inevitable disruptions.[2]

- *Master planning strategies*: Every design should have planned zones for future growth. These can appear as a dotted line on the site plan, or may be developed as constructed but unoccupied shell space, or as structural capacity to allow for future vertical additions to a building.[2]
- *Loose-fit design*: Many designs make an effort to design precisely to the absolute minimum square footage justified by the program of space requirements, yet such designs are the first to reveal difficulties when new programs appear, or existing programs grow or shrink. The concept of loose-fit is to design with larger spaces that can be used for more than the minimum function originally proposed, and to arrange them in departments or groupings that allow for future adjustments.[2]
- *Adaptable flexibility*: Spaces can be designed to adapt to multiple uses. An example is a patient room that can be adapted for the purpose of simple procedures such as a line insertion. The different function can be accommodated by simply adapting the space because it has been planned to serve a range of possibilities.[2]

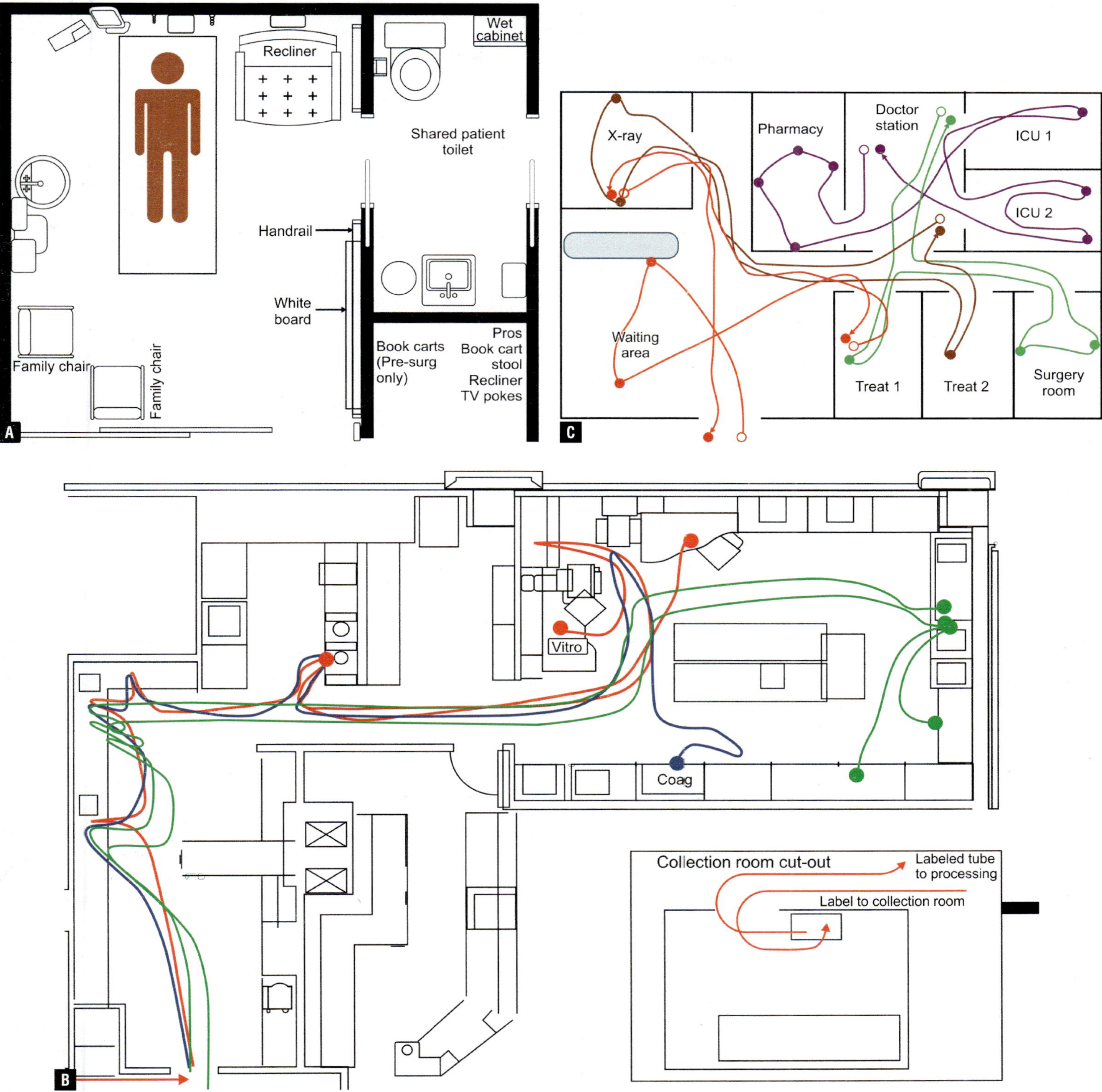

Figs. 4A to C: Spaghetti diagram.

- *Convertible flexibility*: Another type of flexibility is when, with relatively low effort, time, and/or cost, a space can be converted to another use. Examples of this type of flexibility include a storage space with a knockout panel in the slab to allow for a future elevator, or a patient room with plumbing, gasses, and electrical systems in the wall for future conversion to critical care.[2]
- *Robust utilities*: In order to offer flexibility in design, the utility and communication infrastructure of a healthcare facility should be capable of expansion and upgrade. Availability of utility and network capacity simplifies and dramatically reduces the cost of future projects.[2]
- *Plug-and-play infrastructure*: Just as all the utilities of the city are uninterrupted when one property undergoes a construction

or demolition project, a hospital should be designed so that the utility and primary horizontal and vertical circulation infrastructure remains in service while departments, wings, or entire buildings are added or removed.[2]

DEVELOPMENT OF STANDARDS

Standardization within healthcare organizations and design practices also may contribute to lean processes.[1]

Healthcare System Standards

Many larger, multihospital systems are creating standards with the intention of using them comprehensively. Their goals are to streamline certain processes that are repeated for each and every project, including decision-making for the products specified and purchased.[1]

Functionality of key rooms is considered. The goal for such efforts is to develop a best-practice standard. This creates a room organization and operational model that can be applied to future projects, whether renovation or new construction. This approach streamlines the planning process, eliminating redundant efforts and enabling the healthcare organization to maintain a consistent level of quality, provide a comparable patient experience and operate in a similar manner across the system.[1]

Frequently, the development of standards is tied into a brand initiative. This can result in the design of specific components that patients may encounter throughout their journeys.[1]

Design Practice Standards

The design process can benefit from some standardization as well. Work efforts can be structured so that processes and tasks that contribute value are prioritized and those that do not are eliminated.[1]

Certain information gathered throughout a project also can be translated to future projects as standards, thereby reducing the amount of time needed for research related to specific, common elements.[1]

Throughout the course of a project, designers find many redundant efforts. However, that information is rarely used to inform future work. Healthcare organizations are demanding that professionals bring the expertise forward regarding innovation.[1]

Most projects would benefit from referencing detailed information about the rooms included in a project at the outset. The focus then can shift to the specific needs of the organization, maximizing the time spent on innovation and streamlining the entire process.[1]

Similarly, the analysis typically conducted on life cycle and performance of materials for use on one project should be considered more comprehensively for application on all projects.[1]

One way to achieve this is to develop a comprehensive matrix of products that typically are specified in project work. Performance characteristics for each product can be listed, along with information related to first cost and life cycle cost. Data gathered from various mockup installations also can be useful when products are considered.[1]

These tools enable designers to identify quickly which products are suitable for a specific circumstance, streamlining this part of the design process.[1]

Many hospital organizations reflect back to their previous facility move-in or opening day and wonder why little has changed from the previous facility. Staff is still managing operational fire drills, patient satisfaction has not improved and physicians are still frustrated. It feels like the new facility is haunted by the problems of the old. *With more thoughtful facility design and incorporating lean thinking from master planning through postoccupancy, management can dramatically improve efficiency, space utilization, staff satisfaction and patient outcomes.*

VISUAL MANAGEMENT AND 5S FOR WORKPLACE ORGANIZATION

The 5S, when incorporated in a design project, is often a response to a storage or layout problem identified in the current state analysis. To economize space, teams may consider conducting 5S activities early in the predesign work to determine the appropriate supplies/equipment in conjunction with improving the inventory system.

The 5S:

- Sort
- Straighten
- Scrub
- Standardize
- Sustain

The 5S and workplace organization can also be incorporated in layout redesign to reduce walking, excess motion, delays, and potential errors in any work environment. Once the future state workflow is determined then a team can organize the new space so it supports the work.

Visual management is a concept applied during a 5S activity but can easily stand alone. The goal of visual management, "status at a glance", should be kept in mind throughout the entire design process.

There are more lean concepts that have application to facility design. However, by applying just the above principles to the evaluation of processes in consideration of the new space, teams will be able to reduce waste. The key is to not just apply lean in pockets. Lean thinking should be incorporated throughout the entire design process to maximize opportunity.

FIVE WAYS DESIGN CAN MAKE DOCTORS' VISITS SHORTER

Shorter wait times are a patient satisfier, but certain design configurations can make patient wait times and appointments take longer. In the case of an ambulatory care center, longer appointments mean fewer appointments per day, restricting the "carrying capacity" of the facility. For instance, the same medical office building can complete either 100 or 150 appointments per day, depending on their length. The following design features can help to speed things up.[6]

Multifunction Rooms with Portable Equipment

In many hospitals, providers perform different functions in different spaces. As a result, they struggle with the ebbs and flows of patient volume misaligning with each of the available specialized room types.[6]

Multifunction rooms with portable equipment allow any function to occur in any space. A preoperative testing clinic is a prime example. Ten multifunction rooms with portable equipment offer more flexibility than five electrocardiogram rooms and five lab rooms. Patients do not have to wait for a specialized room to become available when they can use any room.[6]

Number of Exam Rooms Divisible by 3, 4, or 5

As a rule of thumb, the number of exam rooms should not be a prime number. This improves the likelihood that each staff member will care for the same number of patients. For example, with 16 exam rooms and a 1:4 staff ratio, each nurse cares for four patients. With 17 exam rooms, patients assigned to the nurse with five patients will wait longer.[6]

Shared Changing Areas

Design can cut patient wait times by manipulating the distribution of changing rooms. For instance, in an imaging center, separate changing areas for each modality usually result in uneven use. Where appropriate, share changing areas between modalities. This way ebbs and flows in traffic between the different modalities offset one another. This makes more rooms available, so patients are less likely to wait. Furthermore, lockers for patient belongings offset the need to hold a changing room for a patient's return.[6]

Sufficient Storage

Having supplies readily at hand keeps clinicians focused on patient care. In-room storage limits time wasted on hunting and gathering efforts (storage must be right-sized to avoid collecting superfluous items). This also holds true for items as mundane as a standard printer. An in-room printer allows the clinician to print patient discharge information uninterrupted.[6]

Centralized Registration

Many outpatient centers require patients to check in at the main registration desk as well as at their specialist clinic. Further, they require patients to do so on each subsequent visit to the facility. Every registration stop adds 5–10 minutes to the patient's visit. Instead, by locating all of the registration and check-in functions at the main desk and electronically transmitting patient information to each clinic, patients only check in one time. This saves valuable minutes from each visit.

Patient satisfaction drops for each five minutes of waiting time. Saving even one minute per visit adds up to a substantial time and cost savings for a healthcare organization over the course of a year. Given the impact this might have across the lifetime of a facility, the choices that designers make to save time are more critical than ever.

LEAN STRATEGIES THAT CAN STREAMLINE HOSPITAL DESIGN

Simulations and Prototypes

Healthcare facilities are challenged to continually deliver care with fewer resources. There has been a high level of focus on the impact of the physical environment on caregivers' ability to deliver care safely and efficiently. Poorly designed physical environments can reduce the effectiveness of staff to provide care and potentially impact the safety of patients and caregivers.[1]

To achieve a more efficient model of care, the entire team is asked to think beyond their current methods of working. Understanding healthcare processes before actually developing the space can facilitate resolution to the operational issues. In the spirit of lean design, all processes should be driven by the patient's experience.[1]

With this in mind, the goal is to create a model where all aspects of care—caregiver workflow, distribution of supplies and medications and clinical documentation—are pushed to the point of service. Hands-on exercises, including simulation modeling and prototyping, are effective tools that enable caregivers to explore possibilities more freely.[1]

Simulation Modeling

Simulation modeling can quickly assess the impact of change on a given aspect of flow. For one Chicago-area hospital, simulation modeling was a highly effective tool to test an outcome assumption of reducing its operating room case load.[1]

An analysis of the current process in place included evaluating each of the steps in the process, applicable trends, impact of the process on staff and the technologies to be leveraged. The steps that were not considered value-added or that could be combined or automated were changed.[1]

Following the definition of a new process, it was possible to determine how the new facility would be designed. The importance of this exercise was apparent when analyzing the costs associated with delays in case starts. By reducing these costs and the associated process steps by 50%, a savings of four nursing full-time equivalent employees was seen.[1]

Methods such as this enhance communication, one of the key objectives of lean design. All participants feel more invested in the process and are better equipped to provide commentary in an environment that supports all points of view. Additionally, the focus is placed on patients and their needs, identifying the places where redundancies and unnecessary tasks are performed.[1]

Prototyping

To improve nursing efficiency and allow for increased nurse time at the bedside, a greater emphasis has been placed on the design of floor layouts and nurses' stations. Due to the myriad operational models and workplace cultures, there is no singular solution emerging. Prototyping is an effective means to validate assumptions to inform the design of future patient units.[1]

This method can help meet needs quickly and effectively through the use of techniques that test theories related to positive outcomes. Prototyping methods encompass workflow, technology and processes.[1]

Once process standards are established, the physical room prototypes can be constructed in a simple manner so that the workflow can be tested in real conditions. This allows for a variety of assumptions to be validated in a low-risk environment.[1]

Rooms may evolve into a final, finished state where a number of design solutions can be evaluated, such as construction details, standardization of components, finish materials and color palette. This can allow both the design team and the contractor to confirm their assumptions prior to building multiple rooms.[1]

The opportunity to collaborate and to discuss the best solutions can address issues often raised during the construction process, such as constructability, cost and final execution.[1]

Flexible and Modular Design

One of the key principles of lean design is to create as much flexibility, scalability and adaptability as possible.[1]

Flexibility

Much of the planning in healthcare is for an unknown future, incorporating adaptability makes sense. Changes in work processes, equipment and technology can require costly changes to the physical environment. A flexible environment enables adaptation of design, space and the future state of practice over time.[1]

One approach can be to design a patient unit that allows for flexibility for any medical specialty or acuity. Rooms can be sized and configured to be universal rooms, allowing for future flexibility to convert acute beds to a higher intensity of care with minimal renovation. The unit can be organized to support the optimal workflow no matter what the medical specialty and thus be standardized.[1]

Modularity

For outpatient facilities, modular clinic designs can be used that allow for flexibility based upon workflow and scheduling. Shared reception and waiting spaces accommodate visitors comfortably while modules for exam rooms and their associated spaces support a standardized model of care and can flex according to a particular clinic's schedule for a given day.[1]

Taking this another step further, the facility can be designed and built to enable future practices and allow continuous improvement with minimal cost or disruption. When considering the physical impact that modification to the care model can drive, work spaces must be designed to meet these needs, ranging from private spaces to support critical thinking to open, collaborative environments to promote care coordination over various disciplines.[1]

Modular components and systems can enable modifications to be made easily with minimal disruption.[1]

Value and Benefit

The incorporation of lean principles can help a healthcare facility achieve optimal performance by improving strategic, operational and financial outcomes. Patients are put at the forefront of the experience, leading to greater satisfaction. Additionally, patient handoffs and patient moves are minimized, leading to a smoother, more streamlined overall care delivery process.[1]

Likewise, if done in a methodical and well-conceived manner, incorporating lean principles into the design process itself can greatly enhance any healthcare project by improving the quality and efficiency of the outcome.[1]

Results Related to the Project Delivery

When lean thinking is applied to the design process, both the design team and users have a better understanding of operations and vision for the future state. This collective knowledge also has positive implications on the project delivery.

- Reduced lead time of schematic design and design development phases.
- Decreased modifications and change orders; users are confident in the design decisions.
- Appropriate response to new constraints or changes.
- Reduced project cost since plans are not overbuilt to accommodate ineffective processes.

Lean Facility Design Project

Following points are helpful regardless of type, scope, timeline, or objectives.

When to Start: The Earlier the Better

Incorporate lean early in the planning and design process to provide a clear lean vision. It is difficult when lean is "squeezed in" or late in the design phases. When lean is an after thought, challenges may arise with the schedule and it becomes impossible to have all the key players available to participate. If schematic design is underway before lean is integrated there may be too many constraints and decisions in place to re-engineer flow and process.

Prior Lean Experience is an Advantage

With existing lean skills, the facility design work becomes a natural extension of the organization's lean journey. Building on previous experience accelerates this new application of lean. Lean is based on the concept of learn by doing, but previous experience is a great foundation on which to build. Without lean experience the organization must simultaneously learn lean while trying to integrate it into the design project. The owner and design team commitment to lean activities is difficult if either party is new to lean.

Clarify Constraints and Assumptions

An understanding of the constraints and assumptions helps guide the team by providing a framework for the future state. It is important to reiterate with the users that the design will evolve and new architectural or other constraints may arise that require their reconsideration.

Example constraints:

- Square footage
- Number of rooms

Example assumptions:[1,2]

- EMR before move
- Retain existing staffing model

Must Involve the People Who do the Work

Toyota has taught us to recognize the people who do the work as the resident experts. This means including front line staff, leadership, physicians, patients, and ancillary services in the planning and design work. These key players become the team members for lean activities and continue as the user group for design reviews.

Clarity of Operational Direction

In addition to using lean methods to redesign workflow and solve specific layout problems, use lean thinking for high level operational decisions. Strategic direction provides a framework for the future state and clear aim for improvement teams.

Partnership Between the Design Team and Users is Key

Lean is a mechanism for strong collaboration between the design team and users. When integrating lean activities into the design process this partnership becomes even more critical since the deliverables depends upon a symbiotic relationship.

Internal Resource Designated to Support Lean Design Work

It is important to have an internal person(s) on the owner side to coordinate, support and communicate the results of the lean design work. This role should act as a lean coach to the teams and work closely with the design team to ensure the lean activities are synchronized with the project schedule. Additionally, this person can support process improvement work and testing of new systems prior to the move in.

Executive Team Sponsor for Lean Design Work

In addition to a coach, the teams need a champion from senior leadership. This sponsor should breakdown barriers and act as a liaison to the executive team. To be truly effective, this requires active participation and an understanding of the goals and challenges.

Fully Developed Future State Processes

It is critical that there is clarity of future state processes and operations. This information informs the design and guides the users as they approve the architectural plans. Agreement on "criteria for future state" will direct the new work as the design evolves. Future state value stream maps create standard, visual documents of procedural steps for operations in the new workspace.

Example criteria:

- Standardization
- Flexible space
- Privacy for patients
- Separate patient flow from staff work area.

The Work is Just Beginning

The reality of any construction project is that the planning and design is just the beginning.

As the build moves forward, the organization has an opportunity to continue lean improvements to further optimize their systems. These opportunities include:

- Fix broken processes before move in
- Mockup spaces and test key flows
- Trial and refine future state ideas in existing space.

Ultimately, adherence to the gold standard of lean thinking, improving quality and decreasing waste, is the mantra that can lead an organization to a successful experience replacing or creating a new physical space. The rigor and diligence required to reap the merits of this work will reward owners and the design team many fold in a facility that truly supports improved delivery of care.

CONCLUSION

A lean hospital is physically designed to minimize waste for patients and for all who work inside its walls. It is designed with direct input from staff to support efficient workflows and value streams, rather than forcing departments and employees to adjust their work to the space. A lean hospital focuses more on what is functional and effective for the patients and staff rather than glossing over bad processes with marble entryways and lobby fountains. Lean hospitals use collaborative and iterative design and build practices like integrated project delivery.

REFERENCES

1. www.hfmmagazine.com
2. www.aahid.org
3. mospace.umsystem.edu
4. hospitalbuild.lifesciencemagazines.com
5. docplayer.net
6. www.healthcaredesignmagazine.com

OTHER REFERENCES

- Grunden N, Hagood C. Lean-led hospital design: Creating the Efficient Hospital of the Future 1st Edition. 2012.
- Graban M. Lean Hospitals-improving quality, patient safety, and employee engagement, 2011.
- Mersereau E, Jimmerson C. Improving healthcare delivery using Lean thinking for facility design. 2011.
- The Joint Commission. Health care at the crossroads: Guiding principles for the development of the hospital of the future.
- May, Matthew E. The elegant solution: Toyota's formula for mastering innovation. New York, N: Free Press. 2006.
- Jimmerson, Cindy. Value stream mapping for healthcare made easy. New York, N : Productivity Press. 2009.
- Going Lean in Health Care. IHI innovation series white paper. Cambridge, MA: Institute for Healthcare Improvement, 2005. (available on www.IHI.org)
- Lean Healthcare Exchange: www.leanhealthcareexchange.com
- Green Belt Lean Certification for Facility Design: www.leanhealthcarewest.com/Page/Green Belt Lean Certification Programs
- General information regarding Lean for Facility Design: www.leanhealthcarewest.com/Page/Lean for Facility Design Services
- Caldwell D, Martin D. Five Ways Design Can Make Doctors' Visits Shorter. 2016.
- Joselyn M. Stroupe. It's the process.

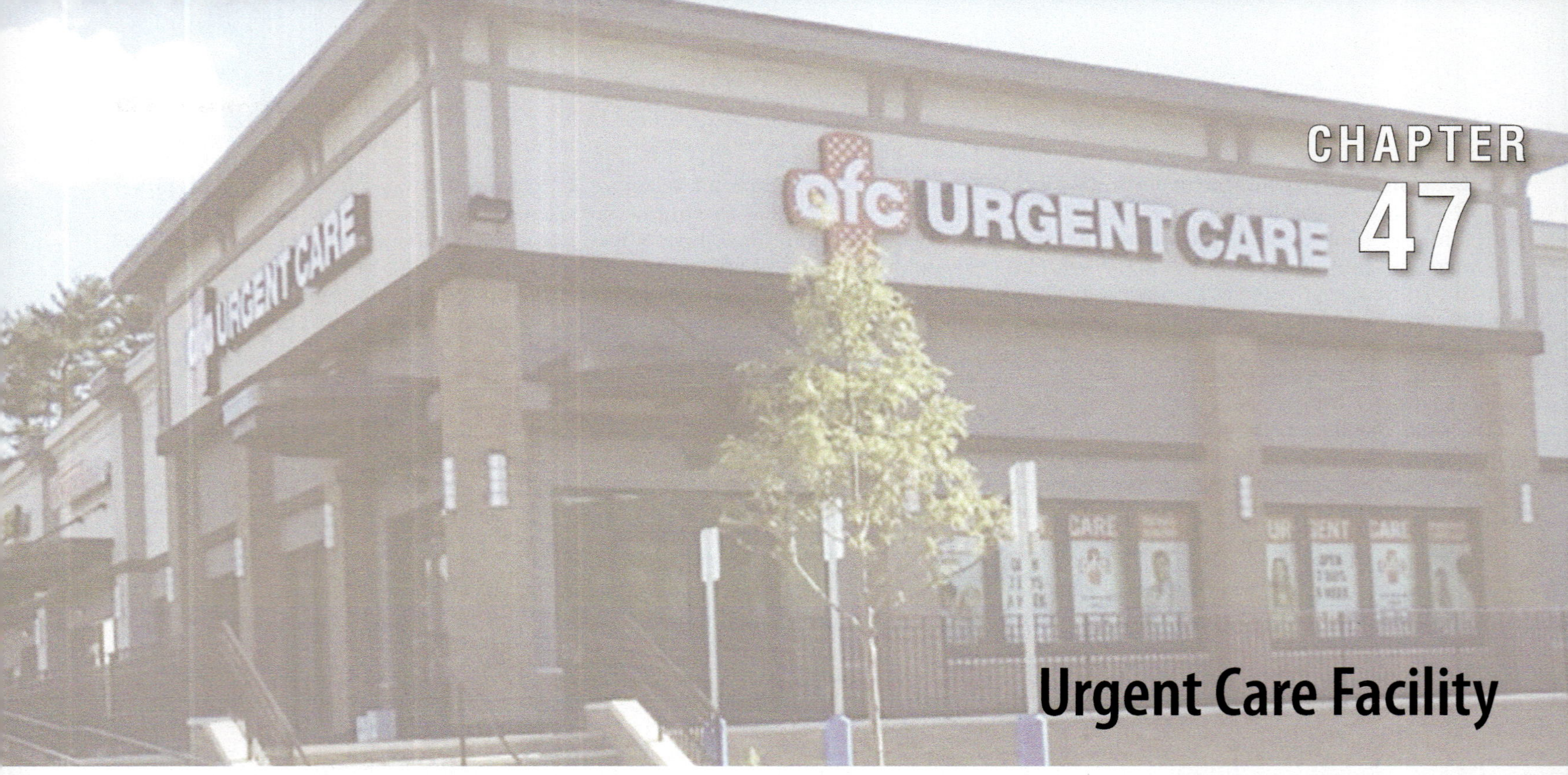

CHAPTER 47

Urgent Care Facility

Vijay Kumar Tadia, Rajesh Gupta, Shakti Kumar Gupta, Sunil Kant, R Chandrashekhar

The urgent care medicine (UCM) is the provision of immediate medical service offering outpatient care for the treatment of acute and chronic illness and injury. It requires a broad and comprehensive fund of knowledge to provide such care. UCM concentrates on the evaluation and treatment of acutely arising conditions in all age groups.

—*American Academy of Urgent Care Medicine (AAUCM)*

URGENT CARE FACILITY

- There is no universal definition.
- It can provide services that fall in between primary care and emergency department (ED).
- It can also include some primary care services and could branch into other areas, e.g. weight loss, allergy care, wellness, etc.
- Urgent Care Association of America describes it as, "The delivery of ambulatory medical care outside of a hospital ED on a walk-in basis, without a scheduled appointment".
- Generally focused on episodic, acute care rather than on long-term management of chronic illness or preventive care.

HISTORY

Over the last two decades, urgent care facilities (UCFs) have proliferated, growing to 9,000 facilities in the United States.[1,2] The recent, rapid expansion of UCFs is often attributed to such factors as long wait times for primary care appointments, crowded EDs and patient demand for more accessible care, including after-hours appointments.

The UCFs provide care on a walk-in basis, typically during regular business hours, as well as evenings and weekends, though not 24 hours a day. UCFs commonly treat conditions seen in primary care practices and retail clinics. In contrast to EDs, UCFs generally are not equipped to deal with trauma, provide resuscitation or admit patients to a hospital—all reasons for seeking ED care. UCFs are typically staffed by physicians, generally with backgrounds in primary care or emergency medicine, and some also have nurse practitioners or physician assistants working under physician supervision.

The UCFs first emerged in the 1970s but did not take root, in part, because the industry lacked a sufficient marketing strategy to draw consumer interest. Since then, patient demand for more convenient access to care reportedly has increased, prompting renewed growth in UCFs. Historically, UCFs often were independently owned, standalone facilities, but the landscape of UCFs has changed considerably. Large UCFs chains operate in some regions of USA. Also, hospital systems are establishing UCFs to expand their service area and referral base. UCFs visits generally cost less than ED visits, though they tend to be on par with primary care office visits. *In India, Aapka Urgicare has ventured into urgent care facility space.*[3]

Reasons for the Proliferation of Urgent Care Facilities[4]

These are:
- Growth spurt began in mid-1990s and has continued
- Acceptance by the public
- Lack of access to primary care (no access or delayed access)
- Overcrowding in ED
- Long wait times at other providers (EDs especially)
- Convenience of longer hours and walk-ins
- Emphasis on high-quality care
- Increased healthcare consumerism spurred by high-deductible plans.

Common Characteristics of Urgent Care

- Walk-in or unscheduled care
- Many UCFs also offer call-ahead options and online appointment-making.
- Extended hours, including weekends and evenings.
- Provide an array of services beyond primary care.

- Customer service approach to providing care.
- Occupational health services often provided.

Services Provided by Urgent Care Facilities

- Primary care
- On-site radiology
- Simple fractures and lacerations
- Intravenous hydration
- On-site lab testing
- Medications—prepackaged pharmaceuticals and pain management
- Occupational medicine and worker's compensation
- Other services may include immunizations, travel medicine, and sports and school physicals.

Future of Urgent Care

The growth and development of UCM should be of no surprise to anyone. Fueled by frustration over long waits in the emergency room (for non-emergency care), and a reduction in available primary care appointments (often resulting in patients waiting for weeks to see their primary care physician), a new growth spurt for the urgent care industry began in the mid-1990s and continues today. The public's desire for immediate access to medical care has been the driving force behind this monumental growth.[5]

For many patients, UCFs are the main place to go for care—especially on weekends or evenings when their primary-care physicians do not have office hours. Urgent care centers are a boon for patients in other ways. The wait time to see a provider is typically half an hour or less, compared to a multi-hour wait time in many EDs. Employers, insurers and other payers also benefit from UCFs, which charge only a fraction of what an ED visit would cost. And employees can get back to work sooner instead of spending half the day in the ED.[6]

The extended hours and immediate availability of care at UCFs provides convenience for patients. As the specialty of UCM grows, the public is learning that urgent care is a better choice over the emergency room for their immediate, non-life-threatening healthcare needs.[5,6]

PLANNING AND DESIGNING CONSIDERATIONS

Patient Privacy

Each facility design ensures appropriate levels of patient acoustic and visual privacy and dignity throughout care process.

Parking[7]

- The UCFs should provide parking capacity sufficient to satisfy the needs of patients, personnel, and the public.
- Additional spaces should be provided for emergency vehicles.
- Designated street, public and shared lot spaces reserved for use of UCF
- All required parking spaces should be near the urgent care entrance.

Access

Facility should be accessible to handicapped individuals.

Entrance

- At grade level
- Clearly marked
- Located so patients need not go through other activity areas.

Signage

- The facility should post interior or exterior signs that clearly indicate the type and level of care offered and the hours of operation.
- The facility should post the address of the nearest 24-hour emergency facility (hospital).

Examination Rooms

- At least two urgent care examination rooms.
- Provision should be made to preserve patient privacy from observation from outside an examination room through an open door.

General Purpose Examination/Observation Room

If an examination room is used as an observation room, it should be located immediately accessible to the nurse or control station and a toilet room (Fig. 1).

Space Requirements

- Space requirements.
  - Each examination/observation room should have a minimum clear floor area of 80 sq ft.

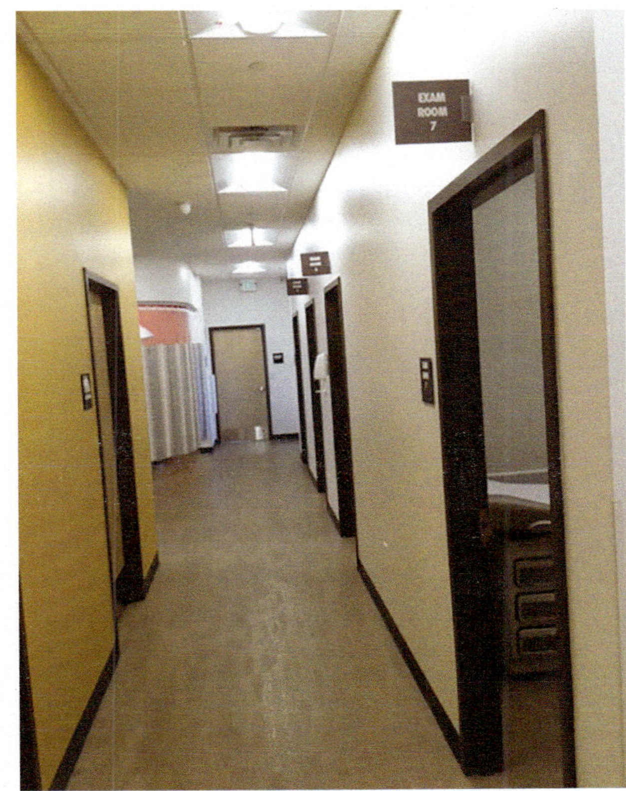

Fig. 1: Location of general purpose examination/observation room.

- The size of the exam room should accommodate a minimum clearance of 2 ft 8 inches at each side and at the foot of the examination table.
  or
- A room arrangement in which an examination table placed at an angle, closer to one wall than another, or against a wall.
- Clearance zone with minimum clearance 2 ft 8 inches at each side and at foot of alternate location.

- If the space is also used as a procedure room, Procedure Room requirements must also be met.
- A handstation should be provided.
- Accommodations for written or electronic documentation should be provided.
- *Ventilation*:
  - Minimum 6 air changes per hour
- *Power*:
  - Minimum 8 receptacles
  - Minimum 4 receptacles convenient to head of exam table.

Special Purpose Examination Room (Fig. 2)

- Provision made to preserve patient privacy from observation from outside exam room through open door.[7]
- Space requirements[7]
  - Minimum clear floor area 100 sq ft
  - Room size permits minimum clearance 3 ft 6 inches at side, head, or foot of exam table, bed, or chair that corresponds with care provider's expected work position.
  - Minimum clearance 1 ft at all sides of exam table, bed, or chair other than work position.
- Hand washing station
- Documentation area for written or electronic documentation
- *Ventilation*:
  - Minimum 6 air changes per hour
- *Power*:
  - Minimum 8 receptacles
  - Minimum 4 receptacles convenient to head of exam table.

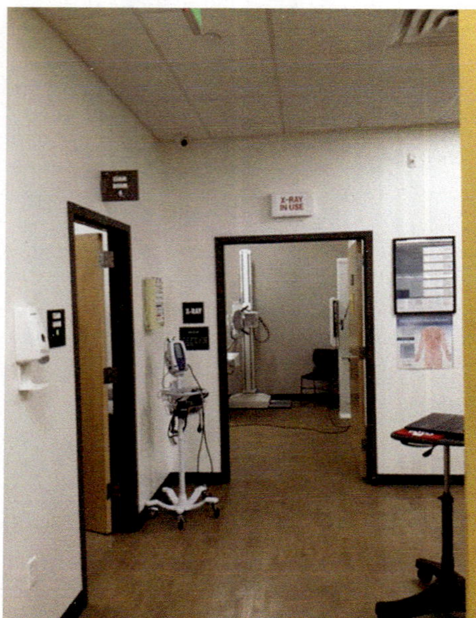

Fig. 2: Special purpose examination room.

Urgent Care Procedure Room[7]

When a procedure room is provided, it should meet the following requirements.

- The maximum number of patients to be accommodated in the procedure room at any time should be one.
- Space requirements
  - Each procedure room should have a minimum clear floor area of 80 sq ft.
  - Room size should permit a room arrangement with a minimum clearance of 3 ft 6 inches at each side, head, and foot of the examination table.
    or
  - Room arranged with exam table placed at an angle, closer to one wall than another, or against wall.
    - ◊ Alternate location shown for exam table.
    - ◊ Clearance zone with minimum clearance 3 ft 6 inches at each side and at foot of alternate location.
- A scrub station or a hand washing station should be located at each procedure room.
- Documentation area for written or electronic documentation should be provided.
- *Power*:
  - Minimum 8 receptacles
  - Minimum 4 receptacles convenient to head of exam table.

Observation Facilities

- Facilities should be provided for holding urgent care patients until they can be discharged or transferred to an appropriate hospital.
- Use of one or more examination or procedure rooms for this purpose should be permitted or include dedicated patient observation positions.

Facility Requirements

Size, type, and equipment should be as required for anticipated patient load and lengths of stay.

Functional Requirements

- Direct visual observation of each patient should be provided from the nurse station, except where examination or procedure rooms are used for patient holding. In the latter case, a limited view from the nurse/control station to the doors of the examination or procedure rooms should be permitted.
- *Each observation position should have the following*:
  - Patient privacy
  - Access to patient toilets
  - Secure storage for patients' valuables and clothing.
- Support areas for observation facilities
- *Ventilation*:
  - Minimum 10 air changes per hour
  - Exhaust.
- Each patient observation position is enclosed with floor to ceiling partitions to assure minimum sound transmission.

Medication Safety Zones[7]

Where medication is prepared or dispensed, medication safety zones should be provided as defined in this section for preparing, dispensing, storing, and administering medications.

- A medicine preparation room or area, self-contained medication dispensing unit, automated medication-dispensing station, or other system approved by the authority should be permitted to serve as a medication safety zone.
- Medication safety zones should be located out of circulation paths to minimize the potential for distraction and interruption.
- Work space organization for medication safety zones should be designed so that staff can access information and perform required tasks.
- Work counters should provide space to perform the required tasks.
- Task-specific lighting levels for healthcare settings.
- Medication preparation room/area
  - Work counter
  - Hand washing station
  - Lockable refrigerator
  - Locked storage for controlled drugs.
- *Ventilation*:
  - Minimum 4 air changes per hour.
- *Sharps containers*:
  - Placed at height that allows users to see top of container.
  - Space to prepare medicines in addition to any self-contained medicine-dispensing unit.
  - Self-contained medication dispensing units
    - ◊ Located at nurse station, in clean workroom or in an alcove.
    - ◊ Lockable unit to secure controlled drugs.
    - ◊ Hand washing station or hand sanitation located next to stationary medication-dispensing units.
- Bedpan storage and cleaning facilities
- Nourishment area (if patients will be held for more than 4 hours)
  - Hand washing station located in or directly accessible.
  - Food preparation sink (only when meals are not prepared in nourishment area).
  - Work counter
  - Storage
  - Fixtures and appliances for beverages and/or nourishment.
- *Ventilation*:
  - Minimum 2 air changes per hour.

Support Areas for Diagnostic and Treatment Areas

- Nurse control and workstation
  - A nurse control and workstation should accommodate charting, files, and staff consultation activities.
  - It should be located to permit visual control of the clinical area and its access.
  - Communication links with the examination room, procedure room, reception control, laboratory, radiology, and on-call staff should be provided.
- Clean supply storage room
  - Ventilation
    - ◊ Minimum 4 air changes per hour
    - ◊ Positive pressure.
- Soiled workroom
  - Hand washing station
  - Clinical flushing-rim sink
  - Ventilation
    - ◊ Minimum 10 air changes per hour
    - ◊ Exhaust
    - ◊ Negative pressure.

  or
- Soiled holding room
  - Ventilation
    - ◊ Minimum 10 air changes per hour
    - ◊ Exhaust
    - ◊ Negative pressure.

Sterilization Equipment[7]

- Means of sterilization provided for nondisposable supplies
  - Sterilization equipment in facility

    or
  - Arrangement to obtain such services from a source approved by the department.

    or
  - No means of sterilization provided if only disposable supplies are used.
- Emergency equipment storage
  - Readily accessible
  - Under staff control.
- Wheelchair and stretcher storage
  - Located in clinical area.

Imaging Services

- Space should be provided to accommodate the imaging services the facility provides.
- Details requirements for diagnostic radiography facilities are given below.

DIAGNOSTIC RADIOGRAPHY FACILITIES

General

- Room design and equipment siting should accommodate manufacturer's operational, service, and safety clearances for the imaging equipment used.
- Shielded control alcove (see Fig. 4)
  - Shielded control alcove or room
    - ◊ Each examination/procedure room containing non-portable radiation-emitting imaging equipment should include a fixed shielded control alcove or room to minimize radiation exposure of technologists and others. Movable imaging equipment affixed to rails, tracks, or booms should not be considered portable.
    - ◊ This alcove or room should include a shielded view window designed to provide a full view of the examination/procedure table and the patient at all times, including a full view of the patient when the table is tilted or the chest X-ray is in use.
  - For mammography machines with built-in shielding for the operator, omission of a shielded control alcove should be permitted when approved by the certified radiation physicist or authority having jurisdiction.

Radiography Room

- Radiography rooms should be sized to accommodate the services provided.
- A hand washing station should be provided in the procedure room.

Radiography/Fluoroscopy Room

- Radiography/fluoroscopy rooms should be sized and configured to accommodate the services provided.
- A hand washing station should be provided in the procedure room.
- A separate toilet room with hand washing station should be provided with direct access from each dedicated fluoroscopy room. Patients should be able to leave the toilet room without re-entering the fluoroscopy room.

Mammography Room

- Visual privacy of patients should be provided. Views into the mammography room by the public or other patients should be prevented when the room is in use.
- A hand washing station should be provided in the procedure room.
- Changing room(s) for mammography patients should be immediately accessible to the waiting area and procedure room(s).
  - Patient changing rooms
    - ◊ Changing rooms that are immediately accessible to imaging examination/procedure rooms should be provided.
    - ◊ Each room should include a seat or bench and mirror.
    - ◊ Provisions for hanging patients' clothing and securing valuables should be provided either in the patient changing room or in shared secured storage.
  - Combination of mammography changing room(s) with changing areas for other imaging services should be permitted.

Support Areas for Imaging Facilities

- Spaces or rooms for reviewing images and for administrative work should be provided as required to support the imaging services provided.
- *The following facilities should be provided as the imaging technology requires*:
  - Film and media processing facilities
  - Storage for exposed film.

Support Areas for Patients[7]

- Changing rooms or booths.
  - Where changing rooms or booths are provided, a toilet room should be immediately accessible.
  - Include seat or bench and mirror.
  - Provisions for hanging patients clothing and securing either in patient changing room or in shared secured storage.
- *Toilet rooms*: Toilet rooms with hand washing stations should be directly accessible to procedure room(s) if procedures provided at the facility require patient access to toilets.
- Separate changing rooms are not required if imaging is used only for emergency procedures.
- *Ventilation*:
  - Minimum 6 air changes per hour
- Nurse call system
  - Emergency staff assistance station.

Laboratory Services

If facilities for laboratory services are provided, the following requirements need to be met. Facilities for laboratory services provided on-site should be located in or immediately accessible to the outpatient facility.

Laboratory Testing/Work Area[7]

- When lab tests are performed on-site, a separate, dedicated room should be provided.

  or
- If only few tests are performed, lab room or open lab area can be provided.
- Work area
  - Space should be provided to accommodate all tests provided on-site.
  - Work areas should be sized to meet equipment specifications and lab technician needs.
  - Should have the following:
    - ◊ Work counter
    - ◊ Sink(s)
    - ◊ Access to tele/data service
    - ◊ Electrical service.
- Hand washing station(s) should be provided.

Support Areas for the Laboratory[7]

- Storage cabinet(s) or doset(s)
- Specimen collection facilities
  - In facilities where urine or feces specimens are collected, a toilet room with staff controlled access should be provided.
  - A hand washing station should be available in the specimen collection area.
  - In facilities where collection for drug screening is performed, the hand washing station should either be directly outside the toilet room and under staff control or in the toilet room if the water is controlled by shutoff valves outside the room and directly accessible to staff (Fig. 3).
  - Blood collection facilities should have:

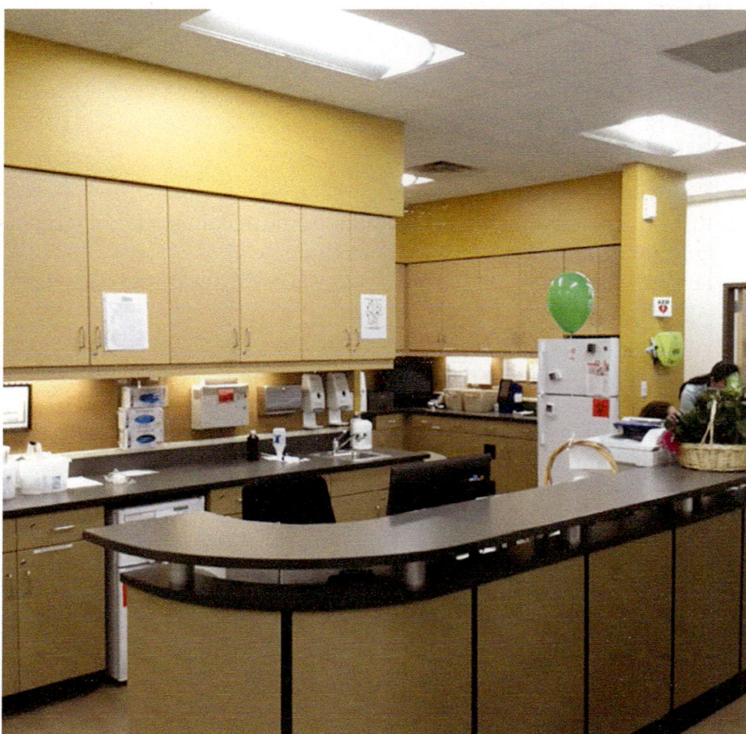

Fig. 3: Support areas for the laboratory.

  - ◊ Work counter
  - ◊ Seating space for patients
  - ◊ Hand washing station
  - ◊ Reclining chair or gurney for patients who become unsteady.
- Ventilation
  - ◊ Minimum 10 air changes per hour.

Equipment[3]

The Urgent Care Association of America (UCAOA) has suggested major medical equipment that any UCF must have. This list is given below:[6]

- X-ray (digital preferred)
  For: Diagnostics—Chest, head, body, extremities.
- Developer—90 seconds
  For: Wet process chemical development of X-rays.
- Controller
  For: Digital system to control X-ray unit.
- Hematology unit (optional)
  For: Blood samples, WBC, RBC, platelets, differentials.
- ECG (EKG)
  For: Cardiac diagnostics.
- MCG Ultrasound (optional) (from Cardiac Analytics)
  For: Diagnosis CAD in office (for carotid/cardiac, abdominal, DVT) along with cart.
- Spirometer
  For: Measures lung capacity.
- Hyfrecator
  For: Electric device to remove skin lesions, also used for cauterization of veins.
- Cryogenics
  For: Used to freeze off dermatological occurrences.
- Microscope
  For: Used to look at serum, stools, urine, sputum.
- Centrifuge
  For: Used to produce lab samples for study.
- Autoclave
  For: Sterilizes instruments.
- Surgical lights (2)
  For: High intensity light for minor procedures.
- Exam lights
  For: High intensity, small lights for examinations.
- Audiometer
  For: Tests hearing (workman comp contracts require).
- Crash cart
- Oxygen regulator and tanks
  For: Emergencies.
- IV poles
  For: Administering D5W/NS, etc. and meds.
- Kick bucket (stainless steel with 4 wheels)
- Baum Meters (10) (wall mounted and portable blood pressure units)
- Electronic thermometers (4)
  For: Ear canal readings.
- Surgical instruments, assorted
- Assorted miscellaneous lab and clinical minor equipment and supplies
- Scales (one adult, one pediatric)
- Otoscopes/Ophal (wall mounted, cordless halogen)
- Power table
  For: Minor surgery and specific exams (obese patient/handicap).
- Exam tables (with electric and drawers)
- Exam stools
  For: Physicians to examine patients.
- Staff seating (mix of ergonomic seats)
- Staff desks (all executive style)
- Patient seating (ergonomic modern)
- Patient furniture (mix of tables and lamps)
- Telephone system (console with speakerphones)
- Security system (full alarm with security camera and recording capabilities)
- Televisions (13 inches cable ready—in exam rooms)
- DVD player (to interface with TVs)
- Cabinets
  For: drugs and supplies.
- Fax machine
- Photocopier
- Scale calculators
- File cabinets
- Miscellaneous equipment
- Signs—Internal (various required signs and placards)
- Signs—External (one or two signs, lighted or backlit - plastic or wood)
- Safe
- Computer system
- Scanners (2)
  For: Scanning of documents; capable of scanning health insurance cards and insert into electronic health records (EHR).
- EHR
- Digital camera (2)
  For: To insert picture of patients into medical records; To document patient dermatology or other conditions.

GENERAL SUPPORT FACILITIES

Environmental Services Room[7]

- A minimum of one environmental services room per floor should be provided.
- *Each environmental services room should be provided with the following*:
  - A service sink or floor-mounted mop sink
  - Provisions for storage of supplies and housekeeping equipment
  - A hand washing station or hand sanitation dispenser
- *Ventilation*:
  - Minimum 10 air changes per hour
  - Exhaust
  - Negative pressure.

Public and Administrative Areas

Public and administrative areas should conform to the requirements given below:

Public Areas

The following should be provided:

- Vehicular drop-off and pedestrian entrance
  - A minimum of one entrance should be reachable from grade level.
  - Accessibility
    - ◊ Access to wheelchairs and stretchers should be provided at the urgent care entrance.

 ◊ If a platform is provided for ambulance use, a ramp for wheelchairs and stretchers should be provided in addition to steps.
- *Reception*: A reception and information counter, desk, or kiosk should be provided.
- Waiting space(s)
- Public toilets
  - Toilet room(s) for public use should be readily accessible from the waiting area without passing through patient care or staff work areas or suites.
- Local telephone access
  - Access to make local phone calls should be provided.
- Provisions for drinking water
  - Access to drinking water should be provided.
- Wheelchair storage
  - Readily accessible wheelchair storage should be provided.
- Lobby and reception
  - Reception and information functions may be combined or separate.
  - These areas should meet the following requirements:
    - ◊ Reception and information areas should provide direct visual control of the urgent care entrance and access to the treatment area and the lobby.
    - ◊ If provided, nurse/control stations and triage area(s) should be in direct communication with medical staff.
    - ◊ A public toilet with hand washing stations should be provided.
    - ◊ Access to make local phone calls should be provided.
- Waiting area
  - This should include provisions for wheelchairs.
  - This should be separate from the area provided for scheduled outpatient services:
    - ◊ *Diagnostic imaging waiting area*: In the UCF diagnostic imaging waiting area requires special consideration to reduce the risk of airborne infection transmission, public waiting areas shall be designed, ventilated, and maintained with available technologies such as enhanced general ventilation and air disinfection techniques similar to inpatient requirements for Airborne Infection Isolation (AII) rooms.
- *Ventilation*:
  - Minimum 12 air changes per hour
  - Exhaust ventilation

    or
  - Recirculating ventilation system with HEPA filter.

Administrative Areas[7]

- Interview space
  - Provision for acoustical privacy
  - Readily accessible to waiting area.
- Multipurpose room for staff conferences (may be used for consultations).
- General or individual offices
- Medical records
  - Provisions should be made for securing medical records of all media types used by the facility.
  - To maintain confidentiality of records, the medical records area should be either restricted to staff movement or located so it is remote from treatment and public areas.
- Storage for staff personal effects (locking drawers, cabinets, or lockers) which is readily accessible to individual work areas.

Architectural Details and Mechanical, Electrical, and Plumbing

Corridor Width[7]

- Minimum 48 inches corridor width or compliance of corridor width with National building code.
- Corridors include turning spaces for wheelchairs.

Ceiling Height[7]

- Minimum 7 ft 10 inches (with certain exceptions)
- Minimum 7 ft 6 inches in corridors
- Minimum 7 ft 6 inches in normally unoccupied spaces
- Minimum height 7 ft 6 inch from lowest protruding element of equipment in radiography rooms.

Doors and Door Hardware[7]

- Door type
  - All doors between corridors, rooms, or spaces subject to occupancy should be of the swing type or shall be sliding doors.
  - Sliding doors
    - ◊ Use of manual or automatic sliding doors should be permitted where fire and other emergency exiting requirements are not compromised.
    - ◊ When sliding doors with breakaway features are used in the full open position, they should be permitted to temporarily restrict the minimum corridor width required by applicable building codes.
    - ◊ Sliding doors in patient care areas should not have floor tracks.
- *Door openings*: The door opening sizes given are the minimum clear width and height.
  - The minimum clear door opening for rooms where wheeled-bed stretchers will be used should have these dimensions:
    - ◊ 48 inches in width
    - ◊ 84 inches in height

    Or
  - The door does not provide stretcher access
    - ◊ Door to room used by patients minimum clear width 36 inches.
- *Door swing*: Doors should not be permitted to swing into corridors except doors in behavioral health units and doors to nonoccupiable spaces (e.g. environmental services rooms, electrical closets) and doors with emergency breakaway hardware.
- Door hardware
  - Door hardware should comply with local requirements.
  - Lever hardware should be provided.
- Patient toilet facilities
  - *Door opening*: Where a toilet room opens onto a public area or corridor, visual privacy should be maintained.
  - Door hardware
    - ◊ Doors to patient use toilets in patient care and treatment areas should have hardware that allows staff emergency access.
    - ◊ Doors to patient toilet rooms in outpatient psychiatric facilities should be permitted to have hardware that allows staff to control access.

Hand Washing Stations[7]

- Anchored to support vertical or horizontal force of 250 lbs.
- *Counter-mounted sinks*:

- Countertops made of porcelain, stainless steel, or solid mineral surface materials
- Plastic laminate countertops
  - ◊ At minimum substrate marine-grade plywood with impervious seal.
- No storage casework beneath sink
- Provisions for drying hands at all hand washing stations except hand scrub facilities
  - Hand drying device does not require hand contact.
  - Hand drying provisions enclosed to protect against dust or soil.
- Liquid or foam soap dispensers.

Grab Bars[7]

- Anchored for concentrated load of 250 lbs.
- Bariatric design
  - Length of rear wall grab bars 44 inches.

Surfaces[7]

Flooring and Wall Bases

- Selected flooring surfaces cleanable and wear-resistant for location.
- Smooth transitions between different flooring materials.
- Flooring surfaces, including those on stairways, stable, firm and slip-resistant.
- Floors and wall bases materials in all areas subject to frequent wet cleaning are not affected by germicidal cleaning solutions.
- Monolithic floors and wall bases in procedure rooms
  - Integral coved base minimum 6 inches high.

Walls and Wall Protection[7]

- Wall finishes washable
- Wall finishes in vicinity of plumbing fixtures smooth, scrubbable and water-resistant.
- Wall surfaces in areas routinely subjected to wet spray or splatter are monolithic or have sealed seams.
- No sharp protruding corners
- Corner guards durable and scrubbable.

Heating, Ventilation, and Air-conditioning Systems[7]

Outdoor Air Intakes

- Located minimum 25 ft from cooling towers and all exhaust and vent discharges.
- Bottom of air intake is at least 6 ft inch above grade
  - Roof mounted air intakes:
    - ◊ Bottom minimum 3 ft inch above roof level.

Filtration[7]

- Filter banks conform to standards

Air distribution systems:

- Ducted return or exhaust systems.

Space ventilation:

- Spaces ventilated as per norms
- Air movement from clean areas to less clean areas
- Minimum number of total air changes indicated either supplied for positive pressure rooms or exhausted for negative pressure rooms.
- Recirculating room HVAC units
  - Each unit serves only single space.
  - Minimum MERV 6 filter for airflow downstream of cooling coils.

Acoustical considerations:

- Equipment location or acoustic provisions limit noise associated with outdoor mechanical equipment to 65 dBA at building façade.

Ventilation and space-conditioning:

- All rooms and areas used for patient care have provisions for ventilation.
- Natural ventilation only allowed for nonsensitive areas via operable windows.
- Mechanical ventilation provided for all rooms and areas in facility in accordance with accepted norms.

ELECTRICAL SYSTEMS[7]

Electrical Distribution and Transmission

Switchboards locations:

- Located in areas separate from piping and plumbing equipment.
- Not located in rooms they support
- Accessible to authorized persons only.
- Easily accessible
- Located in dry, ventilated space free of corrosive gases or flammable material.
- Emergency electrical service conforms with standards.

Lighting:

Portable or fixed examination light in exam rooms and treatment rooms.

Electrical receptacles

- Receptacles in patient care areas conform to standards.

ELECTRICAL RECEPTACLES

Duplex grounded-type receptacles should be installed in all areas in sufficient quantities for tasks to be performed as needed. Receptacles in patient care areas. Receptacles should be provided according to Table 1.

Call Systems

Nurse call stations should be provided as required in Table 2.

Plumbing Systems[7]

Heated potable water distribution systems:

- Systems serving patient care areas are under constant recirculation.
- Non recirculated fixture branch piping does not exceed 25 ft in length.
- No dead-end piping
- Water-heating system has supply capacity at minimum temperatures and amounts.
- Hand washing stations supplied as required above
  or

Table 1: Electrical receptacles for patient care areas in urgent care facilities.

Electrical receptacles for patient care areas		
Location	***Number of single receptacles***	***Receptacle locations***
Diagnostic and treatment area		
General examination rooms	8	4 convenient to head of exam table
International imaging (inducing cardiac catheterization, angiography)	12	8 convenient to table placement with at least one on each wall
Operating rooms	18	12 convenient to table placement 2 on each wall
Phase II recovery area	4	Convenient to stretcher or chair
Endoscopy procedure rooms	8	

Table 2: Locations for nurse call devices in urgent care facilities.

Locations for nurse call devices				
Location	***Patient station***	***Emergency staff assistance station***	***Code cell station***	***Nurse master station***
Diagnostic and treatment areas		•	•	
International imaging (including cardiac catheterization, angiography)				
Operating rooms		•		
Phase postanesthesia recovery area		•		
Phase II recovery area	•	•		
Endoscopy procedure room		•		
Electroconvulsive therapy procedure room and recovery area		•		
Support areas				
Nurse/control station				•

- Hand washing stations supplied at constant temperature between 70°F and 80°F using single-pipe supply.

Plumbing Fixture

Materials used for plumbing fixtures non-absorptive and acid resistant.

Hand Washing Station Sinks[7]

- Basins reduce risk of splashing to areas where direct patient care is provided, sterile procedures are performed and medications are prepared.
- Basin minimum 144 sq inch
- Minimum dimension 9 inches
- Made of porcelain, stainless steel, or solid mineral surface materials.
- Water discharge point of faucets at least 10 inches above bottom of basin
- Anchoring for sinks withstands minimum vertical or horizontal force of 250 lbs
- Fittings operated without using hands for sinks used by staff, patients and public
  - Blade handles or single lever
    - ◊ Minimum 4 inches long
    - ◊ Provide clearance required for operation

  or
  - Sensor-regulated water fixtures
    - ◊ Meet user need for temperature and length of time water flows
    - ◊ Designed to function at all times and during loss of normal power.

Table 3: Station outlets for oxygen, vacuum, and medical air systems in urgent care facilities.[5]

Location	*Oxygen*	*Vaccum*	*Medical Lr*
Airbrone infection isolation room	0	0	–
Cast room	0	0	–
Cardiac catheterization room	2	2	13
Birthing room	13	13	–
Procedure room	1	1	–
Outpatient operating room	2	3	1
Phase postanesthesia recovery area	1	1	–
Phase recovery area	0	0	–
Endoscopy procedure room	1	3	–
Endoscopy recovery stations	0	0	–
Endoscopy instrument processing room decontamination area	–	–	–
Electromotive therapy procedure room	13	13	–

Clinical Sinks

- Trimmed with valves that can be operated without hands.
- Handles minimum 6 inches long
- Integral trap wherein upper portion of water trap provides visible seal.

Medical Gas and Vacuum Systems[5]

Station outlets should be provided as indicated in Table 3.

- *Medical gas systems*: If piped medical gas is used, the installation, testing, and certification of nonflammable medical gas and air systems should comply with the statutory requirements.
- *Vacuum systems*: Where a central clinical vacuum system is provided design and installation should be in accordance with acceptab e standards.

Communication Systems[5]

- Locations for terminating telecommunications and information system devices should be provided.
- A space shall be provided for central equipment locations. Special air-conditioning and voltage regulation should be provided when recommended by the manufacturer.

Fire Alarm System

A fire alarm system should be installed as per requirements.

Elevators[7]

- Outpatient facility located on more than one floor or on floor other than an entrance floor at grade level.
- At least one elevator
  or
- Outpatient facility located on entrance floor at grade level.
- A sample design of an UCF is shown in Figure 4

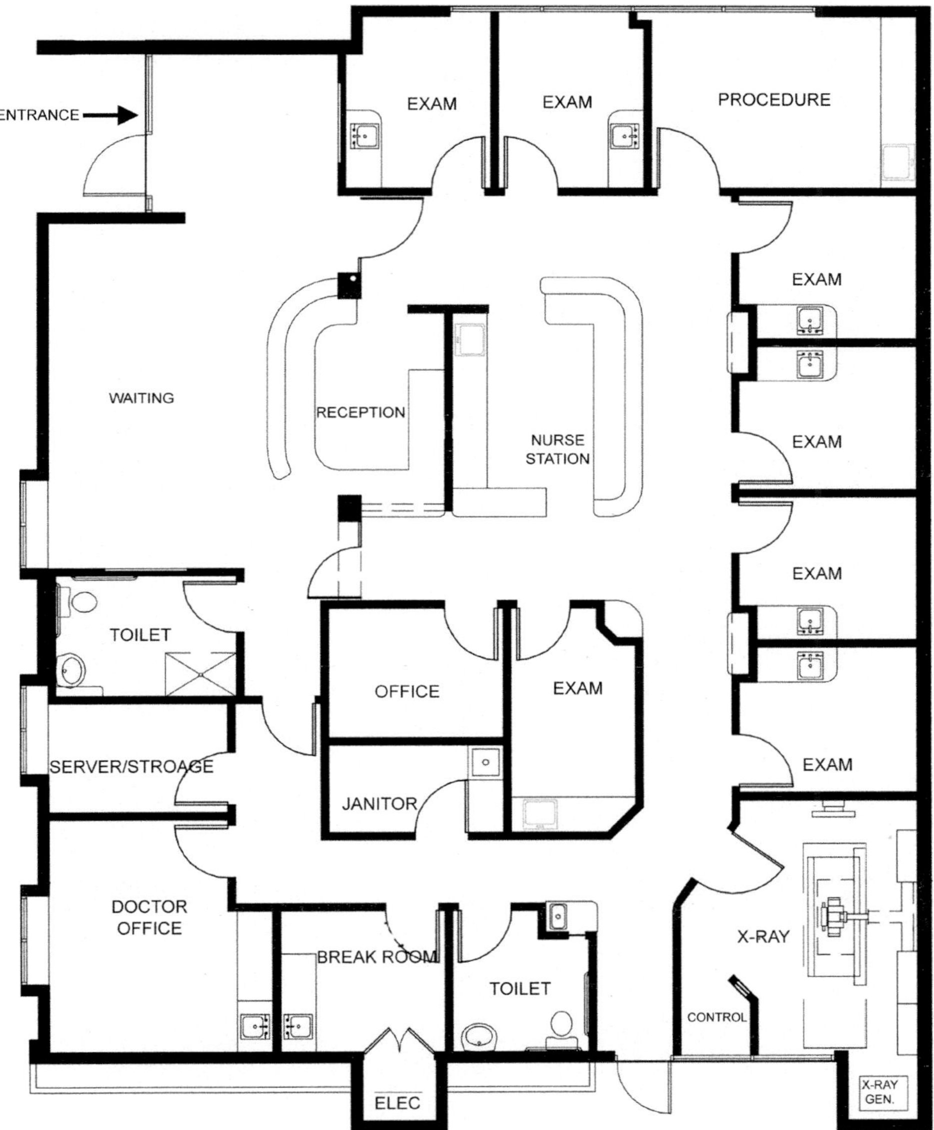

Fig. 4: Design of an urgent care facility.

REFERENCES

1. New York State Dept of Health Ambulatory Services Urgent Case. Background paper albany. New York 2013.
2. urgentcaredoctorjacksonville.com
3. www.hschange.org
4. www.healthlawyers.org
5. aaucm.org
6. www.jvir.org
7. www.mass.gov

OTHER REFERENCES

- The Joint Commission Accreditation Ambulatory Care: Accreditation Handbook for Ambulatory Care. 2010.
- Yee T, Lechner AE, Ellyn R. Boukus. The Surge in Urgent Care Centers: Emergency Department Alternative or Costly Convenience?, 2013.
- Looney KH, Mollie K. O'Brien, Jon Sundock: Urgent Care Centers and Free-Standing Emergency Rooms: A Necessary Alternative Under the ACA.
- Urgent Care Association of America, The Case for Urgent Care, Naperville, Ill. (Sept. 1, 2011).
- Weinick S, Robin M, Renée M. Betancourt. No Appointment Needed: The Resurgence of Urgent Care Centers in the United States, California HealthCare Foundation, Oakland, Calif. 2007.

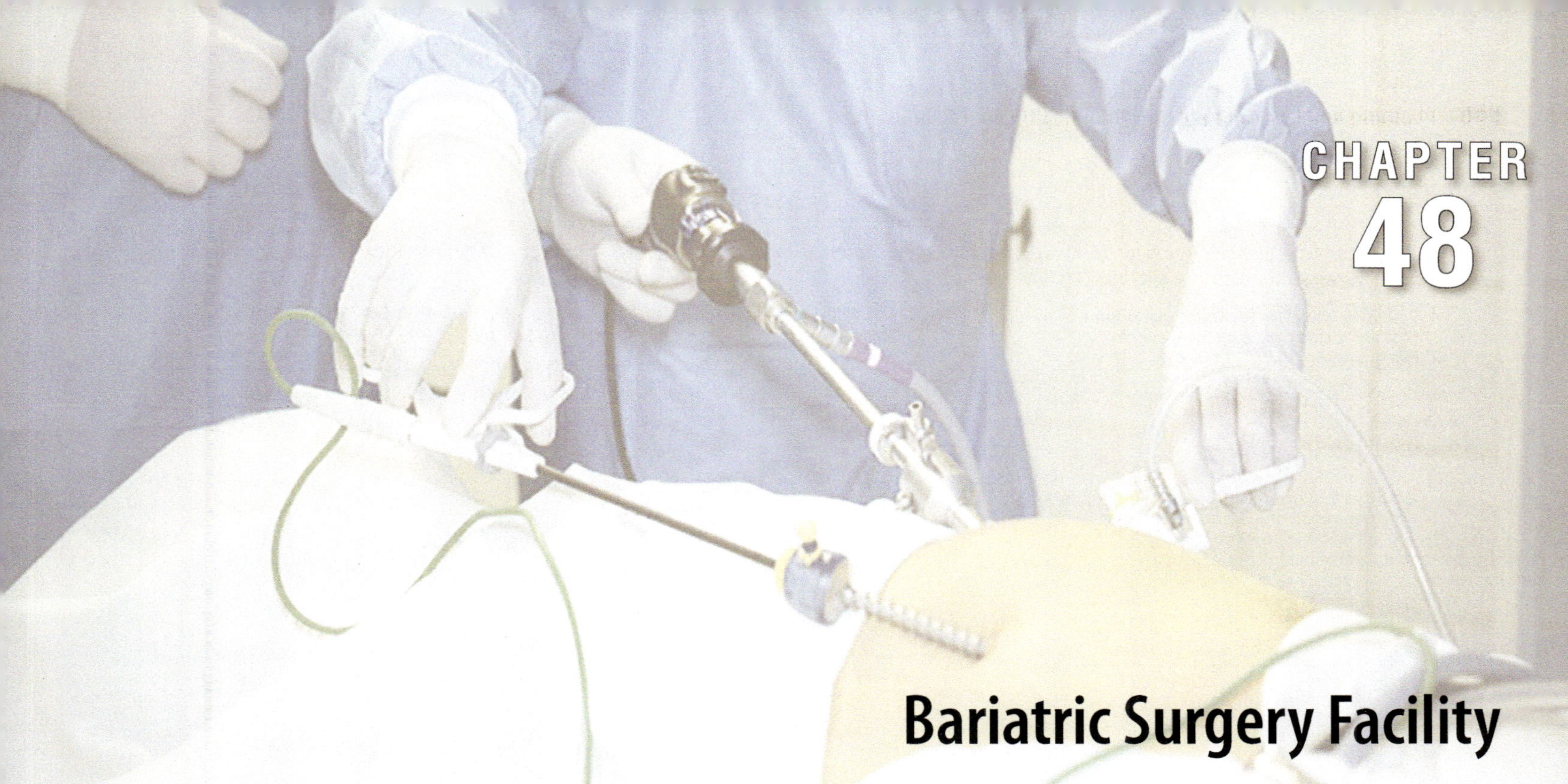

Bariatric Surgery Facility

Kanika Jain, Samarpita Dutta, Shakti Kumar Gupta, Sunil Kant, R Chandrashekhar

INTRODUCTION

Obesity is an epidemic which has plagued the world especially the developed nations. In the current times, it is a significant health problem globally with over one billion adults being overweight. The prevalence of the epidemic is in the same magnitude across both sexes, age groups and race. Thirteen percent of the world's total population has been reported to be obese in the 2014 global estimates of the WHO. It has been reported that more than 50% of the obese population in the world live in ten countries (listed in order of number of obese individuals)—USA, China, India, Russia, Brazil, Mexico, Egypt, Germany, Pakistan, and Indonesia. While the United States of America accounted for 13% of obese people worldwide in 2013, China and India jointly accounted for 15%.[1]

Being obese does not only mean being overweight, it also means that the individual who is obese should be considered as a person with special needs. WHO defines an adult to be obese, if the body mass index (BMI) of any individual is greater than or equal to 30. One cannot care for an obese patient in a similar manner as a normal individual. These patients have special emotional and physical needs. They are found to suffer from a number of chronic ailments such as hypertension, diabetes, sleep apnea, hyperventilation, osteoarthritis, cancers, etc. which warrants admission of such patients time and again. Further, it has been noted that the attendants of such cases are also obese and have special needs as well. Healthcare facilities across the globe are facing the daunting challenge to reconstruct, redesign or construct spaces appropriate to take care of a bariatric patient. The enhanced need to provide safe and quality care for such patients and healthcare workers has emerged as a significant issue for healthcare providers worldwide.[2]

Majority of the healthcare organizations have not yet recognized the special needs of these patients. The hospital administrator is also duty bound to safeguard the health of his employees from any occupation-related injury and therefore, the need to cater to bariatric patients with special facilities and protocols. They pose increased risk to the providers because of their physical structure causing injury and difficulty in maintaining hygiene.

PLANNING PREMISES

Obese patients impact hospitals in two ways: first, by electing to undergo surgical intervention procedures that result in weight reduction, and second, by routine use of healthcare facilities for either acute care (medical or surgical units), emergency care (emergency rooms or critical care units), long-term care (palliative or nursing home units), or ambulatory care provided at the outpatient department. All of these sites need to ensure that current and future development plans are addressing the needs and making the appropriate provisions to provide a safe and efficient care environment for the patients and healthcare workers.[2,3]

The Facility Guidelines Institute (FGI) was one of the first to offer guidance when it published the 2010 edition of the Guidelines for Design and Construction of Health Care Facilities with recommendations for bariatric accommodations. These guidelines remain the most widely adopted source of information for the industry.[3] The following design considerations need to be considered while planning a bariatric facility.

The Route

Healthcare facilities have to be designed holistically. Hence, while conceptualizing space for bariatric patients, due consideration needs to be given to every aspect of the patient's movement within the healthcare facility from entry to exit that is redesigning everything from access doors, entry points, passageways widths, waiting area space, etc.

Constructability

Healthcare architects and builders need to understand that certain facilities like ceiling lifts, grab bars, widened corridors to allow passage to bariatric patients. Facilities need to be strengthened to accommodate the needs of these patients by adding steel plates to reinforce garb bars designed to hold up to 350 kg, etc. (Fig. 1).

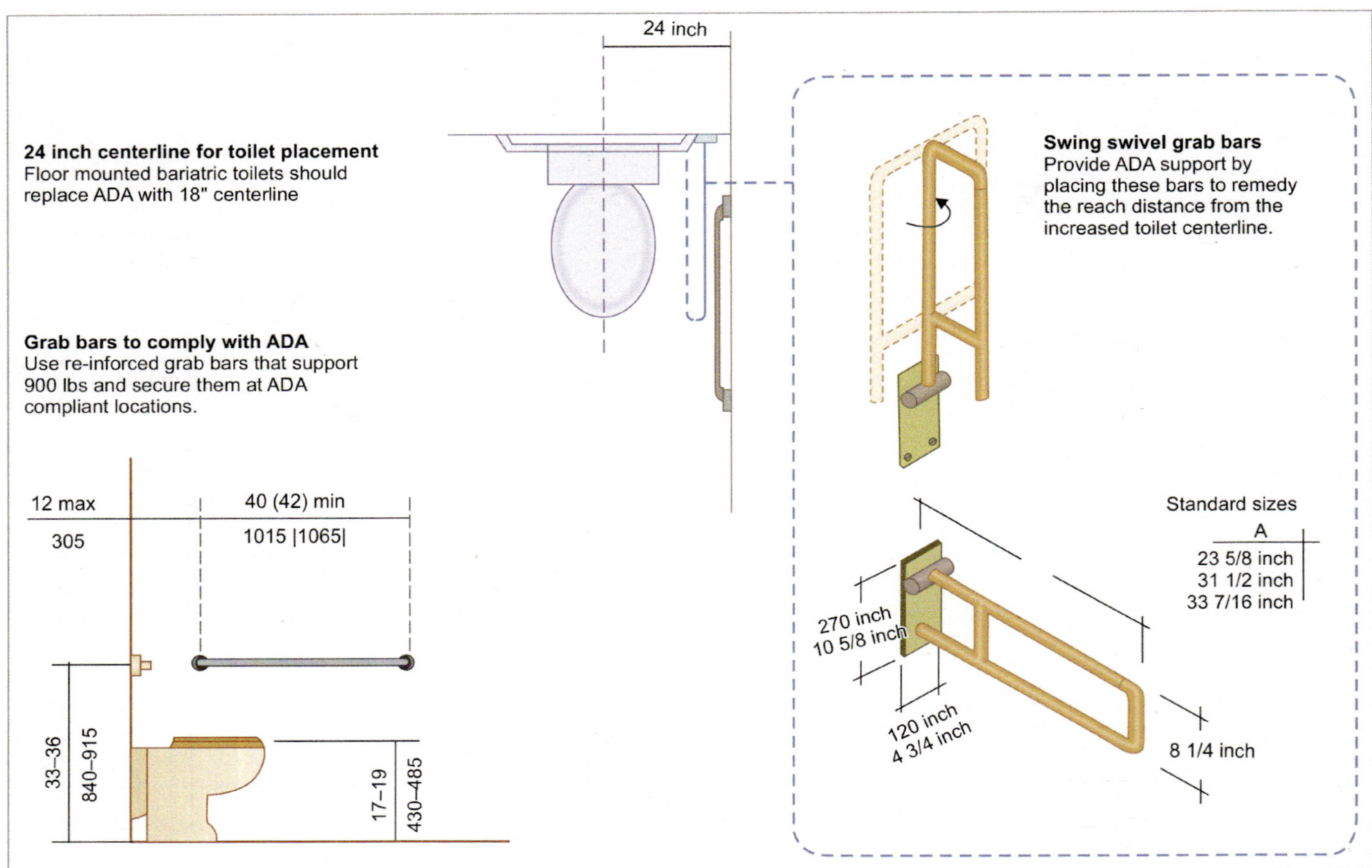

Fig. 1: Grab bars and toilet placement for a bariatric patient.

Making it Feel Seamless

The most challenging aspect of designing spaces for bariatric patients is not allowing it to stand out rather the rooms and other amenities should appear as similar as possible to the one designed for non-bariatric patients. It should feel inclusive and part of the overall aesthetics.

Sensitivity

Patient sensitivity is an essential consideration in designing for bariatric patients. Designs should be such that should not alienate or restrict patients.

Patients

The following advantages are noted for the patients when they are provided with adequate space for mobilization and care:[2]

- Increase in heart/lung capacity and blood circulation
- Reduced risk of pneumonia, thrombosis, and other illnesses
- Improved mobility and quality of life
- Reduced risk of slips/falls
- Reduced spatial disorientation
- Reduced risk of depression.

HEALTHCARE FACILITIES AND HEALTHCARE PROVIDERS[2]

Appropriate facilities and processes will ensure:

- Increased patient and employee satisfaction
- Patients/residents have a reduced need for assistance
- Reduced strain-related injuries and increased staff productivity
- Reduced turnover of staff
- Reduced cost and enhanced quality of nursing.

BARIATRIC SAFE HANDLING PROGRAM

Essential components of a bariatric safe patient handling program should include the following:

- Space and environment considerations
- Equipment needs
- Patient care protocol.

Space and Environment Considerations

Design is a critical tool in the care of and the improved long-term clinical outcomes for bariatric patients. Design concerns include appropriate facilities and space, proper equipment and furnishings. Identification of all the patient care activities is essential prior to determining space requirements. Patient care activities should include the following:

- Provision of care on the bed (positioning, repositioning, skin and wound care, feeding, bathing, etc.)
- Provision of care besides the bed
- Transfer of the patient from the bed to wheelchair, stretchers, commodes, etc.
- Mobilizing the patient within the room or to any other area
- Provision of assistance to the patient for various activities such as rising from the seated position, etc.

When designing space, accommodation for the task that requires the most space is what should be considered. The space necessary for the provision of care to a bariatric patient can be determined by:[2,4]

- A description of the patient population—physical and mental capacities, medical conditions.
- *Type of care to be provided:* In case of critical care setting, in addition to leaving space on the sides and foot end of the bed to allow adequate space for movement of staff and equipment, space has to be left at the head end of the bed as well.
- *Type and size of equipment:* The equipment space must provide for the ability to move the patient, bed, stretchers, lift devices, mobility devices, and seated devices in an ergonomic pathway that limits turns and twisting of equipment while under load to prevent exceeding safe work limits for spinal loading for the healthcare providers.
- How and where patients are transported (patient flow)?

The ultimate design goal when designing for the bariatric patient is to provide opportunities and encouragement for increased mobility, independence and strength. A turning radius of 72 inches of clear floor space is recommended between furnishings, walls, and equipment in order to facilitate equipment maneuvers.[4]

Design Factors for Bariatric Patients

The essential design factors for the various spaces in a bariatric or healthcare facility, includes the following:[4]

- Entrances and routes
- Patient rooms and bathrooms
- Diagnostic and treatment spaces
- Lobbies and waiting areas.

Entrances and Routes

Designing the space for bariatric patients should start from the entrance in the facility itself making it accessible for the patient. Ramps, staircases, lifts and corridors across the hospital should be made wide enough to accommodate bariatric wheelchairs, trolleys, etc.

As per the Facilities Guidelines Institute, 2010 revised guidelines,[4] the corridors within the organization should be wide enough to accommodate a 39 inch by 49 inch wide wheelchair (700 lbs/317 kg capacity) with a 6 ft turning radius factor door width and elevator capacity to make common areas more easily accessible for a patient, equipment and caregivers. Most hospital elevators have an average weight capacity of 2,000–3,000 lbs (906–1,359 kg) a capacity that may be exceeded when the weight of the bariatric patient, bed, transport staff, and specialized equipment are added together.

Bariatric Patient Room

As recommended by the the Bariatric Room Design Advisory Board (BRDAB), Room for a bariatric patient should have the following dimensions:

- Optimal width: 14 ft
- Depth: 15 ft (corridor to exterior wall).

Extra space required includes space required for specialized equipment and furniture such as bariatric beds, wheelchairs, oversized attendants couches and chairs, etc. Additional space is also required to facilitate mobility needs of both the patient and medical team. Bariatric beds are customized to accommodate weights in excess of 350 kg and are wider than the usual patient care beds helping one to increase patient safety and comfort and mitigate risk of injury to caregivers and patients (Fig. 2). These beds should be such that they can be converted to chair positions to facilitate safe patient transfer and have built in scales. Bariatric chairs have expanded widths up to 36 inches, as do the other pieces of bariatric equipment. The beds available for these types of patients can now be expandable up to 54 inches wide and typically 88 inches long. The space at the end of the bed must also be adequate to allow for the capabilities of the newer beds, including technologies such as sitting the patient in an upright position.[2,4]

Space Design for Critical Care Rooms

In addition to the design considerations recommended in a routine bariatric acre room, while planning for space in critical areas it is essential to plan for a well-positioned ceiling track system and repositioning sheet.

Critical Care Room Width

The width of the room is defined from the wall at the "side" of the bed to the wall at the other side of the bed. The recommended minimum room width in the critical care setting for safe patient handling and care of the bariatric patient is a minimum of 168 inches (14 ft) when using a ceiling lift, and 204 inches or 17 ft if floor lift is in use (Figs. 3 and 4).[2]

This space does not include the additional items fitting in the room, such as cupboards or specialty equipment. Additionally, the space assumes that when the seating chairs or lifts are not being used, they are removed from the area.[2]

Critical Care Room Length

The recommended minimum room length for provision of care to the bariatric patient in a critical care environment is 162 inches, 13.5 ft. This does not include furnishing or storage or intensive care equipment space for such things as monitors.

Room length in acute care shifts the need of the head space to the end of the bed:

- About 88 inches for maximum bed length
- About 36 inches for equipment or patient seated in a wheelchair
- About 39 inches for worker space.

The recommended room length for provision if care of the bariatric patient in acute care is a minimum 163 inches or 13 ft 7 inch.

Door width: Door width of 60 inches is recommended to allow passage of a 48 inch or 54 inch wide patient bed.

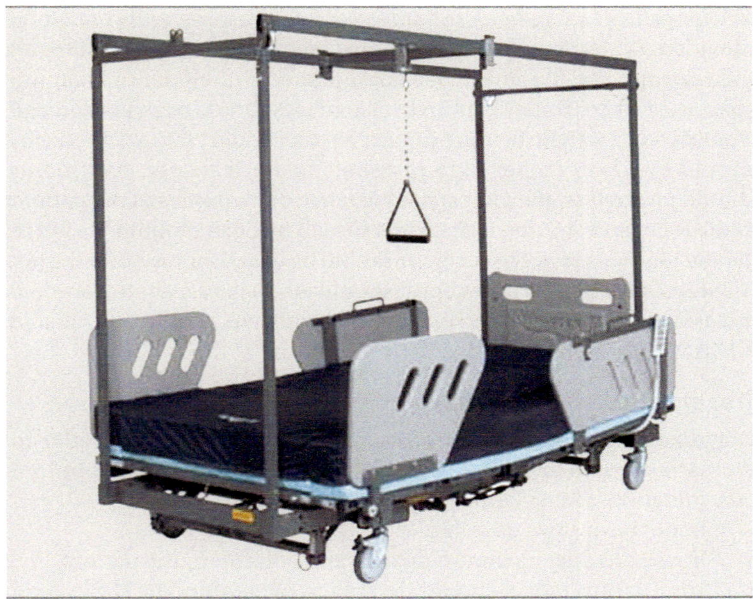

Fig. 2: Bed for a bariatric patient.

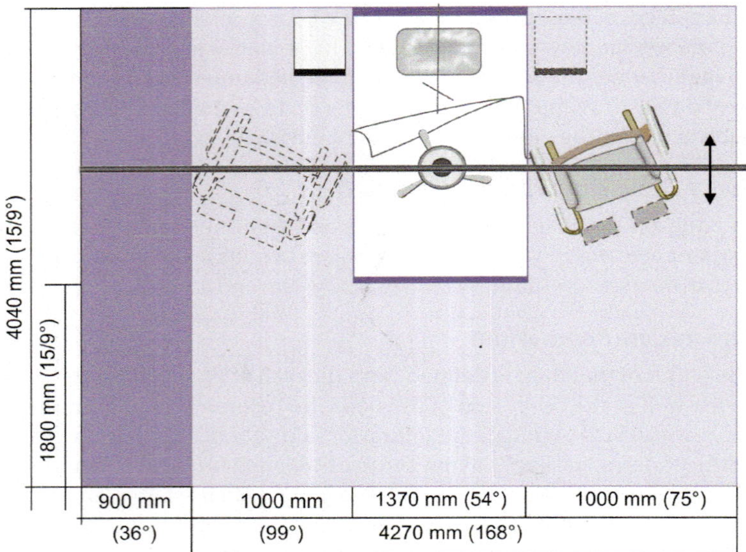

Fig. 3: Optimum space required for enabling wheelchair movement in a bariatric patients room.

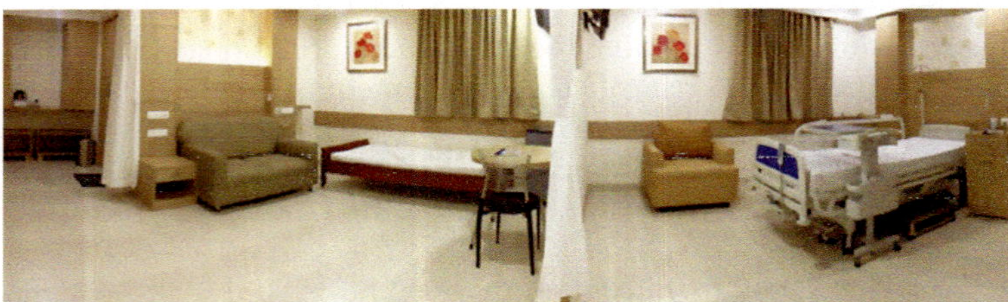

Fig. 4: Bariatric patients room.

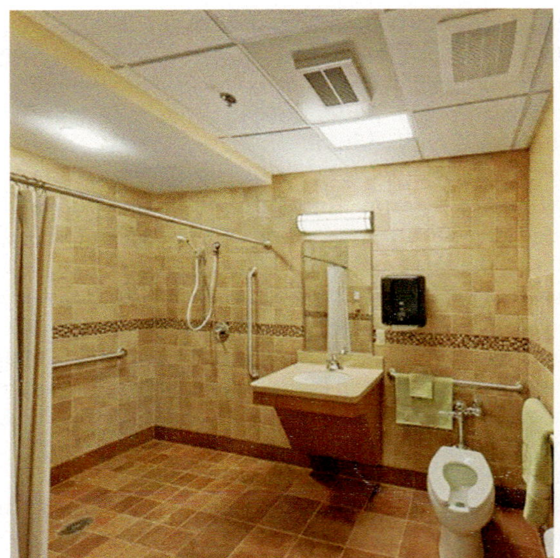

Fig. 5: Layout of a bathroom for a bariatric patient.

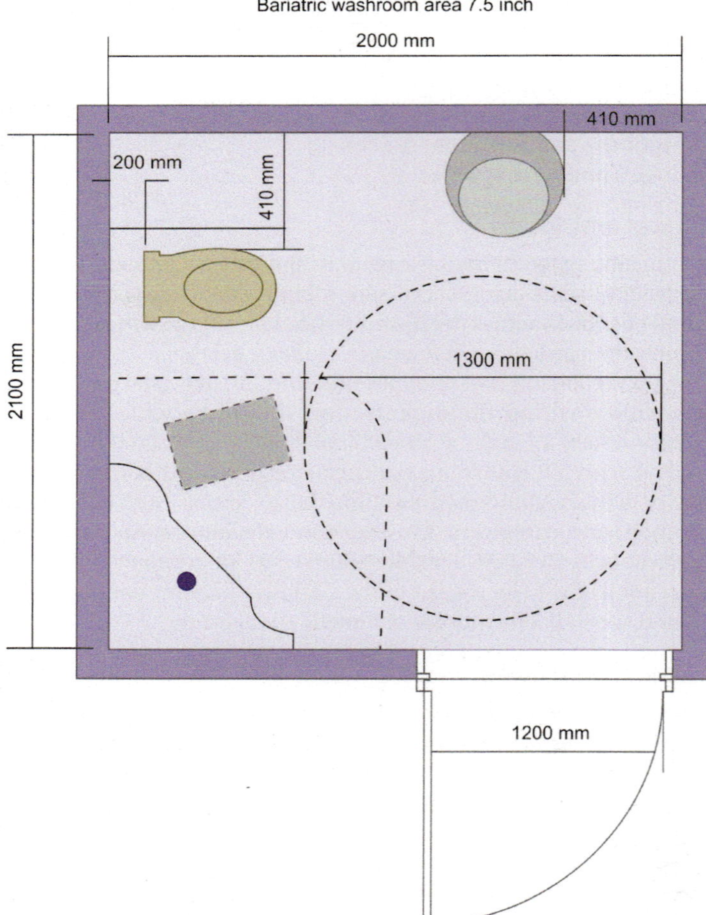

Fig. 6: Bariatric washroom design.

The Bariatric Patient Bathroom (Figs. 5 and 6)

The BRDAB recommends the bariatric patient bathroom of at least 45 sq ft (6480 sq inch) in size. Design guidelines suggest that the minimum centerline for toilets should be 24 inch from the wall. The BRDAB preferred a pair of unequal-leaf swinging doors—with one leaf 42 inches wide, the other 18 inches. This positioning will help provide maximum clear opening with the least overall width while giving more wall space to supporting functions. A minimum of a 6 ft turning radius must be provided. Bariatric patient washrooms are recommended to have all toilet fixtures and the sink to be floor mounted as they allow maximum space clearance. Toilet seats for such patients should be oversized and should have a weight-bearing capacity of more than 350 kg. Toilet seats should be 17–19 inches high to enable patients to rise. Bathrooms should be sized to allow for staff assistance on two sides of the patient at the toilet and shower. Dispensers should be flush mounted to aid in clearance and safety. The receptor should be tested for load bearing per ANSI Z124.1.2-2005. The receptor should also have a front transitional edge for easy access. Multiple reinforced grab bars should be available and rated for 1,000 pounds each.

Treatment and Diagnostic Spaces

Diagnostic and treatment room space requirements are similar to the patient room spaces. The following points need to be kept into consideration while planning for such spaces:[4]

- Should be easily accessible.
- Should provide maximum privacy and comfort to the patient.
- Examination tables should be able to accommodate more than 45 kg of weight.
- Tables should be electronically powered for patient transfers.
- Weighing scales up to—1000 kg
- Clear floor area—150 sq ft minimum
- Treatment table clearance—5 ft at sides and foot

- Portable or built-in lift—400 kg. minimum
- Furniture, plumbing fixtures, casework—floor mounted and rated at 450 kg/1,000 lbs.

Lobbies and Waiting Areas

It is pertinent to plan and order for furnishing especially seating in the waiting areas and lobby in any bariatric facility as obese patients face a problem in sitting in standard sized chairs because of lack of adequate space. Chairs being provided should be greater in width than the standard chairs and the arms must have a grasp point on the front of the arm, providing a stable platform or push point. A seat that pitches forward assists the patient with a safe exit from the chair.[4]

Interiors, Aesthetics and the Need for Protection

Higher loads and increased movement of specialized equipment required for the care of the obese render the bariatric spaces prone to greater wear and tear. Wall cladding which is preferably thicker and rigid (either for the full wall or for wainscoting) should be considered. High load bearing hand rails should be considered. Hand rails should have the proper grip radius for both patient comfort and safety. Patients and equipment moving through doorways can lead to heavy wear on the door surface, jamb, handle and frame. Protection options include fully clad doors, door frame guards, kick plates and handle protectors.[2,4]

Wall guards complete the wall protection package by absorbing impact from wheelchairs and lower equipment surfaces, such as carts, gurneys, and diagnostic equipment.[2,4]

Two options for wall construction in bariatric installations are:[2,4]

- About 20 gauge metal framing with vertical studs spaced 16 inch on center. Horizontal metal strapping to be 16 gauge × 6 inch wide. A layer of ½ inch plywood to be mechanically fastened to the metal framing followed by 5/8 inch gypsum board.
- About 20 gauge metal framing with vertical studs spaced 16 inches on center. Horizontal wood strapping to be 2 × 6 board. A layer of ½ inch plywood to be mechanically fastened to the metal framing followed by 5/8 inch gypsum board.

Selection should be based on impact resistance, with particular attention paid to the design and construction of the inner retainer.

Miscellaneous rooms and their design considerations: The premise for deciding upon the design considerations for areas such as examining rooms, radiology, operating room and the morgue is equipment space, worker space and by task. Process mapping should be the tool which should help decide the overall facility plan. The mapping would consider the pathways and areas that the patient would attend during an admission through discharge or death. Consideration must also be given to transporting the patient/resident through halls and doorways with adequate width, and elevators with the appropriate capacity and space. Planning in the event of a death is important in facilities that will need to transport and temporarily house the body in a morgue. Morgue stretchers, body containers, and refrigeration areas are not usually equipped to manage the weight capacities required by bariatric patient/residents.[2,4]

Equipment Considerations (Figs. 7A to D)

Bariatric Wheelchairs

Typical dimensions for bariatric wheelchairs are 35–39 inches in width by 26 inches in depth in comparison to the standard wheelchairs which are typically 26 inches wide by 26 inches deep. In selecting bariatric wheelchairs, it is important to check the ergonomics for easy movement with increased weight load.

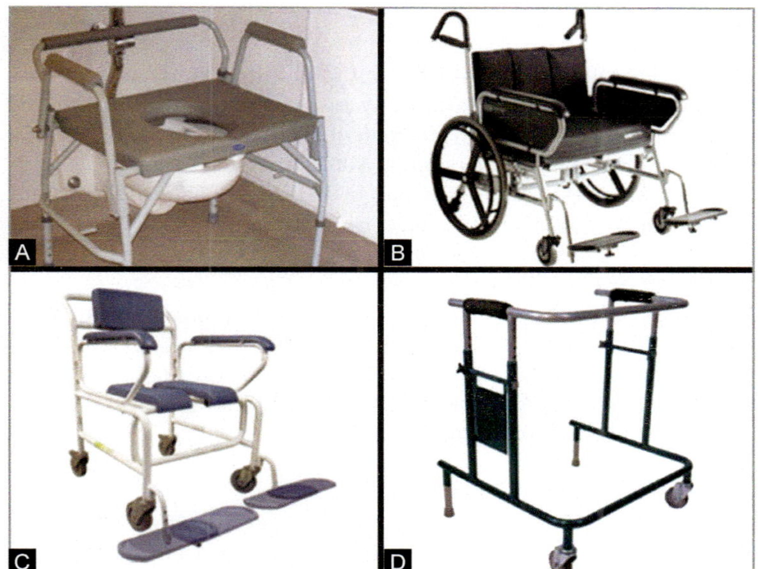

Figs. 7A to D: Equipment required for bariatric patients.

Stretchers

Bariatric stretchers are available with weight capacities up to 700 pounds (318 kg). The use of powered high/low stretchers may be advantageous to facilitate patient transfer and positioning. Stretchers with integrated scales should be considered for patients with poor mobility.

Examination Table

Standard patient examination tables have weight capacities of up to 400 pounds (182 kg), and examination tables for bariatric patients have weight capacities up to 800 pounds (363 kg). The use of powered high/low examination tables should be considered for heavier patients due to their reduced mobility. Powered tables should be able to lower to as little as 18 inches from the floor to facilitate the transition from a wheelchair onto the examination table.

Air Mattresses for Patient Transfer

These mattresses enable air assisted safe patient lateral transfer thereby minimizing the risk of injury to the patient as well as to the care provider. They also prevent any skin shearing and bruising. The mattresses available in the market are also radiolucent and MRI compatible for artifact-free imaging.

Weighing Scales

Special bariatric weighing scales have weight capacity above/up to 800 pounds (363 kg). Scales with higher weight limits are typically electronic, which require batteries or 115V power to operate. Wheelchair-accessible scales allow the patient to sit on a chair during weighing, and have ramps to aid in the positioning of the wheelchair. If standing platform scales are used, facilities should consider selecting models with built-in hand rails to stabilize patients during weighing. Some scales also have additional features such as BMI and body fat percentage calculators.

Physiologic Monitors and Sphygmomanometers

Sphygmomanometers and monitors need to be supplied with extra-large cuff sizes so that they may fit bariatric patients and accurate readings may be obtained.

Diagnostic Imaging System

Primary considerations for imaging systems for bariatric patients includes the bore size, table capacity and image quality. Bore size is a critical factor when evaluating the potential use of an imaging device for extremely obese patients, as standard bore sizes may be insufficient for an extremely obese patient. The weight-bearing capacity of the system and the image quality need to be considered.

Operating Room Tables

In the operation theater weight and size of operating room tables must be sufficient to accommodate the individual patient while still maintaining full articulation capabilities. In addition, side extenders and foot boards are recommended. Bariatric operating room tables are available with weight-bearing capacity of up to 1,000 pounds (454 kg).

Overhead Lifts/Slings/Hoists

Patient lifting and transportation needs to be aided with slings/hoists and lifts to minimize injuries and ensure safety of patient and hospital staff. Three types of hoists may be used—electric mobile hoists, hydraulic mobile hoists and gantry hoists which are available in different sizes. Due to the nature of a bariatric patient's condition, a hoist and sling must be selected with the appropriate safe working load (SWL) to ensure compatibility and longevity.

Deep vein thrombosis (DVT) pumps: Special emphasis may be laid on provision of DVT pumps in these facilities because the condition of deep vein thrombosis in these patients, although rare, is a preventable complication.

Patient Care Protocol

A written protocol for care of the bariatric patient is needed before operationalizing the facility. This may be utilized during training of staff and their induction on being posted to this facility.

Prehospital Care

This may be considered for facilities which provide pre- hospital care to such patients. To provide emergency services to these patients, ambulances may be specially equipped with wide doors with suitable stretcher and other equipments to suit the need of bariatric patients. These are significantly more expensive than normal ambulances. Some bariatric ambulances are actually classified as heavy vehicles and require a special license to drive. Acquiring the license is normally part of bariatric patient training provided by the hospital or health provider, in addition to dealing with the heavy and specialized equipment used in bariatric ambulances.[5]

Preparation of Patient Room

In preparation of the room, space is of utmost concern. Apart from adequately sized furniture, patient bed, mattress, etc. other things to be in place are scales to measure the height and weight of the patient, BP cuffs, etc. A bariatric patient kit should be made available consisting of 2 large patient gowns, a large bed-pan, 2 large sliding sheets, a bariatric cuff and other items as needed.

Planning for Admission and Discharge

Care of bariatric patient starts from the time of admission and sometimes even before, just with receiving the patient from the transport vehicle. Appropriately sized stretchers or wheelchairs should be available in case the patient is brought to the emergency. Discharge of these clients should be handled in a smooth functional manner. Patient should be counseled for appropriate care of self after discharge. Wheelchairs and trolleys needed for their transport should be taken care of and also ambulance services for their transport till home if it is in the scope of services of the hospital.

Patient Assessment Plan

The first step in caring the patient is patient assessment. The purpose is to identify the risks to the patient and adequately plan the resources to reduce those risks. In addition to the recommended risk assessment other critical issues to assess include:[6]

- Patient's required level of assistance
- Weight-bearing capability
- Height and weight
- Conditions likely to affect transfer or repositioning techniques—these may include hip or knee replacements, paralysis, amputations, contractures, osteoporosis, respiratory and cardiac conditions, skin conditions.[6]

Plan for Patient Mobilization

Mobilization is an important aspect of patient rehabilitation and needs to be focused on. Firstly, the patient and the attendants need to be briefed about the hospitals mobilization plan for bariatric clients. Secondly, care has to be taken whether patient is fit for self-mobilization or needs support. If the patient is capable of self-mobilization, then appropriate equipment to support such as walking aids and sit-to-stand frames should be provided. However, if the patient is unable to move himself, then appropriate facilities for transfer or shifting need to be in place such as slings or hoists. Transfer trolleys also need to be checked for their maximum handling capacities.

Other Support Services

There are other services such hospital linen which need to be considered for bariatric patients and should be available in different sizes and adjustments. The hospital dietary services should be able to provide a well-balanced diet for these patients depending on their physical conditions and existing comorbidities.

CONCLUSION

For quality care for bariatric residents, administrators need to understand the relationship between space, equipment, patient care, patient size, and furnishings. Space and capacity planning throughout healthcare facilities must be given consideration in order to safely and properly care for the increasing numbers of these patients. Including front-line HCWs in bariatric space design is essential.[2]

Emerging power devices for transport items, such as beds, stretchers, and wheelchairs, will eliminate the number of workers and possible worker space required. Appropriate space is a critical step and urgent priority in improving the safety of the bariatric patient and the HCW during patient handling and nursing care tasks.[2]

REFERENCES

1. newsmanager.commpartners.com
2. www.wales.nhs.uk
3. www.healthcaredesignmagazine.com
4. www.mediteksurgical.ca
5. macslift.com
6. www.ace.co.nz

OTHER REFERENCES

- World Health Organization. Obesity and overweight [Internet]. Available from: http://www.who.int/mediacentre/factsheets/fs311/en/
- Chastain S, Barbara A, and Chisholm D, Phil E. (2008). The shortest path to recovery. Page Southerland Page. Retrieved from:http://www.pspaec.com/perspectives/The_Shortest_Path.pdf
- Cohen, Martin H., et al. (April 2010). Patient handling and movement assessments: A white paper. Facilities Guidelines Institute.
- Facilities Guidelines Institute. (2010). Guidelines for design and construction of healthcare facilities.
- Facilities Guidelines Institute. (2010). Patient Handling and Movement Assessments (PHAMA): A White Paper.
- Kroll K, Karen K. (January 2005.) Evidence-based design in healthcare facilities. Building Operating Management.
- Lawson E, Bryan A. (2005). Evidence-based design in healthcare. Business Briefing: Hospital Engineering & Facilities Management.
- Malone N, Eileen, Dellinger B, Barbara D. (May 2011). Furniture design features and healthcare outcomes. The Center for Health Design.
- Pelczarski E, Kathryn K. (March 2007). Basic concerns in bariatrics. Healthcare Design Magazine.
- Special handling and movement challenges related to bariatrics. (August 2007). Retrieved from: http://www.visn8.va.gov/patientsafetycenter/safePtHandling/BariatricsToolkit.pdf
- Wignall D, Doug S. (March 2008). Design as a critical tool in bariatric care. Journal of Diabetes Science and Technology, 2(2), 263-267.
- Williams A, David S. (March 2008). Design with dignity: The design and manufacture of appropriate furniture for the bariatric patient population. Bariatric Nursing and Surgical Patient Care. 3(1), 39-40.

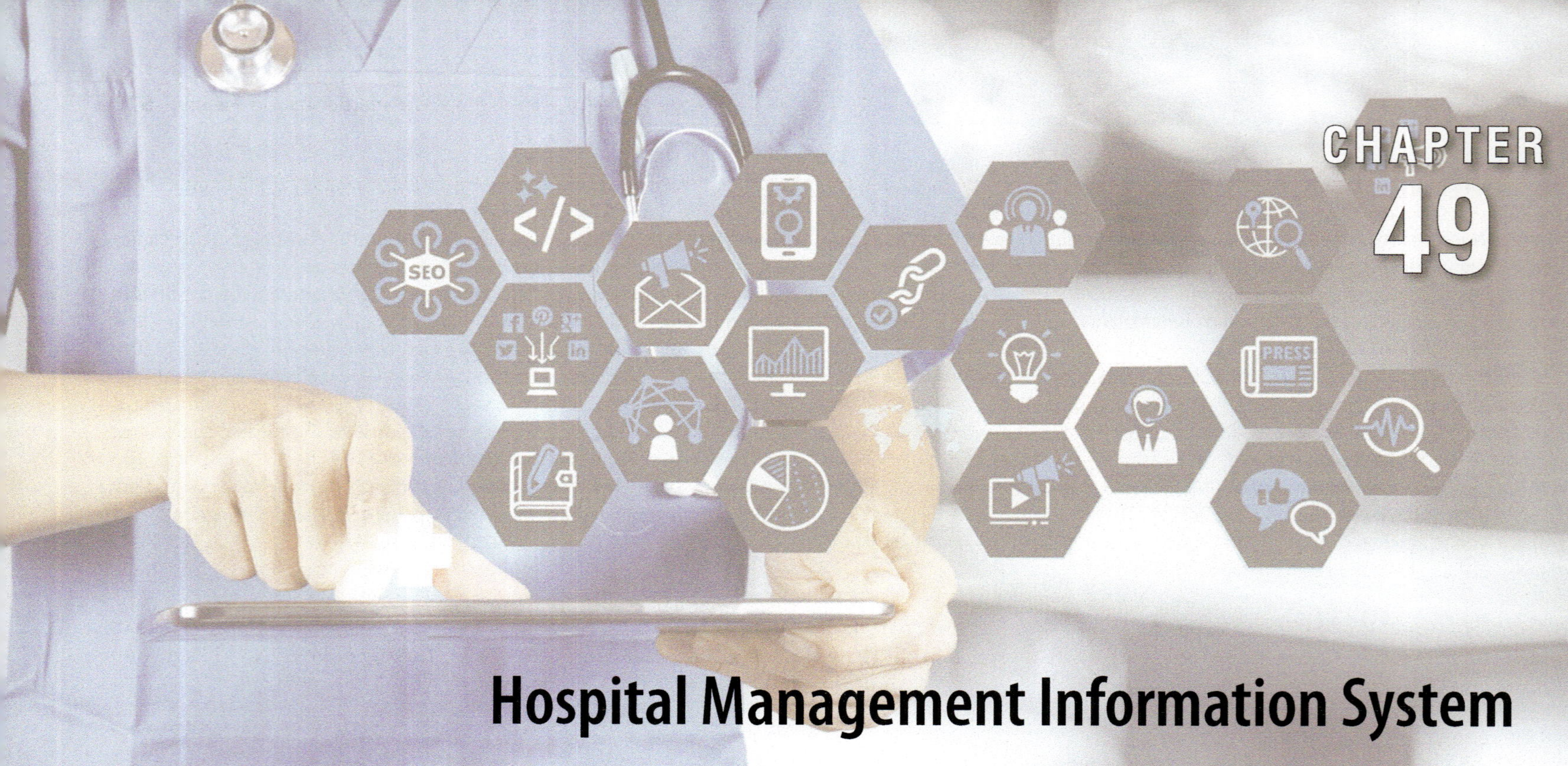

Hospital Management Information System

Vijay Kumar Tadia, Shrish Kumar, Shakti Kumar Gupta, Sunil Kant, R Chandrashekhar

"For years health care has missed out on the huge benefits that information technology has bestowed upon the rest of the economy"[1]

—Bill Gates

The decision to invest in a technology of such magnitude as Hospital Management Information System (HMIS) is an arduous task for the management of the hospital and it has substantial financial implications. What makes the things complicated is the fact that such a technology is not that popular in India. The perceived notions of high cost and inertia of staff towards adoption of a new technology further complicates the already uncertain environment. Despite of the so many advantages of the use of information technology, still many healthcare organizations think twice before investing in such a technology.

The HMIS forms an important part of modern hospital-based care. Information and communication technology (ICT) makes health systems function efficiently and effectively. In healthcare, data is critical and deploying technology facilitates the usage of data. Apart from improving the ability to collect, store, and analyze health data across the organization, this also helps the patients in a long run, whenever they access the hospital. Health management information systems interfaces technology with the existing combination of people and procedures that make up the management of a healthcare system. Regular information systems do not provide intelligent data but HMIS does. It helps people involved in the process analyze information and produce meaningful results. HMIS represents the IT infrastructure—the hardware and software. It helps streamline the functioning of the hospital by automating processes and aiding proper management of data. All activities, from registration of the patient to preparation of discharge summary, including online entry of diagnosis and prescription by the doctor in the examination room, maintenance of drug inventory in pharmacy, stores, maintenance of linen accounts, laundry, diet, laboratory services, etc., are managed through the HMIS. The HMIS are distinct from regular information systems in that HMIS is used to analyze other information systems applied in operational activities in the organization and this term is commonly used to refer to the group of information management methods tied to the automation or support of human decision making, e.g. decision support systems, research tools and executive information systems.[2]

DEFINITION(S)

The HMIS has been understood and described in a number way. It is also known as the information system, the information and decision system, the computer-based information system. The HMIS has more than one definition, some of which are given below:[3]

- The HMIS is defined as a system which provides information support for decision making in the hospital setup.
- The HMIS is defined as an integrated system of healthcare seeker, healthcare provider and integrated computer technology for providing the information to support the operations, the management and the decision making function in the healthcare institution.
- The HMIS is defined as a system based on the database of the organization evolved for the purpose of providing information to the people in the hospital.[4]
- The HMIS is defi ned as a computer-based information system.

The physical view of the HMIS can be seen as assembly of several subsystems based on the databases in the organization. These subsystems range from data collection, transaction processing and validating, processing, analyzing and storing the information in databases. The subsystem could be at a functional level or a corporate level. The information is evolved through them for a functional or a department management and it provides the information for the management of business at the corporate level. The HMIS is a product of a multi-disciplinary approach to the business management. It is a product which needs to be kept under a constant review and modification to meet the corporate needs of the information.

The HMIS is for the people in the organization. The HMIS model may be the same but it differs greatly in the contents. The HMIS, therefore, is a dynamic concept subject to change, time and again, with a change in the business management process. It continuously interacts with the internal and the external environment of the business and provides a corrective mechanism in the system so that the change needs of information are dealt with effectively. The HMIS, therefore, is a dynamic design the primary objective of which is to the information the information for decision making and it is developed considering the organizational fabric, giving due regard to the people in the organizational the management functions and the managerial and the managerial control. The HMIS model of the organization changes over a time as the business passes through several phases of developmental growth cycle. It supports the management of the business in each phase by giving the information which is crucial in that phase.

Benefits of HMIS[5]

- It helps in maintaining a totally secured database of patients and business information. This information is readily available.
- It helps in improved healthcare delivery by providing medical personnel with better data access, faster data retrieval, higher quality data and more versatility in data display.
- It helps in improving efficiency, both on the cost and the clinical care perspective. This is achieved by avoiding duplications, repetitions, delays, missing records and confusions.
- It helps to force orderliness and standardization of the patient records and procedures in the healthcare facilities and increasing accuracy and completeness of medical records of patient.
- It helps in gathering information to meet management challenges.

PLANNING AND DESIGN CONSIDERATIONS

- *Location and layout:* Location of IT department can be in administrative section depending on the strength of bed size of hospital. the size of IT department and in addition to the server or data storage unit. It needs to take into account computers desk facility that needs to be provided and a server room with sufficient temperature control for heat emission due to continuous working of server. The area required can vary in accordance with the number of master computers and the space that server room occupies.
- *Internal facility:* Facilities like telephone, fax and software's like virtual private network (VPN).
- *Hardware and software:* Giving due regard to the technical and operational feasibility, the economics of investment is worked out. Then the plan of procurement is made after selecting the hardware and software. One can take the phased approach of investment starting from the lower configuration of hardware going over to higher as development takes place. The process is to match the technical decision with the financial decision. The system development schedule is linked with the information requirement which in turn, is linked with the goals and objectives of the organization. The selection of the architecture, the approach to the information system development and the choice of hardware and software are the strategic decision in the design and development of the HMIS in the organization. The organizations which do not care to take proper decisions in these areas suffer from over-investment, under-utilization and are not able to meet the critical information requirement.

It is important to note the following points:

- The organization's strategic plan should be the basis for the MIS strategic plan.
- The information system development schedule should match with the implementation schedule of the business plan.
- The choice of information technology is a strategic business decision and not a financial decision.

Having narrowed down the hardware configurations to two or three options, the technical evaluation considers the performance-related issues such as reliability, dependability, performance on the volume scale, security, integrity and autonomy, etc. All the options may not equally satisfy the evaluation standards set by the organization on these factors. The performance-related issues will help fine tune the configuration details such as the memory, the number of ports, the specific input and output devices and the hardware infrastructure. Technical evaluation also helps to break down the hardware on a time scale, i.e. the minimum required in the initial stage and subsequent add-ons, expansions and upgrades on a time scale. The information technology is constantly under development and the scale on which such improvement takes place is phenomenal. Hence, it is necessary to select the latest technology in all areas of information processing. The investment is protected, if the Information Technology choice is scalable, upgradeable and also expandable with the growth of the business. Technical evaluation and the information technology approach should confirm to the information processing needs of the organization. The issues like the centralized versus distributed, the online versus the batch versus the real time, the network versus the mini or the superman are also evaluated. Technical evaluation also helps in narrowing down the hardware choices as all the vendors may not satisfy the requirement of the organization.

Budget: Budget allocation for complete system including hardware, software and implementation cost.

ORGANIZATIONAL STRUCTURE

Head of IT/Chief Engineer of IT is responsible to the Chief Executive Officer of hospital and IT experts under him (See Flowchart 1).

Steps in the Process of an In-house HMIS Development

Forming a project team: The project envisaged should have a project team that would look after the goal of networking. The team that was prepared included:

- Project coordinator
- Project leader
- Project team.

Project coordinator: A senior member from the hospital administrative hierarchy has to be entrusted with this task. His/her functions include:

- Drawing a clearly laid plan for the computerization with deadlines.

Flowchart 1: Organizational structure.

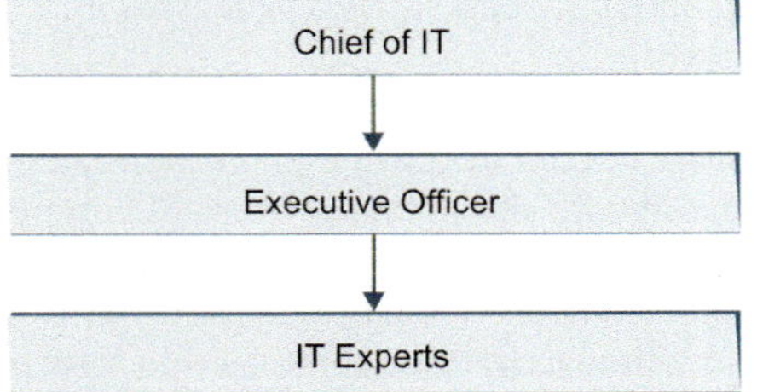

- Supervising and reviewing the progress made by the team.
- Making sure that resources are available for the project at all the times.

Project leader: He is usually the member of the computer department. The functions of the leader are same as the coordinator, but he remains in close proximity to the team than the latter. He/she provides constant guidance in terms of scheduled targets and internal review of the work done.

Project team: This included the following people:
- Programmers
- Maintenance engineers
- Data entry people
- Representatives from each department in the hospital.

Their role is to plan the activities within the overall plans of the project. They serve as the link between the users and the IT consultant.

Collection of the user requirement specification (URS): This is the first step in the process of computerization. The URS are also known as the system requirements specification (SRS). Each department involved in the computerization process is given a URS questionnaire for the inputs. The contents of URS include:
- Data flow diagrams with brief description covering activities, sub-activities, linkages, input, and output in a schematic form giving interfaces and interlinkages with other systems.
- Coding structure and logics giving the structure of each and every element that needed to be coded in the system.
- Input/Screen formats covering
  - Functional description
  - Screen level information giving description of each and every field.
  - Field level checks and controls
  - Authorization and security checks for each of the forms.
  - Modification/hold/updating routine.
- Reports, the reporting frequency, contents of the reports, compilation logic, users of the report, input-output linkages.

This URS report from the blueprint of the final hardware and software configurations that are purchased later.

Preparation of a system design document (SDD): The step after URS preparation is to make a detailed and technical SDD. This process is mainly carried out by the specialists from the computer facility of the hospital, and the expert from IT consultancy involved in the project.

Data that is collected from the URS is analyzed and then put to use. The following are the issues tackled in the SDD:
- Screens with edit checks, attribute sheets, method of accepting data and its storage.
- Report formats with process sheets for their mode of retrieval
- Database file structures
- Data flow diagrams
- Processes and their logic
- Inter-relationship between various processes
- Security features
- Recovery procedures of backups.

With the blueprint of URS and the SDD in hand, the management decides to go ahead with the actual process of computerization and HMIS development. The HMIS is made secure by passwords for authorization, data is saved on magnetic drives, electronic trail system helps to pinpoint where a particular transaction took place. The main server room is well protected against fire hazard and unauthorized access is not possible to that area.

Enterprise Solution Architecture

Flowchart 2 is depicted the enterprise solution architecture.

Solution Mapping for Healthcare Processes and Activities for Hospital Management Information System

Role of Masters

- Entities
- Process policies—controls the flow of the system
- Activity policies—controls what users can do within a screen.

One-point Ownership for a Master

- Corporate level—things that are common across the enterprise.
- Line of business level—things that are common within a line of business.
- Unit level—things that can be controlled by the unit head.

Impact

- If a master is controlled by the corporate or line of business, if a unit wants a new master record or wants a change in the existing master, they have to approach the corporate or line of business.
- Workflows across units and line of business—if there is a workflow across two centers, the relevant masters have to be common.
- Consolidation of data will be limited by the level at which a master is
- Standardization across the enterprise.

Decision Making Process

The salient features are:
- Does it impact consolidation?
- Does it impact workflow?
- How frequently new or edit is required?
- Is it practical for the corporate or line of business head to maintain the master?
- Are there geographical differences?
- Are people moving across units/line of business—in which case, such people have to be common?
- Common customers/suppliers impacting invoicing, collections and payments.
- Who will create and who will approve?

Systems and Modules in HMIS

System and Modules

Systems in HMIS are as follows:
- *Patient management system:* That takes care of patient registration, appointment scheduling, admission discharge transfer, patient relations, etc.
- *Wards management system:* That takes care of wards, nursing staff, bed management, etc.
- *Space management system:* That takes care of the OP rooms; consult rooms and operations theaters, etc.
- *Resource management system:* That takes care of all staff deployment, right from the staff to the nurses and doctors.
- Clinical records management system
- Laboratory information system
- Radiology information system
- Pharmacy management system
- Housekeeping/laundry management system
- Equipment maintenance system (EMS)

Flowchart 2: Enterprise solution architecture.

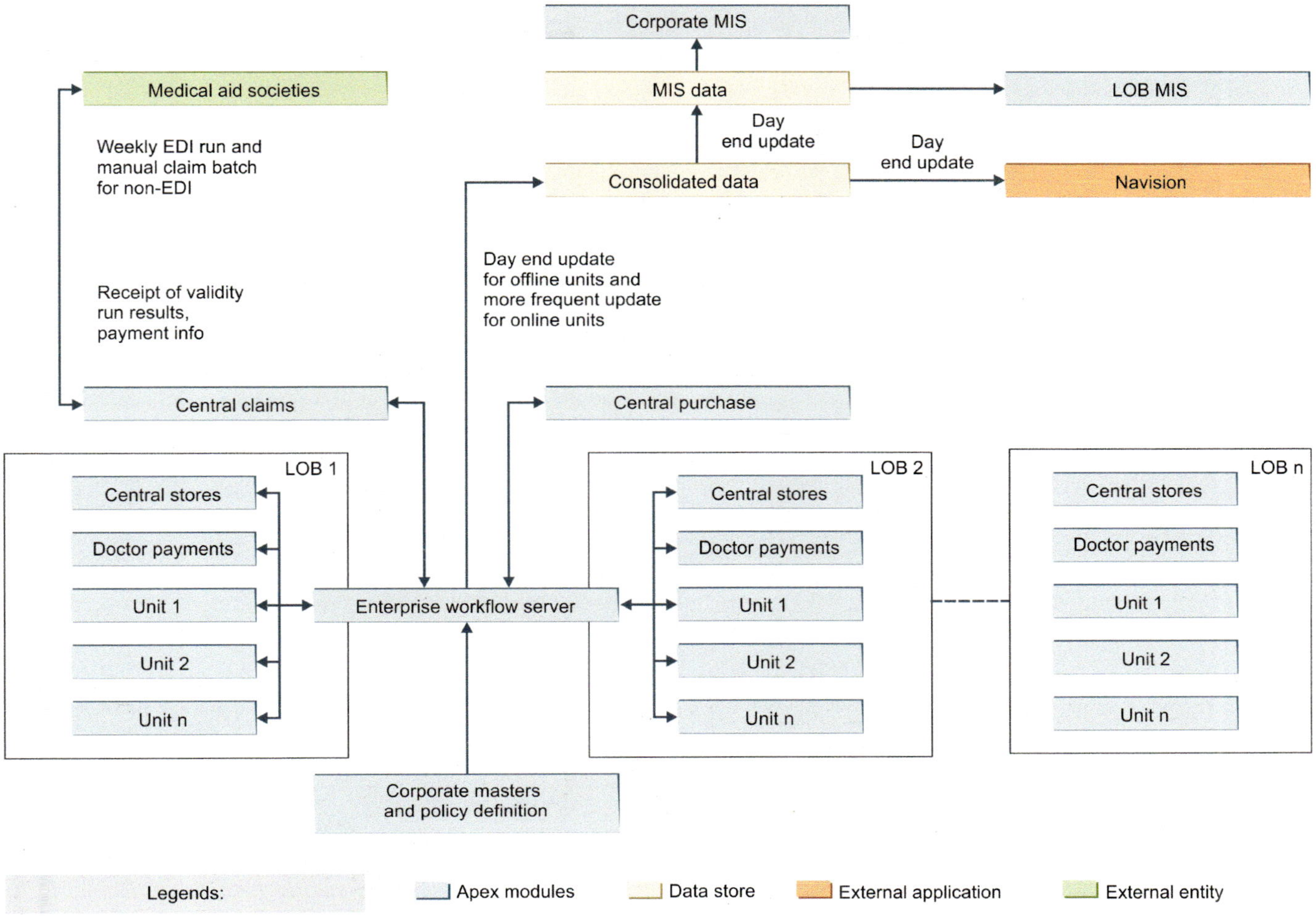

Corporate MIS
MIS data
LOB MIS
Medical aid societies
Day end update
Day end update
Consolidated data
Navision
Weekly EDI run and manual claim batch for non-EDI
Receipt of validity run results, payment info
Day end update for offline units and more frequent update for online units
Central claims
Central purchase
LOB 1
Central stores
Doctor payments
Unit 1
Unit 2
Unit n
Enterprise workflow server
LOB 2
Central stores
Doctor payments
Unit 1
Unit 2
Unit n
LOB n
Central stores
Doctor payments
Unit 1
Unit 2
Unit n
Corporate masters and policy definition
Legends: Apex modules; Data store; External application; External entity

(LOB: line of business)

- Financial accounting and billing system
- Insurance and contracts management
- Hospital administration
- Roster management.

Modules in the system of HMIS are as follows:

- Master patient index (MPI)
- Admission, discharge, transfer (ADT)
- Emergency
- Outpatient clinics (all specialties)
- Reservation (appointment)
- Medical record
- Pharmacy and drug stores
- Laboratory information system (LIS)
- Clinical pathology
- Radiology information system (RIS)
- Radiotherapy (nuclear medicine)
- Operation theaters
- Order management
- Nursing station
- ICU
- Blood bank
- Price list
- Service packages
- Medical insurance account
- Patient billing
- Cashier
- Account payable and receivable
- Dietary service
- Physician account
- Purchasing
- Inventory management
- General ledger
- Fixed assist
- Human resources
- Payroll
- Governmental insurance.

The HMIS addresses the entire administrative, financial and medical functional areas of modern multispeciality hospital. The package enables improved patient care, patient safety, increase service quality and efficiency and reduced costs. It provides easy access to critical information, thereby enabling management to make better medical and financial decisions on time. It provides the benefits of streamlining operations, enhanced administration and control, improved response, cost control and improved profitability.

Overview of HMIS Modules

Figure 1 is depicted the overview of HMIS modules.

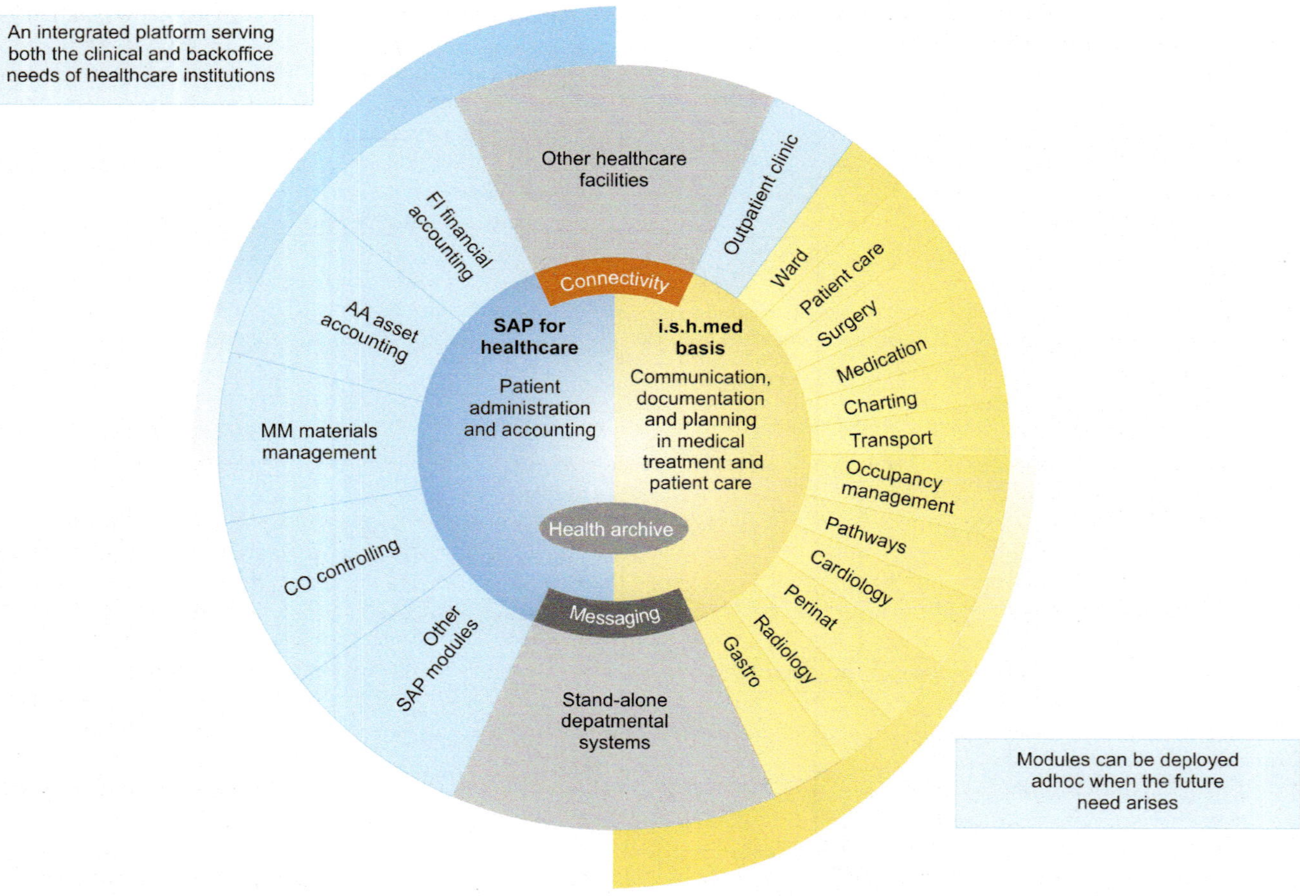

Fig. 1: Overview of HMIS modules.

MODULES IN HMIS

Module 1: Outpatient Department

OPD Management System

Login form for authorization:

- Before the form is filled for registration, the staff has to login into system.
- Patients registration form.
- Prescription to the patient (IPD/OPD).

Objectives of OPD Management System[6,7]

- Increase customer satisfaction by providing high quality reports and prescriptions as quickly as possible.
- Increase cash flow thus helping business grow by integrating the electronic medical record and billing with the clinical so that the patient treatment cycle gets completed faster and more patients can be treated in less time.
- The OPD management system allows defining each user's level of access to the system
- The audit trail log tracks all entries into the system including the information entered, a timestamp, and the employee code of the person making the entry.
- Daily backups of the database are taken.
- Highly secured, user friendly, reliable and seamlessly integrated web-based information system.
- Clinic practitioners, pharmacists and pathologists can share the patient's clinical information providing better service to their consumers.
- It automates the process of collecting and retrieving patient information.
- Integration of patient identification, data consistency, and transparency.
- Access to dozens of online resources and tools to customize and build your own systems.

Module 2: IPD Module

This function, patient IPD admission, facilitates the process of patient admission and the allocation of beds to patients. The system identifies the patient as either a new IPD patient, or an intern referred from hospital OPD/CMO. This function gives information on vacant beds in a hospital. Occupancy status on that particular position can be ascertained while allocating the bed. The main function, patient admission, facilitates the admission of patients according to requirements, considering the type of admission and the patient's condition. The admission of a patient can be direct, or be a referral from a consultant or hospital. The category of the patient can be company, self, government schemes, insurance or MLC, depending on which the admission procedure is completed. Once the patient is admitted to the hospital, the room charge starts from the time of admission. The case paper of the patient is printed from the system and is sent to the proper nursing station. Once the admission of the patient is completed, an IPD identification number is created by the system for that particular admission of the patient. The IPD admit card is also printed along with the case paper. The system informs, with audio-visual alerts, the respective nursing station of the admission of the patient under them, allowing them to prepare room for the patient. In the case of MLC, the system stores the details of the police station, as well as the name of the official informed about the medical legal case.[8]

Patient Transfer

This function of the hospital management system is to facilitate the transfer of a patient from one room to another within the hospital. With this function, the patient's actual position can be updated online so that internal functions such as billing, investigation and surgery can be planned. The position of the patient is very important since charges for surgery procedures and investigations are related to room category.[8]

Inpatient Department Investigation Cases

This module of the hospital management system deals with all kinds of investigations suggested by doctors. The function enables the entry of investigations/procedures for a particular patient. The entered investigations are rooted through the billing/cash office and once the patient pays for the investigations, the entries of the same go to their respective diagnostics centers. This flow is not compulsory for IPD patients since the billing for IPD patients is done at the time of discharge. Investigation requisition is created and printed with function and the same is available at respective diagnostics centers for the preparation of reports.[8]

Diagnostic Centers

This module enables the retrieval of the patient's investigation and procedure record from different locations, i.e. IPD, OPD, casualty. The module covers a laboratory system for pathology, radiology, cardiology, neurology, and chest medicine. Prescriptions written by doctors are routed through a billing system to the respective diagnostic centers.[8]

Deposits, Advances, Refunds, Discounts and Concessions

This function of the hospital management system facilitates all types of payments received from the patient. This function plays a vital role in payment recovery from patients throughout their stay.[8]

The advances from the patient depend on the type of admission and the patient category is prompted by the system. The interim bill versus advances ratio is also maintained in order to carry out recovery planning.[8] Advances and deposits accepted by the billing/cash counter are directly posted into accounts. Refund cases are considered when excess advances have been paid. The accounts official authorizes this transaction, after which a refund is processed. In the case of company category patients, the ratio analysis between the interim bill and the amount stated in the authority letter from the company is compared for further action. If a patient is to be given a discount, then the amount is authorized and the discount is processed. The discount categories are flexible and can be changed by the administrator.[8]

Reports

Following are the main reports/outputs:[8]

- *Patient list—admitted/discharged:* This report gives information on admitted/discharged patients during a certain time period. This facilitates keeping track of the admissions versus discharges ratio.
- *Bed occupancy reports:* This report gives information on bed occupancy at any given time room category-wise.
- *Ward allocation reports:* This report gives allocated room reports for tracking of patients.
- *Interim bill versus advance report:* This report gives the ratio of interim bill vs. advances paid by the patient with the percentage of payment.
- *Admission/discharge register:* The admission and discharge register is maintained by the system. This report gives details regarding patient admissions and discharges during specific period.
- *Patients/by doctor:* This report categorizes patients by attending physician at any point of time.
- *Appointment list:* The appointments for consultants are maintained on the system.
- Performed operation list.
- Patient follow-up report.
- Prescriptions discharge card

Module 3: Operation Theater

Surgery (Flowcharts 3 to 6)

The process from ordering till post-surgery documentation is shown in the following Figure 5. This document focuses only on the scheduling process.

When a doctor orders a surgery for a patient, a clinical order (service request) needs to be created in the system for an existing patient. Along with the clinical order for surgery, a clinical order for a preanesthesia check-up (PAC) is created if required along with this if blood bag if required blood bag or component is reserved.

The doctor will have access to the planning grid for direct scheduling of the surgeries. The operating theatre (OT) manager continuously have to check if the ordered surgeries can be performed and update the OT plan.

Additional services can be ordered and scheduled within the same clinical order.

After the doctor has created the clinical order for the surgery the patient or a relative has to appear at the patient relations department (PRD) in order to confirm the OT-booking and pay a deposit within 24 hours. When the surgery appointment is settled the OT-booking gets confirmed by PRD. If the patient is not able to confirm the OT-booking or is not able to pay for it, the OT-booking will be cancelled or rescheduled by the PRD and the doctor gets informed.

The OT-manager handles the final OT scheduling, which is happening in two levels. Three days before the surgery, the OT manager has to finalize the OT plan which will be released after the latest update 1 day before the surgeries will take place. In case the surgery needs to be rescheduled, the OT-manager handles the rescheduling of the surgery appointment. Rescheduled surgery appointments appear in a list in the PRD for further processing.

Surgery Complications (Fig. 2)

Surgery Documentation

For the surgery documentation, the following forms of the documentation will be performed:

- Presurgery documentation
- Postsurgery documentation

The presurgery documentation is a bunch of tasks that have to be performed. In order to have an overview of the tasks and the status of the tasks, a situation for the presurgery documentation will be provided. The situation has to be assigned to the surgery manually. This can be done easily by using the surgery view of the clinical workstation (CWS).

The postsurgery documentation includes and ends with the documentation of the patient in the recovery room. The postsurgery documentation is not including the documentation of the patients on the ward or ICU. In order to support the documentation, process the function of a situation will be used. By using a situation predefined steps will guide the user. The different CWS will show the status of the

Flowchart 3: Surgery process: overview.

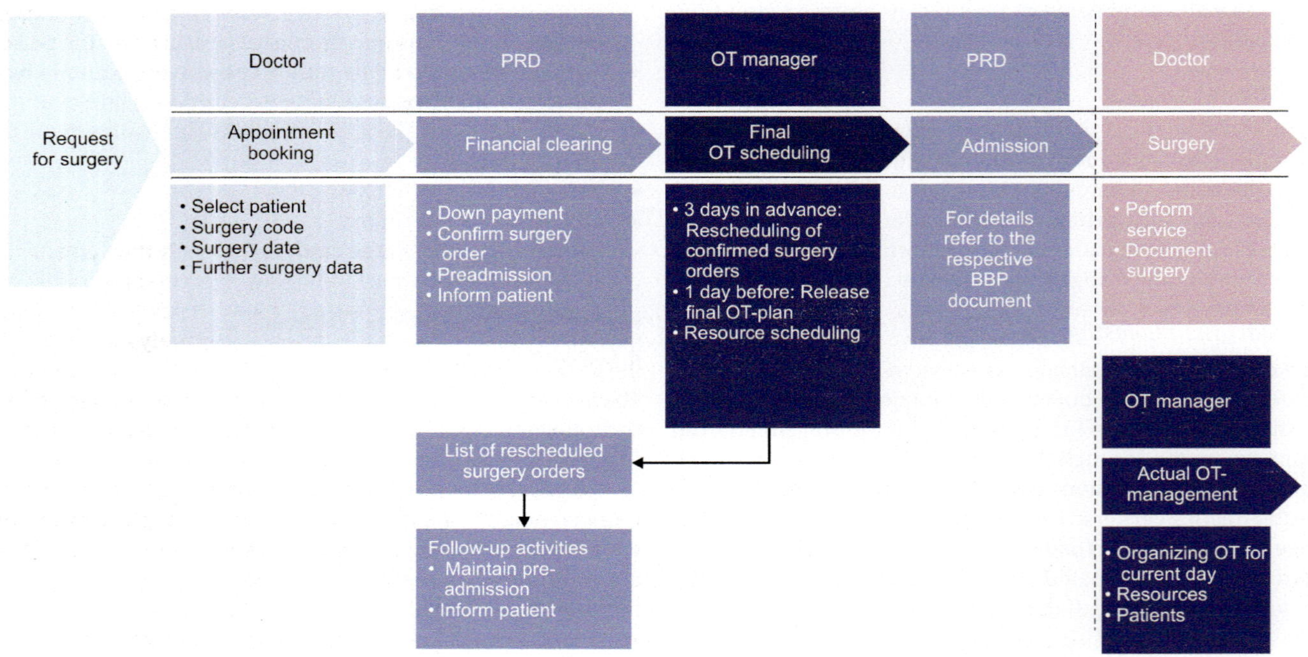

Flowchart 4: Surgery process: financial clearing.

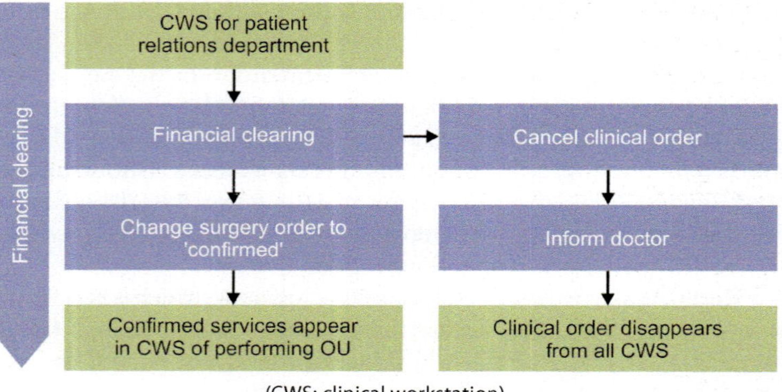

(CWS: clinical workstation)

Flowchart 5: Surgery process: final surgery scheduling.

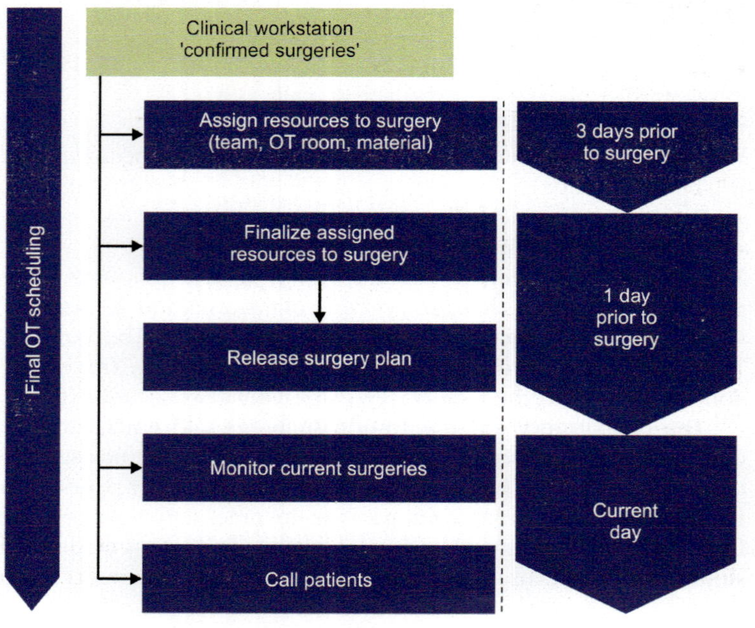

Flowchart 6: Surgery service order.

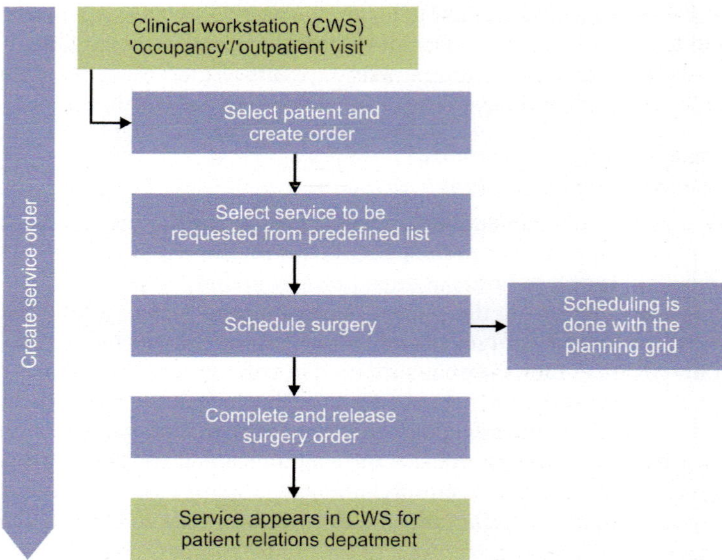

documentation and further details of the patient and surgery. Further on it gives access to all required functions related to the surgery.

Module 4: Laboratory Information System

Everybody wants quicker and accurate laboratory investigations today, thus faster reporting makes your laboratory ahead of others. There are no delays of billing cycles so you receive money faster from your collection centers than anybody else. All types of pathology and radiology reporting are possible. Works on intranet (access within the hospital) as well as internet, which works consist of unlimited LAN terminals license, it's a complete package for making hi-tech automated pathology laboratory. LIS is capable to send report to collection center via internet; It consists of electronic signature and report delivery at doorstep anywhere in the world using internet. It has got SMS sending facility. Report can

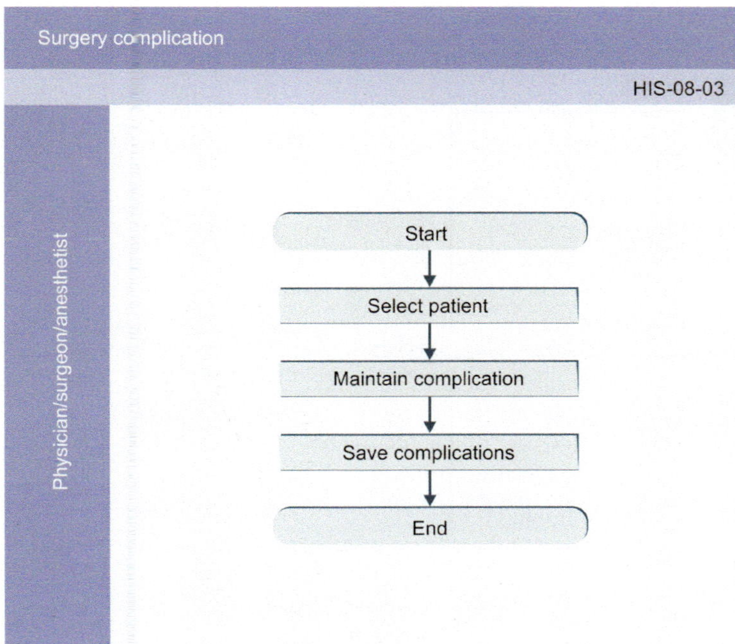

Fig. 2: Surgery complications.

be delivered directly to patient's doorstep using internet. Specimens are accepted by barcodes. It has got barcode scanning and printing facilities. AMC services includes—Online hosting of software, high speed data center as well as maintaining the server, Hospital need not worry about software crashing, database backup, etc.[6]

Web-based Laboratory Information System Flowchart[7]

Flowchart 7 is depicted the web-based LIS Flowchart.

Detailed Work Flow

- *Pathology laboratory on-line requisition entry:* The collection center/ referring doctor fills out an on-line requisition form and sends the barcoded specimen (s) vials to the pathology laboratory.[7]
- *Sample:* When the specimens vials arrive at the lab, the barcoded vials are scanned, samples are accepted or rejected for a specific reason.
- *Demographics:* All other patient demographics are acquired through the patient registration or unique identification number.
- *Pathology laboratory starts case/accession:* Upon receipt of the specimen from the collection center/ referring doctor or individual patient, a unique sample identification number is allocated to the specimen. The technician will then process the specimens and prepare them for review by the pathologist. LIS has a "Work Sheet" used to track the status of each specimen.[7]
- *Clinical work, transcription and sign out report:* Once the samples are tested, the clinical work can be performed. The technician enters the results and completes the report, uploads images and any relevant document (i.e. clinical, insurance details, etc.).[7]
- *Post sign out report:* Upon completion of the technicians work, the pathologist reviews the report and signout the report from any location whether it is another laboratory, a hospital, home, etc.[7]
- *Report is authorized and ready for delivery:* Once the case has been finished and the doctor has signed out (authorized) the report, it is ready for the printing. LIS generates automatically HTML/PDF format of the report. The report is ready and can be emailed, faxed to the referring physician, or the physician may log into LIS to view the report online. The entire reporting process is done electronically, automatically, and instantly. Report delivery is made electronically. There are no couriers or shipping companies involved.[7]

Development of an In-house Diagnostic Information System

The diagnostic information system (DIS) is the central stage where crucial investigations are carried out on patients and is a vital component of any hospital. The logistic requirements in terms of equipment and manpower are demanding. The need of timely information regarding diagnostic results, availability of equipment and consumables cannot be over emphasized. All the laboratories are connected to the hospital wide network, which enables the sharing of data and images with the rest of the hospital. Facilities are being provided to record and project investigations for live display in the hospital auditoria. Research is an integral part of the culture at both the hospitals. It is imperative that clinicians should be able to retrieve patient care details swiftly and accurately.

Product overview: The overview of the DIS is as follows:
Aims and objectives of the system:
- Raising the requisition from any terminal in the hospital.
- Documentation for the requisition
- Generation of memo for billing
- Collection of samples
- Receiving of the samples in the departments
- Testing the samples in the respective departments
- Recording the preliminary and finalized reports
- Integration with the electronic medical record and discharge summary
- Integration with the hospital tumor registry.

Modules of the product: The following modules are covered in the product:
- Requisition
- Generating a memo
- Appointments
- Sample collection
- Department receiving center
- Examination signal
- Reporting
- Requisition status
- MIS queries.

Overview of the Modules of the Product

- Requisition
- Generating a memo
- Appointments
- Sample collection
- Department receiving center
- Reporting
- Requisition status
- MIS queries.

Requisition

Requisition for a particular test for a patient is raised on the advice of the concerned doctor. Each requisition is attached to a unique requisition

Flowchart 7: Web-based laboratory information system flowchart.

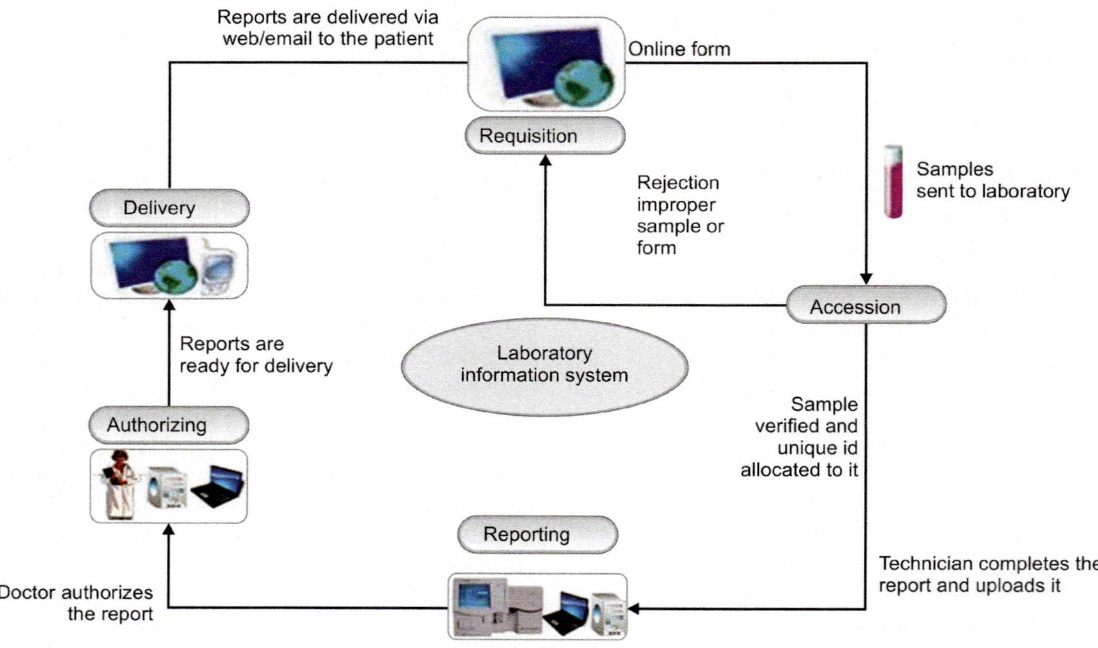

number. The requisition number indicates the department and modality in which the test will be conducted, the year in which the requisition is being generated and the serial number of the test in that year. Also, a pathology number (Path number) is generated for all the pathology tests that are requested.

One requisition number may be used for conducting more than one examination in a department for microbiology and biochemistry requisitions.

Memo Generation

Memos are generated for all the raised requisitions. The memos indicate the amount to be paid to the hospital for each service requested. The outpatient memos are generated for outpatients and can be paid individually. The inpatient memos are generated for admitted patients and are included in final or interim bill.

Appointments

Appointments are issued for each requisition raised for the patient. The date, time, location and the instructions are specified for each service specified in the requisition.

Sample Collections

In sample collection center, technician collect the samples and send to the respective departments. The collection center in which the sample is collected, the department and modality to which the sample will be sent, and the case number of the patient whose sample is collected are noted down.

In sample collection center, all the requisitions whose memos are paid are displayed. As and when the sample is collected, the corresponding requisition is ticked by the technician.

Sample receiving center: Receives the samples and an internal number is generated. The requisition number is ticked in the receiving department.

If a biochemistry sample is collected, path number has to be entered.

Examination completion signal is generated by ticking the corresponding requisition number.

Reporting is done by the concerned doctor/pathologist. All the observations are marked and preliminary report for each examination done is written by the doctors after seeing the examination details. The examination details are available and the preliminary report is entered which is immediately available for the authorized person to finalize. The finalized reports are printed and attached to the case file.

Requisition status: The status of any requisition can be found out from anywhere in the hospital through the on-line system.

The status of all the requisitions between two given dates or the requisitions of a specific case number can be found. The status indicates the stage of the requisition, which could be appointment, memo generated, payment paid, sample collected, sample received, report written and also path number if allotted.

MIS queries: These are generated to list the details of all the patients for whom requisitions are raised between given dates, surgical pathology reports generated between given dates, NIP and referral cases, doctor wise details of the requisitions.

Flowchart of the Diagnostic Information System

Flowchart 8 is depicted the DIS.

Functional Requirements

- All the screens are designed as per the following standard architecture:
  a. *Initial panel and answer back panel:* The initial panel will be used to key in a "KEY FIELD", so that linked data/Basic can be retrieved from the database.

     Answer back panel is the panel where respective data will be displayed from related database tables on receiving the "KEY FIELD".

Flowchart 8: Diagnostic information system.

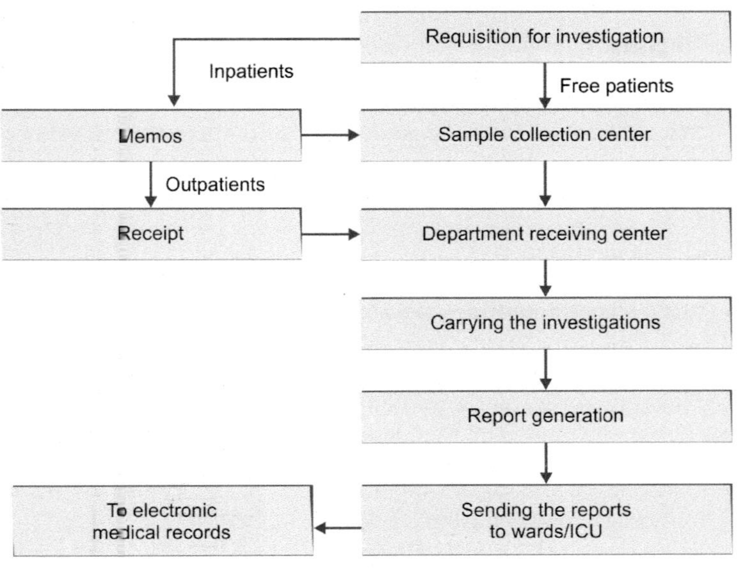

b. *Entry panel:* Entry panel is the panel in which the user will enter the information. Tool tip help should be provided when the mouse is moved to the specific field.

c. *Command panel:* Command panel is the panel where user will give the instruction for next operation. Tool tip help should be provided when the mouse is moved to the specific button.

- *Message box:* This box will display the help messages related to the field where the cursor is currently positioned. The message box will also provide messages as may be appropriate such as:
  - New record successfully added
  - New record could not be added
  - Record successfully modified
  - Record could not be modified
  - Record deleted
  - Record cannot be deleted
  - Record committed
  - Record commitment failed
  - Printing completed
  - Printing error
  - Transaction could not be saved
  - Last transaction cancelled.

Module 5: Electronic Medical Record (EMR)

- MRD is one of the most suitable department for computerization of its entire function.
- It is a computerized legal medical record in an organization like hospital.

Essential Features of EMR Software

- Easy to use
- System should not be slow
- Reliable
- Secure
- Should meet exact needs
- Operating system should be familiar
- Easily upgradable for future needs
- Should be able to integrate with other systems in hospital.

Advantages

- Space saving
- Paper less
- Faster and more efficient
- More convenient data trail
- Information is readily available at medical audits
- Automatic assignments of ICD numbers.

Disadvantages

- High implementation cost
- Privacy concerns
- Challenges in implementation
- Training to utilize system
- Security.

Analysis of Medical Records

- Daily average OP attendance
- Daily indoor admissions
- Daily deaths
- Bed-turnover
- Average length of stay
- Number of surgeries done
- Demography of patients
- Confinements
- Investigations
- Autopsies
- Daily bulletins
- Morbidity statistics
- Mortality statistics
- Seasonal and annual prevalence of disease
- Epidemiologic patterns: Statistics of end-results
- Administrative data
- Monthly bulletins
- Annual reports
- Various statements to the media.

Statistical Bulletin

Generated from MR of the month under review, with comparative data from last month and corresponding month of last year.

- Bed occupancy rate
- Total number of patient admitted
- Average length of stay
- Bed turnover rate
- Mortality data
- Total number of patient discharged: Daily census of patient
- Total IP service days in the month: Demography of patient
- Performance statistics
- Confinements/abortions
- Surgeries performed
- Investigations: laboratory, radiology, ECG, etc.
- Specialized procedures, e.g. USG, endoscopy
- Family welfare statistics
- National health programs performance statistics.

Module 6: Pharmacy Management System

Pharmacy management system offers a modular integrated solution for their information needs.

Importance of Pharmacy Management System

Sale of drugs, cash management and management of stocks of drugs and medical accessories at an optimum level at any point of time is the key focus in any pharmacy/medical store, system addresses these aspects very carefully. It caters to both independent pharmacies as well as pharmacies in a hospital. The system takes care of effective management of fast/slow moving items, drugs with expiry dates in near future are taken care of by the system. Reports and queries related to Brand-wise, profit margin-wise, sales cycle-wise analysis of revenues generated from drugs form the highlight of the product.[6]

- During the peak time, i.e. at rush hours all the PCs (Personal Computers) can be operated for sales. This will help in serving a customer in quick time and will also ensure that no customer goes away.
- Since every PC can perform all the operation for standard daily operation, activity can be split between the different PCs connected through LAN.
- One PC for purchase entries and creating purchase orders. The second PC can be allocated for accounts and generating daily reports such as expiry, sales, products, and customer history.

  Owner can have one independent PC with using password facility and also can have control on cash management, sales and purchases, expiry goods and daily reports.
- Thus, the LAN version helps in carrying out number of operations simultaneously from any of these machines as well as comfort for owners to operate from an independent machine to access all information/reports as per the need.

Sales[6]

- Issue and sale of drugs
- Bills/receipt generation/printing
- Comprehensive price list update facility
- Monitoring sale/issue of controlled drugs
- Comprehensive drug database
- Drug formulations
- Dosage and contraindication
- Manufacturer/Supplier details.

Inventory[6]

- Stock levels
- Purchase and inventory management
- Purchase order,
- Goods receipt note
- Invoice
- Stock updates based on receipts and issues
- Date-expired items list by batch
- Batch for withdrawal
- Stock replenishment plan
- Consumption patterns
- Stock movement report.

Accounting[6]

- Cash book
- Bank book
- Accounts receivable
- Accounts payable
- Inventory-related valuation reports for bank and balance sheet.

Queries/Report[6]

- Extensive querying/reporting on
- Revenue generated from drugs
- Brand-wise, doctor wise
- Margin-wise and volume-wise: Analysis of quantity and value of stocks: ABC and FSN analysis.

Admin[6]

- Define new user
- Add/edit/delete user
- Add/remove authorities of user.

Added Features[6]

- Elaborate sorting and search facilities.
- "Single Click" or "Hot Key" facilities for the most frequently used operations.
- Data backup and restore, login security system to ensure that only authorized to use software.
- Sales/Inventory/Drug database
- International standards extensive drug database
- Shorter learning curve for the employees
- Easy-to-use graphical user interface
- Computer-based tutorial
- Integrated and robust design.

Add on Barcode Module[6]

Especially created module for barcode printing, this module gives chemist shop the following advantages:

- Reduces the dependency of skilled manpower totally as any person can do the billing.
- The billing is done at a greater speed thus reducing the billing time substantially.
- Human error of keying wrong medicine or description gets completely eliminated and ensures the medicine is charged with the right price.
- The labeling work can be done at off-period time.
- Barcode facility becomes a critical tool for serving number of customer in peak period particularly for the pharmacies having monthly turnover in excess of 5 lacs.

Module 7: Picture Archival and Communication System

A picture archiving and communication system (PACS) is a medical imaging_technology which provides economical storage of, and convenient access to, images from multiple modalities (source machine types). Electronic images_and reports are transmitted digitally via PACS; this eliminates the need to manually file, retrieve, or transport film jackets. The universal format for PACS image storage and transfer is Digital Imaging and Communications in Medicine (DICOM). Non-image data, such as scanned documents, may be incorporated using consumer industry standard formats like Portable Document Format (PDF), once encapsulated in DICOM. A PACS consists of four major components: The imaging modalities such as X-ray computed tomography (CT) and magnetic resonance imaging (MRI), a secured network for the transmission of patient information, workstations for interpreting and reviewing images, and archives for the storage and retrieval of images and reports. Combined with available and emerging web technology, PACS has the ability to deliver timely and efficient access to images, interpretations, and related data. PACS breaks down the physical and time barriers associated with traditional film-based image retrieval, distribution and display.[9]

Uses

- *Hard copy replacement:* PACS replaces hard-copy based means of managing medical images, such as film archives. With the decreasing price of digital storage, PACSs provide a growing cost and space advantage over film archives in addition to the instant access to prior images at the same institution. Digital copies are referred to as soft-copy.
- *Remote access:* It expands on the possibilities of conventional systems by providing capabilities of off-site viewing and reporting (distance education, telediagnosis). It enables practitioners in different physical locations to access the same information simultaneously for teleradiology.
- *Electronic image integration platform:* PACS provides the electronic platform for radiology images interfacing with other medical automation systems such as HIS, EMR, Practice Management Software, and RIS.
- *Radiology workflow management:* PACS is used by radiology personnel to manage the workflow of patient exams.

Integration[9]

A full PACS should provide a single point of access for images and their associated data. That is, it should support all digital modalities, in all departments, throughout the enterprise.

In: Patient identification and orders for examination. These data are sent from HIS to RIS via integration interface, in most of hospital, via HL7 protocol. Patient ID and orders will be sent to modality (CT, MR, etc.) via DICOM protocol (Worklist). Images will be created after images scanning and then forwarded to PACS server.[10]

Diagnosis report is created based on the images retrieved for presenting from PACS.

Server by physician/radiologist and then saved to RIS system.

Out: Diagnosis report and images created accordingly. Diagnosis report is sent back to HIS via HL7 usually and images are sent back to HIS via DICOM usually if there is a DICOM viewer integrated with HIS in hospitals (In most of cases, Clinical Physician gets reminder of diagnosis report coming and then queries images from PACS server).[10]

Snapshots of Module

Snapshots of module given below will help in giving an overview, of what all information are being taken at various instances.

- Login form
- Patient entry form
- Prescription entry form
- Patient diagnosis history form
- Patient injection history form
- Patient receipt entry form
- Accumulated receipt form
- Patient receipt query form
- Gastroscopy test form
- Biochemistry test form
- Colonoscopy test form
- Blood test form
- Stool test form
- Sonography test form
- X-ray form
- Urine test form
- Test reports form
- Search by name form
- Search by date form.

Login Form

Refer Figure 3.

Patient Entry Form

Refer Figure 4.

Prescription Entry Form

Refer Figure 5.

Patient Diagnosis History Form

Refer Figure 6.

Patient Injection History Form

Refer Figure 7.

Patient Receipt Entry Form

Refer Figure 8.

Accumulated Receipt Form

Refer Figure 9.

Patient Receipt Query Form

Refer Figure 10.

Gastroscopy Test Form

Refer Figure 11.

Login Form
Enter User Name admin
Password ########
Forgot Password
Change Password

Fig. 3: Login form.

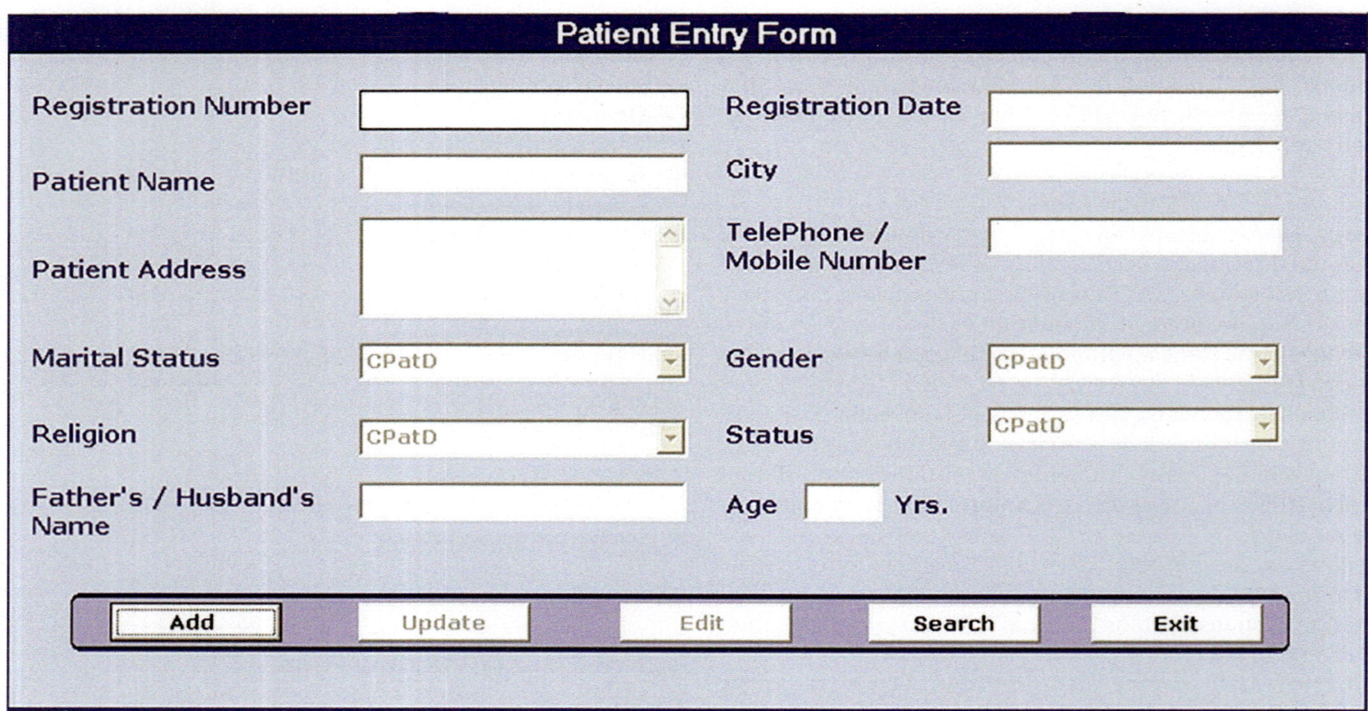

Fig. 4: Patient entry form.

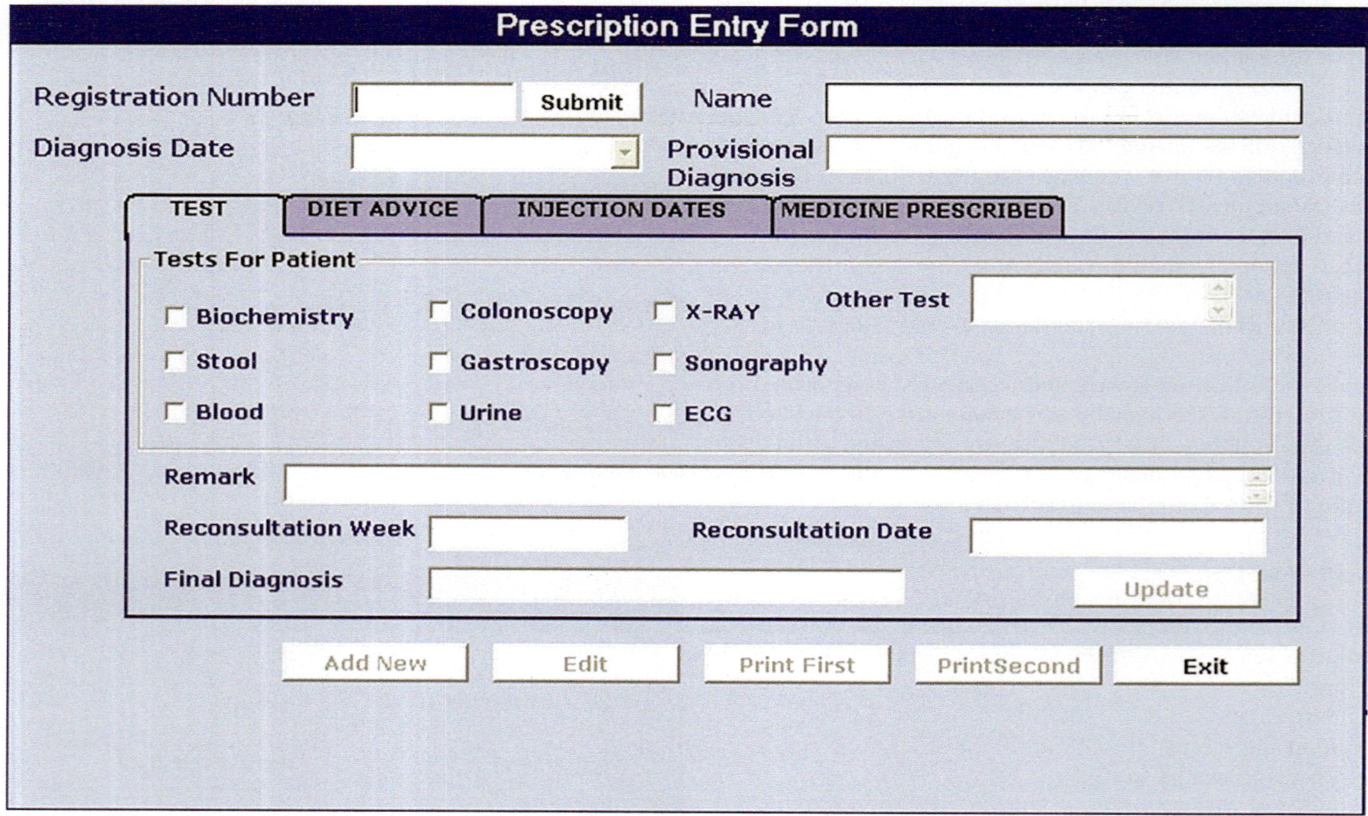

Fig. 5: Prescription entry form.

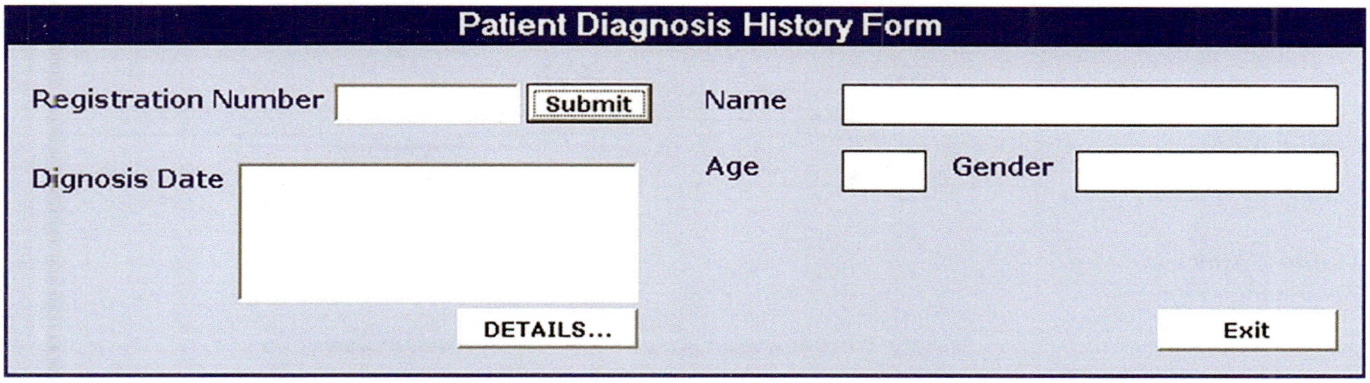

Patient Diagnosis History Form

Registration Number Submit Name

Dignosis Date Age Gender

DETAILS... Exit

Fig. 6: Patient diagnosis history form.

Patient Injection Entry

Registration Number Submit Name

Diagnosis Date Age Gender

Injection Date

Injected Address

Injection Status

Injection Date	Status

Exit

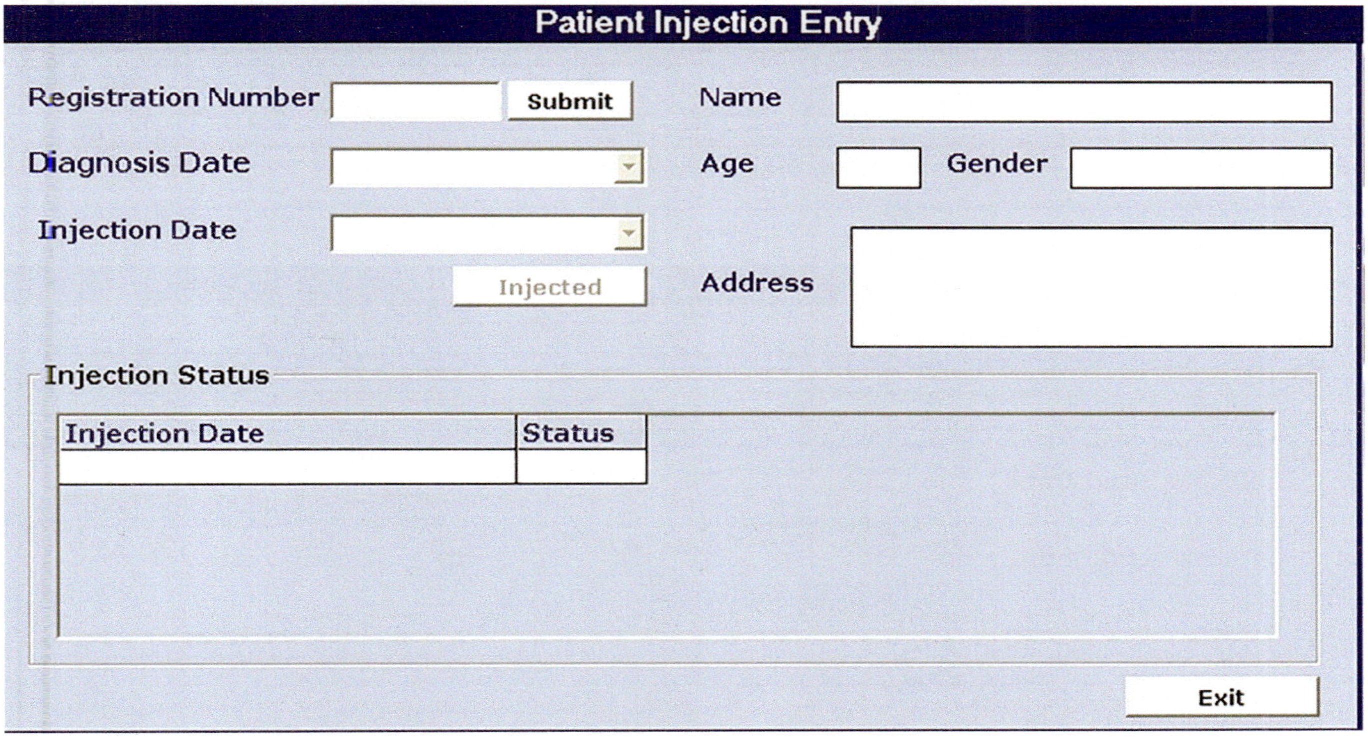

Fig. 7: Patient injection history form.

Biochemistry Test Form

Refer Figure 12.

Colonoscopy Test Form

Refer Figure 13.

Blood Test Form

Refer Figure 14.

Stool Test Form

Refer Figure 15.

Sonography Test Form

Refer Figure 16.

X-ray Form

Refer Figure 17.

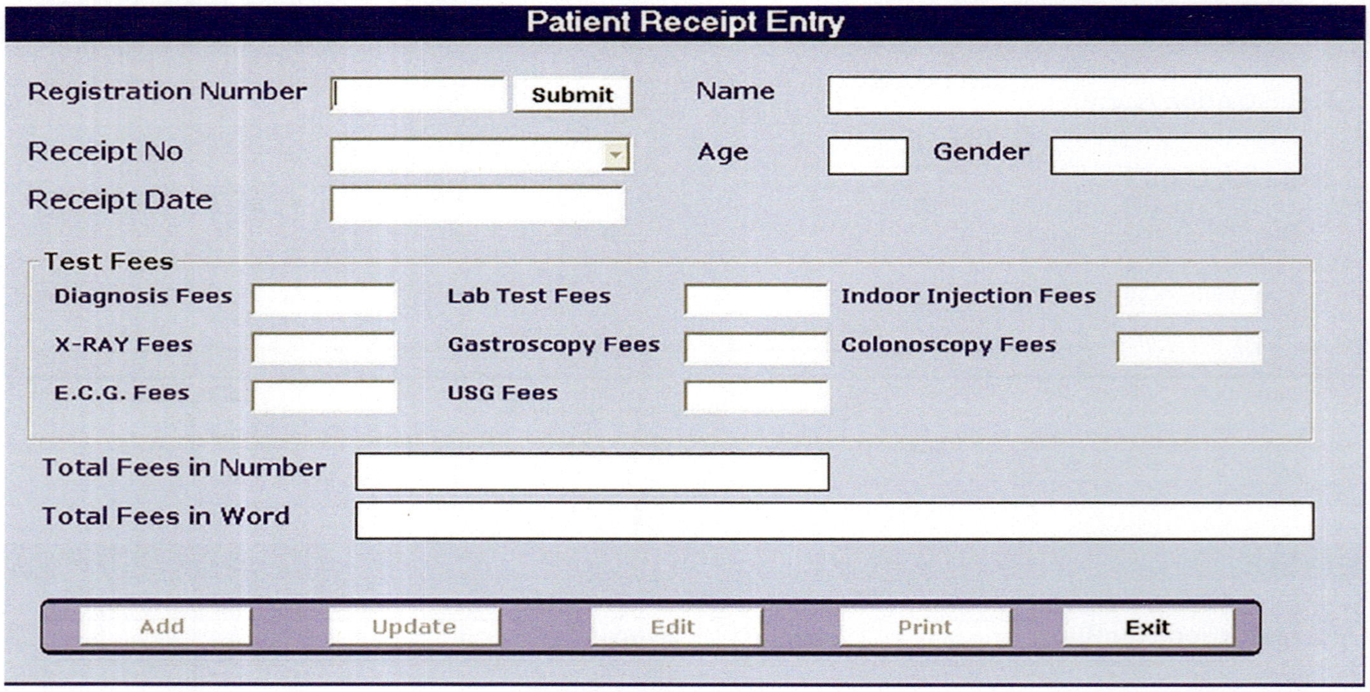

Fig. 8: Patient receipt entry form.

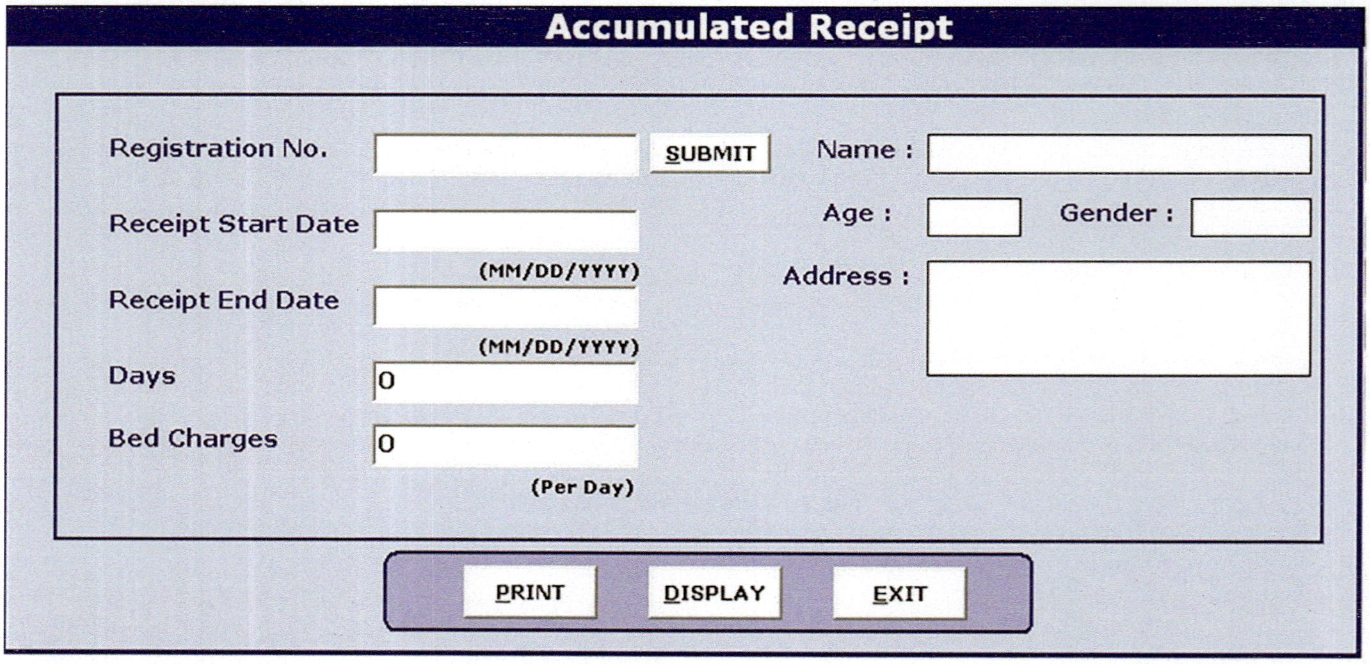

Fig. 9: Accumulated receipt form.

Urine Test Form

Refer Figure 18.

Test Reports Form

Refer Figure 19.

Search by Name Form

Refer Figure 20.

Search by Date Form

Refer Figure 21.

Patient Receipt Query

Registration Number [ ] Submit Name [ ]

Receipt Date [ ] Age [ ] Gender [ ]

Total Fees in Number [ ] Address [ ]

Dignosis Fees [ ]

Total Fees in Word [ ]

Complete Receipt Details.... Exit

Fig. 10: Patient receipt query form.

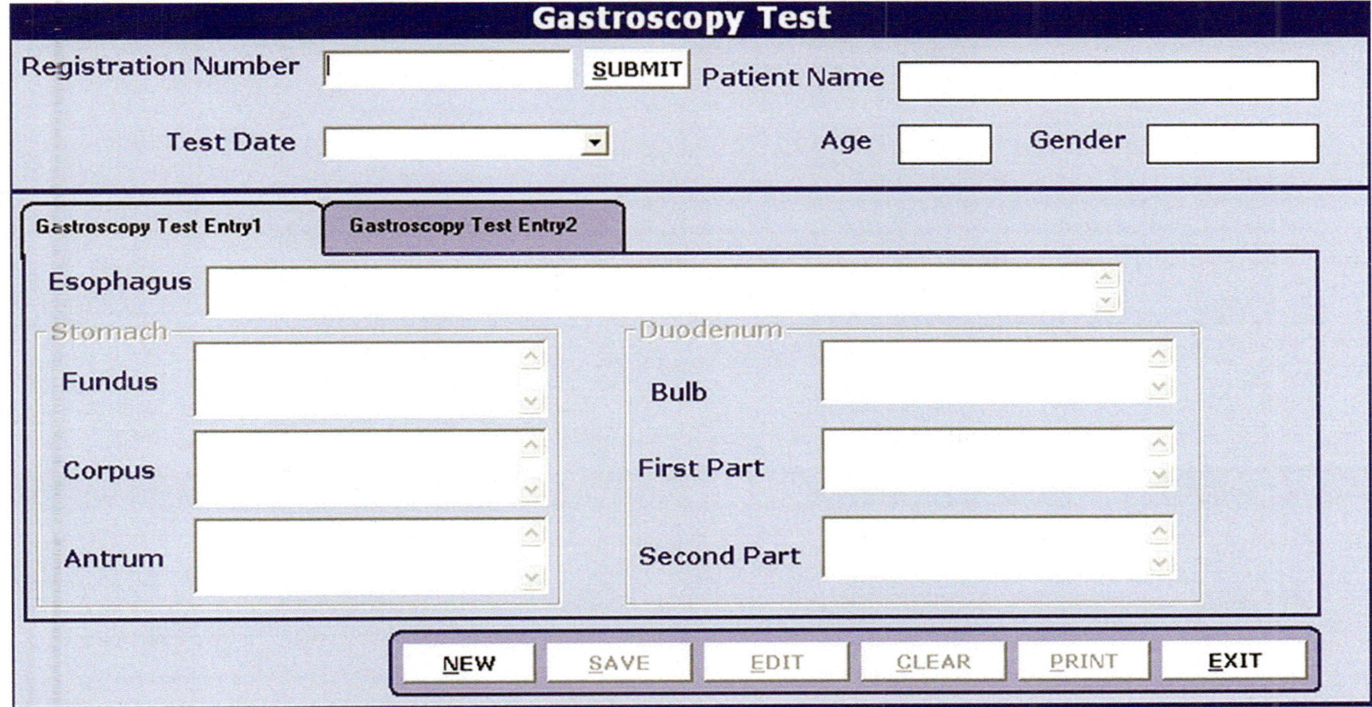

Gastroscopy Test

Registration Number [ ] SUBMIT Patient Name [ ]

Test Date [ ] Age [ ] Gender [ ]

Gastroscopy Test Entry1 | Gastroscopy Test Entry2

Esophagus [ ]

Stomach
Fundus [ ]
Corpus [ ]
Antrum [ ]

Duodenum
Bulb [ ]
First Part [ ]
Second Part [ ]

NEW SAVE EDIT CLEAR PRINT EXIT

Fig. 11: Gastroscopy test form.

Management Information System for a Corporate Hospital

Individual units can be provided with on-line reports based on Microsoft Excel. The requirements of the units with each line of business have to be documented in the individual line of business solution mapping document. The MIS would be organized by legal, cluster and line of business structures. It should be possible to compare between line of business as well as see the trend within a line of business. It should be possible to drill down to the unit level from each of the structures. MIS would provide the following information:

- Gross margin giving details of net income, materials consumption, doctors' variable fees and outsourcing charges.
- Throughput analysis:
  - Counts and value for each area within each unit, e.g. in clinic, the breakup of consultation, review, additional procedures; in hospital, the breakup of casualty, theater, etc., In pharmacy, the breakup of prescription, cosmetics and OTC.
  - By payers, e.g. cash, medical aid, other corporates.
  - By referral, e.g. External referring doctors, internal referring doctors, ambulance, etc.
- Activity analysis for the following:
  - Patient feedback
  - Referral feedback
  - Admission
  - Surgeries
  - Discharges
  - Purchases against purchase orders
  - Collections
  - Material consumption
  - Doctors payable

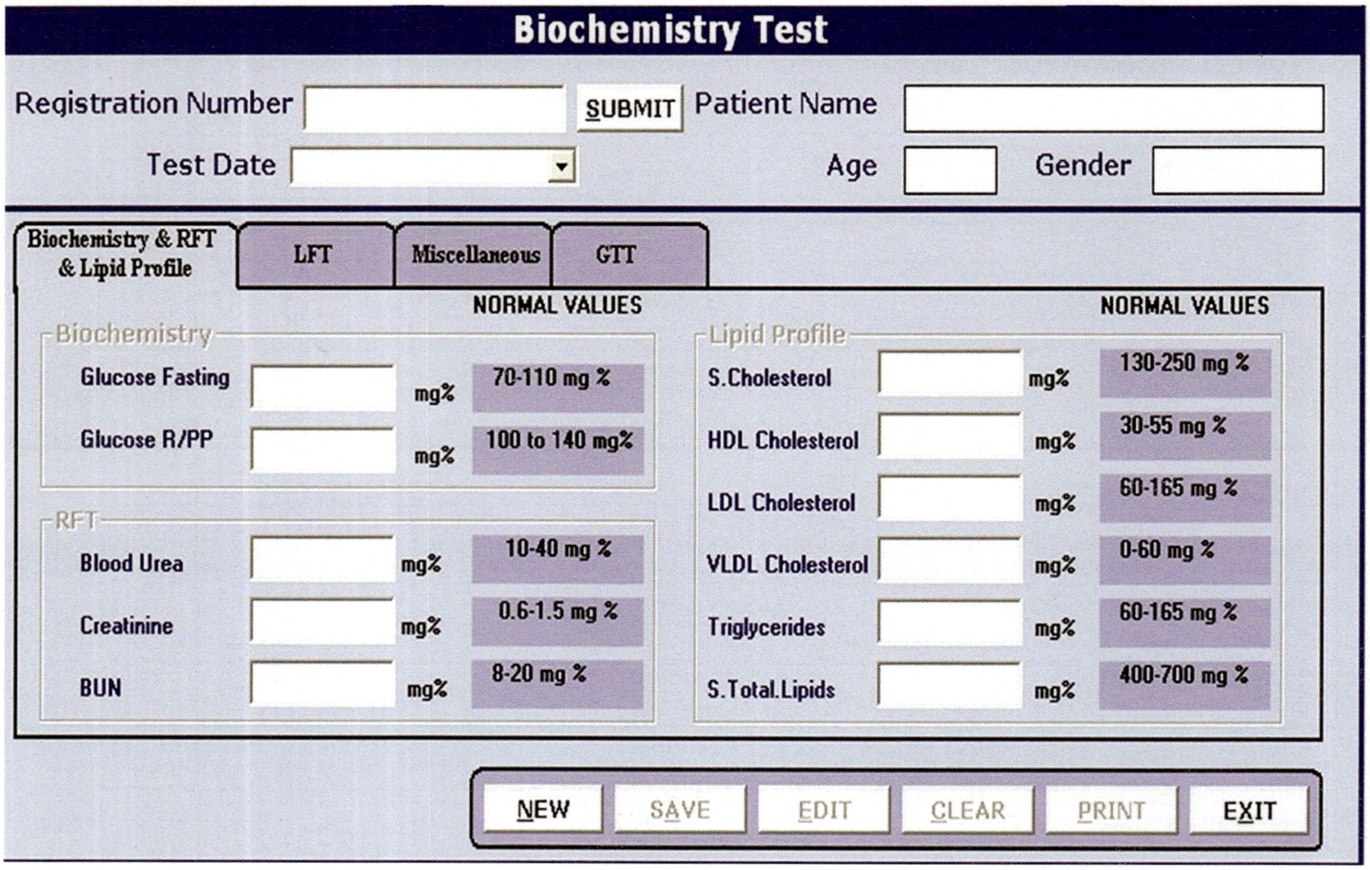

Biochemistry Test

Registration Number [ ] SUBMIT Patient Name [ ]

Test Date [ ] Age [ ] Gender [ ]

Biochemistry & RFT & Lipid Profile | LFT | Miscellaneous | GTT

Biochemistry			NORMAL VALUES
Glucose Fasting		mg%	70-110 mg %
Glucose R/PP		mg%	100 to 140 mg%
RFT			
Blood Urea		mg%	10-40 mg %
Creatinine		mg%	0.6-1.5 mg %
BUN		mg%	8-20 mg %

Lipid Profile			NORMAL VALUES
S.Cholesterol		mg%	130-250 mg %
HDL Cholesterol		mg%	30-55 mg %
LDL Cholesterol		mg%	60-165 mg %
VLDL Cholesterol		mg%	0-60 mg %
Triglycerides		mg%	60-165 mg %
S.Total.Lipids		mg%	400-700 mg %

NEW SAVE EDIT CLEAR PRINT EXIT

Fig. 12: Biochemistry test form.

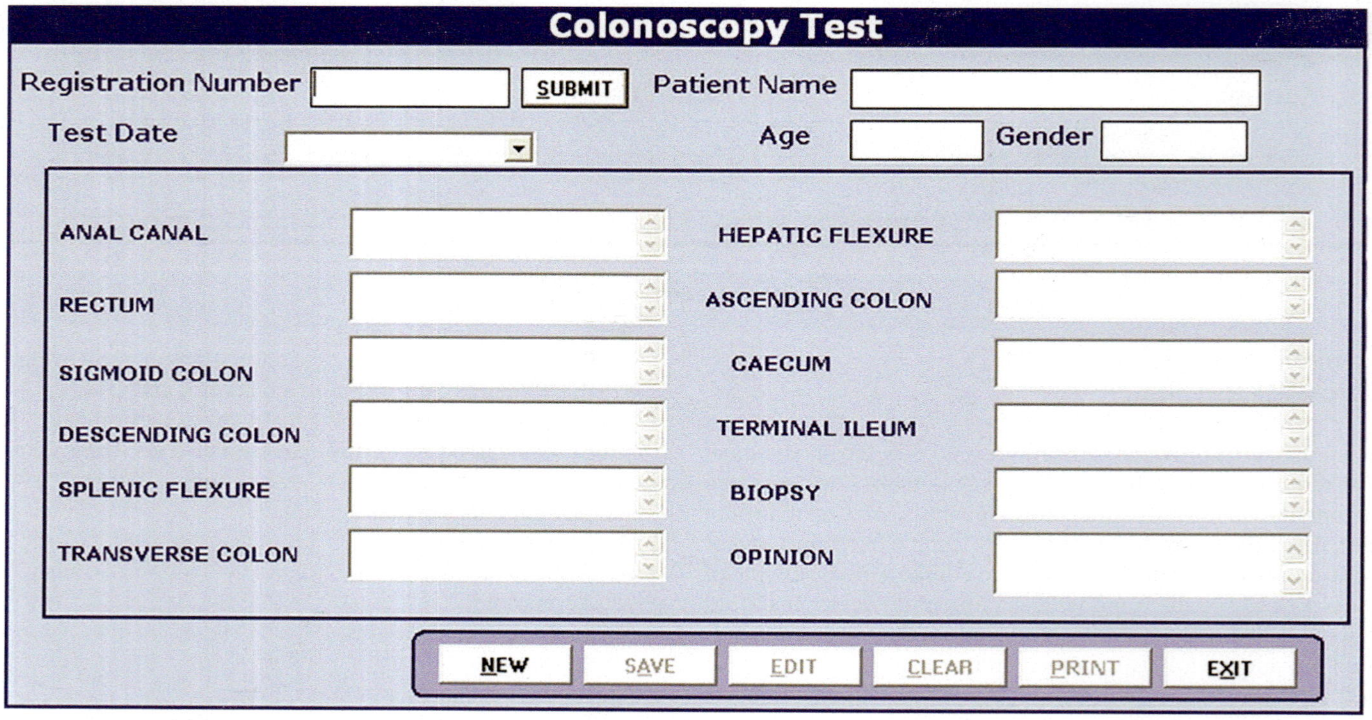

Colonoscopy Test

Registration Number [ ] SUBMIT Patient Name [ ]

Test Date [ ] Age [ ] Gender [ ]

ANAL CANAL	HEPATIC FLEXURE
RECTUM	ASCENDING COLON
SIGMOID COLON	CAECUM
DESCENDING COLON	TERMINAL ILEUM
SPLENIC FLEXURE	BIOPSY
TRANSVERSE COLON	OPINION

NEW SAVE EDIT CLEAR PRINT EXIT

Fig. 13: Colonoscopy test form.

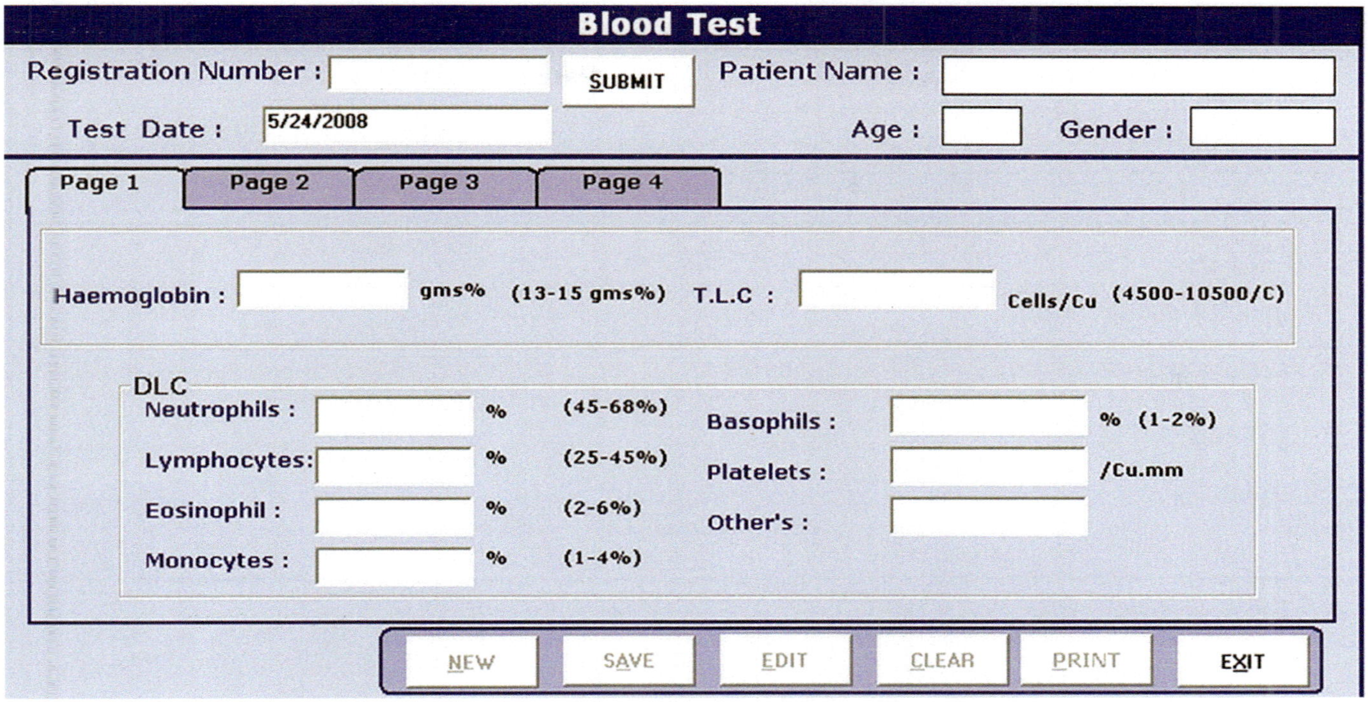

Blood Test

Registration Number : [ ] SUBMIT Patient Name : [ ]

Test Date : 5/24/2008 Age : [ ] Gender : [ ]

Page 1 | Page 2 | Page 3 | Page 4

Haemoglobin : [ ] gms% (13-15 gms%) T.L.C : [ ] Cells/Cu (4500-10500/C)

DLC

Neutrophils :	%	(45-68%)	Basophils :		% (1-2%)
Lymphocytes:	%	(25-45%)	Platelets :		/Cu.mm
Eosinophil :	%	(2-6%)	Other's :		
Monocytes :	%	(1-4%)			

NEW SAVE EDIT CLEAR PRINT EXIT

Fig. 14: Blood test form.

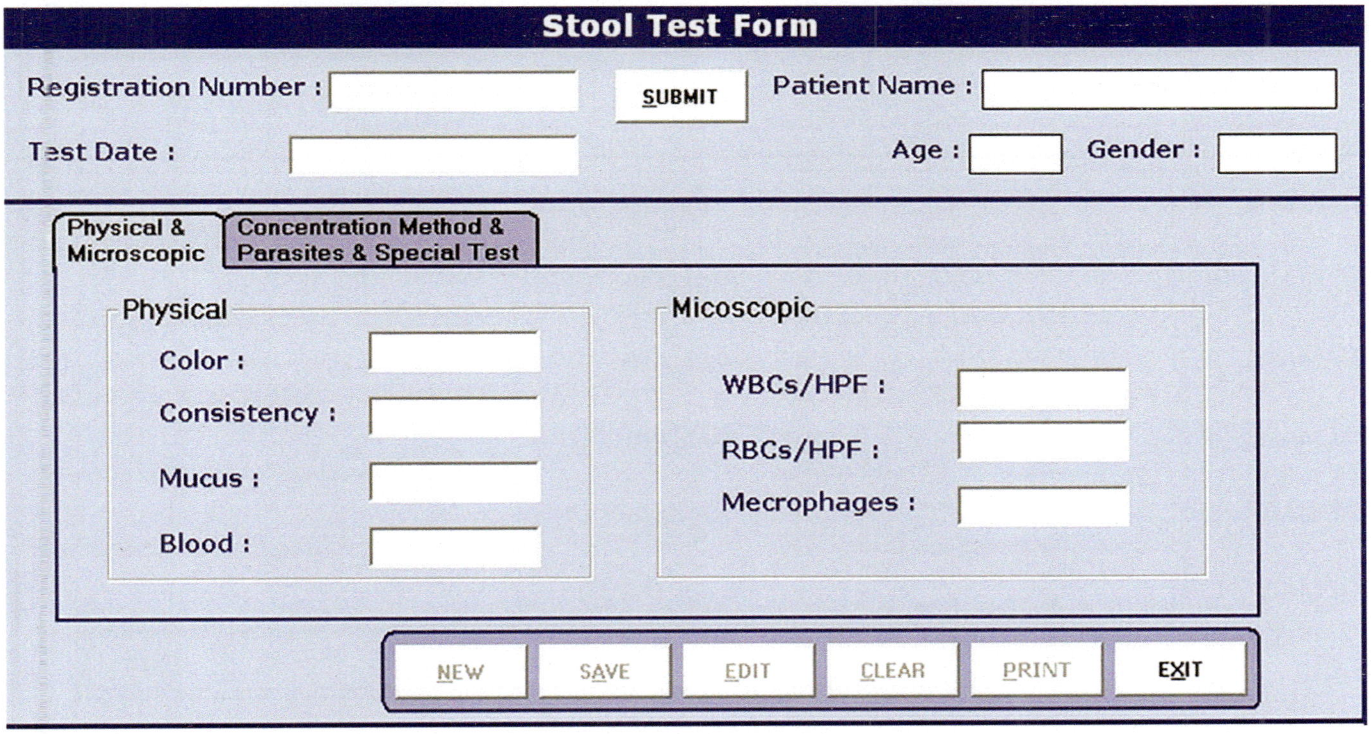

Stool Test Form

Registration Number : [ ] SUBMIT Patient Name : [ ]

Test Date : [ ] Age : [ ] Gender : [ ]

Physical & Microscopic | Concentration Method & Parasites & Special Test

Physical

Color :

Consistency :

Mucus :

Blood :

Micoscopic

WBCs/HPF :

RBCs/HPF :

Mecrophages :

NEW SAVE EDIT CLEAR PRINT EXIT

Fig. 15: Stool test form.

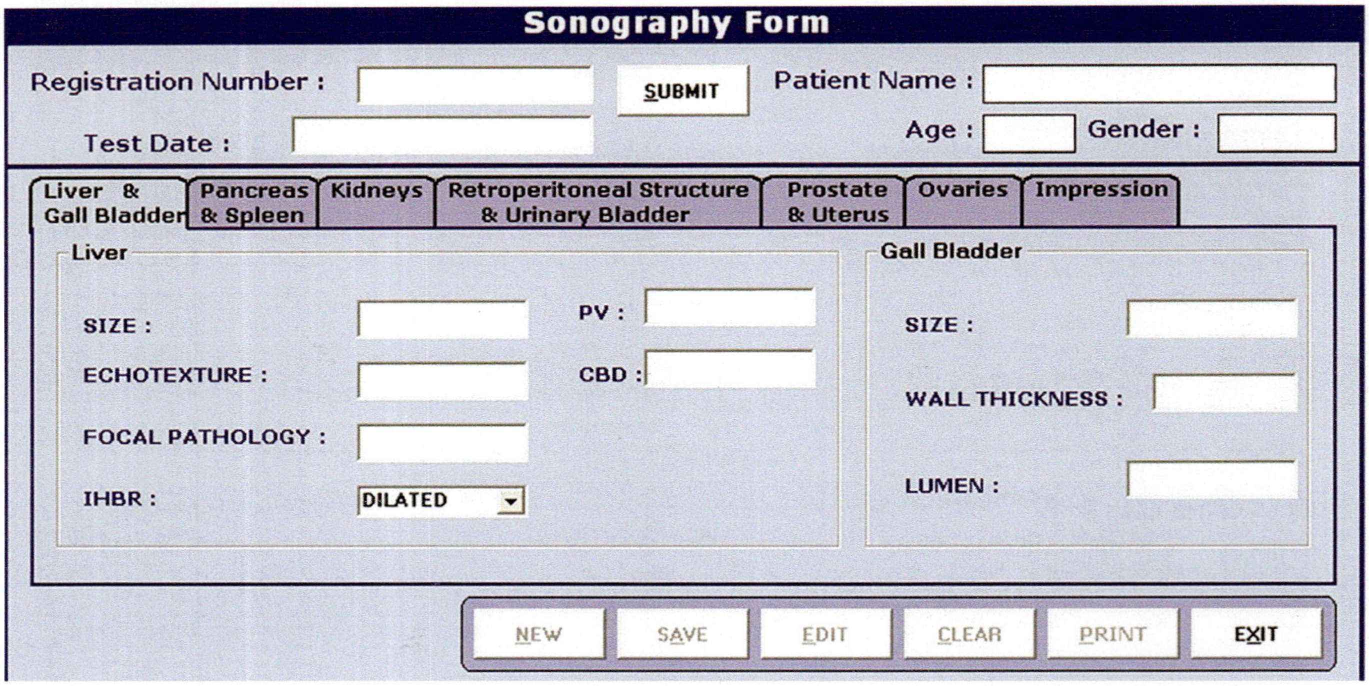

Sonography Form

Registration Number : SUBMIT Patient Name :

Test Date : Age : Gender :

Liver & Gall Bladder | Pancreas & Spleen | Kidneys | Retroperitoneal Structure & Urinary Bladder | Prostate & Uterus | Ovaries | Impression

Liver

SIZE : PV :

ECHOTEXTURE : CBD :

FOCAL PATHOLOGY :

IHBR : DILATED

Gall Bladder

SIZE :

WALL THICKNESS :

LUMEN :

NEW SAVE EDIT CLEAR PRINT EXIT

Fig. 16: Sonography test form.

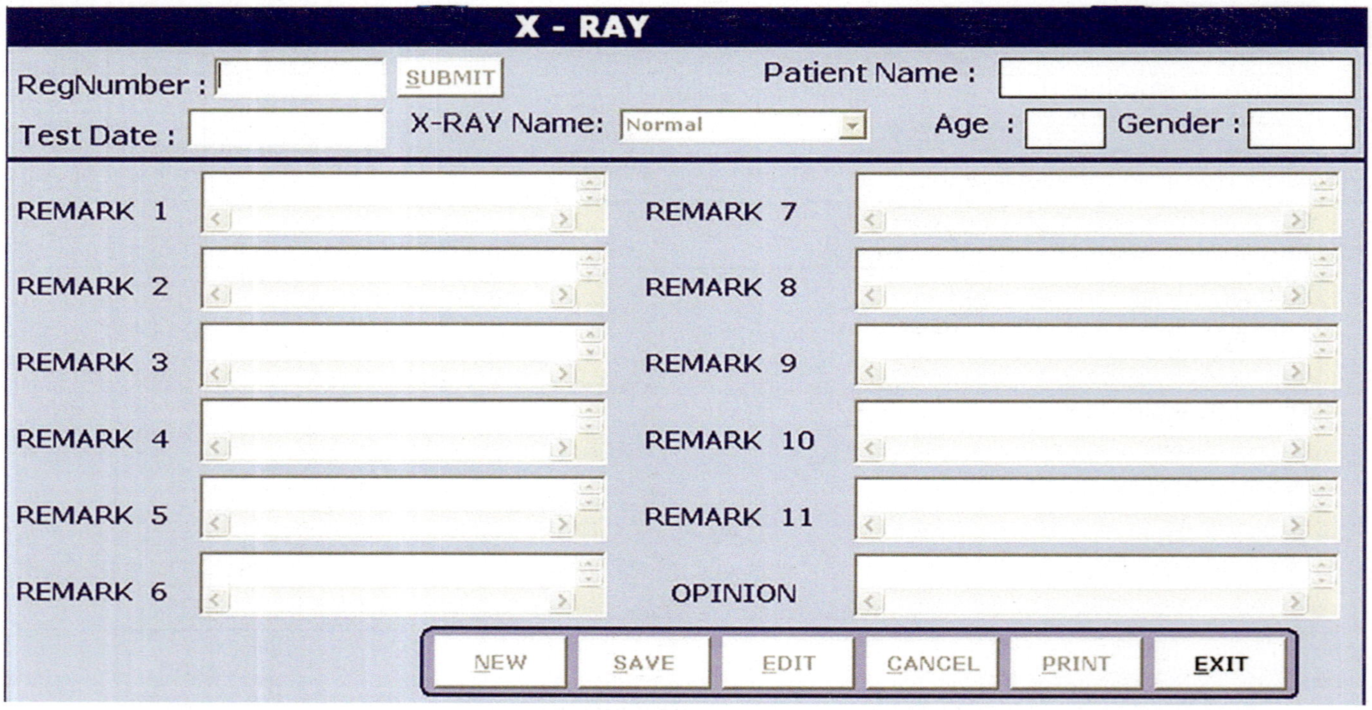

X - RAY

RegNumber : SUBMIT Patient Name :

Test Date : X-RAY Name: Normal Age : Gender :

REMARK 1 REMARK 7

REMARK 2 REMARK 8

REMARK 3 REMARK 9

REMARK 4 REMARK 10

REMARK 5 REMARK 11

REMARK 6 OPINION

NEW SAVE EDIT CANCEL PRINT EXIT

Fig. 17: X-ray form.

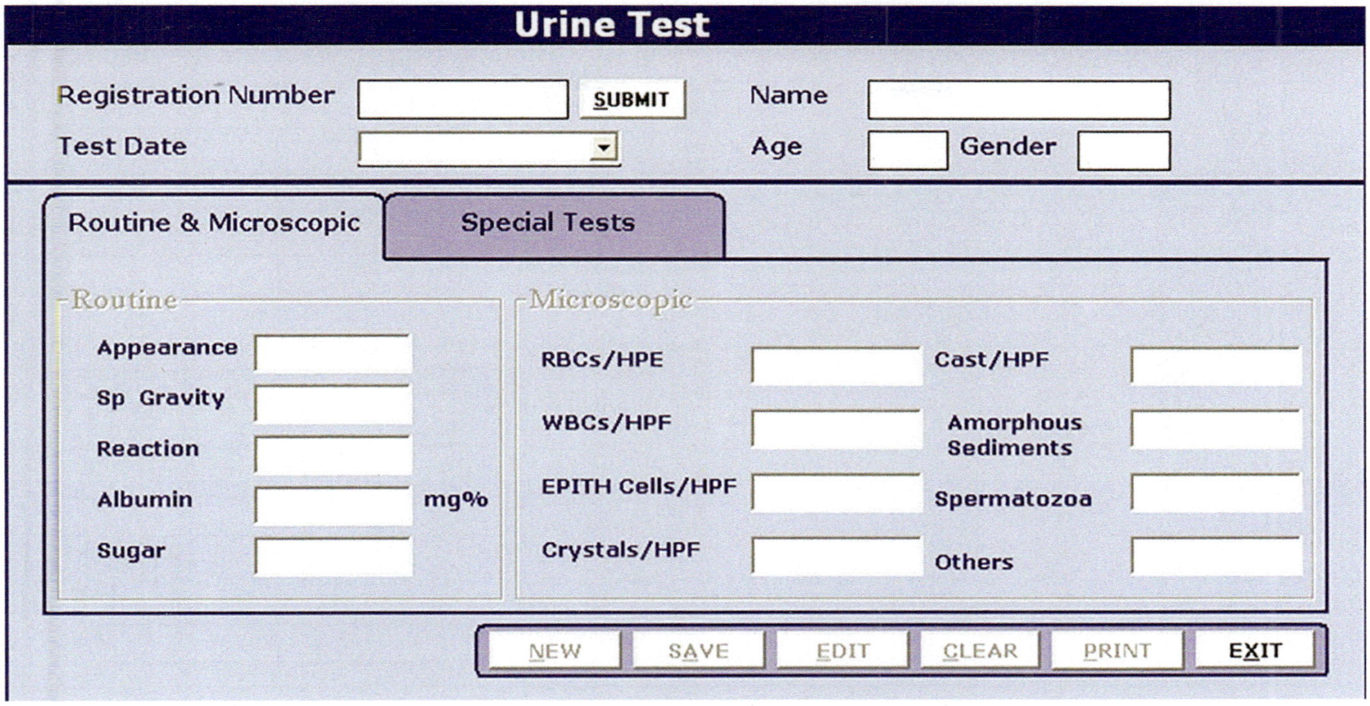

Urine Test

Registration Number [ ] SUBMIT Name [ ]
Test Date [ ] Age [ ] Gender [ ]

Routine & Microscopic | Special Tests

Routine

Appearance [ ]
Sp Gravity [ ]
Reaction [ ]
Albumin [ ] mg%
Sugar [ ]

Microscopic

RBCs/HPE [ ] Cast/HPF [ ]
WBCs/HPF [ ] Amorphous Sediments [ ]
EPITH Cells/HPF [ ] Spermatozoa [ ]
Crystals/HPF [ ] Others [ ]

NEW | SAVE | EDIT | CLEAR | PRINT | EXIT

Fig. 18: Urine test form.

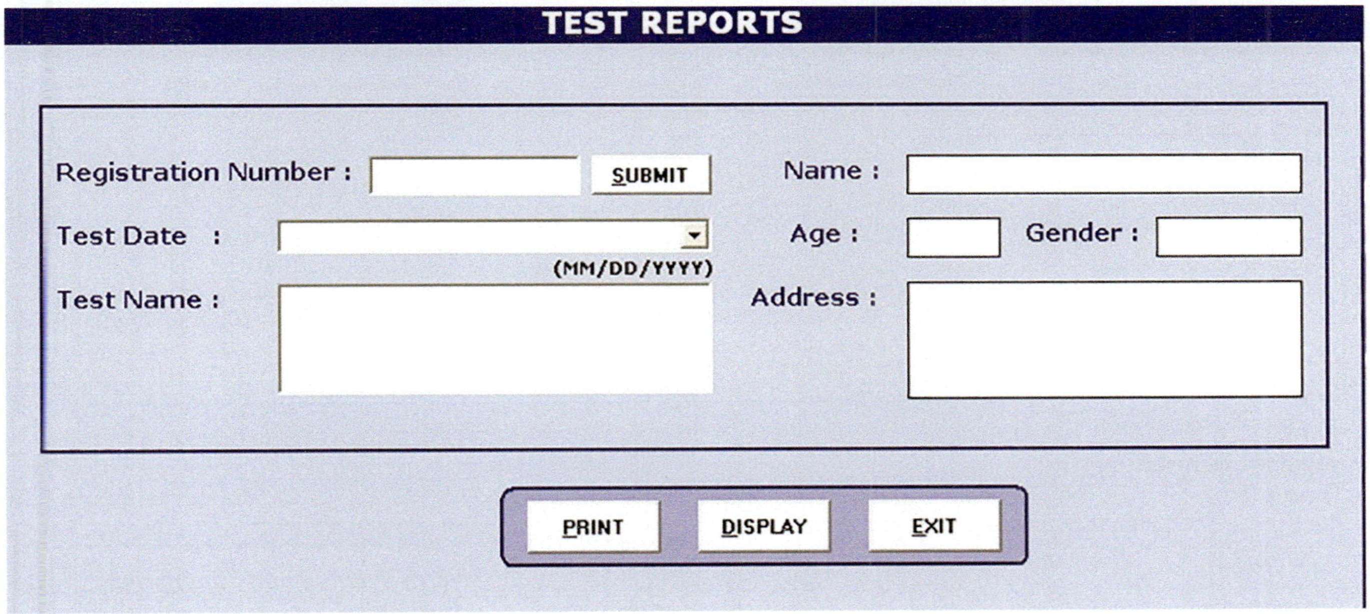

TEST REPORTS

Registration Number : [ ] SUBMIT Name : [ ]
Test Date : [ ] (MM/DD/YYYY) Age : [ ] Gender : [ ]
Test Name : [ ] Address : [ ]

PRINT | DISPLAY | EXIT

Fig. 19: Test reporters form.

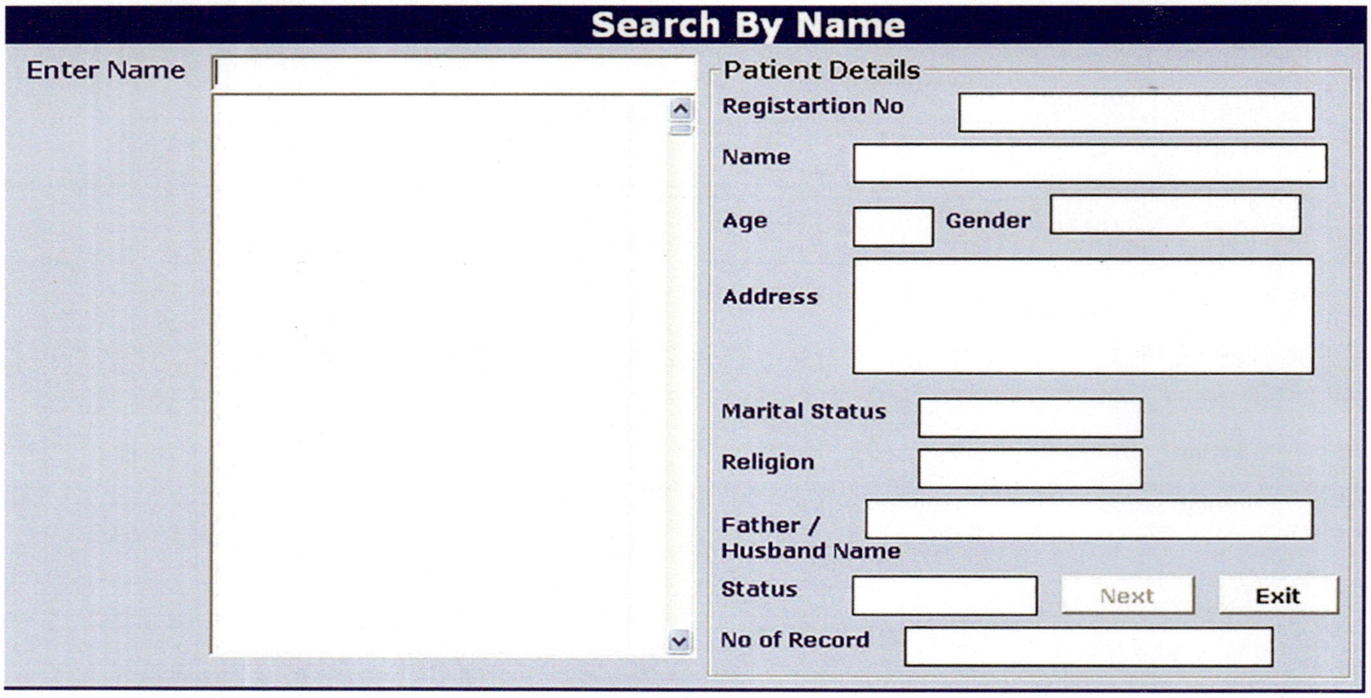

Search By Name

Enter Name

Patient Details

Registartion No

Name

Age Gender

Address

Marital Status

Religion

Father / Husband Name

Status Next Exit

No of Record

Fig. 20: Search by name form.

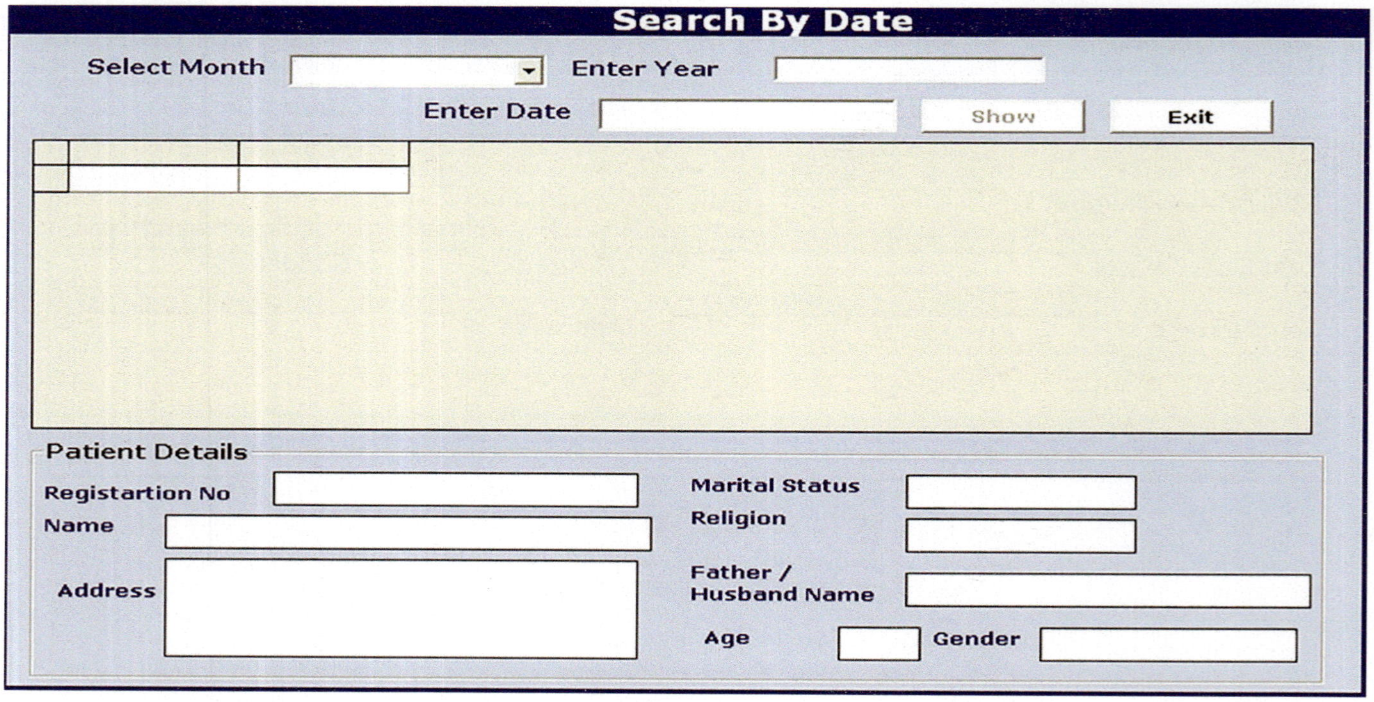

Search By Date

Select Month Enter Year

Enter Date Show Exit

Patient Details

Registartion No

Name

Address

Marital Status

Religion

Father / Husband Name

Age Gender

Fig. 21: Search by date form.

- Outsourcing
  - ◊ Hours of locum
  - ◊ Tests in laboratory
  - ◊ Reporting in imaging
  - ◊ Orders outsourced by dental and optometry
- Home deliveries by pharmacy and optometry
- Sentinel events
- Analysis by diagnosis in clinic, hospital and microbiology
- Anonymized reports for HIV patients—count with geographical area and the drug utilization
- Anemic patients having Hb <8 for female and Hb <10 for males—count and geography
- Analysis of CD4 test giving number of patients in different ranges of value of result.

• Analysis of exception activities:
  - Blocked time for doctors
  - Service cancellations
  - Discounts given after invoicing
  - Refunds
  - Cash purchases
  - Returns from patients
  - Returns from units to central stores
  - Returns to suppliers
  - Stock adjustments
  - Destruction of materials
  - Out of stock.
• Analysis of exceptions within activities:
  - Appointments not met
  - Short payments
  - Discounts given in a bill
  - Claim rejections
  - Write offs
  - Change of doctor
  - Change of type of consultation
  - Birth
  - Diagnosis
  - Morbidity
  - Mortality
  - Retests done in laboratory
  - Spoilages in imaging
  - False calls in ambulance
  - Discharges done without invoicing
  - Services provided without requisite authorization letters
  - List of doctors whose license is due to expire
  - List of practices whose license is due to expire.
• Productivity analysis:
  - Consulting doctors
  - Bed utilization
  - Theater utilization
  - Equipment utilization
  - Computer operator
  - Turnaround time for services.
• Ratio analysis:
  - Appointment to walk in
  - Ambulance conversion
  - Casualty conversion
  - Referral conversion
  - Average length of stay of patients in hospital
  - Stock to sales trend.
• Process flow:
  - Receivable with aging
  - Stock movement
  - Stock (with aging)
    - ◊ Good stock
    - ◊ Expired stock
    - ◊ Stock nearing expiry
    - ◊ Stock below minimum level
  - Unbilled income
  - Unbilled receivables
  - Deposit shortfall in hospital.

REFERENCES

1. ashrm.org
2. www.tnhsp.org
3. www.gjimt.ac.in
4. www.scribd.com
5. www.igrandee.com
6. www.birlamedisoft.com
7. www.netbloodbank.com
8. www.futurismtechnologies.com
9. aimspune.com
10. fr.scribd.com

OTHER REFERENCES

• Littlejohns P, Wyatt JC, Garvican L. Evaluating computerised health information systems: hard lessons still to be learnt, British Medical Journal. 2003;326.
• Heeks R. Failure, Success and Improvisation of Information Systems Projects in Developing Countries, 2002.
• AbouZahr C, Boerma, T. Health information systems: the foundations of public health, Bulletin of the World Health Organisation. 2005;83:8.
• Datapro Research Corporation, Delarn, NJ 08075, USA: Applications overview: Medical and Healthcare, Computer Applications in hospital (ISHA), 1979.
• Christensen WW, Stearns EI. Microcomputers in Health Care Management. Aspen Publishers, 1990.
• Gupta SK, Kant S, Chandrashekhar R, Satpthy S. Modern trends in planning and designing of hospitals: Principles and practice. Jaypee Brothers Medical Publishers (P) Ltd, 2001.
• Hübner-Bloder G, Ammenwerth E. Key Performance Indicators to Benchmark Hospital Information Systems – A Delphi Study. Methods of Information in Medicine, 2009.
• Joshi SK. Quality Management in Hospitals. Jaypee Brothers Medical Publishers (P) Ltd, 2009.
• Kelkar SA. Hospital Information Systems: A Concise Study. PHI Learning Private Limited, 2010.
• http://www.inmedica.com

CHAPTER 50

COVID-19: Planning Premises and Design Considerations for Healthcare Facilities

Khalid Mehmood, Saroj Kumar Patnaik, Shakti Kumar Gupta, Sunil Kant, R Chandrashekhar

INTRODUCTION

COVID-19 is an infectious disease that is caused by a newly discovered virus—severe acute respiratory syndrome coronavirus-2 (SARS-CoV-2), which belongs to the family of the coronaviruses. Majority of people who get infected with this COVID-19 virus may either remain asymptomatic or experience very mild-to-moderate respiratory symptoms ranging from mild fever, cough, and sore throat to shortness of breath, recovering without the need of any special treatment. Elderly and people with comorbid medical problems like the cardiovascular disease, diabetes, chronic respiratory disease, cancer and immunocompromised patients are prone to suffer and develop serious illness. Best ways to contain the spread and to slow down transmission is to be well informed about the COVID-19 virus, the disease it can cause and how it spreads. To protect from infection, washing hands regularly and more frequently or using an alcohol based rub frequently and avoid touching face. As we are aware that the COVID-19 virus spreads primarily through droplets of saliva or discharge from the nose when an infected person coughs or sneezes, so it's important that we all practice respiratory etiquette (e.g., by coughing into a flexed elbow).[1] Social distancing, early detection and prompt case tracing, appropriate and timely quarantine are effective measures for containment.

The COVID-19 pandemic has often been compared with global influenza outbreaks in an attempt to put this new threat in a historical context. According to WHO data, seasonal flu causes 3–5 million cases of severe illness and 290,000–650,000 deaths from respiratory disease each year.[2] H1N1, the virus that caused the swine flu pandemic of 2009/10, infected 11–21% of the global population (750 million–1.4 billion people) and caused around 280,000 deaths from respiratory disease and cardiovascular disorders; about two thirds of those deaths occurred in people aged 18–64 years.[3,4]

COVID-19 INFECTION

The SARS-CoV-2 virus is capable of surviving in aerosols for hours and also on surfaces including stainless steel, glass, plastic and cardboard for days.[5] It can transmit during the asymptomatic incubation phase and also up to two weeks after the onset of symptoms.[6] Each infected person may transmits the virus on to an average of three others.[7] The incubation period is approximately 5–6 days (range 1–14 days). Clinical presentation varies from asymptomatic, subclinical infection and mild illness to severe or fatal illness. Deterioration often during the second week of illness in clinical condition can occur rapidly.[7] Viral load may be 60 times greater in people with severe symptoms compared with mild asymptomatic cases. Death is generally due to pneumonia and possibly hyper inflammation associated with cytokine storm syndrome.[8]

Planning and Designing of a COVID-19 Healthcare Facility/Center[9-12]

The COVID-19 pandemic appeared like a global storm, taking not only the lives but also the livelihood of people. Today, the entire world is struggling with this global crisis with the healthcare industry and its frontline warriors, the healthcare work forces, are facing numerous challenges to fight this deadly pandemic. India is one of the developing nations, with a population of >1.38 billion and the government has taken various initiatives to address the challenge. Several temporary facilities were established across the globe to cater to the increase number of cases among the affected population. While these were the makeshift arrangements, they too deserve detailed attention in line with any other healthcare facility. Despite their special medical needs, these facilities faced and still are facing and trying to overcome the challenges of constraints in optimal resource allocation, diversification, conservation and utilization. Many fast track and emergency facilities including temporary structures were setup for treating thousands of COVID-19 patients. In the present scenario, apart from addressing the increased requirement of immediate response and treatment centers, through the temporary facilities, it is equally important to have basic facilities and to adopt healthy and sustainable practices within the centers with good indoor environment quality to address the health and wellbeing of COVID patients, health care workers, minimize the chances of spread of infection while at the same time conserving the resources.

Hospital building being a complex infrastructural identity, requires for its construction, the in-depth perspective, scientific knowledge, holistic approach and continued improvements. The hospitals are constructed as per guidelines, such as those of the American Institute of Architects (AIA), National Health Services (Guidelines of UK), Indian Public Health Standards (IPHS), and Scales of Accommodation for Hospitals for the Armed Forces, iHFG (Indian Health facilities guidelines) There has been a metamorphic change in perspectives, planning and implementing the infrastructural requirements in the COVID encompassing environment.

The main defining factor for the inevitable changes is the peculiar characteristics of the COVID-19, which is characterized by its unpredictable virulence, communicability, a very high component of asymptomatic carriers and many unknown significant facts, making everyone including the patients, visitors, staff and others visiting the hospital as potential COVID carriers and almost every surface/object in a hospital being a potential contaminated one. Though the new challenges faced by hospital administrators are herculean, it does not mean to say that the existing planning and designing of the hospitals are faulty and inappropriate. Hospital designing has been revolutionized through the continuous improvement of numerous processes in the recent past and today's hospitals do cater to infection control measures and the other satisfying aspects of patient care provisioning for better clinical outcomes among patients and to improve their satisfaction level by being user friendly. Provisioning of heating, ventilation, and air conditioning (HVAC) systems, fire and electrical safety, expansion capabilities and isolation facilities have been an inseparable part of effective hospital planning, for a long time.

Hospital buildings should have evidence-based design (EBD) and meticulous planning to incorporate the Green concepts viz. use of natural resources like lighting and ventilation, be resilient and adaptable for expansion of services. Use of technology should also be optimized to automate different processes, thereby relieving the stress and challenges imposed on the constrained resources, especially in a pandemic situation like of COVID-19.

GENERAL CONSIDERATIONS

The essentials of planning and designing re-emphasize introduction of safety and efficiency while considering the infrastructural requirements to develop a COVID care facility.

- *Day Lighting*: Apart from providing psychological well-being to patients, it is essential for natural sanitization of spaces. Appropriate building widths and East-West orientation are some variables which enable day lighting in hospital spaces. Depending on requirements, solar tunnels can also be utilized.
- *Natural Ventilation*: It is safer and cost-effective method than artificial HVAC, supplemented by conventional means, if required. Centralized courtyard landscapes provide natural evaporative cooling. Industry ceiling circulators are also effective. Place the patients in adequately ventilated single rooms if possible. For naturally ventilated general ward rooms, this is considered to be 60 litres/second per person. When single rooms are not available, people suspected of having a particular infection, e.g., COVID-19 can be cohorted together.

  Cohort is not recommended tested and confirmed with people who are suspected of infection.
- *Decentralized Microservice Zones*: This apart from preventing hospital acquired infections will enable maintenance and servicing to be easier and faster.
- Nonporous material, is used that is wipeable, cleanable and minimally affected by frequent cleaning, spraying of disinfectants and fumigation and products such as acrylic mineral fiber (Corian) PVC, UPVC, polycarbonate high pressurized laminates are suitable. The surfaces including floors, walls, and roofs are appropriately designed for easy cleaning and less dust/dirt accumulation. Coving is provided wherever necessary to facilitate cleaning and prevent dust accumulation.
- Human contact with likely contaminated areas, is reduced by providing touch free control of lighting, temperature controls, sensor based taps, automatic doors, switchable privacy glass and foot operated latches and handles.
- Flexibility, to convert regular beds into intensive care beds, expansion capacity in emergency conditions and compartmentation into negative pressure areas in wards, as and when required.
- Shared staff spaces like spaces at workstations, locker rooms, restrooms are to be redesigned with provision of smaller and multiple spaces.

For the ease of understanding and better conceptual learning, the content of the topic subject has been broadly arranged, organized and put forth under different subheads to address the key areas of concern in planning and designing of a COVID environment enabled Fast-track and Emergency COVID-19 Healthcare Facility.

The following are the key areas of concern:
- Site selection
- Layout
- Modular structures for temporary COVID-19 facilities
- Hygiene practices
- Ventilation parameters

- Energy efficiency
- Water conservation
- Waste management
- Interior furnishings
- Facilities for health workforce

An understanding of these areas is of key concern. It would be helpful for both the upcoming and existing healthcare facilities to address the implementation challenges, optimally utilize the available constrained resources, exploring the possibility of adopting measures over and above the bare minimum guidelines and to achieve the purpose of preventing the large scale spread of infection.

Site Selection

While selecting the site for building a temporary facility for treating the COVID-19 infected patients, take the site selected for temporary facility should preferably be near to or at least easily approachable from an existing hospital. The site should not be close to residential and commercial zones.

Layout

Importance of an ideal layout and design of the temporary COVID facilities lies in the fact that it plays a significant role in avoiding the spread of infections both within and outside the facility. As these temporary facilities are meant for management of patients who are tested COVID positive, so proper zoning is required to avoid cross infection between the patients with mild and severe symptoms and the healthcare work force.

The layout design incorporates the need to facilitate unidirectional movement of patients and healthcare workers offering treatment to patients, in each zone, to avoid cross infection within the facilities.

The layout design is made in such a way that it caters to the requirements of the different categories of patients and has the provision of separate zones for each of these categories. Temporary COVID facilities are divided into three categories on the basis of type of COVID patients to be treated and infrastructural requirements.

- Level-I: Quarantine facilities
- Level-II: Isolation facilities
- Level-III: Critical Care facilities

Level-I: Quarantine Facilities

The Level-I (temporary) COVID facilities are meant for providing care to symptomatic COVID patients who have only mild symptoms and do not require Oxygen or any Mechanical Ventilation support. Patients are moved to the short stay ward where distances and natural ventilation are as per the assured standards. Patients with mild-to-moderate illness can wait here for few hours till the laboratory results are received; receive health promotion sessions and treatment. The patient is moved to the observation room in case there is need to keep the patient under observation for additional more hours. Patients who are tested negative can be discharged or referred to another healthcare facility if other medical care is required. Mild and moderate cases are referred to the community facility for isolation and follow up.

Level-II: Isolation Facilities

The Level-II COVID facilities are equipped with isolation rooms/cabins/chambers with appropriate oxygen supply for the management of patients who need oxygen support for their treatment. Patients who don't need intensive care are treated at such facilities. Severe cases are moved directly to the severe case ward. Medical care is provided and samples are taken. This ward is composed of individual, self-contained rooms with hybrid ventilation.

Level-III: Critical Care Facilities

The Level-III COVID facilities are equipped at par with an intensive care unit (ICU), for providing intensive care and monitoring to critically ill patients with the help of mechanical ventilators.

Critical cases are moved directly to the critical case ward. Medical care is started and samples are taken. It is composed of individual self-contained rooms with hybrid ventilation.

A recommended layout design for a standalone 75-bedded temporary COVID facility is illustrated in Figure 1.

It is recommended that the COVID facility layout has two separate areas, one for the patients and one for the healthcare workforce. Further the area for patients is divided into three zones, i.e., Mild (Quarantine), Moderate (Isolation), and Critical (ICU) areas according to the severity of illness of the patients.

The layout design accommodates two different types of areas:

- Patients and Visitors area
- Healthcare Workforce area

Patients and Visitors Area[13,14]

The sub-areas needed for the functioning of the patients and visitors area are briefly described as under:

- *Entry with Biocontainment unit*: Provide separate entrance for the entry of patients and the visitors. Sanitization points at the entrance to ensure that people are disinfected before entering the facility and entrance is spacious enough to avoid overcrowding. Appropriate measures for checking Mask and non-contact thermal scanning of all the patients and visitors before entering the facility.
- *Reception*: The information desk with the designated authority is located in the reception area. The receptionist provides appropriate information to the patients and guide them to the concerned areas such as waiting room, sampling room and wards. The receptionist communicates regularly with the staff about the patient flow to avoid confusion/mishaps.
- *Screening/Triage area*: Triage is the preliminary area where patients are screened and tested for the virus. It is divided into two distinctive zones: Staff zone, and Patients' zone (high-risk zone). One meter distance fence should be there to separate the staff and patients. Patients are examined and investigated in individual booths. Double fencing or a Plexiglas barrier may be used for separation. Separate hand washing points (soap and water)/ Sanitizer for patients and staff. Part of an existing building or a temporary structure like a tent may be used for screening. Clinically triage all patients at admission for early recognition of possible COVID-19 infection and immediately isolate people with suspected infection in an area separate from other patients. The facility may be kept completely open (no doors) to allow a proper natural ventilation. Flow of patients, services and facilities in the screening area of a severe acute respiratory infection (SARI) treatment Center is shown in Figures 2 and 3.

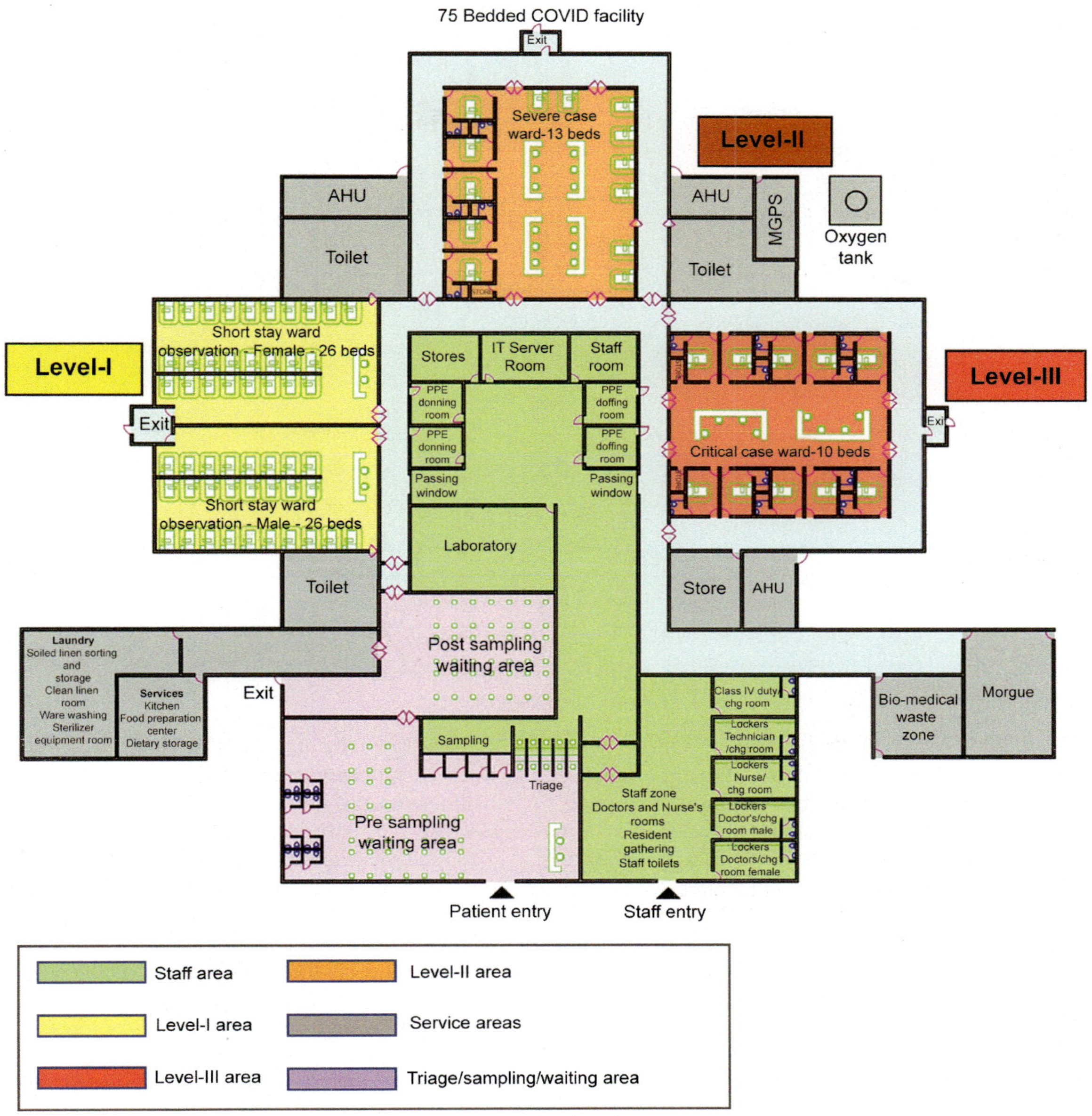

Fig. 1: Showing basic layout of COVID Center.

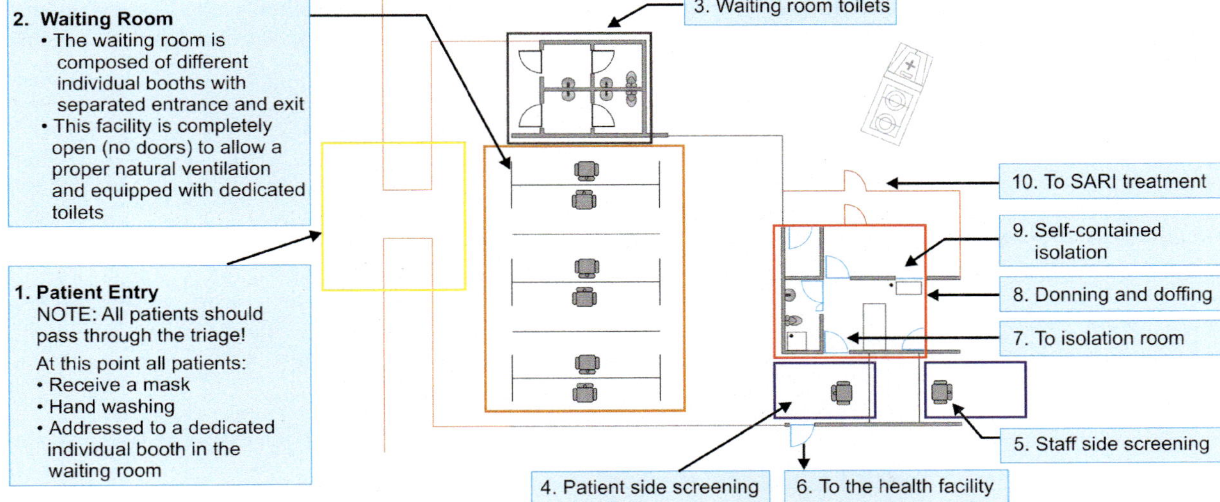

Fig. 2: Services and facilities in the screening area of a Severe Acute Respiratory Infection (SARI) treatment Center.

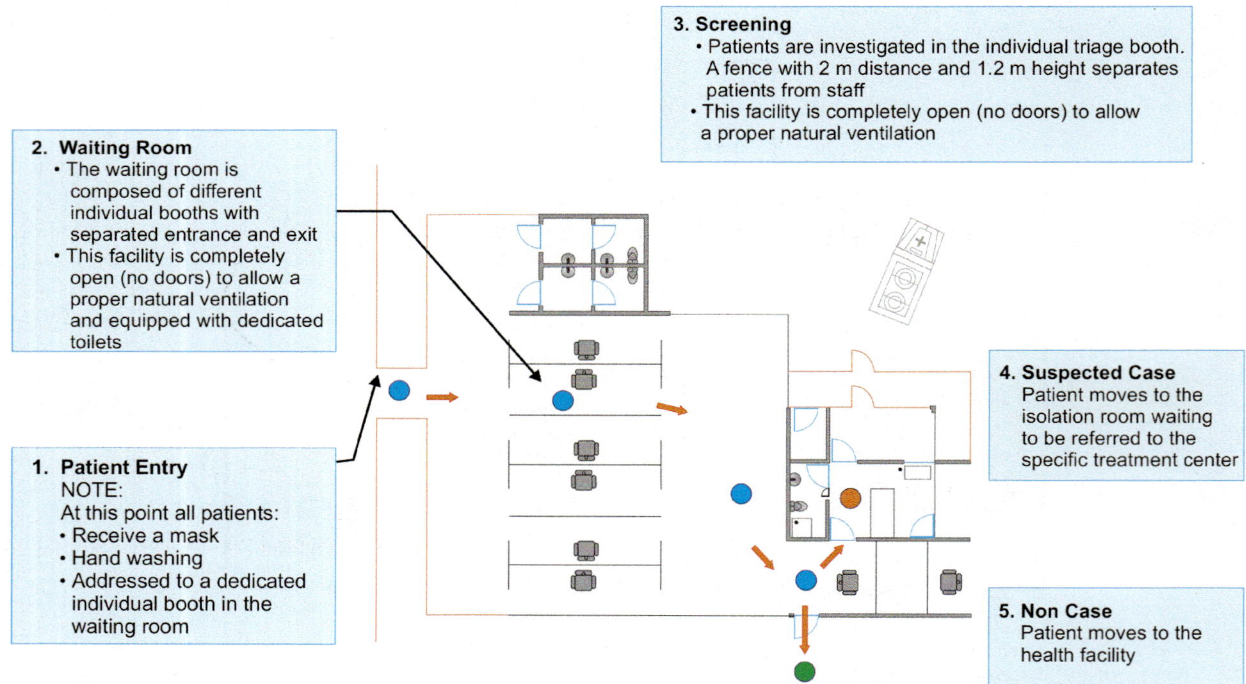

Fig. 3: Flow of patients in the screening area of a Severe Acute Respiratory Infection (SARI) treatment Center.

- *Waiting room*: The waiting room should be spacious enough with capacity for adequate seating arrangements, after maintaining minimum physical distance of 6 feet between adjacent seats, good ventilation, cleaned and disinfected regularly to avoid infection spread. It is composed of different individual booths with separate entrance and exit and equipped with dedicated toilets. The facility should be kept completely open (no doors) to allow a proper natural ventilation.
- *OPD consultation room*: it must incorporate elements for video conferencing solution with facilities for virtual OPD consultation, so that, maximum Doctor to patient interface is through Audio/Video Controls.
- *Sampling room (Fig. 4)*: The sample room should be planned and activated to deal with situations like COVID-19, wherein samples from symptomatic and asymptomatic patients are collected and sent for testing. The sampling room may be an individual booth with hybrid ventilation. Multiple booths for collecting samples should be provided. The sampling areas are Air conditioned or ventilated as recommended in Ventilation Parameters. Each booth should be properly labelled to avoid error and allow proper flow of the patients.
- *Wards*: The ward facility is provided in each of the three zones including mild, moderate and critical zones according to the severity of illness and medical conditions of the patients. The beds in wards are placed at a distance of 6 feet from each other. (Details of Indoor air Quality is explained in ventilation parameters). Fabric ducts can be used, which are fast and flexible to erect. Use transparent partition between the patients' beds and the nursing station to enable visual contact and regular monitoring of patients should be done. Light fixtures to be used must be of appropriate grade. It signifies degree of protection provided against intrusion of solid parts (including human parts such as fingers, dust and water in electrical enclosure). It has 2 numerals. First number signifies protection against ingress of solid objects (Graded 0-no protection to 6-dust tight) and second number signifies protection against liquids (Graded 0-no protection to 8 protection against effects of continuous immersion in water). In wards requiring cleaning with water jets Gd 6 fixtures should be utilized which provide protection against water entering when water jets are utilized for cleaning. Typical layout of isolation ward and isolation room is depicted in Figure 5.

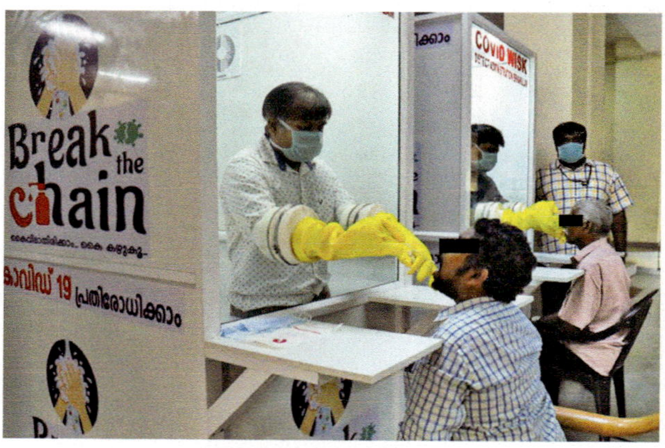

Fig. 4: Sampling room.

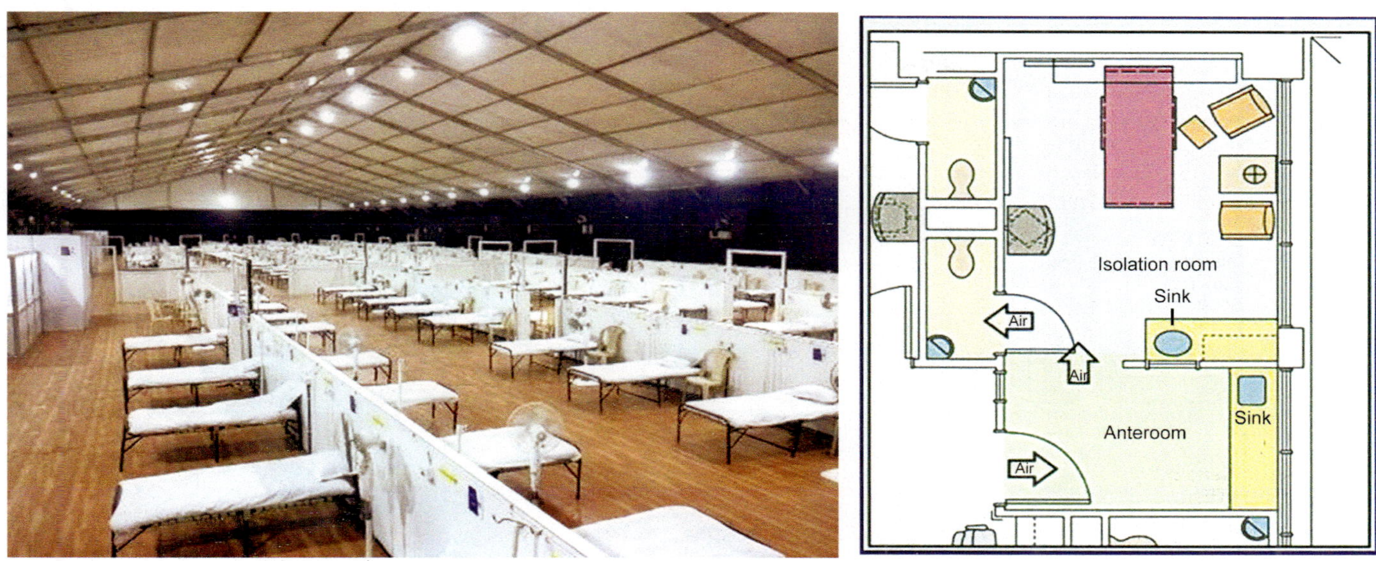

Fig. 5: Typical Layout of Isolation ward and Isolation room.

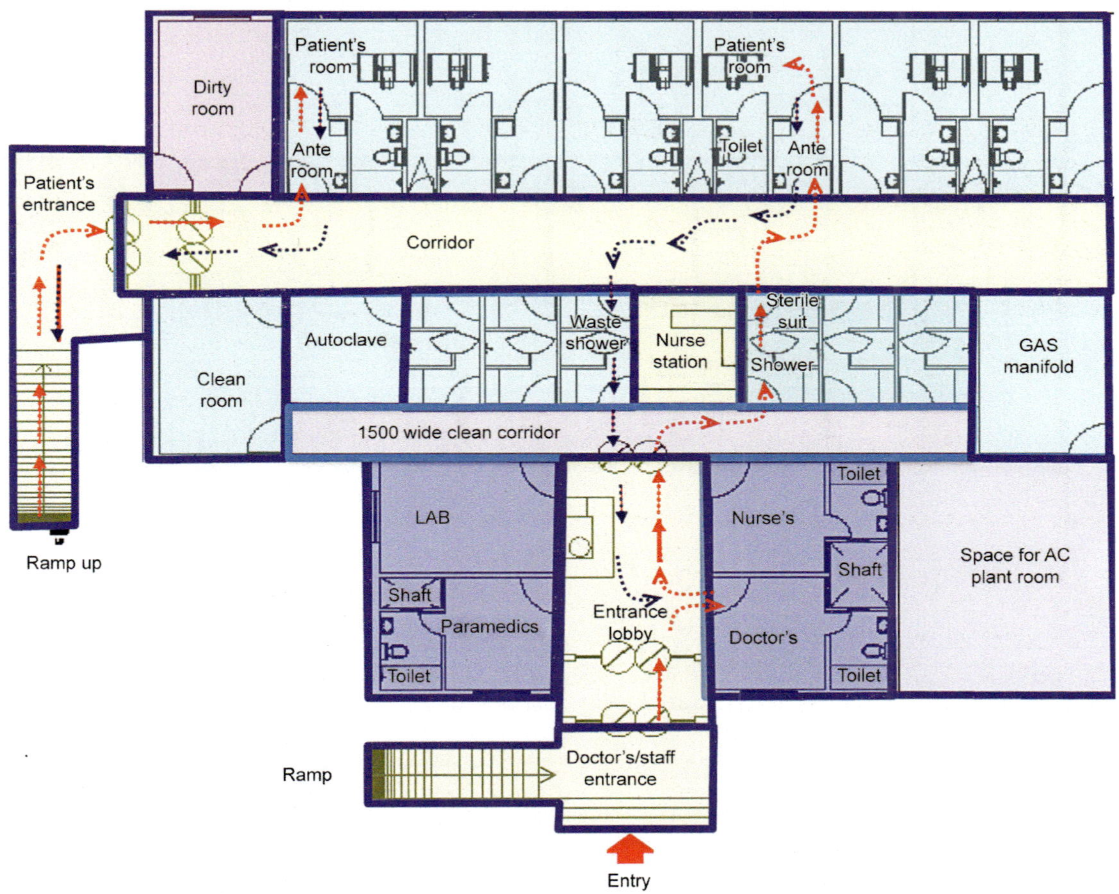

Fig. 6: Standard layout of Independent Block of COVID Ward.

Moderate and severe areas should be properly equipped with the required medical gases supplied through manifold room by pipeline. Dedicated areas for Oxygen plant and storing of medical gases need to be located near Level-II and Level-III zones.

An area of 16–22 m^2 should be allocated for each ward bed so as to ensure adequate physical distancing. Layout of Independent Block of COVID Ward is depicted in Figure 6, and a Typical COVID ward design on EBD is shown in Figures 7 to 10 and a Standard Containerized Four Bedded COVID Ward is depicted in Figure 11.

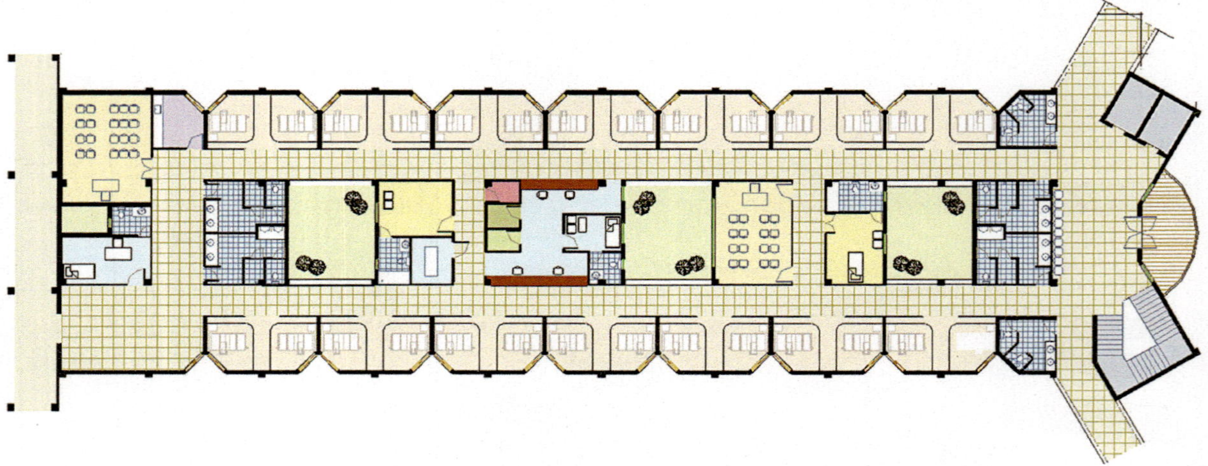

Fig. 7

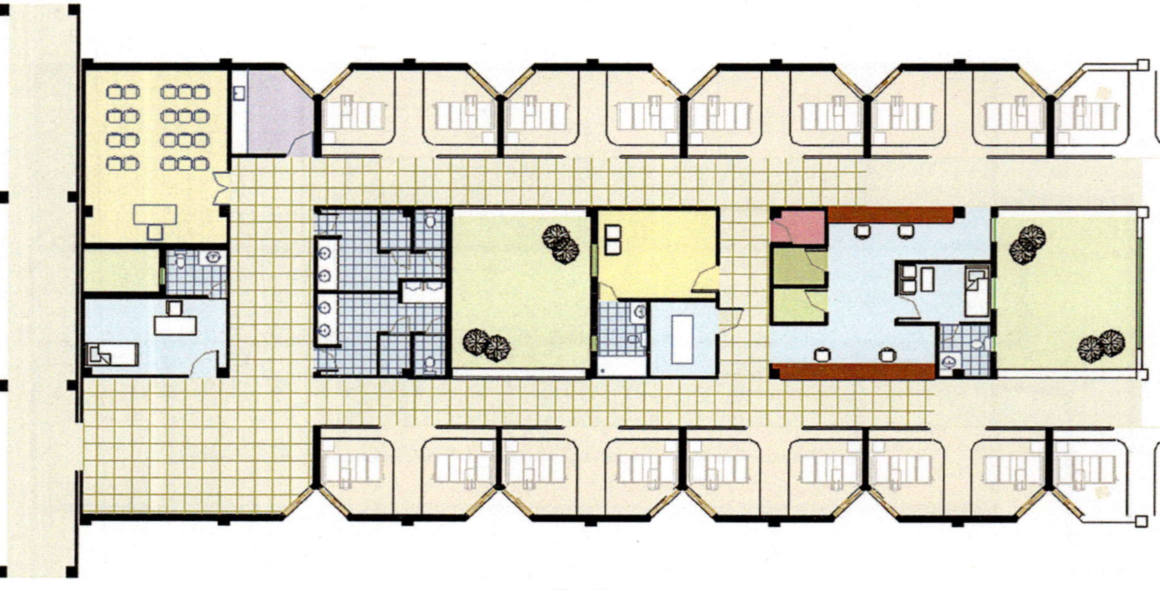

Fig. 8

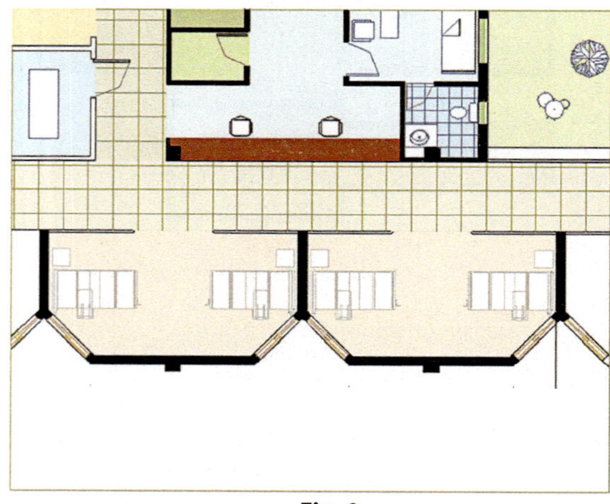

Fig. 9

Figs. 7 to 9: Typical COVID ward design on evidence-based design.

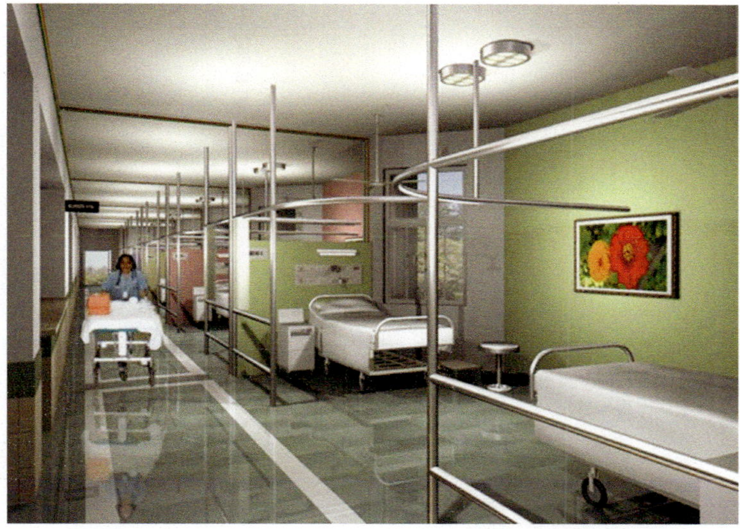

Fig. 10: Suggested view of typical COVID ward on evidence-based design.

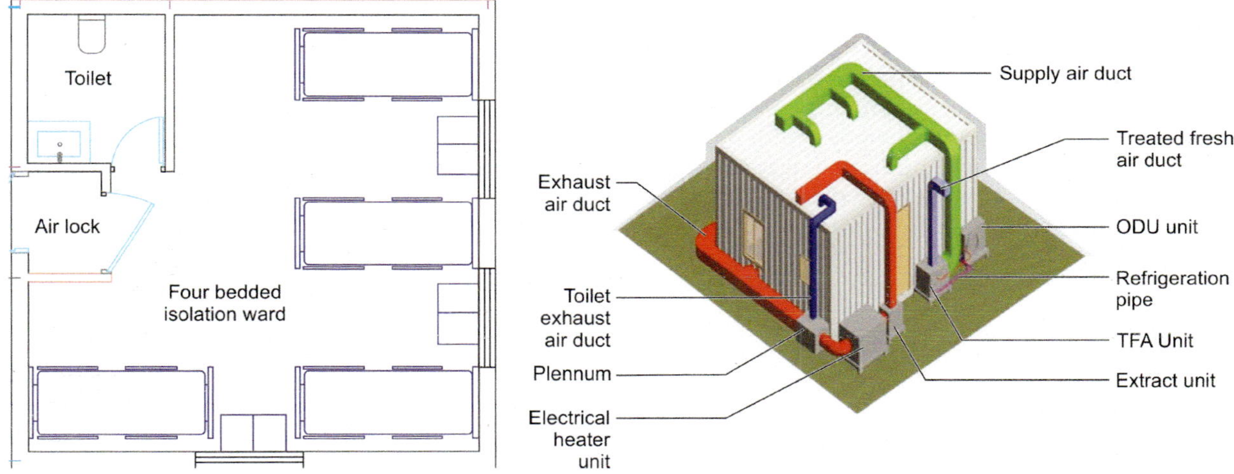

Fig. 11: Standard containerized four bedded COVID ward.[17]

- *Washrooms*: Dedicated washrooms for the patients and staff with regular sanitization and cleaning of washrooms. Adequate facilities such as hand wash areas, showers, water closets and tissues should be provided. As far as possible touch free/sensor based fixtures in toilets should be done.
- *Discharge room*: Patients who do not fit the case definition and are referred back home/other centers or patients who are recovered and tested negative are directed to the discharge room. It should be provided with good ventilation and other required facilities such as washrooms, hand washing points at the entrance and exits.
- *Pharmacy*: A designated area for pharmacy within the facility where required medicines and personal protective items are available and easily stored should be provided.
- *Morgue*: A dedicated isolated area with highly restricted entry away from the patient and staff areas for respectful keeping and storing of the dead bodies should also be provided.

Healthcare Workforce Area

- *Entrance for staff*: Separate entrance for staff with regular thermal scanning of staff entering the facility is required to monitor the temperature and sanitization points to avoid infection spread should be provide. Staff entry through visibility of reception area should be provided so that only authorized people enters the facility. There should be availability of Hand hygiene points with availability of soap, availability of running water or alcohol hand rub in all rooms. Entrance should be spacious enough to avoid overcrowding. Natural ventilation should be ensured with wide open windows. Shelves for staff members' personal items should be available.
- *Changing/Retiring rooms*: Adequate spacious male and female changing rooms to avoid overcrowding during shift changes with locker facility to store personal items and shelves for scrubs, boots or closed shoes for cleaners should be provided. Adequate natural ventilation or use air extractors and a wind tower should be ensured. These rooms may be utilized as retiring facilities during prolong stay/duty hours like night shifts.
- *Disinfection room*: Disinfectant chambers should be provided through which staff need to pass through before coming in and going out from premises to contain the spread of infection.
- *Donning and Doffing areas*:
  - *Donning area*: The area designated for healthcare workforce to put on their personal protective equipment (PPE) (Fig. 12) such as gown, mask, eye protection and gloves before entering to the patient zone.

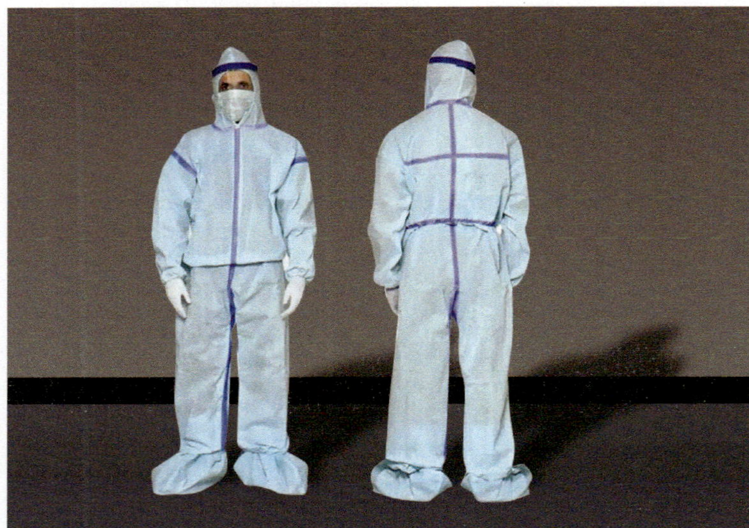
Fig. 12: Personal protective equipment (PPE).

- *Doffing area (Fig. 13)*: The area designated for healthcare workforce, for removing the PPE kits after treating the patients/ completion of shift duties. Physically isolated Donning and Doffing Areas, should be provided as Doffing area is a highly contaminated zone and it cannot be mixed with any other activity. The Donning areas are to be located near the patient area and the Doffing areas are to be located nearest to the exit from the patient area for the staff.

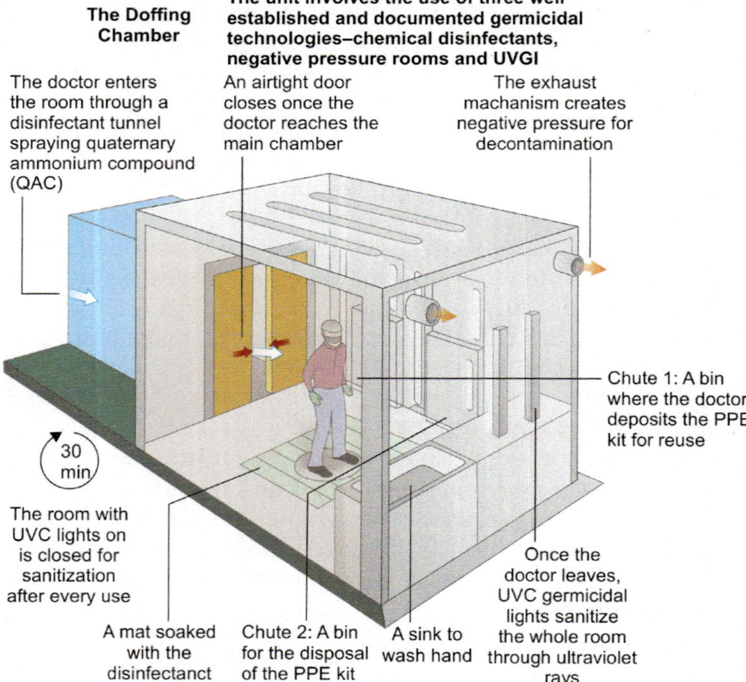

Fig. 13: Doffing area.

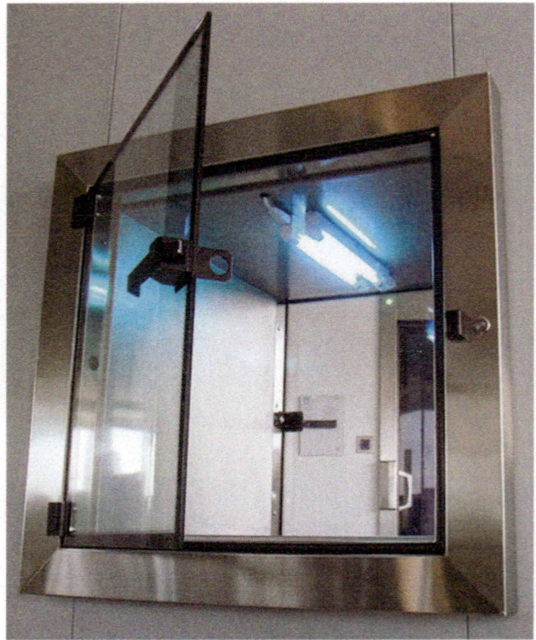
Fig. 14: Passing window.

- *Passing window (Fig. 14)*: A double door passing window should be provided at the entrance of the COVID area to avoid unnecessary movement and mixing of the staff. Items like Medicines, Food, Linen, etc., maybe passed through the passing window and received by the staff working inside the COVID area without the entry of pharmacy/ laundry/food and beverage staff into the COVID area.

  Similarly, all items to be passed out of the COVID area, should be sent out through the double door passing window without the need of any COVID duty staff to come out of the area.
- *Doctor rooms and Nursing stations*: Designated rooms for doctors and Nursing Stations should be provided, so that they can perform their other duties when they are not working directly with patients. Nursing Stations should be recommended at every level of the facility for regular and direct monitoring of the patients.
- *Laboratory area*: A dedicated area should be provided for laboratory testing of the collected samples with entry for authorized hospital staff only.
- *Hand washing points*: Multiple hand washing and sanitization points should be provided at all levels of the layout in the facility for better hygiene of the healthcare workforce.
- *IT Server room*: IT systems should be provided in the facility to capture all patient data in digital format rather than paper form. A designated room should be provided in the staff area for IT server. The data can be accessed by senior staff/doctors outside the COVID areas as well and treatment protocols can be modified accordingly. A video calling facility in wards, for the patients to commute with their family members, should also be provided as they are restricted to meet physically. It facilitates patient to feel better psychologically.

Plan for Surge Capacity Contingency

Areas such as parking, auditorium and waiting halls should be designed so as to be convertible into patient care areas. Surge capacity entails human resources and also, logistics and infrastructure management for optimization.

Mobile/Modular Structures for Temporary COVID-19 Facilities

Temporary structures should be built within minimum possible time with the best of medical facilities. Site work and construction should be planned simultaneously to reduce time. It can be expanded depending upon the requirements and each level is expanded by adding the modular facilities without compromising on the design for avoiding cross infection. The possibility of using mobile modular structures, as it can be installed in any open area available or as an extension to the existing facility should be explored. Railway yards, Hospital vicinity like parking lot, Auditoriums, Shopping Mall, Hostels, Colleges, etc., may be utilized for developing the modular facility constructed using prefabricated materials that is assembled at the site. The required infrastructure should be installed in the modular structures such as

- **Electrical:** Main utility power, individual unit level cabling, lights and electric points including 6A and 15A switches. All the points to be checked for polarity and continuity.
- **Plumbing:** Water supply plumbing lines, drainage to sewer, plumbing fixtures. Supply potable water to avoid any infections.
- **Ventilation:** Ducts to deliver and remove air, high-efficiency particulate air (HEPA) filtration, wet scrubber, fans in the individual units, exhaust fans, ultraviolet (UV) portable disinfectant.
- **Other facilities:** Other facilities that are to be provided in the individual modular unit include clinical wash hand basin, suitable extract fan, transfer grille to en suite door, en suite facility and fully glazed doors with integral privacy blinds, to allow staff observation and patients views out (Fig. 15).

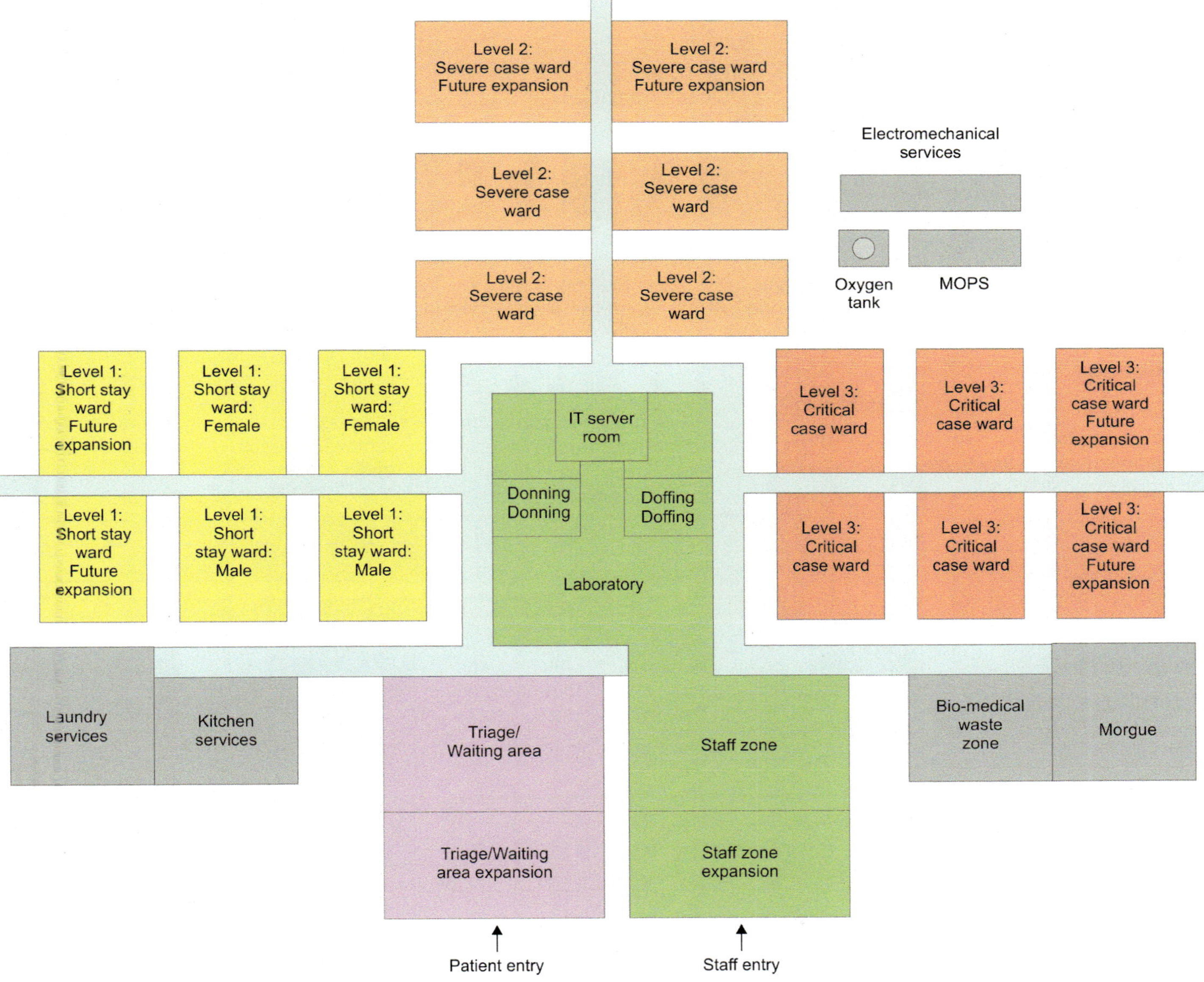

Fig. 15: Showing layout of modular expandable COVID facility.

Railway Coaches

The Ministry of Railways took several initiatives in developing railway coaches as temporary COVID care facilities; to meet the increasing demand of no. of beds with the increase in number of COVID infected people across the country. The coaches are used for treating mild cases that can be clinically assigned to the COVID care facilities as per the guidelines issued by the Ministry of Health. Coaches were converted into six to eight bays or cabins for patients and toilets were converted to bathrooms. The coaches were provided with oxygen cylinders and power plug sockets for medical equipment (Fig. 16).

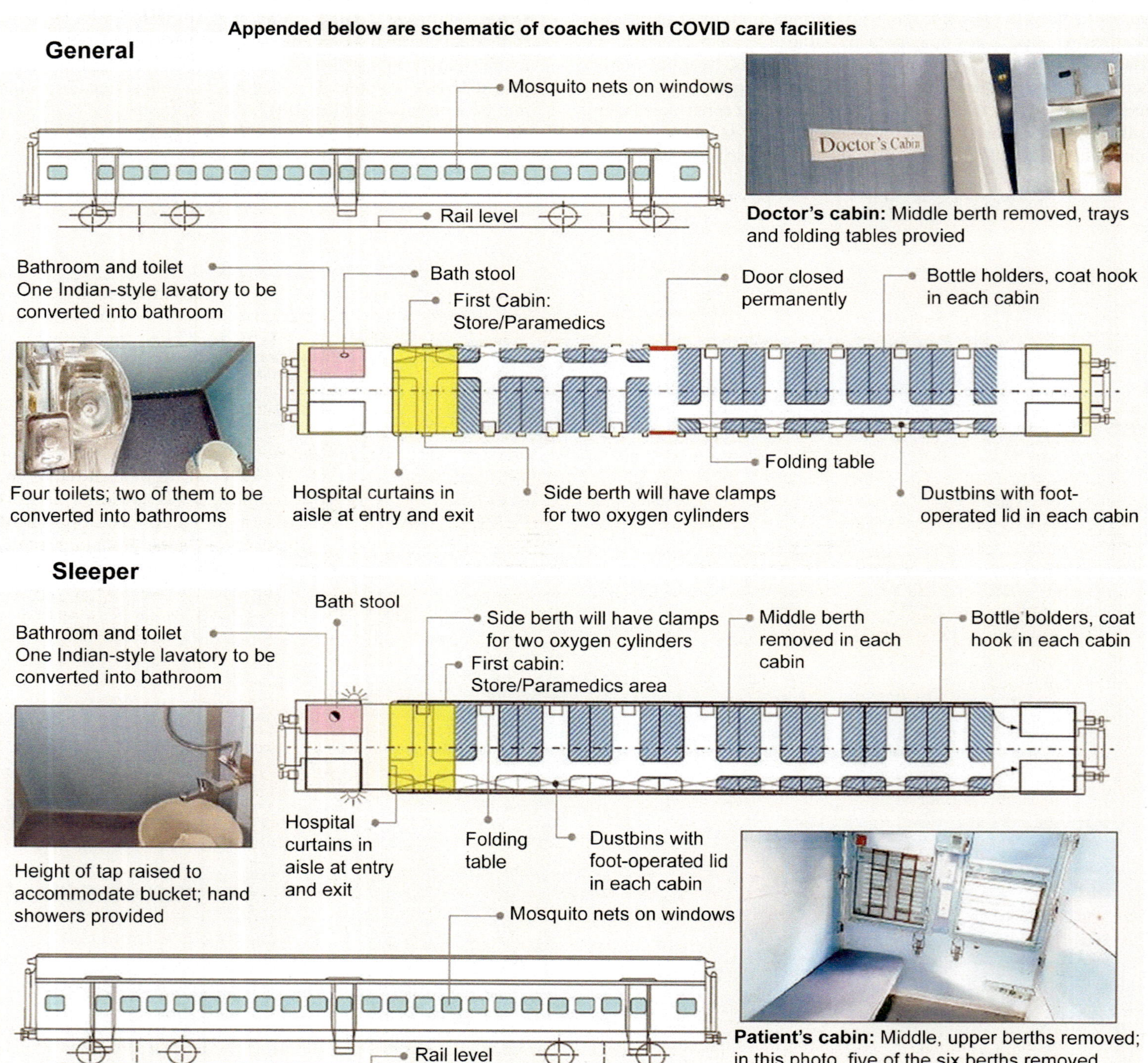

Fig. 16: Showing schematic of Railway Coach converted to Temporary COVID Care Center.

Note: For more details on railway coaches, please refer to 'Guidance document on appropriate suspect/confirmed cases of COVID-19' issued by Ministry of Health and Family welfare and Ministry of Railways developed document on 'COVID Care coaches of Indian Railways'.

Hygiene Practices

Good hygiene remains one of the corner stone for combating COVID-19. Considering the various possibilities of spread within the premises, there is a need for significantly enhancing hygiene measures beyond regular practices. Hygiene measures are adopted at the individual level and specific measures are implemented at all the spaces and surfaces where in the occupants are likely to come in contact. The following measures need to be considered for implementation of hygiene in hospitals:

- Provide signages/posters/floor markings for social distancing.
- Sensor based automatic doors from the entrance to all areas.
- Use antimicrobial copper on high touch surfaces like door handles, over patient tables, intravenous (IV) pole, Monitor pen, Bed rail, visitor chair arms, etc. (Copper based Door handles see Fig. 17)
- *Patients/Health workforce occupied area*:
  - Use entryway mats in all the entry and exit points.
  - Provide multiple hand wash/sanitization stations
  - Regularly check temperature and other COVID symptoms
  - Carryout regular surface cleaning and disinfection of materials and equipment with appropriate sanitizers
  - Regularly change linen materials
  - Monitor proper cleaning of plates, cups, glasses and cutlery in cafeteria and kitchen
  - Periodically sanitize high touch surfaces like workstations, door handles/knobs, handrails, lift doors and buttons.
- *Housekeeping protocols*: Clean restrooms with GreenPro/ecolabelled housekeeping chemicals, hourly cleaning of the high touch surfaces such as door handles/knobs and flush buttons, etc., keep soap solutions/sanitizers and tissue papers near wash basins, mop once in 4 hours all regularly occupied spaces with ecolabelled cleaning chemicals or soap water.

It should be ensured that all finishes, furniture and patient care equipment are effectively cleaned and are compatible with the facility's requirement as mentioned in Table 1.

Table 1: Recommended characteristics for selecting finishes and furniture for SARI (COVID-19) healthcare facility.[9,10,15,16]

Characteristic	Selection guidance
Cleanable	• Avoid items with hard-to-clean features, such as crevasses • Do not use carpets in patient care areas • Select material that can withstand repeated cleaning
Easy to maintain and repair	• Avoid materials prone to cracks, scratches or chips, and quickly patch or repair if they do occur • Select materials that are durable or easy to repair
Resistant to microbial growth	• Avoid materials that hold moisture, such as wood and cloth, as these facilitate microbial growth • Select metals and hard plastics
Nonporous	• Avoid items with porous surfaces, such as cotton, wood and nylon • Avoid porous plastics, such as polypropylene, in patient care areas
Seamless	• Avoid items with seams • Avoid upholstered furniture in patient care areas

Ventilation Parameters[18]

Ample growing evidences suggest the likelihood of spread of the disease through the air-conditioning and ventilation systems, warranting the need to detail out and take extreme care to ensure that these indispensable systems, while providing comfort, also work to support the mitigation rather than propagation of the disease. The sketch in Figure 18 shows there are several transmission routes for the COVID-19 virus.

The infectious droplets from infected person's cough or respiration come in a spectrum of sizes. The bigger droplets, typically larger than 5 μ traverse some distance and subsequently settle down on nearby surfaces or floors or may be even directly respired by nearby people. The smaller droplets which are <5 μ float around in the air for longer times, even hours. Depending on the relative humidity of the surrounding air and the velocity of ejection from the cough, these droplets desiccate into smaller particles called 'Droplet Nuclei' aerosols. These aerosols

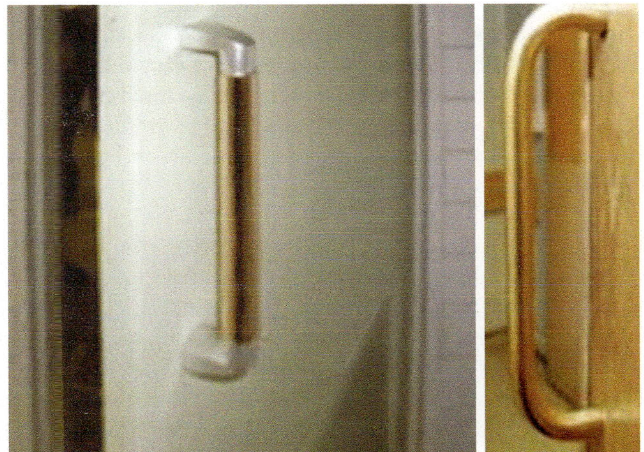

Fig. 17: Showing Copper based Door handles.

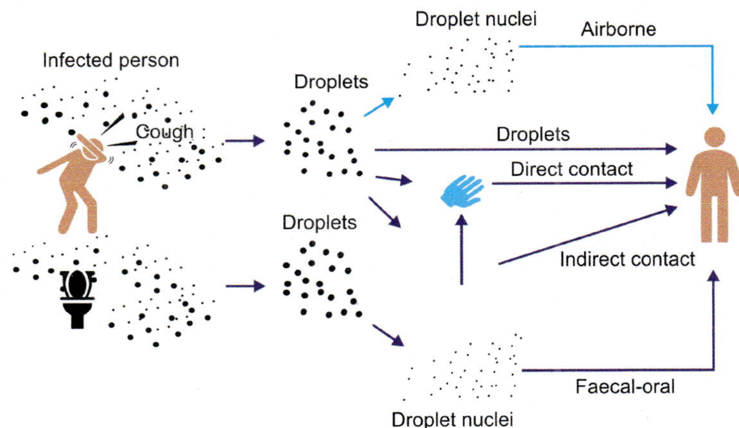

Fig. 18: WHO reported exposure mechanisms of COVID-19 SARS-CoV-2 droplets.

travel considerable distances from the infected person. The HVAC systems need to primarily contend with the aerosolized droplet nuclei. In simplified terms the infection equation can be expressed as:

$$\text{Infection rate} = \text{Viral concentration} \times \text{Exposure time}$$

The HVAC systems need to ensure that the viral concentration is substantially reduced so that the chance of airborne infection is diminished.

To achieve dilution of not only viral concentration, but also the other airborne pathogens, the HVAC system designs needs to work around the following aspects:

- Fresh air and recirculation air change rates.
- Passive filtration using media filters.
- Air purification using ultraviolet germicidal irradiation (UVGI).
- Air distribution and displacement

Apart from dilution of pathogens, the other parameters that need to be controlled are:

- Room pressure gradient
- Relative humidity
- Temperature
- Exhaust
- Energy efficiency

Fresh Air and Recirculation Air Change Rates

Air change rate represents the number of times the entire volume of air in the room is replaced each hour. One of the methods to reduce the exposure of the person to the concentration of toxic chemicals and the number of microbes is by providing ventilation, i.e., introducing clean fresh air into the area. More number of air changes per hour (ACH) reduces the exposure of the patients and the healthcare workers to the toxic chemicals and microbes.

Similarly, in air conditioning systems, certain quantity of air is recirculated in the space through the air filtration system of the air handling unit. The number of times the air gets churned through the filtration system results in more of the particulate matter and the microbes getting filtered out of the air. This recirculation of air is also expressed in ACH.

The chart given in Table 2 is from the CDC and shows the time required for airborne-contaminant removal efficiencies of 99% and 99.9% through air change rates.

The times given in Table 2 assume perfect mixing of the air within the space (i.e., mixing factor = 1). However, perfect mixing usually does not occur in reality. Removal times will be longer in rooms or areas with imperfect mixing or air stagnation. Caution should be exercised in using this table in such situations. For booths or other local ventilation enclosures, manufacturers' instructions should be consulted.

Passive Filtration using Media Filters

Filters can effectively trap particulate contaminants, including microbiological pathogens, and remove them from the air passing through them. Various grades of filters can be used to achieve different degrees of cleanliness. In critical care facilities such as in quarantine, triage and ICU, a proper filtration system generally consists of a pre-filter and a final filter in the air handling unit (AHU). The pre-filter should be placed upstream, ahead of the cooling/heating coil (in the case of air conditioning systems), to remove large particles for a clean heat transfer medium. More importantly, the pre-filter can prolong the life of the final filter placed downstream of the AHU (whether for air conditioning or mechanical ventilation), resulting in a cost-effective operation (Fig. 19).

Table 2: Air change efficiency chart (CDC).[12]

ACH§	Time (minutes) required for removal 99% efficiency	Time (minutes) required for removal 99.9% efficiency
2	138	207
4	69	104
6+	46	69
8	35	52
10+	28	41
12+	23	35
15+	18	28
20	14	21
50	6	8

Air changes per hour (ACH) and time required for airborne-contaminant removal efficiencies of 99% and 99.9%.

+ Denotes frequently cited ACH for patient-care areas.

§ Values derived from the formula:

$$t2 - t1 = -[\ln (C2/C1)/(Q/V)] \times 60, \text{ with } t1 = 0$$

Where,
t1 = initial timepoint in minutes
t2 = final timepoint in minutes
C1 = initial concentration of contaminant
C2 = final concentration of contaminant
C2/C1 = 1 – (removal efficiency/100)
Q = air flow rate in cubic feet/hour
V = room volume in cubic feet
Q/V = ACH

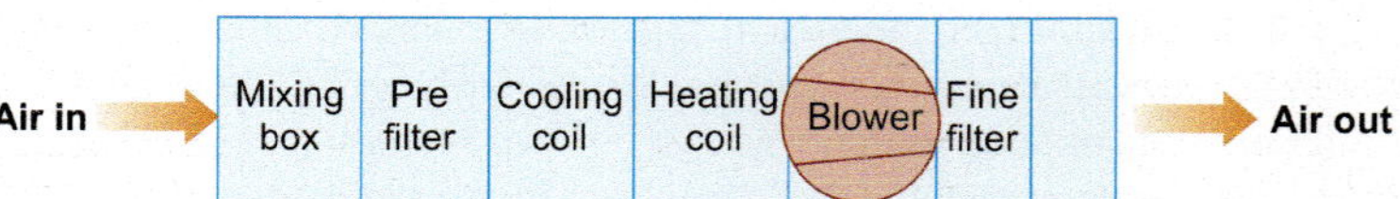

Fig. 19: Two stage filtration in an air handling unit.

Filter classifications: The ASHRAE Standard 52.2 classifies filters used in HVAC application by their minimum efficiency reporting values (MERV). The standard takes into consideration the fractional efficiencies of filters for particles in the size range of 0.3–10 µ. Air filters of MERV13 and above have the potential to remove microbes and other particles ranging from 0.3 µ to 10.0 µ (Table 3).

HEPA filters: High-efficiency particulate air filters trap a vast majority of very small particulate contaminants from an air stream.

The worst case particle size at which the filter efficiency is least is called as the most penetrating particle size (MPPS), and the efficiency of a filter at MPPS is called as the MPPS Efficiency. A HEPA filter has an overall filtration efficiency of above 99.95% at MPPS. For any other particle size, smaller or larger than the MPPS, the filtration efficiency of the HEPA filter would be greater than its MPPS efficiency. The MPPS of a HEPA filter would most commonly fall between 0.10 to 0.30 µ.

Most viruses, including CoVs, range from 0.004–1.0 µ (*Goldsmith CS et al. 2004, ultrastructural characterization of SARS coronavirus*). However, viruses are rarely observed as individual particles, but instead are expelled from the body already combined with water, proteins, salts, and other components as large droplets and aerosols. Thus far, SARS-CoV-2 has been observed in aerosolized particles in a spectrum of sizes, including 0.25–0.5 µ (*Liu Y et al., 2020. Aerodynamic characteristics and RNA concentration of SARS-CoV-2 aerosol in Wuhan*

Table 3: Minimum efficiency reporting values (MERVs) and filter efficiencies by particle size.

Standard 52.2 minimum efficiency reporting value (MERV)	Composite average particle size efficiency, % In size range, µm			Average arrestance, %
	Range 1 (0.3–1.0)	Range 2 (1.0–3.0)	Range 3 (3.0–10.0)	
1	n/a	n/a	E3 < 20	$A_{avg} < 65$
2	n/a	n/a	E3 < 20	$65 \le A_{avg} < 70$
3	n/a	n/a	E3 < 20	$70 \le A_{avg} < 75$
4	n/a	n/a	E3 < 20	$75 \le A_{avg}$
5	n/a	n/a	$20 \le E_3$	n/a
6	n/a	n/a	$35 \le E_3$	n/a
7	n/a	n/a	$50 \le E_3$	n/a
8	n/a	$20 \le E_2$	$70 \le E_3$	n/a
9	n/a	$35 \le E_2$	$75 \le E_3$	n/a
10	n/a	$50 \le E_2$	$80 \le E_3$	n/a
11	$20 \le E_1$	$65 \le E_2$	$85 \le E_3$	n/a
12	$35 \le E_1$	$80 \le E_2$	$90 \le E_3$	n/a
13	$50 \le E_1$	$85 \le E_2$	$90 \le E_3$	n/a
14	$75 \le E_1$	$90 \le E_2$	$95 \le E_3$	n/a
15	$85 \le E_1$	$90 \le E_2$	$95 \le E_3$	n/a
16	$95 \le E_1$	$95 \le E_2$	$95 \le E_3$	n/a

hospitals during COVID-19 outbreak) necessitating high efficiency filtration techniques to reduce the transmission potential of pathogens such as SARS-CoV-2.

HEPA and ULPA filters are classified as per their filtration efficiencies at MPPS. The classification chart of ISO 29463 is given in Table 4.

Air Purification Using UVGI

In HVAC systems, UVGI is being increasingly used for surface sterilization (for cooling coils and condensate drain pans) and as a supplement to filters for air purification. UVC Germicidal Ultraviolet wavelength (254 nm) is effective in impacting the DNA structure and RNA of a microorganism thereby inhibiting reproduction. Microorganisms such as mold, bacteria and viruses will be destroyed with the required concentrations of germicidal irradiation. All viruses and almost all bacteria (excluding spores) are vulnerable to moderate levels of UVGI exposure, but the magnitude of the effect is species-dependent. Out of the UV spectrum, it is the UVC that has the maximum capability to destroy the microorganisms. There are a number of factors to be considered that affect the deployment of UVC:

- *Residence time*: Greater the exposure time (contact time between the contaminant and the UV source), more is the UV energy being delivered to the contaminant resulting in a greater Kill Rate.
- *Intensity*: Greater intensity results in more UV energy being delivered to the contaminant resulting in a greater Kill Rate.
- *Reflection*: Reflection of the UV rays using reflectors on inner surfaces of the AHU or duct can be a helpful tool to considerably increase the effectiveness of the UV rays produced.
- *Relative humidity (Fig. 20)*: It affects the susceptibility of microorganisms in the AHU as well as the duct where it is used. The susceptibility factor for the viruses was higher at 55% RH than that at 85% RH (*Tseng et al.: Inactivation of viruscontaining aerosols by ultraviolet germicidal irradiation, Aerosol Sci Technol 2005*). Microbial susceptibility to UVGI—may increase or decrease, depending on the organism.
- *Temperature*: Temperature affects the UV output of the lamp. Temperatures below 13.3°C (56°F) inside the AHU reduces the output to lower than 50% of the full output.

(Refer ASHRAE 2012 Systems and Equipment Handbook, Chapter 17 for further details)

Another consideration for the lamp selection is the lamp fouling factor when it is covered with dust. There is an advantage of locating the lamps downstream of high efficiency filters to protect them from dust accumulation. Otherwise, the lamps will need to be cleaned from time to time. A point to note is that UVC can disinfect a pathogen only if it can reach it either directly or through reflection. In general, reducing the total number of pathogens reduces the risk of transmission.

UVGI is being used as an engineering control to interrupt the transmission of pathogenic organisms, such as *Mycobacterium tuberculosis* (TB), influenza viruses (including COVID-19 virus), mold, and possible bioterrorism agents (*Brickner 2003; CDC 2002, 2005; General Services Administration 2003*).

Fungal spores are larger than most bacteria and are more resistant to UVGI than most bacteria. For spores, UVC exposure is postulated to result in the formation of lethal photoactive products (*Memarzadeh et al., American Journal of Infection Control, June 2010*). For removal of spores, high efficiency air filtration, viz. MERV14 or superior, would be a better choice. Using a combination of UVGI and high efficiency filters can be an effective solution in certain situations.

Table 4: Classification of EPA, HEPA and ULPA filters.

Filter group Filter Class	Integral value		Local value[ab]	
	Efficiency (%)	Penetration (%)	Efficiency (%)	Penetration (%)
E10	≥85	≤15	---[c]	---[c]
E11	≥95	≤5	---[c]	---[c]
E12	≥99,5	≤0,5	---[c]	---[c]
H13	≥99,95	≤0,05	≥99,75	≤0,25
H14	≥99,995	≤0,005	≥99,975	≤0,025
U15	≥99,9995	≤0,0005	≥99,9975	≤0,0025
U16	≥99,99995	≤0,00005	≥99,99975	≤0,00025
U17	≥99,999995	≤0,000005	≥99,9999	≤0,0001

[a] See 7.5.2 and EN ISO 29463-4.

[b] Local penetration values lower than those given in the table may be agreed between supplier and purchaser.

[c] Group E filters (Classes E10, E11 and E12) cannot and shall not be leak tested for classification purposes.

Note: ISO 29463-1:2017 developed by ISO/TC 142 includes a classification system for high efficiency air filters according to their filtration performance (efficiency or penetration) similar to EN 1822-1

[E series: EPA# efficient particulate air (Filter); h series: HEPA# high efficiency particulate air (filter); U series: ULPA# ultra low particulate air (filter)].

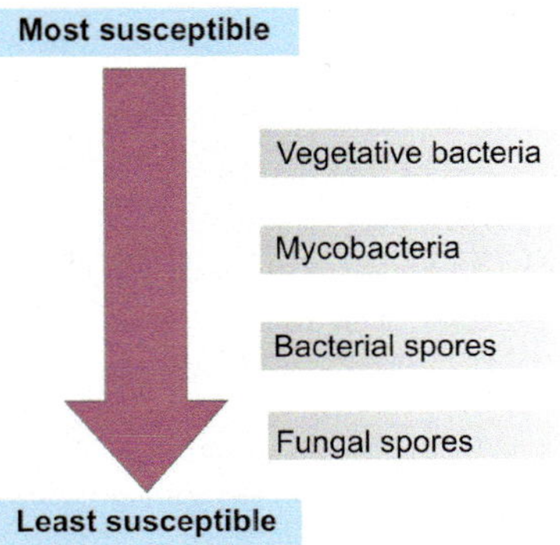

Fig. 20: Susceptibility of microorganisms to ultraviolet germicidal irradiation (UVGI).

Reference: ASHRAE-2008c.

CDC guideline addresses UVGI as a supplemental engineering control and are classified as Category II, 'Suggested for implementation and supported by suggestive clinical or epidemiological studies, or a theoretic rationale'.

UVGI is used in two formats in the Air Conditioning Systems

In AHUs: UVGI directed at environmental surfaces can damage microorganisms present or growing on the surface. Lower-intensity UVGI is effective for surface inactivation because irradiation is applied continuously. UVGI from lamps in AHU plenums has been used successfully to inactivate microorganisms present on airstream surfaces such as on cooling coils and drain pans (*Menzies et al. 1999, 2003*). This helps in keeping the cooling coils and drain pans clean. Since the bio films that normally develop on the heat exchange surface get eliminated, studies have indicated better heat transfer because of the UVGI radiation. Menzies et al. found a significant decline in building-related symptoms associated with use of UVGI in AHUs though significant declines in airborne levels of fungi and bacteria as well as endotoxins were not detected in the workplace.

In Ducts: UV lamps placed in ductwork have been used to inactivate Mycobacterium species and other microorganisms. The residence time of the microbe under UVGI illumination is an important factor while considering the UVGI lamp design inside the duct. This is achieved by installing the UV lamps parallel to the airflow inside the ducts (Figs. 21 and 22).

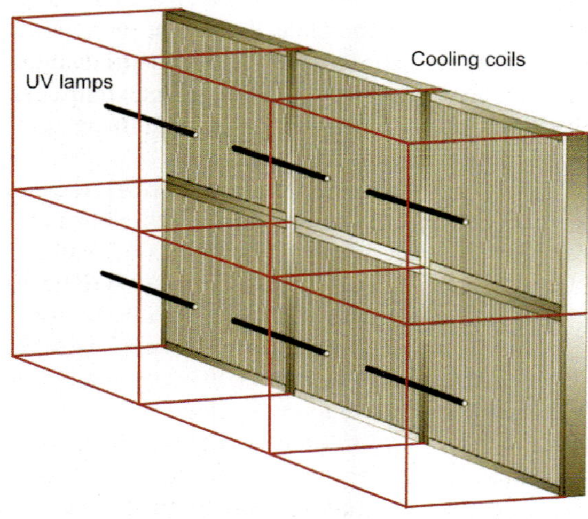

Fig. 21: UVGI lamps for irradiating cooling coil.

Diagram from Ultraviolet Germicidal Irradiation Handbook: Wladyslaw Kowalski, Springer Publication.

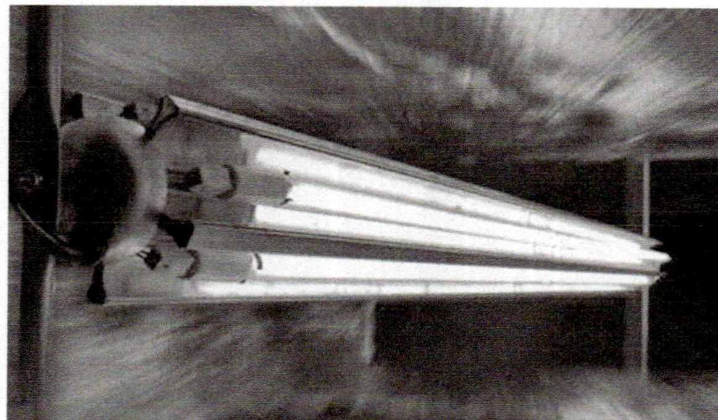

Fig. 22: Multiple UV lamp fixture for installation in ventilation ductwork.

Photograph of Sanuvox from Ultraviolet Germicidal Irradiation Handbook: Wladyslaw Kowalski, Springer Publication.

Safety Requirements for UVC

Inadvertent exposure to UVC can be dangerous for humans. Doors, covers and lamp mounting brackets that give direct access to UV radiation lamp systems shall be equipped with an interlocking mechanism that removes power from the UV radiation lamp system when the door is open or cover removed.

Further, polymeric cabinet, structural, and current carrying parts and wiring which are subjected to irradiance from a UV lamp system will need to be shielded from the UVC light or be constructed of a material that is capable of withstanding UVC exposure levels expected in the product without degrading.

Apart from air conditioning systems, UVGI lamps can be fitted in rooms to intercept microbes inside the room where they may be generated by occupants, thereby controlling infection at the source. When used in rooms, the systems are called **Upper Room UV systems** (Fig. 23). The Upper Room UV systems create a germicidal zone of UV rays. This zone is confined to the upper portion of the room. Air that enters this zone gets disinfected. Upper air UV disinfection is considered to be the most practical method of airborne infection control in resource limited locations since they are passive (no moving parts), have modest costs, and consume very low energy unlike air conditioning and mechanical ventilation systems which can be prohibitive. Safety issues associated with Upper Room are addressed in the CDC/NIOSH and recommend REL of 0.006 J/cm^2, or 60 J/m^2 (at 254 nm) for 8 hours of exposure.

The UV reflectance hazards for Upper Room (and Lower Room) systems should not be ignored and care should be taken to ensure there are no highly UV-reflective ceiling paints or materials in locations that may direct reflected UV rays towards the eyes or skin.

Air Distribution

It is not only air filtration and differential pressure that is important for infection control but how the air is introduced into the room and then how it sweeps away the contaminants is also important. The air supply has to reach each part of the space to improve dilution and remove the pollutants from the space. A few examples will make the concept clear.

- Airborne infectious isolation (AII room), also called the negative isolation room, the people in the outside corridor and the healthcare workers will need to be protected from the patient. The room is thus kept under negative pressure. The healthcare worker should be safe when attending to the patient and the latter's respiration should be directly exhausted. The air pattern shown in Figure 24 just do that. The clean air from the supply air duct comes first on the healthcare worker and thence to the patient and then exhausted from the nearby exhaust grille.

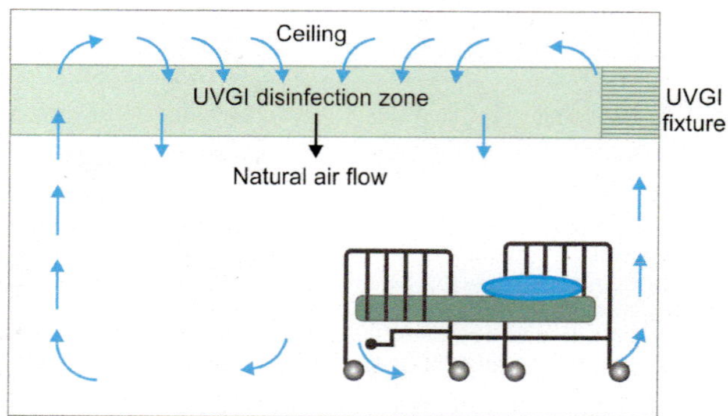

Fig. 23: Upper-room ultraviolet system (schematic from ScienceDirect).

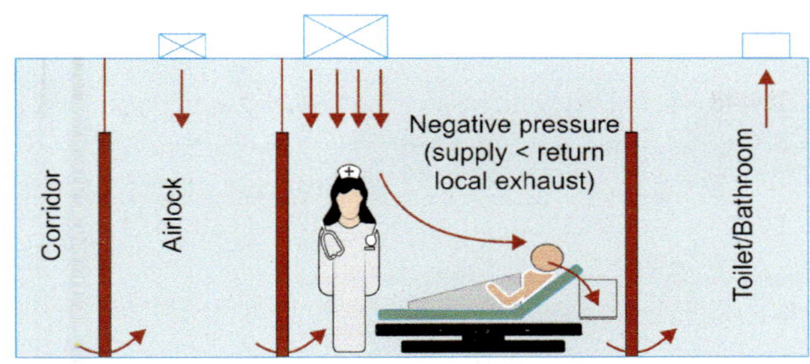

Fig. 24: Air distribution pattern for a (negative pressure) airborne infection isolation (AII) room.

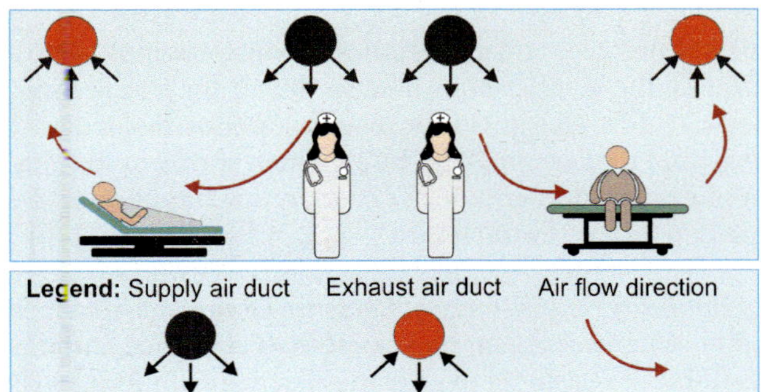

Fig. 25: Air distribution pattern for an ICU.

- In infectious intensive care unit (ICU) (Fig. 25) the air pattern will have to ensure that the aisles have clean air and so do the patients. The respiration from the patients will have viral load which will have to be swept away by the room air directly into the exhaust without mixing in the room air.
- Air patterns for window, Wall mounted and Cassette split air conditioners.

  (*As recommended in IMA-HBI-ISHRAE COVID-19 Guidance Document for Air-conditioning and Ventilation in Healthcare Facilities*).

Considering that the virus spreads through coughing and sneezing by an infected patient, it is important to ensure that the draft of air from the AC unit is not directed to the occupants. It is recommended to direct the supply air into the occupied zone in such a way that a high velocity draft is avoided. Window and wall mount split AC units and cassettes have setting to direct the air flow. See the illustrated Figures 26 and 27 for reference.

The air patterns in rooms dealing with **quarantine and triage in emergency rooms**, need to be from clean to dirty axis, as part of design considerations, as this impacts the transmission of disease.

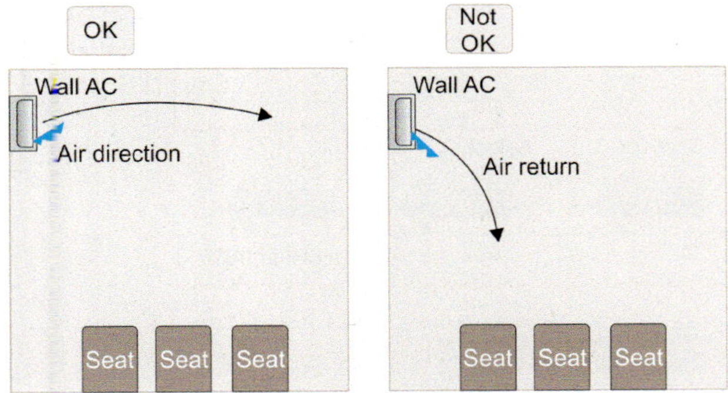

Fig. 26: Air pattern for wall mounted AC units.

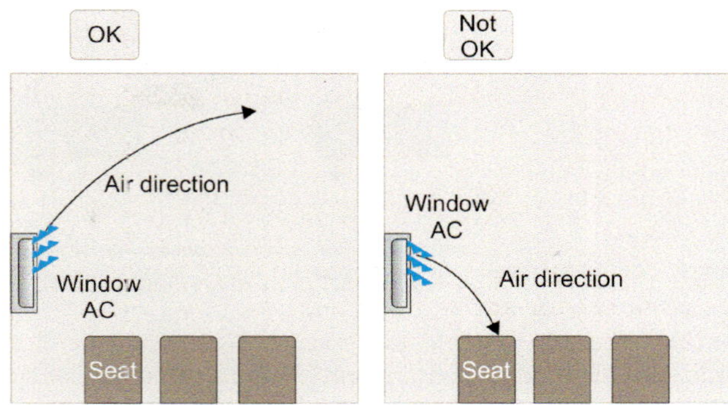

Fig. 27: Air pattern for window AC Units.

Some Important Points Regarding Air Distribution with Ducted Systems

- False ceiling returns are not acceptable because of the fact that the plenum above the false ceiling is not cleanable and thus can be a place where pathogens can grow.
- In recirculatory AHUs or ducted split units, the units shall not be shared between different rooms/zones because infection in one room/zone may get conveyed into the other rooms/zones.

General Notes on Maintenance of HVAC Systems

Location of AC equipment and its servicing: All AC equipment require servicing from time to time, whether it is to attend to the parts or for cleaning the filters which puts the unitary equipment viz. wall units, window AC units, ducted splits and cassettes, at a disadvantage in areas with contagion, as the technicians are at considerable risk in such areas and servicing with PPE suits can be very inconvenient.

Cleaning of filters: Filters, whether of recirculatory AHUs, unitary AC units or of exhaust units, are likely to have high viral load and cleaning these filters put the technician to high level of risk, so the use of filter cleaning booths is advocated, which are to be located in a designated safe area and the technicians attending to the filter cleaning activity need to wear appropriate PPE. Sewage treatment of the water used for cleaning must be taken care of.

Disposal of HEPA filters: The replacement of HEPA filters must be done by trained personnel wearing the necessary PPE and disposal of these filters to be done in accordance with "Bio medical waste" regulations.

Cleaning of UVGI lamps: The UVGI lamps fitted in the AC systems function well only if they are not covered with dust and maintenance schedule in the facility must include cleaning of these lamps.

Condensate drain for AC equipment: Water from the condensate drain of AC equipment must be treated for viral load before discharge into sewage and it is not to be recycled for any usage.

Maintenance of all equipment: All HVAC equipment are required to be serviced and maintained as per the recommendations of the respective manufacturers.

Room Pressure Gradient

Although the quantity of air distributed to the space and the air patterns are important from air quality view point, space pressurization is even more important. The quantity of air in supply, return, fresh and exhaust

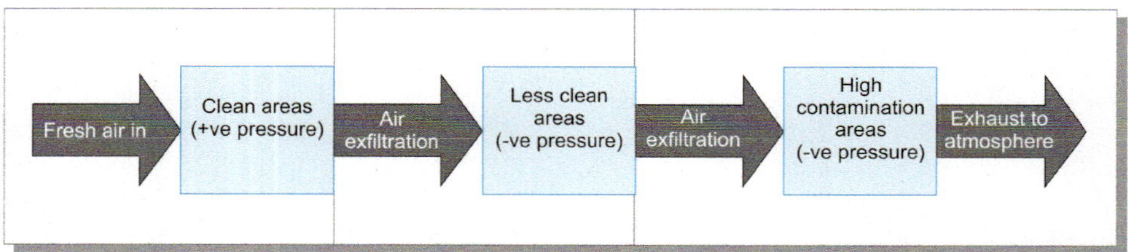

Fig. 28: Pressure gradient to achieve air exfiltration from clean to contaminated rooms.[9,10]

air should be balanced so that air travels from the cleanest space to the dirtiest space or from least contaminated to highly contaminated areas (Fig. 28).

In COVID healthcare facilities, the administrative areas, doctors' rooms, nursing stations, reception areas may be considered among the cleaner areas. The triage and quarantine areas have higher levels of contamination and the ICUs, isolation rooms, washrooms, changing rooms and doffing areas have the highest levels of contamination. Accordingly, the room pressure gradient has to be planned as shown below:

The ASHRAE Standard 170-2017 recommends the pressure gradients for the various areas/rooms in a hospital and indicates the areas that need positive, negative or neutral pressure with respect to the surroundings. In particular the isolation rooms and ICUs pressure gradient has to be lower than –2.5 Pa compared to the adjoining areas. Introduction of an airlock (also called ante room) outside these critical rooms (isolation rooms and ICUs) can significantly improve the barrier effectiveness when doors get opened and the pressures are equalized. The illustration in Figure 29 "ASHRAE Design Guide" for Clean rooms makes the concept clear.

Relative Humidity

Moisture in the air is the first arm of defense of our immune system. Studies have shown that our body cannot fight with the respiratory particles or pathogens as adequately when we're in a dry environment. Further, the infectivity of the bacteria too increases with low humidity. Relative humidity of at least 40% is considered the threshold.

All microorganisms need water to grow initially. Very high humidity leads to higher levels of dust mites and fungi, which exacerbate respiratory conditions symptoms, cough, wheeze and asthma. Immunosuppressed or immunocompromised patients are at increased risk.

Effect of humidity on airborne transmission of cough aerosol: Small particles get generated during the course of coughing and sneezing and to a lesser extent by even talking and breathing. Particle size distributions of coughed materials encompass a broad spectrum of diameters, from very small to large droplets. It is known that most of the viable particles ranging from 0.65 to 3.3 μm in the cough-generated aerosols are immediately respirable (*KP Fennelly et al. "Cough-generated Aerosols of Mycobacterium tuberculosis: A New Method to Study Infectiousness," American Journal of Respiratory and Critical Care Medicine*).

While big particles and droplets from cough promptly fall to ground and surfaces, the smaller ones float in the air for a long time. Small particles <5 μ (droplet nuclei or residue) are formed from droplets (usually within milliseconds) in the air which shrink in size due to the process of evaporation and desiccation in low humidity and remain suspended in air for several hours.

Effect of Humidity on Virulence of Bacteria: Organisms that have been exposed to dry environment have increased virulence and increased rates of antibiotic resistance even in the absence of antibiotics (Fig. 30).

Apart from virus, there is a correlation of humidity with the growth of various pathogens as given in the Sterling chart (Fig. 31).

All things considered, the humidity level of 40% ~ 60% is considered to be the most suitable environment for humans and decreases problems from pathogens.

Temperature

As recommended in IMA-HBI-ISHRAE COVID-19 recommends temperature range of 24–30°C for comfort conditioning, in case the job requires use of special clothing, e.g., PPE for healthcare staff, temperature lower than 24°C may be considered to ensure sufficient dissipation of heat released from body through heavier clothing.

Exhaust

Another important aspect is how to deal with the used air or exhaust air. It is especially true when dealing with all infected patient areas viz. triage, quarantine and critical when dealing with ICUs, isolation rooms and patient area washrooms. Hospital exhausts can have inordinate load of pathogens and we have to be careful where we exhaust the air. The exhaust air must be protected for containment by at least MERV10 grade filters. The exhaust air from isolation rooms and ICUs is most likely to contain a high viral load and hence a suitable technique should be deployed to prevent the spread of infections. Treatment of exhaust air can be done preferably by HEPA H13 (EN1822-1) filter class or equivalent. It is preferable to install them at the primary point of air

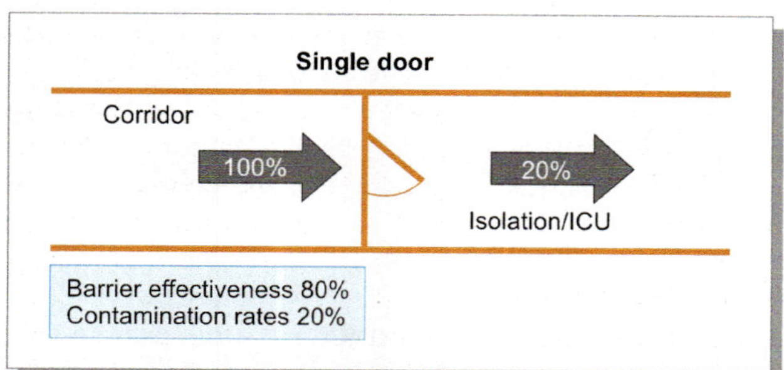

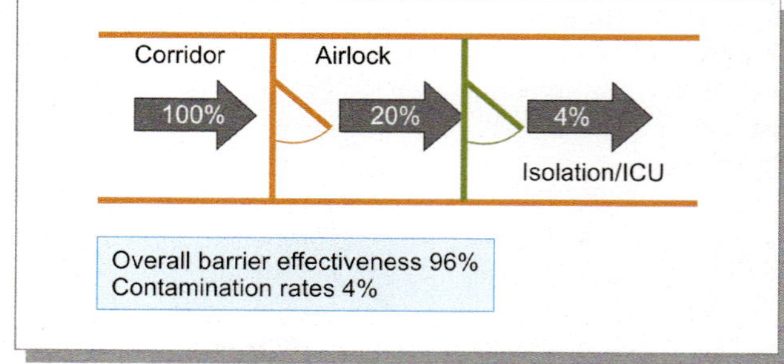

Fig. 29: Advantage of using airlock for contamination control.

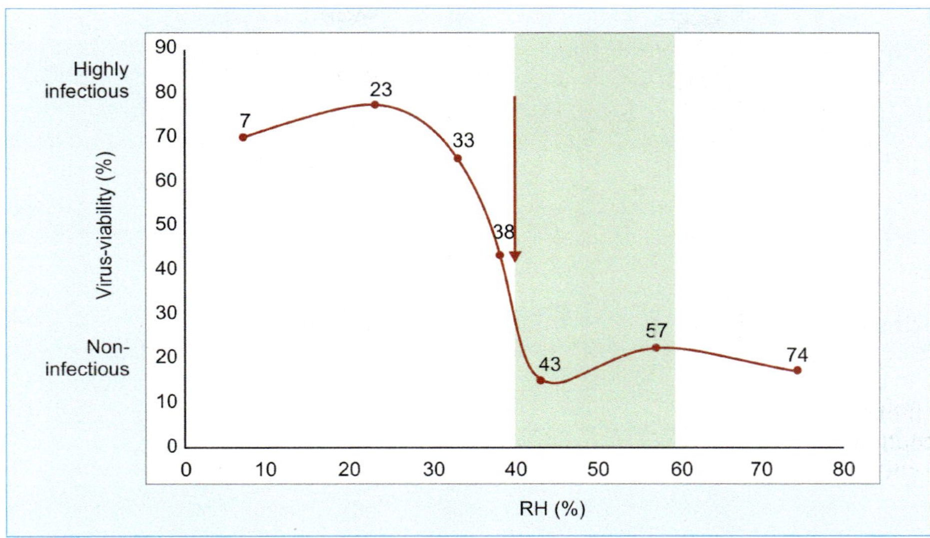

Fig. 30: Stephanie Taylor, Presenter, "Optimize Occupant Health, Building Energy Performance and Revenue through Indoor-Air Hydration," ASHRAE.

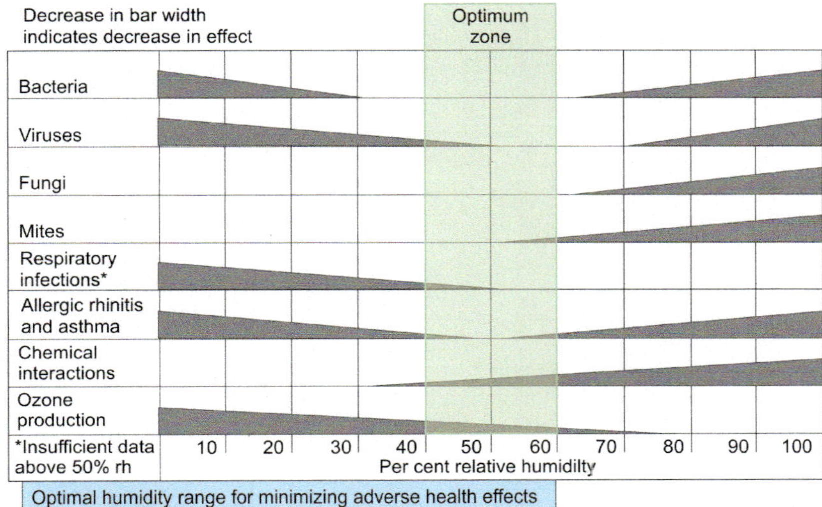

Fig. 31: Criteria for human exposure to humidity in occupied buildings, EM Sterling, 1985 ASHRAE Transactions CH85-13-1.

extraction in the room and the exhaust blower shall be at the discharge end of the exhaust duct in order to maintain a negative pressure in the exhaust duct.

Another acceptable method is treatment of exhaust air by Chemical disinfection. This can be done by bubbling the exhaust air through a "Diffused air aerator tank" (preferably of non-metallic material) holding a 1% sodium hypochlorite solution.[2]

When both the above methods are not viable, the exhaust air shall be let off into the atmosphere through a high velocity upward plume at a height of 3 meter above the tallest point of the building, thereby lowering the viral load concentrations to insignificant levels by dilution. This exhaust discharge shall be well away from other air intake points and populated places.

Two other options available for treatment of exhaust air are UV irradiation and Heating (*MER Darnell et al. Observed that, an exposure time of 45 min at a temperature of 75°C resulted in complete inactivation of SARS-CoV*). Similarly, irradiation with UVC of 254 nm wavelength, with an exposure time of 15 minutes at irradiation intensity of 4016 μW/cm² resulted in complete inactivation of SARS-CoV.

The HVAC guidelines that are adapted from the IGBC Green guidelines are depicted in Tables 5 to 15.

Upper Room UV Systems can be a Beneficial Addition for Air Purification.

Energy Efficiency

HVAC systems mostly work 24×7 and thereby consume a lot of energy. It is important to avoid profligate designs so as to adopt the energy efficiency as an important parameter. While choosing various components of the HVAC system, wherever possible, choose environment friendly options. As detailed in previous section of this chapter, the Level-I, Level-II or Level-III facilities may have access to varied resources and affordability.

Finally, there are converted facilities, which are functioning hospitals and nursing homes converted to COVID hospitals.

To provide comfort and sweep out pathogens in the healthcare facilities, various options available to date are Natural ventilation, Mechanical ventilation, Air conditioning with unitary equipment viz. wall units/window air conditioners or cassettes or with AHU systems

Table 5: HVAC essentials for ICU.[9]

Temperature °F [°C]	*Relative humidity %*	*Room pressure with respect to surroundings*	*Minimum fresh air ACH*	*Minimum recirculation air ACH*	*Only AHU*	*Unitary AC + Fresh Air/ Exhaust Modules*	*Mechanical ventilation*	*Natural ventilation*	*Remarks*
70°F~75°F [21~24]	40~70%	> (–) 2.5 Pa	12	Nil	Only AHU	Unitary AC + Fresh Air/ Exhaust Modules acceptable for converted hospitals only	N/A	N/A	-
Filtration					MERV7 + MERV14 for AHU	Coarse Filters of AC units and (MERV7 + MERV14) for Fresh Air Module	N/A	N/A	H13 HEPA/Chemical treatment/Plume for Exhaust for both AHU based and Unitary AC systems
					UVGI for Cooling coil for AHU option				UVGI for Cooling coil for AHU option

Table 6: HVAC essentials for negative isolation room and quarantine facilities.[9]

Room type	*Temperature °F [°C]*	*Relative humidity%*	*Room pressure with respect to surroundings*	*Minimum fresh air ACH*	*Minimum recirculation air ACH*	*Only AHU*	*Unitary AC + Fresh Air/Exhaust Modules*	*Mechanical ventilation*	*Natural ventilation*	*Remarks #*
Airborne infectious isolation (AII), also called negative isolation room	70°F~75°F [21~24]	40~70%	> (–) 2.5 Pa	12	Nil	Only AHU	Unitary AC + Fresh Air/ Exhaust Modules acceptable for converted hospitals only	N/A	N/A	UVGI for cooling coil for AHU
	Filtration					MERV7 + MERV14 for AHU	Coarse filters of AC units and (MERV7 + MERV14) for Fresh Air Module	N/A	N/A	H13 HEPA/ Chemical treatment/ Plume for exhaust for both AHU based and unitary AC systems
Quarantine	70°F~75°F [21~24]	40~70%	Negative	2	12	AHU	Unitary AC + Fresh Air/ Exhaust Modules acceptable for converted hospitals only	Mechanical ventilation with minimum 12 ACH fresh air supply	Natural ventilation (supply air 160 L/s per person)	
	Filtration					MERV7 + MERV14 for AHU	Coarse Filters of AC units and (MERV7 + MERV14) for Fresh Air Module	(MERV7 + MERV14) for supply air	N/A	• All exhausts to be to safe place • Upper room UVGI recommended for all options • UVGI for cooling coil for AHU option • Duct mounted UVGI for supply air for AHU

Table 7: HVAC essentials for TRIAGE lab facilites.[9,10]

Room type	Temperature °F [°C]	Relative humidity %	Room pressure with respect to surroundings	Minimum fresh air ACH	Minimum recirculation air ACH	Only AHU	Unitary AC + Fresh Air/Exhaust Modules	Mechanical ventilation	Natural ventilation	Remarks
Triage	70°F~75°F [21~24]	40~70%	Negative	2	12	AHU	Unitary AC + Fresh Air/Exhaust Modules (for Converted Hospitals only)	Mechanical ventilation with minimum 12 ACH fresh air supply	Natural ventilation (supply air 160 L/s per person)	
			Filtration			MERV7 + MERV14 for AHU	Coarse Filters of AC units and (MERV7 + MERV14) for Fresh Air Module	(MERV7 + MERV14) for fresh air supply	N/A	• All exhausts to be to safe place • Upper room UVGI for all options • UVGI for cooling coil for AHU option • Duct mounted UVGI for supply air for AHU option.
Laboratory	70°F~75°F [21~24]	N/R	Negative	2	6	AHU	Unitary AC + Fresh Air/Exhaust Modules	Mechanical ventilation with minimum 12 ACH fresh air supply	N/A	
			Filtration			MERV7 for AHU	MERV7 for Fresh Air	MERV7 for fresh air supply	N/A	• All exhausts to be to safe place • UVGI for cooling coil for AHU option

Table 8: HVAC essentials in lab, residents room and dining facilities.[9]

Room type	Temperature °F [°C]	Relative humidity %	Room pressure with respect to surroundings	Minimum fresh air ACH	Minimum recirculation air ACH	Only AHU	Unitary AC + Fresh Air/ Exhaust Modules	Mechanical ventilation	Natural ventilation	Remarks
Laboratory, glass washing and laboratory, sterilizing	70°F~75°F [21~24]	N/R	Negative	2	10	AHU	Unitary AC + Fresh Air Modules	Mechanical Ventilation with minimum 12 ACH fresh air supply	N/A	
			Filtration			MERV7 for AHU	MERV7 for Fresh Air	MERV7 for fresh air supply	N/A	All exhausts to be to safe place
Resident gathering/ Activity/ Dining	70°F~75°F [21~24]	N/R	N/R	4	4	AHU	Unitary AC + Fresh Air Modules	Mechanical ventilation with minimum 12 ACH fresh air supply	Natural ventilation (supply air 160 L/s per person)	UVGI for cooling coil for AHU option
			Filtration			MERV7 for AHU	MERV7 for Fresh Air	MERV7 for fresh air supply	N/A	• All exhausts to be to safe place • Upper Room UVGI Recommended for all options • UVGI for cooling coil for AHU option • Duct mounted UVGI for supply air for AHU option

Table 9: HVAC essentials for physio therapy and change rooms.[9]

Room type	*Temperature °F [°C]*	*Relative humidity %*	*Room pressure with respect to surroundings*	*Minimum fresh air ACH*	*Minimum recirculation air ACH*	*Only AHU*	*Unitary AC + Fresh Air/ Exhaust Modules*	*Mechanical ventilation*	*Natural ventilation*	*Remarks*
Physical therapy	70°F~75°F [21~24]	N/R	Negative	2	6	AHU	Unitary AC + Fresh Air Modules	Mechanical ventilation with minimum 12 ACH fresh air supply	Natural ventilation (supply air 160 L/s per person)	
			Filtration			MERV7 for AHU	MERV 7 for Fresh Air	MERV7 for fresh air supply	N/A	• All exhausts to be to safe place • Upper Room UVGI Recommended for all options • UVGI for cooling coil for AHU option • Duct mounted UVGI for supply air for AHU option
Main entry/ External change room	70°F~75°F [21~24]	N/R	Positive	2	12	AHU	Unitary AC + Fresh Air/ Exhaust Modules	Mechanical ventilation (minimum 12 ACH supply)	N/A	
			Filtration			MERV7 for AHU	MERV7 for Fresh Air	MERV7 for fresh air	N/A	• All exhausts to be to safe place • Upper Room UVGI Recommended for all options • UVGI for cooling coil for AHU option • Duct mounted UVGI for supply air for AHU option

Table 10: HVAC essentials in donning and doffing areas.[9]

Room type	*Temperature °F [°C]*	*Relative humidity%*	*Room pressure with respect to surroundings*	*Minimum fresh air ACH*	*Minimum recirculation air ACH*	*Only AHU*	*Unitary AC + Fresh Air/ Exhaust Modules*	*Mechanical ventilation*	*Natural ventilation*	*Remarks*
(Entry to COVID Zone)/ Change room/ Donning area	70°F~75°F [21~24]	N/R	Positive	2	12	AHU	Unitary AC + Fresh Air/ Exhaust Modules	Mechanical ventilation (minimum 12 ACH supply)	N/A	
			Filtration			MERV7 for AHU	MERV7 for Fresh Air	MERV7 for fresh air	N/A	• All exhausts to be to safe place • Upper Room UVGI recommended for all options • UVGI for cooling coil for AHU option • Duct mounted UVGI for supply air for AHU option
Change room/ Doffing area	70°F~75°F [21~24]	N/R	Positive	2	12	AHU	Unitary AC + Fresh Air/ Exhaust Modules	Mechanical Ventilation (minimum 12 ACH fresh air supply)	N/A	
	Filtration					MERV7 for AHU	MERV 7 for Fresh Air	MERV7 for Fresh air	N/A	• H13 HEPA/Chemical treatment/Plume for exhaust for both AHU based/Unitary AC systems/Mechanical ventilation systems • Upper room UVGI recommended for all options • UVGI for cooling coil for AHU option • Duct mounted UVGI for supply air for AHU option

Table 11: HVAC essentials in doctors/nurses room and food preparation center.[9]

Room type	Temperature °F [°C]	Relative humidity %	Room pressure with respect to surroundings	Minimum fresh air ACH	Minimum recirculation air ACH	Only AHU	Unitary AC + Fresh Air/ Exhaust Modules	Mechanical ventilation	Natural ventilation	Remarks
Doctors' room/ Nurses' room	70°F~75°F [21~24]	N/R	Positive	2	6	AHU	Unitary AC + Fresh Air Modules	Mechanical ventilation (minimum 12 ACH fresh air supply)	N/A	
			Filtration			MERV7 for AHU	MERV7 for Fresh Air	MERV7 for fresh Air	N/A	• All exhausts to be to safe place • UVGI for cooling coil for AHU option • Duct mounted • UVGI for supply air for AHU option
Food preparation center	70°F~75°F [21~24]	N/R	Negative	2	10	AHU	Unitary AC + Fresh Air/ Exhaust Modules	Mechanical Ventilation (minimum 12 ACH fresh air supply)	N/A	
			Filtration			MERV7 for AHU	MERV7 for fresh Air	N/A	N/A	• UVGI for cooling coil for AHU option • Duct mounted • UVGI for supply air for AHU option

Table 12: HVAC essentials in laundry, janitor's closet, dietary, clean linen and wash room.[9]

Room type	Temperature °F [°C]	Relative humidity %	Room pressure with respect to surroundings	Minimum fresh air ACH	Minimum recirculation air ACH	Only AHU	Unitary AC + Fresh Air/ Exhaust Modules	Mechanical ventilation	Natural ventilation	Remarks
Ware washing/ Laundry/Soiled linen/Bedpan	N/R	N/R	Negative		10 [exhaust only]	N/A		Mechanical ventilation (10 ACH exhaust only)	N/A	
Room/ Janitor's closet/ Bathroom/ Sterilizer Equip room			Filtration					MERV7	N/A	
Dietary storage	70°F~75°F [21~24]	N/R	N/R	2	10	AHU		Mechanical ventilation (minimum 10 ACH fresh air supply)	N/A	
			Filtration			MERV7 for AHU		MERV7	N/A	UVGI for cooling coil for AHU option
Clean linen room	70°F~75°F [21~24]	N/R	Positive	2	10	AHU	Unitary AC + Fresh Air/ Exhaust Modules	Mechanical ventilation (10 ACH supply)	N/A	
			Filtration			MERV7 for AHU	MERV7 for Fresh Air	MERV7 for fresh air	N/A	UVGI for cooling coil for AHU option
Wash room	N/R	N/R	Negative		10	N/A	Exhaust fan only	Exhaust fan only	N/A	
			Filtration			N/A	N/A	Please refer Remarks#1	N/A	H13 HEPA/ Chemical treatment/Plume

Table 13: HVAC essentials in various areas.[9,10]

Function of space	Temperature °F [°C]	Relative humidity %	Room pressure with respect to surroundings	Outside air (minimum ACH)	Recirculation air [minimum ACH]
Food preparation center	70°F~75°F [21~24]	N/R	Negative	2	10
Ware washing	N/R	N/R	Negative		10 [exhaust only]
Dietary storage	70°F~75°F [21~24]	N/R	N/R	10	Nil
Laundry, general	N/R	N/R	Negative	10	Nil
Soiled linen sorting and storage	N/R	N/R	Negative	10	Nil
Clean linen room	70°F~75°F [21~24]	N/R	Positive	2	10
Bedpan room	N/R	N/R	Negative	10	Nil
Bathroom	N/R	N/R	Negative	10	Nil
Janitor's closet	N/R	N/R	Negative	10	Nil
Sterilizer equipment room	N/R	N/R	Negative	10	Nil

Table 14: Negative pressure isolation room parameter.[9,10]

S. No.	Room name	Ventilation frequency	Area
1.	Ward toilet	12 times/h	Heavily contaminated
2.	Ward	12 times/h	Contaminated area
3.	Patient corridor	6 times/h	Semi-contaminated area
4.	Buffer room	6 times/h	
5.	Treatment room	6 times/h	Semi-clean area
6.	Medical staff corridor	6 times/h	
7.	Medical staff office, Dressing room	6 times/h	Clean area

Table 15: Advantages and disadvantages of different types of ventilation system used in hospitals.[9,10]

	Mechanical ventilation	Natural ventilation	Hybrid (mixed-mode) ventilation
Advantages	• Suitable for all climates and weather with air-conditioning as climate dictates • More controlled and comfortable environment	• Suitable for warm and temperate climates-moderately useful with natural ventilation possible 50% of the time. • Lower capital, operational and maintenance costs for simple natural ventilation • Capable of achieving high ventilation rate	• Suitable for most climates and weather • Energy-saving • More flexible
Disadvantages	• Expensive to install and maintain • Reported failure rate in delivering the required outdoor ventilation rate • Potential for noise from equipment	• Easily affected by outdoor climate and/ or occupant's behavior • More difficult to predict, analyse and design • Reduces comfort level of occupants when hot, humid or cold • Inability to establish negative pressure in isolation areas, but may be provided by proper design; depends on situation • Potential for noise intrusion • High-tech natural ventilation shares some of the limitations and disadvantages of mechanical ventilation	• May be expensive • May be more difficult to design

with filtration, and the development and maintenance costs increase in the same order.

Natural ventilation: It depends on favorable climate conditions like no risk of heat stress or no air pollution. It also depends on cross ventilation and convection principles and the facility need to have the required attributes to make this a feasible option.

Mechanical ventilation: It is an option where the climate is favorable but natural ventilation is not practical in terms of availability of the necessary cross ventilation. It is acceptable in certain areas viz. quarantine, triage, resident gathering/activity/dining and physical therapy rooms. It is a practical option in service areas viz. washroom, janitor room and store rooms.

The type of mechanical ventilation used depends on the climate. For example, in warm and humid climates, infiltration may need to be minimized or prevented to reduce interstitial condensation (which occurs when warm, moist air from inside a building penetrates a wall, roof or floor and meets a cold surface). In these cases, a positive-pressure mechanical ventilation system is often used. Conversely, in cold climates, exfiltration needs to be prevented to reduce interstitial condensation, and negative-pressure ventilation is used.

For rooms with locally generated pollutants, such as bathrooms, toilets and kitchens, a negative-pressure system is often used.

Mechanical fans drive mechanical ventilation. Fans can either be installed directly in windows or walls, or be installed in air ducts for supplying air into or exhausting air from a room.

A mechanically ventilated AII room as described by the United States Centers for Disease Control and Prevention (CDC), should have special features in air handling and airflow direction:

- It should achieve a negative-pressure differential >2.5 Pa (0.01 inch water gauge) in the isolation room or have an airflow differential >56 l/s (125 cfm) exhaust versus supply.
- Achieve a clean-to-dirty airflow.
- Have sealing of the room, allowing approximately 0.046 m^2 (0.5 sqft) leakage.
- Supply air has to be more than 12 ACH for a new building, or more than 6 ACH for an existing building (equivalent to 40 l/s for a room measuring 4 × 2 × 3 m for an old building), and
- An exhaust to the outside, or use of a HEPA filter if room air is recirculated.

When the AII room is air-conditioned and is at negative pressure, outside air will infiltrate into the room. If the outside air is warm and humid, it will lead to interstitial condensation. This can be taken care of by having proper vapor barrier paints for the walls and the ceiling. Having a positive pressure airlock at entry to the AII room will also help.

***Air conditioning with unitary equipment*:** It is an economical option where mechanical ventilation cannot provide necessary comfort. Unitary equipment like wall units, window air-conditioners or cassettes can be used for air-conditioning. But the shortcoming of providing such systems is that the requisite air filtration is not there and there is no provision of fresh air. It can be used in quarantine, triage, and patient waiting areas, doctors' and nurses' rooms. Separate provision for inducting fresh air can be made and where necessary provide room pressure gradient by exhaust modules.

***Air conditioning with AHUs*:** It incorporates the necessary air filtration and is the only option for critical areas viz. isolation rooms and ICUs. It is also the preferred option for quarantine and triage. The AHUs can induct fresh air and also create the necessary pressure gradients. Although, it is a good option for air conditioning need of other areas but the economy of using the same has to be evaluated first.

IGBC recommends that after setup of the system; ensure complete flush out of the system for about 72 hours, so that all the pollutants including the dust particles and volatile organic compounds (VOCs) are completely flushed out.

***Hybrid or mixed-mode ventilation*:** Hybrid or mixed-mode ventilation depends on natural driving forces to provide the desired (design) flow rate, and uses mechanical ventilation when the natural ventilation flow rate is too low.

When natural ventilation alone is not suitable, exhaust fans can be installed to increase ventilation rates in rooms housing patients with airborne infections. If the environment in the room causes thermal discomfort, spot cooling or heating systems and ceiling fans may be added. Another possibility is the installation of whirlybirds (whirligigs/wind turbines) that do not require electricity and provide a roof-exhaust system increasing airflow in a building.

Advantages and disadvantages of different types of ventilation systems that may be utilized in Hospitals is shown in Table 15.

Energy Efficiency

Although healthcare facilities are energy intensive but good energy management practices can reduce energy consumption to the tune of 30–40% and can reduce the operational expenses. Focus on achieving energy efficiency without compromising on the quality of healthcare facilities to the patients. The energy consumption of HVAC systems is very high and take steps to ensure that the installed systems are energy efficient. Measures that need to be considered for implementation of energy efficient equipment in the Emergency COVID facilities are:

Air conditioning system:

- Use of CFC free refrigerant HVAC systems.
- Install Halon free fire suppression systems.
- Use unitary air-conditioners with BEE 3-star rating (or) air-conditioners with a COP equivalent to 3.1.

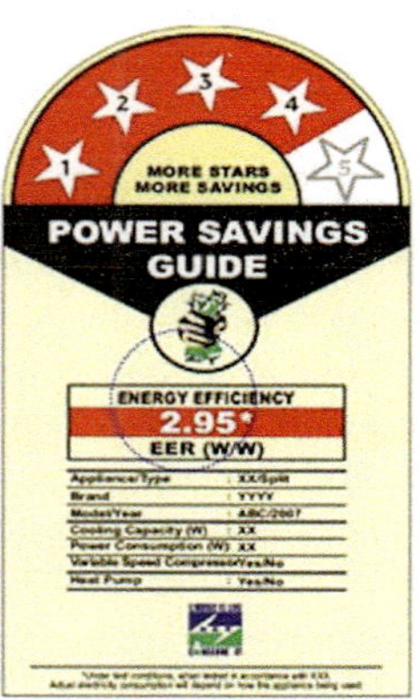

Lighting:

- Use efficient lighting fixtures such as LEDs/CFLs.

Other equipment:

- Use fans with efficiency equivalent to BEE 3-star rating or more.
- Install Pumps and Motors in the building with efficiency equivalent to BEE 3-star rating or more.
- Use efficient hot water systems such as solar hot water systems or BEE star rated geysers.

New COVID Healthcare Facilities

Air-conditioned Healthcare Facilities

Design the facility to comply with Energy Conservation Building Code (Revised Version May, 2008) (or) ASHRAE Standard 90.1-2013 (without amendments) through one of the following approaches:

- Performance based approach (Whole building simulation).
- Prescriptive approach.

  (The total annual energy consumption of the building should not exceed the total base case energy consumption computed, as per ECBC (or) ASHRAE Standard 90.1-2013).

***Performance based approach (Whole Building Simulation)*:** Demonstrate compliance of the facility performance by whole facility simulation, as per the baselines outlined in ECBC (or) ASHRAE Standard 90.1-2013 (without amendments). Simulation is to be carried out at comfort temperatures of 24 +/– 2°C.

***Prescriptive approach*:** The project should meet the applicable criteria as established in prescriptive measures of ECBC (or) ASHRAE Standard 90.1-2013 (without amendments).

Non Air-conditioned Healthcare Facilities (Prescriptive Approach)

Non air-conditioned facilities are those which are not serviced and will not be serviced in the future, either through central air-conditioned systems or unitary air-conditioners. Air-conditioning may be considered for critical areas, not >10% of the total regularly occupied area. Spaces with unitary air-conditioners shall comply with IEQ Mandatory Requirement-1 (Fresh Air Ventilation, Non air-conditioned buildings criteria). Non air-conditioned buildings shall meet the following prescriptive measures, as applicable:

- ***Building envelope***: The project must ensure that the following building envelope measures meet the baseline criteria.
  - Solar Heat Gain Coefficient (SHGC).
  - Window Glazing U-value (only if WWR >40%).
  - Overall Wall Assembly U-value.
  - Overall Roof Assembly U-value.
- ***Lighting***: The Lighting Power Density (LPD) in the building interior, exterior and parking areas shall be reduced by minimum 10% over ECBC base case.

(General Notes)

- Projects which use on-site renewable energy sources (such as solar energy, wind power, biomass, etc.) can subtract renewable energy generated, from the total energy of the proposed case.
- Projects installing solar hot water systems can assume electrical heating in the base case.
- Energy efficient materials, products and equipment that are certified by IGBC under Green Product Certification Programme or by a third-party agency approved by IGBC can be used by the project to show compliance.

Existing Healthcare Facilities

- **EPI approach:** Demonstrate that the annual energy consumption in the facility is within the Energy Performance Index (EPI) limits as mentioned in the Table 16.
- **Performance based approach (whole building simulation):** Demonstrate compliance of the facility performance by whole building simulation, as per the baselines outlined in ECBC (or) ASHRAE Standard 90.1-2010 (without amendments). Simulation is to be carried out at comfort temperatures of 24 + 2°C.

Room Design

The room design for the various rooms in the hospital with recommendations on the expectation, as per the standard and options where possible in terms of air conditioning with unitary equipment viz. wall units, window air conditioners and cassettes, natural ventilation and mechanical ventilation are elaborated under the room design. Various areas require temperature and relative humidity settings (where air conditioned), air change rates for fresh air and re circulation, filtration, room pressure differential to prevent cross contamination between areas and air flow patterns to sweep away the pathogens from where they are generated to exhaust points. Also, an important aspect of air distribution in the room is that there should not be turbulence. Turbulence vitiates the concept of air patterns and result in contamination spreading over the place. The placement of grilles and diffusers and the sizing should be such that there are no air drafts. Typically at occupancy level, air velocities should be around 0.2 m/s [*ASHRAE 55*].

Table 16: Source; Implementing Energy Efficiency in Buildings (A report by UNDP, BEE).

Climatic zone	*EPI range*
Warm and humid	275
Composite	264
Hot and dry	261
Moderate	247

Fabric Ducts: As an alternative use Fabric Ducts as against the normal sheet metal ducts. These can be used for supply as well as exhaust/return air, available with antimicrobial and fire rating, cleanable in washing machines and as a sustainability initiative, some manufacturers offer fabrics out of recycled polyester. Fabric ducts have a number of air diffusion options which include linear vents, nozzles, orifices, and porous fabrics. These options can be used to achieve uniform air flow, necessary air throw and low turbulence. Moreover, these ducts can be procured and installed in relatively short time.

Recommendations for Ventilation in the COVID Facility

Intensive Care Units

ISHRAE COVID-19 document recommends Relative Humidity of 40~70% and this is acceptable as against 40~60% mentioned in ASHRAE Standard 170-2017.

WHO recommends 6~12 ACH, preferably 12 ACH with no recirculation of air. ASHRAE Standard 170-2017 allows for recirculation of air if there is HEPA in the return. Filtration recommended is MERV7 for first stage and MERV14 or better for second stage for supply air. Exhaust to atmosphere must be with minimum H13 grade HEPA filter (EN1822-1).

Converted facilities: In existing nursing homes/hospitals being converted into COVID facilities, many of the ICUs are based on local air circulating, air-conditioning units such as room air-conditioners, wall splits and cassettes units, which are not recommended because of various reasons:

- Maintenance of the units has to be done in the patient area
- Filtration is inadequate
- There is no provision of fresh air or exhaust

Following steps can be taken to alleviate the inside conditions till the time it is not practical to go for an upgrade:

- Introduce an inline fan for inducting fresh air of minimum 2 ACH. Use two stage filtrations with minimum MERV7 and MERV14 rated filters. Since directly inducting fresh air into the room can lead to condensation in the room especially during monsoon, make sure that the fresh air is led to the return air grill portion of the air-conditioning unit.
- Keep the room at a negative pressure of a minimum 2.5 Pa. When the area is under negative pressure, the adjoining room should be maintained at the same level of hygiene as the ICU as air from this area will infiltrate into the ICU.
- Exhaust unit is needed to achieve the [-] 2.5 Pa in the area with respect to the adjoining areas.
- Exhaust to atmosphere must be with H13 or equivalent grade HEPA filter.

Airborne Infectious Isolation Room (Also called Negative Isolation Room) (Figs. 32 and 33)

ISHRAE COVID-19 document recommends Relative Humidity of 40~70% and this is acceptable as against 40~60% mentioned in ASHRAE Standard 170-2017. WHO recommends 6~12 ACH, preferably 12 ACH with no recirculation of air. Filtration recommended is MERV7 for as first stage and MERV14 or better as second stage for supply air. The exhaust to atmosphere must be with minimum H13 grade HEPA filter (EN1822-1).

Additional recommendation: UVGI for AHU cooling coil is a useful option to keep the cooling coil and drain pan clean of biofilm.

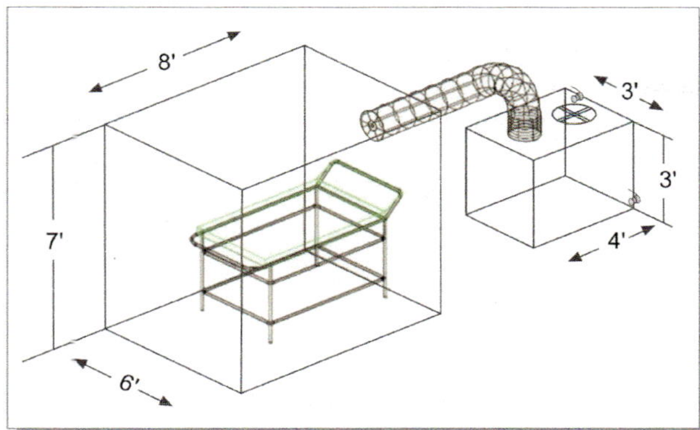

Fig. 32 : solation enclosure with Chemical disinfection for exhaust air. (*Dimensions are only indicative*).

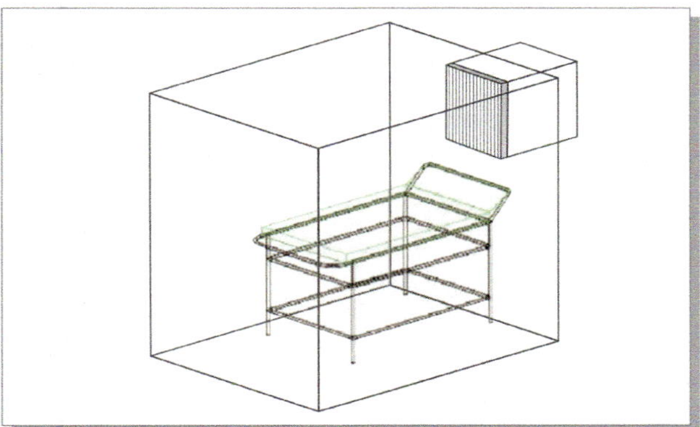

Fig. 33: Isolation enclosure with HEPA filtration for exhaust air.

Converted facilities: Make-shift Isolation Enclosures may have to be built when existing nursing homes/hospitals are being converted into COVID facilities

(Reference: IMA-HBI-ISHRAE covid-19 Guidance Document for Air-conditioning and Ventilation in Healthcare Facilities).

In resource constrained setting, several COVID-19 patients requiring isolation may be required to be admitted to a single large room. This presents a significant risk to the healthcare workers as well as a possibility for environmental spread of virus laden particles.

For such instances, make-shift patient isolation enclosures can provide the necessary protection for the healthcare workers. This could be a temporary cubicle or tent constructed out of a skeleton structure (plastic or metal) with a plastic sheet or canvas covering. The tent should be covered on all sides excepting the front, where PVC strip curtains or a similar arrangement may be provided. Arrangements for light and a fan may be provided for the comfort of the patient.

The cubicle or tent shall be provided with an exhaust blower to extract the air from inside the enclosure and exhaust out into the atmosphere after suitable treatment. Exhaust air treatment can be done as mentioned earlier. The exhaust blower shall be so sized that a negative pressure of >2.5 Pa is maintained inside the enclosure.

Quarantine and Triage

The ASHRAE Standard 170 recommends that in case of recirculation of air through AHU, there has to be HEPA filter in the return. The filtration in the AHU will be in two stages: MERV7 + MERV14 or better.

In case local unitary equipment is used viz. wall units, window air-conditioners or cassettes, use of fresh air is mandatory. Fresh air has to be introduced towards the return air of the units so that the chance of condensation is reduced. The room exhausts have to be suitably placed to ensure that the exhaust air does not affect thoroughfares or susceptible areas.

These areas may be mechanically ventilated. If this is done, it has to be ensured that a minimum of 12 ACH of fresh air is supplied in the room and the pressure relationship is negative with respect to surroundings. Here too, the room exhausts have to be suitably placed to ensure that the exhaust air does not affect thoroughfares or susceptible areas.

In case natural ventilation is adopted, the WHO recommends an average natural ventilation rate of 160 L/s/patient.

Additional recommendation: Considering the high viral loads that may be present in these areas, use of Upper Room UV Systems can be a beneficial addition for air purification.

UVGI for AHU cooling coil for air conditioning with AHU, keeps the cooling coil and drain pan clean of biofilm.

Laboratory

Filtration recommended is MERV7

In case local unitary equipment are used viz. wall units, window air conditioners or cassettes, use of fresh air is mandatory. Fresh air has to be introduced towards the return air of the units so that the chance of condensation is reduced. The room exhausts have to be suitably placed to ensure that the exhaust air does not affect thoroughfares or susceptible areas

These areas may be mechanically ventilated. If this is done, it has to be ensured that a minimum of 12 ACH of fresh air is supplied and the pressure relationship is negative with respect to surroundings. The filtration in the fresh air supply AHU will be: MERV7 or better. Here too, the room exhausts have to be suitably placed to ensure that the exhaust air does not affect thoroughfares or susceptible areas.

Resident Gathering/Activity/Dining and Physical Therapy Rooms

For AHU, use MERV7 filter is recommended.

In case local unitary equipment are used viz. wall units, window air conditioners or cassettes, use of fresh air is mandatory. Fresh air has to be introduced towards the return air of the units so that the chance of condensation is reduced. The room exhausts have to be suitably placed to ensure that the exhaust air does not affect thoroughfares or susceptible areas.

In case natural ventilation is adopted, the WHO recommends an average natural ventilation rate of 160 L/s/patient.

These areas may be mechanically ventilated. If this is done, it has to be ensured that a minimum of 12 ACH of fresh air is supplied in the room and the pressure relationship is negative with respect to surroundings. Here too, the room exhausts have to be suitably placed to ensure that the exhaust air does not affect thoroughfares or susceptible areas.

Additional recommendation: Considering the high viral loads that may be present in these areas due to high occupancy, use of Upper Room UV Systems can be a beneficial addition for air purification.

UVGI for AHU cooling coil for air conditioning with AHU will keep the cooling coil and drain pan clean of biofilm.

UVGI in supply air duct for air conditioning with AHU, for air disinfection will further improve the indoor air quality.

Entry to COVID Zone external change room

Filtration with AHU system has to be with MERV7 filters for supply air areas.

In case local unitary equipment are used viz. wall units, window air conditioners or cassettes, use of fresh air is mandatory. Fresh air has to be introduced towards the return air of the units so that the chance of condensation is reduced.

These areas may be mechanically ventilated. If this is done, it has to be ensured that a minimum of 12 ACH of fresh air is supplied in the room. The filtration in the fresh air supply AHU must be MERV7 or better. The room exhausts have to be suitably placed to ensure that the exhaust air does not affect thoroughfares or susceptible.

***Additional recommendation*:** Considering the high viral loads that may be present in these areas, use of Upper Room UV Systems can be a beneficial addition for air purification.

UVGI for AHU cooling coil for air conditioning with AHU, will keep the cooling coil and drain pan clean of biofilm.

UVGI in supply air duct for air conditioning with AHU, for air disinfection will further improve the indoor air quality.

Change Room Suite for PPE Donning and Doffing

Filtration with AHU system has to be with MERV7 filters for supply air. The change room area is critical for the safety of the healthcare workers, as the donning area has to be clean and the doffing area has a possibility of high viral load.

A diagram (Fig. 34) showing the recommended air infiltration/exfiltration direction and pressure gradient, to ensure a clean to dirty axis is given below. The direction of doors should be made note of to ensure that pressure aids in keeping the doors closed.

In case local unitary equipment is used viz. wall units, window air conditioners or cassettes, use of fresh air is mandatory. Fresh air has to be introduced towards the return air of the units so that the chance of condensation is reduced.

These areas may be mechanically ventilated. If this is done, it has to be ensured that a minimum of 12 ACH of fresh air is supplied in the room and the pressure relationship is negative with respect to surroundings.

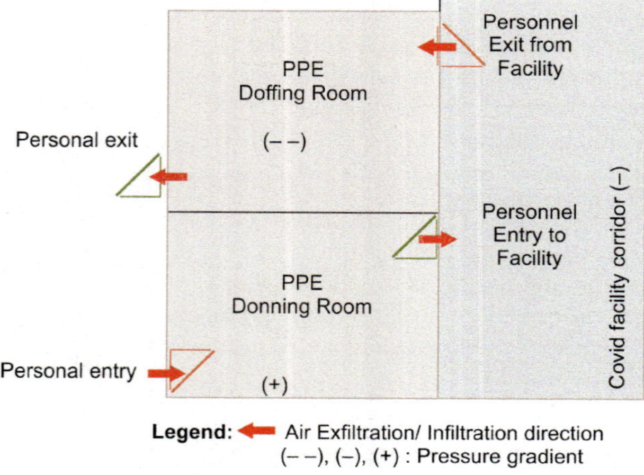

Fig. 34: Pressure gradient criteria for change room suite (donning and doffing areas).

***Additional recommendation*:**

- Considering the high viral loads that may be present in these areas, use of upper room UV systems can be a beneficial addition for air purification.
- The exhaust air from the doffing area will need to be discharged into atmosphere with minimum H13 grade HEPA filter (EN1822-1).
- UVGI for AHU cooling coil for air conditioning with AHU, will keep the cooling coil and drain pan clean of biofilm.
- UVGI in supply air duct for air conditioning with AHU, for air disinfection will further improve the indoor air quality.

Doctors' and Nurses' rooms

Filtration with AHU system has to be with MERV7 filters for supply air.

These areas may be mechanically ventilated. If this is done, it has to be ensured that a minimum of 12 ACH of fresh air is supplied in the room and the pressure relationship is negative with respect to surroundings.

In case local unitary equipment are used viz. wall units, window air conditioners or cassettes, use of fresh air is mandatory. Fresh air has to be introduced towards the return air of the units so that the chance of condensation is reduced.

***Additional recommendations*:**

- UVGI for AHU cooling coil for air conditioning with AHU, will keep the cooling coil and drain pan clean of biofilm.
- UVGI in supply air duct for air conditioning with AHU, for air disinfection will further improve the indoor air quality.

Service areas

The Service Areas need to be mechanically ventilated. For the food processing area (kitchen), air conditioning may be considered because of heat considerations. In case of AHU for air conditioning or in the case of mechanical ventilation system, the supply air filtration can be MERV7.

In case local unitary equipment are used viz. wall units, window air conditioners or cassettes (for Food Preparation and Clean Linen Room), use of fresh air is mandatory. Fresh air has to be introduced towards the return air of the units so that the chance of condensation is reduced.

***Additional recommendation (Fig. 35)*:** For air-conditioned space in Food Preparation Center, Dietary Storage and Clean Linen Storage:

- UVGI for AHU cooling coil for air conditioning with AHU, will keep the cooling coil and drain pan clean of biofilm.
- UVGI in supply air duct for air conditioning with AHU option for air disinfection will further improve the indoor air quality.

Wash Rooms

Wash rooms can have high viral load in the exhaust. The exhaust must have a minimum of 10 air changes. It is necessary to ensure that the exhaust to atmosphere don't get into thoroughfares and occupied areas. If this is not possible, examine if it can be dispersed high into the air, 3 meters above the highest point of the building while taking care that this doesn't get into air intakes of adjacent buildings. If even this is not possible, exhaust air has to be filtered through HEPA filters of minimum grade H13 (EN1822-1) before discharging into atmosphere.

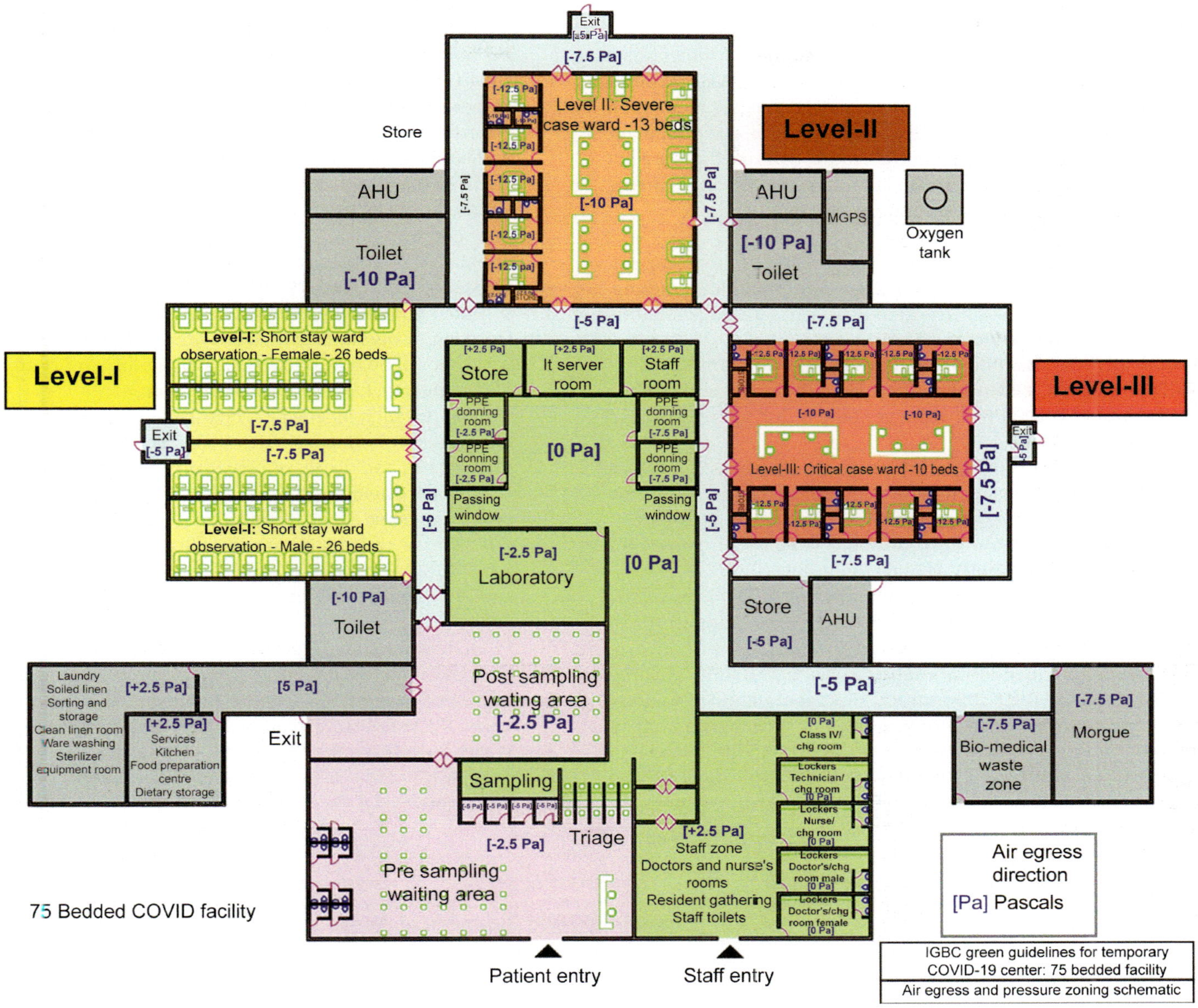

Exit
[-7.5 Pa]
Store
AHU
Toilet
[-10 Pa]
Level II: Severe case ward -13 beds
[-12.5 Pa]
[-10 Pa]
[-7.5 Pa]
Level-II
AHU
MGPS
Oxygen tank
[-10 Pa]
Toilet
[-5 Pa]
[-7.5 Pa]
Level-I
Level-I: Short stay ward observation - Female - 26 beds
[-7.5 Pa]
Exit
[-5 Pa]
[-7.5 Pa]
Level-I: Short stay ward observation - Male - 26 beds
[+2.5 Pa] Store
[+2.5 Pa] It server room
[+2.5 Pa] Staff room
PPE donning room [-2.5 Pa]
PPE donning room [-2.5 Pa]
[0 Pa]
PPE donning room [-7.5 Pa]
PPE donning room [-7.5 Pa]
Passing window
Passing window
[-5 Pa]
[-5 Pa]
Level-III
[-10 Pa]
[-10 Pa]
Level-III: Critical case ward -10 beds
[-12.5 Pa]
Exit
[-7.5 Pa]
[-7.5 Pa]
[-2.5 Pa] Laboratory
[0 Pa]
[-10 Pa] Toilet
Store [-5 Pa]
AHU
Laundry Soiled linen Sorting and storage Clean linen room Ware washing Sterilizer equipment room
[+2.5 Pa]
[+2.5 Pa] Services Kitchen Food preparation centre Dietary storage
[5 Pa]
Exit
Post sampling wating area [-2.5 Pa]
[-5 Pa]
[-7.5 Pa] Bio-medical waste zone
[-7.5 Pa] Morgue
Sampling
[0 Pa] Class IV/ chg room
Lockers Technician/ chg room [0 Pa]
Lockers Nurse/ chg room [0 Pa]
Lockers Doctor's/chg room male [0 Pa]
Lockers Doctor's/chg room female [0 Pa]
[-2.5 Pa]
Triage
Pre sampling waiting area
[+2.5 Pa] Staff zone Doctors and nurse's rooms Resident gathering Staff toilets
75 Bedded COVID facility
Air egress direction
[Pa] Pascals
Patient entry
Staff entry
IGBC green guidelines for temporary COVID-19 center: 75 bedded facility
Air egress and pressure zoning schematic

Fig. 35: Air egress and pressure zoning schematic.

Water Conservation

Experts' opinion indicates that, COVID-19 is not a waterborne disease. However, while consuming or using water, the associated sanitary fixtures and their surfaces can be a potential source of infection.

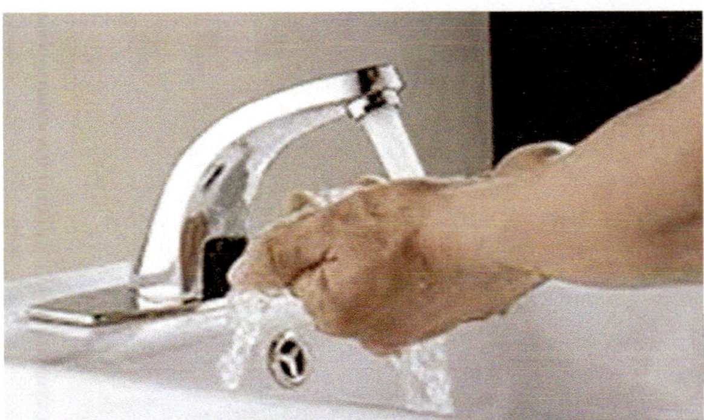

IGBC recommends the following measures to reduce the spread of infection through sanitary fixtures:

- **Fixtures in existing buildings and new buildings**
  - Install sensor-based plumbing fixtures for Faucets, water closets and urinals.
  - Use sensor-based hand dryers and paper towels in washrooms, kitchen/canteen.
  - Use sensor based or foot operated drinking water dispensers.
  - Use Long handle (Surgical) faucets which can be operated by elbow in washrooms/kitchen/dining areas.
- **Before starting operations**
  - Carry out chemical cleaning of water storage tanks.
  - Carry out flushing of water carrying pipes with clean water.
- **Check the quality of potable water regularly and take corrective measures.**

Waste Management (Fig. 36)

COVID facilities have to deal with biomedical waste and consumer waste during various types of Hospitals operations. Since COVID facilities have extensive requirement of personal protective equipment such as masks, gloves, gowns, PPE kits, etc., the quantum and volume of waste to be handled also increases. Furthermore, if the used kits are not disposed off in a proper recommended manner it may lead to further infections and increased risk of community spread.

The Central Pollution Control Board of the Ministry of Environment, Forest and Climate Change has recently issued guidlines for handling, treatment and disposal of waste generated during treatment, diagnosis and quarantine. The salient features are:

- *Isolation facilities*: Healthcare facilities having isolation wards for COVID-19 patients need to follow these steps to ensure safe handling and disposal of biomedical waste generated during treatment of COVID-19 patients
  - It should be kept in separate colour coded bins (with foot operated lids) 2/bags/containers in wards and maintain proper segregation of waste as per BMWM Rules, 2016 as amended and Central Pollution Control Board (CPCB) guidelines for implementation of BMW Management Rules.
  - As precaution double layered bags (using 2 bags) should be used for collection of waste from COVID-19 isolation wards so as to ensure adequate strength and no-leaks.
  - A dedicated collection bin labelled as "COVID-19" must be used to store COVID-19 waste and kept separately in temporary storage room prior to handing over to authorized staff of Common Bio-Medical Waste Treatment Facility (CBWTF). Biomedical waste collected in such isolation wards can also be lifted directly from ward into CBWTF collection van.
  - In addition to mandatory labelling, bags/containers used for collecting biomedical waste from COVID-19 wards, should be labelled as "COVID-19 Waste". This marking would enable CBWTFs to identify the waste easily for priority treatment and disposal immediately upon the receipt.
  - A separate records of waste generated from COVID-19 isolation wards should be maintained .
  - Dedicated trolleys and collection bins in COVID-19 isolation wards should be used . A label "COVID-19 Waste" to be pasted on these items also.
  - The (inner and outer) surface of containers/bins/trolleys used for storage of COVID-19 waste should be disinfected with 1% sodium hypochlorite solution daily.
  - Opening or operation of COVID-19 ward and COVID-19 ICU ward should be reported to the State Pollution Control Board and respective CBWTF located in the area.
  - Used PPEs such as goggles, face-shield, splash proof apron, plastic coverall, Hazmat suit, nitrile gloves must be segregated into red bag and disposed off within 72 hours.
  - Used mask (including Triple layer mask, N95 mask etc.), head cover/cap, shoe-cover, disposable linen gown, non-plastic or semi-plastic coverall in must be collected in the yellow bags.
  - Used masks, tissues and toiletries, of COVID-19 patient shall become biomedical waste and shall be segregated in yellow bag.
  - PPEs doffed by healthcare workers accompanying deceased body of COVID-19 patient to crematorium / graveyards should be treated as biomedical waste and disposed as per provisions under SWM Rules, 2016 and BMW Management Rules, 2016.
  - Waste handlers must be provided training about infection prevention measures such as hand hygiene, respiratory etiquettes, social distancing, use of appropriate PPE, etc.

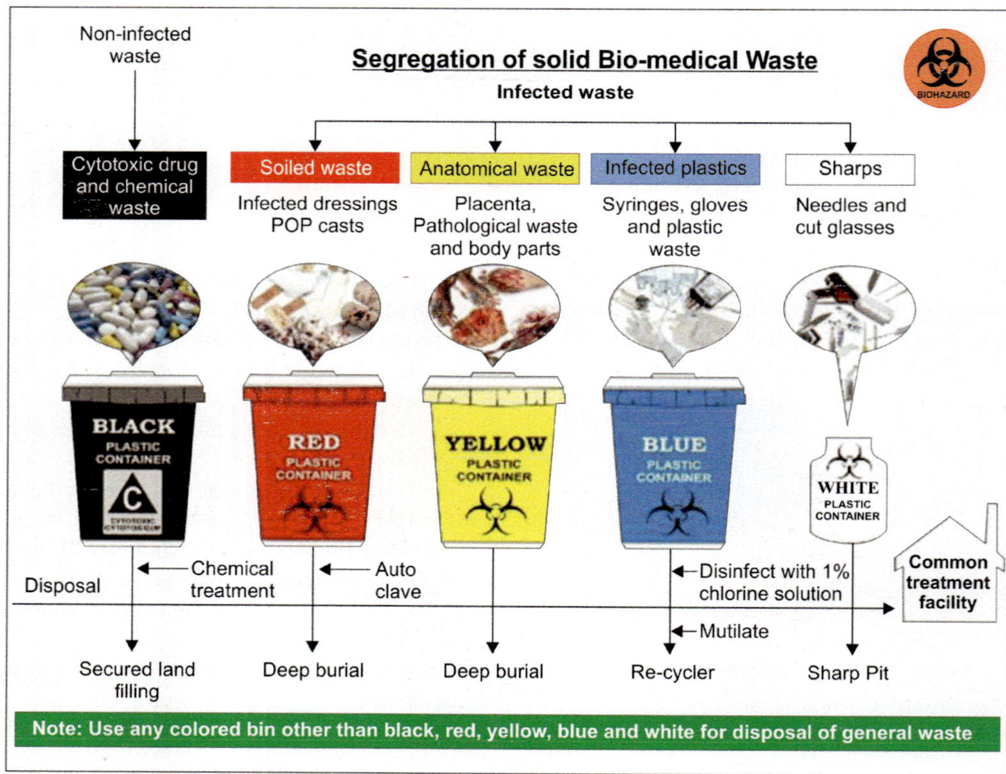

Fig. 36: Color coded bins for segregation of bio-medical waste.

- Sample collection centers and laboratories for COVID-19 suspected patients
  - Opening or operation of COVID-19 sample collection centers and laboratories must be reported to concerned SPCB. Similar guidelines applicable for the isolation wards should be applied suitably in case of test centers and laboratories. Pre-treatment of transport media, plastic vials, vacutainers, tubes, plastic vials, pipette tips must be undertaken as per BMWM Rules, 2016 and collect in red bags.
- Duties of Common Bio-medical Waste Treatment Facility (CBWTF) with reference to COVID-19: The healthcare facility management, through an effective tender, can ensure that the CBWTF operator follows the directives given by CPCB with respect to COVID-19. Some of these are enumerated below:
  - CBWTF operators need to report to SPCBs/CPCB about receiving of waste from COVID-19 isolation / COVID-19 Testing Centers;
  - Workers should be provided with adequate PPEs including three layer masks, splash proof aprons/gowns, nitrile gloves, gum boots and safety goggles;
  - Dedicated trolleys should be used to collect COVID-19 ward waste.
  - Vehicle should be sanitized with sodium hypochlorite or any appropriate chemical disinfectant after every trip.
  - COVID-19 waste should be disposed-off immediately upon receipt at facility.
  - Operators of CBWTF are to maintain separate record for collection, treatment and disposal of COVID-19 waste. They are also required to provide special training to their workers to handle COVID-19 waste.
  - CBWTF operator are required to register on 'COVID19BWM' Tracking App developed by CPCB for entering the data of COVID-19 biomedical waste received and disposed.
  - Provide training to waste handlers on infection prevention measures, hand hygiene, respiratory etiquettes, social distancing, use of PPE, etc. via videos and demonstrations etc. translated in local language.

Interior Furnishings

Interior layout, furnishings and high touch surfaces can be potential sources of infection in the COVID healthcare facilities.

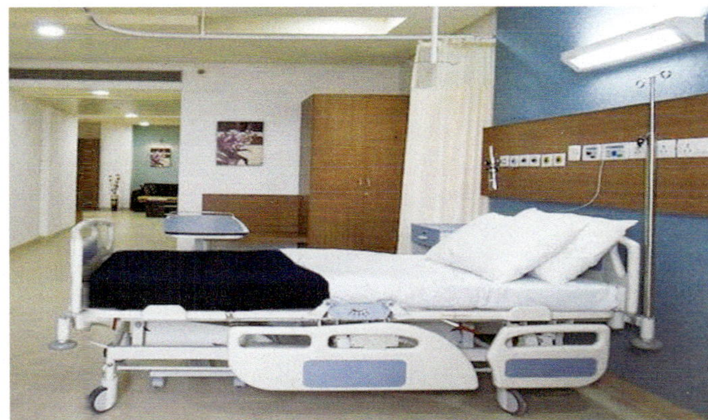

Following measures are recommended to be incorporated in the layout designing to minimize the risk of infection:

- Abundant day lighting in design.
- Maintain 6 feet distance in arrangement of beds, furniture layouts for workforce and furniture layout in common areas.
- Address Color psychology through appropriate color selection for the interior wall, surfaces, paintings, linens, bed sheets, curtains, etc.
- Use materials with recycled content and that are recyclable.
- Select materials for interior furnishings that are antibacterial, easy to maintain, resistant to microbial growth, nonporous and seamless.

Facilities for Healthcare Workforce

Healthcare workers being the frontline warriors are the one who are most exposed people and thereby run the risk of high probability of infection. Hazards include direct exposure to the infected patients, long working hours, psychological stress and fatigue. It is recommended to provide the following facilities to reduce the risk of infection spread amongst the healthcare workforce:

- Provide adequate kits and protective items for healthcare workforce like Masks, PPE kits, Face shields, Gloves, sanitizers, etc. (Fig. 37).
- Provide stress relieving breakout spaces like facilities for mental relaxation (Fig. 38).
- Provide basic facilities such as bathrooms in donning and doffing areas.
- Provide dormitories for workforce.
- Optimize staff working timings appropriately.

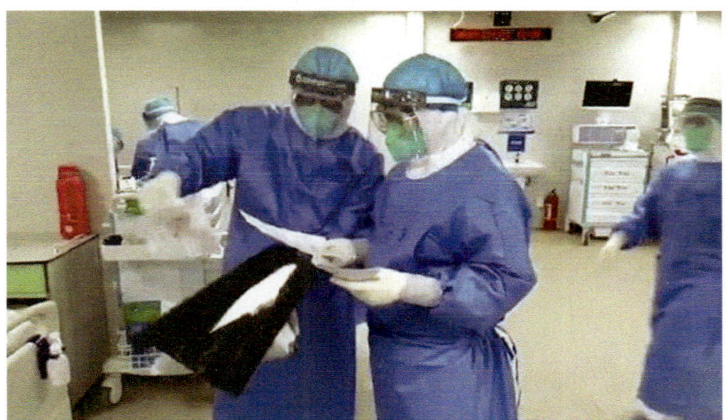

Fig. 37: Protective kits for healthcare workforce.

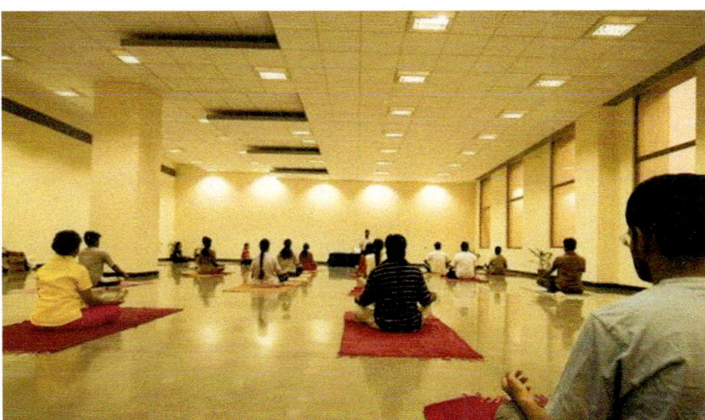

Fig. 38: Facilities for healthcare workforce.

REFERENCES

1. https://www.who.int/health-topics/coronavirus
2. World Health Organization. Influenza (seasonal). November 2018. Available from: https://www.who.int/en/news-room/fact-sheets/detail/influenza-(seasonal)
3. Kelly H, et al. The age-specific cumulative incidence of infection with pandemic influenza H1N1 2009 was similar in various countries prior to vaccination. PLoS One. 2011;6(8):e21828.
4. Dawood FS, et al. Estimated global mortality associated with the first 12 months of 2009 pandemic influenza A H1N1 virus circulation: a modelling study. Lancet Infect Dis. 2012;12(9):687-95.
5. Van Doremalen N, et al. Aerosol and surface stability of SARS-CoV-2 as compared with SARS-CoV-1. N Engl J Med 2020; 17 March.
6. Rothe C, et al. Transmission of 2019-nCoV infection from an asymptomatic contact in Germany. 2020;382(10):970-1.
7. European Centre for Disease Prevention and Control. Coronavirus disease 2019 (COVID-19) in the EU/EEA and the UK – ninth update. 23 April 2020.Available from: https://www.ecdc.europa.eu/sites/default/files/documents/covid-19-rapid-risk-assessment-coronavirus-disease-2019-ninth-update-23-april-2020.pdf
8. Mehta P, et al. COVID-19: consider cytokine storm syndromes and immunosuppression. Lancet. 2020;395(10229):1033-4.
9. IGBC's Green Guidelines for Fast Track and Emergency Facilities for Treating COVID-19 – Aug 2020.
10. ASHRAE Standards 52.2, 170-2017, 90.1 Guidelines.
11. ISO 29463.
12. CDC Guidelines for Environmental Infection Control in Health-Care Facilities.
13. Severe Acute Respiratory Infections Treatment Centre WHO doc Mar 2020.
14. Atkinson J, Chartier Y, Pessoa-Silva CL, Jensen P, Li Y. Natural ventilation for infection control in health-care settings. Geneva: World Health Organization; 2009.
15. WHO Minimum requirement for infection prevention and control programmes.
16. WHO's Severe Acute Respiratory Infections Treatment Centre (SARI).
17. COVID19 TATA Isolation Wards – Public document.
18. ISHRAE Covid document

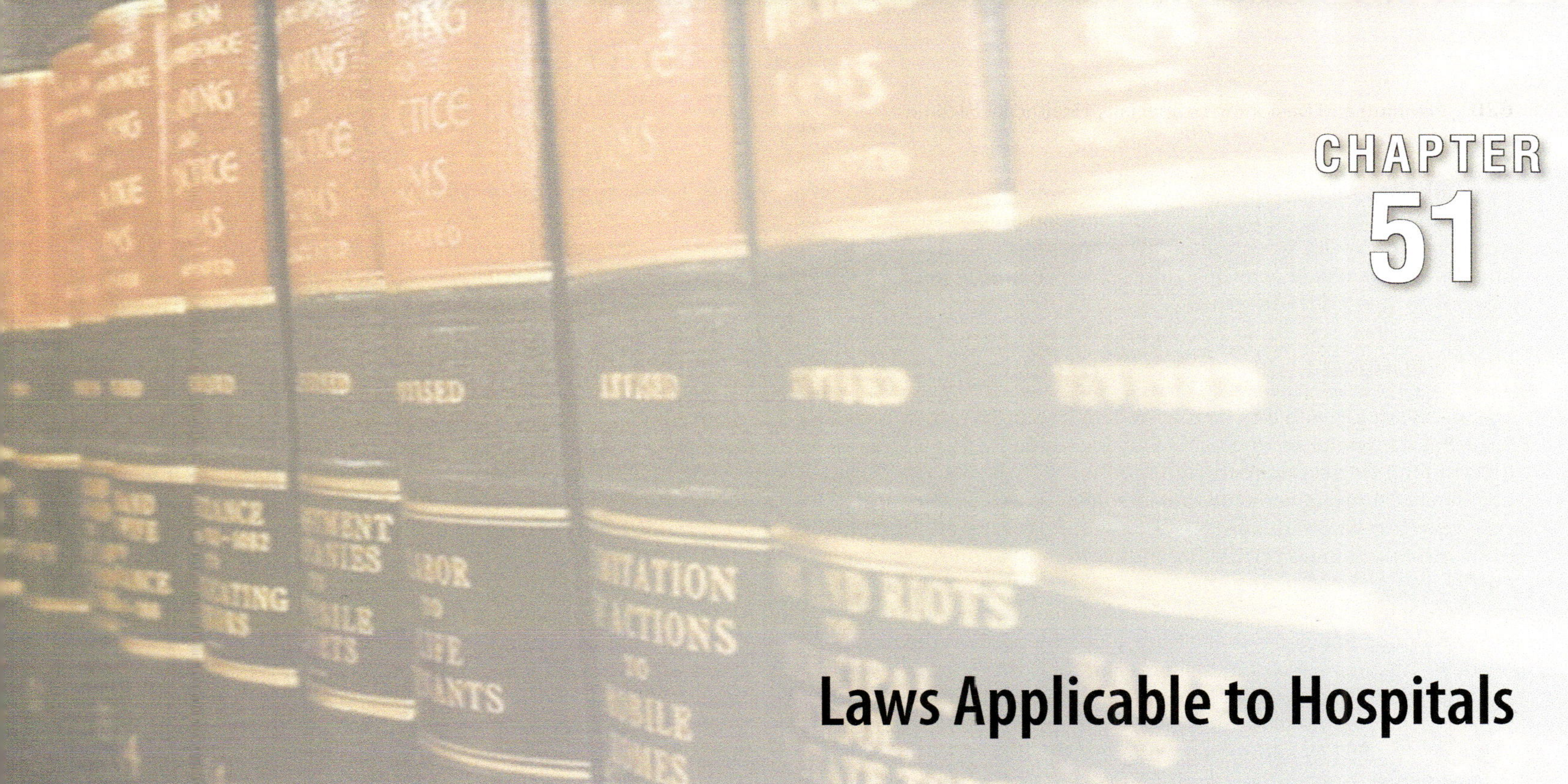

CHAPTER 51

Laws Applicable to Hospitals

Khalid Mehmood, Sunil Seth, Shakti Kumar Gupta, Sunil Kant, R Chandrashekhar

Healthcare in India features a universal healthcare system run by the constituent states and territories. Law is an obligation on the part of society imposed by the competent authority, and noncompliance may lead to punishment in the form of monetary fine or imprisonment or both.

The earliest known code of laws called the code of Hammurabi governed the various aspects of health practices including the fees payable to physician for satisfactory services. The first ever code of medical ethics called the Hippocratic Oath was laid down 2500 years ago, in the 5th century BC, by Hippocrates—the Greek physician. The modern version of Hippocratic Oath (called the declaration of Geneva), devised by the WHO after the Second World War and is accepted by international medical fraternity.

The process of establishment of healthcare system during the colonial rule also necessitated creation of legislative framework for practitioners of medicine. As the number of doctors qualified in Indian medical colleges increased, creation of laws for them became necessary.

The Medical Council of India, a national level statutory body for the doctors of modern medicine, was constituted after the enactment of Indian Medical Council Act 1933. MCI has now been replaced by National Medical Commission. The first legal recognition and registration for the Indian systems of medicine came when the Bombay Medical Practitioner' Act was passed in 1938. Laws governing the commissioning of hospital are the laws to ensure that the hospital facilities are created after due process of registration; the facilities created are safe for the public using them, have at least the minimum essential infrastructure for the type and volume of workload anticipated and are subject to periodic inspections to ensure compliance.

There are other laws pertaining to governing to the qualification/practice and conduct of professionals, sale, storage of drugs and safe medication, management of patients, environmental safety, employment and management of manpower, medico-legal aspects and laws pertaining to safety of patients, public and staff within the hospital premises. There are laws governing professional training and research, business aspects, licences/certifications required for hospitals, etc. A hospital administrator should be aware about all these laws, regulations, policies, procedures, reports and returns and keep abreast with the latest amendments to be on the safe side of law and provide quality care to the patients.[1]

TELEMEDICINE AND INDIA[2]

India being a very vast country which is densely populated, telemedicine plays a very important role in enabling medical services being made accessible and deliverable to the remote areas as well, more so since the concentration of medical health care facilities is found more in the cities than in rural India, which constitutes majority of the national population. Indian Space Research Organisation (ISRO) made a modest beginning in telemedicine in India with a Telemedicine Pilot Project in 2001, linking Chennai's Apollo Hospital with the Apollo Rural Hospital at Aragonda village in the Chittoor district of Andhra Pradesh.

In India, the telemedicine service comes under the jurisdiction of the Ministry of Health and Family Welfare and the Department of Information Technology.

Due to the prevalent pandemic caused by widespread COVID-19, there appeared challenges to provide healthcare services to people in need – especially in the wake of social distancing coupled with the high risk of catching the COVID-19 infection. It was the need of the hour to regulate and promote Telemedicine as a tool available for patients suffering from other ailments to consult and seek timely medical advice, at the same time, also help the RMP's to effectively manage patients and deliver timely consultation as and when desired and required – without requiring the patient to visit the hospital and/or clinic.

Thus with the lockdown in force all over the country, use of Telemedicine consultation helped both the patient as well as doctors from preventing the spread of highly contagious COVID-19 disease and reduce the risk of exposing vulnerable patients as well as health workers to the COVID-19 virus.

TELEMEDICINE GUIDELINES MARCH 25, 2020[2,3]

The Ministry of Health and Family Welfare ("MoHFW") on March 25, 2020, has issued the Telemedicine Practice Guidelines ("Guidelines") for enabling Registered Medical Practitioners ("RMPs") to provide healthcare using telemedicine. 'Telemedicine' is the delivery of health care services, where distance is a critical factor, by all healthcare professionals using information and communication technologies for the exchange of valid information for diagnosis, treatment and prevention of disease and injuries, research and evaluation, and for the continuing education of healthcare providers, all in the interests of advancing the health of individuals and their communities.

The Guidelines have been adopted as an amendment to the Indian Medical Council (Professional Conduct, Etiquette and Ethics) Regulations, 2002 by adding regulation 3.8 titled as 'Consultation by Telemedicine'. In accordance with these regulations, the consultation through telemedicine by the RMPs under the Indian Medical Council Act, 1956 will be permissible in accordance with the Guidelines. The Guidelines in its scope covers the telemedicine consultations provided in India only. Some of the key directives are as follows:

- Appropriateness and Sufficiency
- Identification of the RMP and the Patient
- Patient Consent
- Prescribing Medicines

The Digital Information Security in Healthcare Act ('DISHA') is proposed to be enacted to provide for electronic health data privacy, confidentiality' security and standardization and provide for establishment of National Digital Health Authority and Health Information Exchanges.

DIGITAL HEALTH LAWS AND REGULATIONS[4,5]

According to the WHO, e-Health is the use of ICT (information and communication technologies) for health. The Ministry of Health and Family Welfare, in order to take up the digital India initiative ahead, has started various e-Governance initiatives in Healthcare sector in India, named as e-Health division, with a vision to deliver better healthcare services in terms of access, quality, affordability, lowering of disease burden and efficient monitoring of health entitlements to citizens. Information Technology Act, 2000 ("IT Act"): Under the IT Act, the following rules have been enforced which triggers in the e-Health sector: The Information Technology (Reasonable security practices and procedures and sensitive personal data or information) Rules, 2011 ("SPDIR") and The Information Technology (Intermediaries Guidelines) Rules, 2011 ("Intermediary Guidelines"): The SPDIR mandates a body corporate or person who, on behalf of the body corporate, collects, receives, possess, stores, deals or handles information of the provider of information, including sensitive personal data shall provide a privacy policy for handling of or dealing of the afore-mentioned information.

The New Telecom Policy, 1999[6]

All service providers who render "Application Services"-which includes telemedicine services - using telecom resources provided by telecom service providers, are required to be registered as an 'Other Service Provider' ("OSP") with the Department of Telecommunications.

INTELLECTUAL PROPERTY RIGHTS[7,8]

e-Healthcare facilities/platforms give way to innovations, developments, trademarks and content generation and the protection of the same is a high priority in today's market. Intellectual Property laws enable the entities to protect their ideas, innovations and developments in various forms, few of which are:

1. **Copyrights:** To protect the contents/data placed on the platform under the Copyright Act, 1957,
2. **Patent:** To protect an invention, the Patent Act, 1970 has come in force.
3. **Trademarks:** To protect the words, taglines or logos with which any person would identify. The 'mark' of an e-Health application or device could be registered as a trademark under the Trademark Act, 1999.

DIFFERENCES BETWEEN ORDINANCE, BILL, LAW AND ACT[9]

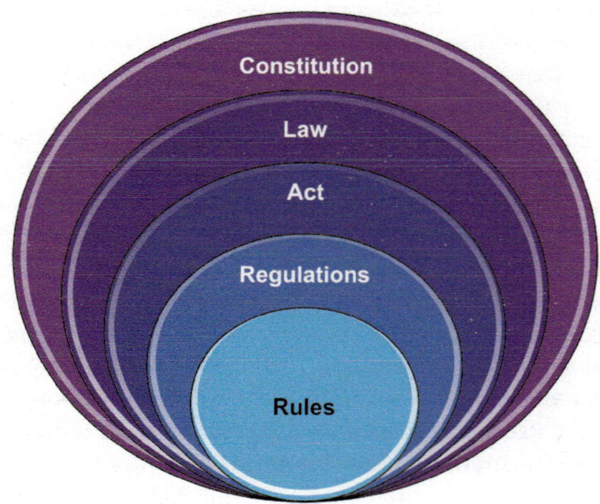

Bill

It can be considered as an initial stage of an act. It is a proposal to make a new law and usually, is in the form of a document which summaries what is the policy behind the proposed law and what is to be the proposed law. It can be introduced by government itself or proposed by a member of the Parliament. It is first placed in the lower house of the parliament and after discussions, once it has been passed; it goes to the Upper house for approval. Once it gets passed by the upper House it is sent to the President for his assent. Finally, a bill becomes a law (Act) of the land once it has been passed by the parliament and also got assent from the President.

ACT

Once the Bill has been passed by the legislature, it is sent to the President or the Governor, as the case may be for the approval. By receiving his assent, it becomes an Act. An Act is a law which is made by the legislature like Parliament or State Legislative Assembly.

Law

The term 'law' in general applies/refers to the set of regulations or rules to be followed. Law can be in the form of an act, ordinance, order, by-laws, rule, regulation etc. An act is a subset of law. Anything which has the power to confer legal rights, obligations, liabilities etc. is law. Law can be any Provisions of all valid Acts passed by the legislature, Acts and codes from pre-independence India, Ordinances passed by a Governor of a State or the President of India, Decisions of the High Courts or Supreme Court , Authorized orders, notices, rules, etc made by government bodies.

Ordinances

Ordinances are temporary laws that are circulated by the President of India on the recommendation of the Union Cabinet. They can only be delivered when the Parliament is not in session. They enable the Indian government to take immediate legislative action. At times, when the legislature of the Union is not in session and there is a need to make legislation (Act) in emergency. In such cases, the government refers a proposal to the President or Governor, and if they approve of them, it becomes an Ordinance. Legally, an ordinance is the equal to Act. It can be seen as a temporary law till its expiry or till it is repealed or it is approved by the legislature.

In short, if the governor assents to the bill, it becomes an Act for the state which passed it and in such cases, if the government sends a proposal to the President or Governor, and if they approve of it, it becomes an Ordinance. Legally, an ordinance is the equivalent of an Act; but is not passed by the legislature.

The laws enlisted below are applicable to Hospitals and as a hospital administrator, medical architecture and hospital consultant one needs to be well versed with their Implications for hassle free day to day operations and smooth running of hospital services. These are the passing references about various Acts and for detailed information and knowledge about each, one can read and go through the Bare Acts.

Laws Governing the Commissioning of Hospital

S. No.	*Name of Act/Rule*	*Year*
1.	Indian Telegraph Act	1885
2.	Government Buildings Act	1899
3.	Building and Other Construction Workers (Regulation of Employment and Conditions of Service) Act	1908
4.	The Registration Act	1908
5.	Red Cross Society (Allocation of Property) Act	1936
6.	Bombay Lifts Act	1939
7.	Delhi Lift Act	1942
8.	Bombay Nursing Homes Registration Act	1949
9.	Delhi Nursing Home Registration Act	1953
10.	Companies Act	1956
11.	Electricity Rules	1956
12.	St John Ambulance Association (India) Transfer of Funds Act	1956
13.	Bombay Nursing Homes Registration (Extension and Amendment) Act	1959
14.	The Society Registration Act	1860
15.	Atomic Energy Regulatory Body Approval for Radiology/ Nuclear Medicine Services under the Atomic Energy Act	1962
16.	Delhi Fire Prevention and Fire Safety Act	1986
17.	Fire Safety Rules	1987
18.	Atomic Energy (Safe Disposal of Radioactive Wastes) Rules	1987
19.	Municipality to Local Authority (74th Constitutional Amendment Act)	1992
20.	Karnataka Medical Registration (Amendment) Act	2003
21.	Bombay Nursing Homes Registration (Amendment) Act	2005
22.	Delhi Fire Service Act	2007
23.	The National Capital Territory of Delhi Laws (Special Provisions) Second Bill	2011
24.	Clinical Establishments Bill	2010
25.	Radiation Protection Certificate for Radiology Department from BARC	–

Laws Governing the Qualifications/Practice and Conduct of Professionals

S. No.	*Name of Act/Rule*	*Year*
1.	Indian Medical Degrees Act	1916
2.	Indian Nursing Council Act	1947
3.	The Dentists Act	1948
4.	The ICN Code of Ethics for Nurses	1953
5.	Indian Medical Council Act	1956
6.	Kerala Anatomy Act	1957
7.	Karnataka Anatomy Act	1957
8.	The Apprenticeship Act	1961
9.	The Dentists (Code of Ethics Regulation)	1976
10.	All India Council for Technical Education (AICTE)	1987
11.	Rehabilitation Council of India Act	1992
12.	Delhi Nursing Council Act	1997
13.	Kerala Co-operative Hospital Complex and the Academy of Medical Sciences (Taking Over the Management) Act	1997
14.	Rehabilitation Council of India (Amendment) Act	2000
15.	Indian Medical Council (Professional Conduct, Etiquette and Ethics) Regulations,	2002
16.	Dental Council of India Regulations	2006
17.	Kerala Professional Colleges or Institutions (Prohibition of Capitation Fee, Regulation of Admission, Fixation of Non-Exploitative Fee and Other Measures to Ensure Equity and Excellence in Professional Education) Amendment Act	2007
18.	**National Medical Commission (NMC) Act, 25th September, 2020**	**2020**
19.	Registration of Medical Practitioners with State Medical Councils	–
20.	AICTE Physiotherapy Rules	–

Laws Governing Storage/Sale of Drugs and Safe Medication

S. No.	Name of Act/Rule	Year
1.	Sale of Goods Act	1930
2.	Drugs and Cosmetic Act	1940
3.	Central Excise Act (for Permit to Use and Store Spirit)	1944
4.	The Drug and Cosmetics Rules (Amendment 2005)	1945
5.	Pharmacy Act	1948
6.	The Drugs Control Act	1950
7.	Central Sales Tax Act	1956
8.	Homoeopathy Central Council Act	1973
9.	Drug and Cosmetic Act Amendment	1982
10.	Narcotics and Psychotropic Substances Act	1985
11.	Blood Bank Regulations Under Drugs and Cosmetic (2nd Amendment) Rules	1999
12.	Homoeopathy Central Council (Amendment) Act	2002
13.	VAT Act	2005
14.	License for Possession and Use of Rectified/Denatured Spirit	–
15.	Retail Drug License	–
16.	IPC Section 274 (Adulteration of Drugs)	–
17.	IPC Section 275 (Sales of Adulterated Drugs)	–
18.	IPC Section 276 (Sales of Drug as Different Drug or Preparation)	–
19.	IPC Section 284 (Negligent Conduct with Regard to Poisonous Substances)	–

Laws Governing Biomedical Research

S. No.	Name of Act/Rule	Year
1.	Breeding of and Experiments on Animals (Control and Supervision) Amendment Rules	2005
2.	Constitution of Committee for the Purpose of Control and Supervision of Experiments on Animals (CPCSEA)	–

Laws Governing Management of Patients

S. No.	Name of Act/Rule	Year
1.	Birth and Death and Marriage Registration Act	1886
2.	Guardians and Wards Act	1890
3.	The Epidemic Disease Act	1897
4.	Drugs and Magic Remedies (Objectionable Advertisements) Act	1954
5.	Delhi Registration of Birth and Deaths Act	1969
6.	MTP Act	1971
7.	MTP Rules	1971
8.	Delhi Municipal Corporation (Malaria and Other Mosquito Borne Disease) Bye-Laws	1975
9.	Lepers Act	1975
10.	Ear Drums and Ear Bones (Authority for Use for Therapeutic Purposes) Act	1982
11.	Eyes (Authority for Use for Therapeutic Purposes) Act	1982
12.	The Mental Health Act	1987
13.	Pre-Natal Diagnostic Techniques (PNDT) Act	1994
14.	Transplantation of Human Organs and Tissues Act	1994
15.	Transplantation of Human Organs and Tissues Rules	2014
16.	Pre-Conception and Pre-Natal Diagnostic Techniques (PCPNDT) (Prohibition of Sex Selection) Rules	1996
17.	**Epidemic Diseases (Amendment) Bill**	**2020**
18.	Rules for Insurance Cover for the Sterilization Cases	–
19.	Law of Contract, Section 13 (Consent)	–

Laws Governing Medico Legal Aspects

S. No.	Name of Act/Rule	Year
1.	Indian Evidence Act (Disclosure of Privileged/Confidential Patient related Information before a Court of Law)	1872
2.	Law of Privileged Communications	1872
3.	Law of Torts	1986
4.	Consumer Protection Act	1986
5.	Protection of Human Rights Act	1993
6.	IPC Section 52 (Interpretation of Good Faith)	–
7.	IPC Section 80 (Accident in doing a Lawful Act)	–
8.	IPC Section 89 (Act done in Good Faith for benefit of Child or Insane person by or by consent of Guardian)	–
9.	IPC Section 92 (Act done in Good Faith for benefit of a Person without Consent)	–
10.	IPC Section 93 (Communication made in Good Faith)	–
11.	IPC Section 269 (Negligent Act likely to spread Infection of Disease dangerous to Life)	–

Laws Governing The Safety of Patients, Public and Staff within the Hospital Premises and Environmental Protection

S. No.	Name of Act/Rule	Year
1.	DMC Sanitation and Public Health Bye Laws	1959
2.	The Water (Prevention and Control of Pollution) Act	1974
3.	(Procedure for Transaction of Business) Rules	1975
4.	The Water (Prevention and Control of Pollution) Rules	1975
5.	The Water (Prevention and Control of Pollution) Cess Rules	1977
6.	Air (Prevention and Control of Pollution) Act	1981
7.	The Air (Prevention and Control of Pollution) Rules	1982
8.	The Air (Prevention and Control of Pollution) (Union Territories) Rules	1983
9.	Environment Protection Act	1986
10.	The Environment (Protection) Rules	1986
11.	Biomedical Waste (Management and Handling) Rules and amendment thereof	1998
12.	Sewerage and Drainage Act	1999
13.	The Noise Pollution (Regulation and Control) Rules	2000
14.	The Noise Pollution (Regulation and Control) (Amendment) Rules	2002
15.	The Water (Prevention and Control of Pollution) Cess (Amendment) Act	2003
16.	The Noise Pollution (Regulation and Control) (Amendment) Rules	2006
17.	The Noise Pollution (Regulation and Control) (Amendment) Rules	2010
18.	IPC Section 278 (Making Atmosphere Noxious to Health)	–

Laws Governing the Safety of Patients, Public and Staff within the Hospital Premises

S. No.	Name of Act/Rule	Year
1.	The Indian Fatal Accidents Act	1855
2.	Explosives Act	1884
3.	The Indian Boilers Act	1923
4.	The Prevention of Food Adulteration Act	1954
5.	The Arms Act	1959
6.	The Insecticide Act	1968
7.	Radiation Protection Rules	1971
8.	Gas cylinder Rules	1981
9.	The Radiation Surveillance Procedures for the Medical Application of Radiation	1989
10.	The Protection of Human Rights Act	1993
11.	The Atomic Energy Act	2001
12.	Vaccination (Repeal) Act	2001
13.	The Petroleum Act	1934
14.	The Cigarettes and Other Tobacco Products Act	2003
15.	The Disaster Management Act	2005
16.	Prohibition of Smoking in Public Places Rules	2008
17.	The Tamil Nadu Medicare service Persons and Medicare Service Institutions (Prevention of Violence and Damage or loss of Property) Act	2008
18.	Karnataka Prohibition of Violence Against Medicare Service Personnel and Damage to Property in Medicare Service Institutions Act	2009
19.	IPC Section 336 (Act endangering life and personal safety of others)	–
20.	IPC Section 337 (Causing hurt by act endangering life and personal safety of others)	–
21.	IPC Section 338 (Causing grievous hurt by act endangering the life and personal safety of others	–
22.	National Building Code	2016

Laws Governing the Employment of Manpower

S. No.	Name of Act/Rule	Year
1.	Negotiable Instruments Act	1881
2.	The Workmen's Compensation Act	1923
3.	Official Secrets Act	1923
4.	Indian Trade Union Act	1926
5.	The Payment of wages Act	1936
6.	Weekly Holidays Act	1942
7.	Industrial Disputes Act	1947
8.	Employees State Insurance Act	1948
9.	Minimum Wages Act	1948
10.	ESI (Central) Rules	1950
11.	Employees Provident Fund and Miscellaneous Provisions Act	1952
12.	Citizenship Act	1955
13.	The Employment Exchanges (Compulsory Notification of Vacancies) Act	1959
14.	TDS Act	1961
15.	Maternity Benefit Act	1961
16.	The Payment of bonus Act	1965
17.	The Public Provident Fund Act	1968
18.	The Payment of Gratuity Act	1972
19.	Equal Remuneration Act	1976
20.	Child and Adolescent Labour (Prohibition and Regulations) Act	1986
21.	Scheduled Caste and Scheduled Tribe (Prevention of Atrocities) Act	1989
22.	Persons With Disabilities (Equal Opportunities, Protection of Rights and Full Participation) Act	1995
23.	Information Technology Act	2000
24.	Information Technology (Amendment) Act	2008
25.	Workmen's Compensation (Amendment) Act	2009

Laws Governing Professional Training and Research

S. No.	Name of Act/Rule	Year
1.	MCI rules for Internship Training	–
2.	National Board of Examinations Rules for DNB Training	–
3.	Nursing Council of India Rules for Starting School/College of Nursing	–
4.	ICMR Rules Governing Medical Research	–

Laws Governing the Business Aspects of Hospital

S. No.	Name of Act/Rule	Year
1.	Indian Contract Act	1872
2.	Charitable and Religious Trusts Act	1920
3.	Sale of Goods Act	1930
4.	The Insurance Act	1938
5.	Copyright Act	1957
6.	Gift Tax Act	1958
7.	Income-tax Act	1961
8.	Customs Act	1962
9.	The Public Liability Insurance Act	1991
10.	The Public Liability Insurance Rules	1991
11.	Cable Television Network (Regulation) Act	1995
12.	The Foreign Exchange Management Act (FEMA)	1999
13.	Rules for Display of Red Cross Insignia	–
14.	Vehicle Registration Certificate	–
15.	Wireless Operation Certificate from Post and Telegraphs	–

LICENCES/CERTIFICATIONS REQUIRED
(Applicable to Hospitals in NCT, Delhi)*

S. No.	Licences Required	Issuing Authority and Frequency
1.	Registration under (Section-5) of Delhi Nursing Home Act, 1953	DHS, Govt of Delhi, Karkardooma (Yearly)
2.	Incorporation of Hospital as Company	Registrar of Companies
3.	Allotment of Land	State DI/SIDC/Infrastructure Corporation/SSIDC
4.	NOC and Consent under Water and Air Pollution Control Acts	State Pollution Control Board

Cont'd...

Cont'd...

S. No.	Licences Required	Issuing Authority and Frequency
5.	Approval of construction Activity and Building Plan	a. Town and Country planning b. Municipal and Local Authorities c. Chief Inspector of Factories d. Pollution Control Board e. Electricity Board
6.	Sanction of Electricity Power	State Electricity Board
7.	Boiler Inspection Certificate	Chief Inspector of Boilers
8.	Upgrading of Bed Strength	Before implementation
9.	NOC from Delhi Fire Service	Initially
10.	Certification of Inspection of Electrical Installation/Substation	Initially
11.	NOC from MCD-compliance of Municipal Bye-laws by the Hospital	Initially
12.	Indemnity Insurance Policy	Yearly
13.	Standard Fire and Special Perils policy	Yearly
14.	Registration under (Section-7) of Contract Labor Act, 1970	Labor Commissioner, Govt of NCT, Delhi (Yearly)
15.	License for Operating Lifts under Section-5 and 6 and Rules 4 and 5	Inspector of Lifts, Govt of NCT, Delhi
16.	License under Air (Prevention and Control of Pollution) Act 1981	Department of Environment, Govt of Delhi
17.	Registration for Operation of X-ray Facility (Under AERB Registration)	AERB, Anushakti Nagar, Mumbai (Every 02 years)
18.	License to Operate Blood Bank (under Rule 122-G of Drug and Cosmetics Act, 1940)	Office of the Drug Controller (Every 05 years)
19.	Drug License for Medical Store	Office of the Drug Controller (Every 05 years)
20.	Drug License for IPD (Indoor Patient Department) Pharmacy	Office of the Drug Controller (Every 05 years)
21.	Drug License for OPD (Outdoor Patient Department) Pharmacy	Office of the Drug Controller (Every 05 years)
22.	Authorization for Generation of Biomedical Waste	DPCC, Govt of NCT, Delhi (Renewal yearly)
24.	Contract for Disposal of Biomedical Waste	Yearly
25.	Income-tax Exemption Certificate	Chief Commissioner IT, Govt of NCT, Delhi (03 yearly)
26.	License for Animal Rearing	
27.	Licence for Dhobi Ghat	

Cont'd...

Cont'd...

S. No.	Licences Required	Issuing Authority and Frequency
28.	License for storage of Petrol/ Diesel on Form-XV under the Petroleum Rules 2002	Joint Chief Controller of Explosives, Faridabad (02 yearly)
29.	Registration under State Sales Tax Act, and Central and State Excise Act	Sales Tax Department, Central and State Excise Department
30.	FEMA Licence under Foreign Exchange Management Act (FEMA)	General permission of RBI
31.	Licence Foreign Collaboration and Industrial Form FC-IL - Composite Form	
32.	Environmental Clearance (EC)	Ministry of Environment (Initially)
33.	License for the Manufacture/Sale/ Preparation/Exposure/Storage of Articles of Food and Drinks Under Section-24	
34.	License for Dangerous and Offensive Trade Under Section-327	
35.	Renewal/Grant of Lodging House License in NDMC	
36.	Registration under Rule-34, MTP Act, 1971	Deptt. of Family Welfare, Govt of Delhi (One time)
37.	Registration under PNDT Act, 1994	Appropriate Authority (under PNDT Act) Govt of NCT of Delhi (05 yearly)

*The list is merely an overview of various Licences, registrations and certifications, clearances etc. For complete and detailed information on any of the above mentioned licences, any recent and upto date changes please visit/contact your nearest Health/Appropriate Authority, as most of these licences are Amended by the State and Central Govt/Competent Authorities/Regulatory Bodies, according to the need of the hour.

REFERENCES

1. Shah D: Laws Applicable to Medical Practice and Hospitals in India, May 8, 2017.
2. https://www.mohfw.gov.in/pdf/Telemedicine.pdf
3. ISRO Telemedicine Initiative. Televital.com.
4. https://www.who.int/ehealth/about/en/
5. Rule 4 of the SPDIR.
6. https://main.trai.gov.in/sites/default/files/ACTO_21052019.pdf
7. Section 2(o) of the Copyright Act, 1857.
8. Rule 5 of Guidelines for Examination of Computer Related Inventions, 2015.

INDEX

Page numbers followed by *b* refer to box, *f* refer to figure, *fc* refer to flowchart, and *t* refer to table.

A

B

F

G

H

I

K

L

P

T

U

V

W

X

Y